Principles
of
Medical
Pharmacology

Principles of Medical Pharmacology

SIXTH EDITION

EDITED BY

HAROLD KALANT, M.D., Ph.D.

Professor Emeritus
Department of Pharmacology
University of Toronto Faculty of Medicine

WALTER H. E. ROSCHLAU, M.D.

Professor Emeritus
Department of Pharmacology
University of Toronto Faculty of Medicine

New York   Oxford   •   OXFORD UNIVERSITY PRESS   •   1998

Oxford University Press

Oxford   New York
Athens   Auckland   Bangkok   Bogota
Bombay   Buenos Aires   Calcutta   Cape Town
Dar es Salaam   Delhi   Florence   Hong Kong   Istanbul
Karachi   Kuala Lumpur   Madras   Madrid
Melbourne   Mexico City   Nairobi   Paris
Singapore   Taipei   Tokyo   Toronto

and associated companies in
Berlin   Ibadan

Library of Congress Cataloging-in-Publication Data
Principles of medical pharmacology /
Harold Kalant, Walter H.E. Roschlau.—6th ed.
p.   cm.   Includes bibliographical references and index.
ISBN 0-19-510024-7   1. Pharmacology.
I. Kalant, Harold.   II. Roschlau, Walter H. E.
[DNLM: 1. Pharmacology.   QV 4 P957 1997]
RM300.P74   1997   615'.7—dc20   DNLM/DLC
for Library of Congress   96-29399

The editors wish to thank the publishers and authors for their generous permission to use the following figures and tables:

Figure 9-5: Adapted from Figure 1; P. Seeman and H.H.M. Van Tol: "Dopamine receptor pharmacology." Trends in Pharmacological Science 1994; 15:264–270. Elsevier Science Ltd., Oxford, England

Figure 25-2: Adapted from Figure 1; J.F. Butterworth and G.R. Strichartz: "Molecular mechanism of local anesthesia—a review." Anesthesiology 1990; 72:711–734. J.B. Lippincott Company, Philadelphia, Pennsylvania.

Figure 26-4: Adapted from Figure 1; H. Kalant: "Research on alcohol metabolism: a historical perspective." Keio Journal of Medicine 1991; 40 (3):113–117. Keio University School of Medicine, Tokyo, Japan.

Figure 28-4: Adapted from Figure 133; L. Heimer: "The Human Brain and Spinal Cord. Functional Neuroanatomy and Dissection Guide." 2nd ed., 1985. Springer-Verlag New York, Inc., New York, New York.

Figure 35-1: Adapted from Figure 4; W.A. Catterall: "Molecular properties of voltage-gated ion channels in the heart." In: H.A. Fozzard et al., eds. The Heart and Cardiovascular System—Scientific Foundations. 2nd ed., 1991, Chapter 37. Lippincott-Raven, Philadelphia, Pennsylvania.

Figure 35-3: Adapted from Figure 1; R.E. Ten Eick, D.W. Walley, and H.H. Rasmussen: "Connections: Heart disease, cellular electrophysiology and ion channels." FASEB Journal 1992; 6:2568–2580. Federation of American Societies for Experimental Biology, Bethesda, Maryland.

Figure 37-5: Adapted from Figure 7; M.R. Rosen and P.T. Schwartz, eds.: "The Sicilian Gambit. A new approach to the classification of antiarrhythmic drugs based on their actions on arrhythmogenic mechanisms." Circulation 1991; 84:1831–1851. American Heart Association, Dallas, Texas.

Figure 39-3: Adapted from Figure 1; S.G. Young: "Recent progress in understanding apolipoprotein B." Circulation 1990; 82:1574–1594. American Heart Association, Dallas, Texas.

Tables 39-1 and 39-6: Adapted from Tables 1 and 6; H.N. Ginsberg, Y. Arad, and I.J. Goldberg: "Pathophysiology and therapy of hyperlipidemia." In: M.J. Antonaccio, ed. Cardiovascular Pharmacology. 3rd ed. 1990:485–513. Lippincott-Raven, Philadelphia, Pennsylvania.

Table 39-5: Adapted from Table 36-4; M.S. Brown and J.L. Goldstein: "Drugs used in the treatment of hyperlipoproteinemias." In: A.G. Gilman, T.W. Rall, A.S. Nies, P. Taylor, eds. Goodman and Gilman's The Pharmacological Basis of Therapeutics. 8th ed. Elmsford: Pergamon Press 1990:879.

Figure 41-3: Adapted from Figure 11; B.A. Stanton: "Molecular mechanisms of ANP inhibition of renal sodium transport." Canadian Journal of Physiology and Pharmacology 1991; 69:1546–1552. NRC Research Press, National Research Council of Canada, Ottawa, Ontario.

Figures 66-1, 66-2, and 66-3: Adapted from Figures 1, 2, and 3; R.E. Grymonpre, P.A. Mitenko, D.S. Sitar, F.Y. Aoki, and P.R. Montgomery: "Drug-associated hospital admissions in older medical patients." Journal of the American Geriatrics Society 1988;36:1092–1098. Waverly (Williams & Wilkins), Baltimore, Maryland.

Figures 66-5, 66-6, and 66-7: Adapted from Figures 1, 2, and 4; G.R. Wilkinson: "The effect of age and liver disease on the disposition and elimination of diazepam in adult man." Journal of Clinical Investigation 1975; 55:347–359. Society for Clinical Investigation, Rockefeller University Press, New York, New York.

Table 70-3: Adapted from Table 3; T.H. Shepard: "Teratology testing: I. Development and status of short-term prescreens. II. Biotransformation of teratogens as studied in whole embryo culture." In: S.M. MacLeod, A.B. Okey, S.P. Spielberg, eds. Developmental Pharmacology. New York: Wiley-Liss 1983:152.

Figure 70-10: Adapted from Figure 1; H. Kappus: "Overview of enzyme systems involved in bioreduction of drugs and in redox cycling." Biochemical Pharmacology 1986;35:1–6. Elsevier Science Inc., New York, New York.

3 5 7 9 8 6 4 2

Printed in the United States of America
on acid-free paper

The Department of Pharmacology
dedicates
the sixth edition of this book to
the memory of
WILLIAM ALLAN MAHON
(1929–1997)
A major contributor to the development of
Clinical Pharmacology in Canada,
an outstanding teacher,
long-time friend and colleague,
member of the Book Committee,
and a constant voice of good sense,
good science and good humor

Preface
to the Sixth Edition

This book had its origin over 35 years ago in the form of detailed lecture notes that were prepared by Drs. E.A. Sellers, H. Kalant, and W. Kalow. These notes were distributed by faculty members of the Department of Pharmacology, University of Toronto, to students in Medicine, Dentistry, and Pharmacy, and later to undergraduate Arts and Science students enrolled in specialist programs in pharmacology and toxicology. The lecture assignments to individual staff members changed from year to year, so that the notes gradually came to reflect the combined approaches of the whole Department. In addition, as the growing Department came to include steadily more clinicians with cross-appointments in Pharmacology, the content acquired a correspondingly better balance between clinical and basic pharmacological components.

In 1975, the notes were edited to provide greater uniformity of organization and style, and were combined into the first edition of this textbook. It was intended as a working text for students, not as an exhaustive reference work or an advanced treatise for senior clinicians and researchers, whose needs are better met by a variety of specialized publications. The illustrations were simple line drawings, and the list of suggested readings at the end of each chapter was not intended to provide detailed documentation of every point in the chapter, but only to provide additional sources of information for those readers who were interested in learning more about the subjects covered in the chapter.

The book has evolved, matured, and expanded through five editions preceding the present one, un-der the overall supervision of the departmental Book Committee, and a progression of editors:

1st edition, 1975: P. Seeman and E.M. Sellers

2nd edition, 1976: P. Seeman and E.M. Sellers

3rd edition, 1979: P. Seeman, E.M. Sellers, and W.H.E. Roschlau

4th edition, 1985: H. Kalant, W.H.E. Roschlau, and E.M. Sellers

5th edition, 1989: H. Kalant and W.H.E. Roschlau.

The first four editions were published by the Department itself, with the technical assistance of the University of Toronto Press. The 5th edition was published by B.C. Decker Inc., Toronto and Philadelphia, and later by Mosby-Year Book, Inc.

Despite these many changes, the *primary purpose and general character of the book* have remained the same. It continues to be a textbook of pharmacology rather than of therapeutics, although the increasingly rapid growth of knowledge and the steadily closer interdependence of basic and clinical aspects of the subject have made this distinction less sharp than it once was. It has also become necessary to include many very recent advances that seem likely to become clinically important in the immediate or near future.

The present edition, the 6th, retains this general didactic approach, but has undergone some *major changes of content and style.* Many chapters have been greatly expanded or completely rewritten, and new overview chapters or sections on signal transduction mechanisms and on the functional organization of the central nervous system, cardiovascular system, and gastrointestinal system have been included. The illustrations have been completely redrawn, and in this process the artist worked very closely with the editors and authors. It is hoped that the new illustrations will add to the appearance, clarity, and didactic value of the book.

An important new feature is the *short case histories* that appear at the beginning of each chapter in the sections on the pharmacology of the various organ systems. These sketches are not intended to serve as the primary material for medical curricula built on "case-based learning." Histories of the latter type, by their very nature, must be much more detailed, multidisciplinary, and longer than would be appropriate for a textbook of pharmacology. Rather, these histories should help the student see the clinical importance of basic pharmacological principles. We hope that the presentation of these histories at the *beginning* of the respective chapters, rather than at the end, will raise the reader's level of interest in, and alertness to, the basic pharmacology, and that it will therefore be read with closer and more critical attention. No questions and answers are provided to accompany these case histories because course instructors will probably have their own individual approaches to using the material, for which a "catechism" would be inappropriate.

Consistent with their adoption by the health care systems in many countries, *système international (SI) units* are used as much as possible in this edition, but are accompanied in most instances by the traditional units with which many teachers and clinicians continue to be more comfortable. As in previous editions, drugs are discussed under their non-proprietary (i.e., official or "generic") names, but examples of the most common proprietary names are also given for convenience. *North American spelling and nomenclature* are used throughout; in those very few instances in which United States and Canadian official nomenclature differs (e.g., U.S. "epinephrine" and Canadian "adrenaline"), both names are indicated in the text.

This is the first edition published by Oxford University Press, and the publishers have made an important contribution to the accuracy and quality of the text by arranging for independent reviews of all chapters in the manuscript stage. Valuable comments and suggestions by the reviewers are gratefully acknowledged by the editors and authors.

The editors express their gratitude to the chapter authors for the care, cooperation, and patience they have shown in revising, updating, and improving the text; to the departmental Book Committee for its support and encouragement, and to Prof. D. Kadar for detailed and vigilant reading of much of the text; to Mr. Jeffrey House, Vice President of Oxford University Press, for his enthusiastic support and promotion of this project; to Ms. Nancy Wolitzer, Mr. Sean Finnegan, and other members of the publisher's editorial staff, for their thorough and helpful work-up of the material; to Ms. Diana Clark and Ms. Merrylee Greenan for their capable preparation and processing of the manuscript; and to Mr. Stephen Mader for his expert design and execution of the illustrations, and for his patience, cooperation and initiative in the many revisions they have undergone.

Finally, the Department wishes to record its gratitude to the authors who, continuing the tradition that has existed since the first edition of this book, have generously donated their efforts for the benefit of the Department and its graduate students. All royalties from the sale of the book go to a special fund for the support of educational and scholarly activities not covered by the regular departmental budget.

Toronto   The Editors
Spring 1997

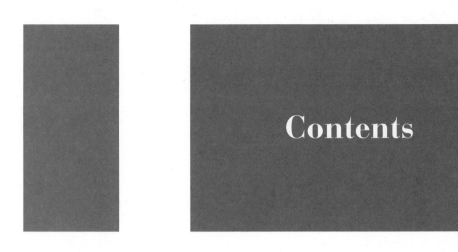

Contents

II AUTONOMIC NERVOUS SYSTEM AND NEUROMUSCULAR JUNCTION

III CENTRAL NERVOUS SYSTEM

VII   GASTROINTESTINAL SYSTEM

VIII   ENDOCRINE SYSTEMS

IX   ANTI-INFECTIVE CHEMOTHERAPY

X   ANTINEOPLASTIC CHEMOTHERAPY, IMMUNOPHARMACOLOGY

XI   SPECIAL TOPICS OF PHARMACOLOGY

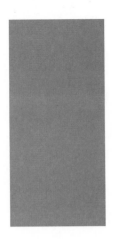
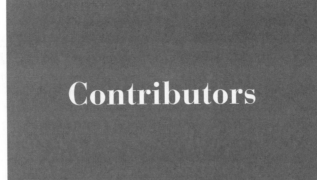

Contributors

UWE ACKERMANN, PH.D.
Professor
Department of Physiology
Faculty of Medicine
University of Toronto

MARGARET J. BAIGENT, PH.D.
Associate Professor (Retired)
Department of Nutritional Sciences
Faculty of Medicine
University of Toronto

JOSEPH M. BRANDWEIN, M.D.
Assistant Professor
Department of Medicine
Faculty of Medicine
University of Toronto

W. McINTYRE BURNHAM, PH.D.
Professor
Department of Pharmacology
Faculty of Medicine
Director
Bloorview Epilepsy Research Program
University of Toronto

USOA BUSTO, PHARM.D.
Associate Professor
Faculty of Pharmacy
University of Toronto
Scientist
Addiction Research Foundation of Ontario

F.J. LOU CARMICHAEL, M.D., PH.D.
Associate Professor
Departments of Anesthesia and Pharmacology
Faculty of Medicine
University of Toronto

PAUL DORIAN, M.D., M.SC.
Associate Professor
Departments of Medicine and Pharmacology
Faculty of Medicine
University of Toronto

LASZLO ENDRENYI, PH.D.
Professor
Department of Pharmacology
Faculty of Medicine
University of Toronto

ELIZABETH L. FORD-JONES, M.D.
Associate Professor
Department of Pediatrics
Faculty of Medicine
University of Toronto

CHRISTINE FORSTER, PH.D.
Associate Professor
Departments of Medicine and Pharmacology
Faculty of Medicine
University of Toronto

SUSAN R. GEORGE, M.D.
Professor
Departments of Medicine and Pharmacology
Faculty of Medicine
University of Toronto

GERALD J. GOLDENBERG, M.D., PH.D.
Professor
Departments of Medicine and Pharmacology
Director
Interdepartmental Division of Oncology
Faculty of Medicine
University of Toronto

DENIS M. GRANT, PH.D.
Associate Professor
Departments of Pediatrics and Pharmacology
Faculties of Medicine and Pharmacy
University of Toronto
Senior Scientist
Research Institute, The Hospital for Sick Children, Toronto

LARRY A. GRUPP, D.SC.
Associate Professor
Department of Pharmacology
Faculty of Medicine
University of Toronto
Senior Scientist
Addiction Research Foundation of Ontario

DANIEL A. HAAS, D.D.S., PH.D.
Associate Professor
Department of Anesthesia
Faculty of Dentistry
Department of Pharmacology
Faculty of Medicine
University of Toronto

PATRICIA A. HARPER, PH.D.
Assistant Professor
Departments of Pediatrics and Pharmacology
Faculty of Medicine
University of Toronto
Scientist
Research Institute, The Hospital for Sick Children, Toronto

EVA JANECEK, B.SC.PHARM.
Senior Clinical Tutor
Faculty of Pharmacy
University of Toronto

DEZSÖ KADAR, B.SC.PHARM., PH.D.
Professor
Department of Pharmacology
Faculty of Medicine
University of Toronto

HAROLD KALANT, M.D., PH.D.
Professor Emeritus
Department of Pharmacology
Faculty of Medicine
University of Toronto
Director Emeritus
Biobehavioral Research
Addiction Research Foundation of Ontario

WERNER KALOW, M.D.
Professor Emeritus
Department of Pharmacology
Faculty of Medicine
University of Toronto

SHITIJ KAPUR, M.D.
Research Scientist, PET Centre
Clarke Institute of Psychiatry
University of Toronto

JAY S. KEYSTONE, M.D., M.SC.
Professor
Departments of Medicine and Pharmacology
Faculty of Medicine
University of Toronto
Director
Tropical Disease Unit
The Toronto Hospital

JATINDER M. KHANNA, PH.D.
Professor
Department of Pharmacology
Faculty of Medicine
University of Toronto

GIDEON KOREN, M.D.
Professor
Departments of Pediatrics, Pharmacology, and Medicine
Faculties of Medicine and Pharmacy
University of Toronto
Director
Division of Clinical Pharmacology & MotheRisk
The Hospital for Sick Children, Toronto

A. JOSÉ LANÇA, M.D., PH.D.
Assistant Professor
Department of Pharmacology
Faculty of Medicine
University of Toronto

LAURA A. MAGEE, M.D., M.SC.
Assistant Professor
Departments of Medicine and Pharmacology
Faculty of Medicine
University of Toronto

WILLIAM A. MAHON, M.D.
Professor Emeritus
Departments of Medicine and Pharmacology
Faculty of Medicine
University of Toronto

ANA E. MARQUEZ-JULIO, M.D.
Assistant Professor
Department of Medicine
Louisiana State University
New Orleans, Louisiana

MICHAEL A. MCGUIGAN, M.D., C.M., M.B.A.
Associate Professor
Departments of Pediatrics, Pharmacology, and Health
    Administration
Faculty of Medicine
University of Toronto
Medical Director
Ontario Regional Poison Control Centre
The Hospital for Sick Children, Toronto

JANE MITCHELL, PH.D.
Assistant Professor
Department of Pharmacology
Faculty of Medicine
University of Toronto

MALCOLM J. MOORE, M.D.
Associate Professor
Departments of Medicine and Pharmacology
Faculty of Medicine
University of Toronto

CLAUDIO A. NARANJO, M.D.
Professor
Departments of Pharmacology, Psychiatry, and
    Medicine
Faculty of Medicine
Head
Psychopharmacology Research Program
Sunnybrook Health Science Centre
University of Toronto

ALLAN B. OKEY, PH.D.
Professor and Chair
Department of Pharmacology
Faculty of Medicine
University of Toronto

CECIL R. PACE-ASCIAK, PH.D.
Professor
Departments of Pediatrics and Pharmacology
Faculty of Medicine
University of Toronto
Senior Scientist
Research Institute, The Hospital for Sick Children,
    Toronto

DAVID S. RIDDICK, PH.D.
Assistant Professor
Department of Pharmacology
Faculty of Medicine
University of Toronto

EVE A. ROBERTS, M.D.
Associate Professor
Departments of Pediatrics, Medicine, and
    Pharmacology
Faculty of Medicine
University of Toronto

MYROSLAVA K. ROMACH, M.D.
Assistant Professor
Department of Psychiatry
Faculty of Medicine
University of Toronto

WALTER H.E. ROSCHLAU, M.D.
Professor Emeritus
Department of Pharmacology
Faculty of Medicine
University of Toronto

PHILIP SEEMAN, M.D., PH.D.
Professor
Departments of Psychiatry and Pharmacology
Faculty of Medicine
University of Toronto

BERNARD P. SCHIMMER, PH.D.
Professor
Banting & Best Department of Medical Research and
    Department of Pharmacology
Faculty of Medicine
University of Toronto

EDWARD M. SELLERS, M.D., PH.D.
Professor
Departments of Pharmacology, Medicine, and
    Psychiatry
Faculty of Medicine
University of Toronto

JOHN W. SEMPLE, PH.D.
Associate Professor
Departments of Pharmacology and Medicine
Faculty of Medicine
University of Toronto
Staff Scientist
St. Michael's Hospital, Toronto

NEIL H. SHEAR, M.D.
Associate Professor
Departments of Medicine, Pharmacology, and
    Pediatrics
Faculties of Medicine and Pharmacy
Director
Program in Clinical Pharmacology/Pharmacy
Sunnybrook Health Science Centre
University of Toronto

DANIEL S. SITAR, B.SC.PHARM., PH.D.
Professor
Departments of Medicine and Pharmacology &
    Therapeutics
Faculty of Medicine
University of Manitoba
Winnipeg, Manitoba

LAWRENCE SPERO, PH.D.
Professor
Department of Pharmacology
Faculty of Medicine
University of Toronto

WILLIAM C. STURTRIDGE, D.D.S., M.D., PH.D.
Associate Professor
Departments of Medicine and Pharmacology
Faculties of Medicine and Dentistry
University of Toronto

JACK UETRECHT, M.D., PH.D.
Associate Dean
Faculty of Pharmacy
Professor
Departments of Pharmacology and Medicine
Faculties of Medicine and Pharmacy
University of Toronto

SHARON L. WALMSLEY, M.D.
Assistant Professor
Department of Medicine
Faculty of Medicine
University of Toronto

JERRY J. WARSH, M.D., PH.D.
Professor
Departments of Pharmacology and Psychiatry,
    Institute of Medical Science
Faculty of Medicine
Head
Section of Biochemical Psychiatry
Clarke Institute of Psychiatry
University of Toronto

PETER G. WELLS, PHARM.D.
Professor
Department of Pharmacology
Faculties of Medicine and Pharmacy
University of Toronto

CATHARINE WHITESIDE, M.D., PH.D.
Professor
Department of Medicine
Faculty of Medicine
University of Toronto

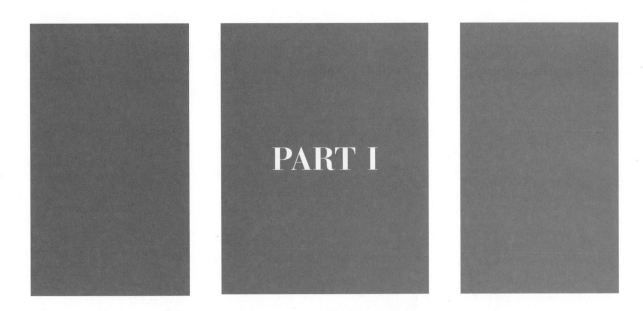

PART I

GENERAL PRINCIPLES
OF PHARMACOLOGY

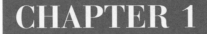

CHAPTER 1

Introduction to General Pharmacology

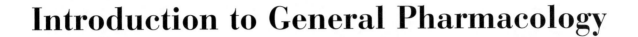

H. KALANT

WHAT IS PHARMACOLOGY

The word **pharmacology** is derived from the Greek words *pharmakon* (a drug or poison) and *logos* (word or discourse) and means "the science (discourse) that deals with the fate of drugs in the body and their actions on the body." It overlaps extensively with **pharmacy** (the science of preparation of drugs) and with **therapeutics** (the treatment of disease, by drugs and other means). Some of the areas of overlap are mentioned below.

Pharmacology is both a basic and a clinically applied science. As a basic science, it deals with the fate and actions of drugs at various levels (molecular, cellular, organ, and whole-body, in any animal species), drawing on knowledge, concepts, and techniques derived from biochemistry, physiology, biophysics, and other divisions of biological science. As an applied science, it deals with the same questions, but in the specific context of the human species and the use of drugs in the treatment of disease. This book includes both elements of the subject.

WHAT IS A DRUG

No definition of "drug" yet offered is entirely satisfactory. Perhaps the nearest we can come to one is the following: A drug is any substance, other than a normal constituent of the body or one that is required for normal bodily function (e.g., food, water, oxygen), that, when applied to or introduced into a living organism, has the effect of altering body function(s). This alteration may prove useful in the treatment of disease (therapeutic application) or it may cause disease (toxicity), but these outcomes are quite a separate matter from the definition of "drug."

Cold and hay-fever remedies bought off a supermarket shelf, penicillin given on prescription, and LSD (lysergic acid diethylamide) bought illicitly on the street are all drugs. Vitamin C in orange juice is a food, but pure ascorbic acid injected in large doses to alter fibroblast activity is a drug. Hydrocortisone secreted by the adrenal cortex is a hormone, but when administered in large doses to suppress inflammatory or immune responses it is a drug. These actions may be useful in treating such diseases as rheumatoid arthritis or asthma, or they may cause Cushing's disease.

Pharmacology is not concerned primarily with what the drug may be used for but with what actions it has and what fate it encounters in the living organism.

SCOPE AND SUBDIVISIONS OF PHARMACOLOGY

How pharmacology is divided and how it overlaps with pharmacy and therapeutics are best illustrated by showing schematically what happens when a drug enters the body (Fig. 1-1).

1. Whether the drug is given as a tablet or capsule by mouth, as a vapor or aerosol by inhalation, or as a crystalline suspension by subcutaneous injection (or in any other form), it must first go into free solution at the site of administration. A special

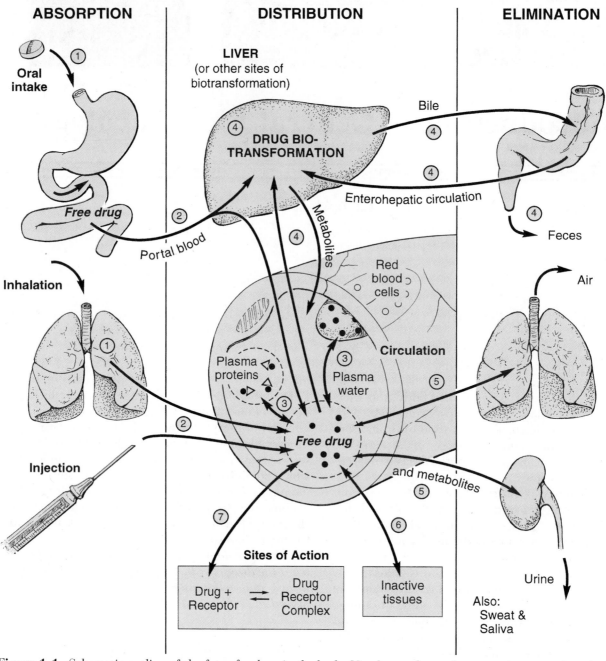

ABSORPTION   **DISTRIBUTION**   **ELIMINATION**

Oral intake

①

LIVER
(or other sites of biotransformation)

④ **DRUG BIO-TRANSFORMATION**

Bile ④

④ Enterohepatic circulation

Free drug ②

Portal blood

④ Metabolites

④ Feces

Inhalation

Red blood cells

①

Circulation

③

Air

Plasma proteins ▷ ◁

③

Plasma water ⑤

②

Free drug

and metabolites ⑤

Injection

⑦

⑥

Urine

Sites of Action

| Drug + Receptor | ⇌ | Drug Receptor Complex | | Inactive tissues |

Also:
Sweat & Saliva

Figure 1-1. Schematic outline of the fate of a drug in the body. Numbers refer to the successive steps described in this section.

formulation of the drug may be needed to protect it against destruction by gastric acid or by other degradative processes elsewhere. Preparation of the drug form, and adjustment of its physical properties so that the drug will dissolve at the desired rate, and in the right location, are problems of **pharmacy.**

  2. The dissolved drug must be absorbed into the portal blood if it is given by mouth; it will be directly absorbed into the systemic circulation if it is given by injection or by inhalation, or if it is applied to skin or mucous membranes. Absorption of the drug can involve a variety of different mechanisms that enable it to cross cell membranes, not only in the gastrointestinal tract but in all tissues. The absorption of a drug is strongly influenced by its molecular size, lipid solubility, ionization, and other physicochemical properties. These questions are discussed in detail in Chapter 2. From the portal blood, some of the drug is taken up by the liver, but some goes on into the systemic circulation. This is considered in detail in Chapter 7. The study of drug absorption and uptake by the liver is part of **pharmacology.**

Bioavailability of a drug, i.e., the proportion of an administered dose that eventually reaches the systemic circulation in unchanged form, depends on both (1) and (2) and therefore is of concern to **both pharmacy and pharmacology.** It is considered in Chapter 5.

3. Once in the systemic blood, the free drug dissolved in the plasma water may be reversibly taken up into red cells or reversibly bound to plasma proteins.

4. It may be taken up into the liver or other tissues where it can be converted into metabolites of the original drug. These may be eliminated in the bile, and thus reach the intestine, where they can either be excreted in the feces or be reabsorbed and carried in the portal blood back to the liver (enterohepatic circulation). Alternatively, the metabolites (and the original drug itself) may pass back from the liver into the general circulation and be carried to all other organs and tissues.

5. Among these other organs is the kidney, where both the drug and its metabolites may be filtered by the glomerulus or secreted by the tubule into the urine. However, depending on the concentration, the degree of ionization of the drug at the pH of the urine, and other factors, some of the drug may be reabsorbed from the urine by the tubule and pass back into the blood. This is discussed in greater detail in Chapter 7. Another organ to which the drug is carried is the lung. If the drug or its metabolite is volatile, it can pass from the blood into the alveolar air and be eliminated in the breath. This is particularly important for terminating the action of volatile anesthetics (see Chapter 24) and is also the basis of the Breathalyzer test for blood alcohol level (see Chapter 26).

6. Among the tissues and organs through which the drug passes, some are not affected by it and therefore simply act as reservoirs that form part of the drug's volume of distribution. This influences the equilibrium concentration of drug in the plasma after administration of a specified dose.

All of the processes mentioned in (2) to (6) determine the rate at which the concentrations of the drug and its metabolites in the plasma and tissues rise and fall as well as the maximum concentrations reached after a given dose. Together, these factors influence the speed of onset and duration of drug effects. The study of the time course of drug concentration, and of the factors affecting it, is called **pharmacokinetics.** It is discussed in detail in Chapter 5. The pharmacokinetic features of a drug determine the dosage schedule that is used clinically (see Chapter 6) and therefore influence the **therapeutic program.**

7. Most (but not all) drugs bind to relatively specific receptors on the surface or in the interior of the tissue cells on which the drugs act. The binding of a drug to its receptor may initiate biochemical or biophysical changes that lead to its characteristic effects on body functions, and the drug is called an **agonist** at that receptor. In other cases, a drug may bind to a receptor without initiating any change, but it may prevent another substance from gaining access to the receptor where it normally acts; many drugs function in this way as **receptor blockers** or **antagonists.** In a small number of cases a drug may bind to a receptor and produce changes *opposite* to those produced by other agonists; it is then called an **inverse agonist** (see Chapter 27).

The study of these mechanisms of drug action is called **pharmacodynamics,** and the quantitative study of the relations among drug dose, concentration, and magnitude of effect is called **pharmacometrics.** These topics are discussed in Chapters 8 and 9. The ability of a drug to combine with its receptor depends on specific features of the drug's molecular structure. Therefore the study of pharmacodynamics overlaps with the field of **pharmaceutical chemistry,** which deals with the chemical synthesis of drugs and the study of their **structure–activity relationships.**

In addition to these basic divisions of the subject matter of pharmacology, there are other sets of divisions based on different criteria. For example, pharmacology may be divided according to:

1. The organ system of primary interest, e.g., neuropharmacology, cardiovascular pharmacology, renal pharmacology
2. The techniques used, e.g., biochemical pharmacology, molecular pharmacology, behavioral pharmacology, immunopharmacology
3. The purpose or application to which the knowledge is put, e.g.,
   - Clinical pharmacology, the study of pharmacokinetics and pharmacodynamics in patients receiving drugs for the treatment of disease;

therefore it also includes the effect of disease on the action and disposition of the drug
- Pharmacogenetics, the study of genetic factors causing variation in the response to drugs
- Toxicology, the study of drugs that are acting as poisons rather than as agents for the treatment of disease; it includes specialized subdivisions such as forensic toxicology, clinical toxicology, industrial and environmental toxicology, and behavioral toxicology
- Agricultural pharmacology, the use of drugs for pest control

DRUG CLASSIFICATIONS

Classification Based on Origin

Throughout human history there have been keen observers who, by chance observation or by systematic trial and error, have recognized the interesting or useful drug effects of certain substances. But such individuals have been the exception; most "drug" use through the centuries has been based on symbolic or magical thinking. For example, a plant with liver-shaped leaves was used to "treat" illnesses thought to arise in the liver.

With the growth of modern science over the last three centuries, systematic observation of the effects of exogenous substances on the body has given rise to techniques for screening possible new drugs. At first, the substances screened were natural materials gathered by botanists, anthropologists, and explorers. Later, chemists extracted and purified the active ingredients of these natural materials, and later still they synthesized wholly new compounds that did not exist in nature, but that, by analogy with natural compounds, might be expected to have drug effects.

On the basis of their origin, drugs may be placed in the following four broad categories.

Natural preparations or galenicals

These are relatively crude preparations obtained by drying or extracting plant or animal materials (e.g., digitalis leaf, tincture of belladonna, and desiccated thyroid). This type of medicine, originally prepared by medicine men or priest-physicians, and later by apothecaries or physicians, dates back to prehistoric times. An early careful and systematic description of all known such drugs was written by the Greek physician Galen (A.D. 130–200), who practiced in Rome. In Galen's honor such drugs later became known as "galenicals." Even now, new drugs are found from such materials, but they are no longer likely to be used as galenicals; pharmaceutical chemistry is more likely to carry them immediately to the next stage.

Pure compounds

These are isolated from natural sources by physical and chemical extraction and purification procedures. A number of classical examples are shown in Table 1-1. The first to be isolated was morphine, which Sertürner purified from opium in 1805. Many important drugs have come from natural sources, even in the last few years. Modern examples include penicillin and numerous other antibiotics that derive from a variety of molds and fungi, and various anticancer and antileukemic chemotherapeutic drugs such as vinblastine and vincristine that are obtained from certain varieties of periwinkle plant.

Semisynthetic substances

These are obtained by chemical modification of the pure compounds obtained from natural sources. For example, acetylating two hydroxyl groups in morphine yields diacetylmorphine (heroin). Changing a side-group in penicillin yields oxacillin. Inserting a fluorine atom in the adrenal steroid hydrocortisone yields fludrocortisone. Many such semisynthetic modifications result in dramatic improvements of the parent compounds with respect to potency, specificity, and duration of action.

Table 1-1 Some Examples of Drugs Derived from Plant Materials in Various Parts of the World

Plant Material or Galenical Preparation	Pure Compound	Original Source
Tincture of belladonna	Atropine	Orient (ancient)
Coca leaves	Cocaine	Peru, Bolivia
Curare	d-Tubocurarine	Amazon Basin
Digitalis leaf, tincture	Digoxin, etc.	England
Ephedra	Ephedrine	China
Calabar bean	Eserine	West Africa
Opium	Morphine	Greece (ancient)
Tobacco	Nicotine	North and Central America
Cinchona bark	Quinine	Peru
Rauwolfia	Reserpine	India

Purely synthetic compounds

This is the most recent class. The first barbiturate was synthesized in 1902. Most drugs are now synthetic. Some of these substances were synthesized for other purposes, and medical uses were discovered accidentally. For example, disulfiram was invented as an agent to vulcanize rubber: The observation that rubber-factory workers got very bad reactions when they drank alcohol led to its use as an antialcoholism drug. In contrast, other drugs (e.g., dimercaprol [BAL], an antidote for arsenic or mercury poisoning) have been synthesized deliberately on the basis of predicted chemical properties. Still others have been synthesized on the basis of knowledge gained from the study of semisynthetic modifications of existing compounds. By learning which molecular features are necessary for which drug actions, pharmaceutical chemists are increasingly able to "custom design" a molecule to produce or enhance a desired pharmacological effect, while minimizing undesired effects.

Classification Based on Use

Most textbooks of pharmacology, particularly those intended for students and practitioners of medicine, dentistry, pharmacy, nursing, and other health sciences, classify drugs according to organ system (upon which they exert their most prominent actions) or therapeutic use (to which they are put). For example, drugs are classed as antibiotics, antiarrhythmic agents, diuretics, and anticonvulsants. There are some valid arguments against this method of classification: Almost every drug has more than one effect and acts in more than one tissue, and different drugs may produce a similar therapeutic effect by quite different means. Nevertheless, this is still the most commonly used system of classification, and in deference to tradition and clinical usefulness, it is also employed in this book.

DRUGS AND SOCIETY

Human society comes into contact with drugs in many different ways:

1. Medical prescription or therapeutic use. This is the exposure that receives most attention in medical teaching, but it is by no means the most common.

2. Over-the-counter sale, without prescription. These drugs are also intended primarily for "therapeutic" purposes, even though their use is most commonly not under medical supervision. A huge range of drugs (cough remedies, analgesics, topical antiseptics, local anesthetics, antihistamines, hypnotics, and so forth) can be bought in this way. Many are quite potent and are seriously toxic if used improperly.

3. Nonmedical use. Alcohol, cannabis, and a wide range of other psychoactive substances (i.e., that affect mood, perception, psychomotor performance, and emotional responses) dominate this category. Some are legally available, some are diverted from legal production to the illicit market, and some are manufactured illegally. All such use carries the potential risk of abuse, with the attendant problems of toxicity and dependence (see Chapter 72).

4. Industrial use. Many preservatives, artificial flavorings, colorings, and fillers are added to processed foods and even to pharmaceutical preparations. Though each is kept to a level considered safe in any individual product, very little is known about cumulative totals, or interactions between substances, and what these may contribute to low-grade toxicity in the consumer.

5. Agricultural use. Widespread use of pesticides has contributed greatly to increased agricultural productivity in many parts of the world. However, pesticides, weed-killers, and herbicides (together with industrial wastes, automobile exhaust fumes, and other products of human industry) contribute to total environmental toxicity.

6. Accident. Apart from the obvious cases of accidental poisoning, which come to hospital emergency rooms, and deliberate suicidal or homicidal poisonings, which are dealt with by forensic toxicologists as well as hospitals, there are natural accidents. For example, a certain fungus growth on peanuts can generate a very potent carcinogen (aflatoxin); another fungus growth on rye generates ergot alkaloids, which on occasion cause serious poisoning.

Exposure to drugs by all these means has become far more common as a result of population growth, chemical inventions, improved means of communication, and industrialization. Apart from the accident category, the other forms of exposure all carry certain benefits and certain hazards, but the optimum balance of benefits versus risks is often hard to define. It depends to a large extent on the scale of social values. This is particularly true of the third, fourth, and fifth categories, but is also true of the first and second.

Therefore most societies control the availability,

quality, and permitted uses of drugs. Such controls are generally pragmatic, rather than theoretical. To a large extent they are handled by government administrative regulation, but certain broad principles and policies are laid down in legislation, which differs to some extent from country to country.

DRUG STANDARDS AND REFERENCES

The rapid progress in the chemical industry in the past half-century has altered the nature of pharmacy, pharmacology, and therapeutics. Because most drugs used nowadays are potent pure chemicals, they must be prepared and used under strict controls. Therefore, their definition and standardization are regulated by law in terms of name, purity, potency, and preparation, and so is their distribution to the public.

Not only the active drugs themselves, but also the forms in which they are dispensed, must be carefully controlled if the effectiveness of drug treatment is to be assured. For application in drug therapy, most chemicals have to be put into tablets; capsules, ampoules, aerosols, ointments, solutions, or suppositories. The drug must have the highest purity compatible with chemical stability and economic feasibility. It must have appropriate crystal size. It must be compatible with ingredients usually necessary to give bulk to a tablet, to regulate its hardness, cohesiveness, and its rate of disintegration in gastric or intestinal juice. The tablet may have to be protected from light and may have to withstand storage in tropical climates. It may require a corrective for taste. It should not explode in the patient's stomach (as have some tablets used in the treatment of tuberculosis). Above all, it must release the drug in such a manner that the drug will be absorbed at a suitable rate. There are equivalent problems in compounding drug vehicles other than tablets. All this is the domain of **pharmacy,** and all of it is subject to controls and standards.

The standards are published in **pharmacopoeias** such as the *British Pharmacopoeia (B.P.)*, the *U.S. Pharmacopeia (U.S.P.)*, the *Codex Français*, and the *International Pharmacopoeia*. These books are revised periodically and supplements to them may be issued between editions. A drug listed in a pharmacopoeia is termed an "official" drug because it enjoys official recognition by a government. Canada has no pharmacopoeia of its own, but other pharmacopoeias that have official status may be used.

There are also a number of reference books that are widely used in North America (although they do not have official status in every province of Canada):

Pediatric Dosage Handbook. American Pharmaceutical Association.

European Pharmacopoeia.

U.S. National Formulary (N.F.). American Pharmaceutical Society.

American Medical Association Drug Evaluations.

Accepted Dental Therapeutics (A.D.T.). Published annually by the American Dental Association. Convenient and useful for dentists, it includes information on (1) drugs of recognized value in dentistry, (2) drugs of uncertain status more recently proposed for use by dentists, and (3) some drugs now generally regarded as obsolete.

Physician's Desk Reference. Published annually by Medical Economics. For American practitioners, the **PDR** lists and describes FDA-approved prescribing information, including indications, contraindications, effects, dosages, routes, and methods.

Compendium of Pharmaceuticals and Specialties (C.P.S.). Published annually by the Canadian Pharmaceutical Association. For Canadian practitioners, this publication is very useful; it describes many of the prescription drugs available in Canada and their uses, contraindications, adverse reactions, and doses.

DRUG NOMENCLATURE

Many names given to drugs are often confusing to those who are not familiar with the nomenclature system. When a drug is first synthesized and subjected to initial screening, it is usually referred to, in the scientific literature, by its chemical name or by a code number indicating the manufacturer and test document file number (e.g., R015-4513, EN-2234A). When it reaches the stage of clinical testing, it usually receives a more convenient but unofficial short name. After it comes into general use, it may receive other names indicative of different levels of medical or official approval. When a pharmaceutical company finally receives permission to bring the new drug onto the market, usually a proprietary (trade or brand) name is given to it. The use of this name is protected by law and is restricted to the firm that introduces the preparation; it carries the symbol ®. Thus, the same drug may be known (unfortunately) under several different names at the same time.

1. Chemical name
2. Nonproprietary drug name (sometimes called "generic name")
   - Official names (in pharmacopoeias)
   - Approved names (not yet in pharmacopoeias)
     - U.S. Adopted Name (USAN; Joint Committee of AMA, U.S. Pharmacopeial Commission, and American Pharmaceutical Association)
     - Canadian Proper Names
     - Approved names, British Pharmacopoeial Commission
3. Proprietary name: manufacturer's trade name, registered by the owner, somewhat like a copyright
4. Common name

Examples:

1. *Chemical names:* 1-methyl-4-phenyl-4-carbethoxypiperidine; 1-methyl-4-phenylisonipecotic acid ethyl ester
   Official names: pethidine (B.P.), meperidine (U.S.P.), isonipecaine (I.P.)
   Proprietary names: Demerol, Dolantin, Dolantol.
2. *Chemical name:* ortho-acetoxybenzoic acid
   Official names: acetylsalicylic acid (B.P.), aspirin (U.S.P.)
   Proprietary names: Aspirin (in Canada only), Empirin, Entrophen, and many more.

It is in the financial interest of the manufacturer to popularize and use the trade name only, because the patent (the exclusive right to sell the drug) will last only 17 years in the United States, but the trade name registration (the right to sell a drug by a given name) lasts for at least 50. Even when exclusivity ends, the value of brand name recognition goes on, and may be significant. The time from patenting to marketing is usually 8–10 years, and the cost of development is typically in the hundreds of millions of dollars per drug. In addition, the patent may not be valid because someone else may have published an article or own a patent with close to the same idea. If the drug is really very good, it will also be produced in a country that does not have reciprocal patent laws, e.g., Italy, Argentina, or Hungary. It is easy to appreciate why a company that has spent millions of dollars for drug development will encourage the use of its own brand, or proprietary, name. As a rule, the trade name is chosen to be simple and euphonious, while the nonproprietary name tends to be difficult and to not suggest its use or chemical

nature. A combined **Committee on Nomenclature of the American Medical Association, American Pharmaceutical Association, and U.S. Pharmacopeial Commission** has made good progress in correcting this situation, and thus the United States Adopted Name (USAN) is easier to remember and suggests the nature of the drug. The names, chemical structures, and uses of newly introduced drugs are published in the *Journal of the American Medical Association (JAMA)*.

We recommend the use of official, USAN (U.S.A.), proper (Canada), or approved (U.K.) names, which are used in most reputable journals and which are almost always the same because of international cooperation in naming. If a drug becomes official, the USAN, proper, or approved name will almost certainly become the official name.

The use of trade names leads to an artificially complex vocabulary, which hinders medical communication. The same product is often produced by several reliable manufacturers, all using different brand names; and the use of trade names encourages high pricing.

In fairness to pharmaceutical firms it must be pointed out that there have been occasional instances in which nonbrand preparations have failed to be reliable. Certain trade name preparations adhere to standards that may be higher than those called for by pharmacopoeial specification. Unreliability of certain types of drugs can be extremely serious. It may be desirable, therefore, to depend on the reputation of the company producing them. This can be done by specifying the brand or the company when writing a prescription.

OTHER SOURCES OF INFORMATION

The material in this book is only a *starting point* in learning about drug actions and drug use. All medical students should consider, and have access to, other reference sources. For anyone with a special interest in drugs or drug research, there are numerous useful scientific journals. For example:

- *Drugs*
- *Pharmacological Reviews*
- *Journal of Pharmacology and Experimental Therapeutics*
- *British Journal of Pharmacology and Chemotherapy*
- *European Journal of Clinical Pharmacology*

- *Canadian Journal of Physiology and Pharmacology*
- *Clinical Pharmacokinetics*

Most of the major medical journals continue to present drug information in the form of editorials or reviews.

The Medical Letter on Drugs and Therapeutics represents a specialized effort to provide practicing physicians and medical students with unbiased data and critical information on newly introduced drugs. It compares new drugs with older agents and critically analyzes claims put forth by manufacturers.

The information presented is concise and usually very up to date. For those who wish to know more about the origins and history of drugs, two very interesting older books are listed under Suggested Reading.

SUGGESTED READING

Efron DH, Holmstedt B, Kline NS, eds. *Ethnopharmacologic search for psychoactive drugs.* Washington, DC: U.S. Department of Health, Education and Welfare, 1967.

Holmstedt B, Liljestrand G, eds. *Readings in pharmacology.* New York: Macmillan, 1963.

CHAPTER 2

Drug Solubility, Absorption, and Movement Across Body Membranes

P. SEEMAN AND H. KALANT

In Chapter 1, a general outline of the fate of drugs in the body was given, beginning with absorption from the site of administration and going on to distribution throughout the body, including the sites of action, biotransformation, and elimination (see Fig. 1-1). All these processes together determine the speed of onset of drug action, its intensity, and its duration.

When a drug is used therapeutically, it is usually desirable to get an adequate concentration to the site of action as quickly as possible, and to maintain that concentration as continuously and evenly as possible. To achieve this, one must understand how the route and rate of administration are chosen, and what factors affect the speed with which the drug reaches its sites of action and elimination.

ROUTES OF DRUG ADMINISTRATION

Topical

The simplest mode of administration is direct local application of the drug to the place where it must act. Such local application is called "topical" (from the Greek *topos* = a place). This most often means direct application to an accessible body surface. Examples include the use of ointments, creams, lotions, powders, or sprays applied to the **skin; eye** drops and ophthalmic ointments; **nose** drops and sprays; **ear** drops; and solutions or sprays for use in the **mouth, throat, rectum, vagina,** and **urethra.**

However, drugs applied to mucous membranes can often be absorbed rapidly enough to produce actions in the rest of the body. When cocaine was first used as a local anesthetic, it was widely adopted in rectal and urologic surgery and used in large amounts that gave rise to many poisonings, including fatal ones. "Topical use" refers to the application of sufficiently small volumes and low concentrations to ensure that the drug acts *only* at that site.

Occasionally, drugs are injected directly into **body cavities** for local action at those sites. For example, corticosteroids may be injected into a joint or a bursa for treatment of a sharply localized arthritis or bursitis not caused by infection. Antibiotics may be injected into the pleural space or into an abscess cavity for treatment of a local pocket of infection surrounded by fibrous tissue that prevents the antibiotic from getting there via the bloodstream. **Intrathecal injection** is employed to administer drugs directly into the cerebrospinal fluid (CSF) bathing the central nervous system, bypassing the blood–brain barrier and the blood–CSF barrier. The doses injected in such cases are enough to produce fairly high local concentrations, but not so large as to produce significant levels in the circulating blood when the drug diffuses away from the site of injection.

Percutaneous

Drug absorption through the intact skin is proportional to the lipid solubility of the drug (the epidermisbehaves as a lipoid barrier; the dermis is freely permeable). Absorption can be enhanced by suspending the drug in an oily vehicle. This is generally not an efficient method for delivering drugs to the systemic circulation. However, a few lipid-soluble drugs are now marketed for percutaneous administration, such as nitroglycerin ointment to treat angina pectoris, scopolamine plasters to prevent motion sickness, nicotine patches to aid cessation of smoking, and patches for administration of male and female sex hormones.

Even though the skin is an effective barrier that hinders the transport of almost all substances, there are very few substances to which it is *totally* impermeable. Even a heavy metal like mercury can be absorbed to some degree through the skin. Indeed, absorption through the skin is an important route of poisoning in humans and animals following accidental exposure to foreign chemicals such as insecticides containing parathion, malathion, or nicotine.

Gastrointestinal Tract

Oral mucosa (sublingual)

A number of drugs can be absorbed through the thinner portions of the oral mucosa. A familiar example is nitroglycerin in the form of small tablets that are placed under the tongue (sublingual). The drug is rapidly absorbed, giving rapid relief of anginal attacks. Drugs absorbed sublingually or buccally are not exposed to gastric and intestinal digestive juices, and are not subject to immediate passage through the liver (i.e., no prior transformation) before entering the systemic circulation. Many drugs, however, are not capable of penetrating the oral mucosa in significant amounts and others are too irritating to be held in the mouth.

Stomach and intestine (oral, per os, p.o., PO)

Absorption from the upper gastrointestinal tract depends on many factors, such as pH, gastric emptying, intestinal motility, solubility of solid drugs, concentration of drug solutions, stability of drugs in gastrointestinal fluids, and binding to gastrointestinal contents.

The relatively large blood supply of the stomach and small intestine, combined with the opportunity for prolonged contact of a drug with the relatively large epithelial surface, aids the absorption of most drugs. The length of time a substance remains in the stomach, however, is the greatest variable affecting the extent of gastric absorption. The rate at which the stomach empties its contents into the small intestine is influenced by the volume, viscosity, and composition of those contents; by physical activity and the position of the body; by the ingested drugs themselves; and by many other factors. Only when a drug is taken with water on a relatively empty stomach is it likely to reach the small intestine fairly rapidly (Fig. 2-1).

Rectal mucosa (suppositories, enemas)

Drugs that escape absorption in the small intestine may continue to be absorbed during their passage through the colon. Moreover, the terminal segment of the large intestine, the rectum, can serve as a useful site for drug administration, particularly when the oral route is unsuitable because of unconsciousness, or nausea and vomiting, or because the drugs have objectionable taste or odor or are destroyed by acid or digestive enzymes. This route also protects susceptible drugs from the biotransformation reactions occurring in the liver (see Chapter 4), because the blood draining the lower part of the rectum passes into the inferior vena cava via the internal pudendal veins rather than through the portal vein and liver. However, absorption by this route is often irregular and incomplete, and some drugs cause irritation of the rectal mucosa.

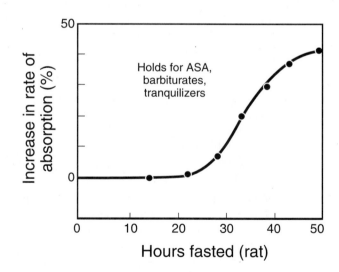

Figure 2-1. Relationship of drug absorption rate to presence of gastrointestinal contents in rats. ASA = acetylsalicylic acid (Aspirin).

Pulmonary Epithelium

Gases, vapors, and aerosols can be inhaled and absorbed through the alveolar surface or the bronchial mucosa, giving rapid access to the circulation. The drugs may be intended for local action (e.g., antiasthmatic agents) or for action elsewhere in the body (e.g., general anesthetics, amyl nitrite for angina pectoris).

Injection

This is also called "parenteral administration" (from the Greek *para* = beside, i.e., not *in*, and *enteron* = gut). The main advantages are more rapid and more predictable absorption, and more accurate dose selection. General disadvantages are the need for strict asepsis, the possibility of pain, and some difficulty in self-administration of drugs by injection. Moreover, injectable drugs are usually more expensive.

Subcutaneous injection (s.c., SC, subcut.)

Only nonirritating drugs can be administered in this way. Large volumes may be painful because of tissue distention. This route provides even and slow absorption, producing sustained drug effects. Vasoconstrictors, such as epinephrine, can be added to the drug solution to decrease the rate of absorption from a subcutaneous injection site. Conversely, the enzyme hyaluronidase breaks down mucopolysaccharides in connective tissue and thus aids the spread of drug solutions injected subcutaneously, leading to much faster absorption.

Intramuscular injection (i.m., IM)

Aqueous solutions are rapidly absorbed from deep intramuscular injection sites. Slow and even absorption becomes possible if the drugs are suspended or dissolved in oil, which forms a depot in the muscle. Irritating substances or large volumes may cause pain, and drugs dissolved in strongly acidic or alkaline solutions can cause sterile abscesses if injected intramuscularly.

Intravenous administration (i.v., IV)

Rapid injection permits the desired blood concentration of a drug to be obtained accurately and immediately, without variation due to irregular absorption or passage through the liver.

However, once the drug is injected, its rapid removal is impossible. Infection, vascular injury, and extravasation of drug into tissues surrounding the injection site are also possible consequences.

Slow infusion (over 20 minutes or more), in addition to the general advantages of intravenous administration, allows the level of the drug in the blood to be "titrated" by proper adjustments of flow rate and drug concentration. Infusions are particularly useful to maintain constant blood levels of drugs over extended periods of time. This lessens the risk of irrevocable administration of an overdose. However, expertise is required to minimize the risk of vascular injury, infection, and accidents (such as severing of infusion lines, bleeding, and air embolism).

Intra-arterial injection (i.a.)

This method is occasionally employed to direct small volumes of drug solutions at high concentrations to specific target tissues or organs, increasing the drug uptake at those sites but minimizing the effects elsewhere by subsequent drug dilution in the general circulation (see Chapter 11).

Injection into body cavities

The peritoneum provides a large absorption surface that permits rapid entry of drugs into the circulation. Therefore **intraperitoneal (i.p., IP) injection** is a common laboratory procedure, but it is seldom used clinically because of the risk of infection, intestinal or vascular injury, and adhesions.

CHOICE OF ROUTE

Regardless of the route of administration, a drug must be absorbed, reach its site of action, and interact in some way with the target tissue. These processes occur at very different speeds, depending on the route of administration. This question will be dealt with in detail in Chapter 5, but Figure 2-2 illustrates the order of magnitude of the times required following oral administration.

The choice of route may depend on therapeutic objectives. For example, intravenous injection or inhalation may be selected to produce a rapid, intense, but rather short-lived effect, whereas oral dosage

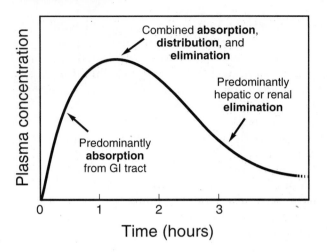

Figure 2-2. Components of the concentration-time curve after oral drug administration.

may be better and more convenient for long-lasting effects of relatively moderate and even intensity.

The choice of routes is sometimes limited by the properties of the drug. Barbiturates (anesthetic or hypnotic agents) and phenytoin (anticonvulsant), for example, dissolve only in rather strongly alkaline solution. If they have to be given by injection for rapid effect, they can be injected intravenously (the blood buffers the pH of the drug solution) but not intramuscularly or subcutaneously. EDTA (ethylenediamine tetraacetic acid—a chelating agent for treating heavy-metal poisoning) is poorly absorbed from the gastrointestinal tract and is therefore generally given by intravenous injection or infusion. Ordinary penicillin G is rapidly inactivated by gastric HCl. Therefore, if given by mouth, it must be given in huge doses to allow for the high percentage destroyed. In serious infections, this may introduce too much uncertainty, and the penicillin is more likely to be given by intramuscular or intravenous injection to ensure that high-enough blood levels are reached.

MOLECULAR PROPERTIES AND DRUG DISTRIBUTION

Once a drug has been administered, its uptake and distribution depend largely on the physical properties of the drug. It must usually pass from the site of administration across capillary walls into the circulation, and from the circulation it must again cross capillary walls to reach the site(s) of action (Fig. 2-3). Even if the drug is applied topically, it will often have to cross cell membranes to reach specific

intracellular sites of action, such as an enzyme or a nuclear receptor.

The ability of the drug to cross capillary walls, cell membranes, and other barriers to free movement depends to a large extent upon its solubility in aqueous and lipid phases, and upon its molecular size and shape.

Drug Solubility

To be pharmacologically active, a drug must have some solubility within the body fluids. Although the water molecule as a whole is electrically neutral, it acts as a partial dipole because the O region of the molecule has a slight preponderance of negative charge (electrons) while the two H regions are preponderantly positive. Drugs that are positively or negatively charged can therefore associate readily with water molecules, and are water-soluble (i.e., hydrophilic). In general, any chemical substituent group, when attached to a drug molecule, will affect the electron distribution within the drug and make that molecule either more water-soluble (and less lipid-soluble) or less water-soluble (and more lipid-soluble, or lipophilic).

The absolute solubility of a drug is usually less important than its relative solubility in lipid and water. When a drug molecule arrives at the cell membrane, this relative solubility determines whether it is more likely to stay in the water phase or to permeate into the fatty material of the cell membrane. Relative solubility of a drug is measured by its partition coefficient between oil and water, or between water and an organic solvent such as chloroform or hexane. The oil/water partition coefficient (P) is the ratio of the drug concentration (C) in the oil phase to that in the water phase:

$$P_{\text{oil/water}} = \frac{C_{\text{oil}}}{C_{\text{water}}}$$

Using radioisotopically labeled drug, it is also possible to measure the partition coefficient of a drug after equilibration between an aqueous buffer and a cell membrane preparation obtained by homogenizing and fractionating a tissue sample:

$$P_{\text{m/buffer}} = \frac{C_{\text{membrane}}}{C_{\text{buffer or water}}}$$

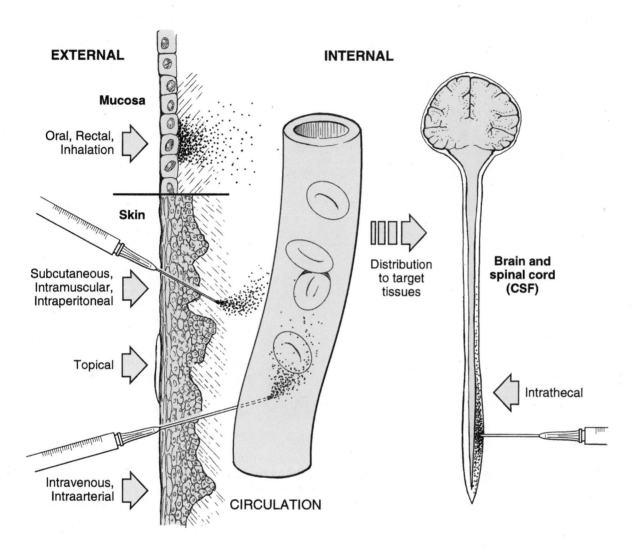

Figure 2-3. Routes of drug administration, in relation to biological barriers to drug diffusion.

The membrane/buffer partition coefficients of various drugs can also be estimated arithmetically by using the $P_{m/b}$ values of the "parent drug" structures and the P factors of common substituent groups shown in Table 2-1. If the partition (P) factor for a substituent is greater than 1, this means that the substituent increases the solubility of the drug in the membrane (or in fat, or oil, or in octanol) by the factor listed in the table. However, if the P factor of the substituent is less than 1, the substituent reduces the solubility of the drug in the membrane (or oil) phase.

For example, *iso*-butanol is:

$$CH_3—CH—CH_2OH$$
$$|$$
$$CH_3$$

and its $P_{m/b}$ will be

$$=P_{m/b} \text{ (methane)} \times (P_{CH_3})^3 \times P_{branch} \times P_{OH}$$
$$=0.6 \times 3^3 \times 0.63 \times 0.07 = 0.71$$

This is quite close to the measured $P_{octanol/water}$ of 0.65.

Molecular Mechanisms of Drug Absorption

Of the following eight molecular mechanisms of drug passage across membranes, only the first four are of major significance:

- Passive diffusion of water-soluble drugs
- Passive diffusion of lipid-soluble drugs

Table 2-1A Membrane/Buffer Partition Coefficients of Some Basic Structures

Parent Structure		$P_{m/b}$
CH_4 (methane)		0.6
Benzene ring	⬡	25
Cyclohexane	⬡	16

Table 2-1B Partition Factors of Substituent Groups in Drug Molecules

Substituent Group	Partition Factor	
	If on Aromatic Parent	If on Aliphatic Parent
—I	×13	×10
—Br	× 7.3	× 6
—Cl	× 5	× 2.5
—CH_2 or —CH_3	× 3	× 3
—F	× 1.4	× 0.7
—SH	× 1.3	× 0.9
—OCH_3	× 0.95	× 0.34
—NO_2	× 0.53	× 0.14
=S=O	× 0.3	× 0.3
—COOH	× 0.52	× 0.2
—OH	× 0.2	× 0.07
—C≡N	× 0.27	× 0.15
—NH_2 or —NH— or —NH_3^+	× 0.06	× 0.064
—C=O	× 0.09	× 0.062
= (double bond)	×0.5	
Branching in C chain	×0.63	
Ring closure	×0.9	

- Active transport
- Pinocytosis/phagocytosis
- Facilitated diffusion
- Passive filtration
- Adsorption of drugs to cell contents
- Drug passage via gap junctions

Each of these mechanisms is explained below.

Molecular Size

Most drugs, excluding peptides, have molecular weights of the order of 250–450 Da. Among the lightest are the anesthetic gas nitrous oxide, and ethanol, which have molecular weights of 44 and 46 Da, respectively. The muscle relaxant *d*-tubocurarine (curare) is exceptionally heavy and has a molecular weight of about 700 Da. Small peptides like ADH (antidiuretic hormone) are in the 1000–2000 Da range. Insulin, a small protein, has a molecular weight of 6000 Da; that of albumin is 65,000 Da, while the heavier proteins may range into the hundreds of thousands or the millions of daltons (such as botulinum toxin). Thus, compared to the protein molecules, which are the main building blocks of the body, most drug molecules are small.

Passive Diffusion of Water-Soluble Drugs

The passive diffusion of water-soluble drugs into cells largely depends on the molecular size of the drug. This is because the aqueous channels of the cell membrane are only about 8–10 Å wide and will restrict passage of any molecules larger than those with molecular weights of 150–200 Da. These channels in the cell membrane belong to a large family of specific proteins (aquaporins), each of which con-

sists of six transmembrane domains surrounding the central pore. Most of them allow only water to pass through, but at least one (aquaporin 3) also permits passage of small water-soluble molecules such as urea and glycerol (Fig. 2-4). Since most drugs are either lipid-soluble or have molecular weights greater than 150–200 Da, passive diffusion through these channels is not the major mechanism of drug permeation.

Drugs that are highly water-soluble have low $P_{m/water}$, with values less than 2. Examples of such highly water-soluble drugs that appear to enter cells by simple passive diffusion through aqueous channels are shown in Table 2-2.

The permeation rate of water-soluble drugs falls as the molecular weight of the drug becomes larger (Fig. 2-5). A puzzling exception is the mechanism of tetracycline permeation, since the substance is quite water-soluble but has a high molecular weight.

Passive Diffusion of Lipid-Soluble Drugs

The majority of lipid-soluble drugs permeate cell membranes by passive diffusion between the lipid molecules of the membrane (see Fig. 2-4). The per-

Table 2-2 Examples of Water-Soluble Drugs That Enter Cells Through Aqueous Channels in the Membrane

Drug	MW (Da)	$P_{m/b}$
Salts (e.g., Li_2CO_3)	~70	0.0002
Caffeine	194	0.17
Ephedrine	165	1.6
Low-MW diuretics (e.g., furosemide)	~100	
Ascorbic acid (vitamin C)	176	0.02
Sulfanilamide	172	0.03
Hydrogen peroxide	34	0.02
Nicotinamide (vitamin B_3)	122	0.02
Saccharin	183	1.7
Amino acids	100–150	0.02

meation rate of a lipid-soluble drug depends on the following factors:

- Concentration (or dose) of drug
- Oil/water partition coefficient of drug
- Concentration of protons (cH^+)
- Surface area of the absorbing membrane

Unlike the situation with highly water-soluble drugs, the permeation rate of lipid-soluble drugs does not vary systematically with the size of the molecule. However, extremely large drug molecules of around 1000 Da or more can be absorbed only by pinocytosis.

Dependence on the concentration (or dose) of the drug

The overall rate of drug permeation increases if the amount of drug administered is increased; this simply means that "the more you give, the more is absorbed." However, the relation between dosage and absorption is not simple. Some drugs are absorbed in direct proportion to the amount given, while other drugs have a nonlinear relation. This may create serious difficulties in trying to regulate the drug dosage for a particular patient.

Role of the oil/water (or membrane/buffer) partition coefficient

The oil/water partition coefficient of a drug is the principal factor determining the absorption of drugs

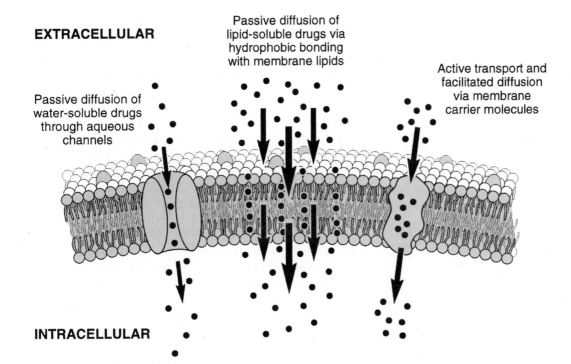

Figure 2-4. Pathways of drug permeation across cell membranes. Aqueous channels occur within the central pores of specific proteins (aquaporins).

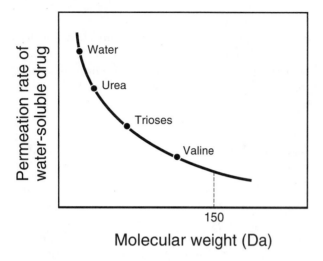

Figure 2-5. Relation between size of water-soluble drugs and rate of permeation. Those above 150 Da permeate extremely slowly and need other mechanisms to traverse the membrane barriers.

in the body. In general, the higher the value of $P_{oil/water}$ or $P_{m/water}$ of a drug, the more rapidly it will be absorbed across cell membranes and tissue barriers. There are many examples of this general rule in homologous series of drugs, such as barbiturates permeating the colon, or sedative-hypnotics (e.g., carbamates) permeating the stomach epithelium (Fig. 2-6).

The situation is not simple, however, since the small intestine (where the bulk of drug absorption occurs, because of the large surface area involved) shows an optimum $P_{oil/water}$ value for maximum rate

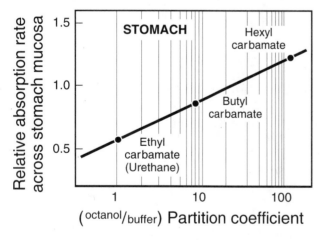

Figure 2-6. The more lipid-soluble sedatives permeate more easily across the stomach mucosa.

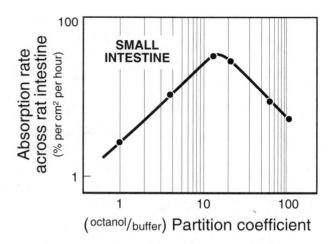

Figure 2-7. "Cut-off" phenomenon for lipid-solubility as a factor increasing the absorption rate of a drug (see Fig. 2-8 for the explanation).

of absorption (Fig. 2-7). This optimum is explained by the fact that there is a hydrophilic barrier that drugs must pass through before they can permeate across the cell membrane itself. This hydrophilic barrier consists of the unstirred water between the microvilli and immediately next to the surface sugar coat (glycocalyx) of the cell membrane (Fig. 2-8). In order to permeate a tissue barrier such as the intestinal mucosal epithelium, a drug must therefore have some water solubility as well as some lipid solubility. If it has a very high lipid solubility and very low water solubility, it will be blocked by the water barrier even though its extremely high lipid solubility would otherwise enable it to cross the membrane itself very readily. The point at which this "cut-off" of drug absorption occurs will vary with the cytologic features of the membrane involved. For the colon and gastric mucosa, in which the glycocalix is not nearly as thick as in the small intestine, it does not occur until the partition coefficient of the drug is at least 1000. For human skin, it lies somewhere between 100 and 1000 (Fig. 2-9).

The chemical force that causes lipid-soluble drugs to move readily across membranes is termed the hydrophobic force (or bond). It is not that the membrane and the drug have any particular attraction to one another, but water "repels" the lipid-soluble drug, thus driving it into the membrane. Since the cell membrane is extremely thin (75 Å), it becomes fully loaded with drug molecules in a few milliseconds. Some of the drug molecules in the membrane then spill over into the water on the other side of the membrane, i.e., into the cytoplasm, and the permeation process is thus completed.

Dependence of drug absorption on pH and drug protonation

The net electrical charge on a drug molecule is very important in determining the rate of its absorption across cell membranes and tissue barriers. Almost all drugs can be classed as uncharged drugs, organic acids, or organic amines (tertiary and quaternary). Organic acids and organic amines are markedly affected by pH.

For example, a tertiary amine type of drug can exist in two forms, with or without a proton attached, that are in equilibrium with each other:

STOMACH   INTESTINE
(Low pH = High cH$^+$)   (High pH = Low cH$^+$)

$$\underset{\text{(protonated, charged)}}{\overset{R}{\underset{R}{\underset{|}{\overset{|}{N^+}}}}\overset{R}{\underset{H}{}}}\quad\rightleftharpoons\quad\underset{\text{(unprotonated, uncharged)}}{R-N\overset{R}{\underset{R}{}}}$$

In a medium containing very few free protons (i.e., high pH or low cH$^+$), such as the fluid in the lumen of the duodenum, the tertiary amine will not be protonated, and it will be uncharged, as shown on the right. This uncharged form of the tertiary amine has a high oil/water partition coefficient and readily permeates membranes. But in a medium containing many free protons (i.e., low pH or high cH$^+$), such as the gastric juice, the tertiary amine is protonated, resulting in a net positive charge for the molecule. This charged form of the tertiary amine has a low oil/water partition coefficient and, therefore, has a low rate of permeation through the mucosa.

The importance of cH$^+$ in determining drug absorption is illustrated dramatically by an experiment described by Travell in 1940. He noted that large doses of strychnine (a tertiary amine), given by stomach tube to a cat, produced no toxic effects if the stomach fluid was kept at a high cH$^+$ of about 10^{-2} moles of protons per liter (pH 2). However, when the contents of the stomach were made alkaline (pH 8), the strychnine molecules lost their protons, became uncharged, permeated the mucosa, and killed the cat.

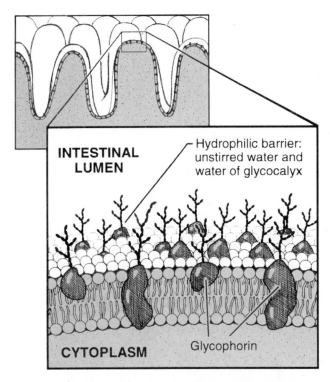

Figure 2-8. The cell membrane surface of the small intestine is extensively covered with a rich glycocalyx (i.e., surface sugar coat). The membrane glycophorins (i.e., protein–sugar molecules) are heavily hydrated with water molecules "frozen" to the sugar hydroxyls. The ice-like water forms a hydrophilic barrier that accounts for the existence of a limiting value of lipid solubility for efficient permeation, shown in Figure 2-7.

In the case of an organic acid, the same general principles apply. The organic acid molecules also can exist in two forms, as shown:

STOMACH   INTESTINE
(Low pH = High cH$^+$)   (High pH = Low cH$^+$)

$$R-COOH\quad\rightleftharpoons\quad R-COO^-$$

(protonated, uncharged)   (unprotonated, charged)

The protonated organic acid, however, is a neutral molecule and thus permeates the tissues readily, whereas the charged form does not. Hence, organic acids such as barbiturates, phenytoin, acetylsalicylic acid, dicumarol, phenylbutazone, sulfonamides, and thyroxine have a higher absorption rate in the stomach where the cH$^+$ is high.

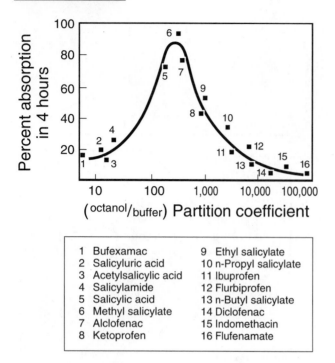

1	Bufexamac	9	Ethyl salicylate
2	Salicyluric acid	10	n-Propyl salicylate
3	Acetylsalicylic acid	11	Ibuprofen
4	Salicylamide	12	Flurbiprofen
5	Salicylic acid	13	n-Butyl salicylate
6	Methyl salicylate	14	Diclofenac
7	Alclofenac	15	Indomethacin
8	Ketoprofen	16	Flufenamate

Figure 2-9. Rate of diffusion of various nonsteroidal anti-inflammatory agents across unbroken skin in humans, as a function of the octanol/buffer partition coefficient. Absorption "cut-off" corresponds to a coefficient of about 240.

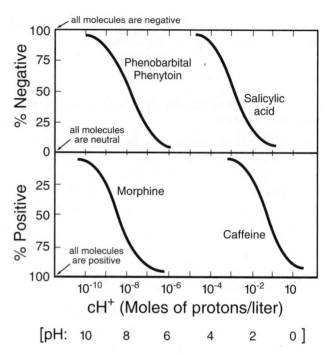

Figure 2-10. Organic amines are positively charged (i.e., protonated) at high concentrations of protons (i.e., high cH^+ or low pH). Organic acids are also protonated at high cH^+, which makes them become uncharged.

The form of the drug (i.e., charged or uncharged) in the tablet, vial, or ampoule does not matter. Rather, it is the degree of ionization of the drug in the gastrointestinal contents or other body fluid that matters, and this depends upon the relation between the pH (i.e., $-\log[H^+]$) of the fluid in question and the pK_a of the drug. K_a is the acidic dissociation constant, i.e., the equilibrium constant for the dissociation that yields free hydrogen ions:

$$-\overset{\overset{\textstyle O}{\|}}{C}-OH \quad \overset{K_a}{\rightleftharpoons} \quad R-\overset{\overset{\textstyle O}{\|}}{C}-O^- + H^+$$
Acidic drugs

$$R-\overset{+}{N}H_3 \quad \overset{K_a}{\rightleftharpoons} \quad R-NH_2 + H^+$$
Basic drugs

Obviously this dissociation will be affected by the cH^+ in the medium in which it is occurring (Fig. 2-10). High cH^+ (low pH) will drive the equilibrium to the left, in accordance with the law of mass action. The higher the pH of the fluid, the higher is the ionization of acidic drugs and the lower that of basic

drugs; the lower the pH, the lower is the ionization of acidic drugs and the higher that of basic drugs. Put in other terms, basic drugs tend to accept protons, and to give them up only when the cH^+ of the surrounding fluid is very low. Therefore the K_a of basic drugs is low, and the pK_a (i.e., $-\log K_a$) is high. Conversely, acidic drugs (by definition) give up protons readily, so their K_a values are high or their pK_a values are low. The pK_a of a drug can be calculated from the Henderson-Hasselbalch equation. When the pK_a of a drug equals the pH of the surrounding fluid, equal numbers of ionized and unionized molecules of the drug will be present, i.e., **the pK_a = pH at which 50% ionization occurs.** Table 2-3 gives some examples of the effect of the pH of the stomach contents on the absorption of various drugs.

Dependence on surface area available for absorption

It should be obvious that more drug is absorbed if there is more area available for absorption. In certain diseases, such as regional ileitis, the surgeon may have to remove much of the inflamed intestine, thus

Table 2-3 Effect of Local pH on Drug Absorption from Stomach

Drug	% Absorbed in Presence of 0.1 M HCl $cH^+ = 10^{-1}$ M	% Absorbed in Presence of $NaHCO_3$ $cH^+ = 10^{-8}$ M
Salicylic acid	60	13
Thiopental	46	34
Caffeine	24	>24
Morphine	0	16

drastically reducing the surface area available for absorption of nutrients, vitamins, and drugs.

For any substance that can penetrate the gastrointestinal epithelium in measurable amounts, the small intestine represents the greatest area for absorption. This is true whether the molecule is charged or uncharged. For example, ethanol can be absorbed to some extent by the stomach, but it is absorbed about eight times faster from the small intestine (Table 2-4). Phenobarbital is absorbed 17 times more rapidly from the intestine than from the stomach.

The great epithelial area of the intestine provided by the many villi and microvilli is much larger than the surface of the gastric mucosa. This great intestinal area more than compensates for the effect of the high pH on the ionization of organic acids. It follows, therefore, that the rate at which the stomach empties its contents into the intestine markedly affects the overall rate at which drugs reach the general circulation after oral administration. The absorption of tertiary amines, which constitute the majority of commonly used drugs, would be particularly dependent on the speed with which they arrive in the

Table 2-4 Dominant Role of Surface Area in Drug Absorption

Drug	% Absorbed from Stomach in 1 Hour	% Absorbed from Small Intestine in 10 Minutes
Ethanol	38	64
Phenobarbital	17	52

intestine. But for all drugs, it is essentially valid to say that the overall rate of gastrointestinal absorption is inversely related to the rate at which the stomach empties. That is why so many agents are administered on an empty stomach with sufficient water to ensure their rapid passage into the intestine.

Active Transport of Drugs

Although the principal mechanism for drug permeation is passive diffusion, more and more examples of active transport of drugs across cell membranes are being discovered. Active transport is defined as a process that moves the drug against the concentration gradient, that can be blocked by inhibiting metabolism or by reducing adenosine triphosphate (ATP) levels, and that can be saturated. It can carry drugs out of the cell or into the cell. By these criteria, the following drugs are among those actively transported:

- Penicillin by the renal tubule
- 5-Fluorouracil by the intestine
- Nitrogen mustard and melphalan by lymphocytes
- Digitalis glycosides by the liver
- Pentazocine, narcotic antagonists by leukocytes (Fig. 2-11)

Pinocytosis and Phagocytosis of Drugs

Drugs with large molecular weights, generally 1000 Da or more, enter cells or cross tissue barriers by

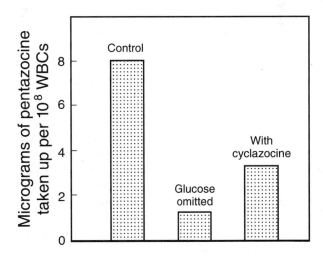

Figure 2-11. Active uptake of pentazocine by white blood cells (WBCs) is dependent upon an energy supply (glucose), and can be inhibited by cyclazocine, which competes for the same transport mechanism.

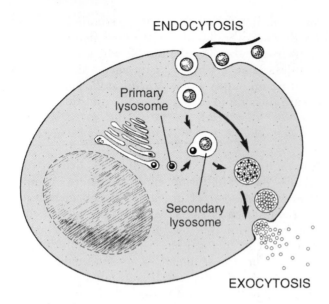

ENDOCYTOSIS

Primary
lysosome

Secondary
lysosome

EXOCYTOSIS

Figure 2-12. Pinocytosis or endocytosis of proteins results in a secondary lysosome, which in turn fuses with a primary lysosome. After hydrolysis within the fused vesicle, the products may be released by exocytosis.

means of pinocytosis or phagocytosis (Fig. 2-12). Substances normally absorbed in this manner include proteins, various bacterial toxins, milk antigens, and other antigens. Drugs tightly bound to plasma proteins can also enter in the same way. These substances enter the lysosomal system and may be digested within the lysosome (Fig. 2-12). If large amounts of the foreign substance enter, however, it may overwhelm the lysosomal protective mechanism and enter the circulation by exocytosis.

Facilitated Diffusion of Drugs

Diffusion along a transmembrane concentration gradient is, for some substances, facilitated by the presence of relatively selective carrier molecules in the membrane. These carrier molecules combine with the substances in question, forming complexes that can diffuse more rapidly across the membrane than the free substances themselves but that dissociate on the other side of the membrane to release the free substances into the cell. Drugs that permeate by facilitated diffusion include:

- Amino acids into brain (e.g., L-dopa)
- Adenosine-like compounds
- Nucleotide antimetabolites (used in cancer or antiviral chemotherapy)

Passive Filtration of Drugs

This is an important mechanism for drug elimination by the kidney glomerulus. Only the free, or unbound, drug and metabolites are available for glomerular filtration.

Adsorption of Drugs to Cytoplasm

Most drugs, once having entered the cell, adsorb reversibly to cell proteins and lipids, just as they do to plasma proteins. Since the concentration of cell proteins is very high, the cytoplasmic concentration of the drug can achieve a level many times higher than that in the plasma. Drug adsorption, however, is *not* a drug transport mechanism, but rather, a drug reservoir mechanism. As with plasma proteins, this drug reservoir serves to smooth out the time course of drug action so that the drug is not quickly biotransformed and excreted.

Drug Passage via Gap Junctions

There are gap junctions between epithelial cells of the same tissue, endothelial cells of the same tissue, and mesothelial cells of the same tissue (such as smooth muscle cells). Small molecules (<500 Da) can move from cell to cell through these gap junctions. The membranes of the connected cells contain cylindrical protein structures called **connexins** (analogous to the aquaporins), and aqueous channels run through them across the thickness of the membrane. The gap junction is formed by the exact alignment of the connexins of the two cells so that their two channels form one continuous passage between the cytoplasmic compartments of the two cells (Fig. 2-13).

TYPES OF TISSUE BARRIERS TO DRUGS

Table 2-5 summarizes the types of tissue barriers to drug permeation.

Epithelial Barriers

The epithelial membranes of the skin, gastrointestinal lumen, cornea, and urinary bladder all seal off the outside world from the body tissues and fluids. The epithelial cells in these membranes are all joined to one another by occluding zonulae, which are continuous tight junctions made up of rows of membrane particles of one cell that are fused to rows of membrane particles of the adjacent cell. Thus, these zonu-

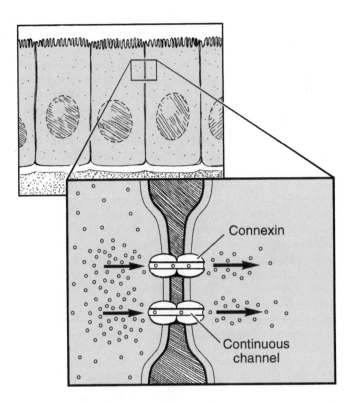

Figure 2-13. Cell-to-cell passage of drugs through gap junctions, as demonstrated by Loewenstein in fruit-fly salivary glands.

lae completely block off the intercellular spaces (Fig. 2-14).

Because these membrane particles form a continuous closed junction around the cell (somewhat similar to a necklace of pearls), drug molecules are forced to permeate the cell membrane by virtue of their lipid solubility, and to go *through* the cell rather than *between* the cells. Large molecules, as explained previously, must be pinocytosed in order to traverse the barrier. The basement membrane, adjacent to all epithelial cells, is composed of a loose carbohydrate–protein matrix and offers no resistance to drug permeation.

Capillary Barriers to Drugs

There are three types of capillary structures in the body:

- Capillaries with maculae
- Fenestrated capillaries: in kidney, pituitary, and exocrine glands
- Capillaries with occluding zonulae: all capillaries in the brain except those in the choroid plexus, median eminence, area postrema, pineal gland, and pituitary gland

Capillaries with maculae

These include the vast majority of capillaries in the body. Such macular capillaries are found throughout

---

Table 2-5 Summary of Types of Tissue Barriers to Drug Permeation

Tissue	Barrier	Permeability
Outside world: gastrointestinal mucosa, skin, cornea, lung, urinary bladder	Occluding zonulae (continuous tight junctions)	Complete blockage of intercellular spaces; drugs must permeate cell membranes
Capillaries except:	Maculae	Open intercellular spaces
glomeruli, excretory and secretory organs	Fenestrae	Free passage of drugs with MW <45,000 Da
blood–brain barrier	Occluding zonulae	Drugs permeate membranes
CSF barriers: choroid plexus cells → CSF	Occluding zonulae	Difficult passage
CSF → brain	No barrier	Very easy passage
Placenta	Limited by blood flow	Slow equilibration
Peritoneum	Maculae	Free passage

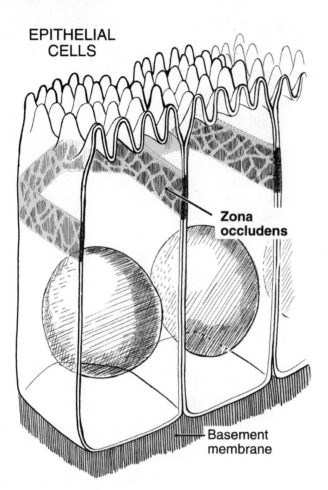

EPITHELIAL CELLS

Zona occludens

Basement membrane

Figure 2-14. The continuous tight junctions between adjacent cells in membranes separating the outside world from the body space are composed of "necklaces" of membrane proteins.

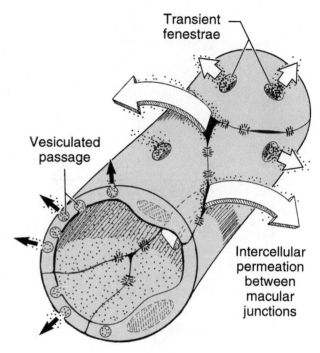

Transient fenestrae

Vesiculated passage

Intercellular permeation between macular junctions

Figure 2-15. Solute and drug permeation across capillary walls occurs via intercellular spaces and transient windows or fenestrae.

the body—in muscles, skin, peritoneum, gastrointestinal tract, bone, liver, heart. They possess macular junctions between the endothelial cells (Fig. 2-15). Such maculae do not form a continuous belt but exist only as patches of membrane particles on one cell membrane fused to corresponding sets of particles on the second cell membrane. Hence, there are intercellular spaces around these maculae.

In addition to the intercellular spaces, these capillaries are rich in pinocytotic vesicles. Some of these vesicles transiently extend through the entire cytoplasm, forming a transient window (fenestra) or open channel from the capillary lumen all the way to the basement membrane. All drugs, regardless of solubility, readily pass through these transient fenestrae and the intercellular spaces. Drug molecules larger than 100,000 Da must be pinocytosed and

transported by movement of the vesicles across the cells.

Tissues with fenestrated capillaries

The excretory and secretory organs generally have fenestrated capillaries. Such tissues include the kidney glomeruli (Fig. 2-16), thyroid, pituitary, salivary glands, and pancreas. The fenestrae or "windows" through the cytoplasm of the cell may be covered by a few angstroms of nonmembrane material, which essentially offers no barrier to any drug or solute existing free and unbound in the plasma. The basement membrane only holds back molecules larger than about 45,000 Da.

Tissues with occluded capillaries: the blood–brain barrier

The only capillaries in the body that have their intercellular spaces completely occluded by occluding zonulae are the brain capillaries. As mentioned briefly above, almost all brain capillary endothelial cells are connected to one another by these occluding zonulae, which thus constitute the "blood–brain barrier" (Fig. 2-17). There are five regions of the brain,

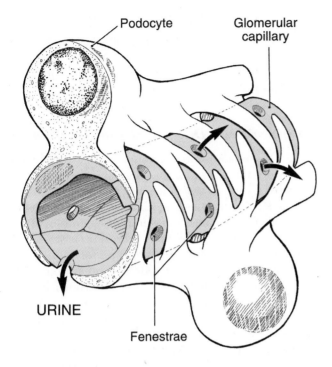

Figure 2-16. Capillaries in the kidney glomerulus are of the fenestrated type.

however, where no occluding zonulae exist, and consequently these regions are relatively permeable to drugs present in the blood. These regions are:

- The pituitary gland
- The pineal body
- The area postrema
- The median eminence
- The choroid plexus capillaries

The area postrema contains the vomiting control center, and since the capillaries there are fenestrated, the vomiting center readily monitors the circulating levels of foreign substances such as toxins and drugs. It is clearly advantageous for the area postrema to be readily exposed to substances in plasma. However, the rest of the brain capillaries with occluding zonulae protect the brain from circulating toxins, drugs, and harmful solutes.

Another important feature of the blood–brain barrier is that these brain capillaries have very few vesicles; consequently, there are no transient fenestrae.

Cerebrospinal Fluid Barriers to Drugs

The cerebrospinal fluid (CSF) is secreted by the epithelial cells of the choroid plexus, which are in

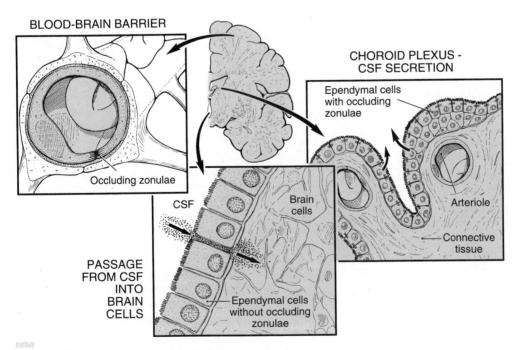

Figure 2-17. Blood–brain and CSF–brain barriers.

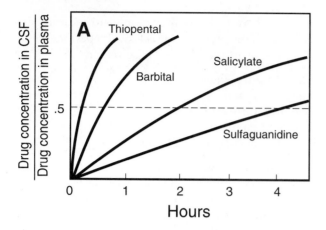

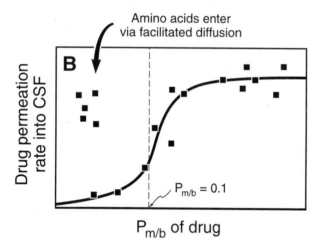

Figure 2-18. A. Effect of lipid solubility of drugs (e.g., thiopental, barbital) on rate of equilibration between CSF and plasma. B. General relation between drug permeation rate and the membrane/buffer partition coefficient. Thus, some amino acids (e.g., L-dopa) have partition coefficients below 0.1 and would not enter the brain were it not for the fact that the brain capillaries have special facilitated diffusion mechanisms for these drugs.

contact with the brain ventricular spaces. These epithelial cells are connected by occluding zonulae (see Fig. 2-17). Therefore only lipid-soluble drugs normally get into the CSF from the blood (Fig. 2-18).

The CSF is separated from the brain tissue by epithelial cells lining the ventricles, and these cells are not connected by occluding zonulae (see Fig. 2-17, bottom). Hence, the CSF–brain barrier is extremely permeable, offering unrestricted passage of drug molecules between the CSF and the brain cells. Clinically, advantage may be taken of this fact. For example, penicillins are not very lipid-soluble and,

therefore, penetrate poorly from the blood into the brain. However, a high concentration of penicillin in the brain (e.g., for treating a brain infection or abscess) can be obtained by intrathecal injections directly into the CSF.

Permeation of Drugs Across the Placenta

Because there is a limited amount of maternal blood flowing into the placenta, the shortest time for equilibration of a drug between mother and fetus is on the order of 10–15 minutes (see Chapter 65). This delay can be useful, because it permits the mother to be anesthetized during the final stages of labor, with enough margin of safety (about 10 minutes) to avoid a serious depression of the baby's breathing after birth. (It is also worth noting that newborn babies are more resistant to general anesthesia, so it takes more than the usual amount of the anesthetic to depress their breathing.)

The following are illustrative half-times for equilibration of various drugs between maternal blood and fetal cord blood:

Streptomycin

Anesthetics	8 minutes
Secobarbital	8 minutes
Sulfadiazine	1 hour
Curare	4 hours
Penicillin	10 hours
Streptomycin	18 hours

Until proven otherwise, it is safe to assume that all drugs cross the placenta and that all drugs enter the breast milk. Children of morphine-addicted mothers may be born with depressed respiration and pinpoint pupils. Antipsychotic drugs are transferred across the placenta, and if the mother is on rather high dosage, the offspring may be born with extrapyramidal signs (see Chapter 28). Erythromycin and tetracyclines cross the placenta in appreciable amounts and also appear in breast milk.

Drug Permeation Across the Peritoneum

The cells of the peritoneum and of the capillaries in the peritoneum are connected by macular ("spot") junctions. Hence, drugs and other solutes injected intraperitoneally have rapid and unrestricted access to the bloodstream. All drugs, whether lipid-soluble or not, whether charged or uncharged, readily permeate between the cells. Large molecules, however, must be carried across the peritoneum by pinocytosis.

Drug Permeation Across the Lung

As with all epithelial barriers to the outside world, the alveolar cells are also held together by continuous occluding zonulae. The cells are exceedingly rich in vesicles and the cytoplasm is very thin. Therefore, there are probably many transient fenestrae formed by the momentary fusion of vesicles on both sides of the cell. This would account for the ready alveolar permeation of a water-soluble compound like nicotine.

General anesthetics have no difficulty crossing the lung barrier since these drugs are quite lipid-soluble.

SUGGESTED READING

Brown D, Katsura T, Kawashima M, et al. Cellular distribution of the aquaporins: a family of water channel proteins. Histochem Cell Biol 1995; 104:1–9.

Davson H, Zloković B, Rakić L, Segal MB. An introduction to the blood-brain barrier. London: Macmillan, 1993.

Houston JB, Upshall DG, Bridges JW. A re-evaluation of the importance of partition coefficients in the gastrointestinal absorption of nutrients. J Pharmacol Exp Ther 1974; 189:244–254.

Leo A, Hansch C, Elkins D. Partition coefficients. Chem Rev 1971; 71:525–616.

Mattocks AM, El-Bassiouni EA. Peritoneal dialysis: a review. J Pharm Sci 1971; 60:1767–1782.

Schanker LS. Physiological transport of drugs. In: Harper NJ, Simmonds AB, eds. Advances in drug research. London: Academic Press, 1964:71–106.

Van Lieburg AF, Knoers NV, Deen PM. Discovery of aquaporins: a breakthrough in research on renal water transport. Pediatr Nephrol 1995; 9:228–234.

Yano T, Nakagawa A, Tsuji M, Noda K. Skin permeability of various non-steroidal anti-inflammatory drugs in man. Life Sci 1986; 39:1043–1050.

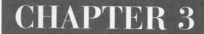

CHAPTER 3

Drug Distribution

L. ENDRENYI

The administration of a drug to a patient is often analogous to sprinkling salt all over one's plate in the hope that enough of the salt will land on the potatoes. In fact, most of it will land on other parts of the meal. In understanding drug distribution one has to consider the pattern of "scatter" of the amount of drug in the body, as indicated schematically in Figure 3-1.

The body fluids act as solvents and carriers for the great majority of drugs so that they reach their sites of action dissolved in the water that bathes the cells. The crudest division of the total body water is into intracellular and extracellular water; extracellular water is subdivided into plasma water and interstitial fluid. However, some parts of the extracellular water, such as the inaccessible water in bone and the slowly accessible water in tendon and cartilage, are not reached by drugs; therefore, the distribution volumes to be discussed are not necessarily identical to the volumes truly occupied by water in the body. In short, the distribution compartments discussed here are usually physiological rather than anatomical entities (Fig. 3-2).

TERMINOLOGY

Actual Volume of Distribution

This is the anatomical volume accessible to the drug. For example, a charged compound, which cannot enter cells, will have as its volume of distribution the extracellular space of about 12 liters. A nonpolar compound will spread through the total body water of about 40 liters (about 60% of the weight of a 70-kg man). Very few therapeutic drugs are confined to such a simply identified space as plasma.

Apparent Volume of Distribution

The apparent volume of distribution is a calculated value. First, recall the simple relationship between mass (amount of drug), volume, and concentration. Let them be designated by M, V, and C, respectively. Concentration is mass per unit volume, i.e.,

$$C = M/V$$

Knowing any two of these quantities, one can always calculate the third. For example, to calculate a volume when the mass of a drug and a concentration are given:

$$V = M/C$$

The apparent volume of distribution of a drug can be determined by injecting the drug intravenously. If a plot of the logarithmic concentration versus time yields a straight line, extrapolation to zero time gives the theoretical initial serum concentration of the drug (C_0), assuming instantaneous distribution (Fig. 3-3). (For greater detail see Chapter 5.)

Once an apparent volume of distribution is known for a particular drug, the amount of drug that must be given to achieve a desired concentration can be determined. It is important to realize that this approach is a mathematical convenience that works quite well in practice but says virtually nothing about where the drug really is in the body.

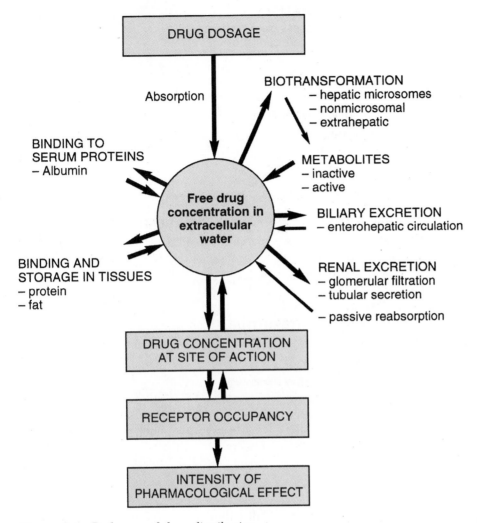

Figure 3-1. Pathways of drug distribution.

SITES OF DRUG DISTRIBUTION

Total Body Water

Ethyl alcohol is the most commonly consumed drug that equilibrates with the total body water (TBW), although the pharmacological effects experienced are due to the fact that some molecules attach to susceptible structures. If, for the sake of simple arithmetic, a lean young man weighing 70 kg has a total body water of 50 liters (70% of body weight), then a 15-g drink of alcohol (i.e., 0.21 g/kg) would give a concentration of 15 g/50 L of total body water. This is the same as 30 g/100 L, or 0.3 g/L. Since alcohol does not bind significantly to plasma proteins, and plasma is about 93% water, one can therefore expect a concentration in plasma of 0.28 g/L.

However, the body water in an obese elderly female is usually only about one-half of her body weight. If she also weighs 70 kg, she will have only 35 liters of body water. Therefore the same dose of 15 g of alcohol (i.e., 0.21 g/kg) would produce, in her, an alcohol concentration of 0.40 g/L, or more than 40% higher than it did in the 70-kg lean man.

Antipyrine is another drug that spreads throughout the total body water without concentrating in any one area. It is an old synthetic analgesic, and this drug, as well as some of its derivatives, is now often used to determine the volume of total body water. If a known amount of the drug is injected intravenously into the subject and the plasma concentration is measured after equilibrium is reached, the total water in which the drug is now diluted can be calculated.

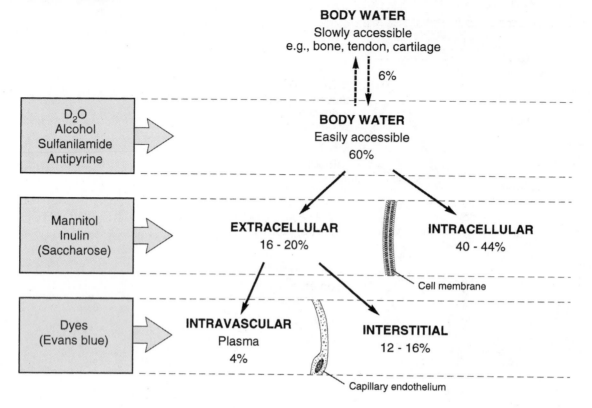

Figure 3-2. Various spaces (compartments) and volumes of distribution (approximate, as percent of total body mass, assuming average body fat). The boxes on the left show agents that typically distribute into the respective compartments. Consequently, these substances are used as indicators for measuring the apparent volumes of these spaces.

Extracellular Water

The cell membrane acts as a diffusion barrier, but most capillary walls are permeable to all but very large molecules (see Chapter 2). For such substances, therefore, the plasma and interstitial fluid can be regarded as a unit called the extracellular fluid (ECF). Since many drugs act at the cell surface, but are inert once inside the cell, drug distribution in extracellular fluid is pharmacologically very important.

Mannitol is a sugar alcohol that is often used to measure extracellular fluid volume because it does not enter cells, is not transformed in the body, but is readily excreted through the kidney by glomerular filtration.

In a study of mannitol distribution, 50 g of the substance was administered to a 70-kg man. From repeated observations, referenced to plasma water, an extrapolated initial concentration of 4.46 g/L of water was measured. Consequently, the apparent volume of distribution was $50/4.46 = 11.2$ liters, which is 16% of the body weight, or 160 mL/kg. In a series of investigations of healthy adult males, the mannitol distribution volume averaged 160 mL/kg but ranged from 141 to 187 mL/kg. Hence the concentration of a drug that distributes in extracellular space may vary considerably from person to person, even if all other factors are equal.

Many drugs spread through extracellular fluid in less time than it takes them to penetrate cell membranes. There is, therefore, an initial transient period when their extracellular concentration is high compared to their intracellular concentration. If these drugs act on the cell surface, their onset of action will, therefore, be more rapid than if their site of action is within the cell.

Blood

Even within the blood, the distribution of a drug could be uneven. Thus, while a proportion of the

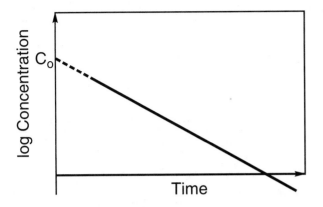

Figure 3-3. Determination of a drug's apparent volume of distribution. $V = \text{Dose}/C_0$ (see text).

drug molecules could be dissolved in water, others could be attached to various constituents of blood. These intravascular distribution processes will be considered briefly.

Intravascular distribution

Drug concentrations are typically measured in plasma and/or serum. Unless the drug is equally partitioned between cells and plasma, drug concentrations will be dependent on the protein concentration and/or the hematocrit value (i.e., the proportion, by volume, of red blood cells in the whole blood).

Since the distribution of ethanol between plasma and cells is a passive one, it follows that the ethanol content of a tissue is determined by its water content. This has important consequences for blood analysis, as cells contain less water than plasma. The average water contents are about 68% and 94%, respectively. Since cells occupy about half of the blood volume (hematocrit $\simeq 0.5$), the whole blood contains about 81% water. The commonly accepted conversion factor for calculating plasma ethanol from blood ethanol is 1.16 ($= 94/81$), although this will obviously vary with the hematocrit value. Hence a whole blood alcohol value of 50 mg/100 mL implies a plasma ethanol concentration of about 58 mg/100 mL.

The situation becomes even more complex if variations in plasma composition are taken into account. A volume of 100 ml of human blood plasma contains 4–9 g protein, about 0.1 g sugars, and 0.4–0.6 g lipids, which, after a fatty meal, may rise to over 1 g/100 mL. Hence the normal variation in plasma water is from about 89% to about 96%.

Serum and plasma protein binding

Most drugs are carried from their sites of absorption to their sites of action and elimination by the circulating blood. Some drugs are simply dissolved in serum water, but many others are partly associated with blood constituents such as albumin, globulins, lipoproteins, and erythrocytes. For the great majority of drugs binding to serum constituents, **albumin** is quantitatively the most important macromolecule and often accounts for almost the entire drug binding. For example, intravenously injected Evans Blue binds so strongly to plasma albumin that almost the whole dose is retained in the plasma, and its plasma concentration provides a measure of plasma volume. Some basic drugs bind extensively to α_1-acid glycoproteins.

Plasma protein binding influences the fate of drugs in the body. Only the unbound or free drug diffuses through capillary walls, reaches the site of drug action, and is subject to elimination from the body. Since drug binding to albumin is readily reversible, the albumin–drug complex serves as a circulating drug reservoir that releases more drug, as free drug is biotransformed or excreted. Thus, albumin binding decreases the maximum intensity, but increases the duration of action of many drugs.

Misleadingly small distribution volumes can be obtained for highly bound drugs when their total concentration (bound + unbound) is measured in the plasma. However, it is the free drug in the plasma water that equilibrates with the rest of the body. Consequently, the volume of distribution should be evaluated, for meaningful interpretation, from the concentration of the unbound drug.

Protein binding of drugs is dealt with specifically in the section of this chapter entitled Plasma and Serum Protein Binding of Drugs.

Body Fat

Adipose tissue is capable of storing large amounts of lipid-soluble drugs. Since blood flow to fat is relatively low per gram of tissue, a long period of time will be required for equilibrium to be achieved between the concentrations of unbound drug in plasma and in fat. In the reverse direction, drug stored in fat may require a long time to be removed completely from the body. Thus, body fat generally becomes an important site of storage after prolonged exposure to a lipid-soluble drug or chemical. For example, the insecticide DDT is now stored in the body fat of nearly every living creature on earth. Some wild animals have died suddenly from the DDT released when their fat depots were depleted by starvation.

Tissue Binding

If the tissue concentration of a drug is higher than its concentration in the plasma free water, tissue localization has occurred. If the binding site has a large capacity for the drug, the presence of the binding site is equivalent to an increase in the effective volume of distribution of the drug. The end result can be a marked prolongation of the life of the material in the body. One example is radioactive strontium (^{90}Sr). It is so strongly bound to sites in the bone (which is relatively poorly perfused anyway) that it has a tissue half-life of years.

Enterohepatic Circulation as a "Reservoir"

Enterohepatic circulation is another potential site of drug distribution. Phenolphthalein, for example, which is used as a popular laxative, is rapidly extracted from the body by the liver, excreted via the biliary system into the gut, and then reabsorbed across the intestinal mucosa into the blood. The circulating quantity of phenolphthalein thus acts as a reservoir, and the drug stays in the body for days instead of the few hours for which it would persist without this recirculation. Unfortunately, little is known of the relative rates of biliary excretion and the intestinal reabsorption of drugs, so the general significance of the enterohepatic cycle as a drug reservoir is difficult to assess. Enterohepatic circulation is discussed in greater detail in Chapter 7.

PLASMA AND SERUM PROTEIN BINDING OF DRUGS

Affinity and Extent of Binding

The interaction of a drug with a binding site on a protein is a reversible reaction obeying the law of mass action. The total measured drug concentration in serum is the sum of the unbound and bound drug concentrations (Fig. 3-4).

In the reaction shown in Figure 3-4, k_1 and k_2 are the rate constants of the forward and reverse reactions. The processes of association and dissociation of drug and protein have half-times of a few milliseconds.

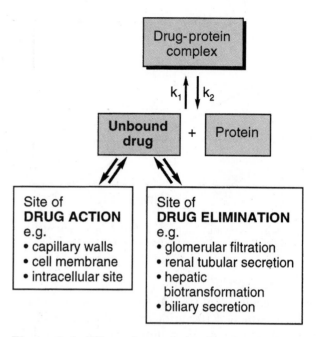

Figure 3-4. Effect of protein binding on drug disposition. Only the unbound drug is available for eliciting an effect and for elimination (see text).

The affinity between a drug and its binding sites is accurately expressed as the concentration ratio of the drug in the bound form to the product of unbound drug and albumin:

$$\frac{[\text{Drug–protein complex}]}{[\text{Unbound drug}] \times [\text{protein}]} = \frac{k_1}{k_2}$$

The ratio of the rate constants k_1/k_2 is the association constant (K_a), and its units are liters per mole. The greater the affinity between drug and protein, the larger is the K_a. Affinity is more frequently expressed in terms of the dissociation constant (K_d). This is equal to k_2/k_1, its units are moles per liter, and it is inversely proportional to the affinity. The dissociation constant equals the free drug concentration at which 50% of the corresponding binding sites on the protein are saturated. The relation between association and dissociation constants is exemplified by warfarin (an anticoagulant) binding to albumin with a K_a of 1.6×10^5 L/mole and a K_d of 6.2×10^{-6} moles/L.

At high drug concentrations, almost all binding sites on the protein molecule become saturated. When a drug binds with different affinities at several different kinds of site in the protein molecule, several different equilibria are involved. Each of these is characterized by a dissociation constant. The maximum possible binding capacity of a protein for a given drug equals the molar albumin concentration multiplied by the number of binding sites for that drug.

Figure 3-5 illustrates the effect of three variables

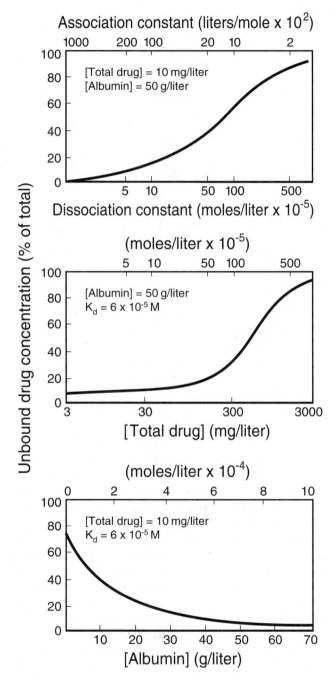

Figure 3-5. Effect on drug–albumin interaction of changes in dissociation constant (top), total drug concentration (middle), and albumin concentration (bottom). Albumin has a molecular weight of 69,000 Da; the assumed molecular weight of the drug is 300 Da (see text).

on the free concentration of a hypothetical drug, with a molecular weight of 300 Da, binding to a single site on albumin. At any given drug and albumin concentrations, the unbound fraction of the total drug rises with decreasing affinity (increasing dissociation constant, K_d). With any given affinity, the fraction of free drug rises when the total drug concentration increases or when albumin concentration falls. If the albumin concentration is in the normal range, the binding affinity is very high (K_d very low), and total drug concentration is low, practically all the drug in the serum will be present in the bound complex. Even with very high binding affinity and normal albumin concentration, the binding capacity becomes saturated at high drug concentrations, and the free drug concentration rises rapidly.

A glance at the two lower panels of Figure 3-5 makes it obvious that statements about "the percentage of drug bound to serum albumin" are of limited value unless the concentrations of drug and albumin are stated. When they are specified, the statement applies only to that situation. However, at low drug concentrations, the fractions of the drug being either bound or unbound approach their limiting values. These are important characterizations of the extent of binding of the drug to plasma proteins under the given conditions.

The considerable differences among normal persons in the affinity of some drugs to serum proteins are not yet fully understood. Age appears to be one factor, with binding relatively low in neonates and perhaps in old age. Appreciable sex differences in affinity have not been found. Temperature, pH, and ionic strength can affect the number of binding sites and their dissociation constants in vitro, and even clinically encountered variations in these factors may be of importance. Competition for plasma protein binding sites by endogenous substances, such as free fatty acids or other organic acids, may play a role.

Protein Binding and Drug Distribution

Whatever the route of administration, almost all therapeutic agents reach their sites of action via the systemic circulation. Only the fraction of the drug in the bloodstream that is not bound to plasma proteins can leave the circulation, distribute throughout the body, and reach the sites of action. Because the equilibrium between bound and free drug is constantly maintained, some of the drug–albumin complex continuously dissociates as free drug diffuses out of the blood through capillary membranes.

Once drug distribution is complete, the free drug

concentration throughout the extracellular water will equal that in serum water. It is not the total drug, but rather the free drug concentration in the serum that correlates with the concentration at the sites of action. It does not usually matter in this regard whether the active site is at the cell surface or lies intracellularly.

For highly albumin-bound drugs the free drug concentration in serum is only a small percentage of the total concentration. For example, during phenylbutazone therapy the total serum concentration of the drug is nearly 100 times higher than its concentration in serum water and extracellular fluid. With such extensive binding, most of the drug in the body may at all times be sequestered in the drug–albumin complex. The exact fraction that is free depends on the specific drug, on drug and albumin concentrations, and on any interference with binding by endogenous substances or other drugs.

An important example of the difference between total drug concentrations in the serum and in extravascular fluids is furnished by cerebrospinal fluid (CSF). Indeed, it was the much lower concentration of some sulfonamides in CSF than in serum that called attention to the reversible binding of drugs by serum proteins. The concentration in CSF of a sulfonamide that is 75% bound to serum albumin is only one-fourth of the total drug concentration in serum. Similarly, the CSF concentration of phenytoin in subjects with normal serum albumin averages only about 10% of the total serum level when the latter is in the therapeutic range. What is true for CSF also applies to other less easily obtained extravascular fluids. However, to the extent that they contain albumin, their total drug concentration will be higher than that of CSF.

Protein Binding and Drug Elimination

The kidneys remove drugs and their metabolites from the blood by glomerular filtration and/or by tubular secretion. The first process is dependent on diffusion; the second often involves an active transport mechanism. Drug binding to albumin has entirely different effects on glomerular and tubular excretion of drugs.

Since albumin does not appreciably pass through the glomerular membrane, neither does drug bound to albumin. In contrast, the free fraction of almost all drugs is readily filtered. The concentration of drugs in the glomerular filtrate generally equals the free drug concentration in the serum. Thus, as blood passes through the glomeruli, no change occurs in the free drug concentration except for the minute effect of the increased unbound albumin concentration. It follows that there is little stimulus for dissociation of the drug–albumin complex, and that *albumin-bound drug is completely protected from glomerular filtration*. In addition, binding to serum albumin can further decrease the rate of elimination of drugs that are lipid-soluble at the pH of tubular fluid by increasing their back-diffusion from the glomerular filtrate into blood.

The rate of glomerular filtration of a drug is therefore inversely proportional to the extent of drug–albumin binding. Glomerular elimination of highly albumin-bound drugs can be extremely slow. This is most important for drugs that are also slowly biotransformed and poorly excreted by the renal tubules. For example, diazoxide is primarily eliminated by glomerular filtration, but its 90% binding to serum albumin renders this route relatively ineffective and results in a half-life of approximately 30 hours. The slow elimination from the body of some benzothiadiazide diuretics and sulfonamide anti-infectives partly reflects their extensive binding to albumin and their consequent slow filtration by the glomeruli.

Unlike their crucial effect on glomerular filtration, drug–albumin interactions have variable effects on, and do not generally limit, the **tubular elimination** of drugs. Only free drug can be secreted by the tubules but, in contrast to the diffusion-controlled glomerular filtration, the more rapid active tubular secretion decreases the serum concentration of free drug. Because equilibrium between free and bound drug is always maintained, a decrease in the concentration of free drug immediately causes dissociation of some of the drug–albumin complex and thus makes further drug available for tubular elimination. The interaction between drug and albumin is so rapidly reversible that any free drug withdrawn from serum by active transport mechanisms is instantly replaced. As a consequence, even drugs such as certain penicillins, which are more than 90% bound to serum albumin at therapeutic concentrations, can be removed almost completely from the blood by tubular secretory mechanisms during a single passage through the kidneys (see also Chapter 7).

The importance of binding to albumin is generally analogous in the case of **hepatic biotransformation** of drugs. Drugs that enter the hepatocyte by simple diffusion are protected from biotransformation to the extent of their binding to serum albumin. As albumin binding increases, drug available at any one time at the site of hepatic biotransformation decreases. Coumarin anticoagulants, phenylbutazone, and certain sulfonamides are among the drugs for which the rate of hepatic transformation has been shown to be inversely proportional to the extent of their albumin binding.

On the other hand, hepatic biotransformation or biliary secretion of drugs that are concentrated in the hepatic cell by active transport mechanisms may not be limited by albumin binding. Free drug molecules withdrawn from the serum are immediately replaced by more free drug resulting from the dissociation of the drug–albumin complex. This explains the rapid hepatic clearance of some highly albumin-bound substances such as sulfobromophthalein and propranolol. The quantitative aspects of hepatic metabolism are considered in greater detail in Chapter 7.

Protein Binding and Pharmacological Actions

Only free drug can reach the sites of action and exert a pharmacological effect. (See Table 3-1 for a partial list of drugs that are extensively bound in human serum.) Binding to serum albumin decreases the maximum intensity of action of a single dose of most drugs because it lowers the peak drug concentration achieved at the sites of action. The magnitude of this decrease is directly proportional to the fraction of the administered dose bound to serum albumin. If 50% of the dose becomes albumin-bound, the attainment of any given peak intensity of pharmacological action will require approximately twice the dose that would be necessary in the absence of any albumin binding.

Because albumin binding slows the elimination of drugs that are removed from the serum by glomerular filtration or by diffusion to the hepatic biotransformation site, it increases the duration of action of a single dose of such drugs. The duration of action of some diuretics, sulfonamides, and tetracyclines tends to correlate with the degree of their albumin binding. However, this may be due only in part to a direct effect of albumin binding. The amount of such drugs bound to tissue proteins may correlate with the extent of their binding to albumin, and a high degree of such **binding at inactive tissue sites** would also lead to a long half-life and duration of action. In contrast to its effect on "passively" eliminated drugs, binding to plasma proteins can facilitate the transport of drugs within the bloodstream. Therefore, it may shorten the duration of action of drugs that are actively transported into renal tubular or hepatic cells, just as it can decrease their half-lives.

Table 3-1 Approximate Drug Binding in Human Serum (Examples of Highly Bound Drugs)

Drug	% Free
Anticoagulants	
Warfarin	0.5
Bishydroxycoumarin	1
Anti-infectives	
Cloxacillin	5
Oxacillin	8
Doxycycline	10
Sulfadimethoxine	10
Sulfisoxazole	10
Anti-inflammatory	
Fenoprofen	1
Phenylbutazone	3
Oxyphenbutazone	3
Indomethacin	10
Salicylic acid	18
Cardiovascular	
Digitoxin	5
Propranolol	7
Diazoxide	9
Quinidine	15
Central nervous system	
Diazepam	1
Amitriptyline	4
Imipramine	4
Chlorpromazine	4
Chlordiazepoxide	5
Nortriptyline	6
Desipramine	8
Phenytoin	10
Thiopental	15
Diuretics and uricosurics	
Probenecid	1
Furosemide	3
Chlorothiazide	5
Sulfinpyrazone	5
Ethacrynic acid	10
Oral hypoglycemics	
Tolbutamide	5
Tolazamide	6
Chlorpropamide	13
Miscellaneous	
Clofibrate	5

Clinically Important Aspects of Serum Protein Binding

- Free drug concentration is lower, pharmacological activity is decreased, and drug clearance by glomerular filtration and passive processes is decreased in the presence of protein binding.
- One highly protein-bound drug may be competitively displaced by another highly bound drug. The pharmacological effect of the displaced drug will increase, as will its renal clearance.
- Endogenous substances with high affinity for protein binding sites (e.g., bilirubin, fatty acids) may displace a highly bound drug.
- In disease states characterized by hypoalbuminemia (e.g., hepatic failure or nephrotic syndrome) the concentration of free, active drug will be higher at any given total concentration.

DRUG DISTRIBUTION FOLLOWING RAPID INTRAVENOUS INJECTION

The general conditions described above apply to the distribution of a drug some time after its administration (say, at steady state). The following considerations apply to the *time course* for approaching these conditions.

The concentration in blood following a rapid intravenous injection is at its highest value initially and then falls ultimately to zero (Fig. 3-6). The time course of drug concentrations can be divided into three stages: initial dilution, distribution, elimination (renal and metabolic). (See also Chapter 5.)

Initial Dilution

A drug rapidly injected in a small volume will, for approximately two or three circulation times, be distributed in a "bolus" within the circulation (Fig. 3-7). If the drug has a very narrow margin of safety and acts on receptors within sensitive, vital systems, serious toxicity may occur if injection is too rapid (e.g., isoproterenol and cardiac arrhythmias; thiopental and medullary respiratory depression). Generally, drugs should be injected slowly (e.g., diazepam at less than 2.5 mg/min). Conversely, for a few drugs with a high threshold, rapid bolus injection may be required to initiate a response. A special situation applies if the rapidly injected drug is highly protein-bound. During the "bolus" phase, drug binding sites on albumin will be saturated, and free drug concen-

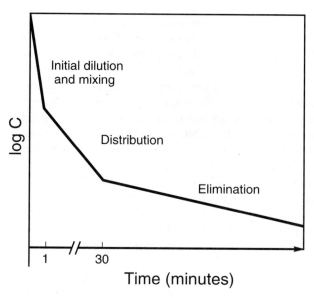

Figure 3-6. Time course of drug concentration following intravenous drug injection.

tration will be much higher relative to total drug concentration than after complete redistribution has occurred. Highly protein-bound drugs for which such kinetics may be important include quinidine, phenytoin, and diazoxide.

Redistribution

If the drug is injected rapidly, the total dose is distributed in only a small volume of blood. As this blood

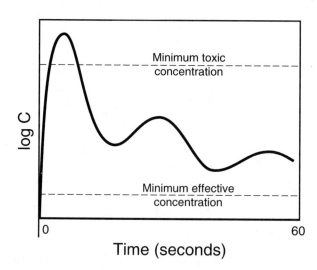

Figure 3-7. Mixing of drug after rapid intravenous injection (i.e., dissipation of bolus effect over two or three circulation times).

moves through the lungs and out into the body, the drug mixes in a larger volume of blood, and when this blood reaches the capillaries the drug is distributed by diffusion to the extracellular space (and into cells if it can cross the cell membrane). After about 15 minutes or so, the drug will be distributed fairly evenly throughout the extracellular fluid space. There are some exceptions to this—the drug will not reach the average concentration in poorly perfused tissues.

Different tissues in the body have different blood perfusion rates. Hence, drugs reach equilibrium quickly in some tissues and more slowly in others. The effects on different groups of tissues can be demonstrated by inhaling a constant concentration of halothane (a general anesthetic) and measuring the time course for the amount taken up by the whole body. As shown in Figure 3-8, the uptake of halothane by the whole body generally can be subdivided into three phases: a rapid-uptake phase, which reflects the uptake of halothane by the **vessel-rich group of tissues** (VRG) (brain, heart, liver); a phase of intermediate rates, which shows the uptake of halothane by the **muscle group of tissues** (MG); and a very slow phase, which reflects the uptake of halothane into the **vessel-poor group of tissues** (VPG) (fat, skin, bone, ligaments, teeth, hair). After exposure to the drug is stopped, the rates for the declining amount of halothane demonstrate again the presence of the three tissue groups. (Note the qualitative similarity of the picture shown in Fig. 3-8 to that illustrated in Fig. 3-6.)

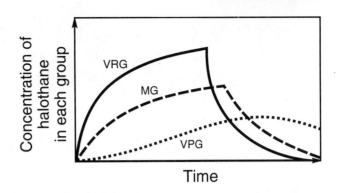

Figure 3-9. Concentration of halothane in various tissue groups while undergoing redistribution (cf. Fig. 3-8).

It is the organs and tissues of the vessel-rich group that are the targets in most drug therapy, and the rate of onset of drug action in them can be very fast. But it is important to remember that blood flow can be different in various parts of the same organ. For example, the blood flow to the gray matter of the brain is almost four times as high as to the white matter, so drugs that are able to cross the blood–brain barrier reach the cortex and brain nuclei much faster than the rest of the brain.

The muscle group fills up with drug more slowly than the vessel-rich group, and because of relative concentrations, drugs that have initially gone to vessel-rich organs can be carried out of them again by the circulation and moved on to relocate in the muscle and fat groups of tissues. This **redistribution** is shown in Figure 3-9 in a general way, and various specific examples are given in succeeding chapters.

SUGGESTED READING

Koch-Weser J, Sellers EM. Importance of drug-protein binding. N Engl J Med 1976; 294:311–316 (part 1), 526–531 (part 2).

Levy R, Shand D, eds. Clinical implications of drug-protein binding. Clin Pharmacokinet 1984; 9(Suppl 1):1–104.

Oie S. Drug distribution and binding. J Clin Pharmacol. 1986; 26:583–587.

Pratt WB, Taylor P. Principles of drug action. 3rd ed. New York: Churchill Livingstone, 1990.

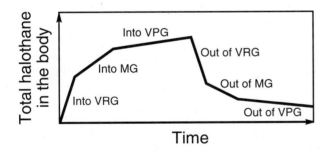

Figure 3-8. Uptake and distribution of a drug (halothane) in various tissue groups depending on blood perfusion rates (see text). VRG = vessel-rich group; MG = muscle group; VPG = vessel-poor group.

CHAPTER 4

Drug Biotransformation

D. S. RIDDICK

We live in a chemically hostile world in which we are exposed each day to a wide variety of foreign chemicals via inhalation, ingestion, and percutaneous absorption. These foreign chemicals, or xenobiotics, include therapeutic and recreational drugs, environmental contaminants, and dietary constituents. Fortunately, we possess a diverse array of enzymes that are able to act on xenobiotics in a manner that hastens their elimination from our bodies. **Drug biotransformation** refers to the chemical transformation of a xenobiotic within a living organism, usually by enzyme-catalyzed reactions.

BIOLOGICAL SIGNIFICANCE

All foods that animals eat contain traces of potentially toxic chemicals. This is particularly true of plants, which lack excretory mechanisms and therefore accumulate metabolic excretory products in vacuoles inside their cells. Many plants produce alkaloids that are potent pharmacological agents. When the plants are eaten as food, those toxic or pharmacologically active materials that have high lipid solubility are the most likely to be absorbed from the gastrointestinal tract and the least likely to be excreted in their original form. They may be filtered at the glomerulus and reabsorbed from the renal tubule, or excreted in the bile and reabsorbed from the intestine, remaining in the body for long periods of time. The same is true for drugs and environmental contaminants.

The kidneys of terrestrial animals conserve water by producing a highly concentrated urine. This favors reabsorption of lipid-soluble chemicals in the renal tubule by increasing the concentration gradient from lumen to blood. Higher animals possess enzymatic machinery that converts lipid-soluble xenobiotics into more polar and hence more water-soluble products. This permits more efficient excretion in a limited volume of water in the urine or bile.

Drug biotransformation reactions have three potential consequences with respect to pharmacological activity. (1) **Activation.** An inactive precursor may be converted into a pharmacologically active drug, e.g., the insecticide parathion (inactive) is converted by the liver into paraoxon (active, toxic); L-dopa (inactive) is converted to dopamine (active) in the basal ganglia. In this case, L-dopa is a pharmacologically inactive prodrug that is converted enzymatically in vivo into a pharmacologically active molecule. (2) **Maintenance of activity.** A pharmacologically active chemical may be converted into another active chemical, i.e., an active metabolite, e.g., diazepam (active) is converted to oxazepam (active). (3) **Inactivation.** An active drug may be converted to inactive products, e.g., pentobarbital (active) is converted to hydroxylated metabolites (inactive). The products of biotransformation are usually more water-soluble than the original drugs: that is the only feature common to all of these reactions.

In the discussion that follows, we will refer to several enzymes of drug biotransformation. It is important to point out that, in many cases, the same enzymes that biotransform xenobiotics are also involved in the biotransformation of endogenous chemical substances. For example, the synthesis and/or degradation of steroid hormones, cholesterol, eicosanoids, bile acids, and bile pigments utilizes enzymes that are also involved in drug biotransformation.

Thus, there is a close relationship between drug biotransformation and fundamental homeostatic processes.

DRUG BIOTRANSFORMATION REACTIONS

Drug biotransformation reactions are commonly grouped into two phases: **phase I** and **phase II.** Phase I processes include oxidation, reduction, and hydrolysis reactions that may increase, decrease, or not alter the pharmacological activity of a drug. In general, phase I reactions introduce or unmask a functional group (hydroxyl, amine, sulfhydryl, etc.) that makes the drug more polar. Phase II processes consist of synthetic or conjugation reactions in which an endogenous substance (e.g., glucuronic acid, glutathione) combines with the functional group derived from phase I reactions to produce a highly polar drug conjugate. Most phase II reactions result in a decrease in the pharmacological activity of the drug. Many drugs undergo the sequential process of phase I reaction followed by phase II reaction. However, there are many exceptions. The product of phase I biotransformation may be sufficiently polar to be eliminated directly without the need for a phase II reaction. A parent drug may possess a functional group that can be conjugated directly via a phase II reaction without the need for a phase I reaction. In addition, phase II reactions may precede phase I reactions. Finally, a parent drug may be eliminated unchanged without the need for any biotransformation. These relationships are summarized in Figure 4-1.

Virtually every tissue has some ability to carry out drug biotransformation reactions. However, the most important organ of biotransformation is the **liver.** The gastrointestinal tract, lungs, skin, and kidneys also display substantial drug biotransformation activity. The fact that the gastrointestinal tract and liver are major sites of drug biotransformation means that many drugs that are administered orally will be extensively biotransformed before they reach the systemic circulation. This **first-pass effect** can severely limit the oral bioavailability of some drugs. In addition, intestinal microorganisms are capable of catalyzing drug biotransformation reactions. For example, a glucuronide conjugate of a drug may be excreted via the bile into the intestine where gut bacteria may convert the conjugate back into free drug. The free drug may then be reabsorbed from the intestine and reenter the liver via the portal vein. In the liver, the free drug may once more be conjugated with glucuronic acid and secreted into the bile, and this process of **enterohepatic circulation** may begin again.

At the subcellular level, enzymes of drug biotransformation are located in the endoplasmic reticulum, mitochondrion, cytosol, lysosome, and to a limited extent, the nuclear envelope and plasma membrane. The major site of drug biotransformation within hepatocytes and other cells is the membranes of the smooth endoplasmic reticulum. When a tissue is homogenized and subjected to differential centrifugation, the membranes of the endoplasmic reticulum form vesicles called **microsomes.** The microsomal fraction is able to carry out many drug biotransformation reactions in vitro.

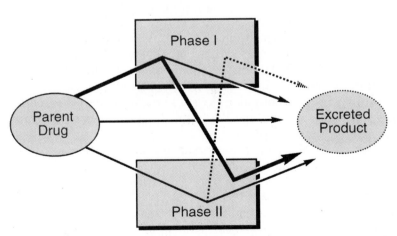

Figure 4-1. Summary of possible sequential relationships between phase I and phase II reactions of drug biotransformation.

Phase I Reactions

Oxidation

Oxidations are the most important category of drug biotransformation reactions in quantitative terms. The microsomal mixed-function oxidase (MFO) system is capable of catalyzing a wide variety of oxidation reactions. This microsomal drug-oxidizing system requires the participation of two distinct proteins embedded in the phospholipid bilayer of the endoplasmic reticulum membranes. First, a member of a hemoprotein superfamily termed the **cytochromes P450** functions as the terminal oxidase in this pathway. The name cytochrome P450 is derived from the fact that the reduced form (ferrous) of this hemoprotein binds carbon monoxide, forming a complex that has a unique absorption spectrum with a maximum at 450 nm. Second, a flavoprotein termed **NADPH–cytochrome P450 reductase** serves to transfer reducing equivalents from the cofactor NADPH (nicotinamide adenine dinucleotide phosphate, reduced) to the hemoprotein. The activity of this enzymatic system requires the reducing cofactor NADPH and molecular oxygen. Typically, this system functions as a monooxygenase in that one atom of oxygen is incorporated into the drug substrate and the other atom of oxygen contributes to the formation of water. The overall balanced equation for a typical monooxygenase reaction is as follows:

$$RH + O_2 + NADPH + H^+ \rightarrow ROH + H_2O + NADP^+$$

In this scheme, RH represents an oxidizable drug substrate and ROH represents the hydroxylated product of the reaction.

A simplified scheme of the cytochrome P450–catalyzed oxidative cycle is shown in Figure 4-2. The numbers in the cycle correspond to the major steps described below:

1. The drug (RH) binds to cytochrome P450 to form a binary complex. Initially, the hemoprotein is in its oxidized ferric form (Fe^{3+}). The binding of substrate to cytochrome P450 results in specific changes in the hemoprotein absorption spectrum. Depending on the nature of the spectral change, drugs can often be classified as "type I" or "type II" substrates. Type I substrates bind to a lipophilic substrate pocket of the cytochrome P450 protein and tend to shift electron distribution of the hemoprotein in a way that permits subsequent easy electron transfer between the reductase and the cytochrome. How-

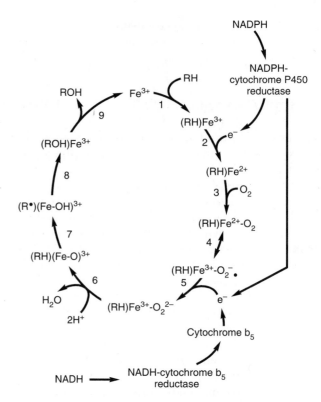

Figure 4-2. The catalytic cycle for a cytochrome P450–mediated hydroxylation reaction. Fe represents the heme iron, RH the substrate, and ROH the hydroxylated product.

ever, type II substrates bind directly to the heme iron of cytochrome P450, resulting in an interaction that tends to retard the subsequent reduction of cytochrome P450.

2. The reducing cofactor NADPH donates an electron to the flavoprotein NADPH–cytochrome P450 reductase, which in turn reduces the substrate-bound cytochrome P450 to its ferrous form (Fe^{2+}). The reductase utilizes both flavine–adenine dinucleotide (FAD) and flavine mononucleotide (FMN) as electron-shuttling prosthetic groups.

3. Molecular oxygen binds to the ferrous iron of the cytochrome P450–substrate complex to generate a ternary product.

4. An electronic rearrangement is thought to occur, although the precise oxidation states of the oxygen and iron in these intermediates are not well characterized.

5. A second electron transfer occurs. There are at least two possible sources of this reducing equivalent. The flavoprotein NADPH–cytochrome P450 reductase can transfer an electron from NADPH as in step 2. Alternatively, an electron may be donated by the cofactor NADH and shuttled via the flavoprotein NADH–cytochrome b_5 reductase and the hemoprotein cytochrome b_5 to cytochrome P450. This second electron is required to activate the bound oxygen.

6. In a poorly understood step, the oxygen–oxygen bond is split with the uptake of two protons. The result is the release of water and the generation of an "activated oxygen," perhaps an iron–oxene species $(Fe–O)^{3+}$.

7. Hydrogen abstraction from the substrate is thought to occur, resulting in the production of transient hydroxyl and substrate carbon radical species.

8. Recombination of the hydroxyl and carbon radicals occurs to give the product (ROH).

9. Dissociation of ROH restores the cytochrome P450 to its initial ferric state.

The cytochrome P450 catalytic cycle does not function with perfect efficiency. In the presence of particular drug substrates that are "difficult" to biotransform, such as ethanol, the catalytic cycle becomes "uncoupled." That is, the utilization of reducing equivalents is dissociated from product formation. As a result, potentially toxic reactive oxygen species (superoxide anion, hydrogen peroxide) can be liberated in the process of cytochrome P450 catalysis.

The phospholipid of the endoplasmic reticulum membrane is a key component in the monooxygenase reaction. The precise function of the lipid is not clear, but it has been suggested that the lipid is required for substrate binding, electron transfer, or facilitating the interaction between cytochrome P450 and its reductase. There appear to be between five and 20 molecules of cytochrome P450 per molecule of reductase in liver microsomes, and thus the process of heme reduction (i.e., the reductase activity) is generally thought to be the rate-limiting step in drug oxidation reactions.

The cytochromes P450 appear to be the most versatile biological catalysts known to date, being capable of catalyzing over 60 different types of reactions on literally hundreds of thousands of substrates. Although the initial reaction product of most cytochrome P450–catalyzed reactions is the corresponding hydroxylated derivative, a wide range of products is formed from many drug substrates. In many cases, the initial hydroxylated derivative is unstable and promptly breaks down into the recognized end-product. Figure 4-3 illustrates some of the diverse oxidation reactions that can be carried out by cytochromes P450.

The cytochrome P450 system can handle a diverse array of chemical substrates for two reasons. First, there are multiple molecular forms of cytochrome P450 present in any given species. Second, many cytochrome P450 species are capable of biotransforming a large number of substrates. Thus, the microsomal cytochrome P450 system combines the properties of enzyme multiplicity and low substrate specificity. The existence of multiple forms of cytochrome P450 was firmly established during the 1970s and 1980s by classical protein biochemistry techniques. Individual purified cytochromes P450 were distinguished on the basis of spectral properties, molecular masses as determined by electrophoretic mobilities, substrate selectivities, and immunoreactivities with polyclonal and monoclonal antibodies. cDNAs encoding multiple forms of cytochrome P450 proteins have been rapidly isolated and sequenced during the 1980s and 1990s. Molecular cloning techniques have led to the adoption of a standardized nomenclature system based on amino acid sequence similarity and divergent evolution. Each cytochrome P450 protein is identified by the root symbol "CYP" followed by an Arabic number denoting the gene family, a capital letter designating the gene subfamily, and an Arabic number representing the individual gene (e.g., CYP1A1).

In general, cytochrome P450 proteins with greater than 40% sequence identity are included in the same family, and those mammalian sequences with greater than 55% identity are included in the same subfamily. There are currently more than 481 cytochrome P450 genes and 22 putative pseudogenes that have been described in 85 eukaryotic and 20 prokaryotic species. Of the 74 gene families so far described, 14 families exist in all mammals examined to date. These 14 families comprise 26 mammalian subfamilies. The diversity of the human cytochromes P450 is illustrated in Figure 4-4. At least 36 apparently functional cytochrome P450 gene products have been identified in humans along with an additional nine apparently nonfunctional pseudogenes. Pharmacologists are mainly interested in the products of gene families 1, 2, and 3, as these enzymes are involved in drug biotransformation. Members of gene families 4, 5, 7, 8, 11, 17, 19, 21, 24, 27, and 51 play important roles in the biotransformation of endogenous chemical substances.

The molecular cloning approach has led to an increased understanding of the evolutionary relationships among members of the cytochrome P450 superfamily. The cytochromes P450 display a wide phylogenetic distribution: these enzymes have been detected in organisms ranging from bacteria to hu-

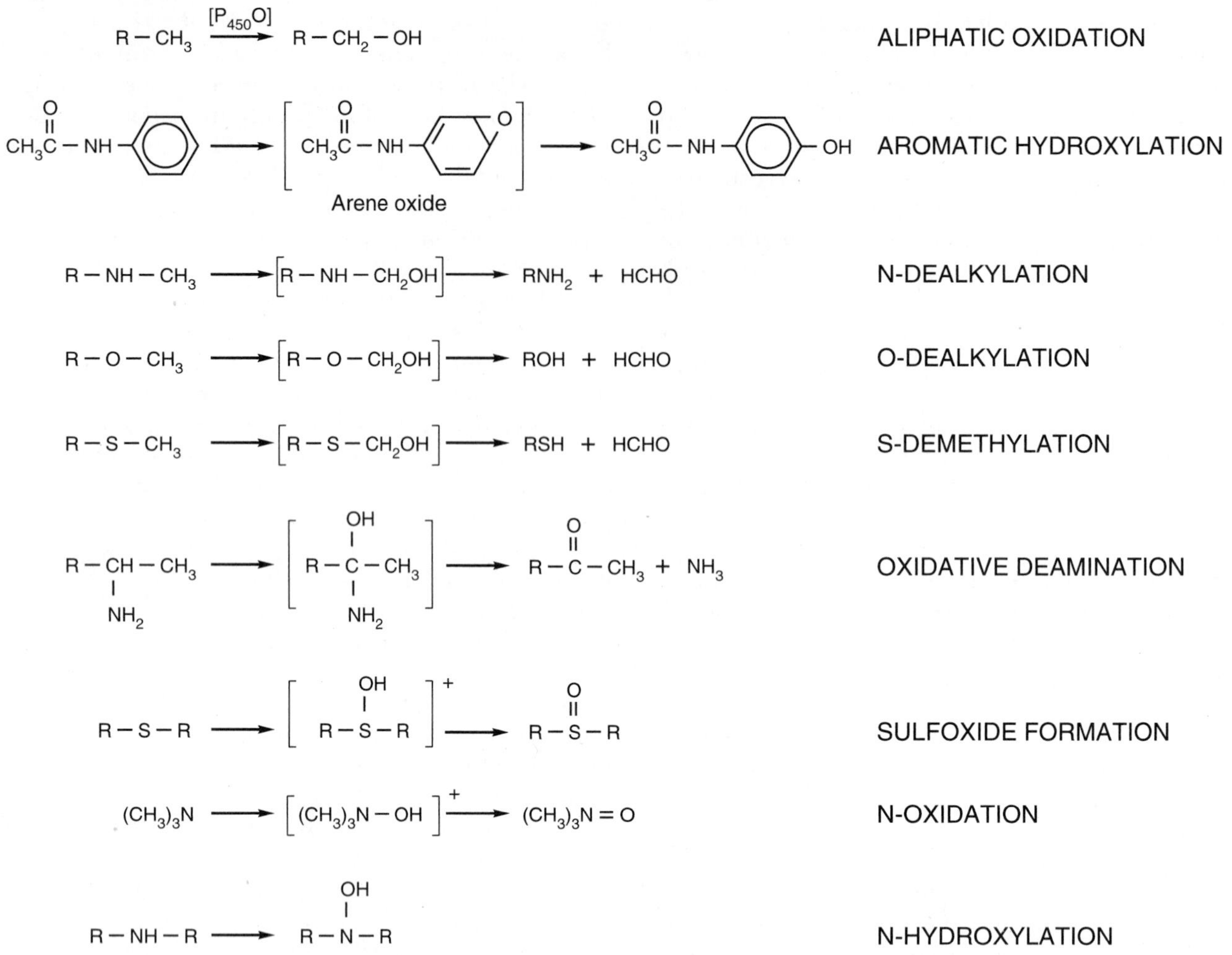

$$R-CH_3 \xrightarrow{[P_{450}O]} R-CH_2-OH \qquad \text{ALIPHATIC OXIDATION}$$

AROMATIC HYDROXYLATION

Arene oxide

$$R-NH-CH_3 \longrightarrow [R-NH-CH_2OH] \longrightarrow RNH_2 + HCHO \qquad \text{N-DEALKYLATION}$$

$$R-O-CH_3 \longrightarrow [R-O-CH_2OH] \longrightarrow ROH + HCHO \qquad \text{O-DEALKYLATION}$$

$$R-S-CH_3 \longrightarrow [R-S-CH_2OH] \longrightarrow RSH + HCHO \qquad \text{S-DEMETHYLATION}$$

OXIDATIVE DEAMINATION

SULFOXIDE FORMATION

$$(CH_3)_3N \longrightarrow [(CH_3)_3N-OH]^+ \longrightarrow (CH_3)_3N=O \qquad \text{N-OXIDATION}$$

N-HYDROXYLATION

Figure 4-3. A limited sample of the diverse oxidation reactions catalyzed by cytochromes P450.

mans. The steroidogenic cytochromes P450 are probably among the "oldest" members of the superfamily. They are necessary in early organisms for maintenance of membrane integrity. Xenobiotic-transforming cytochromes P450 probably evolved from the steroidogenic enzymes as an adaptive response to detoxify dietary chemicals. Much of the diversification of cytochrome P450 forms may have been driven by "animal–plant warfare" in which animals evolved a battery of enzymes to handle the array of toxic chemicals produced by various plant species.

A major distinction between cytochromes P450 relates to the nature of the electron transport process utilized. As described earlier, the eukaryotic microsomal system utilizes the flavoprotein NADPH-cytochrome P450 reductase to transfer electrons directly from NADPH to the hemoprotein. However, most bacterial and eukaryotic mitochondrial cytochromes

P450 utilize a ferredoxin reductase and a nonheme iron–sulfur protein to transfer electrons from NADPH to the hemoprotein. Unlike the eukaryotic cytochromes P450 which are integral membrane proteins, the bacterial cytochromes P450 are soluble, and thus it has been possible to obtain X-ray crystallographic data from four bacterial enzymes to date. These crystal structures have been instrumental in generating proposed three-dimensional models of mammalian cytochromes P450. The combination of crystallographic and molecular biological approaches, such as site-directed mutagenesis and construction of chimeric enzymes, has ushered in the present era's study of protein structure–function relationships.

Not all oxidation reactions are catalyzed by cytochromes P450. The microsomal **flavin-containing monooxygenases** (FMO) catalyze NADPH-depen-

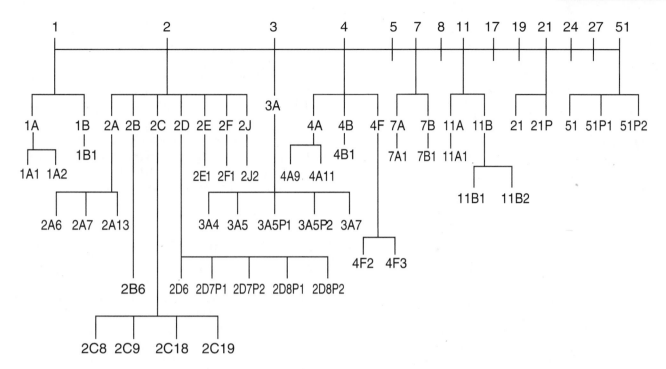

Figure 4-4. Multiplicity and nomenclature of the human cytochromes P450. Each gene product is designated by an Arabic numeral indicating the family (1, 2, 3, 4, 5, 7, 8, 11, 17, 19, 21, 24, 27, 51), a capital letter indicating the subfamily (A, B, C, D, E, F, J), and an Arabic numeral indicating the specific enzyme. P indicates a nonfunctional pseudogene.

dent oxygenation of nucleophilic phosphorus, nitrogen, and sulfur atoms present in a wide variety of xenobiotics including thioether- and carbamate-containing pesticides and numerous therapeutic agents (e.g., ephedrine, phenothiazines, *N*-methyl-amphetamine). Molecular cloning has identified a single gene family composed of five genes *(FM01, FM02, FM03, FM04, FM05)* that have been identified in a variety of mammalian species including human, pig, rabbit, rat, and guinea pig.

Another important drug-oxidizing system appears to involve **prostaglandin-synthase-dependent co-oxidation.** In the normal process of eicosanoid turnover, prostaglandin G_2 is reduced to prostaglandin H_2 by the hydroperoxidase activity of the enzyme prostaglandin synthase. Along with this reduction reaction, many xenobiotics including acetaminophen, phenytoin, and benzo*[a]*pyrene can be co-oxidized. This pathway appears to be of considerable toxicological importance as it often leads to the generation of toxic reactive metabolites. Other enzymes that catalyze oxidation of xenobiotic chemicals include the following: **alcohol dehydrogenase, aldehyde dehydrogenase, xanthine oxi-** **dase, monoamine oxidase, and diamine oxidase.**

Reduction

Several drugs are biotransformed by reductive pathways. Microsomal and cytosolic enzymes catalyze the reduction of **azo** linkages (RN=NR′; e.g., Prontosil), **nitro** groups (RNO_2; e.g., chloramphenicol), and **carbonyl** groups (RCOR′; e.g., haloperidol). Although these pathways have been recognized for several years, our understanding of the enzymes that catalyze these reactions is limited.

Interestingly, the cytochrome P450 and NADPH–cytochrome P450 reductase enzymes that catalyze oxidation reactions are also involved in reduction reactions. The examples of doxorubicin and halothane biotransformation illustrate this point. Doxorubicin and many other antineoplastic agents contain a quinone moiety that can undergo a one-electron reduction catalyzed by NADPH–cytochrome P450 reductase, resulting in the formation of a semiquinone free radical (Fig. 4-5). The semiquinone radical can be oxidized back to the quinone with

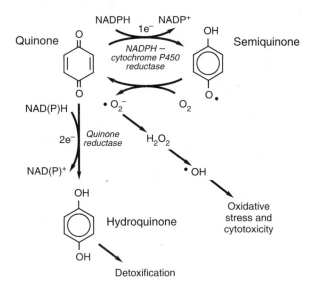

Figure 4-5. Pathways of biotransformation of quinone-containing drugs (e.g., doxorubicin). One-electron reduction initiates the process of "redox cycling," leading to oxidative stress and cytotoxicity. Two-electron reduction is a detoxification pathway leading to the formation of the hydroquinone derivative. Doxorubicin can also be reduced at a side-chain position (catalyzed by carbonyl reductase) to yield its major metabolite, doxorubicinol.

concurrent generation of superoxide anion. The production of superoxide anion and other reactive oxygen species promotes oxidative stress, lipid peroxidation, and DNA damage; these effects are partially responsible for the antitumor property of the drug. Quinone-containing drugs can also undergo a two-electron reduction catalyzed by the enzyme **quinone reductase** or **DT-diaphorase,** resulting in the production of the hydroquinone derivative. This process generally represents a detoxification pathway.

Biotransformation of the anesthetic halothane under anaerobic conditions involves a cytochrome P450–catalyzed reductive dehalogenation reaction. This pathway is thought to be responsible for the hepatotoxicity of this drug. The reaction mechanism is distinct from the cytochrome P450–catalyzed oxidation pathway in the following way. Under anaerobic conditions, no oxygen is present; as a result, the electrons derived from NADPH are not utilized to activate oxygen, but, rather, contribute directly to the formation of halothane radical species. This type of reduction reaction may be of particular importance in centrilobular hepatocytes and cells in the center of solid tumors that display very low oxygen tensions.

Hydrolysis

Drugs containing ester functions (RCOOR'; e.g., procaine, succinylcholine) are hydrolyzed by a variety of nonspecific **esterases** in liver, plasma, gastrointestinal tract, and other tissues. Amides (RCONHR'; e.g., procainamide, lidocaine) are hydrolyzed by **amidases;** most of this biotransformation occurs in the liver. Finally, **peptidases** in plasma, erythrocytes, and many other tissues biotransform polypeptide drugs (e.g., insulin, growth hormone).

Phase II Reactions

In general, phase II reactions involve the coupling of a drug or drug metabolite with an endogenous substance. These reactions require the participation of specific transferase enzymes that are localized in the microsomal or cytosolic fractions and high-energy activated endogenous substances. Most conjugation reactions result in detoxification; however, several examples of bioactivation by phase II enzymes are now known. The most important phase II reactions are described below.

Epoxide hydration

A number of olefins and aromatic compounds can undergo phase I oxidative biotransformation to an epoxide intermediate; in the process, an oxygen atom is inserted across a carbon–carbon double bond. Drugs such as carbamazepine and carcinogens such as benzo[*a*]pyrene are biotransformed by cytochromes P450 to epoxide derivatives. Epoxides are reactive electrophilic species that can bind covalently to proteins and nucleic acids leading to cytotoxicity. One means by which epoxides can be detoxified is via the nucleophilic attack of water on one of the electron-deficient carbon atoms of the oxirane ring, a reaction catalyzed by the enzyme **epoxide hydrolase** (also known as epoxide hydrase or epoxide hydratase). The product of this enzymatic reaction is a dihydrodiol derivative; nonenzymatic rearrangement of an aromatic epoxide leads to the production of a phenol. As noted for other drug biotransformation enzymes, there is more than one molecular form of epoxide hydrolase. Both microsomal and cytosolic forms of this enzyme have been characterized in liver and other mammalian tissues.

The classification of epoxide hydrolase as a phase II enzyme is not universally accepted. Like other enzymes that carry out conjugation reactions, epoxide hydrolase catalyzes the conjugation of an endogenous substance (water) with a drug metabolite (epoxide).

Glucuronidation

One of the most important phase II reactions involves conjugation of drugs with the endogenous substance glucuronic acid. Many functional groups are subject to glucuronidation including hydroxyl (e.g., morphine, acetaminophen), carboxyl (e.g., clofibrate, benzoic acid), amine (e.g., meprobamate), and sulfhydryl (e.g., 2-mercaptobenzothiazole) groups. The reaction mechanism for the formation of a glucuronide conjugate with benzoic acid is shown in Figure 4-6. Free glucuronic acid will not couple with drugs; however, uridine diphosphate-glucuronic acid (UDP-GA) will. UDPGA is formed from glucose-1-phosphate in a two-step process that occurs in the cytoplasm. The conjugation of glucuronic acid to the drug substrate is catalyzed by a member of the **UDP-glucuronosyltransferase** superfamily. The result is the production of a glucuronide conjugate of the drug in which the C-1 atom of glucuronic acid now has the β configuration. Glucuronide conjugates can be excreted via the bile or urine; intestinal microorganisms that contain the enzyme β-glucuronidase may hydrolyze the conjugate and initiate the process of enterohepatic circulation. Many endogenous substances including bilirubin, bile acids, and steroids are also subject to glucuronidation.

Multiple forms of UDP-glucuronosyltransferase exist. These enzymes are present in highest concentration in the liver, but are also found in the kidney, small intestine, lung, skin, adrenals, and spleen. The enzymes are located in the endoplasmic reticulum. A nomenclature system for the UDP-glucuronosyltransferases has been proposed, based on divergent evolution and sequence similarity. At least 26 distinct cDNAs in five mammalian species have been sequenced. By analogy to the cytochrome P450 nomenclature system, the existence of two families (*UGT1* and *UGT2*) has been proposed. The *UGT2* family consists of subfamilies *UGT2A* and *UGT2B*. At present, at least 10 human UDP-glucuronosyltransferases have been sequenced.

Glutathione conjugation

The **glutathione *S*-transferases** catalyze the enzymatic conjugation of xenobiotics with the endogenous tripeptide glutathione (glutamylcysteinylglycine, GSH). Xenobiotics with a suitably electrophilic center (e.g., epoxides, arene oxides, nitro groups, hydroxylamines) can be subject to nucleophilic attack by glutathione. Indeed, glutathione conjugation reactions can proceed nonenzymatically. Figure 4-7 illustrates that the products of glutathione conjugation reactions undergo further modification to yield mercapturic acid derivatives as final elimination products. Xenobiotics that undergo biotransformation catalyzed by glutathione *S*-transferases include ethacrynic acid and bromobenzene. In most cases, glutathione conjugation represents an important detoxification process; however, some xenobiotics (e.g., 1,2-dihaloalkanes and halogenated alkenes) are toxic only after conjugation with glutathione or cysteine.

The glutathione *S*-transferases are encoded by at

$$\text{Glucose-1-P} + \text{UTP} \longrightarrow \text{UDP-Glucose} + \text{PP}$$

$$\text{UDP-Glucose} + 2\text{NAD}^+ + \text{H}_2\text{O} \longrightarrow \text{UDPGA} + 2\text{NADH} + 2\text{H}^+$$

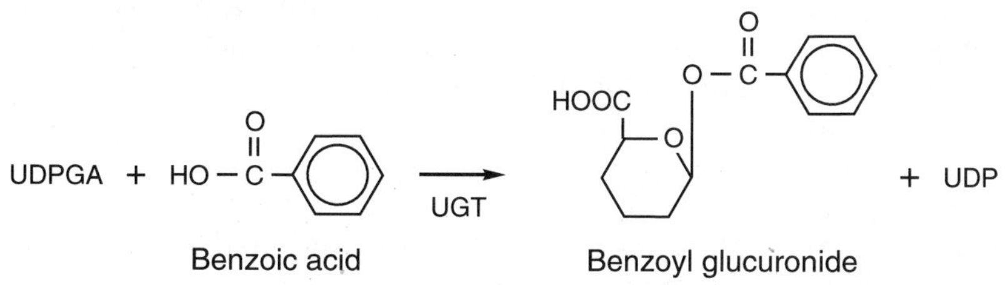

Figure 4-6. Reaction sequence for glucuronic acid conjugation of benzoic acid. UDPGA represents uridine diphosphate-glucuronic acid, UGT represents UDP-glucuronosyltransferase, and PP represents pyrophosphate.

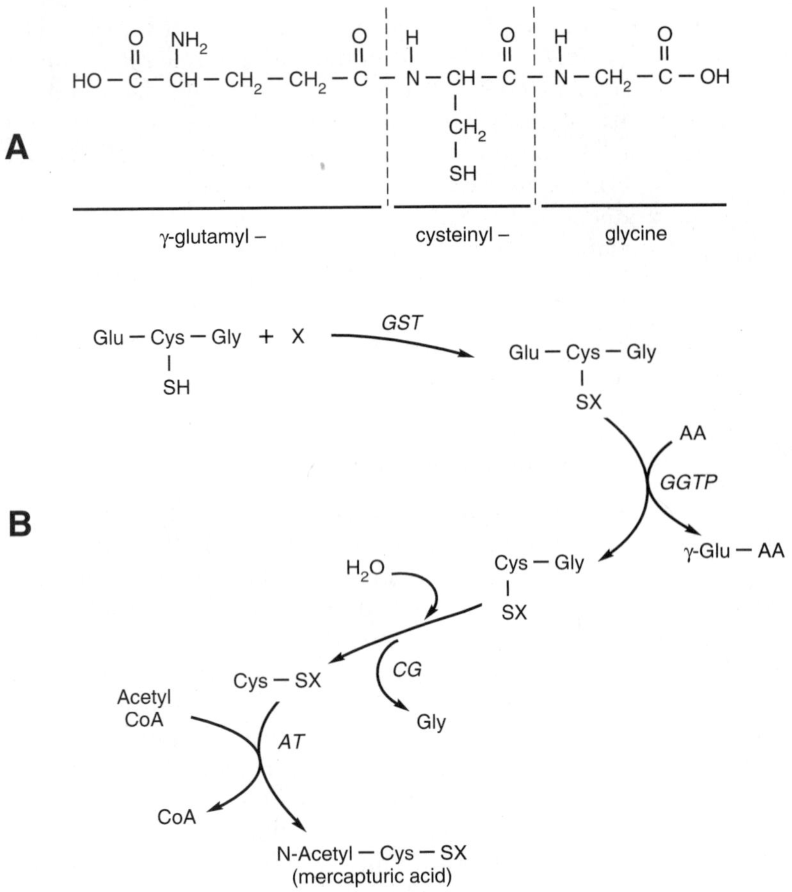

Figure 4-7. Glutathione conjugation catalyzed by glutathione S-transferase. A. Structural formula of glutathione.
B. Pathways of mercapturic acid formation. X is an electrophilic drug metabolite or epoxide reacting with glutathione. Enzymes catalyzing the successive steps are glutathione S-transferase (GST); γ-glutamyl transpeptidase
(GGTP); cysteinyl glycinase (CG); acetyltransferase (AT).

least six different gene families; five of the families
encode cytosolic enzymes (alpha, mu, pi, sigma,
theta), whereas the sixth encodes a microsomal form.
The catalytically active cytosolic enzymes are homo-
or heterodimers consisting of two protein subunits
derived from the same class. A new nomenclature
system has been adopted for the human glutathione
S-transferases in which each gene product is given a
capital letter designation (A, M, P, T for alpha,
mu, pi, theta, respectively) and an Arabic numeral
indicating the order in which the protein subunits
are characterized within a class (e.g., GSTA1). Allelic
variants are indicated by a lowercase letter. Any two
members within a class display greater than 50%
amino acid identity. The family of human glutathione
S-transferases currently consists of at least 13 different gene products: GSTA1, A2, A3, M1a, M1b, M2,
M3, M4, M5, P1, T1, T2, and microsomal.

The glutathione S-transferases appear to be of
particular interest in the field of cancer chemotherapy. The increased and/or differential expression of
one or more glutathione S-transferases in tumor cells
has been implicated as a contributing factor in the
resistance of such cells to drugs such as doxorubicin
and melphalan (see Chapter 60).

Sulfation

Many phenols, alcohols, and hydroxylamines can
undergo sulfation reactions catalyzed by **sulfotransferases.** Inorganic sulfate must first be activated to
3'-phosphoadenosine-5'-phosphosulfate (PAPS) in a

$$ATP + SO_4^{2-} \xrightarrow{\text{Sulfurylase}} \text{Adenosine-5'-Phosphosulfate (APS)} + PP$$

$$APS + ATP \xrightarrow{\text{APS Kinase}} \text{3'-Phosphoadenosine-5'-Phosphosulfate} + ADP$$
$$\text{(PAPS)}$$

$$PAPS + ROH \xrightarrow{\text{ST}} RO - SO_3H + \text{3'-Phosphoadenosine-5'-Phosphate}$$

Figure 4-8. Reaction sequence for sulfate conjugation of an alcohol. ROH represents the substrate for the sulfation reaction, ST represents sulfotransferase, and PP represents pyrophosphate.

two-step process (Fig. 4-8). A member of the sulfotransferase family then catalyzes the formation of the sulfate ester. Compounds that undergo sulfation reactions include acetaminophen, salicylamide, methyl-dopa, ethanol, and many steroid hormones.

The sulfotransferases are cytosolic enzymes found in many tissues including liver, kidney, gut, and platelets. The classification of sulfotransferase enzymes is not as advanced as it is for some of the other enzyme families. To date, the sulfotransferases have been classified mainly on the basis of substrate selectivity; however, recent molecular cloning techniques have led to the sequencing of 19 cytosolic sulfotransferase cDNAs, four of which encode human enzymes. Mammalian sulfotransferases are classified into three major groups: phenol sulfotransferases, estrogen sulfotransferases, and hydroxysteroid sulfotransferases. The phenol sulfotransferases have been the most extensively studied class from the viewpoint of drug biotransformation. Humans possess at least two forms of phenol sulfotransferase, one of which is thermolabile and catalyzes the conjugation of dopamine and other phenolic monoamines, whereas the other form is thermostable and carries out the sulfation of simple phenols.

Acetylation

Cytosolic enzymes known as **N-acetyltransferases** catalyze the transfer of acetate from acetyl coenzyme A to primary aromatic amine and hydrazine functional groups to yield acetamides and hydrazides (Fig. 4-9). Examples of chemicals that undergo acetylation include sulfonamides, isoniazid, procainamide, *p*-aminobenzoic acid, caffeine, and a variety of aromatic amine carcinogens. In humans, three *N*-acetyltransferase (NAT) gene loci exist, but only two functional gene products exist, NAT1 and NAT2, which display 81% amino acid identity.

An acetylation polymorphism was described in the human population during the 1950s following the introduction of isoniazid therapy for tuberculosis. Population studies demonstrated that humans could be segregated into two distinct modes of a frequency distribution of isoniazid elimination rate. Recent molecular investigations have revealed that individuals showing impaired acetylation of isoniazid (and several other drugs) possess a variant allele at the *NAT2* locus. To date, more than eight variant *NAT2* alleles that correlate with acetylator phenotype have been detected in human populations.

N-Acetylation of aromatic amine procarcinogens is generally thought to be a detoxification pathway; however, it is clear that acetyltransferases may also play an important role in bioactivation of potentially carcinogenic aromatic amines. An example is the acetylation of the hydroxylamine produced by the cytochrome P450–catalyzed *N*-oxidation of 2-aminofluorene; the product is an unstable acetoxy ester of increased carcinogenicity.

Methylation

A variety of drugs and endogenous chemicals are biotransformed by **methyltransferase** enzymes that utilize *S*-adenosylmethionine as the methyl donor (Fig. 4-10). Most of the methyltransferases are cytosolic enzymes. Catechol *O*-methyltransferase catalyzes the methylation of phenolic hydroxyl groups found in endogenous and exogenous catecholamines. A hydroxyindole *O*-methyltransferase has also been reported in the pineal gland. *N*-Methylation of numerous amines occurs. Histamine *N*-methyltransferase catalyzes the methylation of histamine and related compounds in the liver, whereas phenylethanolamine *N*-methyltransferase carries out the methylation of norepinephrine in the adrenal gland. At least two *S*-methyltransferases have been characterized: thiopurine *S*-methyltransferase catalyzes the methylation of purine derivatives such as 6-mercap-

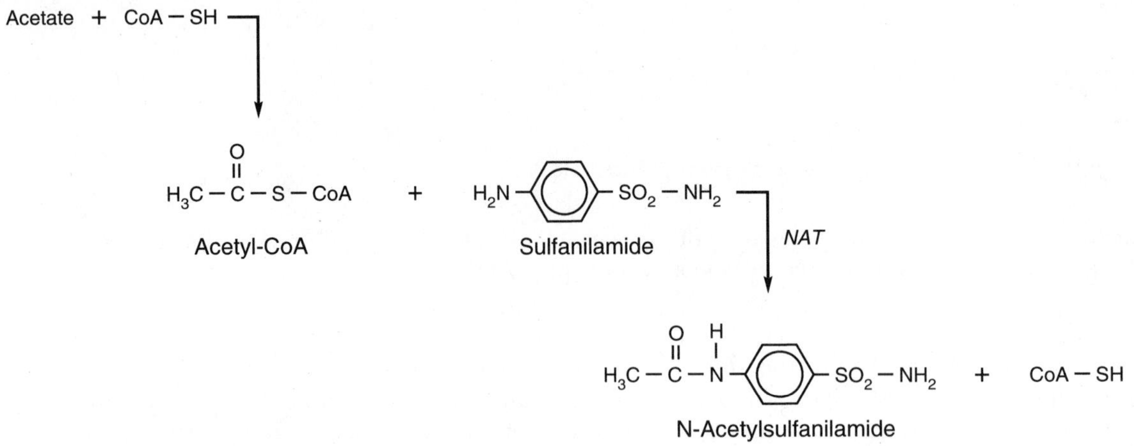

Figure 4-9. Acetylation of an exogenous amine with endogenous acetate catalyzed by *N*-acetyltransferase (NAT). Coenzyme A is abbreviated CoA–SH.

topurine (Fig. 4-10) and azathioprine, whereas thiol *S*-methyltransferase acts on nonpurine agents including captopril and D-penicillamine.

Glycine conjugation

Aromatic carboxylic acids such as benzoic acid (Fig. 4-11) and salicylic acid can be inactivated by conjugation with the endogenous amino acid glycine. In this scheme, the inert carboxylic acid is activated to its acyl coenzyme A derivative prior to amide formation with the amino function of the donating amino acid. Such reactions are commonly catalyzed by transacylases found in hepatic mitochondria. Other amino acids can be utilized for conjugation including glutamine and taurine.

DRUG BIOTRANSFORMATION AND ADVERSE DRUG REACTIONS

Many adverse drug reactions can be traced to an improper balance between bioactivation and detoxification reactions. A classic example involves hepatic necrosis caused by the analgesic acetaminophen. When used at normal therapeutic doses, acetaminophen undergoes glucuronidation and sulfation, reactions that terminate the actions of the drug and hasten its elimination. Some acetaminophen is bioactivated via a cytochrome P450–catalyzed reaction to *N*-acetylbenzoquinonimine. Under normal circumstances, this reactive intermediate can be detoxified by conjugation with glutathione. Thus, a favorable

balance exists between bioactivation and detoxification. However, when acetaminophen is administered in excessive doses, the glucuronidation and sulfation pathways become saturated. More acetaminophen biotransformation is channeled through the cytochrome P450–mediated bioactivation pathway. Detoxification of the reactive metabolite depends on the presence of adequate levels of glutathione. With time, glutathione becomes depleted faster than it can be regenerated. At this point, detoxification cannot keep pace with bioactivation. The reactive metabolite is able to bind covalently to cellular protein thiols and initiate hepatotoxicity. It is possible to prevent hepatotoxicity and death by the administration of *N*-acetylcysteine within 8 to 16 hours following acetaminophen overdose. The antidote serves to reestab-

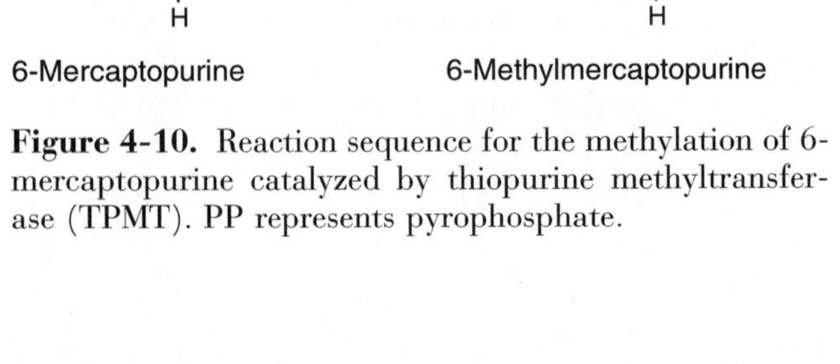

Figure 4-10. Reaction sequence for the methylation of 6-mercaptopurine catalyzed by thiopurine methyltransferase (TPMT). PP represents pyrophosphate.

lish a favorable balance between bioactivation and detoxification.

Many adverse drug reactions that were previously labeled "idiosyncratic" (to indicate that they occurred in a small fraction of the population for no apparent reason) now appear to be caused by genetic deficiencies in various enzymes of drug biotransformation (e.g., CYP2D6, CYP2C19, NAT2). Several adverse drug reactions appear to have an immunological component. In certain cases, drugs (e.g., dihydralazine, tienilic acid, aromatic anticonvulsants) may be bioactivated by cytochromes P450 to reactive metabolites that bind covalently to proteins. The drug–protein adduct may be perceived by the host as "foreign," leading to the production of autoantibodies that may play a role in toxicity.

INDUCTION AND INHIBITION OF DRUG BIOTRANSFORMATION

Many drug-biotransforming enzymes are able to increase in amount and activity in response to certain substances known as inducers. In many cases, an inducer is also a substrate for the enzyme that it induces; however, some substrates are not good inducers and some inducers are not good substrates. In the field of drug biotransformation, most is known about the induction of members of the cytochrome P450 superfamily, although individual forms of epoxide hydrolase, UDP-glucuronosyltransferase, and glutathione *S*-transferase are also inducible. Many molecular mechanisms for enzyme induction have been characterized. The most common means of regulation is **increased DNA transcription;** however post-transcriptional mechanisms such as RNA processing, mRNA stabilization, translational efficiency, and protein stabilization have been identified as important in the regulation of expression of cytochromes P450.

CYP1A1 and CYP1A2 are induced by halogenated aromatic hydrocarbons (e.g., dioxins, PCBs) and polycyclic aromatic hydrocarbons (e.g., 3-methylcholanthrene, benzo[*a*]pyrene). Several hydrocarbons present in cigarette smoke are potent inducers of CYP1A1 and CYP1A2. These types of chemicals bind to a cytosolic receptor protein known as the aromatic hydrocarbon (AH) receptor, which mediates an increase in the rate of transcription of the genes encoding CYP1A1 and CYP1A2. This has great toxicological importance as CYP1A1 and CYP1A2 play important roles in the bioactivation of aromatic hy-

drocarbons and aromatic amines to toxic, mutagenic, and carcinogenic metabolites. This may be of particular importance in extrahepatic sites such as the lung. Exposure of humans to hydrocarbon inducers is known to increase the clearance of antipyrine, acetaminophen, phenacetin, caffeine, and theophylline.

A broader spectrum of induction of hepatic drug-biotransforming enzymes is produced by barbiturates such as phenobarbital. Phenobarbital causes proliferation of the hepatic endoplasmic reticulum, and increases in NADPH–cytochrome P450 reductase, several phase II enzymes, and several forms of cytochrome P450 (e.g., CYP2A1, 2B1, 2B2, 2C6, 3A1, and 3A2 are all induced in the rat). CYP2B1 is the classical phenobarbital-inducible enzyme in rat liver; however, the mechanism by which barbiturates increase the rate of transcription of this gene is still not understood. Phenobarbital increases the biotransformation of many drugs in humans, including phenytoin, warfarin, chlorpromazine, digitoxin, and cyclophosphamide.

Isoniazid or chronic ethanol administration increases the levels of CYP2E1, an enzyme that is important in the oxidation of alcohols and the bioactivation of carcinogenic nitrosamines. Induction of CYP2E1 by these chemicals occurs mainly via protein stabilization. Glucocorticoids, macrolide antibiotics, anticonvulsants, and rifampin induce members of the CYP3A subfamily. This is of tremendous importance, as species of CYP3A are the major contributors to the hepatic biotransformation of a broad array of therapeutic agents in humans (as diverse as cyclosporin A, erythromycin, nifedipine, diazepam, and ketoconazole). The hypolipidemic drug clofibrate induces CYP4A enzymes that are involved in the hydroxylation of several fatty acids and eicosanoids. A recently cloned member of the steroid hormone receptor superfamily, termed the peroxisome-proliferator-activated receptor (PPAR), appears to mediate the induction of CYP4A forms by clofibrate and related chemicals.

Induction of drug-biotransforming enzymes can be an important cause of drug interactions. Phenobarbital and ethanol serve as two important examples. Phenobarbital and phenytoin are both used in the treatment of epilepsy. Phenobarbital can induce the enzymes responsible for phenytoin biotransformation, thus lowering the steady-state plasma concentrations of phenytoin and altering the ability of phenytoin to control seizures. Chronic ethanol consumption induces CYP2E1 and leads to enhanced biotransformation of acetaminophen, isoniazid, and

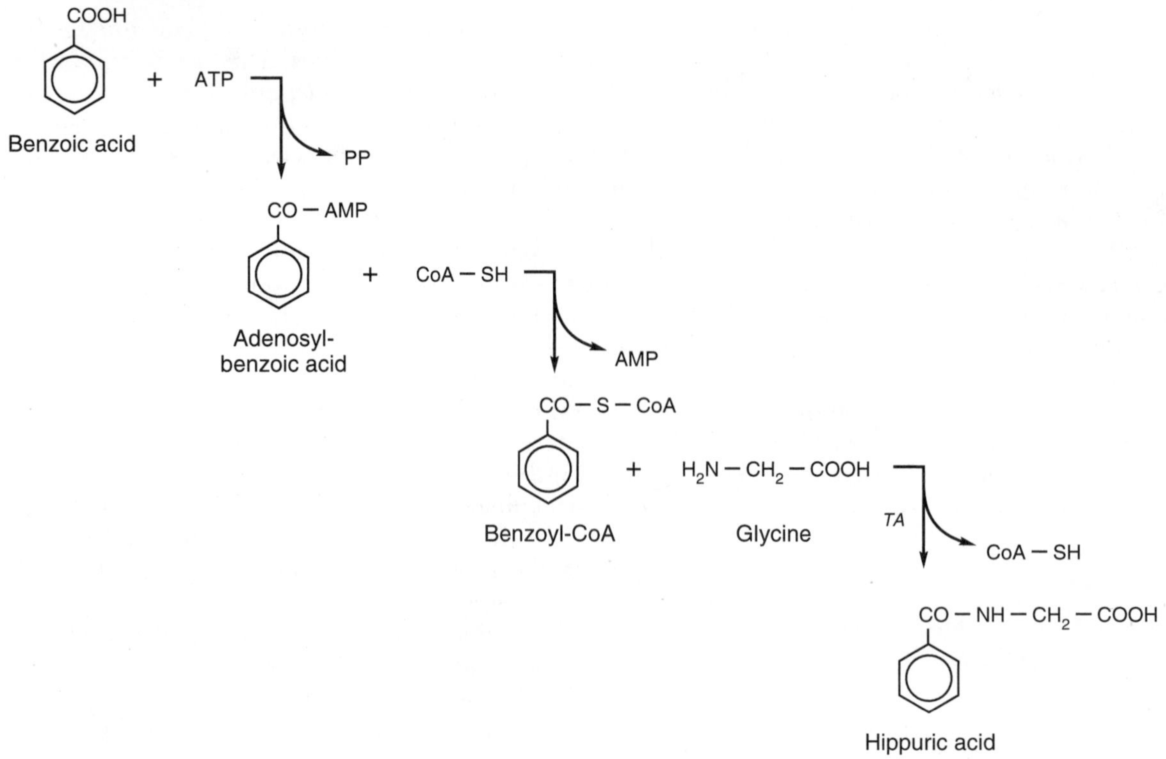

Figure 4-11. Conjugation of the endogenous amino acid glycine with exogenous benzoic acid catalyzed by a transacylase (TA). PP represents pyrophosphate and CoA–SH represents coenzyme A.

carcinogenic nitrosamines. Chronic ethanol users are at greater risk for acetaminophen-induced hepatotoxicity because of the increased rate of generation of reactive metabolites of acetaminophen. Some examples of drugs that are known to induce drug biotransformation in humans are listed in Table 4-1.

In view of the large numbers of drugs that share the same enzymatic sites of biotransformation, it is not surprising that interactions among them are very common. In general, acute interactions tend to be inhibitory, i.e., one drug competes with another for an enzyme binding site, and each thus inhibits the biotransformation of the other. Several mechanisms are available for the inhibition of cytochromes P450 by xenobiotics. Imidazole-containing drugs such as cimetidine and ketoconazole coordinate tightly to the heme iron and thereby inhibit the biotransformation of other drugs and endogenous chemicals. Macrolide antibiotics and several other drugs are biotransformed by cytochromes P450 to intermediates that form a tight complex with the heme moiety and thus prevent the further participation of the enzyme in drug biotransformation reactions. Many other drugs

function as mechanism-based or suicidal inactivators of cytochromes P450 in that the chemical is biotransformed by the enzyme to a reactive intermediate that irreversibly inactivates the enzyme via a covalent interaction with the protein (e.g., chloramphenicol) or heme (e.g., ethinyl estradiol, secobarbital, spironolactone) moiety.

The number of therapeutic agents that can inhibit drug biotransformation is extremely large, and inhibition of drug biotransformation is a very important cause of drug interactions. Oral contraceptives containing estrogens and progestins inhibit the hepatic biotransformation of several drugs.

Coadministration of ethanol with certain drugs can decrease the clearance of the drug and lead to an exaggerated pharmacological effect. Ketoconazole or erythromycin can inhibit the CYP3A-mediated biotransformation of the antihistamine terfenadine, leading to elevated plasma levels of terfenadine and increased risk of development of a serious ventricular arrhythmia termed "torsade de pointes." A final interesting example involves the interaction between dihydropyridine calcium-channel blockers and grapefruit juice. It appears that grapefruit juice con-

Table 4-1 Examples of Xenobiotics that Function as Inducers or Inhibitors of Drug Biotransformation in Humans

Inducers	Inhibitors
Benzo[a]pyrene	Allopurinol
Chlorcyclizine	Chloramphenicol
Clofibrate	Cimetidine
Dexamethasone	Dicumarol
Ethanol	Disulfiram
Ethchlorvynol	Erythromycin
Glutethimide	Ethanol
Griseofulvin	Ethinyl estradiol
Isoniazid	Ketoconazole
Phenobarbital	Nortriptyline
Phenylbutazone	Phenylbutazone
Phenytoin	Secobarbital
Rifampin	Spironolactone
	Troleandomycin

tains certain bioflavonoids that can inhibit the CYP3A-mediated biotransformation of drugs such as felodipine, thereby increasing the systemic bioavailability of these drugs. Some examples of drugs that inhibit drug biotransformation in humans are listed in Table 4-1.

OTHER FACTORS AFFECTING DRUG BIOTRANSFORMATION

Species and Strain

Species differ with respect to biotransformation reactions both qualitatively and quantitatively. Cats are deficient in UDP-glucuronosyltransferase activity, and as a result they are very susceptible to the pharmacological actions of morphine. A bromocyclohexenyl derivative of barbituric acid was developed in an attempt to generate a short-acting barbiturate in humans. The drug was found to be rapidly biotransformed in dogs; however, when administered to human volunteers, the drug was found to be very slowly biotransformed and to produce a prolonged hypnosis. Species differences in drug biotransformation emphasize the problems that may be encountered in drug development because of the fact that experimental animals may be poor models for human drug biotransformation.

Differences in biotransformation between various strains of animals are also common. The Gunn rat is deficient in the UDP-glucuronosyltransferase responsible for bilirubin conjugation, making this strain a valuable experimental model for clinical conditions characterized by unconjugated hyperbilirubinemia. Certain inbred mouse strains (e.g., C57BL/6N) respond to treatment with 3-methylcholanthrene with an induction of CYP1A1, whereas other strains (e.g., DBA/2N) do not.

Age

Drug-biotransforming enzymes display interesting developmental patterns of expression both before and after birth. The implication is that individuals may be at increased risk of drug toxicity or suboptimal therapy at particular ontogenic stages. In general, neonates and geriatric patients display reduced drug biotransformation capacity and increased susceptibility to the toxic effects of some drugs. For example, in premature infants and during the first week or two of life in normal infants, there is a deficiency in glucuronidation and renal function. Chloramphenicol is eliminated mainly as a monoglucuronide conjugate; therefore, when chloramphenicol is administered to newborns without proper dose adjustments, life-threatening hematological toxicity can occur. The result is often a combination of pallor and cyanosis, the hallmarks of the "gray baby syndrome." Although it is more difficult to make generalizations about elderly populations, age-related decreases in hepatic biotransformation have been documented for many drugs, especially those biotransformed by cytochromes P450 (see Chapters 65 and 66).

Genetic Factors

Individuals differ in their ability to biotransform many drugs, and part of this variation may be due to genetic factors. Pharmacogenetics is the study of unusual drug responses that have a hereditary basis (see Chapter 12). Mutations in genes coding for drug biotransformation enzymes are important causes of variations in drug response in human populations. For example, the identification of variant alleles at the *NAT2* gene locus accounts for the slow acetylation of drugs such as isoniazid observed in about 50% of Caucasian populations. Similarly, genetic defects at the *CYP2D6* locus result in impaired biotransformation of numerous therapeutic agents including debrisoquin, sparteine, dextromethorphan, several β-adrenoceptor antagonists, and tricyclic antidepressants. Recently, defects in the *CYP2C19* gene have been found to account for impaired hydroxylation of the anticonvulsant mephenytoin.

Sex and Hormonal Factors

Many enzymes of drug biotransformation are under strict control by specific endocrine factors. Sex differences in drug biotransformation are pronounced in rats; adult male rats show higher rates of biotransformation of many drugs than females do. Many of these differences are due to the fact that rats express sex-specific forms of cytochrome P450. Gonadal steroids contribute to these sex differences, but the major hormonal determinant appears to be the sex-dependent patterns of growth hormone secretion from the pituitary gland. Sex differences in drug biotransformation in humans are not as pronounced as in the rat, but male and female patients have been found to biotransform many drugs (e.g., propranolol, benzodiazepines, salicylates) at different rates. Pregnancy, adrenal insufficiency, diabetes, and hypothyroid conditions have all been shown to alter drug biotransformation capacity.

Diet

Both macronutrient and micronutrient dietary components have been found to affect drug biotransformation. It is difficult to make generalizations about the effects of diet on drug biotransformation because individual enzymes may display unique responses to dietary factors. For example, fasting causes a characteristic increase in CYP2E1 levels and activity. In general, diets that are low in protein or deficient in essential fatty acids result in decreased cytochrome P450–mediated biotransformation. Many vitamins (e.g., vitamins A, B_1, B_2, C, E, K) and minerals (e.g., calcium, magnesium, iron, copper, zinc, iodine) can also have complex effects on drug biotransformation capacity.

In addition, many non-nutrient dietary components may affect drug biotransformation. Tryptophan pyrolysis products found in charcoal-broiled meats are inducers of CYP1A1 and CYP1A2 and are also potential carcinogens. There is also evidence that the ability of specific compounds found in vegetables to prevent chemical carcinogenesis is related to their effects on procarcinogen biotransformation. For example, chemicals found in cruciferous vegetables such as broccoli and brussels sprouts (e.g., indole 3-carbinol) and allium vegetables such as garlic (e.g., diallyl sulfide) appear to reduce the formation of procarcinogen biotransformation products that can bind covalently to DNA.

Disease States

Liver cirrhosis and liver cancer are associated with decreased hepatic biotransformation capacity, particularly with respect to cytochrome P450–dependent pathways. Such effects may be due to decreased expression of drug-biotransforming enzymes and/or alterations in liver architecture and altered hepatic blood flow. Many tumor cells display reduced cytochrome P450 content and increased levels of phase II biotransformation enzymes, making them particularly resistant to chemical insult, including the action of cytotoxic antineoplastic agents (see Chapter 60).

Infectious diseases and inflammatory conditions are often associated with reduced hepatic drug biotransformation. Interferons and cytokines that are produced following activation of host defense mechanisms appear to mediate the suppression of drug biotransformation.

METHODS FOR THE STUDY OF DRUG BIOTRANSFORMATION

Modern investigations of drug biotransformation are conducted in experimental systems that range in complexity from an isolated enzyme to an intact animal or human subject.

Studies of drug pharmacokinetics in vivo provide valuable information about the overall fate of a drug in an intact biological system. Measurement of the disappearance of parent drug from plasma cannot distinguish between processes of distribution and biotransformation. It can be very informative to identify and measure specific biotransformation products (i.e., metabolites) in plasma, urine, and/or bile. If the rate of disappearance of parent drug equals the rate of appearance of metabolites, this is good evidence that drug disappearance is due to biotransformation. However, this in vivo approach does not reveal the sites and mechanisms of drug biotransformation. With the use of noninvasive-probe drug assays, it is now possible to phenotype human subjects with respect to the function of specific hepatic enzymes of drug biotransformation. For example, the measurement of specific metabolites of caffeine in urine can be used as an indication of CYP1A2 catalytic function in humans. This is possible because

CYP1A2-mediated caffeine 3-demethylation is a major pathway for caffeine elimination in humans.

At the organ level, most interest in drug biotransformation has focused on the liver. In vitro liver perfusion studies have yielded important information concerning the kinetic and spatial aspects of drug biotransformation. Within the liver, hepatocytes contain the highest concentrations of drug-biotransforming enzymes and it is possible to study drug biotransformation in freshly isolated and cultured hepatocytes. A problem with the use of cultured hepatocytes is that the cells tend to show a loss of differentiated hepatocyte functions (including cytochrome P450–mediated drug biotransformation) during in vitro culture. Similarly, many immortal hepatoma cell lines are deficient in cytochrome P450 function.

Biotransformation of drugs is commonly studied in subcellular fractions, especially microsomes and cytosol. For example, hepatic microsomes supplemented with exogenous NADPH contain all the enzymatic machinery required to carry out the oxidative biotransformation of numerous drugs. Using protein biochemistry techniques, it is also possible to purify a specific drug-biotransforming enzyme and study its function in isolation. An individual cytochrome P450 enzyme can be reconstituted with purified NADPH–cytochrome P450 reductase and phospholipid to yield a functional monooxygenase system. With the advent of molecular cloning techniques, it is now common to express the cDNA for a single drug biotransformation enzyme in a variety of cellular systems, including mammalian and insect cells, yeast, and bacteria. This approach can be particularly powerful as it allows the study of a single enzyme in isolation within a cellular environment.

It must be kept in mind, however, that in vitro drug biotransformation reactions are usually studied under optimal conditions of substrate and cofactor concentrations, temperature, pH, and so forth. The rate of reaction may therefore be quite different from that seen under the influence of rate-limiting factors in vivo.

DRUG BIOTRANSFORMATION IN THE DRUG DEVELOPMENT PROCESS

During the process of developing a new therapeutic agent for clinical use, it is essential to characterize the routes and rates of biotransformation of the compound. Traditionally, this has involved the char-

acterization of the metabolites produced in experimental animals. However, species differences in drug biotransformation render rodents poor experimental models for human biotransformation. Thus, it is desirable and indeed possible to study the biotransformation of new drugs by human enzymes before administering the drug to patients. It is of considerable interest to identify the human enzyme(s) responsible for the biotransformation of a drug so that adverse drug reactions resulting from drug interactions or genetic defects can be understood and predicted. Using the cytochromes P450 as an example, it is possible to use four major in vitro approaches in combination in order to determine which particular enzyme carries out the biotransformation of a drug.

First, studying the biotransformation by a purified or cDNA-expressed human enzyme can tell whether that enzyme has the inherent capability to transform the drug. Second, using a human liver microsomal preparation, it is possible to determine the effect of cytochrome P450 isozyme-selective chemical inhibitors on the reaction of interest. For example, furafylline will inhibit the biotransformation of the drug if CYP1A2 is involved in the reaction. Third, many antibodies that are directed against a drug biotransformation enzyme can serve as isozyme-selective inhibitors. Thus, if anti-CYP1A2 antibody inhibits the reaction to a large extent, then this is good evidence that CYP1A2 makes an important contribution to this reaction in human liver. Finally, if a panel of human liver microsomal samples is available from a number of donors, it is possible to perform correlation analyses. For example, if the rate of biotransformation of the drug of interest correlates with the level of CYP1A2 protein or catalytic activity in a number of human liver samples, then it would appear that CYP1A2 is an important contributor to this reaction. In this manner, advances in protein biochemistry and molecular biology are having an impact on the development of therapeutic agents and on improvement in human health.

SUGGESTED READING

Alvares AP, Pratt WB. Pathways of drug metabolism. In: Pratt WB, Taylor P, eds. Principles of drug action: the basis of pharmacology. 3rd ed. New York: Churchill Livingstone, 1990: 365–422.

Beetham JK, Grant D, Arand M, et al. Gene evolution of epoxide hydrolases and recommended nomenclature. DNA Cell Biol 1995; 14:61–71.

Burchell B, Nebert DW, Nelson DR, et al. The UDP glucuronosyltransferase gene superfamily: suggested nomenclature based on evolutionary divergence. DNA Cell Biol 1991; 10:487–494.

Falany CN. Molecular enzymology of human liver cytosolic sulfotransferases. Trends Pharmacol Sci 1991; 12:255–259.

Gibson GG, Skett P. Introduction to drug metabolism. 2nd ed. London: Chapman & Hall, 1994.

Gonzalez FJ. Human cytochromes P450: problems and prospects. Trends Pharmacol Sci 1992; 13:346–352.

Guengerich FP. Cytochrome P450 enzymes. Am Sci 1993; 81:440–447.

Hayes JD, Pulford DJ. The glutathione S-transferase supergene family: regulation of GST and the contribution of the isoenzymes to cancer chemoprevention and drug resistance. Crit Rev Biochem Mol Biol 1995; 30:445–600.

Lawton MP, Cashman JR, Cresteil T, et al. A nomenclature for the mammalian flavin-containing monooxygenase gene family based on amino acid sequence identities. Arch Biochem Biophys 1994; 308:254–257.

Mannervik B, Awasthi YC, Board PG, et al. Nomenclature for human glutathione transferases. Biochem J 1992; 282:305–306.

Nelson DR, Koymans L, Kamataki T, et al. P450 superfamily: update on new sequences, gene mapping, accession numbers and nomenclature. Pharmacogenetics 1996; 6:1–42.

Okey AB, Riddick DS, Harper PA. Molecular biology of the aromatic hydrocarbon (dioxin) receptor. Trends Pharmacol Sci 1994; 15:226–232.

Ortiz de Montellano PR, ed. Cytochrome 450: structure, mechanism, and biochemistry. 2nd ed. New York: Plenum Press, 1995.

Porter TD, Coon MJ. Cytochrome P450: multiplicity of isoforms, substrates, and catalytic and regulatory mechanisms. J Biol Chem 1991; 266:13469–13472.

Tukey RH, Johnson EF. Molecular aspects of regulation and structure of the drug-metabolizing enzymes. In: Pratt WB, Taylor P, eds. Principles of drug action: the basis of pharmacology. 3rd ed. New York: Churchill Livingstone, 1990: 423–467.

Vatsis KP, Weber WW, Bell DA, et al. Nomenclature for N-acetyltransferases. Pharmacogenetics 1995; 5:1–17.

Weinshilboum R. Methylation pharmacogenetics: thiopurine methyltransferase as a model system. Xenobiotica 1992; 22:1055–1071.

CHAPTER 5

Pharmacokinetics

L. ENDRENYI

RATIONALE AND BACKGROUND

Aims of Pharmacokinetics

Pharmacokinetics is the quantitative description of the rates of the various steps of drug disposition. These steps include (1) the absorption of drugs, which enables them to reach the systemic circulation, (2) their distribution to various organs and tissues in the body, and (3) their elimination by biotransformation and excretion.

The rates of these processes have two main uses. First, they are by themselves of great interest to pharmacologists because they characterize in some detail the fate of a drug in the body, and thus permit the factors that determine this fate to be studied. Second, physicians use pharmacokinetic data for calculating and selecting the routes, doses, and frequencies of drug administration.

Such pharmacokinetic assessments are particularly essential in the view of clinicians when, for a given drug, the doses eliciting toxic side effects are not much higher than those required for therapeutic action. Care must also be exercised when there is large variation in the responses of different patients to a given dose of a drug. The variability can appear in several forms: There may be a wide spread among the responses of different people; the responses to some drugs may be separated into two or more distinct groups, based on genetic differences; and rare idiosyncratic responses may occur. In all these cases, a pharmacokinetic study of an individual patient is desirable in optimally adjusting the drug dose.

Relation of Dose, Plasma Drug Concentration, and Effect

A particular amount (dose) of an administered drug will produce an effect according to the following sequence:

Dosage
↓
Concentration in plasma water
↓
Concentration at site of action
↓
Intensity of effect

The intensity of drug action is most often related to the concentration of the drug at the site of action ("receptor"). Similarly, the duration of the drug effect is related to the greater or lesser persistence of its presence at this site. The concentration at the receptors changes, in turn, as the drug enters, is distributed in, and leaves various parts of the body, and as it undergoes biotransformation (metabolic degradation) reactions.

Pharmacodynamic investigations examine the intensity and the time courses of responses to drugs. Unfortunately, some clinical responses (e.g., effectiveness of sleep induction, or decrease in chronic skeletal pain) are difficult to characterize quantitatively. Therefore, we frequently assume that the intensity of pharmacological action correlates better with the concentration of free drug in plasma than with the dose, and evaluate in **pharmacokinetic** studies the time course of drug concentrations in the plasma (and in other body fluids) following various routes of drug administration. As an important application, the efficacy of drug therapy can be improved, and toxicity decreased, by using plasma drug concentrations as an aid in adjusting drug dosage.

In some situations, however, the relation between plasma concentration and effect is difficult to interpret—e.g., in the case of irreversibly acting drugs (phenoxybenzamine); acute, chronic, or cross tolerance (barbiturates); combinations of drugs with synergistic or antagonistic actions (barbiturate + amphetamine); and presence of active metabolites (e.g., diazepam and desmethyldiazepam).

Methodology of Pharmacokinetics

Whenever the fate of a drug in the body is described qualitatively or quantitatively, a hypothetical **model** of the body is assumed. Figure 5-1 illustrates a fairly general model characterizing the fate of drugs in the body. (Note the similarity to Figures 1-1 and 3-1, which illustrate the same concepts with slightly different emphasis.)

Such a hypothetical model, however, is entirely useless unless it is verified by experimental observations. To achieve this goal, the mathematical consequences of the model are derived first by considering material and rate balances. The predictions of the model must then be compared with experimental observations: Agreement suggests, but does not prove, that the assumptions involving the model have been correct.

KINETICS OF DRUG DISPOSITION PROCESSES

Elimination Following Intravenous Injection: One-Compartment Model

Since first-order drug disposition is the most common (and simplest) pattern, we shall assume it in this model. This means that the rate of the process at any given time is proportional to the concentration at that time. Consequently, after the intravenous introduction of a drug, its concentration (C) in the plasma decreases at a rate that is proportional at all times (t) to the concentration itself. This statement is described mathematically by:

$$\text{Rate} = (-dC/dt) = kC$$

(k is the proportionality or rate constant). If the initial concentration is C_0, the solution of this differential equation is:

$$C = C_0 e^{-kt}$$

(here e is the base of the natural logarithms). The exponentially moderated decrease of the plasma concentration is shown in Figure 5-2A.

In practice, a more convenient form of this equation is obtained by using logarithms to the base 10, rather than natural logarithms:

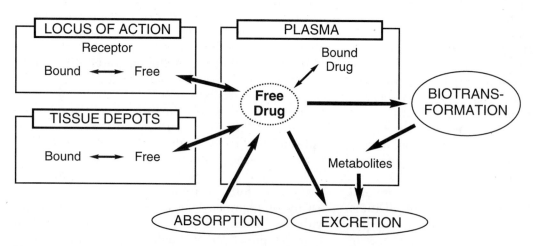

Figure 5-1. Schematic representation of the fate of drugs in the body.

$$\log_{10}C = \log_{10}C_0 - \frac{k}{2.303} \cdot t$$

$(2.303 = \log_e 10$, often written as ln 10). Thus, if we plot the logarithm of the concentrations (log C) against the times of their observation (t), we should obtain a straight line (Fig. 5-2B). The plot provides the values of k and C_0 at once, since the slope of the line equals $-k/2.303$ and the vertical intercept is log C_0.

From the latter and the injected dose (D_0) the **volume of distribution** (V) can be calculated:

$$V = D_0/C_0$$

Another important quantity, the **half-life of elimination** ($t_{1/2}$), can also be evaluated from the elimination rate constant:

$$t_{1/2} = 0.693/k$$

(since $0.693 = \ln 2$). This is the time period during which the concentration decreases to one-half of its previous value.

Example: A 100-mg dose of a drug was injected intravenously and its concentration (in milligrams per liter) in the plasma was observed repeatedly. The logarithms of the concentrations have been plotted against the times (in hours) of their observation. A straight line could be drawn through the points, which had a slope of -0.0751 and an extrapolated intercept of 1.30. Consequently,

$$k = -2.303 \times (-0.0751) = 0.173 \text{ hr}^{-1}$$

and

$$C_0 = \text{antilog } 1.30 = 10^{1.30} = 20 \text{ mg/L}$$

From these, the half-life of elimination is

$$t_{1/2} = 0.693/0.173 = 4.0 \text{ hours}$$

and the volume of distribution

$$V = 100/20 = 5 \text{ liters}$$

The half-life of 4.0 hours means that 4 hours after the injection of the initial 100 mg, only 50 mg is left in the plasma (and in those parts of the body in which the concentration of this drug is in constant proportion to that in the plasma). After 8 hours 25 mg is left; 12.5 mg remains after 12 hours; and so

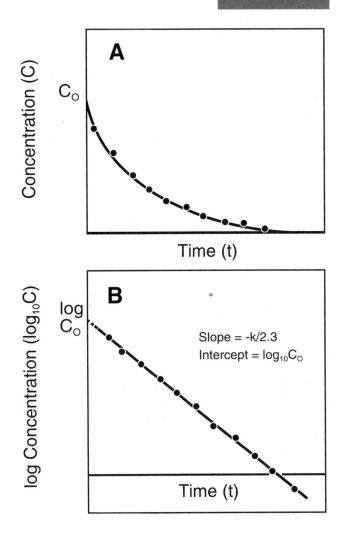

Figure 5-2. Time dependence of a drug concentration in blood after an intravenous injection. The drug concentration is plotted on a linear (A) and on a logarithmic (B) scale.

on. With a distribution volume of 5 liters this is equivalent to concentrations of 20, 10, 5, and 2.5 mg/L at 0, 4, 8, and 12 hours after injection, respectively.

The Model: Such simple results are based naturally on the assumption of a very simple model. A single compartment is hypothesized which may possibly refer to the plasma and to all the tissues and receptors in which the drug is in equilibrium with the free (i.e., unbound) drug molecules in the plasma. Thus in Figure 5-1, illustrating a model for the fate of drugs in the body, the plasma, tissue, and receptor compartments are now pooled. Absorption is omitted since the drug is introduced directly into the bloodstream, and elimination from the plasma includes excretion and possible metabolic degradations. Consequently, we are left with Model 1.

The one-compartment model provides an extremely simple description of the pharmacology of drug disposition and the relevant physiology. Nevertheless, the model is often very useful for characterizing drug kinetics and predicting drug dosages.

Two-Compartment Model

Distribution and elimination

After intravenous injection, curvature can often be detected in the early part of the semilogarithmic elimination plot. This is reasonable because, as already indicated, it takes some time for the drug to be redistributed from the circulating plasma or central compartment to the extracellular space. During this period the logarithmic concentration in plasma decreases more rapidly than in the later, linear, steady-state section of the curve (Fig. 5-3). Therefore, we now assume two compartments (Model 2): a central compartment that may perhaps refer to the plasma, and a peripheral compartment including the extracellular space and, possibly, the tissues and receptors in equilibrium with it.

(A two-compartment system can be described mathematically by two differential equations, the solution of which is the sum or the difference of two exponential terms, provided that the system is "open," i.e., that it has an exit. The final, linear segment of the semilogarithmic elimination plot is always characterized by the term containing the smallest exponent, i.e., the longest half-life.)

One of the most useful applications of pharmacokinetic models involves the prediction of the time course of drug concentrations for compartments and models of drug administration which actually have not been experimentally investigated. For example, drug concentrations are frequently measured only in the central compartment (including usually the

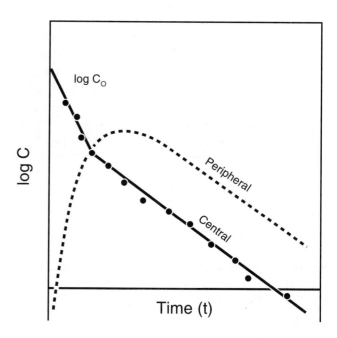

Figure 5-3. Time course of plasma (central) and tissue (peripheral) concentration of a drug following its intravenous injection, in the presence of distribution and elimination.

plasma). Still, if a drug displays two-compartment characteristics, then it is possible to predict the time dependence of its concentration in the peripheral compartment (Fig. 5-3), which is often linked to receptors associated with drug action.

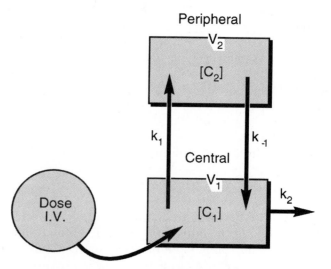

Model 2. Two-compartment open model with rapid intravenous injection.

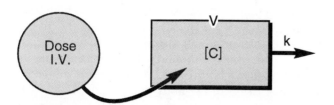

Model 1. One-compartment open model with rapid intravenous injection.

Absorption and elimination

If the drug is administered not intravenously but, for example, orally, intramuscularly, or subcutaneously, then generally its concentration in the plasma will rise during the initial absorption phase and decrease again when (1) the absorption is complete, (2) the drug is in steady state between the plasma and the peripheral compartments, and (3) the rate of concentration decrease is dominated by the elimination processes (Fig. 5-4). In a semilogarithmic scale the final, descending part of the curve is linear (Fig. 5-4B).

The model is identical to Model 1 with the addition of an absorption compartment (Model 3). This is justified because it has been found repeatedly that the rate of absorption is proportional to the unabsorbed amount of drug, so a first-order compartment for absorption may be assumed.

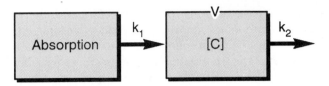

Model 3. Absorption and elimination.

Concentration Dependence of Rates

We have assumed that the rates of various processes are proportional to the drug concentration in the compartment from which the molecules exit. This is usually a reasonable assumption. For example, it is valid for diffusion-controlled processes since the rate of diffusion is proportional to the concentration gradient (the difference of concentrations on the two sides of a membrane or other barrier), and the concentration of the "receiving" side is usually negligibly small in comparison with the concentration in the "donating" compartment. Similarly, the rate of urinary excretion is usually proportional to the concentration of the free drug in plasma water. Certainly, this is true for excretion by glomerular filtration, but in practice it is often valid even for active transfer processes such as tubular secretion or reabsorption, when the drug concentration in the relevant compartment is low enough that the carrier system is not close to being saturated.

However, carrier systems can become saturated at high concentrations. The rate of urinary excretion is then constant, independently of the plasma concentration, and thereby conforms to the features of a zero-order process. A linear plot for the time course of concentrations (Fig. 5-5A) shows a constant rate of decline: In contrast, the slope in the semilogarithmic plot of concentrations (Fig. 5-5B) is not constant in this region but gets gradually steeper. Eventually the concentration decreases sufficiently so that the carrier system is not saturated any more. After passing through an intermediate region, the concentration reaches, at its lower levels, the range of first-order removal.

Some drugs act therapeutically in the transitional range between the regions of purely zero-order and purely first-order kinetics (e.g., phenytoin, dicumarol, salicylic acid). Other substances are physiologically effective within the range of zero-order kinetics (e.g., ethanol). Similar considerations apply to biotransformation reactions or to binding to plasma proteins. At high drug concentrations the catalyzing enzyme or the binding protein (albumin) becomes

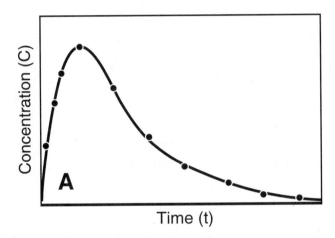

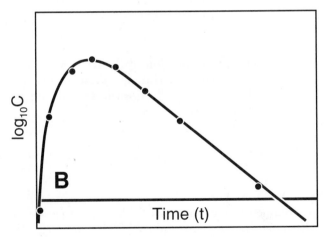

Figure 5-4. Time course of plasma concentration after the oral administration of a drug. The drug concentration is plotted on a linear (A) and on a logarithmic (B) scale.

saturated with substrate (drug) molecules and, therefore, the rate of the appropriate process is independent of the drug concentration. However, at much below saturating concentrations these rates also become proportional to the concentrations.

As mentioned earlier, the rate of absorption is also proportional to the amount of the unabsorbed drug. This is, of course, not so when drug tablets are specially coated to form slow, sustained-release preparations that are absorbed at a rate independent of the amount of drug remaining in the intestinal lumen.

DURATION OF DRUG ACTION

It is usually assumed that a drug evokes some demonstrable effect when its concentration in the central compartment is higher than a minimal threshold level ($C_{\text{effective}}$). Similarly, when the plasma concentration exceeds $C_{\text{therapeutic}}$, a specific therapeutic response is elicited. Drug action is maintained at a detectable level as long as the drug concentration exceeds the minimum effective level.

A useful guideline characterizing the duration of drug action can be established on the basis of these principles. This states that **the duration of drug effects is proportional to the half-life of elimination and to the logarithm of the dose**, provided that the absorption and distribution of the drug are rapid in comparison with its elimination (including biotransformation and excretion) and that these are first-order processes.

Therefore, it is very difficult to obtain increased duration of drug action by increasing the dosage, since the latter must be raised exponentially to attain an only linear increase in the duration.

In order to demonstrate these proportionalities, let us assume one-compartmental elimination, without a distribution phase. If different doses of a drug are introduced by a given route of administration, the semilogarithmic concentration–time profiles will be parallel lines (Fig. 5-6). Furthermore, if the ratios between the consecutively higher doses (i.e., the differences between their logarithms) are constant, then the lines are equally distanced. In the horizontal direction, equal distances between lines, particularly at the concentration level $C_{\text{therapeutic}}$, imply the uniformly gradual increase in the duration of drug action (t_D). Thus, equal increments of duration are paralleled by uniform increments of the logarithm of the dose and, therefore, the two quantities are linearly related.

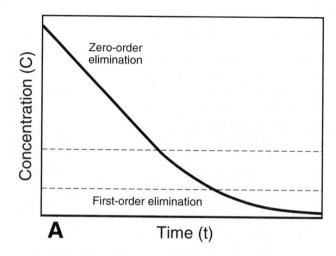

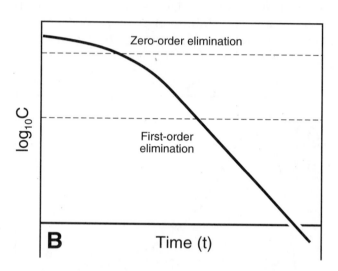

Figure 5-5. Time course of plasma concentration of a drug exhibiting zero-order kinetics at high levels. Linear plot (A) and semilogarithmic plot (B).

An important application of this rule states that **the duration of drug action is extended by one half-life when the dose is doubled.** This conclusion can be formalized as:

$$t_{2D_0} = t_{D_0} + t_{1/2}$$

Example: Let us assume that for the drug considered earlier, with a half-life of 4 hours and an apparent volume of distribution of 5 liters, the therapeutically effective concentration $C_{\text{ther}} = 5$ mg/L. We have already seen that the plasma concentration has fallen to this level 8 hours after the intravenous injection of a dose of 100 mg. If the dose is doubled

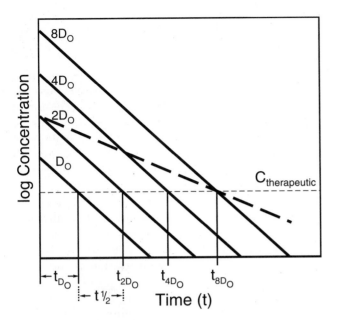

Figure 5-6. Effect of intravenously injected drug doses and biological half-life on the duration of drug action.

to 200 mg, then, according to our rule, the duration of effective drug action is extended to 8 + 4 = 12 hours.

The proportionality of duration with elimination half-life can be similarly illustrated. After all, longer half-lives indicate shallower lines in the semilogarithmic plot (oblique shallow line in Fig. 5-6). Consequently, for a given intercept (initial concentration), the minimal effective concentration is reached after a longer time.

The guidelines characterizing the duration of drug action can also be applied, with very good approximation, in the presence of fast absorption and distribution, because these alter the shape of the concentration profile only slightly. However, caution must be exercised when nonlinear kinetics or extended absorption and/or distribution causes substantial curvature in the semilogarithmic concentration–time plot.

The effect of dosage on duration can be particularly striking if absorption is not fast in comparison with elimination (Fig. 5-7). At low doses, the drug effect appears quite late and lasts only for a short time. Larger doses bring about an earlier appearance of the effects. Also, these are very substantially prolonged.

The above considerations are not applicable when the effects of a drug or chemical are not always proportional to its concentration in the central compartment. For instance, organophosphate insecticides

destroy certain enzymes in the body. Consequently, their effect is prolonged well after their elimination, until the enzymes are resynthesized.

EXTENDING THE DURATION OF DRUG ACTION

Infusion of a Drug

If the drug is introduced at a constant rate, in the form of intravenous infusion or as a sustained-release tablet, its concentration in the plasma increases at a gradually diminishing rate. In the case of an infusion, after awhile a fairly constant concentration is reached. The infusion may be discontinued either before or after reaching the plateau. This is indicated by arrows in Figure 5-8, showing a curve obtained at high infusion rate that is continued to steady state at the plateau and, with identical kinetic constants, another curve that characterizes a lower-rate infusion interrupted before reaching the plateau.

After interruption of the infusion, the time course of drug concentrations follows earlier-described prin-

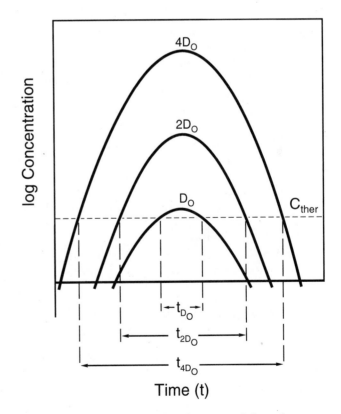

Figure 5-7. Effect of orally administered drug dosage on the duration of drug action. (See text for explanations.)

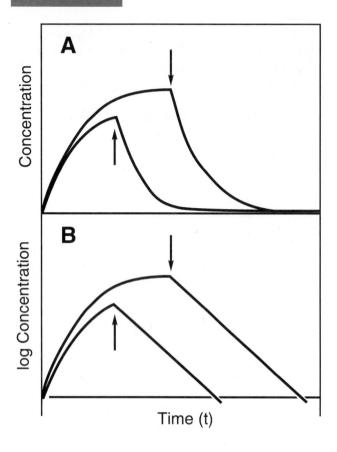

Figure 5-8. Time course of drug concentration during and following intravenous infusion. The arrows indicate the cessation of drug administration. Linear plot (A) and semilogarithmic plot (B). (See text for additional explanations.)

ciples. If redistribution of the drug is essentially complete, then its elimination is characterized by a descending straight line in the semilogarithmic plot (Fig. 5-8B).

In the plot of concentration against time (Fig. 5-8A), the accumulation curve is the inverted mirror image of the elimination pattern.

Applications of the infusion curves in clinical pharmacokinetics are described in Chapter 6.

Repeated Drug Administration: Dosage Regimens

The aim of approximately constant plasma concentration levels can be reached also by repeated application of the drug. We would like the concentration to stay above the threshold level for effective therapeutic action (C_{ther}) but safely below the toxic concentration (C_{tox}) that would begin to cause harmful

side effects. This aim is achieved when appropriate maintenance doses are given repeatedly at the proper dosing intervals.

Figure 5-9 illustrates the time course of drug concentrations following repeated intravenous administrations. A one-compartment model is assumed (rapid distribution in comparison with elimination). Thus, in the semilogarithmic plot (Fig. 5-9A) the descending segments are linear and parallel since all of them are characterized by the same elimination rate constant and half-life. In the concentration–time plot (Fig. 5-9B) the vertical (ascending) lines are of equal length, on the assumption that identical maintenance doses are used. The descending sections are exponential and not linear in Figure 5-9B. The discontinuation of drug administration is indicated by arrows.

When the initial dose equals the maintenance doses, the final, desired concentration range is reached not immediately, but only after several dosage intervals. But the patient is probably sickest and in greatest need of reaching the proper therapeutic drug concentration in the initial phase of the medication. Therefore, it is very desirable to administer a high initial, so-called **loading or priming dose,** and to continue later with the small **maintenance doses** (Fig. 5-9C). These are generally given at regular dosing or **maintenance intervals.**

Absorption and distribution processes alter the concentration profiles only very slightly if they are fast in comparison with elimination. Slower absorption and/or distribution distort the curves in a manner similar to that seen with a single drug administration: In the semilogarithmic concentration–time plot, curvatures downward and upward, respectively, are introduced. In particular, after intramuscular or oral drug intake, the multiple peaks of the concentration profile do not rise suddenly, and are not sharp, in contrast to those seen in the intravenous examples.

A systematic dosage schedule involving repeated drug administration is referred to as a **dosage regimen.** Its components, the loading dose, maintenance doses and dosing intervals, have been described in the preceding paragraphs. Their consideration aids the design of effective clinical drug administration. For example, in attending to two patients with different elimination but identical absorption and distribution rate constants, identical minimum (threshold) plasma concentrations can be maintained if the subject having faster elimination receives the drug more frequently or if his maintenance dose is higher (or both). This is discussed in greater detail in Chapter 6.

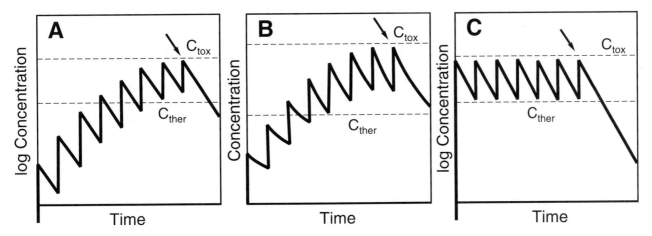

Figure 5-9. Drug concentration following repeated intravenous injections: A. Logarithmic concentration scale. B. Linear concentration scale. C. Repeated injections following a loading dose, logarithmic concentration scale. Arrows indicate cessation of drug administration.

MORE COMPLICATED MODELS

We have considered two kinds of models containing two compartments. In one (Model 2), elimination of the drug starts immediately after administration, even while it gets distributed between the plasma and the peripheral compartments. Thus the two processes take place simultaneously. In the other (Model 3), a drug molecule must be absorbed into the plasma before it can be eliminated from there. The two processes must, therefore, follow each other.

These systems of parallel and consecutive processes (compartments) can of course be extended and also combined with each other. But verification of such models is substantially more difficult mathematically and, especially, experimentally. Usually it is not sufficient to measure drug concentrations in the plasma; samples are required also from the urine and from other parts of the body. Also, the formation of metabolites should be observed.

BIOAVAILABILITY

Definitions

Bioavailability: The percentage of a drug, contained in a drug product, that enters the systemic circulation in an unchanged form after administration of the product. This concept includes not only the amount of drug that enters the body, but also the rate of entry.

Bioequivalence: Comparable bioavailability between related drugs.

Therapeutic equivalence: Comparable clinical effectiveness and safety between similar drugs.

Bioinequivalence: Statistically determined difference in bioavailability between related drugs.

Therapeutic inequivalence: Clinically important difference in bioavailability between similar drugs.

Measurements of Bioavailability

Correlation of drug dose with pharmacological response

This is possible only for drugs with end points that can be readily measured, e.g., anticoagulation by warfarin. It is not a very good measure of bioavailability, since it is also affected by differences in drug–receptor combination and in intrinsic efficacy of the receptor–effector link.

Plasma concentrations

After a **single oral dose** of drug, serial measurements of plasma concentration are obtained. Three parameters of importance are derived from such a procedure (Fig. 5-10):

1. Peak drug concentration
2. Time to peak concentration
3. Area under the concentration–time curve (mg·hours/L) (AUC)

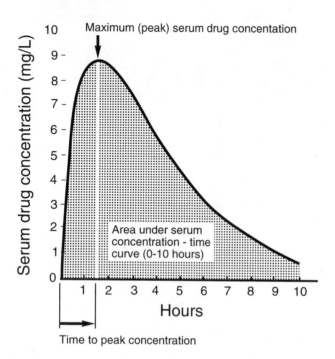

Figure 5-10. Serum concentration–time curve after oral administration of a single dose of a hypothetical drug.

The first two quantities are simple indicators for the **rate** of absorption. An increased rate is suggested by a higher peak concentration and a shorter time required to reach the peak concentration (curve Y in Fig. 5-11A). In contrast, AUC reflects the **extent** of absorption. Consequently, after oral or intramuscular administration of a drug, the bioavailability can be evaluated by comparing the measured AUC with the AUC determined after intravenous injection (i.e., 100% absorption) of the same dose of the drug:

$$\text{Bioavailability} = \frac{\text{AUC (oral)}}{\text{AUC (intravenous)}}$$

Repeated doses of most drugs result in cumulation, and the mean steady-state plasma drug concentrations are a good index of drug bioavailability. Again, it is not the steady-state concentration (C_{ss}) itself, but the ratio of C_{ss} (oral) to C_{ss} (intravenous) that provides the estimate of bioavailability after oral ingestion.

Relative bioavailability

The bioavailability of one orally administered drug (generally a new formulation of an existing drug) is compared with that of an existing reference drug product. It is usually expressed as the ratio of the AUCs for the two preparations.

After the patent of a drug expires, new formulations are often made available. The minimum requirement for the regulatory approval of these so-called "generic" drugs involves a demonstration that their bioavailabilities are identical to that of the original drug (that their relative bioavailability is 1.0, i.e., that they are bioequivalent). In more critical cases, the therapeutic equivalence of the two formulations must be shown.

Urinary excretion

For drugs excreted predominantly unchanged in the urine, bioavailability can be determined by urine collection. For example, consider three formulations of a drug, X, Y, and Z. As shown in Figure 5-11, the cumulative excretion curves reflect the plasma concentration time curves, which in turn reflect the effectiveness of absorption.

Formulations X and Z have the same rate constants of absorption as indicated by the same time to peak concentration. However, Z has a smaller plasma AUC, lower total urinary accumulation, and, consequently, lower bioavailability than preparation X. In contrast, formulations X and Y have identical plasma AUCs and cumulative urinary excretions and, therefore, their bioavailabilities are the same. However, the absorption rate of preparation Y is higher than that of formulation X.

This method cannot be applied to the excretion curves of free drug + total metabolites of a drug that is substantially biotransformed. Any first-pass biotransformation products would appear in the urine, but they should not be included in the estimate of bioavailability because they had never reached the systemic circulation in active form (see First-Pass Effect later in this chapter).

Factors Influencing Bioavailability of Orally Administered Drugs

Formulation of the drug product

As noted in Chapter 1, a drug administered by any route other than intravenous must first dissolve and become available for absorption. Therefore the first important influence upon bioavailability is the formulation of the tablet, capsule, suspension, or solu-

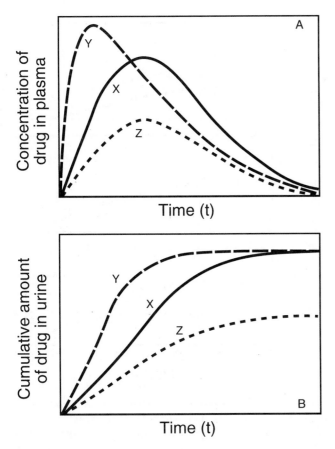

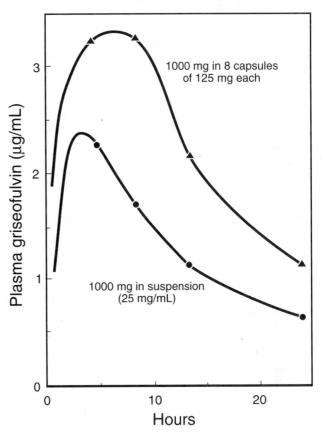

Figure 5-11. Relation between plasma concentration curves (A) and cumulative urinary excretion curves (B) for three different preparations of a drug that is excreted unchanged in the urine. Curve X = slow and complete absorption (100% bioavailability); curve Y = fast and complete absorption (100% bioavailability); curve Z = slow and incomplete absorption (<100% bioavailability).

Figure 5-12. Bioavailability of griseofulvin administered orally to the same subjects as ordinary suspension (lower curve) and as micropulverized form (upper curve).

tion of the drug in the preparation that is taken by the patient.

For many drugs, tablet disintegration time or drug dissolution rate correlates satisfactorily with their bioavailability. Therefore dissolution rates are generally measured and reported. In the case of digoxin, for example, the most rapidly dissolving tablets are equivalent to digoxin solution in bioavailability, but most tablets are less effectively absorbed.

Sometimes bioavailability can be improved drastically by a simple physical change. For example, the antifungal antibiotic griseofulvin is absorbed rather poorly during its passage along the intestine. Grinding it very fine (micropulverization) increases the surface-to-mass ratio, speeding up the dissolution and thus enabling much more of the drug to be absorbed during the intestinal transit (Fig. 5-12).

Interactions With Other Substances in the Gastrointestinal Tract

Gastric absorption of many acidic drugs is increased if the stomach is empty and the pH in the lumen is low. Food will slow gastric emptying, probably raise the pH, and dilute the gastric and small-intestinal contents. Conversely, it is possible to imagine a slowly absorbed drug for which the presence of food could result in more complete absorption. For example, a cationic drug, which would be preferentially absorbed from the small intestine, may be protected from destruction by gastric HCl if mixed with food during its passage through the stomach (see Chapter 2).

Other substances present simultaneously in the intestine may modify the absorption of a drug, as a result of ion neutralization, complex formation, coprecipitation, etc. (see also Chapter 64). For example, mineral oil taken as a laxative can dissolve highly lipid-soluble drugs or vitamins and impair their absorption. In contrast, alcohol weakens the barrier to the passage of iron salts and causes excessive absorption, which may cause disease due to iron-pigment accumulation in the tissues.

Biotransformation in the Intestinal Mucosa or Liver (First-Pass Effect)

The bioavailability of some drugs is low because the drug, after its absorption and transfer to the portal venous blood, is avidly extracted and biotransformed in the liver. Examples of such drugs include hydralazine, lidocaine, organic nitrates, propranolol, morphine, and nortriptyline (see also Chapters 4 and 7).

For some drugs, this can also occur in the intestinal mucosa, immediately after absorption and before the drug can pass into the portal venous blood. This may be an important determinant of the bioavailability of diazepam. The first-pass effect on bioavailability is illustrated in Figure 5-13.

Intramuscular Injection

Skeletal muscle would seem to be a reasonable route for drug administration. However, the bioavailability of intramuscularly administered chlordiazepoxide, digoxin, and phenytoin is variable and low (Fig. 5-13). In part, this is because blood flow through muscle varies greatly according to the muscle chosen for the injection (deltoid > quadriceps femoris > gluteus maximus) and also according to its state of activity (blood flow can be as low as 3 ml/100 g/min at rest, and as high as 30 ml/100 g/min during hard work).

Therapeutic Importance of Bioavailability

Fluctuations and differences in the completeness of absorption can be of major therapeutic importance if a drug exhibits at least one of the following characteristics:

- A given (e.g., twofold) variation in the attained concentration evokes a large change in the response in the therapeutic range (e.g., warfarin).
- The relationship between effect and concentration is clearly nonlinear at the recommended doses (e.g., phenylbutazone, phenytoin, salicylate in high, anti-inflammatory doses).

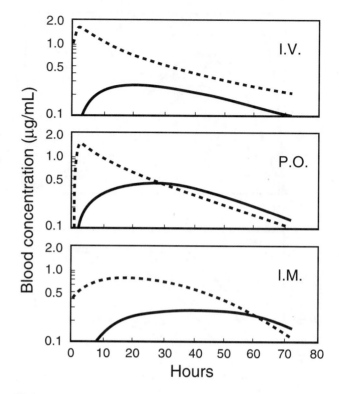

Figure 5-13. Concentration curves of precursor drug (chlordiazepoxide, broken curve) and biotransformation product (desmethylchlordiazepoxide, solid curve) after three different routes of administration. Intravenous injection gives 100% bioavailability; oral administration shows first-pass effect with lower precursor and higher product curves; intramuscular injection gives slow absorption relative to excretion, so both precursor and product curves are lower.

- The difference between concentrations eliciting therapeutic effects and those associated with toxicity is small, resulting in a narrow margin of safety (e.g., digoxin); see Chapter 8.

SUGGESTED READING

Gibaldi M, Perrier D. Pharmacokinetics. 2nd ed. New York: Marcel Dekker, 1982. [More detailed, fairly mathematical.]

Notari RE. Biopharmaceutics and clinical pharmacokinetics. 4th ed. New York: Marcel Dekker, 1987. [An introduction with little mathematics.]

Ritschel WA. Handbook of basic pharmacokinetics—including clinical applications. 4th ed. Hamilton, IL: Drug Intelligence, 1992. [Condensed summary of principles, calculations and clinical implementation.]

CHAPTER 6

Clearance: The Quantitative Basis of Dosage

L. ENDRENYI

TOTAL BODY CLEARANCE

Clearance is a quantitative measure characterizing the rate of removal of endogenous or exogenous substances, including drugs, from the body or from a specific part of the body. Hepatic biotransformation, excretion by the kidneys and bile, exhalation by the lungs, and fecal excretion are the usual routes of drug elimination. The corresponding specific clearances are considered in Chapter 7. Here we will deal with their sum, the total body clearance (TBC), measuring the overall rate of disappearance or elimination of a substance from the whole body.

Clearance is expressed as the volume of body fluid from which a substance (drug) is removed in unit time. Consequently, when concentrations are measured in plasma, the volume of this fluid from which the drug is apparently removed (cleared) in unit time is referred to as the plasma clearance.

In terms of kinetic parameters, i.e., the first-order elimination rate constant (k) and apparent volume of distribution (V), the total body clearance can be expressed as:

$$Cl = kV \quad [\text{mL/min}] = [\text{min}^{-1}] \times [\text{mL}]$$

(Dimensions of the various quantities in this and all following equations are given in square brackets.)

This simple calculation is in agreement with the definition of clearance given above since, as seen in Chapter 5, the rate constant is defined numerically as the fraction of a substance eliminated (cleared) in unit time; its product with the apparent volume of distribution yields the volume from which the drug is apparently removed in unit time.

The volume defined by clearance is often measured by dividing the amount of drug removed in unit time by the concentration of the drug in the relevant body fluid. Usually, however, evaluation of the total body clearance is based on a different kinetic principle. It can be shown that clearance is inversely proportional to the area under a curve (AUC) fitted to concentration readings obtained at different times. If the drug is completely absorbed following its administration, such as after intravenous injection, then

$$Cl = \text{Dose/AUC} \quad [\text{mL/min}] = [\text{mg}]/[(\text{mg/mL}) \times \text{min}]$$

When only a fraction (F) of the dose is absorbed, as is often the case following oral administration, then:

$$Cl = \text{F} \cdot \text{Dose/AUC}$$

For measuring the AUC, the concentrations should be plotted on a linear scale, not a logarithmic one (Fig. 6-1). Also, AUC refers to the complete area under the curve evaluated between the times of zero and infinity following drug administration. Therefore, the curve fitted through the observed values must be extrapolated by an algebraic procedure.

The clearance of drugs is of great importance for kinetic considerations. Its magnitude is independent of modeling assumptions. This is reasonable, since the area under the curve is the same whether we

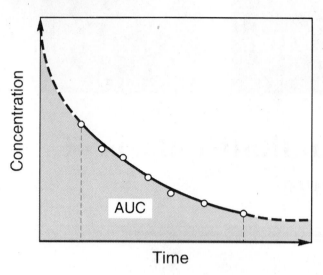

Figure 6-1. Drug concentration in plasma following a single intravenous injection. AUC = area under the curve (shaded). Borders of the experimental range are indicated.

hypothesize the presence of one or two or any number of compartments.

The concept of clearance is biologically meaningful and important. Its study enables pharmacologists to reach conclusions about the effect of hepatic blood flow, renal processes, and protein binding on drug elimination. This is discussed in other chapters.

Furthermore, the steady-state concentration of drugs, which is reached when the rate of intake equals the rate of elimination, is determined by the total body clearance. This question is discussed below in some detail.

DOSAGE FOR INTRAVENOUS INFUSION

Let us consider the rates of input and output processes involving the whole body.

Input could refer to the sum of endogenous production and exogenous intake of a substance. We shall be concerned mainly with the latter. Initially we shall assume that a drug is administered at a constant rate, Q (e.g., by intravenous infusion). The rate is the amount administered per unit time and has units of, say, mg/hr.

The amount of drug in the body at any time is VC, where, as before, V is the apparent volume of distribution and C the concentration in the plasma. The fraction of this amount that is being removed in unit time is given by the elimination rate constant (k). Consequently, the amount eliminated per unit time is kVC.

At steady state, the rate of input is equal to the rate of elimination. Therefore,

$$Q = kVC_{ss}$$

Thus, it is possible to calculate the rate of drug administration (Q) that is required to maintain a desired concentration (C_{ss}).

In terms of clearance,

$$Q = Cl \cdot C_{ss}$$

Consequently, the steady-state concentration is:

$$C_{ss} = Q/Cl \quad [\text{mg/mL}] = [\text{mg/min}]/[\text{mL/min}]$$

This is reasonable since, according to this expression, the steady-state concentration is determined by the ratio of inflow and outflow rates.

(We could consider the analogy of water in a tub [Fig. 6-2] in which both the inflow and outflow faucets are open. The level of water finally attained depends on the rates of both inflow and outflow.)

Since an immediate effect is desired, a **loading dose** of the drug is given by rapid administration (e.g., by injection) to fill the body stores and establish the effective, steady-state plasma concentration. As we have seen, at steady state the amount of drug in the body is VC_{ss}. This is the amount that the loading dose (L) should introduce at once. Consequently,

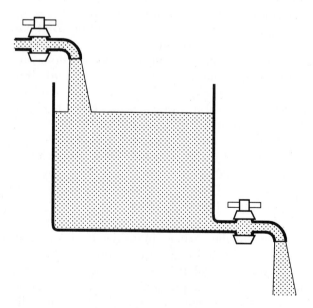

Figure 6-2. Hydrodynamic analogy for drug kinetics: water in the tub.

$$L = VC_{ss} \quad [mg] = [L] \times [mg/L]$$

(The relationships between infusion rate, clearance, and steady-state concentration are used for the convenient evaluation of the clearance. This can be done because the infusion rate is set by the physician or the investigator, and the steady-state concentration can be easily measured. If, in addition, the elimination rate constant or the related half-life is observed, the apparent volume of distribution can also be calculated. This is often the preferred approach.)

Example: lidocaine infusion

Besides being a local anesthetic agent, lidocaine is effective in the treatment of certain cardiac arrhythmias (see Chapter 37). Continuous infusion is indicated in patients in whom the arrhythmia tends to recur and to whom oral therapy cannot be given.

Let us assume the following characteristics of the drug in a 70-kg man:

$C_{ther} = 2.0$ mg/L (therapeutically effective plasma concentration)

$t_{1/2} = 80$ minutes (biological half-life) [where $t_{1/2} = 0.693/k$]

$V_w = 0.70$ L/kg (apparent distribution volume as a proportion of body weight)

Consequently:

$$k = 0.693/80 = 0.0087 \text{ min}^{-1}$$
$$V = 0.70 \text{ [L/kg]} \times 70 \text{ [kg]} = 49 \text{ liters}$$

which indicates that lidocaine is distributed throughout the total body water.

Therefore, the desired infusion rate is:

$$Q = kVC_{ss}$$
$$= 0.0087 \times 49 \times 2.0 = 0.85 \text{ mg/min}$$

Incidentally, the total body clearance is:

$$Cl = kV$$
$$= 0.0087 \times 49 = 0.43 \text{ L/min}$$

The corresponding loading dose is:

$$L = VC_{ss}$$
$$= 49 \times 2.0 = 98 \text{ mg}$$

In practice, a loading dose of 100 mg could be given. The steady-state infusion rate would be about 1 mg/min, and the resulting C_{ss} would be very slightly higher than the target value of 2.0 mg/L.

TIME TO STEADY-STATE CONCENTRATION: PLATEAU PRINCIPLE

Let us assume again that a drug follows first-order kinetics and, for now, that it is administered by continuous intravenous infusion. We have seen that the steady-state concentration (C_{ss}) depends on the rates of both administration and removal of the drug. In contrast, the rate of approach to the steady-state level depends only on the elimination rate constant. Thus, according to the so-called plateau principle, *the time to reach a given fraction of the steady-state concentration is determined only by the elimination rate constant.* In the example of the partially filled tub of Figure 6-2, if a constant level had previously been reached (this could be any level, including an empty tub), and then either of the two faucets is adjusted, the rate at which the new water level is approached depends solely on the setting of the outflow tap.

(The sense of the plateau principle can be appreciated by recalling that the plasma concentration of a drug changes at a rate determined by two simultaneously occurring processes. A constant rate of inflow is assumed by maintaining steady infusion. Thus, the rate of outflow [elimination] completely determines the overall rate of concentration change and, with it, the time course of plasma concentration. The elimination rate, in turn, is defined by the elimination rate constant.)

Envisage five separate infusions of a drug at five different infusion rates $Q5 > Q4 > Q3 > Q2 > Q1$ (Figure 6-3). Since the drug's half-life (or elimination rate constant) does not change, the *time* to reach a plateau will be identical for the five curves. The steady-state *concentration* will depend directly on the corresponding infusion rates.

Attained Fraction of Steady-State Concentration

According to the plateau principle, any fraction of the steady-state concentration depends only on kt, and therefore, the time to reach this fraction depends only on the elimination rate constant, k. The princi-

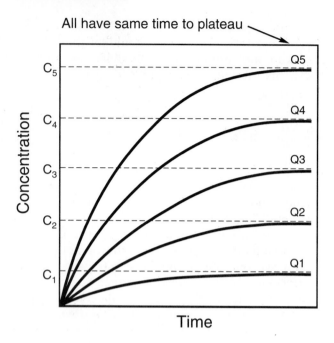

Figure 6-3. Illustration of the plateau principle at five infusion rates ($Q1$ to $Q5$).

ple applies to all shifts from one steady state to another.

The time required to reach a given fraction, $f = 1 - e^{-kt}$, of the steady-state level can be evaluated from the formula, or from the diagram depicting it (Fig. 6-4), or from Table 6-1. The fraction f is called the **fractional attainment.**

From the graph or table, the time to reach 90% of a steady state is $kt = 2.3$.

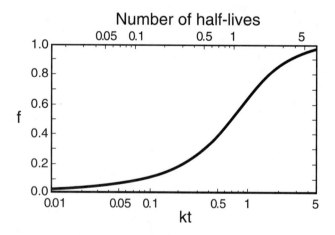

Figure 6-4. Relationship of fractional attainment of the plateau to kt. Recall that $kt = 0.7$ $(t/t_{1/2})$. Consequently, the diagram depicts also the dependence of the fractional attainment on the number of half-lives elapsed.

But
$$k = 0.693/t_{1/2}$$

and therefore:

$$t = 2.3/0.693 \times t_{1/2} = 3.3 \ t_{1/2}$$

Consequently, 90% of the steady-state, plateau concentration is reached during a period of 3.3 half-lives.

Analogous calculations show that:

$$
\begin{aligned}
\text{time to reach 95\% plateau} &= 4.3 \times t_{1/2} \\
\text{99\% plateau} &= 6.6 \times t_{1/2} \\
\text{99.9\% plateau} &= 10.0 \times t_{1/2}
\end{aligned}
$$

For most practical purposes, a useful "rule of thumb" to remember is:

For any drug, time to plateau is roughly 5× half-life.

This approach is quite simplified but nevertheless will give a good ballpark estimate for most drugs.

Two comments should be made at this point about assumptions and applications. First, the plateau principle itself is based on the supposition of first-order kinetics. The quantitative implementation assumes also a single compartment with either intravenous administration or rapid absorption. In spite of these simplifications, the quantitative conclusions can be usefully applied under most practically occurring conditions. Second, the principle and its quantitative consequences can be utilized not only for the simple case of drug infusion but also for other conditions of accumulation and elimination, both in the absence and presence of endogenous substances.

Mathematical Derivation of the Plateau Principle (Optional)

The rate of concentration change is:

$$dC/dt = (\text{rate of drug infusion}) - (\text{rate of drug elimination})$$
$$= (Q/V) - kC$$

Integrating between the initial and the measured plasma concentrations (C_0 and C) observed at times 0 and t, and remembering that the steady-state concentration is:

Table 6-1 Relationship Between the Fractional Attainment *(f)* of New Plateau and *kt* or *t/t$_{1/2}$* *

kt	$t/t_{1/2}$	f	% Fluctuation	f	kt	$t/t_{1/2}$
0.05	0.07	0.049	5.2	0.05	0.05	0.07
0.06	0.09	0.059	6.3	0.10	0.11	0.15
0.08	0.12	0.077	8.3	0.15	0.16	0.23
				0.20	0.22	0.32
0.1	0.14	0.095	10.5	0.25	0.29	0.42
0.2	0.29	0.181	22.1			
0.3	0.43	0.259	35.0	0.30	0.36	0.52
0.4	0.58	0.330	49.3	0.35	0.43	0.62
0.5	0.72	0.394	65.0	0.40	0.51	0.74
0.6	0.87	0.451	82.1	0.45	0.60	0.86
0.8	1.15	0.551	122.7	0.50	0.69	1.00
				0.55	0.80	1.15
1.0	1.44	0.632	172			
1.5	2.16	0.777	348	0.60	0.92	1.32
2.0	2.89	0.865	641	0.65	1.05	1.51
2.5	3.61	0.918	1120	0.70	1.20	1.74
3.0	4.33	0.950	1900	0.75	1.39	2.00
4.0	5.77	0.982	5456	0.80	1.61	2.32
5.0	7.21	0.993	14200	0.85	1.90	2.74
6.0	8.66	0.998				
8.0	11.54	1.000		0.90	2.30	3.32
				0.95	3.00	4.32

$t/t_{1/2}$	kt	f	% Fluctuation	f	kt	$t/t_{1/2}$
				0.98	3.91	5.64
0.5	0.35	0.293	41	0.99	4.61	6.64
1	0.69	0.500	100	0.995	5.30	7.64
2	1.39	0.750	300	0.998	6.21	8.97
3	2.08	0.875	700	0.999	6.91	9.97
4	2.77	0.937	1500			
5	3.47	0.969	3100			
6	4.16	0.984	6300			

% Fluctuation
$$=100(C_{max}-C_{min})/C_{min}$$
$$=100\, f/(1-f)$$

*The relationship displayed in Figure 6–4 is presented here in tabular form. On the left, one can obtain from the number of half-lives $(t/t_{1/2})$ the fractional attainment *(f)* as well as, following repeated injections, the percentage fluctuation of the steady-state concentration. Conversely, on the right, one reads off the number of half-lives required to reach the desired fractional attainment.

$$C_{ss}=Q/kV$$

we obtain the **fractional attainment** *(f)* of the new steady state, defined as

$$f=(C_0-C)/(C_0-C_{ss})=1-e^{-kt}$$

This relationship is shown in Figure 6-4 and listed in Table 6-1.

Note that if we are interested in the time required for complete elimination of the drug, the new C_{ss} = 0 and, therefore, with:

$$f=(C_0-C)/C_0$$

we get again the well-known relationship

$$C=C_0e^{-kt}$$

Thus, the concentration achieved depends on Q and t (k and V are usually constant for a drug in a given person). Note, in addition, that the fraction of the plateau attained (i.e., time to plateau) given by $f = 1-e^{-kt}$ is *independent* of Q.

Application of the Plateau Principle

1. Lidocaine, as mentioned in the example (above) of calculation of loading dose and infusion rate, has a $t_{1/2}$ of 80 min or 1.33 hours. If a continuous infusion was started, it would take $6.6 \times t_{1/2} = 8.8$ hours before plasma concentrations reach 99% of the maximum. This would explain the late appearance of toxicity to the drug.

2. Phenytoin $t_{1/2} = 22$ hours. Time to plateau = 110 hours (by rule of thumb).

3. For drugs administered orally, the same calculations allow us to estimate when a given proportion of maximum cumulation of drug has taken place; e.g., phenytoin by mouth will take 3 days for 90% cumulation.

It will also take this long to eliminate these drugs. Several examples one may wish to think about are tetrahydrocannabinol $t_{1/2} = 50$ hours; diazepam (Valium) $t_{1/2} = 35$ hours; amitriptyline (used in the treatment of depression) $t_{1/2} > 24$ hours; phenobarbital $t_{1/2} = 3.5$ days.

If the dose (or rate of administration) of a drug is changed, the time to reach the new plateau is calculated in exactly the same way as if one started from zero concentration.

DOSAGE REGIMEN FOR REPEATED INTRAVENOUS DRUG ADMINISTRATION

Fluctuation Around Average Steady-State Concentration

The principles described for continuous drug administration apply also to the situation when the drug is given intermittently. The main difference is that now we cannot *exactly* maintain the steady-state concentration. Rather, the concentration will fluctuate around an *average steady-state* value. This average concentration is brought about by the balance of the outflow rate (represented by the clearance) and the average inflow rate.

Consequently, the relationships described earlier remain applicable as long as we consider average concentrations and input rates. When **maintenance doses** of D_m are administered following each **maintenance interval** of T_m, the average rate of drug intake is D_m/T_m. Therefore, the average steady-state concentration is:

$$\overline{C}_{ss} = (D_m/T_m)/Cl$$

Thus, in order to sustain this concentration, a maintenance dose of:

$$D_m = Cl \cdot \overline{C}_{ss} \cdot T_m$$
$$= kV\overline{C}_{ss} \cdot T_m$$

is required.

(Rather incidentally, it can be shown that for the calculation of total body clearance, AUC can be calculated also as the area under the plasma concentration curve segment that is obtained, at steady state, between the administration of consecutive maintenance doses [Fig. 6-5].)

The maintenance dose is proportional to the maintenance interval. This implies that plasma concentrations show larger fluctuation when a drug is administered less frequently (see also Table 6-1).

The proportionality between maintenance dose and maintenance interval raises an important question: How should these two quantities be chosen? The answer will be the result of a compromise between two considerations: the **safety** and the **convenience** of drug administration.

The drug concentration fluctuates around its steady-state average value proportionately to the maintenance dose (Fig. 6-5). Thus, when the maintenance intervals are shortened and the maintenance

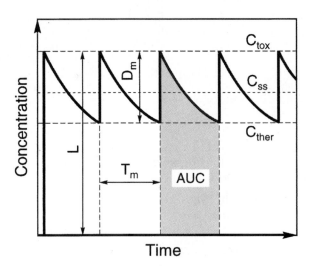

Figure 6-5. Plasma concentration following repeated intravenous injections. L = loading dose; D_m = maintenance dose; T_m = maintenance interval; C_{ther} = therapeutic concentration; C_{tox} = toxic concentration; C_{ss} = steady-state concentration; AUC = area under the curve.

doses are correspondingly reduced, the concentration changes also become smaller. As a result, the safety of drug administration is improved.

However, larger maintenance doses permit longer maintenance intervals, i.e., less frequent administration of the drug. Beyond the obvious convenience, it may increase the probability of a patient's cooperation and compliance with the schedule.

The **maintenance dose** keeps the plasma concentration safely between the minimum therapeutically effective concentration (C_{ther}) and the concentration above which toxic effects would begin (C_{tox}). Therefore:

$$D_m = (C_{tox} - C_{ther})\, V$$

The **maintenance interval** can then be obtained from

$$T_m = D_m/(D_m/T_m)$$

i.e., by dividing the maintenance dose by its ratio to the maintenance interval.

The **loading dose** (L) aims at reaching the maximum of the therapeutic steady-state concentration range immediately following drug administration. Therefore:

$$L = VC_{tox}$$

Two Frequently Applied Dosage Regimens

Two dosing procedures deserve particular consideration; their background is discussed in greater detail in the last section of this chapter. In the first dosing approach, *maintenance intervals equal the half-life* ($T_m = t_{1/2}$). At steady state, the maximum plasma concentration is twice the minimum concentration ($C_{max} = 2C_{min}$); this implies a substantial fluctuation amounting to 100% (see also Table 6-1). It can be demonstrated (cf. last section) that the maximum concentration reached at steady state is twice the maximum concentration obtained after a single drug administration. It follows that *the loading dose should be twice the maintenance dose* ($L = 2D_m$).

The second interesting dosing strategy administers the drug relatively frequently, at maintenance intervals that are less than the half-life of the drug, say, by a factor of at least three ($T_m < t_{1/2}/3$). With this regimen, the plasma concentration at steady state shows only moderate fluctuation. These concentrations are much higher than those seen following a single administration, thereby indicating a substantial accumulation of the drug. As a result, the loading dose should substantially exceed the maintenance dose. Their relationship is approximately given by $L = 1.44\,(t_{1/2}/T_m)D_m$ (see last section).

Practical Dosage Regimens

The calculated ideal maintenance interval should be reduced to a practically manageable value such as 24, 12, 8, 6, or 4 hours, for giving the drug once, or two, three, four, or six times a day. The maintenance dose is adjusted correspondingly. It will be set by taking into account the available dosage forms and the desirability of staying below the toxic and above the minimum therapeutically effective concentration levels (Fig. 6-5).

Thus, drugs that have long half-lives, exceeding 24 hours, will be ingested once daily. Consequently, the dosing interval is less than the half-life, and the initial dose is more than double the maintenance dose.

Drugs having reasonably high safety margins and intermediate half-lives of between 6 and 24 hours could be ingested at intervals approximating their half-lives. Ideally then, the loading dose is twice the maintenance dose. With drugs having a low margin of safety, more frequent administration of lower maintenance doses is required. Occasionally, prolonged-release formulations can be used satisfactorily.

If a drug has a half-life shorter than 6 hours, then it must have a very high safety margin if we wish to consider its repeated administration. The initial dose will equal the maintenance dose. Drugs having a low margin of safety must be administered by continuous infusion.

Example: repeated intravenous administration of aminophylline, a bronchodilator

Let us assume the following characteristics of the drug in a 50-kg, 32-year-old woman:

$C_{ther} = 5$ mg/L (therapeutically effective plasma concentration)

$C_{tox} = 20$ mg/L (toxic plasma concentration)

$\overline{C}_{ss} = 10$ mg/L (approximate average steady-state plasma concentration)

$t_{1/2} = 4.5$ hours (biological half-life)
$V_w = 0.56$ L/kg (apparent distribution volume relative to body weight)

Consequently:

$$k = 0.693/4.5 = 0.154 \text{ hr}^{-1}$$
$$V = 0.56 \times 50 = 28 \text{ liters}$$

Therefore, to get a ballpark figure, the desired approximate rate of drug administration is

$$D_m/T_m = kV\overline{C}_{ss}$$
$$= 0.154 \times 28 \times 10 = 43.1 \text{ mg/hr}$$

where the total body clearance is

$$Cl = kV = 0.154 \times 28 = 4.31 \text{ L/hr}$$
$$= 4.31 \times 1000/60 = 72 \text{ mL/min}$$

The maintenance dose is

$$D_m = (C_{tox} - C_{ther}) V$$
$$= (20 - 5) \times 28 = 420 \text{ mg}$$

The maintenance interval is then evaluated from

$$T_m = D_m/(D_m/T_m)$$
$$= 420/43.1 = 9.7 \text{ hours}$$

Finally, the loading dose is

$$L = VC_{tox}$$
$$= 28 \times 20 = 560 \text{ mg}$$

For a **practical dosing** schedule, the maintenance interval should be lowered from 9.7 hours. If we choose 8 hours, then the maintenance dose would be approximately:

$$D_m \simeq 420 \times (8/9.7) = 346 \text{ mg}$$

However, in this example, preparations for intravenous administration are available in either 250- or 500-mg forms. Therefore, we should consider a maintenance interval of

$$T_m = 6 \text{ hours}$$

This would lead to an approximate maintenance dose of

$$D_m = 420 \times (6/9.7) = 260 \text{ mg}$$

which is close to the actually available dose of:

$$D_m = 250 \text{ mg}$$

The loading dose, establishing immediately the steady-state levels, is

$$L = VC_{max}$$
$$= 28 \times 14.8 = 414 \text{ mg}$$

In practice, therefore, a loading dose of 500 mg would be given. (This yields an initial maximum concentration of 500/28 = 17.9 mg/L, still below the minimum toxic level.) This would be followed by the administration, four times a day, of 250 mg of the drug in 10 mL diluent, which is injected over a 10-minute period.

Note that we have ended up with a dosage schedule in which the maintenance interval (6 hours) was somewhat higher but fairly close to the half-life of the drug (4.5 hours). As a result, the plasma concentration was expected to show over two-fold fluctuation. The loading dose (500 mg) was twice the maintenance dose (250 mg).

REPEATED ORAL ADMINISTRATION

The expressions evaluating dosage regimens for repeated oral administration are almost the same as those discussed for repeated intravenous injections when these aim at reaching an *average* steady-state concentration. The only difference is that for oral administration, *all dosing equations must be multiplied on the right-hand side by the bioavailability (F)*, i.e., by the fraction of a drug dose reaching the systemic circulation.

If we aim again at remaining between the therapeutic and toxic concentration levels, the exact formulae for calculating dosage regimens for repeated oral administration are more complicated and require kinetic information about the relative rates of absorption and elimination.

Fortunately, in many cases it is quite sufficient to apply the expressions given for repeated intravenous administration, since the resulting loading dose and also the maintenance interval and maintenance dose are generally conservative. Indeed, we may recall the following pharmacokinetic observations:

If equivalent doses of a drug are given to a person

by a single intravenous and oral administration, the maximal concentration (C_{max}) attained by the oral route is lower and the time taken to get down to the minimum therapeutically effective concentration (C_{ther}) is usually longer. The latter statement is equivalent to saying that, from about the time of reaching C_{max} by the oral route, the corresponding concentration remains higher than that seen following the equivalent intravenous administration.

These principles are valid also for the case of repeated drug administration. Consequently, because the oral C_{max} is lower and the C_{min} is higher than the equivalent quantities calculated for repeated intravenous dosing, we maintain the plasma concentration safely within the desirable range between C_{tox} and C_{ther}.

In the case of oral administration, all dosing equations must be again multiplied on the right-hand side by the bioavailability (F). This is the reason for talking about "equivalent doses" for the two routes of drug administration.

ACCUMULATION RATIO (OPTIONAL)

The fractional attainment (f) of steady state during the elimination phase provides insight into the degree of accumulation.

Recalling that the loading dose is, for repeated intravenous injections,

$$L = VC_{max}, \text{ where } C_{max} = D_m/(Vf)$$

we get

$$L/D_m = C_{max}/C_0 = 1/f = 1/(1 - e^{-kT_m})$$

Here $C_0 = D_m/V$ is the (extrapolated) initial concentration after a single administration of a dose of D_m.

The ratio of C_{max}/C_0 contrasts the maximum concentrations obtained by repeated and single injections of the same dose, respectively. Therefore, $1/f$ is called the **accumulation ratio.** It characterizes also the ratios of minimum concentrations for repeated and single administrations that are observed at times T_m following the respective maxima.

A good approximation for the accumulation ratio can be obtained by noting that

$$C_{max} \simeq \overline{C}_{ss} + (1/2) \ (D_m/V) = \overline{C}_{ss} + C_0/2$$

Since

$$\overline{C}_{ss} = (D_m/T_m)/kV = C_0/kT_m$$

we have

$$\overline{C}_{ss}/C_0 = 1/kT_m = (1/\ln2)(t_{1/2}/T_m) \simeq 1.44(t_{1/2}/T_m)$$

and

$$C_{max}/C_0 = 1/f \simeq 1.44(t_{1/2}/T_m) + 0.5$$

Similarly, for the minimum concentration:

$$C_{min}/C_0 \simeq \overline{C}_{ss} - C_0/2 \simeq 1.44(t_{1/2}/T_m) - 0.5$$

Note that all three ratios can be approximated by

$$C/C_0 \simeq 1.5(t_{1/2}/T_m)$$

when the drug is given frequently, i.e., when $t_{1/2} > T_m$. (A rule of thumb for this condition should be: $t_{1/2} > 3T_m$.) This is a useful, simple calculating formula.

With frequent dosing, the expressions characterize also the relationship between the loading and maintenance doses since, as we have seen:

$$L/D_m = C_{max}/C_0$$

The exact ratios of C_{max}, $\overline{C}_{ss}$, and C_{min} to C_0 are shown in Figure 6-6. The diagram illustrates also

$$C_{max}/C_{min} = e^{kT_m} = 1/(1 - f)$$

which measures the fluctuation of plasma concentration upon repeated drug administration. The following conclusions are worth noting:

1. In the special case of $T_m = t_{1/2}$, i.e., when the maintenance interval equals the half-life, the accumulation ratio is 2. Consequently,

$$C_{max} = 2C_0$$
$$L = 2D_m$$
$$C_{max}/C_{min} = 2$$

Thus, the maximal concentration reached upon repeated drug administration is double that attained by a single injection. Also, we can observe, under this condition, a twofold fluctuation of the concentration.

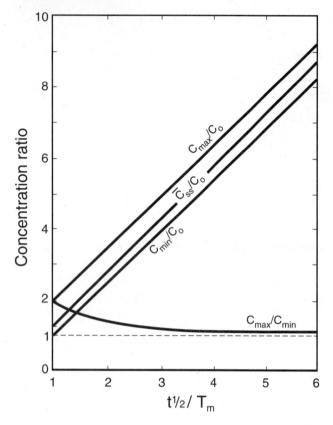

Figure 6-6. Concentration ratios characterizing repeated drug administration. (See text for explanation.)

2. The accumulation ratio increases and the fluctuation decreases with smaller T_m, i.e., when the drug is administered more frequently.

3. In particular, when T_m is very small, the accumulation ratio becomes very large. For instance, we can consider continuous exposure to chemicals in the environment. Even though their intake during a limited period (say, a day) is small, their accumulation could be very substantial.

SUGGESTED READING

Gibaldi M. Biopharmacokinetics and clinical pharmacokinetics. 4th ed. Philadelphia: Lea & Febiger, 1991.

Greenblatt DJ, Shader RI. Pharmacokinetics in clinical practice. Philadelphia: WB Saunders, 1985.

Rowland M, Tozer TN. Clinical pharmacokinetics: concepts and applications. 3rd ed. Philadelphia: Lea & Febiger, 1995.

CHAPTER 7

Drug Clearance by Specific Organs

L. ENDRENYI

ADDITIVITY OF ORGAN CLEARANCES

In Chapter 6, *total body clearance* was defined as the volume of body fluid (usually blood) from which the drug has been completely removed in a unit time. *Clearance by an individual organ* (e.g., the liver or kidney) *refers to the volume of body fluid from which that organ completely removes the drug in a unit of time.*

The total *amount* of a drug eliminated from the body is the sum of the amounts eliminated by the various routes. Correspondingly, the overall *rate* of elimination is the sum of the specific rates of elimination of the drug through the various routes. (This is so since the rate of elimination is the amount of a drug removed in unit time.) For first-order processes, the respective specific organ clearances are also additive and sum up to the total body clearance (*Cl* or TBC, see Chapter 6). This can be seen from the additivity of the corresponding elimination rate constants. The clearances can be thought of as products of the apparent volume of distribution and the respective rate constants.

As an example, consider a drug eliminated in part by hepatic (H) biotransformation and in part by renal (R) excretion. Then, the total amount of the eliminated drug can be considered as a sum of its components:

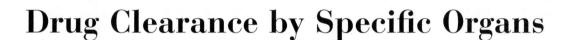

Amount eliminated = amount transformed in the liver + amount excreted by the kidney

The overall rate of elimination can be regarded in the same way:

Rate of elimination = rate of hepatic transformation + rate of renal excretion

Since first-order rate constants are additive, the hepatic and renal constants sum to the elimination constant:

$$k = k_H + k_R$$

The corresponding clearances are obtained by multiplying both sides of this expression by V (the apparent volume of distribution):

$$kV = k_H V + k_R V$$

Consequently the equation:

$$Cl = Cl_H + Cl_R$$

illustrates the additivity of the organ clearances.

In the following sections, drug elimination by various organs, and the corresponding clearances, will be considered briefly.

Organ clearance can also be obtained by *dividing the amount of a drug removed by the organ during a unit time by the concentration of the drug entering the organ.* This second definition is demonstrated below under Perfusion Model.

CLEARANCE BY THE LIVER

Perfusion Model

Consider an organ such as the liver, into which the drug enters at an arterial concentration of C_a, and from which it goes out at a smaller venous concentration of C_v (Fig. 7-1). The blood flow through the organ is Q mL/min. Then, at steady state during 1 minute:

$$\text{Amount of drug entering the organ} = Q \cdot C_a$$
$$\text{amount of drug leaving the organ} = Q \cdot C_v$$
$$\text{amount of drug removed in the organ} = Q \cdot (C_a - C_v)$$

The fraction of drug removed or extracted by the organ from the blood is $(C_a - C_v)/C_a$. This fraction is called the (steady-state) **extraction ratio** *(E)*, which characterizes the effectiveness of the process of removing the drug:

$$E = (C_a - C_v)/C_a$$

A value close to 1 (unity) suggests that most of the drug is quickly and efficiently cleared by the organ; a small extraction ratio, approaching 0, indicates a slow, ineffective process of removal by that organ.

If the blood flow (Q) is multiplied by the fraction (E) of drug extracted by the organ, one should obtain the volume of blood from which the organ removes the drug in unit time. This is the organ clearance as defined earlier. As an example, the hepatic clearance is

$$Cl_H = Q \cdot E$$

In the liver: Q = total hepatic blood flow; C_a = mixed portal venous and hepatic arterial drug con-

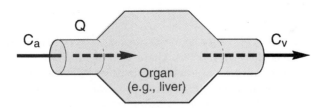

Figure 7-1. Model for organ clearance of drugs. As applied to the liver: Q = total hepatic blood flow; C_a = mixed portal venous and hepatic arterial drug concentration; C_v = hepatic venous drug concentration (see text).

centrations; C_v = hepatic venous drug concentration. Notice that hepatic clearance can be written as

$$Cl_H = Q \cdot (C_a - C_v)/C_a$$

The numerator is the amount of drug cleared by the liver from the blood in 1 minute. This is divided by the concentration of the drug entering the organ. When expressed thus, the clearance is indeed calculated by following the second definition given in the previous section.

For an effectively extracted drug $(E = 1)$, the hepatic clearance approaches the blood flow $(Cl_H \approx Q)$. The liver is admirably set up for extracting large amounts of drugs because of its large size (1500 g), high blood flow (approximately 1 mL/g tissue/min), and unique architecture that brings blood into contact with many cell surfaces. It follows that the hepatic clearance of highly extracted drugs approaches 1500 mL/min. Conversely, low extraction is indicated by hepatic clearance much below 1500 mL/min.

First-Pass Effect

Following oral intake of a drug, only a fraction (F) of the administered amount may reach the systemic circulation. Losses may occur by decomposition or by biotransformation in the gastrointestinal lumen. From there, the drug passes across the membranes of the gastrointestinal tract into the portal vein, then through the liver, and finally into the general circulation. During this so-called first pass, enzymes may transform some of the drug either in the membranes and cells of the gut wall, or in the liver, or perhaps in both locations. For instance, lidocaine is extensively extracted by the liver, while salicylamide undergoes extraction and biotransformation in both intestinal wall and liver.

A substantial loss of a drug can be expected during its first pass through the liver if its hepatic biotransformation is fast and efficient, i.e., if its hepatic extraction ratio is high. Generally, the availability after first passage through the liver can be obtained from:

$$F_H = 1 - E$$

For example, the hepatic extraction ratio of lidocaine, an antiarrhythmic drug, is 0.7. Consequently, the oral bioavailability of the drug is only 30%. This is an upper limit for the oral bioavailability of the drug, since losses during the first pass of the drug can occur not only by hepatic biotransformation but also by other processes. This is one reason for administering the drug by intravenous injection or infusion.

There are a number of **important properties of first-pass drug extraction:**

- It is drug-specific, ranging from zero to complete removal.
- The first-pass effect is often saturable.
- For some drugs it is so effective that at low doses no drug may reach the systemic circulation.
- In liver disease, drugs with high first-pass extraction will become available systemically in higher-than-expected concentrations. This can happen as a result either of impaired function of liver parenchymal cells, or of intrahepatic shunts bypassing the sinusoid and carrying blood directly from the hepatic artery and portal vein to the terminal hepatic vein. Therefore, the drug dose may need to be decreased to prevent toxicity.
- Pharmacological effects may be markedly different after intravenous than after oral administration. For instance, if it is a drug metabolite that is active, oral administration of the drug may be more effective (or toxic) than intravenous injection of the same dose, provided that the biotransformation occurs in the liver.
- Low systemic bioavailability often (but not always) indicates a first-pass effect.
- Complex and unpredictable drug kinetics can be expected as a consequence of the first-pass effect, depending on the relative contribution of intestinal or hepatic binding and/or biotransformation to the phenomenon.

Factors Affecting Hepatic Clearance

Two main factors contribute to the efficiency of hepatic drug clearance:

1. The amount extracted by the liver is expected to increase along with the blood supply, i.e., when the **blood flow** (Q) is higher.

2. Transformation in the liver is assisted when the molecular relationships and conditions in that organ are favorable to biotransformation. These conditions can be characterized by a parameter that is called the **intrinsic clearance of the free (unbound) drug** ($Cl_{intr,f}$). The intrinsic clearance increases together with (1) a larger concentration and amount of the catalyzing enzyme in the liver and (2)

a larger affinity between the drug molecule and the enzyme.

If one of the two components, blood flow or intrinsic clearance, is much smaller than the other, then it has controlling influence on the extraction ratio and, therefore, on the hepatic clearance. For instance, if the intrinsic clearance is much lower than the blood flow ($Cl_{intr,f} << Q$), the blood supply is quite ample and its change would, in practice, not affect the hepatic extraction. Alteration of the intrinsic clearance, however, directly modifies the hepatic clearance in such cases. (Low intrinsic clearance can be a consequence of a drug entering the hepatic cells relatively slowly, by simple diffusion. Drugs with low intrinsic clearance include antipyrine and the anticoagulant warfarin.)

In the reverse condition, if the intrinsic clearance substantially exceeds the blood flow ($Cl_{intr,f} >> Q$), the available enzymic activity is relatively in excess and does not limit the overall rate of biotransformation. Hepatic clearance is dependent now on blood flow; a change in the blood flow causes a corresponding alteration of the clearance. (Drugs having high intrinsic clearance are often concentrated in the hepatocytes and thereby allow the enzymatic reactions to be carried out efficiently. Examples of drugs with high intrinsic clearance include acetylsalicylic acid, morphine, and propranolol.)

For drugs exhibiting a low extraction ratio, the hepatic clearance is modified by various factors that affect the intrinsic clearance of the free drug. These factors include:

- The binding of a drug to plasma proteins and other constituents in the blood. Binding reduces the concentration of the free drug and its intrinsic clearance.
- Conditions modifying the activity of the catalyzing enzyme. Inhibitors reduce, and enzyme inducers increase, this activity.

These factors lose importance for drugs having a high intrinsic clearance. In fact, binding to plasma proteins may have, to some extent, an opposite effect. Since proteins efficiently carry the drug molecules within the circulation, binding to them may actually facilitate clearance. Drugs with high intrinsic clearance show a substantial first-pass effect.

Table 7-1 summarizes factors involved in, and influencing, the hepatic clearance of high- and low-extraction drugs.

Table 7-1 Features of, and Representative Drugs with, High and Low Hepatic Extraction

High Extraction	Low Extraction
Hepatic clearance controlled by rate of blood flow	Hepatic clearance controlled by intrinsic clearance (hepatic biotransformation processes)
Strong first-pass effect	Biotransformation limited by diffusion
Plasma protein binding may facilitate clearance	Plasma protein binding reduces clearance
	Sensitive to enzyme inhibition, induction
Amitriptyline, imipramine	Antipyrine
Chlorpromazine	Diazepam
L-Dopa	Digitoxin
Lidocaine	Phenylbutazone
Morphine, methadone, heroin	Phenytoin
Propoxyphene	Theophylline
Propranolol, alprenolol	Tolbutamide
Tyramine	Warfarin

CLEARANCE BY THE KIDNEY

Urinary excretion is a major route for the elimination of many drugs from the body. Generally, the kidney efficiently removes polar (hydrophilic) substances, but not lipophilic drugs. Consequently, before being excreted, many of these drugs undergo either conjugation or hydroxylation reactions that yield more polar products (see Chapter 4).

The functional anatomical units of the kidney are the nephrons (see also Chapter 41). Arterial blood passes first through the glomerulus, which filters some of the plasma water and its contents. Many, but not all, substances are also secreted in the proximal tubules. Most of the water is reabsorbed all along the nephron, in sequence, from the proximal, distal, and collecting tubules. Consequently, only 1–2 mL/min of the filtered water remains in the form of urine for elimination. Many, but not all, solutes can also be reabsorbed by the tubular epithelium and passed into the renal interstitial fluid, and from there back into the plasma.

Thus, renal excretion of drugs is the result of three processes: glomerular filtration, tubular secretion, and tubular reabsorption. Therefore:

Rate of renal excretion = rate of filtration +
rate of secretion − rate of reabsorption

The renal clearance of a substance can be calculated, in accordance with the definition given earlier, by measuring the amount excreted during a time period and dividing it by the length of the period and by the average plasma concentration observed during this interval:

$$Cl_R = \frac{\text{excreted amount/time interval}}{\text{mean plasma concentration}}$$

Similarly to the rate of excretion, the clearance can be subdivided into components representing filtration, secretion, and reabsorption.

Glomerular Filtration

Glomerular filtration is limited by the size of the pores in the capillary endothelium and the ultrafiltration membrane (400–600 Å diameter). Thus, only small molecules are filtered by the glomeruli into the tubular fluid. Large macromolecules, including most proteins, cannot pass through the filter. Consequently, only free drugs, not bound to plasma proteins, can be filtered. Farther down the tubule, most of the filtered water is reabsorbed, together with variable amounts of free drug, which would reassociate with proteins. The end result is that the binding equilibrium remains almost unchanged.

The filtration process is *passive* (i.e., it proceeds *in the direction of the concentration gradient*) and relatively slow; it is limited by the rate of diffusion to and across the filter. Plasma water is filtered at a rate of about 120 mL/min. This is called the glomerular filtration rate (GFR). Inulin, an exogenous polysaccharide, and creatinine, an endogenous N-containing substance, do not bind to plasma proteins and do not undergo tubular secretion or reabsorption to any significant degree. Therefore, they are widely used as indicators of the GFR. An observed inulin or creatinine clearance of substantially less than 120 mL/min suggests impairment of renal glomerular function.

The GFR of about 120 mL/min is also used as a marker of excretion processes in healthy subjects. A renal clearance in excess of 120 mL/min points to tubular secretion of a substance in addition to its glomerular filtration. A renal clearance less than 120 mL/min indicates net tubular reabsorption (following, or in addition to, filtration and secretion).

Tubular Secretion

The cells of the proximal convoluted tubules *actively transport* certain substances from the plasma to the tubular urine. The transfer of drugs occurs here *against the concentration gradient:* The drugs become relatively concentrated within the tubular lumen.

Active transport processes are characterized by:

1. Energy requirement. They do not occur if the cell metabolism is impaired. Uncouplers of oxidative phosphorylation, such as dinitrophenol, which inhibit the synthesis of ATP by the cell, block active transport.

2. Saturation kinetics. In most cases the process can be described by simple Michaelis-Menten–type kinetics in which the combination of the molecule to be transported (D) and the carrier system (C) occurs first: CD is translocated and dissociation occurs afterward. As in enzymatic reactions, the carrier system recognizes the transported molecules in a stereospecific fashion. When all the carrier molecules are in the CD form, maximal velocity of transport, called T_m, is attained. Since the cell membrane contains limited amounts of carrier molecules, in the presence of two substances $(D_1$ and $D_2)$ transported by the same carrier, D_1 acts as an inhibitor of the transport of D_2 and vice versa. In general, the more slowly a substance is transported (i.e., the longer it occupies the carrier), the more effectively this substance inhibits the transport of another one.

Active tubular secretion is a relatively fast process that clears practically all of the drug, bound to plasma proteins or free, from the blood. Actually only the unbound drug is transported across the tubular epithelium. However, as the free drug is removed from the plasma, its equilibrium with the protein-bound entity is disturbed, and the complex dissociates, replacing some of the unbound substance. The result is the apparent (but not physically simultaneous) removal of nearly all of the drug during the passage of the blood along the peritubular capillaries.

There are at least two transport mechanisms, one for acidic, the other for basic substances (Table 7-2). It is the ionized molecules that are transported.

Para-aminohippuric acid (PAH), an exogenous organic acid, is virtually completely filtered and secreted, but not reabsorbed. Since, following inges-

Table 7-2 Examples of Drugs and Drug Metabolites That Are Actively Secreted into the Renal Tubules

Acids	Bases
Penicillin	Quaternary ammonium
Chlorothiazide	compounds
Salicylic acid	(e.g., choline, tetraethyl-
Phenolsulfonphthalein	ammonium, *N*-methyl-
Diodone (urographic	nicotine, *N*-methylnico-
medium)	tinamide)
Carinamide	Guanidine derivatives
Probenecid	Tolazoline
Cinchophen	Quinine
p-Aminohippuric acid and	Mepiperphenodol
other glycine conjugates	
Glucuronic acid conjugates	
Sulfuric acid conjugates	

tion, it is located in the plasma (partially bound to proteins), its renal excretion provides a measure of renal plasma flow. Typically it is around 600 mL/min.

Tubular Reabsorption

The importance of renal tubular reabsorption of organic substances as a homeostatic process is clear when one considers that most nutrients and vitamins present in plasma gain access to the glomerular filtrate. Consider, for example, the case of glucose. Under normal conditions virtually all the glucose filtered is reabsorbed, so no glucose appears in the urine unless the capacity of the transporting mechanisms is exceeded, as occurs in the advanced diabetic state or after large infusions of glucose. The fact that glucose, an uncharged substance, is reabsorbed into the blood against a large concentration gradient (tubular fluid:plasma) indicates that an **active transport process** is responsible for the absorption.

Not all the reabsorption of organic molecules is accomplished by active transport processes. Many compounds undergo **passive reabsorption**. These substances leave the filtrate to enter the tubular cells and should be able to leave the cell again, in the direction of the blood. Thus, at least two lipidic cell membranes have to be crossed. As described in Chapter 2, lipid-soluble substances are able to cross cell membranes and are thus passively reabsorbed. Charged molecules, in general, are not able to cross the tubular epithelial cell membranes and are thus excreted in the urine. (Note, however, that this does not mean that all uncharged molecules will be reabsorbed. Molecules such as sucrose, that are not charged but are not lipid-soluble either, are not passively reabsorbed.)

Factors that have to be considered in the passive reabsorption of substances from the tubular filtrate are the volume of the filtrate formed per minute (and thus the rate of movement down the tubule and the degree of probability of contact with the membrane) and, most importantly from the clinical point of view, the pH of tubular fluid. Acidification of urine by different means results in a greater proportion of an acidic molecule A^- being in the uncharged HA form, thus increasing its passive reabsorption at the tubular level. The reverse will occur for basic molecules, which in an acid medium will tend to shift to the BH^+ (charged) form. The pK_a of the substance (i.e., the pH of the aqueous phase at which the numbers of ionized and nonionized molecules are equal) will of course determine the relative proportions of the charged and uncharged forms at any pH. Changes in the pH of the tubular fluid are known to affect markedly the urinary excretion of phenobarbital and salicylate (Table 7-3). Some types of diuretics will render the filtrate acid or alkaline (see Chapter 41). For a large variety of drugs, conjugation with strong acids occurs in the liver. Conjugates that are strong acids, such as glucuronic acid conjugates and sulfuric acid conjugates, will remain dissociated at most physiological pHs attained in the kidney and are therefore readily excreted in the urine.

Competitive Inhibition of Renal Tubular Transport

Some drugs act by interfering with the active transport of other drugs or endogenous substances. For example, **probenecid** competes with penicillin for active secretion by the tubular acid secretion system, thus lengthening the half-life of penicillin and raising its plasma concentration (see Chapter 53). Sulfinpyrazone competitively inhibits the active reabsorption of uric acid and thus increases its elimination from the body (see Chapter 34). In other instances, adverse drug reactions can occur as a result of unintended interactions at the renal transport systems (see Chapter 64).

BILIARY EXCRETION

The biliary excretion of substances involves two steps: (1) their transfer from the plasma across the hepatic cell membrane into parenchymal cells of the liver and (2) their active transport across the membrane separating the liver cell from the bile canaliculus. After transient storage in the gallbladder, the compounds enter the small intestine. From here, they are either excreted into the feces or reabsorbed into the portal circulation. In the latter case, by returning to the plasma, they complete the **enterohepatic cycle**, which can substantially extend the duration of their presence in the body.

The active secretion of drugs into the bile takes place against a concentration gradient and results in the elevation of their biliary concentration. As in the kidney, acids and bases have separate transport systems: Two substances transferred by the same system can inhibit each other's secretion.

The biliary clearance can be calculated by dividing the amount excreted in unit time by the plasma concentration. The amount excreted in unit time is the product of the concentration in bile and of the bile flow. Hence:

$$Cl_B = \frac{\text{concentration in bile}}{\text{concentration in plasma}} \times \text{bile flow}$$

The bile flow is typically 0.5–0.8 mL/min. Consequently, biliary clearance is sizeable only when the drug concentration in the bile is much higher than that in plasma. For example, with a concentration ratio of 1000, the biliary clearance is about 500–800 mL/min.

Generally, polar compounds are able to undergo

Table 7-3 Effect of Degree of Ionization on Rate of Urinary Excretion of Drugs

Drug	pK_a	Urinary Clearance Ratios*	
		Acid Urine	Alkaline Urine
Basic drugs		*(more ionized)*	*(less ionized)*
Quinacrine	7.7	3.0	0.5
Procaine	8.95	2.25	0.25
Mecamylamine	11.2	4.6	0.06
Acidic drugs		*(less ionized)*	*(more ionized)*
Phenobarbital	7.4	0.1	0.7
Salicylate	3.0	0.02	1.6

*Clearance ratios are equal to $\frac{\text{Clearance of substance}}{\text{Clearance of inulin}}$.
Ratios greater than 1 imply net tubular secretion; ratios less than 1 imply net reabsorption.

biliary excretion. Often, such substances are formed in the liver when a drug is transformed to a polar conjugate such as a glucuronide, glycine, or sulfate conjugate. A substantial fraction of the conjugates can be hydrolyzed again to re-form the original drug when reaching the gut, thus allowing it to be reabsorbed under certain conditions.

Another limitation on substances undergoing biliary excretion involves their size. Only those having molecular weights of at least 250 Da appear in the bile. The explanation for this phenomenon is not well understood.

SUGGESTED READING

Bekersky I. Renal excretion. J Clin Pharmacol 1987; 27:447–449.

Morgan DJ, Smallwood RA. Clinical significance of pharmacokinetic models of hepatic elimination. Clin Phamacokinet 1990; 18:61–76.

Plaa GL. The enterohepatic circulation. In: Gillette JR, Mitchell JR, eds. Handbook of experimental pharmacology. Vol. 28. Berlin: Springer-Verlag, 1975:130.

Rowland M, Benet LZ, Graham GG. Clearance concepts in pharmacokinetics. J Pharmacokinet Biopharm 1973; 1:123–136.

Rowland M, Tozer T. Clinical pharmacokinetics: concepts and applications. 3rd ed. Philadelphia: Lea & Febiger, 1995.

Wilkinson GR, Shand DG. A physiological approach to drug clearance. Clin Pharmacol Ther 1975; 18:377–390.

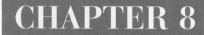

CHAPTER 8

Dose–Response Relationships

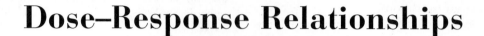

L. ENDRENYI

LOG-DOSE–RESPONSE CURVES

A central question of drug therapy is, "What is the proper dose of a drug that will produce the desired therapeutic action without harmful side effects?" To answer this question, an analysis of the relationship between dose and response is required.

It is customary to contrast these quantities (doses and responses) in diagrams that plot the effect of the drug against the logarithm of the corresponding dose. These diagrams yield **log-dose–response (LDR) curves.**

For example, raising doses of histamine causes gradually increasing contraction of the guinea pig ileum. Very low doses of histamine have practically no effect, and responses can be observed only beyond a threshold dose of about 20 ng. Very high doses of more than about 50 μg have no additional effect and the response remains constant at this maximal ($\geq$ 50 μg) level (Fig. 8-1).

The effect of using a logarithmic dose scale is very important. First, notice that in the example of the histamine response, the horizontal dose scale is indeed logarithmic since the distances between 1 and 10 μg, or 10 and 100 μg are identical. Second, Figure 8-1 indicates that there are only small differences between the responses that are produced by doses of, for instance, 1.0 and 1.1 or even 1.5 μg histamine. The physician is often concerned too much about such minute differences. Rather, one should want to know what the effects are of double, fivefold, tenfold dosages.

PROPERTIES OF LOG-DOSE–RESPONSE CURVES

1. These curves describe the LDR relationship over a wide range of doses.

2. LDR curves are typically S-shaped or "sigmoidal." Their middle section is approximately straight; this facilitates their statistical analysis. This property is used to good advantage in the analysis of bioassays when drug concentrations (doses) are evaluated from the corresponding responses observed in biological samples.

3. Frequently the same effect is produced by different drugs acting with an identical, or at least similar, mechanism. In such cases the LDR curves of the drugs may be expected to run parallel to each other. For example, let us assume that drug A is twice as potent as drug B. Then, in comparison with A, twice as much B is needed to produce some given, identical response. This is true throughout the full range of concentrations. Consequently, in a plot contrasting a response with the corresponding dose, points on the curve characterizing drug B will always lie the same distance to the right of the curve for drug A (Fig. 8-2).

Furthermore, at a given height (i.e., response) of the plot, the dose of drug B will be twice as large as that of drug A (see Fig. 8-2B). In a plot having a linear dose scale (when 20-, 40-, 60-, and 80-mg/kg doses are spaced with equal distance), the response curves for the two drugs are not parallel (see Fig. 2A). In contrast, in the LDR plot (with the logarithmic dose scale) the distance between the curves is constant and equals log 2 = 0.30. Thus, curves of similarly acting drugs are expected to be parallel in the LDR plot.

COMPARISON OF DOSE-RESPONSE CURVES

The strengths of drugs A and B, in the example above, can be compared quantitatively. In this example, when the potency of drug A is double the potency of drug B, we would say that the **relative potency** of drug A with respect to drug B is $R = 2.0$. Of course, this can be stated in other ways, e.g., that drug B is only one-half as potent as drug A, or that the relative potency of drug B with respect to drug A is $R = 0.50$.

In general, if different drugs have parallel LDR curves (as when they act by identical mechanisms), the relative potencies can be evaluated from their horizontal distances. The horizontal concentration scale is logarithmic and therefore the horizontal distance between two curves equals the corresponding value of log R.

Relative potencies are customary measures for comparing relative strengths of different drugs or drug preparations. Their use implies parallelism of LDR curves. In contrast, parallelism is not assumed when the strengths of drugs are compared on the basis of their **equieffective doses**. These are doses of the investigated drugs that give rise to the same magnitude of the designated response. For instance, in Figure 8-2, 20 mg/kg of drug A and 40 mg/kg of drug B are equieffective doses.

AN INTERPRETATION OF THE LDR CURVE: RECEPTOR OCCUPANCY

According to the most common theory of drug action, the drug molecules must attach themselves to receptors in the body before these initiate the process of response (see Chapter 9). Thus, the intensity of drug action is proportional to the occupancy of the receptors or, in other words, to the concentration (square brackets) of the drug–receptor complexes, [DR]:

$$\text{Response} = \alpha[DR]$$

where α is a proportionality constant, also referred to as **intrinsic activity**. The complex is formed from its components and decomposes into them in a dynamic steady state:

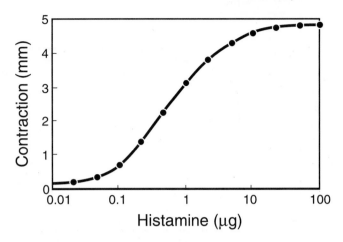

Figure 8-1. Log-dose–response relationships between doses of histamine and muscle contraction (see text).

$D + R$

$$D + R \underset{k_2}{\overset{k_1}{\rightleftharpoons}} DR$$

This picture is quite analogous to the Michaelis-Menten description of simple enzyme reactions, in which an enzyme–substrate complex is in dynamic steady state with its components and forms the reaction product at a rate proportional to the concentration of the complex. It is not surprising, then, that the mathematical descriptions of the two processes are also similar. The dependence of the response on the concentration of unbound drug is characterized by the expression representing a hyperbola:

$$\text{Response} = \frac{\alpha\,[D]\,[R]}{K + [D]}$$

where $K = k_2/k_1$ is the dissociation constant of the drug–receptor complex. This expression is analogous to the relationship between the velocity of an enzyme-catalyzed reaction and the free substrate concentration. It can be converted into a straight-line expression:

$$\frac{1}{\text{Resp}} = \frac{1}{\text{Resp}_{\text{max}}} + \frac{K}{\text{Resp}_{\text{max}}} \times \frac{1}{[D]}$$

where Resp and Resp$_{\text{max}}$ refer to the response and its maximally attainable value, respectively. Figure 8-3 illustrates the histamine data replotted in this way.

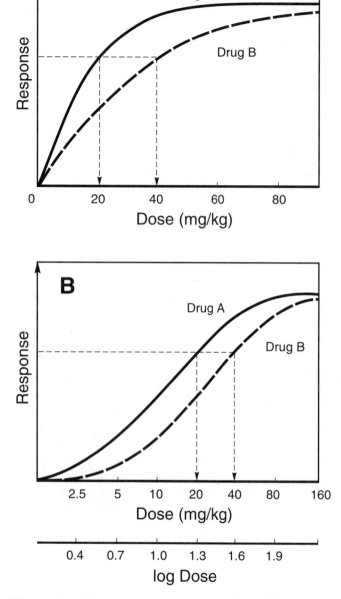

Figure 8-2. Linear dose–response plot (A) and LDR plot (B) of two drugs having different potencies.

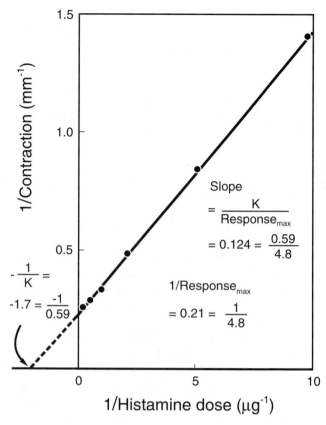

Figure 8-3. Double reciprocal plot for the effect of histamine on muscle contraction (data from Fig. 8-1).

The two formulae are not important; the calculations shown in Figure 8-3 illustrate the essential points: (1) A straight line fitted to observations depicted in the "double reciprocal" plot (or some other similarly linear plots) suggests the applicability of the occupancy theory of drug action, and (2) the dissociation constant and the maximal response can be evaluated from these plots.

ALL-OR-NONE EFFECTS

The example of histamine, which we have just discussed, described a typical graded effect: A slight increase of the dose should bring about a small increase of the response. There are occasions when the available information indicates only that a given dose of a drug either has or has not evoked a certain effect in the various subjects under investigation. Examples for such **quantal** or **all-or-none** responses are the presence or absence of convulsion, death, anesthetic effect, and improvement in a disease state. Usually, either the proportion or the percentage or the actual number of subjects responding to a given dose of the drug is recorded.

Thus, actually only a fraction of the subjects responds to certain drug dosages, while the remaining proportion fails to react. The reason lies in biological variation or diversity, i.e., in the differing sensitivity of the individual subjects to drug action. Individuals range from the very sensitive (hyperreactive) to the least sensitive (hyporeactive) subjects: persons in whom the drug produces its usual effect at unexpectedly low or uncommonly high doses, respectively.

HISTOGRAMS AND CUMULATIVE FREQUENCY PLOTS

When the dosage is varied, the number (or better, the fraction or the percentage) of subjects responding can be plotted against the dose or, preferably, its logarithm. Consider the following example: In each of 60 dogs an investigator gradually increased the rate of intravenous epinephrine infusion until a 35% enhancement of the heart rate was observed. Up to 10 ng/kg/min, this end point was reached in one dog; between 10 and 13 ng/kg/min in two additional dogs; between 13 and 17 ng/kg/min in six more of the animals; and so on. These data are displayed in a so-called histogram, which illustrates the distribution of sensitivities to epinephrine induction of heart rate increases in the various dogs (Fig. 8-4). The histogram is characteristically bell-shaped in similarity to curves describing the so-called **normal distribution** (see below).

The data can be rearranged to give the cumulative number (or fraction) of subjects responding to *all* doses that are lower or equal to the dose under investigation. For example, as before, 35% increase in the heart rate was recorded *up to* an epinephrine infusion rate of 10 ng/kg/min in one dog (1.7%); *up to* 13 ng/kg/min *in a total of* three animals (5.0%); *up to* 17 ng/kg/min *in a total of* nine dogs (15.0%); and so on. The data characterize the **cumulative distribution** of the sensitivities (Fig. 8-5). A curve fitted to them describes the cumulative rearrangement of the normal distribution; the shape of this rearranged distribution is very similar to that of an LDR curve.

It is important to notice that all-or-none responses are observed in individual subjects (or experimental animals) and that the recorded quantity (proportion, percentage, actual number of subjects reacting) is not identical to the response itself. On the other hand, as illustrated in the example of the response to epinephrine, graded effects (e.g., increase in the heart rate) can be converted to quantal responses by selecting a given level of the former (e.g., 35% increase) and observing the number (or fraction, or percentage) of subjects affected to that degree by certain doses of the drug.

In the example, the doses corresponding to consecutive class limits have been increased by a constant ratio, by about 30%. An equivalent statement is that the observations are pooled into groups (classes) defined by limits with logarithmically uniform incre-

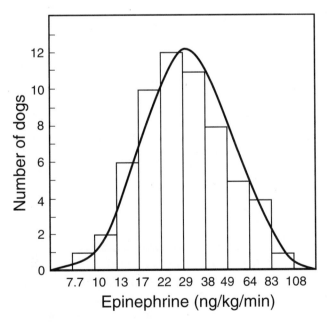

Figure 8-4. Distribution of dogs responding to various infusion rates of epinephrine. (Histogram indicating normal distribution; see text.)

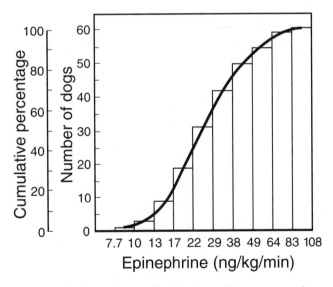

Figure 8-5. Cumulative distribution of dogs responding to various rates of epinephrine infusion. (Data from Fig. 8-4. The fitted curve describes distribution similar to an LDR curve.)

ments, i.e., that the horizontal dose scale is approximately logarithmic.

MEDIAN EFFECTIVE AND MEDIAN LETHAL DOSE

It is possible to evaluate doses to which 20%, 70%, 84%, or any other percentage of the subjects responds. It is customary to calculate such **effective doses,** abbreviated as ED_{20}, ED_{70}, ED_{84}, and especially the **median effective dose** or ED_{50}, which is, of course, the dose that gives rise to the designated response in 50% of the subjects. When drugs have parallel LDR curves, their potencies can be compared through their ED_{50}s; the more potent the drug, the lower is its ED_{50}.

If the response is mortality (e.g., in animal experiments designed to evaluate potency or toxicity), then instead of effective doses we speak of **lethal doses.** For instance, we characterize a dose that gives rise to the death of 50% of the subjects as the **median lethal dose** or LD_{50}. A harmful side effect is manifested in one-half of the subjects at the **median toxic dose** or TD_{50}. Anesthetists talk about anesthetic doses or AD_{50}s, which have the same interpretation as the ED_{50}s.

The strict definition of effective doses, and specifically of the ED_{50}, involves quantal responses: The dosage is sought at which a given percentage (frequently 50%) of the subjects is affected. A looser, less rigorous definition, which is often used in the pharmacological literature, extends the applicability to graded responses. According to this interpretation, the ED_{50} is the dose giving rise to one-half of the asymptotic, maximum (continuous) effect.

LINEAR PROBIT PLOT

As seen earlier, sensitivities of various subjects responding to a given drug dosage are frequently characterized by the normal distribution. For all-or-none responses, the cumulative arrangement of this distribution takes the form of the sigmoidal log-dose–response relationship (see Fig. 8-5). This becomes very useful since properties of the normal distribution have been investigated in great detail.

The considerations described below suggest that straight lines are obtained if the cumulative fractions or percentages of quantal responses are plotted against the logarithm of the dose on normal probability paper (explained in the next section) or in the probit scale. Figure 8-6 illustrates such a plot for the epinephrine data.

BASIS OF THE PROBIT PLOT (OPTIONAL)

The diagram in Figure 8-7 shows the bell-shaped (theoretical) normal distribution and the corresponding cumulative curve that represents the LDR plot. The centers of both curves (coinciding with the peak of the bell curve) occur at the mean. Fifty percent of the subjects respond at this point and the corresponding dose is the ED_{50}.

One of the characteristic features of the normal distribution curve is that two-thirds of the population under study will fall within the range of 1 standard deviation (SD) to each side of the mean or ED_{50}. In other words, the ED_{16} and ED_{84} (i.e., the doses that cause the effect in 16% and 84%, respectively, of all the individuals tested) lie at equal distances of 1 standard deviation below and above the ED_{50}. The ED_{31} and ED_{69} represent 0.5 standard deviation below and above the ED_{50}; the ED_7 and ED_{93} are 1.5 standard deviations, and the $ED_{2.3}$ and $ED_{97.7}$ are 2 standard deviations to each side, and so forth (see Fig. 8-7).

Therefore, one way of converting the sigmoidal

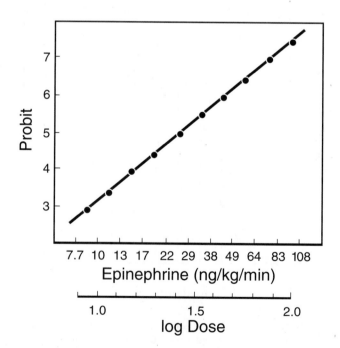

Figure 8-6. Probit plot for responses to epinephrine infusion shown in Figures 8-4 and 8-5.

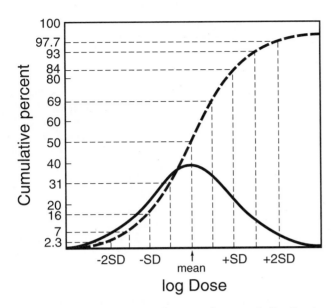

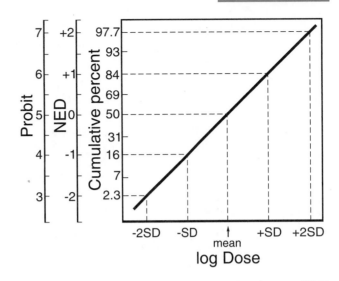

Figure 8-7. Bell-shaped, theoretical normal distribution (with arbitrary vertical scale) and corresponding cumulative curve representing the LDR plot (actual scale).

Figure 8-8. Probit plot for the normal distribution (NED = Normal Equivalent Deviates).

LDR curve to a straight line is to express all the values on the vertical (response) axis in terms of standard deviation units above or below the ED_{50}. The response corresponding to ED_{50} then has a value of 0, the ED_{16} is -1.0, the ED_{84} is $+1.0$, and so forth. (These values are called Normal Equivalent Deviates, or NED.) To avoid the $+$ and $-$ signs, 5 is added to every value, so the response corresponding to ED_{16} (-1) becomes 4; at ED_{50} it is 5, at ED_{84} ($+1$) it is 6, and so on. The units in this scale are called "probability units" or **probits** (Fig. 8-8).

Special "probability papers" and "probit papers" (i.e., preprinted graph papers) are available for plotting the results in probits against the logarithms of the doses, to give a straight line. However, such plots can also be constructed without using special graph papers if the observed cumulative percentages are directly converted into probits with the help of the tabulation given in Table 8-1.

EVALUATION OF DRUG SAFETY

In addition to its therapeutic effect, a drug is likely to have one or more kinds of harmful side effects. Higher doses may even cause death. Each of these responses can be characterized by an LDR curve. In general, the drug is considered to be safe if the LDR region of the harmful side effects is much higher than the therapeutic dose range. This idea is expressed by the

$$\text{Therapeutic index: } TI = TD_{50}/ED_{50}$$

which should be as high as possible for maximal safety.

However, this frequently used index does not characterize sufficiently the *relative* safety of different drugs. Figure 8-9 shows all-or-none LDR curves for the therapeutic and one of the toxic effects of two drugs, A and B. (For convenience only, the responses are illustrated in the probit scale in which straight lines are obtained. For further convenience, parallel lines for therapeutic and toxic responses are assumed. However, the following arguments could be pursued also with nonparallel responses depicted in any diagram.)

The two drugs shown in Figure 8-9 have identical ED_{50} and identical TD_{50} values; consequently they have identical values for the therapeutic index. The relative safeties of the two drugs, however, are quite different: A comparatively high dose of drug B may be beneficial to many or even most patients, but it will also be toxic to some of them (indicated by triangles in Fig. 8-9). Drug A, on the other hand, which has a steeper probit line, does not involve such risks: An almost completely curative dose has nearly none of the toxic effects (indicated by circles in Fig. 8-9). Such differences in drug behavior are characterized by the

Table 8-1 Conversion of Percent to Probit

%	0	1	2	3	4	5	6	7	8	9
0	—	2.67	2.95	3.12	3.25	3.36	3.45	3.52	3.59	3.66
10	3.72	3.77	3.82	3.87	3.92	3.96	4.01	4.05	4.08	4.12
20	4.16	4.19	4.23	4.26	4.29	4.33	4.36	4.39	4.42	4.45
30	4.48	4.50	4.53	4.56	4.59	4.61	4.64	4.67	4.69	4.72
40	4.75	4.77	4.80	4.82	4.85	4.87	4.90	4.92	4.95	4.97
50	5.00	5.03	5.05	5.08	5.10	5.13	5.15	5.18	5.20	5.23
60	5.25	5.28	5.31	5.33	5.36	5.39	5.41	5.44	5.47	5.50
70	5.52	5.55	5.58	5.61	5.64	5.67	5.71	5.74	5.77	5.81
80	5.84	5.88	5.92	5.95	5.99	6.04	6.08	6.13	6.18	6.23
90	6.28	6.34	6.41	6.48	6.55	6.64	6.75	6.88	7.05	7.33

Certain safety factor: $CSF = TD_1/ED_{99}$

It will be low for drug B and much higher for the "safer" drug A. Such quantitative considerations of drug safety apply equally to side effects and to lethality: In the latter case, $CSF = LD_1/ED_{99}$.

Two further remarks can be made: First, a drug may have several therapeutic indices and certain safety factors, one for each comparison of a toxic or lethal response with a therapeutic effect. Second, the LDR curves for various responses to a drug, whether therapeutic, toxic, or lethal, need not be parallel. Indeed, evaluation of therapeutic indices and certain safety factors does not require any assumption of parallelism.

There is an additional complication. The therapeutic and side-effect LDR curves vary from patient to patient. So it is possible, and it occurs with alarming frequency, that a dose that is therapeutic in one patient causes ill effects in another. The physician must be alert to such variations.

SUGGESTED READING

Kenakin TP. Pharmacologic analysis of drug-receptor interaction. 2nd ed. New York: Raven Press, 1993.

Tallarida RJ, Jacob LS. The dose-response relation in pharmacology. New York: Springer-Verlag, 1979.

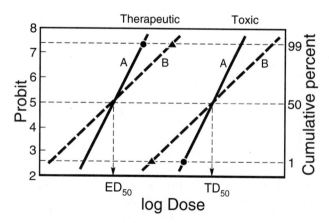

Figure 8-9. Plot illustrating the certain safety factor (see text).

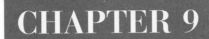

CHAPTER 9

Drug Receptors

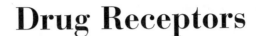

J. MITCHELL AND P. SEEMAN

Many drugs initiate their actions by binding to specific receptors on target cells in the body. Although knowledge of the molecular structure of receptors is very recent, the concept that drugs elicit their effects by binding to molecular receptors was formulated more than a century ago. Paul Ehrlich, working in the late 1800s in the rapidly developing synthetic pharmaceutical industry, experimented with arsphenamine (Salvarsan), which he attempted to develop into a specific antisyphilis drug. To explain the apparent structural specificity of drug action, he introduced the idea that a drug might act as a "magic bullet" directed at a vulnerable "receptor." Although Ehrlich's concepts were not entirely realized, they eventually led to the discovery of sulfonamides for the systemic treatment of bacterial infections by Domagk in 1935 and to the further refinement of the receptor concept as presently understood.

The direct identification of receptors for drugs, hormones, and neurotransmitters by means of radiolabeled ligands began in the mid-1960s. It had become apparent that most receptors have such high affinity for their respective "ligands" (i.e., neurotransmitter, hormone, or drug) that they become saturated when the ligand concentration is in the nanomolar range. Hence, it was necessary to develop methods for preparing radioactive ligands with specific activities sufficiently high to permit detection of the very small amounts of receptors that are present in body tissues. This development was instrumental in both the identification of receptors and development of many new drugs over the last 30 years.

The use of biochemical and molecular biological techniques over the past decade has led to the purification of many receptors and, more recently, to the molecular cloning of literally hundreds of specific receptor genes. Currently we know the molecular sequences of more than a hundred cell-surface and intracellular receptors with which a significant number of therapeutic drugs interact. With this knowledge, it may now be possible to gain more precise information about how drugs bind to specific receptors, and eventually, to design drugs with highly specific binding characteristics.

NATURE OF BIOLOGICAL DRUG RECEPTORS

Regardless of the route of administration, drugs interact with multiple components of the body, but not all of these interactions elicit an effect. Therefore a functional distinction can be made between these components. A **nonspecific binding site** is defined as any body component that a drug binds to without leading to an effect. Drug binding to serum albumin is an example of nonspecific binding. If binding of the drug to the component leads to an effect on the cell or the organism, that component is said to be a **drug receptor.**

Most drug receptors are protein in nature, and many of them are proteins that bind endogenous ligands such as the neurotransmitters, hormones, and growth factors. This chapter deals with the detection and characterization of such receptors; their role in regulatory signaling systems is discussed in Chapter 10.

Not all drugs act on receptors of endogenous ligands; in fact, a range of different biological components may serve as binding sites mediating the actions of drugs. Some of these sites are also proteins, such as the many enzymes that are targets of drug action. These include enzymes in the cells of our own bodies as well as those in the cells of pathogens that infect us. A number of examples of these drugs and their sites and mechanisms of action are given in Table 9-1. There are also many targets of drug action that are not protein in nature, and these include components such as lipids, ions, and water. For example, sterols in fungal and bacterial cell membranes are the targets of polyene and polymyxin antimicrobial agents (see Chapter 54). Divalent metal ions are the targets for chelating drugs, such as dimercaprol for Hg^{2+} or As^{2+} poisoning (Chapter 74), penicillamine for Cu^{2+} in Wilson's disease (Chapter 46), and EDTA for Pb^{2+} poisoning (Chapter 74). Body water may be considered as the target for osmotically active drugs, such as bulk laxatives, osmotic diuretics, and plasma expanders, that all act to change the water content of various body compartments.

DRUG INTERACTIONS WITH SPECIFIC RECEPTORS

The interaction of a drug with a receptor involves various types of chemical forces. Although there are examples of drugs that form covalent bonds with receptors, most drugs bind reversibly to receptors by a combination of electrostatic forces, hydrogen bonds, and Van der Waals forces. To permit these weak, short-range binding forces to act, the ligand and receptor must show molecular complementarity; i.e., the molecular shapes and the locations of their binding groups must fit each other. The requirement for complementarity of binding groups between drug and receptor means that minor alterations of the drug molecule drastically alter the ability of the drug to bind to the receptor. This is reflected in the relative potencies of a series of related drugs as shown in Table 9-2. It can be seen that addition or removal of a single carbon atom alters the potency of acetylcholine analogs by a factor of 10 or more at both muscarinic and nicotinic acetylcholine receptors. Similarly, specific receptors are also stereoselective, showing preference for one optical isomer of a drug. Thus, (−)levo-norepinephrine is 100 times as potent as (+)dextro-norepinephrine. A more complete discussion of pharmacodynamic specificity can be found in Chapter 11.

DRUG–RECEPTOR BINDING

The affinity of a receptor for a drug can be measured experimentally, and the index of this affinity is re-

Table 9-1 Examples of Enzymes as Drug Targets

Drug	Receptor and Mechanism of Action
β-Lactam antibiotics (penicillins and cephalosporins)	Bind to penicillin-binding proteins on bacteria and inhibit transpeptidase reaction required for synthesis of bacterial cell wall
Cardiac glycosides (digitalis)	Inhibit membrane ($Na^+ + K^+$)-ATPase, increase force of contraction in cardiac muscle
Rifampin	Binds to bacterial DNA-dependent RNA polymerase and inhibits RNA synthesis
Fluorouracil	Competes with uracil and becomes incorporated into RNA, blocking RNA processing; also metabolized to ribose and deoxyribose derivatives that inhibit thymidylate synthetase and thus block thymine nucleotides
Sulfonamides	Bind to a bacterial condensing enzyme necessary for the formation of folic acid from p-aminobenzoic acid; bacterial growth is consequently inhibited by lack of folic acid

Table 9-2 Relative Potencies of Acetylcholine Analogs

Analog	Guinea Pig Ileum (Muscarinic Receptor) %	Frog Rectus Abdominis (Nicotinic Receptor) %
Formylcholine	25	10
Acetylcholine	100	100
Propionylcholine	5	400
Butyrylcholine	0.5	150

ferred to as the **association constant, K_a**. If we consider the simplest case, in which a receptor exists in a single state, the affinity of the receptor (R) for a drug (D) can be described by the following equation:

$$D + R \underset{k_2}{\overset{k_1}{\rightleftharpoons}} DR \rightarrow Effect$$

where k_1 is the onset rate constant, reflecting the rate of drug binding to the receptor, and k_2 is the offset rate constant, reflecting the rate of dissociation of the drug–receptor complex. Then the association constant is the ratio of the onset rate constant divided by the offset rate constant:

$$K_a = k_1/k_2$$

with units of molar concentration^{-1}. The **dissociation constant, K_d**, is the reciprocal of the association constant ($1/K_a$), and has units of molar concentration. K_d is the more commonly used index of affinity and is the concentration of drug at which 50% of the receptors are occupied ($C_{50\%occupancy}$). This is equal to the ratio of the offset constant over the onset constant ($K_d = k_2/k_1$). It follows from the equation describing the interaction between a drug and receptor ($D + R \rightleftharpoons DR$) that at equilibrium, the relationship between the concentrations of free drug and drug–receptor complex is given by:

$$K_d = [D_{free}] \times [R_{free}]/[DR]$$

Since
$$K_d[R_{total}] = [R_{free}] + [DR]$$
$$K_d = [D_{free}] \times ([R_{total}] - [DR])/[DR]$$

and by rearranging this equation we get

$$[DR] = [R_{total}] \times ([D_{free}]/K_d + [D_{free}])$$

This equation describes a simple hyperbolic relationship between drug concentration and the concentration of drug–receptor complex, and is analogous to the Michaelis-Menten equation describing the interaction of enzyme with its substrate

$$V = V_{max}[S]/K_m + [S].$$

EXPERIMENTAL DRUG BINDING STUDIES: MEASUREMENT OF DRUG–RECEPTOR AFFINITY

The tissue concentration of most receptors is extremely low, around 10–100 fmoles/mg of tissue. Nevertheless, the dissociation constant of any drug for its receptor can be measured if a radioactively labeled form of the drug can be obtained that has sufficiently high specific activity to be detectable when diluted to nanomolar concentrations. The minimum radioactivity that one can reliably detect in most laboratory detection devices is about 200 dpm (disintegrations per minute). This means that in order to detect receptors in 1 mg of a typical tissue, the radioligand must have a specific activity of at least 200 dpm/10 fmol, or 10 C/mmol (there are approximately 2200 dpm/nCurie). Such high specific activity is feasible for most drugs either by incorporation of tritium (^{3}H) into the drug during synthesis, or in the case of purified peptide drugs, by iodination with radioactive iodine (^{125}I).

Binding assays used to measure drug–receptor interactions are quite simple in principle. Samples of tissue homogenate are mixed with different concentrations of radiolabeled drug in the presence of a physiological buffering system. After incubation of the mixture to reach equilibrium (the time required will depend on the temperature), each sample is processed to separate unbound drug from drug bound to the tissue. This is often performed by filtering the binding assay mixture through a glass-fiber filter such that the tissue will be retained on the filter and the unbound drug will pass through. After sufficient washing to remove unbound drug, the amount of drug bound to the tissue can be measured by counting the radioactivity retained on the filters.

Typical results of a binding assay are shown in Figure 9-1A, where it can be seen that binding increases with addition of increasing concentrations of radioligand. The lack of apparent saturation in this reaction is the result of ligand binding not only to the specific receptors in the tissue but also to nonspecific components such as membrane lipids and other proteins. To distinguish specific binding to the receptor from the nonspecific binding sites, a second set of tissue samples is assayed with the same concentrations of labeled drug but now in the presence of

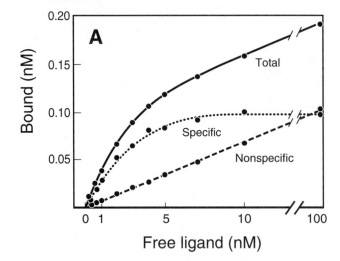

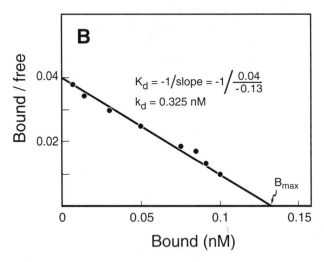

Figure 9-1. Measurement of binding of radiolabeled ligand to tissue homogenate. A. Total binding (solid line), nonspecific binding in the presence of excess unlabeled ligand (dashed line), and specific binding calculated by subtracting nonspecific from total binding (dotted line). B. Scatchard plot of specific binding.

(dashed line) compared to the total binding seen in the absence of cold ligand (solid line). Specific binding of radioligand to the receptors (dotted line) is then calculated by subtracting nonspecific binding from total binding, and the hyperbolic relationship between this specific binding and the free concentration of the drug becomes obvious.

K_d AND B_{max} FROM SCATCHARD ANALYSIS

Since the amount of tissue protein in each sample of the binding assay is known, the data in Figure 9-1A can be regraphed as $[DR]/[D_f]$ (i.e., concentration of specifically bound drug/concentration of free [unbound] drug) on the Y axis and specific binding on the X axis, as suggested by Scatchard (Fig. 9-1B). A straight line in a Scatchard plot indicates a single homogeneous class of binding sites for the drug, with the total number of specific binding sites (R_{total} or B_{max}) given by the X intercept of the line and the dissociation constant given by the negative reciprocal of the slope of the line (slope $= -1/K_d$). Nonlinear Scatchard plots of binding data indicate multiple classes of binding sites and/or cooperative effects between receptors (see below). Analysis of such binding curves is complex but has been facilitated by the availability of computer software that analyzes data obtained from binding assays to obtain estimates of K_d and B_{max} values for these multiple classes of binding sites.

DRUG BINDING TO MULTIPLE RECEPTOR SUBTYPES

Many hormone and neurotransmitter receptors can be further categorized into subtypes based on molecular cloning of multiple cDNAs encoding distinct, but highly related, receptor proteins. The existence of multiple receptor subtypes may permit greater diversity of biological responses (see Chapter 10), and theoretically, greater specificity of pharmacological therapy. Ideally, a perfectly selective drug is one that only binds to a single subtype of receptor. In practice, however, many therapeutic agents are not this selective and bind to several different subtypes of the same receptor and even to different types of receptors, causing unwanted side effects. With the application of molecular techniques many receptor subtypes are now available in recombinant form and

an excess of unlabeled ("cold") drug. Experience indicates that an adequate excess of cold drug is usually between 100 nM and 1 μM (approximately 100 times K_d). The distinction between specific and nonspecific binding sites is based on the higher affinity of the ligand for the specific receptors and the low abundance of these receptors. This means that in the presence of excess cold ligand the specific sites will be saturated and the residual binding of radioligand will be, for all practical purposes, only to the relatively unlimited number of nonspecific sites. As seen in Figure 9-1A, the radioactivity bound to the filters in the presence of cold drug is diminished

are used to test the specificity of binding of both new and existing drugs.

DIFFERENT BINDING AFFINITY STATES OF A RECEPTOR

It has become clear from numerous ligand-binding studies that many, if not most, receptors can exist in more than one state. These states are manifested as more than one affinity for a given agonist. For example, the β-adrenergic receptor has a high-affinity state with a K_d of 100 nM and a low-affinity binding state with a K_d of 10,000 nM for norepinephrine. The agonist high- and low-affinity states exhibited by all G protein-coupled receptors (see Chapter 10) can readily be demonstrated when a competition binding experiment is performed using a radiolabeled antagonist competing with unlabeled agonist, compared to the same labeled antagonist competing with an unlabeled antagonist. This type of study is illustrated for the β-adrenergic receptor in Figure 9-2. A number of reagents have been found to alter the binding curves for agonists on G protein-coupled receptors. An example of this effect is shown in Figure 9-2, where the presence of the guanine nucleo-

tide guanosine triphosphate (GTP) shifts the agonist competition curve to the right but has no effect on the antagonist competition curve. Other agents that affect agonist–receptor interactions include Mg^{2+}, Cl^-, and Na^{2+} ions. It is now known that these agents exert their effects on receptors by regulating the interaction of G proteins with the receptors.

A number of different molecular models have been proposed to explain the allosteric effects of G proteins on receptors. In the early 1980s the **ternary complex model** was proposed by DeLean et al. to explain the binding properties of β-adrenergic receptors, and it was later extended to other G protein-coupled receptors. This model assumes that the receptor interacts with both ligand and G protein and that the ligand and G protein exert reciprocal effects on the binding of each other to the receptor. In essence, the receptor–G protein complex is assumed to be the high-affinity state of the receptor and the receptor dissociated from the G protein is in the low-affinity state. Hence, agents that decrease receptor affinity for agonists all favor dissociation of receptor from G protein (guanine nucleotides, Na^{2+}, and Cl^-), while Mg^{2+}, which favors the receptor–G protein complex, increases agonist binding affinity. Since agonists that bind to these types of receptor exert their effects on the cell via the G proteins, it is only the high-affinity state of the receptor that is thought to be functional. However, these states are interchangeable and should not be thought of as two different groups of receptors. More recent models have now been proposed to incorporate new information on the effects of G-protein subunit interactions with each other and with receptors, and modeling these systems is quite complex.

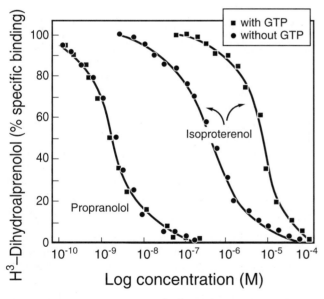

Figure 9-2. Displacement of ^{3}H-dihydroalprenolol (antagonist) by propranolol (antagonist) or isoproterenol (agonist) from a tissue expressing β-adrenergic receptors. The presence of guanosine triphosphate (GTP) has no effect on the antagonist competition curve but shifts the competition curve for the agonist to the right and makes the curve steeper.

EFFECT OF DRUGS ON RECEPTORS

Drugs that act on specific receptors can be classified by their effect on the receptor. **Agonists** are drugs that mimic the effects of the endogenous ligands and evoke a response when bound to the receptor. Depending on their ability to induce the active state of the receptor, agonists may be considered **full agonists**, those drugs that can elicit a maximal response through the receptor (drugs A and B in Fig. 9-3), or **partial agonists**, those that cannot elicit a maximal response even at very high drug concentrations (drug C in Fig. 9-3). A partial agonist is said to have reduced **efficacy** compared to full agonists, i.e., the E_{max} of the partial agonist is lower than that of the full agonists. Efficacy should not be confused with

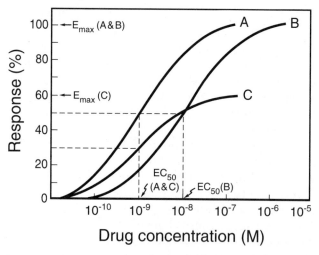

Figure 9-3. Response curves elicited for varying concentrations of three different drugs binding to the same receptor. Drugs A and B achieve the same maximal effect but at different concentrations; drug A is more potent than drug B. Drug C has a potency similar to that of drug A, but the maximal effect achieved by drug C is less than that of A or B, and therefore drug C has a lower efficacy than A or B.

drug **potency,** which is the relationship between the concentration of the drug and its ability to elicit an effect, i.e., the EC_{50} for the drug. In the example given in Figure 9-3, drugs A and C are equipotent (they have the same EC_{50}) and more potent than drug B, whereas drug C has lower efficacy than drugs A and B.

Since it is often desirable to inhibit rather than mimic the actions of endogenous ligands, many therapeutic agents that act on specific receptors are **antagonists.** Antagonists bind to the receptor but do not induce the active state of the receptor and can therefore be considered to have zero efficacy. They do not elicit a response themselves but block the response elicited by the endogenous agonists, and therefore can be considered to have **clinical utility.** Antagonists may be divided into two major classes depending on the type of chemical bonds formed between the drug and the receptor. **Reversible competitive antagonists** bind reversibly to the same site on the receptor as the agonists do and thus compete for the receptor binding site. The presence of a competitive antagonist will result in a shift of the dose-response curve for an agonist at that receptor (Fig. 9-4A). An example of reversible competitive antagonism is the effect of the β-adrenergic receptor antagonist propranolol, which attenuates increases in heart rate and force of contraction caused by epinephrine (Chapter 17). **Irreversible antagonists**

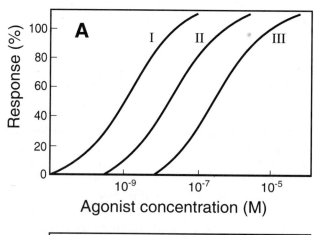

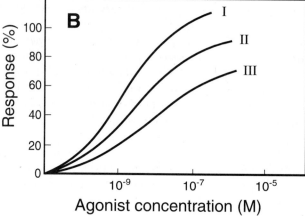

Figure 9-4. Response curves for varying concentrations of an agonist. A. Response curves for agonist alone (I), and in the presence of two concentrations of a *reversible* competitive antagonist (II and III). As the concentration of the antagonist increases, the response curve for the agonist is shifted progressively to the right, increasing the EC_{50} for the agonist, but the maximal effect of the agonist is unchanged. B. Response curves for the same agonist alone (I), and in the presence of two different concentrations (II, III) of an *irreversible* antagonist. Because the antagonist can "permanently" occupy the receptors that it binds to, the maximal effect of the agonist is now reduced.

may also compete with agonists for receptor binding, but either by forming covalent bonds or by virtue of their extremely high affinity for the receptor, they effectively bind irreversibly. Phenoxybenzamine is an example of an irreversible antagonist that forms covalent bonds with α-adrenergic receptors (Chapter 17).

The effect of an irreversible antagonist on the dose-response relationship of an agonist is dependent on the quantitative relationship between receptor occupancy and response. In the case of a linear relationship between receptor occupancy and response in which K_d is the same as EC_{50}, addition of even small doses of an irreversible antagonist will decrease the maximal response that can be elicited by the agonist (Fig. 9-4B). In many cases, however, not all receptors on a cell must be occupied in order to elicit the maximum response of an agonist. This phenomenon, i.e., the existence of **spare receptors,** can be seen in many tissues and means that the K_d measured for an agonist will be higher than the EC_{50} for the same ligand. If there are spare receptors, then the effect of a very small dose of an irreversible antagonist on the dose-response curve of an agonist will appear to be much the same as seen for the reversible antagonist, i.e., the dose-response curve for the agonist will be shifted to the right. Only when the dose of irreversible antagonist is increased to a level that occupies enough receptors to overcome the excess of receptors will the effect of the antagonist be to decrease the maximal response elicited by the agonist.

Drugs may also act by having allosteric effects on the response to an endogenous agonist. This effect may be positive or negative, and results from drug binding either to a site on the receptor distinct from the agonist binding site or binding to an adjoining component of the cell distinct from the receptor. If the effect of the drug is inhibitory then it is classified as a **noncompetitive antagonist.** An example of this type of drug action is seen with some gaseous anesthetics that increase the stimulus threshold required to elicit firing by neurons in the CNS by stabilizing the closed state of ion channels linked to nicotinic cholinergic receptors (see Chapter 13). This effect is thought to be mediated either by drug interactions with sites on the channels that are distinct from the acetylcholine binding site or by less specific drug interactions with membrane lipids that change the function of the channels in the membrane. Other examples of drugs that have allosteric effects on a receptor are the benzodiazepines and barbiturates (Chapter 27). These two groups of sedative-hypnotic drugs also decrease the firing rate of neurons in the CNS, but their action is mediated by enhancing the effect of γ-aminobutyric acid (GABA) on $GABA_A$-receptor-linked chloride channels, causing hyperpolarization of postsynaptic membranes and hence decreased firing of the postsynaptic neurons.

DEFINING THE BINDING SITE AS A BIOLOGICALLY RELEVANT RECEPTOR

In order to establish the relationship between a radiolabeled ligand binding site in vitro and the physiolog-

ical or pharmacological actions of that ligand in vivo, a number of parameters must be compared in the two systems. To define the site, the types of drugs that compete with binding of that labeled ligand need to be determined. These competition experiments result in a list of K_i values for the competing drugs ($K_i \simeq IC_{50}$, i.e., the concentration of competing drug required to inhibit 50% of specific binding of the labeled ligand).

In this type of assay the binding site should demonstrate stereoselectivity: The active enantiomer should have a much lower K_i than the pharmacologically inactive enantiomer. Similarly, a series of related congeners should demonstrate good correlation between their relative potencies in vivo and their K_i values in competition assays. For example, in the case of α-adrenergic receptors the K_i values should increase in the order $(-)$epinephrine $<$ $(-)$norepinephrine $<$ $(+)$epinephrine $<$ dopamine $<$ $(-)$isoproterenol, and if the binding site is a β-adrenergic receptor the order should be $(-)$isoproterenol $<$ $(-)$epinephrine $<$ $(-)$norepinephrine $<$ dopamine $<$ $(+)$isoproterenol.

These criteria are equally relevant whether one is examining a drug binding site in a tissue homogenate or a cloned receptor DNA expressed in a cell system. In either case it is the order of the drug K_i values that characterizes the receptor; the absolute values of these K_is are not important. A further example of this principle is shown in Figure 9-5, illustrating the correlation between the therapeutic potencies of a number of neuroleptic drugs and their respective K_i values for binding to specific subtypes of dopamine receptors. These studies revealed that for most neuroleptics, the overall correlation is best for the D_2-receptors. Under therapeutic conditions, however, clozapine and olanzapine occupy more D_4-receptors than D_2. It is possible that the D_4-receptor is the primary target for these atypical antipsychotic drugs and may explain why clozapine does not elicit parkinsonism as seen with the other antipsychotics (see Chapter 28).

CONCLUSION

Much has been learned about the targets of drug action in the body since the early use of synthetic compounds as drugs a century ago. In particular, the molecular cloning of receptors for many hormones, neurotransmitters, and cytokines, which are the targets of many of our therapeutic agents, has brought a new understanding of drug receptors at the molecular level. Many of the soluble protein receptors, such as

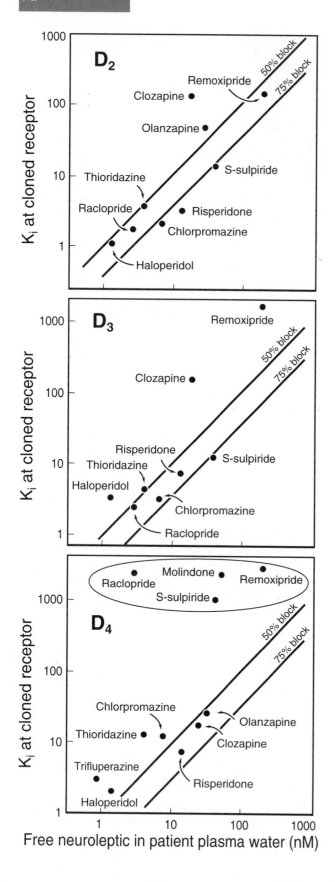

Figure 9-5. Relationship between the dissociation constants (K_i) of various neuroleptics for the cloned dopamine D_2, D_3, and D_4 receptors and the therapeutic concentrations of those neuroleptics, as measured in the plasma or spinal fluid of patients. The diagonal lines show the percentage of receptors occupied by a drug under therapeutic conditions. The K_i values were obtained from experiments using cloned dopamine receptors expressed in different cell lines. (Adapted from Seeman P, Van Tol HHM. *TIPS* 1994; 15:264–270.)

enzymes, are being cocrystallized with their respective drugs, illustrating the precise binding interactions between drug and receptor. This information allows the medicinal chemists to design new drugs with very specific binding characteristics. In the near future we can anticipate that methods to crystallize membrane-bound receptors will emerge and make possible similar studies for these types of receptors.

SUGGESTED READING

Dohlman HG, Thorner J, Caron MG, Lefkowitz RJ. Model systems for the study of seven-transmembrane-segment receptors. Annu Rev Biochem 1991; 60:653–688.

Hulme EC, ed. Receptor-ligand interactions: a practical approach. Oxford: IRL Press, 1990.

Seeman P, Van Tol HHM. Dopamine receptor pharmacology. Trends Pharmacol Sci 1994; 15:264–270.

Tolkovsky AM, Levitski A. Theories and predictions of models describing sequential interactions between receptor, the GTP regulatory unit, and the catalytic unit of hormone-dependent adenylate cyclase. J Cyclic Nucleotide Res 1981; 7:139–150.

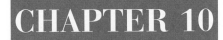

CHAPTER 10

Signal Transduction and Second Messengers

J. MITCHELL

SECOND MESSENGERS

The study of second-messenger systems began with the pioneering studies of Sutherland and Rall in the late 1950s. They found that stimulating cardiac membranes with epinephrine increased the concentration of a water-soluble nucleotide, cyclic adenosine monophosphate (cAMP), and they proposed that the cAMP acted as an intracellular messenger. We now know that stimulation of cells by **first messengers** (hormones and neurotransmitters), which cannot traverse the lipid plasma membrane, results in the regulation of a variety of intracellular compounds (cyclic nucleotides, phospholipids, ions) called **second messengers**. Increases in second-messenger levels inside of cells mimic the physiological effects of the hormones and neurotransmitters that have their receptors on those cells.

SIGNALING MECHANISMS

There are four basic mechanisms by which extracellular ligands regulate intracellular processes, as shown in Figure 10-1. The molecular components of each of these signal transduction systems are quite distinct: (1) The most complex are the **G protein–coupled receptor** systems, composed of a transmembrane receptor that binds a ligand on its extracellular surface and couples to a guanine-nucleotide-binding protein (G protein) on its intracellular surface. The G protein in turn regulates an effector enzyme to generate an intracellular second messenger. (2) The **receptor tyrosine kinase and receptor guanylyl cyclase** systems are composed of transmembrane receptors in which the intracellular portion has enzymatic activity that is allosterically regulated by ligand binding to the extracellular portion of the receptor. (3) The simplest systems are those of the **ligand-gated ion channels,** in which the open state of the transmembrane ion channel is regulated by ligand binding directly to the extracellular side of the channel. (4) Ligands that are sufficiently lipid soluble to cross the membrane can bind to **intracellular receptors;** in this case the receptor–ligand complex then binds to specific DNA sequences within the cell nucleus and regulates gene transcription. These four types of transduction system are described in more detail below.

G Protein-Coupled Second-Messenger Systems

Most hormones and a few neurotransmitters act by regulating intracellular second messengers through G protein-coupled receptors. Table 10-1 is a partial list of the ligands that act by this mechanism and the second messengers that they regulate. The three components of each system—receptor, G protein, and effector enzyme—are either embedded in the plasma membrane or tightly associated with it. The second messengers that are produced by the systems are for the most part water-soluble compounds that are freely diffusible in the cytoplasm.

Before examining each component of these systems in detail, it is useful to consider some of their general properties. If we look at even a partial list of

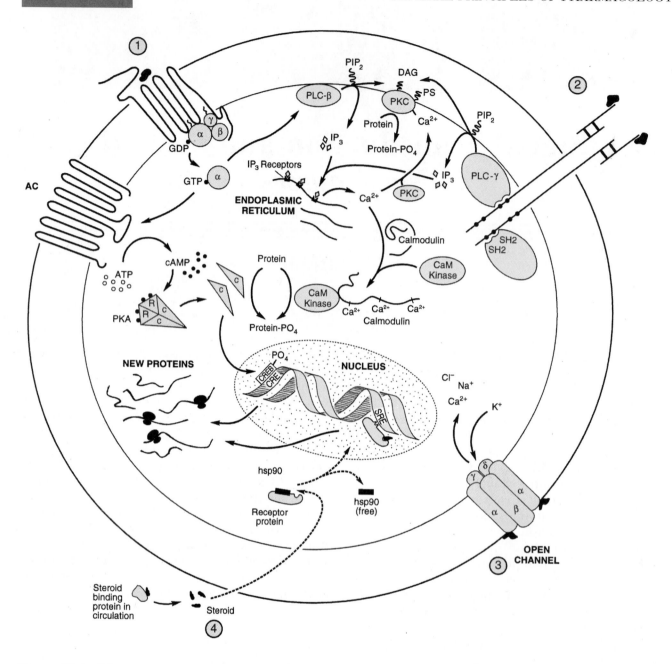

Figure 10-1. Schematic representation of four major signaling mechanisms: (1) G protein–coupled receptors. (2) Receptor tyrosine kinase system. (3) Ligand-gated ion channels. (4) Intracellular receptors. (See text for details.) *Abbreviations:* α, β, γ (mechanism 1) = subunits of G proteins; α, β, γ, δ (mechanism 2) = subunits of ion channel; AC = adenylyl cyclase; ATP = adenosine triphosphate; c = catalytic subunits of PKA; CaM = calmodulin; cAMP = cyclic adenosine monophosphate; CRE = cAMP response element; CREB = cAMP response element-binding protein; DAG = diacylglycerol; GDP = guanosine diphosphate; GTP = guanosine triphosphate; hsp90 = heat-shock protein 90; IP₃ = inositol-1,4,5-tris-phosphate; PIP₂ = phosphatidylinositol-4,5-bisphosphate; PKA = protein kinase A; PKC = protein kinase C; PLC = phospholipase C; PS = phosphatidylserine; R = regulatory subunits of PKA; SH2 = *Src* homology region 2; SRE = steroid response element.

distinct receptors and compare it to the number of second messengers they regulate (Table 10-1), it is clear that many different first messengers regulate a common second messenger, and yet the physiological effect of each first messenger on its target cells is very different. For example, glucagon stimulates cAMP production in liver cells and results in increased carbohydrate breakdown, whereas vasopressin stimulates cAMP in kidney cells, which results in increased water resorption from the nephron. This specificity of a first messenger's actions is the result of two processes: (1) Receptors for a ligand are only present on specific cells, and (2) the expression of proteins that are regulated by the second messengers is also specific to each cell type.

G Protein-coupled receptors

This family of receptors has over 100 distinct members. Each of these proteins is the product of a different gene, yet they all share a conserved structural feature of seven stretches ("domains") of hydrophobic amino acids within the receptor polypeptide. These hydrophobic domains are thought to represent membrane-spanning segments embedded in the membrane in such a manner that the receptor snakes back and forth through the plasma membrane, with one end of the protein protruding outside the membrane and the other end inside the cytoplasm (1 in Fig. 10-1). For this reason, these receptors are often referred to as "serpentine" or "seven transmembrane" receptors.

The endogenous ligands bind to the extracellular side of the receptor. Small ligands, such as the amines, bind to sites within the various transmembrane regions of the receptor, while binding sites for the larger polypeptide ligands, which are less able to penetrate the hydrophobic regions, are on the extracellular loops and amino terminus of the receptor.

The G proteins bind to intracellular segments of the receptor, especially within the third intracellular loop between the fifth and sixth transmembrane regions. The effect of agonist binding on receptor structure is poorly understood, but it likely stabilizes the receptor in a conformation that permits efficient interaction between the receptor and the G-protein trimer. These interactions result in stimulation of the G protein (see below) and subsequent regulation of the effector.

Generally, there are more types of receptors than of endogenous extracellular ligands because multiple subtypes have been found for all but a few of the G protein-coupled receptors. Multiple receptor subtypes for a single ligand were predicted in some cases from pharmacological studies. For example, the differential effect of nicotine and muscarine on cholinergic receptors predicted that there are two distinct classes of acetylcholine receptor, which were named nicotinic and muscarinic receptors. With the recent application of molecular cloning techniques to the field of receptor pharmacology, an even greater number of receptors have been revealed than was anticipated by the pharmacology. For example, five different muscarinic acetylcholine receptors and six different adrenergic receptors are now known. In some cases, multiple receptor subtypes seem responsible for the complex physiological responses to a single ligand, but in many cases we do not yet understand the physiological role of the many receptor subtypes.

When a receptor is stimulated by an agonist, the effect is usually of limited duration. The limitation of receptor stimulation involves a number of processes. Most G protein-coupled receptors have a number of serine and threonine residues in the cytoplasmic loops and carboxyl terminus of the receptor. These residues can be phosphorylated by several kinases, and this phosphorylation may result in diminished interaction between receptor and G protein. This process, known as **receptor desensitization,** allows the cell to respond to a large range of extracellular concentrations of stimuli. After prolonged agonist activation, the number of receptors in the plasma membrane can also be regulated by a process of receptor internalization (followed in some cases by catabolism) known as **receptor down-regulation.** The signals that initiate this down-regulation process are not well understood but appear to be different from those that control receptor desensitization.

G Proteins

The family of G proteins that transduce signals from membrane receptors to effector enzymes and ion channels are known as the heterotrimeric G proteins. Each of these proteins is composed of three distinct subunits, termed α, β, and γ in order of decreasing molecular weight. The α subunit of the trimer binds guanine nucleotides and is the major mediator of the G protein's actions on its effector. The β and γ subunits of the trimer function primarily to support α subunit interactions with the plasma membrane and receptors, but like α subunits they may also regulate effectors directly (see Table 10-2).

The G proteins that participate in transmembrane signaling are all regulated by common mecha-

Table 10-1 Partial List of G Protein–coupled Receptor Systems*

Type of Ligand	Receptor	G Protein	System	Effect
Neurotransmitters				
Acetylcholine	$M_{1,3,5}$	a) $G_{q/11}$	PLC-β	Stimulation
		b) $G_?$	K channel	Closed
	$M_{2,4}$	a) G_i	AC	Inhibition
		b) G_i	K channel	Opened
Dopamine	$D_{1,5}$	b) G_s	AC	Stimulation
	$D_{2,3,4}$	b) G_i	AC	Inhibition
Epinephrine	β_1	a) G_s	AC	Stimulation
		b) G_s	Ca channel	Opened
	β_2	b) G_s	AC	Stimulation
	α_1	a) $G_{q/11}$	PLC-β	Stimulation
		b) $G_?$	PLA$_2$	Stimulation
		c) $G_?$	PLD	Stimulation
	$\alpha_{2a,2b}$	a) G_i	AC	Inhibition
		b) G_o	Ca channel	Closed
GABA	GABA$_B$	a) G_o	Ca channel	Closed
		b) G_i	K channel	Opened
		c) G_i	AC	Inhibition
Glutamate	mGluR$_{1-8}$	a) G_i	AC	Inhibition
		b) $G_{q/11}$	PLC-β	Stimulation
		c) G_i	K channel	Opened
		d) G_o	Ca channel	Closed
Histamine	H_1	d) $G_{q/11}$	PLC-β	Stimulation
	H_2	d) G_s	AC	Stimulation
Serotonin	5HT$_{1a}$	a) G_i	AC	Inhibition
		b) G_i	K channel	Opened
	5HT$_{1c}$	b) $G_{q/11}$	PLC-β	Stimulation
	5HT$_2$	a) G_s	AC	Stimulation
		b) G_o	Ca channel	Closed
Peptide Hormones				
Adrenocorticotropin	ACTH	a) G_s	AC	Stimulation
		b) G_s	Ca channel	Opened
Angiotensin II	AT$_{1a,1b}$	a) G_i	AC	Inhibition
		b) G_q	PLC	Stimulation
		c) $G_?$	PLA$_2$	Stimulation
		d) $G_?$	PLD	Stimulation
		e) G_i	Ca channel	Opened
Glucagon		b) G_s	AC	Stimulation
Opioid	μ, κ, δ	a) G_i	AC	Inhibition
		b) G_o	Ca channel	Closed
Parathyroid Hormone	PTHR	a) G_s	AC	Stimulation
		b) G_q	PLC	Stimulation
Somatostatin	SST, SRIF	a) G_i	AC	Inhibition
		b) G_i	K channel	Opened
		c) G_o	Ca channel	Closed

Table 10-1 (Continued)

Type of Ligand	Receptor	G Protein	System	Effect
Thyrotropin	*TSH*	*a) G_s*	*AC*	*Stimulation*
		b) G_q	*PLC*	*Stimulation*
Vasopressin	*V-1a*	*a) G_q*	PLC	Stimulation
		b) $G_?$	PLD	Stimulation
		c) $G_?$	PLA_2	Stimulation
	V-1b	*b) G_q*	PLC	Stimulation
	V-1c	*b) G_s*	AC	Stimulation
Prostanoids				
Prostaglandins	$PGE_{1,2}$	*b) G_i*	AC	Stimulation
	$PGF_{2\alpha}$	*b) G_q*	PLC	Stimulation
Prostacyclin	PGI_2	*b) G_s*	AC	Stimulation

Abbreviations: AC = adenylyl cyclase; Ca channel = calcium channel; GABA = γ-aminobutyric acid; K channel = potassium channel; PDE = phosphodiesterase; PLA = phospholipase A; PLC = phospholipase C; PLD = phospholipase D.

nisms. The cycle of activation and inactivation of these proteins is depicted in Figure 10-2. In the resting or basal state, the three G-protein subunits are bound together with guanosine diphosphate (GDP) attached to the α subunit. When an agonist binds to its receptor, the associated G protein is altered in some way that causes the release of the GDP. The empty guanyl nucleotide binding site on the α subunit is then occupied by guanosine triphosphate (GTP) that is present in high concentrations in the cytoplasm. The effect of GTP binding is stimulatory to the G protein and the α subunit dissociates from the receptor and G-protein $\beta\gamma$ subunits and binds to the effector. After a few seconds, the intrinsic GTPase activity of the α subunit hydrolyzes the bound GTP to GDP, thereby inactivating itself. The GDP-bound α subunit dissociates from the effector, reassociates with the G-protein $\beta\gamma$ complex, and is then available for another cycle of activation by the receptor.

Functional diversity amongst the different members of the G-protein family is primarily the result of different α subunits, of which more than 20 different ones are now known (Table 10-3). The nomenclature for G proteins was originally based on their function. Thus G_s indicates the stimulatory protein and G_i the inhibitory protein for adenylyl cyclase, and G_t was so named because it was originally called transducin when it was first identified as the stimulatory protein in the retina. This system very quickly

Table 10-2 Regulation of Cloned Mammalian Adenylyl Cyclases

Subtype	G_s Stimulation	PKC Stimulation	$\beta\gamma$ Effect*	G_i Inhibition	Ca^{2+} Effect
I	Mild	No	Inhibition	Yes	Stimulation
II	Robust	Yes	Stimulation	No	None
III	Mild	No	?	?	Stimulation
IV	Robust	No	Stimulation	No	None
V	Robust	Yes	None	Yes	Inhibition
VI	Robust	Yes	None	Yes	Inhibition
VII	Robust	Yes	?	?	None
VIII	Robust	No	?	Yes	Stimulation

*Inhibition or stimulation of G_s activation.

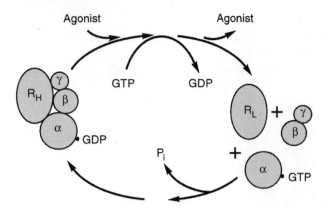

Figure 10-2. G-protein activation–inactivation cycle. *Abbreviations:* α, β, γ = subunits of G proteins; GDP = guanosine diphosphate; GTP = guanosine triphosphate; P_i = phosphate; R_H = high-affinity receptor; R_L = low-affinity receptor.

cones of the retina and activates a cGMP-specific phosphodiesterase. Other G proteins are widely expressed in most tissues of the body and often have multiple functions; for example, G_i is present in most cells, where it inhibits adenylyl cyclase, but it also has direct effects on some ion channels.

The effect of most G proteins on their effectors is stimulatory, but a few act to inhibit their effectors. For example G_o inhibits Ca^{2+} channels in the brain and heart, and adenylyl cyclase is under both positive regulation from G_s and negative regulation from G_i. These two G proteins are regulated by different groups of receptors that are often present on the same cell. Activation of stimulatory receptors and inhibitory receptors at the same time results in an attenuated adenylyl cyclase response in that cell. This dual regulation, in addition to interaction of signal transduction components distal to the G proteins (see below), allows for an integrated response to multiple stimuli on the same cell.

Some G proteins are also targets for pathological agents. $G_s\alpha$ is modified by a toxin produced by the bacterium *Vibrio cholerae*. The modification involves an addition of ADP-ribose to the α_s subunit that results in inhibition of the GTPase activity of the G protein, resulting in persistent activation of $G_s\alpha$.

broke down, however, when G proteins were isolated and cloned without knowledge of their function, and so we also have G_o, G_q, and more recently G_{11}, G_{12}, and so on. Some G proteins are only expressed in defined cell types and have very specialized functions; for example, G_t is found only in rods and

Table 10-3 Families of Mammalian G Proteins*

Family	G Protein	Functions(s)	Expression
G_s	G_s	AC stimulation	Ubiquitous
		Ca channel open	
	G_{olf}	AC stimulation	Olfactory, brain
G_i	G_{i-1}	AC inhibition	Ubiquitous
	G_{i-2}	AC inhibition	Ubiquitous
	G_{i-3}	AC inhibition	Ubiquitous
		K channel open	
	$G_{oA,B}$	Ca channel closed	Brain, heart, endocrine
	$G_{t1,2}$	cGMP PDE stimulation	Retina rods, cones
	G_z	?	Brain
G_q	G_q	PLC-β stimulation	Ubiquitous
	G_{11}	PLC-β stimulation	Ubiquitous
	G_{14}	PLC-β stimulation	
	G_{15}	PLC-β stimulation	Myeloid and B cells
	G_{16}	PLC-β stimulation	Myeloid and T cells
G_{12}	G_{12}	NHE inhibition	Ubiquitous
	G_{13}	NHE stimulation	Ubiquitous

**Abbreviations:* AC = adenylyl cyclase; GMP = guanosine monophosphate; NHE = sodium/hydrogen exchanger; PDE = phosphodiesterase; PLC = phospholipase C.

When the bacterium infects the intestinal cells, the resulting elevation in intracellular cAMP causes the cells to secrete large amounts of water into the gut, resulting in severe diarrhea characteristic of cholera infection. The bacterium *Bordetella pertussis*, which causes whooping cough, secretes a similar toxin that acts on $G_i\alpha$ and $G_o\alpha$, preventing their activation by receptors. With the inhibitory effect of G_i on adenylyl cyclase disrupted by the toxin, cAMP accumulation also increases in cells infected by the pertussis bacterium, resulting in the characteristic cough and immune responses associated with the disease.

Effector enzymes regulated by G proteins

Of the three components that constitute the G protein–coupled signal transduction systems, the effectors have proven the most difficult to study at the molecular level. Only recently have some of these enzymes been isolated and cloned. The adenylyl cyclases and the phospholipases C are the most common targets of hormone and neurotransmitter receptors (Table 10-1). These two systems are well understood and their components are detailed in Figure 10-1. Other enzymes, such as phospholipase A_2, which produces arachidonic acid, are also thought to be regulated by G proteins, but this regulation is less well understood.

Adenylyl cyclases and cAMP as a second messenger. Cyclic AMP (cAMP) is synthesized from ATP by the adenylyl cyclase enzymes embedded in the plasma membrane. These enzymes are large polypeptides thought to contain two clusters of six transmembrane segments separating two similar catalytic domains. There are at least eight forms of adenylyl cyclase. All are stimulated by $G_s\alpha$, but they differ in their sensitivity to inhibition by $G_i\alpha$, stimulation by calcium/calmodulin, and effect of G-protein $\beta\gamma$ subunits (see Table 10-2). These additional regulators allow for the integration of many signals acting on different second-messenger systems within the same cell.

cAMP exerts its effects in cells mainly by activating the cAMP-dependent protein kinases (protein kinase A or PKA). These tetrameric enzymes are composed of two regulatory and two catalytic subunits. The enzymes are activated when two molecules of cAMP bind to each of the regulatory subunits, releasing the catalytic subunits from the tetramer. The released subunits then catalyze the transfer of the terminal phosphate group from ATP to specific serine and threonine residues on their target proteins.

Among these target proteins are enzymes that participate in cellular metabolic pathways and proteins that regulate gene transcription. A well-studied example of a cAMP-activated metabolic pathway is the cascade of enzyme activation leading to breakdown of glycogen in the liver. Activated protein kinase A phosphorylates phosphorylase kinase, which in turn phosphorylates glycogen phosphorylase, the enzyme that breaks down glycogen. The effect of cAMP on gene transcription is mediated by PKA-catalyzed phosphorylation of a protein known as the **cAMP response element–binding protein (CREB)**. CREB binds to specific short DNA sequences known as **cAMP response elements (CRE)**. CREB is bound to the CRE and, when phosphorylated by protein kinase A, it stimulates transcription of genes containing the CRE in their regulatory region.

Phospholipase C and phospholipid second messengers. Members of the G_q family of proteins (Table 10-3) couple various receptors to a group of enzymes known as **phospholipase C-β**. These enzymes belong to a larger family of phospholipases that all use inositol phospholipids as substrates. Signal transduction through this pathway follows a sequence of molecular events similar to that seen for the activation of adenylyl cyclase. Receptor occupation by an agonist activates the G protein, which in turn binds to the phospholipase on the inner surface of the plasma membrane. Once activated, the lipase rapidly breaks down phosphatidylinositol-bisphosphate (PIP_2) to **inositol trisphosphate (IP_3)** and **diacylglycerol**. Both of these molecules can act as second messengers by two different pathways.

IP_3 is a small water-soluble molecule that can rapidly diffuse through the cytoplasm and bind to an IP_3-gated Ca^{2+} channel in the smooth endoplasmic reticulum, resulting in release of stored Ca^{2+} into the cytosol. The rise in cytoplasmic calcium concentration initiates a wave of calcium-dependent reactions in the cell. Many of these reactions are mediated by specific Ca^{2+}-binding proteins, the most ubiquitous being **calmodulin**. Ca^{2+}/calmodulin regulates a number of enzymes including plasma membrane Ca^{2+}-ATPase, which pumps calcium out of the cell, and, as we have seen, some types of adenylyl cyclase (see Table 10-2). Most of the effects of calcium in the cell are the result of activation of a group of protein kinases known as Ca^{2+}/calmodulin-dependent protein kinases. These kinases phosphorylate serines and threonines on a variety of proteins. Once again, the physiological response of any given cell to activation of the phospholipid second messengers is dependent on the Ca^{2+}/calmodulin kinase target proteins expressed in that cell.

The other molecular product of PIP_2 hydrolysis by phospholipase C is diacylglycerol. This lipid molecule remains in the plasma membrane where in concert with phosphatidylserine it activates some members of another family of serine/threonine kinases known as **protein kinase C**. These soluble kinases are translocated to the membrane in response to elevations in cytosolic Ca^{2+} (initiated by the release of IP_3) and are then activated by the combined effect of Ca^{2+}, diacylglycerol, and phosphatidylserine. Once activated, these kinases phosphorylate a cell-specific array of substrate proteins that include many ion channels, receptors, and other kinases that eventually result in increased gene transcription.

Other signal transduction processes regulated by G proteins. In addition to these enzymes, G proteins have more recently been shown also to modulate the activity of many of the voltage-gated ion channels. As can be seen from Table 10-1, many hormones and neurotransmitters regulate both a second messenger and an ion channel by activating a single G protein; for example G_s stimulates both adenylyl cyclase and some types of Ca^{2+} channels. Understanding the mechanisms of interaction of receptors with multiple G proteins and G proteins with multiple receptors will be one of the major challenges of signal transduction research in the future.

Enzyme-Linked Receptors

Receptor tyrosine kinases

This group of receptors mediates signals from a group of endogenous compounds known as **growth factors,** which includes **insulin, epidermal growth factor (EGF), and platelet-derived growth factor (PDGF).** The receptors are composed of single polypeptide chains that traverse the plasma membrane, creating three domains: an extracellular ligand-binding domain, a transmembrane domain, and an intracellular domain that contains the portion responsible for the enzymatic activity of the receptor (2 in Fig. 10-1). Some members of this group of receptors, such as the insulin receptor, exist as dimers of two receptors coupled together by noncovalent bonds. Others, such as the EGF receptor, exist as single units within the membrane and only come together to form dimers in response to ligand binding to each subunit. In either case the binding of the growth

factor to the receptor results in allosteric activation of the tyrosine kinase activity in the cytoplasmic domain of the receptor. The first step in the activation process appears to involve cross-phosphorylation of the two receptor subunits on multiple tyrosine residues within the intracellular domains. This autophosphorylation of the receptor then acts as a signal for binding of other intracellular proteins, which themselves become phosphorylated on tyrosine residues by the receptor and are thereby activated. Once again the specificity of cellular responses to different growth factors is determined by the different combinations of proteins that bind to each growth-factor receptor.

Recently, a large number of proteins that bind to activated growth-factor receptors have been identified. These proteins have varied structures, but they share two highly conserved domains known as **SH2 and SH3** for *Src homology regions 2 and 3* because they were first identified in the proto-oncogene–encoded *Src* protein. The SH2 domain recognizes the phosphotyrosines on the growth-factor receptors, but the function of the SH3 domain is not well understood at present. Characterization of the many proteins containing SH2 and SH3 domains is currently the subject of intense research efforts, and the roles of some of these proteins are now clear. For example, one mechanism by which growth factors regulate cellular growth or differentiation is by activating a cascade of protein kinases known as the **mitogen-activated protein kinases (MAP kinase pathway).** Activation of this pathway is initiated by tyrosine phosphorylation of Grb2 (a protein containing SH2 and SH3 domains). The SH3 domain on Grb2 binds another protein known as mSOS and together the Grb2/mSOS complex activates Ras, a monomeric G protein. Ras has a structure similar to the α subunits of G proteins that interact with the seven transmembrane receptors, and it is activated and inactivated by similar mechanisms (see Fig. 10-2). Hence the interaction of Ras with Grb2/mSOS promotes exchange of GDP for GTP on Ras, thus promoting its activation. The next step in this cascade is less well understood but seems to involve Ras activation of a serine/threonine kinase known as Raf. Raf then activates (by phosphorylation) another kinase, MEK (also known as MAP-kinase kinase), which in turn phosphorylates MAP kinase. MAP kinase can traverse the nuclear membrane, and in the nucleus it phosphorylates a variety of transcription factors. The consequent regulation of gene transcription initiates processes resulting in cellular proliferation or differentiation.

Other proteins that interact with growth-factor receptors are known to regulate intracellular second messengers. For example, members of the phospholipase C-γ family of proteins that regulate intracellular IP$_3$ and diacylglycerol levels in a similar manner to that of the PLC-β family discussed above contain SH2 and SH3 domains and are known to be activated by tyrosine kinase receptors.

The only member of this family of growth-factor receptors that is currently a target for pharmacological agents is the insulin receptor in diabetic patients (see Chapter 50). However, the role of receptor tyrosine kinases in cellular growth, and the association of uncontrolled signaling through these receptors with neoplastic and inflammatory diseases, has created a great interest in the development of agents that will block their activity. For example, mutated *ras* proteins have been found in more than 30% of human cancers. Various agents are being developed to inhibit the activity of mutated *ras* and other proteins in the MAP kinase pathway, as potential therapeutic agents useful in targeting these tumors.

Receptor guanylyl cyclases

The only members of this class of receptors known so far are the receptors for a family of peptide hormones known as the **atrial natriuretic peptides (ANPs)**. These peptides are secreted by cardiac atrial muscle cells in response to increases in blood pressure. ANPs bind to receptors in the kidney, where they induce natriuresis (increased Na$^+$ and water excretion), and in the smooth muscle cells of the vasculature, where they induce relaxation.

The ANP receptor is a single polypeptide that contains an extracellular ANP-binding domain, a single transmembrane domain, and an intracellular guanylyl cyclase catalytic domain. Activation of the receptor results in increased production of cyclic GMP, which in turn activates a serine-threonine kinase, **cGMP-dependent protein kinase (protein kinase G)**. Target proteins for protein kinase G and the signaling cascades that lead to the physiological responses to ANPs have not been well characterized thus far.

Ligand-Gated Ion Channels

The synaptic neurotransmitters bind to a group of receptors on postsynaptic membranes known as the ligand-gated ion channels (3 in Fig. 10-1). Neurotransmitters that bind to this class of receptors/ion channels include acetylcholine, γ-aminobutyric acid (GABA), glycine, and glutamate. Ligand-gated ion channels are important targets for drugs. Indeed, many of the drugs used in the treatment of mental illnesses as well as the sedative-hypnotics act on this group of receptors.

These various ion channels are structurally similar in that each of them is composed of multiple subunits that together form the ion channel through the plasma membrane. Each subunit of the channel is a polypeptide that contains four membrane-spanning domains. The neurotransmitter-binding specificities and ion selectivities are quite distinct for each channel (Table 10-4). The best characterized of this class of receptors is the nicotinic acetylcholine receptor depicted in Figure 10-1(3). This ion channel is composed of five subunits (two α, one β, one γ, one δ) that together form an aqueous pore passing through the plasma membrane. The close apposition of the two α subunits within the membrane forms a "gate" that prevents ions from flowing through the channel. Acetylcholine binds to extracellular sites on the two α subunits, causing a conformational change in these two proteins such that the gate is opened and cations (particularly Na$^+$) flow down their chemical gradient into the cell.

Intracellular Receptors

Ligands that are sufficiently lipid soluble to cross the plasma membrane of cells exert their actions by binding to a group of intracellular proteins known as the **steroid receptor superfamily** (4 in Fig. 10-1). These include the receptors for **glucocorticoids, mineralocorticoids, sex steroid hormones, vitamin D, thyroid hormone, and retinoic acid**. Activation of all of these receptors results in increased transcription of particular genes within the target cell and therefore they have been called **ligand-responsive transcription factors**.

The general structure of a receptor of this class, as depicted in Figure 10-1, is that of a single polypeptide that can be divided into three functional domains. The amino-terminal region of the receptor has a modulatory function and binds a protein known as **hsp90** (a 90-kDa **heat-shock protein**) in the absence of its ligand. The DNA-binding domain of the receptor is in the middle of the protein and contains a structural motif, known as "zinc fingers," that is common to DNA-binding proteins. The ligand-binding domain is in the carboxyl terminus of the receptor. When the ligand binds to the receptor, the hsp90 protein is released, revealing the DNA-binding

Table 10-4 Ligand-gated Ion Channels

Neurotransmitter	Channel (Receptor)	Ion Selectivity	Effect
Acetylcholine	Nicotinic		
Serotonin	$5HT_3$	Cations, primarily Na^+	Excitatory
Glutamate	NMDA,* non-NMDA		
GABA	$GABA_A$	Anions, primarily Cl^-	Inhibitory
Glycine	Gly		

*N-Methyl-D-aspartate; this receptor channel also has an important Ca^{2+} selectivity.

domain and transcription-activating domain of the receptor.

Because the actions of this class of ligands require increased gene transcription, translation, and subsequent protein synthesis, responses are slow, often taking many hours before onset of action. Similarly, the slow turnover of most proteins regulated by these ligands results in a persistent effect following withdrawal of the ligand. Consequently there is no simple temporal correlation between the plasma concentration of hormones or therapeutic agents acting on intracellular receptors and their effects.

SUGGESTED READINGS

Berridge MJ. Inositol trisphosphate and diacylglycerol: two interacting second messengers. Annu Rev Biochem 1987; 56:159–193.

Birnbaumer L, Abramowitz J, Brown AM. Receptor-effector coupling by G proteins. Biochem Biophys Acta 1990; 1031:163–224.

Bourne HR, Sanders DA, McCormick F. The GTPase superfamily: conserved structure and molecular mechanism. Nature 1991; 349:117–127.

Dohman HG, Thorner J, Caron MG, Lefkowitz RJ. Model systems for the study of seven-transmembrane-segment receptors. Annu Rev Biochem 1991; 60:653–688.

Ing NH, O'Malley BW. The steroid hormone receptor superfamily: molecular mechanisms of action. In: Weintraub BD, ed. Molecular endocrinology: basic concepts and clinical considerations. New York: Raven Press, 1995:195–215.

Michell RH. Inositol lipids in cellular signalling mechanisms. Trends Biochem Sci 1992; 17:274–276.

Nishizuka Y. Intracellular signalling by hydrolysis of phospholipids and activation of protein kinase C. Science 1992; 258:607–614.

Saltiel AR. Signal transduction pathways as drug targets. Sci Am 1995; November/December:58–67.

Tang WJ, Gilman AG. Adenylyl cyclases. Cell 1992; 70:869–872.

Taylor SS, Buechler JA, Yonemoto M. cAMP-dependent protein kinase: framework for a diverse family of regulatory enzymes. Annu Rev Biochem 1990; 59:971–1005.

Ullrich A, Schlessinger J. Growth factor signalling by receptor tyrosine kinases. Neuron 1992;9:383–391.

Unwin N. Neurotransmitter action: opening of ligand-gated ion channels. Neuron 1993; 10(Suppl):31–41.

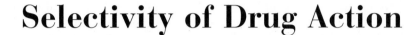

CHAPTER 11

Selectivity of Drug Action

H. KALANT

No drug known is completely specific in the sense of acting exclusively on one type of cell or tissue to produce only one type of effect. However, different drugs do show different degrees of selectivity, and the therapeutic usefulness of a drug is usually related directly to its degree of selectivity. The Australian pharmacologist Adrien Albert set out the principle that most, if not all, drug actions are toxic because the substances act by inhibiting or interfering with one or more cellular functions. Useful drug actions are thus seen as instances of "selective toxicity." Nonselective toxicity is seen as poisoning.

For example, cyanide combines strongly with the ferric iron in various heme proteins, including cytochrome oxidase, and therefore inhibits oxidative metabolism in all tissues. It is therefore clearly a poison. In contrast, penicillin inhibits a bacterial enzyme involved in the formation of bacterial cell walls at concentrations that have no detectable effects on mammalian tissue enzymes. This selectivity permits its use as an antibiotic.

In between these extremes are many drugs that produce desired therapeutic effects at low doses and toxic effects at somewhat higher doses, with varying margins of safety between the two levels. For example, methotrexate (an anticancer drug) in doses of 2.5–5 mg/kg daily has been used to treat severe psoriasis by inhibiting the rapid reproduction of epithelial cells in the psoriatic plaques. But at slightly higher doses it may also inhibit reproduction of mucosal cells in the intestine, leading to ulceration and diarrhea.

Generally, the toxic effects of a drug are separable from its therapeutically useful effects on the basis of differences in (1) their respective mechanisms of

production, (2) their dose–response relationships if the mechanisms are similar, or (3) the sites at which they are produced. Therefore, attempts to increase the utility of a drug are based on either an improved **pharmacodynamic selectivity** (if the mechanisms of toxic and therapeutic effects differ) or on an enhanced **pharmacokinetic selectivity** of distribution to the desired target site.

PHARMACODYNAMIC SELECTIVITY

Molecular Basis of Selectivity

The concept of drug–receptor selectivity is historically an outgrowth of the study of the mechanisms of interaction between enzymes and substrates and inhibitors, and between acetylcholine and other neurotransmitters with their respective receptors. As a general rule, an effective drug molecule has three or more points of attachment to corresponding points on the molecule or group of molecules making up the receptor site. The nature of these points of attachment and their relative positions and distances from each other are all critical to the ability of the drug to combine with the receptor and produce a response. However, very few drugs have molecules that are completely rigid and unable to undergo some degree of change in steric relations among the potential binding groups. Most drugs have at least some single bonds that permit free rotation and thus allow the molecule to assume different conformations.

This is illustrated by **acetylcholine,** its analogs, and its blockers (see also Chapters 14, 15, and 19). The molecule is represented schematically as shown in Figure 11-1A. The groups that are essential for its activity are the charged N^+, the three methyl groups attached to it, the ester linkage, and the spacing of about 7 Å between the N^+ and the carbonyl C. However, the molecule is extremely flexible because of the single bonds that permit free rotation, and numerous conformations of the molecule have been proposed on the basis of different analytical methods; some of these are illustrated in Figure 11-1. Presumably different conformations permit the acetylcholine molecule to fit to the nicotinic and muscarinic receptors and their various subtypes.

Unlike acetylcholine, a number of analogs, such as muscarine and nicotine (for which the receptors were named), muscarone, and various thio-substi-

tuted analogs, have rigid cyclic structures, bulky side-groups, or double bonds that prevent free rotation. Such compounds therefore have much greater selectivity than acetylcholine itself does, for different receptor types. One pair of such rigid analogs with high selectivity for M_1 muscarinic receptors (see Chapters 13 and 20) is illustrated in Figure 11-1B. Research on the development of these rigid analogs has been stimulated by the possible clinical value of selective ligands for the treatment of Alzheimer's disease, without the risk of parkinsonian side effects. The availability of highly selective ligands for different receptors has permitted the rapid progress in receptor pharmacology seen in recent years.

Like acetylcholine, most drugs are able to bind

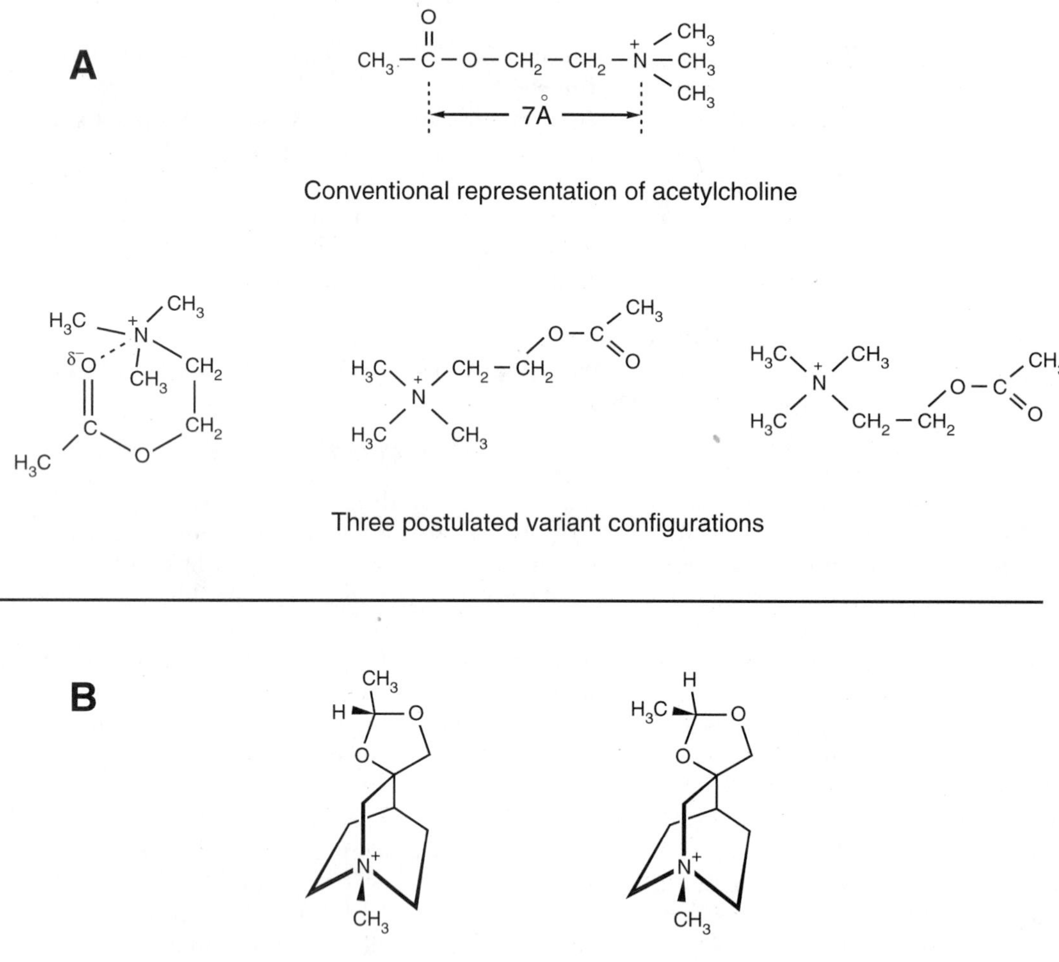

A

Conventional representation of acetylcholine

Three postulated variant configurations

B

Chiral forms of rigid cyclic analogs with highly selective M_1 binding

Figure 11-1. A. Various proposed conformations of the acetylcholine molecule that are possible because of free rotation about single bonds, and that could account for the ability of the same molecule to bind to a variety of different receptors. B. Rigid analogs that are selectively bound by only one subtype of muscarinic receptor.

to more than one receptor, and most receptors are able to bind more than one drug. When a series of different drugs are compared with respect to their abilities to bind to a particular receptor (see Chapter 9), their K_d values as determined from Scatchard plots, or their K_i values for displacement of a labeled ligand, serve as measures of their relative affinities for that receptor. Similarly, a given drug can be compared with respect to its binding to a series of different receptors. If one drug has a K_d or a K_i value several orders of magnitude smaller than those of the other compounds tested, or if it has a K_d or a K_i for one receptor that is several orders of magnitude lower than those for the other receptors, it is considered a highly selective ligand for that receptor, as either an agonist or an antagonist as the case may be.

It has become possible to achieve much higher degrees of such molecular selectivity in the last few years because the application of molecular biology techniques has permitted the isolation, purification, and cloning of large numbers of different receptor types and subtypes (see Chapter 9). This approach makes it possible to recognize whether the different effects produced by the same drug are attributable to actions at the same or different receptor types. By systematic modifications of the molecular structure of the drug, it may then be possible to develop derivatives with different affinities for, and activities at, the different receptors involved. In this way, it may be possible to achieve drugs that can produce the desired effect of the original drug without its undesired side effects. An example is the development of **raclopride**, a highly selective blocker of D_2 and D_3 dopamine receptors. This drug is a potent antipsychotic agent in the treatment of schizophrenia. There is lower risk of troublesome side effects associated with blockade of other receptors (see Chapter 28) when this selective blocker is used.

A variety of structural features contribute to the degree of selectivity of a drug for a receptor, including the size and shape of the molecule, the sizes of its substituent groups, their kinds and degrees of ionic charge, their ability to form hydrogen bonds or covalent bonds, and the presence or absence of planar ring structures that can be held by Van der Waals and similar short-range forces to corresponding planar structures in the receptor. Now that the molecular structures of many receptors are known, attempts are being made to design drugs to fit a particular receptor, rather than having to rely on the relatively inefficient process of synthesizing hundreds or even thousands of variants of the drug and then screening them all to find which have the highest affinity and efficacy. So far, the drug-designing approach is in its infancy, but it will undoubtedly become more successful in the future.

Stereospecificity

Stereospecificity is not an obligatory feature of receptor selectivity, but it may add significantly to it. There are many examples of drugs having optical isomeric forms, only one of which is active. This is consistent with the type of receptor selectivity mentioned above, provided that at least three points of attachment between drug and receptor are required and that all three binding groups are chemically different and attached to either a center or plane of asymmetry. This is illustrated schematically in Figure 11-2.

This seems to be the probable explanation for such examples as the following:

- Atropine is a mixture of *d*- and *l*-hyoscyamine, of which only the *l*-form is active as a muscarinic blocker.
- Morphine has *d*- and *l*-forms, of which only the *l*-form is active as an analgesic.
- Norepinephrine has *d*- and *l*-forms, of which only the *l*-form has significant potency in the elevation of blood pressure and other peripheral vascular effects.
- *d*-Amphetamine is a much more effective central stimulant than *l*-amphetamine, but they are equipotent in producing hallucinations.

Degrees of Selectivity

Despite the promise of rapid development of new drugs with high degrees of selectivity, most of the drugs in current use are still considerably less selective. Since drug–receptor binding depends upon a combination of chemical groupings with different types of bonding possibilities and strengths, and arranged in specific three-dimensional patterns, it is possible to have widely differing degrees of selectivity. A receptor with five critical bonding sites set at several different distances from each other can have vastly greater selectivity than one with only two critical sites and one fixed distance between them.

Thus, at one extreme is tetrodotoxin, a highly specific molecule, which apparently combines only with the sodium channels in nerve cell membranes, acting to block the action potential.

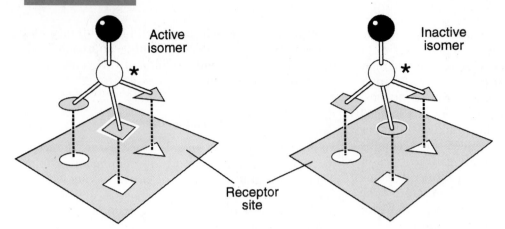

Active isomer

Inactive isomer

Receptor site

Figure 11-2. Schematic representation of complementarity of binding groups between drug and receptor, to account for activity of one optical isomer (left) and inactivity of the other (right). The asterisk marks the asymmetric carbon. The four different substituents are indicated by different shapes; three of these have complementary binding sites on the receptor. If there were only two binding sites, both isomers would be effective, as a result of simply rotating the molecule.

In an intermediate position are drugs that have some basic parts of their molecules in common, while other parts differ. The parts in common may enable them to combine with various types of receptor, but the parts that differ give them some degree of selectivity. For example, the group

$$R-CH_2-CH_2-CH_2-N \begin{array}{c} CH_2- \\ \\ CH_2- \end{array}$$

or

$$R-O-CH_2-CH_2-N \begin{array}{c} CH_3 \\ \\ CH_3 \end{array}$$

seems to enable a molecule to combine to some extent with receptors for histamine, acetylcholine, and possibly catecholamines, and if R is a large cyclic hydrocarbon portion, the drug can function as an antihistaminic, a local anesthetic, a myocardial membrane stabilizer (i.e., an antiarrhythmic agent), and to varying degrees also as an anticholinergic or antiadrenergic agent.

For example, chlorpromazine, procaine, and diphenhydramine are all good local anesthetics, H_1-antihistaminic agents, and reducers of myocardial excitability. In addition, however, the other parts of the molecule contribute to other actions that are not shared by all of these drugs (Fig 11-3):

- Chlorpromazine has an antiemetic effect, some minor cholinergic and adrenergic blocking action, and antipsychotic activity.
- Procaine has a central stimulant action like that of cocaine in that it can act as a convulsant.
- Diphenhydramine is relatively more effective as an H_1-antihistaminic and also as a sedative and a cholinergic blocker.

It is through such mixtures of shared and unshared actions that many drugs have evolved into families of new drugs with preferential increase of one type of action and reduction of another. For example, sulfanilamide, with a combination of antibacterial, hypoglycemic, and carbonic-anhydrase-inhibitor effects, evolved into three separate families of drugs, each one relatively more specific for one or another of these effects (Fig. 11-4).

At the other extreme are drugs that are not believed to act on specific receptor sites at all. General anesthetic agents act by dissolving in a large part of the lipid portion of the cell membrane and interacting with protein inclusions in the membrane. Such drugs have very little stereoselectivity, no strict molecular structural requirements for activity, and are not specific receptor blockers or antagonists. At the same time, they act on a wide variety of different cells and tissues in a similar way, differing only in the relative concentrations needed to affect different types of cells or different functions of the same cell.

Even with such drugs, some minor degree of selectivity is possible. The lipid portion of the cell

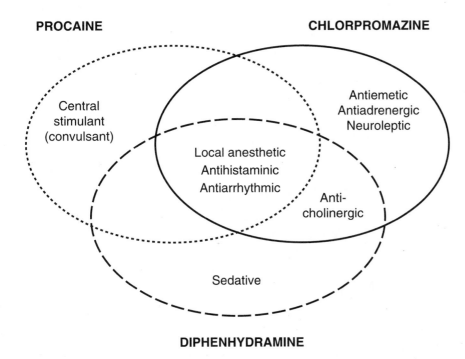

Figure 11-3. Gradations in specificity of actions of three drugs with diethylaminoethanol side-chains. All three share local anesthetic, antihistaminic, and myocardial stabilizing actions. Two share anticholinergic action. Each has other unshared actions.

membrane is not homogeneous, but in fact is quite heterogeneous with respect to the types of lipid immediately adjacent to, and interacting with, the various protein inclusions in the membrane (the "boundary lipids") and those constituting the lipid matrix of the membrane. An anesthetic agent may interact preferentially with certain boundary lipids rather than with the bulk of the matrix lipids and therefore affect the activity of certain receptors or ion channels more than others.

Selective Actions Versus Nonspecific Applications

Sometimes a therapeutic application of a drug does not require a particular mechanism of action, and a variety of drugs with different mechanisms of action may be used to achieve the same therapeutic objective. For example, all immune responses, involving both B and T lymphocytes, are initiated by stimuli that lead to cell proliferation (see Chapter 61). This process, like all growth, whether normal or malignant, requires production of DNA, RNA, and protein. Therefore, treatment of malignant growths, prevention of heterologous transplant rejection, treatment of autoimmune diseases, and control of severe psoria-

sis can all make use of similar drugs. These include inhibitors of DNA synthesis, DNA inactivators (alkylating agents), and corticosteroids. Equally, the toxic effects also reflect nonspecific inhibition of growth and replication in the fastest-growing normal tissues: bone marrow suppression, loss of gastrointestinal epithelium, alopecia (hair loss), and impairment of normal immune mechanisms against viral diseases and malignancies.

PHARMACOKINETIC SELECTIVITY

For those drugs that either do not act selectively on particular receptors or act on receptors that are found on many or all tissues or cell types, some degree of selectivity of action may still exist because of either (1) selective distribution of the drug to an intended target site or (2) metabolic differences that make one tissue more sensitive to the effect of the drug than another.

The difference between molecular selectivity and tissue selectivity may be illustrated by two examples. Atropine is highly selective for muscarinic receptors but produces a very wide range of effects and side effects because muscarinic receptors are found in

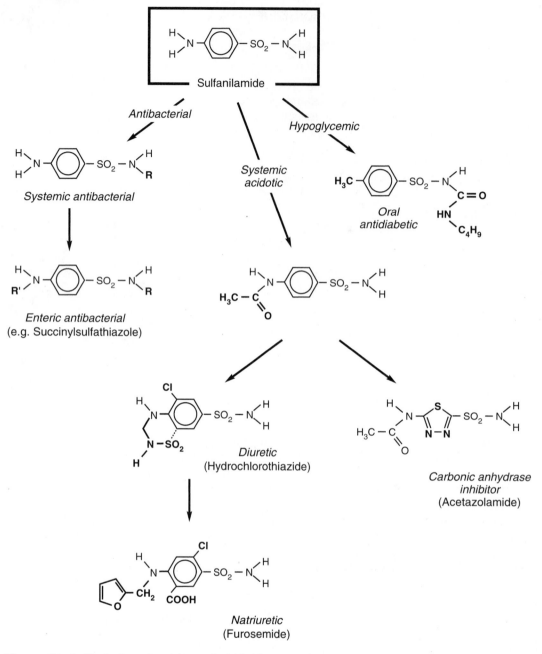

Figure 11-4. Evolution of a drug with multiple actions into separate families of drugs with more specific actions.

many organs and tissues (e.g., eye, GI tract, salivary glands, bladder, and heart). In contrast, general anesthetic agents are nonselective with respect to receptor mechanisms but are relatively selective when administered in the usual fashion, because the circulation delivers a high initial drug concentration to the brain, and nerve cell function is more sensitive than are the functions of nonexcitable cells.

Selectivity Related to Drug Distribution

Many drugs with very low selectivity for either receptors or particular tissue or cell types can still be used effectively to produce a desired therapeutic effect and relatively little toxic effect by being applied selectively to the intended target site. There are a number of ways of achieving selective delivery that are used clinically.

Topical application

This is clearly the most selective route of drug administration. The drug is applied, in the desired concentration, directly at its intended site of action: on a body surface; in the ear, eye, or nose; by irrigation into the bladder; by insertion of suppositories into the rectum or vagina; by inhalation into the bronchi; by injection into a joint cavity, the pleural space, or an abscess cavity. The selectivity results from the fact that any drug absorbed from the site is diluted in such a large volume of circulating blood, and of tissue fluid at other sites, that it is much less likely to have significant effects elsewhere in the body. The usefulness of this approach may be increased by agents that enhance the ability of the drug to penetrate locally into the tissue to which it is applied, or by agents that minimize the drug's escape into the circulation (e.g., vasoconstrictors with local anesthetics).

Intra-arterial or portal venous injection

This achieves selectivity on a similar basis. Certain **antitumor drugs** have very little margin of safety between their effects on cancer cells and on rapidly growing normal cells such as GI epithelium. Selectivity can be achieved in some cases by injecting the drug intra-arterially, just upstream from the cancer, in a concentration that is locally active. But when the drug passes through the tumor site and is diluted in the venous blood, the concentration is too low to affect the rest of the body. This method has been used successfully to treat malignant hepatoma or hepatic metastases by injection into the hepatic artery or into a tributary of the portal vein. A further refinement of this technique is to dissolve the chemotherapeutic agent in an oily carrier such as lipiodol for intra-arterial injection. The oily droplets are trapped in the capillaries of the tumor and facilitate drug uptake into the tumor cells.

Selectivity by ionization

Another example of selectivity based on distribution is that of **atropine** versus **propantheline**. Both are effective blockers of muscarinic receptors, but propantheline does not readily cross the blood–brain barrier because it has a quaternary N, which is a permanent cation. Therefore, it has very little effect on muscarinic sites in the central nervous system compared to atropine, when the drugs are given in doses that produce equal degrees of peripheral effect.

Differential blood flow

Thiopental acts as a depressant on all cells with excitable membranes, including peripheral and central neurons, skeletal muscle, cardiac muscle, and smooth muscle. However, when injected intravenously it is first distributed among the various organs in proportion to their relative blood flows. Since the brain has a very high blood flow, and the drug is highly lipid-soluble, it passes rapidly into the brain and causes anesthesia. As the drug gradually redistributes to other tissues with larger bulk but lower proportional blood flow, the drug passes back out of the brain into the blood and thus ends its anesthetic effect. In contrast, phenobarbital is much less lipid-soluble and does not enter the brain so readily despite the high blood flow. Therefore, it does not exert a rapid initial effect on the brain, and by the time it reaches an anesthetic concentration in the brain it has also reached high levels in other tissues. Thus, it is not suitable for use as an anesthetic, because an effective dose might be toxic to other tissues and would take much too long to be eliminated after the desired period of anesthesia was finished.

Distribution by selective carriers

A drug with low selectivity, either of mechanism or of target, may achieve selectivity of action by being linked to a carrier that does have selective uptake into certain tissues or sites. This is illustrated by several recently developed examples.

Monoclonal antibodies are highly selective for specific epitopes (antigenic portions of a molecule). If such antibodies are raised against a particular epitope forming part of a cell-surface antigen, a drug linked to the antibodies can be delivered selectively to those cells. For example, CD20 is a cell-surface antigen found on 90% of B-cell lymphomas but not on either immature or fully differentiated B cells. ^{131}I was linked to a monoclonal antibody against CD20, and in this way it was possible to deliver radiation specifically to the tumor cells without affecting normal B lymphocytes. Numerous other trials have been made, using antibodies as vehicles for selective delivery of drugs.

Polyamines, such as spermine, carry strong positive charges that cause them to bind electrostatically to DNA. Efforts are currently being made to use polyamines as carriers for drugs that are intended for selective delivery to, and action on, DNA in tumor cells.

Selective concentration by excretion

Many drugs are concentrated in the urine because they are filtered through the glomeruli or actively secreted by the tubules, and poorly reabsorbed farther down. Therefore, they may reach effective concentrations in the tubule or lower urinary tract, even though the concentration in the plasma is too low to produce significant effects in the rest of the body. Examples include the use of **nitrofurantoin** as a urinary antiseptic and of **organomercurials** and **thiazides** as diuretic agents.

This same principle underlies the **selective renal toxicity** of the sulfonamides. These drugs are concentrated in the lumen of the renal tubule as described above. At the same time, the urine becomes acidified by exchange of H^+ for Na^+, and the concentrated sulfonamides crystallize out of the acid urine. The crystals may damage the tubular epithelium.

Selectivity Related to Tissue Differences

Selective cellular binding

Some drugs that are capable of acting on many different types of cell, if present in high enough concentration, show selectivity at ordinary dosage by achieving the effective concentration only in certain cells in which there are binding sites with very high affinity. For example, **quinine** and many other antimalarial agents, though capable of exerting a quinidine-like effect on tissue cell membranes, have a much higher affinity for DNA inside the malarial parasites. Therefore, they can be used at plasma concentrations that are too low to produce myocardial effects but that permit the accumulation of high-enough concentrations inside the parasites to inhibit reproduction of the plasmodia. **Griseofulvin**, an antifungal antibiotic, can also be toxic to mammalian cells. However, it has selectively high binding to keratin (skin, hair, nails). When given in low doses that do not affect other tissues, it can build up a high-enough concentration in keratinized structures to inhibit growth of the fungi, such as *Trichophyton rubrum*, which cause difficult infections of skin and nails.

Selective uptake

It has been known for many years that certain tissues have the ability to take up and concentrate certain substances to levels far greater than those found in other tissues. For example, the **thyroid gland** has a very high ability to take up and concentrate iodine. This ability is used therapeutically by giving ^{131}I to patients with hyperthyroidism, whose hyperactive glands concentrate the iodine even more than usual, and so receive a concentrated dose of radiation while other tissues are unaffected.

However, this is not the only possible application of this principle. Macular degeneration is a disease of the retina that is characterized by abnormal proliferation of capillaries that impair the function of the retinal light sensors. One novel treatment described recently involved a porphyrin pigment that is taken up selectively by the endothelium of proliferating capillaries but not by that of stable mature capillaries. The retina was then exposed to long-wave red light, causing photochemical activation of the porphyrin pigment to form free radicals that destroyed the affected capillaries without harming the normal ones.

Selective intracellular activation

Some drugs are not pharmacologically active in the form that is given but are biotransformed to active metabolites. If one tissue has a particularly effective mechanism for forming the active product, it may be affected by a precursor drug concentration that is too low to affect other tissues. Two examples are given here to illustrate this principle.

Cyclophosphamide is an inactive cyclic derivative of nitrogen mustard that is activated by hydroxylation of the cyclic amide ring, opening of the ring at the hydroxylation site, and cleavage of the opened ring to form free phosphoramide mustard, the active antitumor agent. The hydroxylation occurs in the liver, but the final cleavage seems to occur preferentially in the tumor cells. In this way, the drug can act on the tumor cells with much less risk to normal tissue cells (see Chapter 60).

Some bacterial infections of the large intestine are susceptible to treatment by sulfonamides, but ordinary sulfonamides are absorbed in the small intestine and leave only low concentrations to be carried into the large bowel. If the dose is raised enough to produce the desired concentration in the bowel, the concentration of absorbed drug in the blood and tissues is high enough to cause toxicity. **Enteric sulfonamides**, such as phthalylsulfathiazole and succinylsulfathiazole, are not absorbed readily and remain in the intestine, but are not active against bacteria because their *p*-amino group is conjugated (see Chapter 56). However, intestinal bacterial hydrolases are able to split off the phthalyl or succinyl groups from the *p*-amino N and form free sulfathiazole, which then exerts an antibacterial activity locally, with much lower risk of systemic toxicity.

Selective tissue vulnerability

A drug may be relatively nonselective in terms of the range of tissues it acts on, yet it may have therapeutic specificity if the cellular function that it affects is more important in one tissue than in the rest. For example, the cardiac glycosides of the **digitalis** family inhibit the $(Na^+ + K^+)$-stimulated ATPase that is involved in the active transport of cations across the cell membrane. This enzyme is present in many, probably all, types of cell. However, in muscle cells the levels of Na^+ and K^+ in the cells affect both the transmembrane potential and the levels of free and membrane-bound Ca^{2+}, and thus influence both the excitability and the contractile force (see Chapter 36). The concentration of digitalis glycoside required to inhibit the enzyme is lower in heart muscle than in skeletal muscle, liver, kidney, and many other tissues.

Also, in other tissues the effect of the same degree of ATPase inhibition is not very obvious; for example, the liver does not contract, or conduct impulses, so the consequences of digitalis action on it are not very visible. Therefore, therapeutic specificity (relatively speaking) is achieved by keeping the drug concentration finely balanced between limits that give the desired effect on contraction, or on atrioventricular (A-V) bundle conduction, but not the undesired effects on myocardial irritability or on brain or other organs. However, when the drug concentration is a little higher, the same biochemical action in higher degree leads to the toxic effects on myocardial excitability (ectopic foci) and on the nervous system.

A different type of selective vulnerability has been used to deliver the anticancer agent doxorubicin (see Chapter 60) to cancer cells while sparing normal cells. The drug has been encapsulated in **stabilized liposomes,** which are microscopic vesicles of lipids coated with an inert polymer. This coating protects the liposomes from being coated with immunoreactive substances and being taken up by circulating macrophages. Therefore the liposomes remain in circulation for a much longer time than uncoated ones (days rather than minutes). This allows them to reach the tumor, where the capillaries are leakier than those in normal tissue. The liposomes pass through the leaky capillary walls and accumulate in the tumor, where they break down and release the doxorubicin in high local concentration.

INDIVIDUAL AND SPECIES DIFFERENCES IN SPECIFICITY OR SELECTIVITY

In some instances a species may be unusually resistant to a drug because of a unique metabolic trait; for example, the rabbit is very resistant to procaine toxicity because of high serum esterase activity. This is merely a biological curiosity, because rabbits are seldom likely to be exposed to procaine. In other cases, however, selective toxicity (i.e., useful drug action) depends upon differences between two species in the same field of drug exposure. Good examples are provided by bacterial–mammalian and insect–mammalian systems.

Interspecies Differences

Bacteria versus host

The usefulness of **penicillin** as an antibiotic depends upon its structural resemblance to *N*-acetylmuramic acid (NAMA), with which it competes for binding to an enzyme that incorporates the NAMA peptide into external cell walls of bacteria (see Chapters 52 and 53). As the bacteria divide and grow, they must produce new cell-wall material to protect themselves against osmotic rupture because, like all plant cells, they have a high internal osmotic pressure. Animal cells do not have external cell walls and do not require them because their internal osmotic pressure is kept isotonic with that of the extracellular fluid. Therefore, penicillin has little or no effect on animal cells at concentrations that are bactericidal by means of osmotic rupture.

Sulfonamides are bacteriostatic because of another species difference between bacteria and mammals. All cells require folic acid as a constituent of enzyme systems involved in methyl- and formyl-group transfer reactions, which are necessary for nucleic acid synthesis and hence for growth and cell reproduction (see Chapter 56). Mammalian cells require preformed folic acid, i.e., it is a vitamin for them. In contrast, many bacteria cannot take up folate but require its precursors, from which they synthesize the folate intracellularly. One of the precursors is **para-aminobenzoic acid** (PABA). The para-aminobenzenesulfonic acid amides (sulfonamides) act as competitive antagonists of PABA. For other species of bacteria (e.g., leprosy bacilli), a similar role is played by **para-aminobenzene sulfones.**

Trimethoprim acts on a related enzyme, dihydrofolate reductase, to inhibit the conversion of dihydrofolate to tetrahydrofolate. This step occurs in mammalian cells as well as in bacteria, but trimethoprim has many thousands of times as great an affinity for the bacterial enzyme as for the mammalian enzyme. It is also preferentially active against the corresponding enzyme in the malaria parasite.

Insects versus mammals

Sometimes advantage can be taken of a similar species difference in enzyme activities to develop selectively toxic insecticides. **Malathion** is an organophosphate cholinesterase inhibitor that is metabolized in the liver to inactive products. This metabolic inactivation is more rapid in birds and mammals than in insects, so an appropriate concentration can be selected that is toxic to insects but relatively safe for higher species.

Genetic Differences Within Species

There are numerous instances of "selective toxicity" as a result of genetic variations within species, that can be either harmful or beneficial or both. One example is **primaquine** sensitivity. As described in Chapter 12, a hereditary deficiency of glucose-6-phosphate dehydrogenase, which occurs with relatively high frequency in various African and Mediterranean populations, renders the affected individuals selectively sensitive to primaquine-induced hemolytic anemia, but at the same time it makes them more resistant to the growth of malarial parasites in the liver.

Developmental Differences Within Individuals

Both desirable and undesirable drug effects may be selectively favored by metabolic differences found at different developmental stages in the same cell type or individual. Most of this chapter has dealt with specificity or selectivity in relation to therapeutic use of drugs. It is worthwhile to note some instances in which **toxic effects** are favored.

Thalidomide was formerly used widely as a sedative and antiemetic for pregnant women. It is metabolized by hydrolysis of the glutarimide ring, and the resulting metabolite is thought to interfere with an enzyme system that goes through a period of maximum activity in the embryo between the fourth and seventh weeks of its development. Therefore, the drug can cause severe defects in the embryo at that time yet is relatively harmless earlier or later (see Chapter 70).

Similarly, the newborn infant has a deficiency in the glucuronide conjugation system until it reaches several weeks of age (see Chapter 4). During the same period, it undergoes a physiological hemolysis from breakdown of fetal erythrocytes during conversion to extrauterine conditions. The excess hemolysis gives rise to more bilirubin than the conjugation system can cope with, and the extra bilirubin is carried in the plasma, bound to protein. During this period, drugs that compete either for limited capacity to conjugate or for protein binding sites cause overload of the bilirubin-carrying capacity, and free bilirubin passes into the brain and may cause **kernicterus.**

CONCLUSION

All therapeutically useful drug action is based on some degree of selectivity, but this may depend upon various factors related to the drug itself, the person to whom it is given, and the manner of administration. The mechanisms of selectivity determine the margin of safety between desired and undesired effects, as well as the range of clinical applications.

SUGGESTED READING

Albert A. Selective toxicity: the physicochemical basis of therapy. 6th ed. London: Chapman and Hall, 1979.

Anderson JH, Warren HW, McArdle CS. Clinical pharmacokinetic advantages of new drug delivery methods for the treatment of liver tumours. Clin Pharmacokinet 1994; 27:191–201.

Berti JJ, Lipsky JJ. Transcutaneous drug delivery: a practical review. Mayo Clin Proc 1995; 70:581–586.

Cuello AC, ed. Cholinergic function and dysfunction. Prog Brain Res 1993; 98:1–458.

Fisher A, Heldman E, Gurwitz D, et al. Selective signalling via unique M_1 muscarinic agonists. Ann NY Acad Sci 1993; 695:300–303.

Gitler MS, De la Cruz R, Zeeberg BR, Reba RC. [^{3}H]QNB displays in vivo selectivity for the m_2 subtype. Life Sci 1994; 55:1493–1508.

Goldstein A, Aronow L, Kalman SM. Principles of drug action. 2nd ed. New York: Wiley Medical, 1974.

Hansen CB, Kao GY, Moase EH, et al. Attachment of antibodies to sterically stabilized liposomes: evaluation, comparison and optimization of coupling procedures. Biochim Biophys Acta 1995; 1239:133–144.

Konno T. Targeting chemotherapy for hepatoma: arterial administration of anticancer drugs dissolved in Lipiodol. Eur J Cancer 1992; 28:403–409.

Lasic DD. Doxorubicin in sterically stabilized liposomes. Nature 1996; 380:561–562.

Seeman P. Dopamine receptors and psychosis. Sci Am Sci Med 1995; 2(5):28–37.

Symons MC. Polyamines to target drugs to DNA. Free Radic Res 1995; 22:1–9.

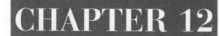

CHAPTER 12

Human Pharmacogenetics

W. KALOW and D. M. GRANT

Pharmacogenetics deals with the influence of heredity on the response to drugs or on their fate in the body. The object of studies in pharmacogenetics is to explain, predict, and control variability in the response to drugs and toxic agents. Although such a definition would in principle include such phenomena as heritable resistance of bacteria to antibiotics and interstrain differences in response to enzyme inducers in mice, this chapter will deal exclusively with human pharmacogenetics, and it will be restricted to matters of clinical relevance. In this context, it is worthwhile noting that the only difference between pharmacogenetic defects and other inborn errors of metabolism is that pharmacogenetic defects tend to be silent in the absence of drug challenge; given the means to detect affected individuals, all of the principles of population genetics are applicable.

Some geneticists use the more general term "ecogenetics" to denote the occurrence of variable responses to any environmental substance, including not only drugs and xenobiotics but also foods and vitamins. However, there are no generally recognized sharp distinctions in terminology. For instance, lactase deficiency, which renders milk an unsuitable nutrient to certain individuals, is considered by some to be an example of pharmacogenetics and by others of ecogenetics. However, although pharmacogenetics is distinct from genetic toxicology (the branch of science concerned with the chemical production of mutations or cytotoxic events), it certainly has the capacity to influence individual risk for the occurrence of such events.

Pharmacogenetics is of special interest for a number of reasons. First, it increases the physician's awareness and anticipation of abnormal drug responses. Second, knowledge of frequently occurring genetic defects that alter drug response will enable drug manufacturers to avoid the introduction of unreliable drugs. Third, genetic defects may be used as experiments of nature to help unravel some mysteries that underlie normal drug responses.

Only an outline of the field can be presented here. This chapter begins with an introduction to classification systems of pharmacogenetics and a brief survey of currently known defects. This will be followed by relatively extensive coverage of a few important examples that have been drawn from the literature on the basis of their clinical importance or because of the level of understanding that has been attained concerning their underlying biochemical and molecular mechanisms.

CORE OF PHARMACOGENETICS AND CLASSIFICATION SYSTEMS

Pharmacogenetics can be subdivided in many different ways.

Functional Subdivision

A recent survey used the following main classifications:

- Disorders characterized by increased sensitivity to drugs
- Therapeutic failures resulting from increased resistance to drugs
- Disorders exacerbated by enzyme-inducing drugs

- Diseases to which chronic drug exposure may contribute
- Disorders of unknown etiology
- Disorders associated with diet
- Reported polymorphisms with clinical disorders not yet demonstrated

Although this is quite cumbersome as a classification scheme, it nevertheless gives an indication of the broad scope of pharmacogenetics. However, in order to develop an understanding of the underlying principles, it is preferable to divide the field on a more systematic basis. Pharmacogenetic disorders may thus be classified along pharmacological and genetic lines (Table 12-1).

Pharmacological Classification

The pharmacological classification distinguishes between alterations in a drug's *pharmacodynamics* (interaction with cellular targets, i.e., drug effect) and alterations in the fate of the drug itself (*pharmacoki-*

Table 12-1 Classification of Pharmacogenetic Defects

Pharmacological

Pharmacokinetic
Mostly affecting drug-metabolizing enzymes; variants tend to have high frequency because variation promotes population survival of toxic catastrophes

Pharmacodynamic
Variation in systems targeted by drugs; the diversity of such systems precludes generalization; monogenic variants of receptors for internal messengers tend to be disease-associated and therefore rare

Genetic

Monogenic
Due to allelic variation at a single gene; measured by counting the carriers of a genetic variant in a population

Multigenic
Due to variations contributed by three or more genes; measured by determining heritability through twin studies

Polymorphic
Frequently occurring monogenic variants; least-common phenotype has a frequency of greater than 1%; planned precautions against adverse reactions are possible

Rare
Infrequently occurring monogenic defects, often unforseeable; a physician always expects the unexpected

netics, usually related to differences in biotransformation).

Genetic Distinctions

The primary genetic classification is between monogenic and multigenic variants.

The observation of monogenic variants, i.e., variants depending on a single gene locus, was the essence of classical genetics and the cradle of much genetic vocabulary. Terms like Mendelian, dominant, recessive, homozygote, heterozygote, and gene frequency all belong only to this part of genetics.

A contrasting aspect of genetic observation is presented by multigenic variation. Many important differences between people are multigenic; i.e., the differences relate to at least three genes, and their combined effects typically allow some environmental influence. A classical example is human adult height, which depends on genetic factors as well as on childhood nutrition.

Monogenic variants

A monogenic variant in pharmacogenetics could be the absence of a particular drug-metabolizing enzyme so that one or another drug is not properly removed from the body. This is typically due to an alteration of the DNA sequence in the gene that codes for this enzyme—in other words, due to an allelic variant of this particular gene. As a consequence, there may be an absence or an alteration of the gene product, the enzyme.

There are mathematical aspects of this kind of variation.

Let us assume there is a functional gene p and a nonfunctional allele q in a given population. This situation may be expressed by the simple equation $(p + q) = 1$. The numerical value of q is referred to as **allele frequency** or gene frequency. As everybody has two versions of each gene (one from the father and one from the mother), any given person may be of genotype pp, pq, or qq; i.e., he or she may be homozygous pp or qq, or heterozygous pq. The **genotype frequencies** in a population are determined by the equation $(p + q)^2 = p^2 + 2pq + q^2$, which is referred to as the Hardy-Weinberg law. For instance, if the allele frequency is $q = 0.1$, it follows that the genotype frequencies are $0.81 + 0.18 + 0.01 = 1$. In words, and using percentages, if 1% of the population carries a double dose of the nonfunctional allele, 18% are heterozygotes with one deficiency gene, and only 81% are fully provided by nature with that enzyme. (Note that the heterozygotes are always more frequent than the rarer of the two homozygotes.) By the widely used definition stated in Table 12-1, this variant is borderline polymorphic.

If the deficiency is functionally evident only in genotype qq, it is recessive; if evident in the heterozygote, it is dominant. If all genotypes are functionally distinguishable, the deficiency is codominant.

Table 12-2 lists prominent examples of monogenic variants in pharmacogenetics. It is not possible to elaborate on all entries, but the list should make it clear that there are many genetically definable causes of aberrant drug responses.

Multigenic variation

Multigenic traits are usually quantitative entities such as stature, IQ, increase in cardiac rate after phenylephrine, or plasma half-life of antipyrine. Usually, environmental factors have a chance of contributing to multigenic traits. Thus, unless a variant is monogenic, it tends to have both environmental and genetic elements. Of these, the genetic component is more readily measured and is defined in terms of heritability. Heritability values in humans are usually derived from studies comparing monozygotic and dizygotic twins. Plasma half-life, clearance, and steady-state concentrations of drugs such as dicoumarol, phenylbutazone, nortriptyline, tolbutamide, and phenytoin generally give heritability values above 50%, even as high as 98% in one set of measurements with antipyrine. Thus there appears to be a substantial element of genetic control in the elimination rate of most drugs that have been investigated properly. However, heritability data in pharmacogenetics are not biological constants, since they are strictly valid only for the population in which they were determined. For example, most of the variation in antipyrine metabolism between nonsmoking healthy adults of the same race and similar eating habits is genetically based, whereas nutrition,

Table 12-2 Monogeneic Traits of Pharmacological or Toxicological Concern*

Variable enzymes of drug biotransformation
†Plasma cholinesterase
  Serum paroxonase
  Monoamine oxidase B
  Catalase
  Alcohol dehydrogenase

Aldehyde dehydrogenase
Dihydropyridine dehydrogenase
Dopamine-β-hydroxylase
Cytochromes P450 and salient substrates:
†CYP1A1—various carcinogens
†CYP2A6—coumarin, nicotine
†CYP2C8—phenytoin
†CYP2C9—warfarin
†CYP2C19—mephenytoin, proguanil
  †CYP2D6—debrisoquin, dextromethorphan
  †CYP2E1—ethanol, solvents
†N-Acetyltransferases (NAT2 and NAT1)
  UDP-glucuronosyl transferase
  Phenol sulfotransferase
  Catechol-O-methyltransferase
  Thiopurine methyltransferase
  Thiol methyltransferase
  Glutathione S-transferase (class μ)

Genes and drug targets
Alterations of enzyme activity or of protein structure as a basis for altered drug responses:
†Hypoxanthine-guanine phosphoribosyltransferase (HGPRT) deficiency or defect (various forms of gout)
†Glucose-6-phosphate dehydrogenase (G-6-PD) deficiencies (hemolytic disorders)
†Malignant hyperthermia (excess Ca^+ release within skeletal muscle fibers due to some anesthetics)
  NADH methemoglobin reductase deficiency (methemoglobinemia)
  Uroporphyrinogen I synthetase deficiency (acute intermittent porphyria)
  Coproporphyrinogen oxidase deficiency (hereditary coproporphyria)
  δ-Aminolevulinic acid synthetase—excessive induction (variegate porphyria)
  Steroid hydroxylase deficiencies (various endocrine vulnerabilities)
  1_α-Hydroxylase of vitamin D precursors—enzyme absence (vitamin D–resistant rickets)
  α_1-Antitrypsin deficiency (emphysema)
  Unstable hemoglobins (various vulnerabilities)

Response differences on a biochemically undefined basis:
  Electroencephalographic differences in alcohol response
  Steroid-induced glaucoma
  Tasting ability for a series of bitter-tasting substances
  Smelling abilities for cyanide, phenylacetic acid, or blossom odors
  Plasma:erythrocyte ratio of lithium
†Diminished receptor occupation of dicumarol-type anticoagulants
†Susceptibility to drug-induced hepatotoxicity demonstrable with lymphocytes in vitro

---

*The purpose of this list is to show the scope of the subject of pharmacogenetics and thereby to lend perspective to the examples (marked †) cited in the text. The porphyrias listed here may all lead to drug-induced, acute neurological crises.

lifestyle, and disease likely contribute substantially to differences in its metabolism among the mixed population attending a large city practice.

SELECTED EXAMPLES OF GENETIC INFLUENCES ON DRUG BIOTRANSFORMATION

Plasma Cholinesterase Variants

A clear example of genetic control of drug metabolism is provided by the cholinesterase variants in human plasma. The most frequent of these variants is called "atypical cholinesterase." The clinically significant cholinesterase variants occur in approximately one in 2000 subjects in Caucasian populations. The plasma cholinesterase is capable of hydrolyzing a number of drugs including cocaine, but its inactivation of the muscle relaxant succinylcholine is of greatest clinical importance. During general anesthesia this drug is given intravenously, and it is therefore immediately and fully exposed to plasma cholinesterase. The fate of the drug thus depends directly on esterase activity. In the presence of atypical cholinesterase, the muscle relaxant action of an ordinary dose of succinylcholine lasts for about an hour instead of only a few minutes (Fig. 12-1).

The biochemical basis of the defect is a very low affinity (i.e., high K_m) of the enzyme for succinylcholine, so the two combine inefficiently (Fig. 12-2). The underlying nucleotide alterations in the cholinesterase gene that lead to the production of the atypical variant and several other mutant forms have recently been defined. However, in spite of these advances the physiological role (if any) of the plasma cholinesterase remains unknown.

Since succinylcholine paralyzes respiratory as well as other muscles, the patient requires artificial respiration until the drug effect wears off. Occasionally there are families with about threefold-higher-than-average cholinesterase activities. In these cases, ordinary doses of succinylcholine have little or no effect.

Acetylation Polymorphism

Genetic control of acetylation was first observed for isoniazid almost 40 years ago, and it has since been shown to affect the elimination of a large number of aromatic amine and hydrazine drugs and environmental chemicals. The capacity for rapid acetylation occurs in families according to a Mendelian pattern

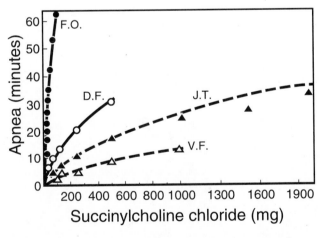

Figure 12-1. Duration of apnea (respiratory muscle paralysis) from succinylcholine administration in four patients with normal and atypical plasma cholinesterase: Patient V.F. has a high level of the usual type of esterase; patient J.T. has a low level of the usual type of esterase; patient D.F. has a mixture of usual and atypical esterase with a preponderance of the atypical one; patient F.O. has atypical esterase. (Adapted from Kalow W. *Pharmacogenetics: Heredity and the Response to Drugs.* Philadelphia/London: WB Saunders, 1962.)

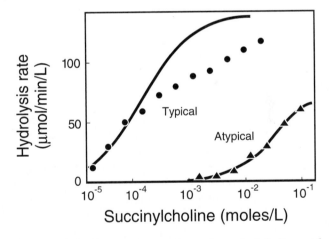

Figure 12-2. In vitro interactions of succinylcholine with plasma cholinesterase, showing the rate of hydrolysis of succinylcholine by human plasma containing either the usual (typical) or the atypical form of the enzyme. For the usual (typical) enzyme, the relation between concentration of drug (dotted curve) and reaction rate (solid curve) grossly deviated from simply theory. Deficient combination between succinylcholine and atypical cholinesterase explains the clinical failure of drug elimination. (Adapted from Kalow W. *Pharmacogenetics: Heredity and the Response to Drugs.* Philadelphia/London: WB Saunders, 1962).

of inheritance with an additive gene dosage effect. As a rule, it can be determined without ambiguity whether a person is a "rapid" or "slow" acetylator, since the blood levels of isoniazid a few hours after intake of a standard dose are four to six times higher in the slow acetylators. Simplified tests for "acetylator phenotype" have been developed which employ measurements of urinary ratios of N-acetylated metabolite to parent drug for compounds including sulfamethazine, dapsone, and, more recently, caffeine. Marked interethnic differences in phenotype frequencies can be observed: Caucasian populations comprise greater than 50% slow acetylators, whereas in Asians (and the genetically related North American indigenous peoples) the proportion of rapid acetylators approaches 90%.

The genetically variable enzyme responsible for producing these phenotypic differences is one of two arylamine N-acetyltransferases (NATs) normally found in significant quantities in the soluble fraction of human liver cells (see Chapter 4). The variable enzyme, known as **NAT2,** catalyzes the N-acetylation of isoniazid and many other drugs (phenelzine, hydralazine, sulfamethazine, sulfapyridine, sulfamethoxazole, procainamide, and dapsone), of drug metabolites (nitrazepam and caffeine), and of several amine carcinogens (benzidine, 2-aminofluorene, 4-aminobiphenyl, and β-naphthylamine). However, the N-acetylation of p-aminobenzoic acid (PABA), p-aminosalicylic acid (PAS), and some of the antibacterial sulfonamides is mediated by the structurally related yet independently expressed **NAT1** enzyme; thus the disposition of such compounds, while potentially also subject to interindividual variation, is unaffected by the classically defined acetylator phenotype. It has recently been shown that both NAT1 and NAT2 are also capable of O-acetylating hydroxylamine metabolites of aromatic amines to produce highly reactive acetoxy esters that can bind covalently to intracellular macromolecules (DNA, proteins) and lead to cellular toxicity or mutations.

Biochemical and molecular genetic studies have demonstrated that defective acetylation in slow acetylators is caused by a marked reduction in the *quantity* of functional NAT2 enzyme protein in the livers of such individuals. Several mutant alleles at the NAT2 gene locus on human chromosome 8 have been cloned and characterized. Each possesses between one and three nucleotide substitutions relative to the so-called "wild-type" (high activity) allele. These mutations may lead to decreased liver NAT2 content, either by reducing translation efficiency of the transcribed mRNA or by decreasing the intrinsic stability of the expressed enzyme. Furthermore,

amino acid substitutions in the expressed protein may decrease its rate of substrate turnover (V_{max}).

A number of adverse drug reactions or diseases associated with acetylator phenotype are summarized in Table 12-3. Although the listed complications are all more frequent in slow acetylators, there are several conceivable instances where the rapid acetylator phenotype may in fact be at greater risk. For example, particularly rapid acetylators may inactivate certain drugs too quickly and be more prone to therapeutic failure at standard doses. In addition, increased formation of reactive metabolites by acetylation, as mentioned above, could lead to a greater occurrence of some types of drug-induced toxicity in rapid acetylators.

Drug Oxidations

The most common forms of drug biotransformation are oxidative reactions of various kinds. Drug-oxidizing enzymes include flavin-containing mono-oxy-

---

Table 12-3 Consequences of Polymorphic Acetylation

Isoniazid (INH)
 Peripheral neuropathy is more common among slow acetylators (and elderly patients)
 Slow acetylators accumulate INH, which in turn inhibits hepatic mixed-function oxidases
 Increased phenytoin toxicity has been described in slow acetylators treated with INH and phenytoin

Hydralazine
 Lupoid reactions are more common among slow acetylators

Procainamide
 Slow acetylators develop lupus earlier and more frequently than fast acetylators

Phenelzine
 Severe adverse reactions (nausea, drowsiness) are more common among slow acetylators

Salicylazosulfapyrimidine
 Side effects of sulfapyrimidine (e.g., hemolysis) are more common among slow acetylators

It has been suggested that a disproportionate number of patients with systemic lupus erythematosus and rheumatoid arthritis are slow acetylators

Occupational bladder cancers in chemical workers were recently reported to have a high prevalence in slow acetylators

An increased incidence of colorectal cancer has been reported in rapid acetylators

genases, alcohol and aldehyde dehydrogenases, xanthine oxidase, and various other oxidoreductases. The most important, however, with respect to the number and variety of drugs affected, are the microsomal mixed-function monooxygenases that have as their terminal element a cytochrome P450 (see Chapter 4). Their reactions have some individually specific features and some characteristics that are common to all. The P450 enzymes are currently subject to intensive investigation at the molecular level. They constitute a superfamily of heme proteins divided into many families on the basis of amino acid sequence similarities, three of which (designated by the nomenclature CYP1, CYP2, and CYP3) are families of drug-metabolizing enzymes. The CYP2 family consists of five subfamilies, which in turn may contain different enzyme proteins. The genes are located on a variety of chromosomes and are expressed independently of each other. Some of these enzymes are constitutive while others are subject to induction, at the level of transcriptional activation, by environmental chemicals.

Clinically, the first evidence for genetically based variation within this system was obtained over 30 years ago when it was observed that intoxication with phenytoin occurred in members of a family that biotransformed this drug by aromatic hydroxylation at an extraordinarily low rate. An equivalent observation was made by Shahidi in a woman in whom large doses of phenacetin had led to substantial methemoglobin formation. The cause of the toxicity was found to be related to an unusual oxidation pathway of phenacetin that produced a methemoglobin-forming metabolite. This unusual pathway predominated because of a familial deficiency in the more common *O*-dealkylation pathway.

A widespread monogenic defect severely affecting the fate of several drugs was first discovered in the late 1970s. The discovery arose from independent studies of two drugs that are metabolized by a P450 now referred to as CYP2D6: (1) In Germany it was found that about 5% of the population was incapable of metabolizing sparteine, an alkaloid with antiarrhythmic and oxytocic properties. In nonmetabolizers, sparteine had a long half-life and accumulated in the body on repeated administration. (2) In an English study of the metabolism of debrisoquin (an antihypertensive drug of the guanethidine class) a severe deficiency of formation of the main metabolite, 4-hydroxydebrisoquin, was found in about 8% of the British population. This explained why the dose of the drug required by different patients during therapy could vary as much as 30-fold. It was later shown that the failures to biotransform sparteine and debrisoquin normally have an identical genetic basis and that the disposition of numerous additional drugs is affected by the same defect (Table 12-4).

Assignment of a given subject to the group of poor or extensive hydroxylators of debrisoquin or

Table 12-4 Drugs Affected by the Debrisoquin/Sparteine Oxidation (CYP2D6) Polymorphism

Antiarrhythmics
Aprindine
Encainide
Flecainide
Mexiletine
N-propylajmaline
Propafenone
Sparteine

β-Adrenoceptor blockers
Alprenolol
Bufuralol
Bunitrolol
Metoprolol
Propranolol
Timolol

Antipsychotics
Haloperidol
Perphenazine
Risperidone
Thioridazine
Zuclopenthixol

Tricyclic antidespressants
Amitriptyline
Clomipramine
Desmethylimipramine
Imipramine
Nortriptyline

Other drugs
Amiflamine
Brofaromine
CGP 15210G
Codeine
Debrisoquin
Dextromethorphan
Guanoxon
Indoramin
Maprotiline
Methoxyamphetamine
Methoxyphenamine
Paroxetine
Perhexiline
Terodiline
Tomoxetine
Tramadol
Tropisetron

sparteine can be achieved by giving a small test dose of either of these two drugs and measuring the ratio of drug and metabolite excreted in urine during the following 8 hours. The use of the cough suppressant dextromethorphan as a safe and widely available alternative for phenotype discrimination has gained wide acceptance in recent years. Inheritance of defective metabolism of these drugs is said to be recessive, since most methods are not sensitive enough to discriminate heterozygous from homozygous extensive metabolizers; poor metabolizers have two copies of defective genes while extensive metabolizers may have one or two functional genes. According to the Hardy-Weinberg law of population genetics, the occurrence of 8% homozygous poor metabolizers in a population implies that 41% of the population are carriers with only half the full enzyme complement. In this sense, the 8% with full-blown deficiency may be like the tip of the iceberg, since clinically significant impairment of drug disposition even in heterozygotes is conceivable.

Biochemical and molecular genetic studies performed in the past decade have provided a wealth of information concerning the mechanisms underlying the debrisoquin/sparteine oxidation defect in humans. It has been determined that the poor metabolizer phenotype is characterized at the protein level in most cases by the absence of a specific isozyme of cytochrome P450, designated as CYP2D6, that is normally encoded from a gene in the CYP2D gene cluster located on human chromosome 22. At the genetic level, cloning and expression studies have so far revealed the existence of nine allelic variants (including wild-type alleles) at the CYP2D gene cluster. A variety of gene mutations, including point mutations in the amino acid coding region, exon/intron splice-site disruptions, and even deletion of the entire CYP2D6 gene have been associated with the poor metabolizer phenotype in human populations.

The potential clinical consequences of defective CYP2D6 function have been widely discussed and debated. For instance, debrisoquin itself is more likely to cause fainting in poor metabolizers because of excessive lowering of blood pressure. Sparteine fell into disuse as an oxytocic agent when it was found that about 7% of women receiving it had severe side effects. In retrospect, it is likely that these 7% were the ones with the oxidation defect. There are also clinical consequences with other drugs listed in Table 12-4. Generally speaking, genetically impaired metabolism of a drug may be clinically important under the following circumstances: (1) The defective meta-

bolic pathway is quantitatively significant in determining the overall fate of the drug in the body. (2) The drug displays a narrow-enough therapeutic range such that alterations in its disposition can lead to drug accumulation to levels above those considered safe. (3) The drug's therapeutic and toxic effects cannot be easily assessed and titrated by clinical monitoring. (4) The drug is widely used in clinical practice. (5) Therapeutic alternatives are limited or absent. Antiarrhythmic agents, β-adrenoceptor antagonists, neuroleptics, and tricyclic antidepressants are among the major therapeutic classes containing currently used drugs that have been claimed to show relevant variations in clinical outcome in patient populations as a result of defective oxidation by CYP2D6.

However, the fate of some drugs is biochemically affected by the CYP2D6 defect, but without any clinically important consequence. The reasons for this may vary. For instance, since the β-adrenoceptor-blocker propranolol undergoes biotransformation by several parallel pathways including oxidation by CYP2D6, other reactions and effective renal elimination can compensate for the CYP2D6 defect. The β-blocker bufuralol, however, is metabolized almost exclusively by CYP2D6, but its metabolite has a similar pharmacological potency; hence the clinical consequences of a defect in metabolite formation are limited.

The biotransformation of quinidine is not noticeably affected by the CYP2D6 defect, but quinidine has a very high affinity for the enzyme and acts as a potent competitive inhibitor of CYP2D6 function. Thus a person receiving quinidine is functionally indistinguishable from a person with genetically defective CYP2D6. Many neuroleptics also cause clinically significant inhibition of CYP2D6. Hence the study of the debrisoquin/sparteine oxidation defect has also revealed and explained a number of drug–drug interactions.

Another polymorphic defect of drug oxidation by a cytochrome P450 isozyme was discovered in the early 1980s and has recently also been investigated at the biochemical and molecular levels. This defect was first shown to impair the 4'-hydroxylation of the S-enantiomer of mephenytoin, an anticonvulsant drug that is now not widely used. However, the metabolism of a number of other currently used drugs is also affected by this defect, including the biguanide antimalarials, omeprazole, diazepam, and some of the barbiturates. About 3–5% of the individuals in Caucasian populations are phenotypically "poor metabolizers" of mephenytoin, while the frequency of this phenotype approaches 20% in Asian populations.

The cytochrome P450 isozyme now known to be affected by the *S*-mephenytoin hydroxylation defect is one of those within the CYP2C subfamily, specifically termed CYP2C19. Livers from individuals of the poor-metabolizer phenotype display reduced levels of CYP2C19 protein in the microsomal fraction. More recently, the molecular defects that produce this phenotype in the majority of cases have been determined for both Caucasian and Asian population groups. A variant gene called *CYP2C19_{m1}*, accounting for about 80% of all defective alleles in both populations, possesses a single-base-pair mutation at the splice junction of exon 5 that produces a premature stop codon. This results in production of a truncated cytochrome P450 protein lacking the necessary heme-binding region that imparts its catalytic function. A second variant allele, *CYP2C19_{m2}*, accounts for the remaining defective genes in Asians but is not present in Caucasians. It also contains a single point mutation that creates a premature stop codon and thus yields a truncated and nonfunctional enzyme.

GENES AND TARGET TISSUES

Genetic control of drug metabolism is only one genetic factor influencing drug response. Many genes confer a special vulnerability or drug resistance on a subject by causing an alteration of a target tissue of a drug. A special category consists of hereditary diseases that include, among other manifestations, altered drug effects. For example, in persons with acute intermittent porphyria, barbiturates may cause fatal paralysis or other neurological dysfunctions; in familial dysautonomia, autonomic stimulants elicit overresponses; in sickle-cell disease, anesthesia or acidifying drugs may provoke a sickling crisis with plugging of capillaries. However, these genetic alterations may give rise to such pathological consequences even in the absence of drugs. In contrast, the following examples concern genes that affect drug response and that have become known *only* because of an abnormal drug response.

Glucose-6-Phosphate Dehydrogenase Deficiency

The most intensively investigated examples have been hemolytic drug reactions related to a deficiency of glucose-6-phosphate dehydrogenase (G-6-PD). The exact mechanism by which G-6-PD deficiency causes red-cell destruction is not established; however, it appears to be related to the cell's inability to maintain the necessary concentration of glutathione in its reduced form. It has been shown that oxidant drugs form H_2O_2 in the red cell and that this oxidizes glutathione. The oxidized disulfide form of glutathione may be attached to hemoglobin. The mixed disulfide-glutathione-hemoglobin complex is unstable and results in hemoglobin changes leading to its oxidation and denaturation (Heinz bodies). These changes result in damage to the erythrocyte membrane and consequent hemolysis.

Approximately 400 million people carry the trait for G-6-PD deficiency, and about 300 enzymic variants are known. All of these variants are inherited as sex-linked traits; many are associated with specific biological sequelae.

There are several variants that are classified as "normal," one variant with increased enzymatic activity, and some variants which cause such severe deficiencies of activity that they lead to hemolytic disease even in the absence of drugs. The role of drugs has been most closely investigated with respect to two G-6-PD types, one being the so-called A⁻ variant in black Americans, and the second, the Mediterranean variant. The A⁻ variant is an unstable enzyme. Young erythrocytes have about the normal level of enzyme activity, but the activity diminishes more rapidly than normal during the lifespan of the red cell. Drug-induced hemolytic reactions are, therefore, self-limited because they cease once the older erythrocytes have been eliminated. The Mediterranean variant conveys a low G-6-PD activity even in young erythrocytes. As a consequence, hemolytic crises when they occur are much more severe, since they do not tend to be self-limiting. A number of agents (e.g., quinine, acetylsalicylic acid) in high doses have caused hemolysis in the presence of the Mediterranean G-6-PD deficiency while they do not do so in the A⁻ variant (Table 12-5). The Canton variant has been shown to be similar to the Mediterranean variant.

The different frequencies of G-6-PD deficiency in different populations are determined by elements of Darwinian selection. G-6-PD deficiency favors survival by increasing resistance to *Plasmodium falciparum* malaria (see Chapters 11 and 57), a factor beneficial only in countries where malaria is endemic, so the gene tends to accumulate in such countries. For several, but not all, variants the main lethal factor is icterus neonatorum (jaundice of the newborn).

Table 12-5 Drugs That May Cause Hemolysis in G-6-PD–Deficient Subjects

Aminoquinolines
  Primaquine
  Pamaquin
  Chloroquine
  Pentaquine

Sulfones
  Dapsone
  Sulfoxone
  Thiazosulfone

Sulfonamides
  Sulfanilamide
  Sulfacetamide
  Sulfafurazole
  Sulfisoxazole
  Sulfamethoxypyridazine
  Salicylazosulfapyridine

Nitrofurans
  Nitrofurantoin
  Furazolidine
  Nitrofurazone

Analgesics
  Acetylsalicylic acid
  Phenacetin (acetophenetidin)
  Acetanilid

Miscellaneous Agents
  Vitamin K (water-soluble analogs)
  Naphthalene (moth balls)
  Probenecid
  Dimercaprol (BAL)
  Methylene blue
  Acetylphenylhydrazine
  Phenylhydrazine
  p-Aminosalicylic acid
  Nalidixic acid
  Neoarsphenamine
  Quinine   } Not shown to
  Quinidine   } be hemolytic
  Chloramphenicol } in blacks

Susceptibility to Drug-Induced Hepatotoxicity Demonstrable with Lymphocytes in Vitro

When a patient presents with a possible idiosyncratic reaction to a drug, such as hepatotoxicity, several questions immediately arise: (1) Are the patient's symptoms indeed caused by the drug? (2) If so, what is the pathophysiology of the toxic reaction? (3) Why did this patient among thousands of exposed individuals suffer a side effect? (4) Is susceptibility to such toxicity inherited? In order to answer questions about drug toxicity experimentally in humans, it is necessary first to have a testable hypothesis on biochemical mechanisms of altered susceptibility and then an assay to assess individual differences in susceptibility that does not expose patients to further drug-related risk.

For example, phenytoin is associated in rare cases with a complex clinical syndrome including fever, skin rash, lymphadenopathy, and hepatotoxicity. It has been postulated that the toxicity is mediated by a reactive arene oxide (epoxide) metabolite of this drug. Lymphocytes from patients who experienced phenytoin hepatotoxicity have shown increased toxicity from arene oxide metabolites of phenytoin in vitro. Furthermore, cells from relatives of the patients also exhibited abnormal dose-response curves to these metabolites, with a family pattern suggestive of an autosomal recessive trait. The data suggest that susceptibility to phenytoin hepatotoxicity is based on a genetically determined deficiency in the detoxification of certain types of reactive metabolites. The biochemical basis of the defect remains to be determined. Such in vitro studies can help significantly in the diagnosis and prediction of idiosyncratic reactions and in determination of their pharmacogenetic basis.

Malignant Hyperthermia

Malignant hyperthermia is a puzzling but rare reaction that usually was fatal until relatively recently. It is a complication of general anesthesia and it occurs on the basis of a genetic predisposition. Failure of muscles to relax after succinylcholine, and an unexplained tachycardia, often herald the onset. There is a rise of body temperature, which rapidly can reach extreme values. In most cases, there is rigidity of some or most skeletal muscles. During the episode, muscle enzymes and proteins are released into the plasma. There is profound hypoxia and metabolic and respiratory acidosis, and the plasma potassium level rises. Early death is often due to cardiac failure, while delayed death may be due to renal failure as a consequence of myoglobinemia.

The cause of the condition is an unusual effect of halothane or other general anesthetics on skeletal muscle. This was proven by pharmacological tests: Muscle biopsy samples obtained from survivors reveal high in vitro susceptibility of the muscle to caffeine-induced contracture, and this caffeine effect is potentiated and partially mimicked by halothane

(Fig. 12-3). The caffeine effect requires high concentrations that could not occur in vivo and thus is strictly a diagnostic tool. Caffeine is known to affect intracellular calcium metabolism by enhancing calcium-induced calcium release from the sarcoplasmic reticulum of muscle cells. Halothane may initiate the hyperthermic attack during anesthesia by causing calcium release as does caffeine, but it has a different though unknown mode of action. The increased calcium concentration in the sarcoplasm can be expected to have a number of biochemical effects, such as increasing ATPase activity by actomyosin, the reticulum, and the mitochondria. Muscular contracture and a hypermetabolic state with lactic acidosis are the consequences, and the resulting huge increase in heat production probably explains the sharp rise in body temperature.

Early recognition of the attack, speedy termination of surgery and anesthesia, cooling of the patient, and correction of the acidosis are among the indicated measures. Intravenous infusion of the muscle relaxant dantrolene has saved lives by terminating the attack.

Malignant hyperthermia also occurs in pigs. The porcine defect has been identified and located within the giant protein, the "ryanodine receptor," which contains the calcium-release channel of the sarcoplasmic reticulum. Thus molecular techniques allow agricultural screening for affected pigs. Humans with a predisposition to malignant hyperthermia sometimes have the same mutation as do affected pigs. However, malignant hyperthermia in humans appears to be genetically heterogeneous, and diagnosis of the predisposition must at present still rely on the formally standardized caffeine-halothane contracture tests using biopsy specimens of skeletal muscle.

Hypoxanthine-Guanine Phosphoribosyltransferase Deficiency

Allopurinol, an analog of hypoxanthine, is used for the treatment of gout. It ameliorates the disease by two different biochemical mechanisms. First, it inhibits the conversion of hypoxanthine and xanthine to uric acid by the enzyme xanthine oxidase; and second, it decreases de novo purine biosynthesis. In some persons with gout, the second effect is absent, and this absence can be correlated with a deficiency of an enzyme called hypoxanthine-guanine phosphoribosyltransferase (total HGPRT deficiency = Lesch-Nyhan syndrome).

Diminished Receptor Occupation of Bishydroxycoumarin-Type Anticoagulants

Another example of decreased drug effect on the basis of alteration of the drug target is the resistance to warfarin in some families. In these cases, it takes 20 times the normal dose to produce the usual therapeutic effect. The biochemical mechanism is likely a diminished affinity of the drug receptor for the anticoagulant (Fig. 12-4). An abnormally rapid metabolic inactivation of the drug is not the cause, although this could conceivably also create a similar drug resistance.

Marker Genes and Drug Response

An example of a completely different nature illustrating the interaction of genes and drugs has been established by statistical means. Women of blood groups A, B, and AB who take oral contraceptives are three times as likely to develop thrombosis as women of blood group O (Table 12-6). This information has not led to any change in use of contraceptive pills. After all, even the relatively greater risk of thrombosis due to the pill associated with blood groups A, B, and AB is small compared to the risks

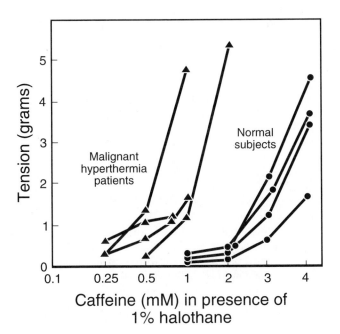

Figure 12-3. Caffeine contracture of muscles biopsied from normal subjects and from malignant hyperthermia patients. (Adapted from Kalow W, Britt BA, Terreau ME, Haist C. *Lancet* 1970; II:895.)

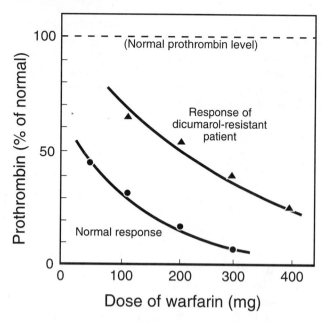

Figure 12-4. Prothrombin responses in normal and dicumarol-resistant patients. (Adapted from O'Reilly RA, Aggeler PM, Hoag MS, Leong LS, Kropatkin ML. *N Engl J Med* 1964; 271:809.)

due to pregnancy and childbirth. However, this study has led to numerous investigations that yield new insights into the puzzling role of the blood-group antigens.

It is certainly not claimed or believed that there

is an immediate and direct interaction between contraceptives and blood-group antigens; more likely there is a complicated series of interrelated events. The significance of this observation lies in the fact that an unexpected genetic risk factor related to a drug effect has been empirically identified and quantitatively evaluated. If numerous such risk factors were known, whether genetic, pathological, or environmental, it might be possible to estimate the clinically significant risks of specific drugs for a given person and thereby improve rational and safe drug therapy.

Some of the specific examples quoted above may be rare, but abnormal drug reactions as a whole are not rare, and many must occur unrecognized. It is clear that genetic factors in such reactions are surprisingly diverse and cannot be neglected in the assessment of drug therapies and iatrogenic disease.

SUGGESTED READING

Balant LP, Gundert-Remy U, Boobis AR, et al. Relevance of genetic polymorphism in drug metabolism in the development of new drugs. Eur J Clin Pharmacol 1989; 36:551–554.

Beutler E. The genetics of glucose-6-phosphate dehydrogenase deficiency. Semin Hematol 1990; 27:137–164.

Beutler E. The molecular biology of G6PD variants and other red cell enzyme defects. Annu Rev Med 1992; 43:47–59.

Britt BA. Malignant hyperthermia—a review. In: Schönbaum E, Lomax P, eds. Thermoregulation: pathology, pharmacology and therapy. New York: Pergamon Press, 1991: 179–292.

Dreyer M, Rudiger HW. Genetic defects of human receptor function. Trends Pharmacol Sci 1988; 9:98–102.

Goldstein J, de Morais S. Biochemistry and molecular biology of the CYP2C subfamily. Pharmacogenetics 1994; 4:285–299.

Gonzalez FJ, Meyer UA. Molecular genetics of the debrisoquine-sparteine polymorphism. Clin Pharmacol Ther 1991; 50:233–238.

Grant DM. Molecular genetics of the N-acetyltransferases. Pharmacogenetics 1993; 3:45–50.

Kalow W. Interethnic variation of drug metabolism. Trends Pharmacol Sci 1991; 12:102–107.

Kalow W, ed. Pharmacogenetics of drug metabolism. New York: Pergamon Press, 1992; 897 pages.

Kalow W, Grant D. Pharmacogenetics. In: Scriver C, Beaudet A, Sly W, Valle D, eds. The metabolic and molecular bases of inherited disease. New York: McGraw-Hill, 1995:293–326.

La Du BN, Bartels CF, Nogueira CP, et al. Proposed nomenclature for human butyrylcholinesterase genetic variants identified by DNA sequencing. Cell Mol Neurobiol 1991; 11:79–89.

Table 12-6 Distribution of Blood Groups, and Frequency of Thromboembolism with Oral Contraceptives

	Blood Groups	
	A + B + AB	O
Number of persons per hundred population:		
Boston	53	47
Sweden	60	40
United Kingdom	54	46
Number of women on oral contraceptives with thromboembolism:		
Boston	46	9
Sweden	49	10
United Kingdom	55	17

After Jick H, Slone D, Westerholm B, et al. *Lancet* 1969; I:539.

MacLennan DH, Phillips MS. Malignant hyperthermia. Science 1992; 256:789–794.

Meyer UA. Molecular genetics and the future of pharmacogenetics. In: Kalow W, ed. Pharmacogenetics of drug metabolism. New York: Pergamon Press, 1992: 879–888.

Nebert DW, Gonzalez FJ. P450 genes: structure, evolution, and regulation. Annu Rev Biochem 1987; 56:945–993.

Spielberg S. Pharmacogenetics: from scientific curiosity to a central theme in drug development and therapeutics. Can J Clin Pharmacol 1995; 2:54–56.

Spielberg SP, Gordon GB, Blake DA, Goldstein DA, Herlong HF. Predisposition to phenytoin hepatotoxicity assessed in vitro. N Engl J Med 1981; 4:959–965.

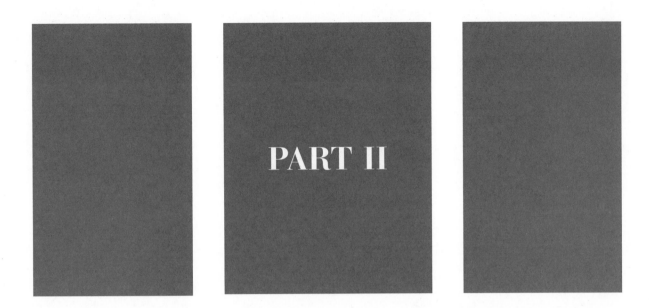

PART II

AUTONOMIC NERVOUS SYSTEM AND NEUROMUSCULAR JUNCTION

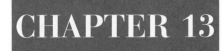

CHAPTER 13

Autonomic Nervous System Neurotransmitters

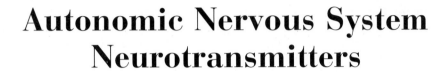

C. FORSTER

Modern concepts of neurohumoral transmission began to emerge almost a century ago, with the discovery by Langley in 1901 that injection of adrenal extracts stimulated sympathetic nerves. It is now known that nerve impulses are transmitted across synapses and neuroeffector junctions, in all parts of the nervous system, by specific chemicals released at axon terminals. The autonomic nervous system consists of all efferent axons leaving the central nervous system, other than those innervating skeletal muscle. They can regulate many physiological activities that are mainly involuntary and not under conscious control. The autonomic nervous system plays a major role in the maintenance of homeostasis in the body; i.e., it controls the steady states of the internal environment by coordinating physiological processes. It regulates the rate and force of contraction of the heart, the caliber of blood vessels, and the muscle tone in the gastrointestinal tract, genitourinary tracts, and bronchioles. It adjusts accommodation of the eye for near and distant vision, and it controls pupil size. It can also modify the secretions of both exocrine and endocrine glands.

Autonomic pharmacology can be defined as the study of those drugs that act either on the autonomic neurons or on receptors in the membranes of target organ cells that are controlled by the autonomic nervous system. Practical examples are pharmacotherapy of hypertension, bronchial asthma, angina pectoris, and many central nervous system disorders (e.g., depression and Parkinson's disease). The drugs may act directly or indirectly on receptors of the system, either to excite or inhibit, or they act indirectly upon the central control or peripheral release of neurotransmitters. In order to understand the selective actions of drugs on the autonomic nervous system, it is essential to have an understanding of its anatomy and physiology. The actions of an autonomic agent can often be predicted if the responses to nerve stimulation are known.

ANATOMY OF THE AUTONOMIC NERVOUS SYSTEM

The autonomic nervous system is composed of control centers located within the central nervous system (CNS) and a peripheral network of afferent and efferent nerves. The hypothalamus is the main locus of integration of this system, but there are other important control centers—for example, in the medulla oblongata—and there are coordinating centers that form the limbic system. The various control centers, however, are not purely autonomic, and there are no important physiological differences between visceral and somatic afferent (sensory) fibers. By convention, the term "autonomic nervous system" is used only in reference to the efferent (motor) neurons supplying the peripheral effector organs. The efferent autonomic nervous system has its origin in nerve cell bodies within the CNS, which give rise to preganglionic fibers (usually myelinated) that are outside the CNS. These synapse in peripheral ganglia with the cell bodies from which the nonmyelinated postganglionic fibers originate that innervate the effector organs.

Structurally and functionally, the autonomic nervous system is further divided into sympathetic and parasympathetic systems. The main pathways of autonomic innervation are shown schematically in Figure 13-1.

In the **sympathetic division** the cells of origin lie in the lateral horns of the thoracic and lumbar portions of the spinal cord, from T-1 to L-3. There are two major groups of sympathetic ganglia—namely, the paravertebral ganglia that lie in a chain close to and on each side of the vertebral column (sympathetic trunk) and the prevertebral ganglia that lie in the abdomen at some distance from the vertebrae (e.g., the celiac ["solar plexus"] and mesenteric ganglia). The adrenal medulla resembles a sympathetic ganglion in that it is innervated by typical preganglionic fibers and is also functionally, anatomically, and embryologically related to the sympathetic ganglia.

The **parasympathetic division** comprises the craniosacral outflow of the autonomic nervous system. The cells of origin are located in the lower brainstem (midbrain and medulla oblongata) and in the sacral portion of the spinal cord from S-2 to S-4. In contrast to the sympathetic ganglia, the parasympathetic ganglia are located very close to, on, or within the innervated organs (e.g., the heart and gastrointestinal tract).

There are important exceptions to most generalizations about autonomic innervation. Nevertheless, in general, sympathetic preganglionic fibers tend to synapse with large numbers of postganglionic fibers; parasympathetic, with few. Sympathetic postganglionic fibers tend to have diffuse distributions, while parasympathetic distribution is more limited and discrete.

There is no true synapse between postganglionic autonomic nerves and their effector organs. The nerve terminals have a characteristic bead-like appearance, the beads or "varicosities" being the sites at which neurotransmitter is released. The released neurotransmitter diffuses 200–1000 Å to reach the effector cell, and effector cells may be simultaneously under the influence of neurotransmitters originating from more than one type of nerve terminal.

PHYSIOLOGY OF THE AUTONOMIC NERVOUS SYSTEM

Most organs are innervated and controlled by both sympathetic and parasympathetic nerves. There are, however, organs that are innervated and controlled by only one division of the autonomic nervous system.

In organs with both sympathetic and parasympathetic nervous control, the effects of the two divisions are usually opposite (e.g., in the heart, bronchi, gastrointestinal tract, bladder, and eye). Both systems are normally active at all times. This basal rate of activity is referred to as sympathetic tone or parasympathetic tone. Thus, the level of function usually depends upon the balance between the tonic activities of two opposing innervations. In certain organs, such as the heart and intestines, there is also an intrinsic control that persists even when the dual external control by the autonomic nervous system is absent. The parasympathetic and sympathetic nerves can override and adjust the activity of the organ to a level above or below that established by the intrinsic mechanisms.

While many organs have dual innervation of individual cells, in some instances the opposing effects of the sympathetic and parasympathetic divisions arise from the fact that they innervate different and functionally opposing cells. In the iris of the eye, for example, the parasympathetic fibers control mainly the circular muscles while the sympathetic fibers control mainly the radial muscles. As a result, increased parasympathetic tone causes constriction of the pupil, and increased sympathetic tone causes dilatation.

In a few organs with dual autonomic control, such as the salivary glands, the effects of the sympathetic and parasympathetic divisions are believed to be complementary. For example, parasympathetic stimulation increases the secretion of the water, electrolyte, and enzyme components of saliva, whereas sympathetic stimulation increases secretion of the mucinous components.

Each division of the autonomic nervous system can exert either an inhibitory or an excitatory effect upon a given organ. The effect upon a particular organ is determined by the characteristic responses of the effector cells in that organ. In many cases, all the cells respond in the same manner; however, in the intestine, the smooth muscle cells of the outer muscular layers relax in response to sympathetic impulses, whereas those of the sphincters contract. Arteriolar smooth muscle provides examples of three possible responses related to the location of the vessel. Sympathetic impulses cause constriction of the arterioles in the skin and viscera, but dilatation of some vessels, particularly in skeletal muscle, and essentially no effect on cerebral arterioles.

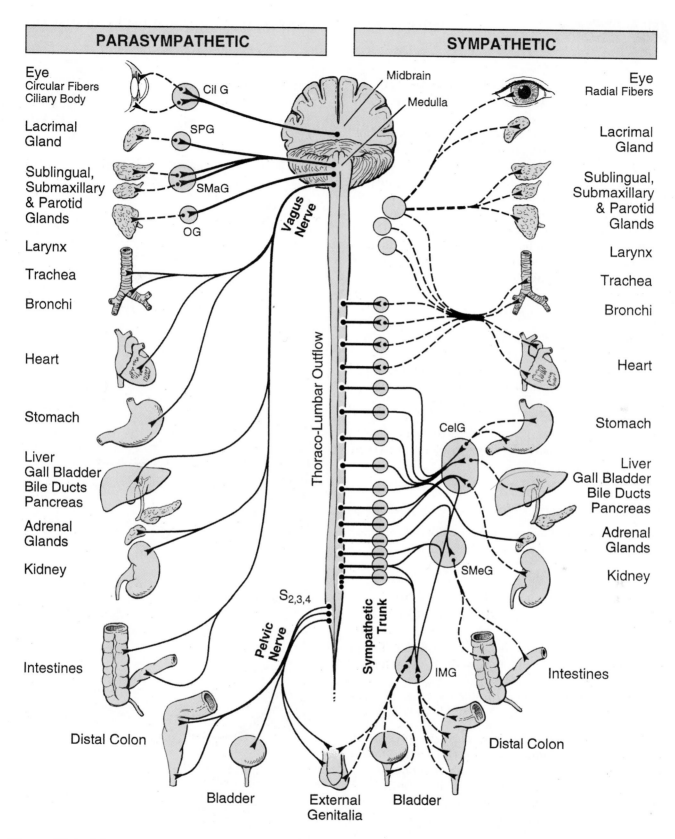

PARASYMPATHETIC

Eye
Circular Fibers
Ciliary Body

Lacrimal
Gland

Sublingual,
Submaxillary
& Parotid
Glands

Larynx

Trachea

Bronchi

Heart

Stomach

Liver
Gall Bladder
Bile Ducts
Pancreas

Adrenal
Glands

Kidney

Intestines

Distal Colon

Bladder

External
Genitalia

Cil G

SPG

SMaG

OG

Vagus Nerve

Pelvic Nerve

S₂,₃,₄

SYMPATHETIC

Midbrain

Medulla

Eye
Radial Fibers

Lacrimal
Gland

Sublingual,
Submaxillary
& Parotid
Glands

Larynx

Trachea

Bronchi

Heart

Stomach

Liver
Gall Bladder
Bile Ducts
Pancreas

Adrenal
Glands

Kidney

Intestines

Distal Colon

Bladder

Thoraco-Lumbar Outflow

Sympathetic Trunk

CelG

SMeG

IMG

Figure 13-1. Schematic representation of the principal pathways by which organs of the body receive parasympathetic and sympathetic innervation. CelG = celiac ganglion; CilG = ciliary ganglion; IMG = inferior mesenteric ganglion; OG = otic ganglion; SMaG = submaxillary ganglion; SMeG = superior mesenteric ganglion; SPG = sphenopalatine ganglion.

TRANSMISSION OF IMPULSES IN THE AUTONOMIC NERVOUS SYSTEM

All preganglionic fibers store and release acetylcholine (ACh) as a chemical transmitter. The postganglionic fibers store and release either acetylcholine or norepinephrine. Both epinephrine and norepinephrine (known in the United Kingdom, Australia, and many other countries as adrenaline and noradrenaline, respectively) are released from chromaffin cells in the adrenal medulla. Fibers in the autonomic nervous system are therefore either cholinergic or adrenergic, depending on which transmitter is released by the particular fiber (Fig. 13-2).

Cholinergic Fibers, Releasing Acetylcholine

1. Preganglionic fibers to all ganglia in the autonomic nervous system and to the adrenal medulla
2. Postganglionic parasympathetic fibers to effector organs
3. Postganglionic sympathetic fibers to sweat glands, and a few sympathetic fibers to blood vessels in skeletal muscle

Adrenergic Fibers, Releasing Norepinephrine

All other postganglionic sympathetic fibers to effector organs.

WHAT ARE THE CRITERIA FOR NEUROHUMORAL TRANSMISSION?

A set of general criteria must be satisfied before a particular substance can be classified as a neurotransmitter.

These criteria apply throughout the nervous system.

1. *Transmitter substances must be present in nerve fibers, particularly the presynaptic terminals, and must be released from there on stimulation.*

A substance that is present in the brain or the spinal cord is not necessarily located in neurons. Nonneural elements (the neuroglia) outnumber neurons about tenfold and may well contain active substances. The fact that an active substance is liberated (usually under nonphysiological conditions) does not provide true evidence for its postulated transmitter status. The latter becomes more likely if it can be

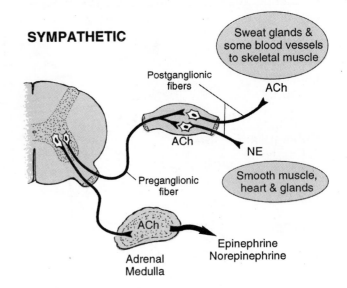

SYMPATHETIC

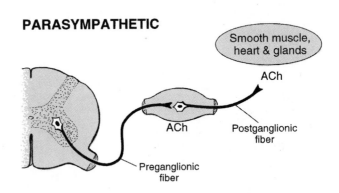

PARASYMPATHETIC

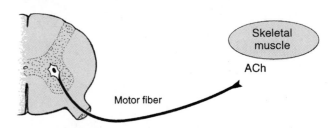

MOTOR (SOMATIC)

Figure 13-2. Classification of autonomic innervation, sites of impulse transmission, and type of transmitter substance. Somatic innervation shown for comparison. ACh = acetylcholine; NE = norepinephrine.

shown that the amount released by stimulation at a physiological intensity is adequate to stimulate or inhibit neighboring neurons or effector cells.

2. *Exogenous application of the presumed transmitter substance to a neuron must produce changes in the neuron that are characteristic of those that occur when it is excited or inhibited by physiological stimuli.*

3. *The pharmacological actions of the putative transmitter and of substances that interact with it must be consistent with its presumed transmitter function (i.e., interaction of agonists and antagonists).*

4. *All enzymes responsible for the synthesis and degradation of the substance must be present in the relevant neurons.*

AUTONOMIC CHOLINERGIC TRANSMISSION

Biosynthesis of Acetylcholine

Acetylcholine is synthesized in the terminals of cholinergic nerves (Fig. 13-3). Acetyl coenzyme A (readily available within the cytoplasm) and choline (transported into the nerve terminal from the syn-apse, as well as from cytoplasmic sources) undergo an acetyl transfer reaction, catalyzed by the enzyme choline acetyltransferase, to form acetylcholine, which is simultaneously transported into vesicles within the nerve terminal varicosities. Each vesicle contains approximately 10,000 molecules of acetylcholine. It is not certain whether all neuronal acetylcholine is packaged within these vesicles, but it is clear that the acetylcholine released from the nerve terminal derives from the vesicles. When the turnover of acetylcholine is high, the transport of choline into the nerve terminal can become the rate-limiting step. Also, for reasons unclear, the most recently synthesized acetylcholine is likely to be the first to be released on stimulation. The vesicles also contain a specific protein called vesiculin, and adenosine triphosphate (ATP).

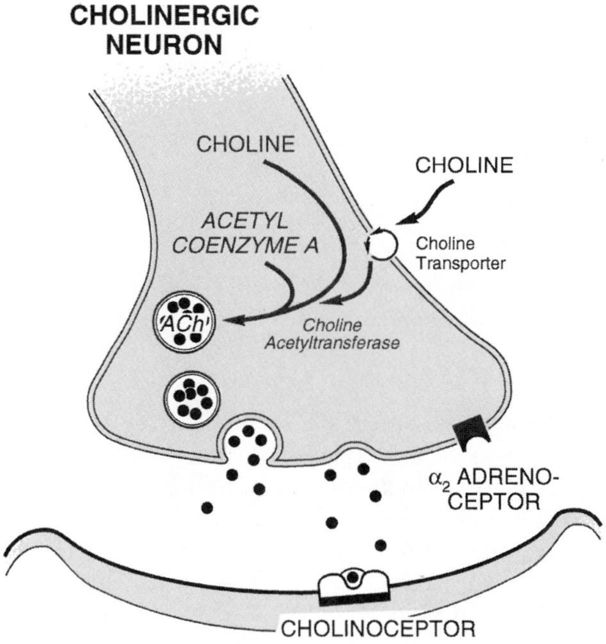

Release of Acetylcholine

When an action potential arrives in the nerve terminal, the vesicles migrate to the nerve varicosity membrane, fuse with it, open to the synaptic cleft, and release their contents (acetylcholine, vesiculin, and ATP). The vesicle is subsequently re-formed by invagination and sealing off of the membrane and moves back into the nerve terminal where it can be replenished with new acetylcholine.

Breakdown of Released Acetylcholine and Choline Reuptake

Acetylcholine is broken down extremely rapidly by the specific enzyme, acetylcholinesterase, which occurs in high concentrations wherever acetylcholine acts as a neurotransmitter, i.e., on both pre- and postganglionic membranes within the autonomic ganglia, on the membranes of parasympathetic nerve terminals, and on pre- and postsynaptic membranes of neuromuscular junctions. Low concentrations are also found in adrenergic neurons. The action of the enzyme begins immediately on release of the transmitter, and 90% of the acetylcholine released may be hydrolyzed before it reaches the postsynaptic membrane, and hence the receptor, to produce the biological effect.

Acetic acid, which is produced during hydrolysis, is rapidly removed into various biochemical pathways (e.g., the Krebs cycle) within the cytoplasm. The choline is actively transported back into the nerve terminal where it can be used to resynthesize acetylcholine.

Figure 13-3. Biosynthesis of acetylcholine (ACh) in cholinergic neurons. Presynaptic α_2-adrenoceptors are found in only some cholinergic neurons (see Table 13-2).

AUTONOMIC ADRENERGIC TRANSMISSION

Biosynthesis of Catecholamines

The neurotransmitter in sympathetic postganglionic nerves is usually norepinephrine. Norepinephrine and its immediate precursor, dopamine, are also found in certain brain areas where they act as neurotransmitters. Epinephrine is produced from norepinephrine in the chromaffin cells of the adrenal medulla and may also be present in some areas of the brain. The primary precursor for the catecholamine biosynthetic pathway is the amino acid L-tyrosine, which is actively transported from the blood into the adrenergic neuron cell bodies and the chromaffin cells. In the cytoplasm of the adrenergic neuron, L-tyrosine is converted to L-dopa (dihydroxyphenylalanine) by the enzyme tyrosine hydroxylase. This is the rate-limiting step in the biosynthesis of catecholamines (see Figs. 13-4 and 13-5). The essential requirements for tyrosine hydroxylase activation are a tetrahydropteridine cofactor, oxygen, and ferrous ion (Fe^{2+}).

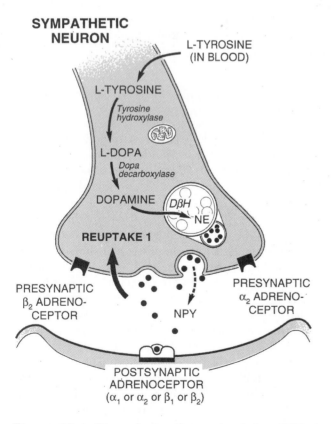

Figure 13-4. Biosynthesis of norepinephrine (NE) in sympathetic nerve terminals. DβH = dopamine-β-hydroxylase; NPY = neuropeptide Y.

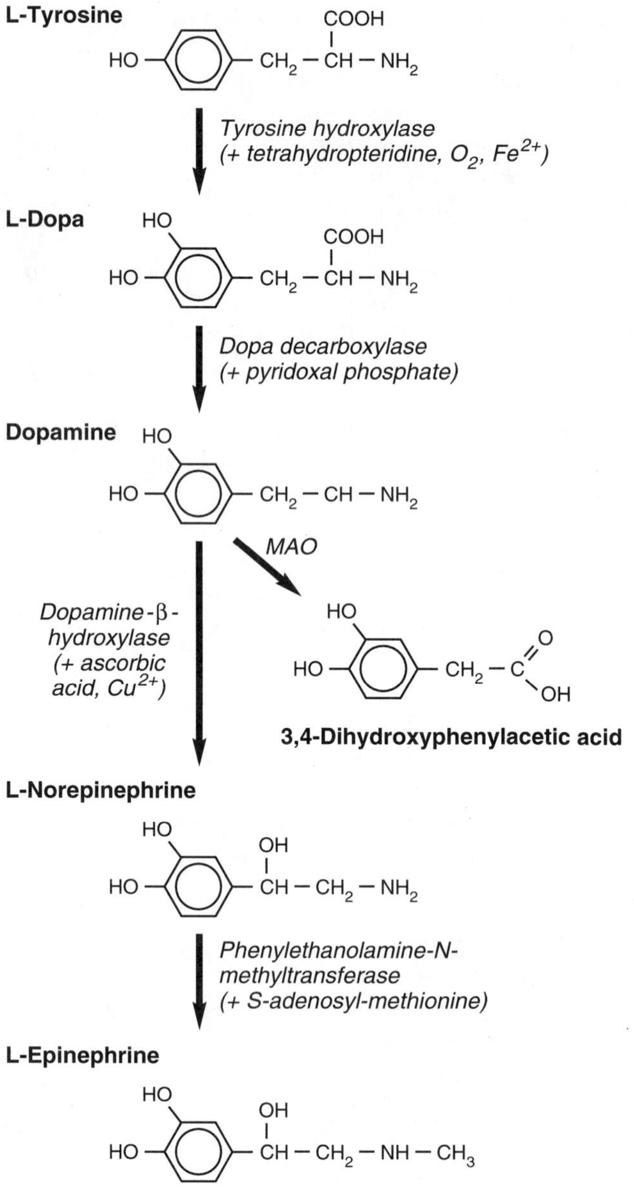

Figure 13-5. Biosynthesis of catecholamines. Essential cofactors shown in parentheses.

L-Dopa is the substrate for another cytoplasmic enzyme, dopa decarboxylase (L-aromatic amino acid decarboxylase), which converts it to dopamine (dihydroxyphenylethylamine). This particular enzyme exhibits a broad substrate specificity. For example, it can produce 5-hydroxytryptamine from 5-hydroxytryptophan. In addition, dopa decarboxylase can convert α-methyldopa to α-methyldopamine, which in turn forms α-methylnorepinephrine, a "false" neurotransmitter. The essential cofactor for the enzyme is pyridoxal phosphate. Once formed, dopamine is either actively taken up by storage vesicles within the nerve terminal or deaminated to 3,4-dihydroxy-phenylacetic acid. In the vesicles, dopamine is converted to norepinephrine by the action of dopamine-β-hydroxylase (DβH). The essential cofactors for DβH are ascorbic acid and cuprous ion (Cu^{2+}; see Fig. 13-5).

Each progressive step in the conversion of L-tyrosine to norepinephrine has been evaluated by using known inhibitors of the various enzymes (Table 13-1). Norepinephrine itself also inhibits the conversion of L-tyrosine to L-dopa by a negative-feedback mechanism involving competition with the tetrahydropteridine cofactor. This process of "end-product" inhibition controls the rate of its own synthesis and also that of dopamine. During increased sympathetic neuronal activity, end-product inhibition is decreased and the synthesis of norepinephrine is enhanced.

In the adrenal medulla, norepinephrine is methylated in the cytoplasm by the enzyme phenylethanolamine-N-methyltransferase (PNMT) to form epinephrine. The rate of synthesis of epinephrine in the chromaffin cells is dependent on glucocorticoids secreted by the adrenal cortex, which are carried in high concentrations directly to the chromaffin cells of the adrenal medulla, where they induce PNMT. In the adult human, epinephrine accounts for approximately 80% of the catecholamines of the adrenal medulla.

Storage of Norepinephrine and Epinephrine

The most important sites for storage of norepinephrine are in granular vesicles, which are highly concentrated in the varicosities of the nerve terminals. There is evidence to suggest that storage vesicles are actually formed in the cell bodies of the neurons and

carried down the length of the axon to the terminal varicosities.

Norepinephrine stored in high concentrations in these granules forms a molecular complex with ATP in a ratio of 4:1 (norepinephrine:ATP). The granules also contain specific proteins (chromogranins) as well as DβH and dopamine. Norepinephrine is also present in free form outside the ATP complex, with which it is in tight equilibrium. Outside the granule there is some free cytoplasmic norepinephrine that probably plays a role in the regulation of synthesis by means of end-product inhibition. There is also evidence that neuropeptide Y (NPY) is released together with norepinephrine and acts as a cotransmitter. The ratio of released NPY to norepinephrine differs in different pathological states and may, therefore, be a key regulator in various pathophysiological events.

Within the granules, norepinephrine is present in at least two different metabolic pools (I and II). Pool I contains material with a rapid turnover: It probably functions as the neurotransmitter. Pool II turns over slowly and contains material of limited physiological significance. An active transport system exists within the granule, helping to maintain a concentration gradient for norepinephrine. This transport system can concentrate norepinephrine against a 200-fold gradient across the granular membrane, and ATP and magnesium are essential for its optimal activity. The transport mechanism is sensitive to the action of certain drugs, such as reserpine (see Chapter 18).

In the chromaffin cells, most of the norepinephrine leaves the granules and is methylated in the cytoplasm to epinephrine, which then reenters the storage granules until released.

Release of Catecholamines

When a nerve impulse is propagated along the postganglionic adrenergic neuron, it releases norepinephrine from the storage granules by exocytosis. The entire contents are released following fusion of the granule membrane with that of the neuronal membrane. A similar process for epinephrine release occurs in the adrenal medulla.

Following norepinephrine release, most (approximately 80%, depending on the size of the synaptic cleft) is retrieved by reuptake (named uptake 1, an L-norepinephrine active-transport mechanism across the axonal membrane) from the synapse into the cytoplasmic pool (see Fig. 13-6). Further active transport occurs against a high concentration gradient from the cytoplasm into the storage granules. This is the most important mechanism by which the

Table 13-1 Inhibitors of Enzymes Involved in the Biosynthesis of L-Dopa, Dopamine, and Norepinephrine

Enzyme	Inhibitor
Tyrosine hydroxylase	Alpha-methyl-p-tyrosine Norepinephrine and dopamine (negative-feedback mechanism)
L-Aromatic amino acid decarboxylase (dopa decarboxylase)	α-Methyldopa Benserazide (RO4-4602)
Dopamine-β-hydroxylase	Disulfiram (Antabuse)

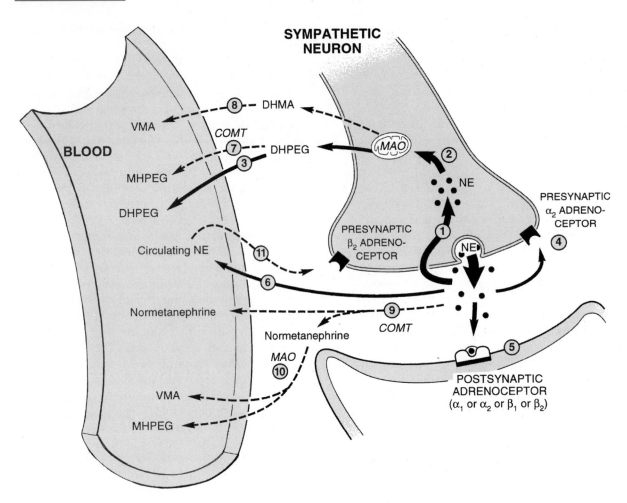

Figure 13-6. Fate of intraneuronal and extraneuronal norepinephrine (NE). The relative importance and order of each step are indicated by differently sized arrows and by numbers. COMT = catechol-*O*-methyltransferase; DHMA = dihydroxymandelic acid; DHPEG = dihydroxyphenylethylene glycol; MAO = monoamine oxidase; MHPEG = methoxyhydroxyphenylethylene glycol; VMA = vanilmandelic acid. (1) Norepinephrine reuptake 1. (2) Intraneuronal metabolism by MAO. (3) Diffusion of DHEPG into circulation. (4) Combination with presynaptic α_2-adrenoceptor. (5) Combination with postsynaptic adrenoceptors. (6) Circulating NE. (7) Extraneuronal metabolism of DHPEG by COMT to MHPEG. (8) Extraneuronal metabolism of DHMA by COMT to VMA. (9) Extraneuronal metabolism by COMT to normetanephrine, followed by MAO (10) to form an intermediate that may be converted to either VMA or MHPEG. (11) Very-low-potency combination with presynaptic β_2-adrenoceptor.

action of norepinephrine is terminated. Both processes are susceptible to drug action (see Chapters 16–18). Some of the released norepinephrine can bind to presynaptic α_2-adrenoceptors that mediate feedback inhibition of further norepinephrine release. Only a small percentage of released norepinephrine goes directly to the circulation. Therefore, the measured concentration of circulating norepinephrine does not correlate with its actual concentration within the sympathetic nervous system, or with the amount of norepinephrine released from sympathetic nerve terminals. The released norepinephrine is

further metabolized or acts on specific postjunctional adrenoceptors to mediate an effect (see below).

Degradation of Catecholamines

Two enzymes are responsible for the degradation of catecholamines: monoamine oxidase (MAO) and catechol-*O*-methyltransferase (COMT). Both enzymes are widely distributed throughout the body. MAO is chiefly associated with the outer surface of mitochondria, in particular those within sympathetic nerve terminals, whereas COMT is located primarily in the synaptic cleft. This distinction is of great importance with respect to the primary metabolic pathways followed by catecholamines. MAO exists in two forms, MAO-A and MAO-B; their pharmacological significance is discussed in Chapter 29.

Norepinephrine within the cytoplasmic pool (but not in the granules) is deaminated by MAO, as is that which is entering by uptake 1. Furthermore, norepinephrine released from the granules by drugs such as reserpine is also deaminated by MAO. The product initially formed by the action of MAO is 3,4-dihydroxyphenylglycol aldehyde (DHPGAL), which is subsequently reduced to dihydroxyphenylethylene glycol (DHPEG). DHPEG subsequently enters the plasma or is further metabolized by COMT to 3-methoxy-4-hydroxyphenylethylene glycol (MHPEG), which is excreted in the urine.

Norepinephrine that is released into the synapse is rapidly O-methylated by COMT, either directly in the synaptic cleft or in adjacent tissue (norepinephrine having undergone a second, extraneuronal, uptake 2) to form normetanephrine. Finally, normetanephrine may be metabolized by MAO, via 3-methoxy-4-hydroxyphenylglycol aldehyde, to 3-methoxy-4-hydroxymandelic acid (MHMA, also called vanilmandelic acid, VMA). This enzymatic degradation of the catecholamines is illustrated in Figure 13-7.

RECEPTORS IN THE AUTONOMIC NERVOUS SYSTEM

In order to elicit a biological response, a drug or neurotransmitter must bind to, and interact with, specific receptors situated on the cell membrane. This interaction produces a drug–receptor (or neurotransmitter–receptor) complex that mediates a series of cellular events leading to a characteristic cellular response (see Chapter 9). Neurotransmitter receptors can be characterized by means of specific agonists that stimulate the receptor, or by antagonists that block or inhibit the response to the specific neurotransmitter.

Cholinergic Receptors (Cholinoceptors)

Although acetylcholine is the neurotransmitter both in autonomic ganglia and at postganglionic parasympathetic nerve terminals, two types of acetylcholine receptor are involved. Dale (1914) was the first investigator to describe the dual function of acetylcholine and to recognize that these separate effects were similar to those of either nicotine or muscarine, respectively. Additional evidence for the dual nature of acetylcholine receptors came from studies with d-tubocurarine, with which the nicotinic effects could be blocked, and with atropine, a selective blocker of muscarinic activity. To date this classification remains the primary subdivision of cholinergic receptors.

Nicotinic Receptors

There are two types of nicotinic receptors—namely, the muscle type and the neuronal type. The activation of both types always causes a rapid increase in cell membrane permeability to Na^+ and K^+, and results in depolarization and excitation. However, the two types are differentiated by the distinct actions of other agonists and antagonists. The neuronal receptor is selectively antagonized by agents such as hexamethonium and trimethaphan, and the selective agonist is dimethylphenyl piperazinium (DMPP). These receptors are located in all autonomic ganglia and on cell bodies of sympathetic and parasympathetic postganglionic fibers.

The muscle type of nicotinic receptor is discussed in Chapter 19. Its selective antagonists are agents such as d-tubocurarine and decamethonium, and a selective agonist is phenyltrimethyl ammonium.

Muscarinic Receptors

Muscarinic receptors are activated nonselectively by acetylcholine, carbachol, and (+)-*cis*-dioxolane. However, five distinct subtypes of muscarinic receptor (designated M_1–M_5) have been identified, which have distinct anatomical locations and distinct pharmacological and molecular characteristics. This diversity was first recognized when the pharmacological actions of pirenzepine were examined. Pirenzepine is unique in that it is the only muscarinic antagonist that selectively inhibits gastric acid secretion.

In this chapter, only M_1-, M_2-, and M_3-receptors are discussed. M_1-receptors appear to be located in ganglia and in some glands; they are selectively activated by a compound known as McN A343 and antagonized by pirenzepine, telenzepine, hexahydrosiladifenidol (HHSiD), and atropine. M_2-receptors are located in the myocardium and smooth muscle; they are selectively antagonized by methoctramine and gallamine. M_3-receptors are located in smooth muscle and secretory glands; they are

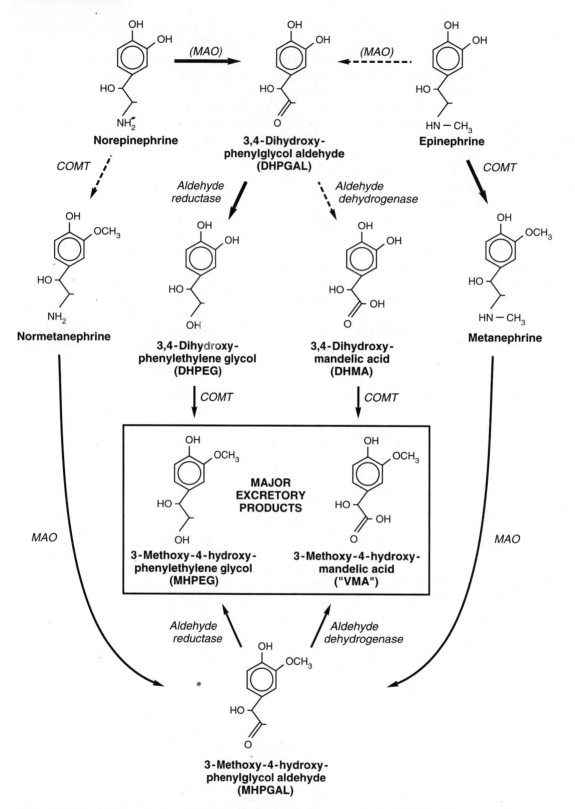

Figure 13-7. Steps in the metabolic degradation of norepinephrine and epinephrine. MAO = monoamine oxidase; COMT = catechol-*O*-methyltransferase; VMA = vanilmandelic acid.

blocked rather selectively by HHSiD, parafluoro-HHSiD, and a piperidine derivative known as 4-DAMP. Currently, it is thought that all three subtypes are located on the vascular endothelium, where they mediate the release of the endothelium-derived relaxing factor (EDRF) nitric oxide. The activation of muscarinic receptors results in their interaction with G proteins. M_1- and M_3-receptors appear to activate G_q and an unidentified G protein that in turn stimulate phospholipase C. This causes the immediate hydrolysis of phosphatidylinositol phosphates to produce inositol trisphosphate (IP_3), which causes release of intracellular Ca^{2+} and hence the cellular response (e.g., contraction of smooth muscle). In addition, this process also causes the production of diacylglycerol (DAG), which activates protein kinase C (PKC), which in turn modulates many ionic and cellular events. M_2-receptors, however, activate a distinct G protein, (G_i), which results in inhibition of adenylyl cyclase. This action could account for the negative cardiac chronotropic and inotropic responses to acetylcholine (see also Chapter 10).

Adrenergic Receptors (Adrenoceptors)

There are two major classes of adrenoceptors, which were first proposed by Ahlquist (1949) on the basis of the ability of epinephrine, norepinephrine, and isoproterenol to regulate various physiological processes. Adrenoceptors are designated as α and β, with further subdivisions into α_1, α_2, β_1, and β_2. The rank order of potency for agonists at α-adrenoceptors is epinephrine > norepinephrine > dopamine > isoproterenol, and for β-adrenoceptors it is isoproterenol > epinephrine > norepinephrine > dopamine. This initial classification was later corroborated by the finding that certain antagonists behave selectively. Phenoxybenzamine is a selective antagonist for α-adrenoceptors, and propranolol is selective for β-adrenoceptors.

α-Adrenoceptors

The recognition of heterogeneity in the α-adrenoceptors arose from the observation that norepinephrine could inhibit its own release from neurons. This feedback mechanism is mediated through prejunctional α-adrenoceptors that are pharmacologically distinct from postjunctional adrenoceptors. The prejunctional adrenoceptors are termed α_2, and the postjunctional adrenoceptors, α_1. Clonidine was one of the first compounds to be described as being more potent at prejunctional adrenoceptors (α_2), whereas

phenylephrine was more potent at postjunctional sites (α_1). Subsequently, selective antagonists were found for the two types: prazosin for α_1- and rauwolscine for α_2-adrenoceptors. The antagonist affinity for α_2-adrenoceptors occurs in a very narrow concentration range.

It is now evident that α_2-adrenoceptors are present also at postjunctional sites. Stimulation of these α_2-adrenoceptors can result in contraction of smooth muscle, platelet aggregation, and release of EDRF from the vascular endothelium.

Both α_1- and α_2-adrenoceptors have been further subdivided. Molecular cloning studies have characterized at least three α_1-adrenoceptors (a, b, and d) that correspond to three pharmacologically identified receptors (A, B, and D), and four α_2-adrenoceptors have been identified. Functionally, these further subdivisions have been more difficult to characterize, but it is now apparent that definitive functional variations can be accounted for by distinct adrenoceptor subdivisions. Selective antagonists for the α_{1A}- and α_{1B}-adrenoceptors have been developed (5-methylurapidil and chlorethylclonidine, respectively). The functional significance of these subdivisions will be highlighted in Chapters 16 and 17.

All α_2-adrenoceptors inhibit adenylyl cyclase by interacting with G_i. Thus, α_2-adrenoceptors cause hyperpolarization. Stimulation of α_1-adrenoceptors increases intracellular Ca^{2+} by activation of phospholipase C through G_q and an unidentified G protein, and hydrolysis of phosphoinositides, resulting in the production of IP_3 and DAG. Diacylglycerol activates protein kinase C, which alters many ionic fluxes. It is likely that the distinct α_1-adrenoceptor subtypes differentially affect these two processes.

β-Adrenoceptors

In the late 1960s, Lands subdivided the β-adrenoceptors into β_1 and β_2 (of which β_1 is located primarily in cardiac tissue and β_2 in all other locations, with some exceptions; see Table 13-2). This division was based on the differences in potency of norepinephrine and epinephrine on the two sites. For example, epinephrine is more potent than norepinephrine on β_2-adrenoceptors. Later, selective antagonists for the two sites were discovered, atenolol and metoprolol for the β_1-adrenoceptor, and ICI 118551 and butoxamine for the β_2-adrenoceptor. Selective agonists for these subtypes are dobutamine for β_1 (in its racemic form with rather mixed α and β effects) and albuterol (salbutamol) for β_2-adrenoceptors.

Recently, a third subtype of β-adrenoceptor has

Table 13-2 Response of Effector Organs to Autonomic Transmitters[a]

Effector Organs	Adrenergic		Muscarinic Cholinergic Responses
	Receptors*	Responses	
Eye			
Radial muscle of iris	α_1	Contr (mydriasis)	—
Sphincter muscle of iris		—	Contr (miosis; strong)
Ciliary muscle	β_2	Relax (slight)†	Contr (strong)‡
Heart			
Heart rate	β_1§	↑	↓
Atrial contractility/conduction	β_1	↑	↓
A-V conduction	β_1	↑	↓ (block)
Ventricular contractility/conduction	β_1	↑	↓
Blood vessels#			
Coronary	$\alpha_1\ \beta_2\ \alpha_2$#	Constr; Dilat (β_2)	
Skin and mucous membranes	$\alpha_1\ \alpha_2$	Constr (strong)	?
Skeletal muscle	$\alpha_1\ \beta_2$	Constr; Dilat (β_2)	Dilat
Cerebral	α_1	Constr (slight)	
Pulmonary	$\alpha_1\ \beta_2$	Constr; Dilat (β_2)	
Abdominal viscera	$\alpha_1\ \beta_2$	Constr; Dilat (β_2)	
Lung			
Bronchial smooth muscle	β_2	Relax	Contr
Bronchial glands		Inhibition (?)	Stimulation
Stomach and intestine			
Motility and tone	$\alpha_1\ \beta_2\ \alpha_2$**	↓	↑ (strong)
Sphincters	α_1	Contr (?)	Relax (usually)
Secretion		Inhibition (?)	Stimulation
Gallbladder and ducts		Relax	Contr
Urinary bladder			
Detrusor muscle	β_2	Relax (usually)	Contr
Trigone and sphincter	α_1	Contr	Relax
Ureter			
Motility and tone	α_1	↑ (usually)	↑ (?)
Uterus	$\alpha_1\ \beta_2$	α_1 = contr †† β_2 = relax	Variable
Skeletal muscle	β_2	Increased contractility; glycogenolysis	—

been identified. This was originally discovered on colon and brown adipose tissue and was termed "atypical" (later termed β_3) because propranolol failed to antagonize its responses to isoproterenol. This adrenoceptor is about 10 times more sensitive to norepinephrine than to epinephrine. Further pharmacological characterization of the β_3-adrenoceptor awaits the development of a selective antagonist. BRL 37344 appears to be a selective agonist for this subtype.

All β-adrenoceptors stimulate adenylyl cyclase through an interaction with a stimulatory G protein (G_s). Stimulation leads to an increase in cyclic AMP, activation of cyclic AMP–dependent protein kinase, and phosphorylation of specific cellular proteins. In the heart, stimulation of β-adrenoceptors causes positive inotropy and chronotropy. There is enhanced phosphorylation of troponin and phospholamban, which in turn raises intracellular Ca^{2+} and thus contributes to the inotropic response. In smooth muscle, accumulation of cyclic AMP leads to relaxation and the membrane becomes hyperpolarized.

Table 13-2 *Continued*

Effector Organs	Adrenergic		Muscarinic Cholinergic Responses
	Receptors*	Responses	
Sex organs, male	α_1	Ejaculation	Erection
Skin			
Sweat glands	α_1	Slight secretion	Profuse secretion
Pilomotor muscles	α_1	Contr	
Spleen capsule	$\alpha_1 \beta_2$	Contr (strong)	
Adrenal medulla		—	Secretion of epinephrine and norepinephrine (*nicotinic effect*)
Pineal gland	β	Melatonin synthesis	—
Posterior pituitary	β_1	ADH secretion	—
Fat cells	β_1	Lipolysis	—
Liver	$\alpha \beta_2$	Glycogenolysis and gluconeogenesis	Glycogen synthesis
Pancreas			
Acini	α_1	Decreased secretion	Secretion
Islet cells	$\alpha_2 \beta_2$	α_2 = decreased secretion β_2 = increased secretion	—
Salivary glands	α_1	Potassium and water secretion (slight)	Potassium and water secretion (profuse)
Lacrimal glands		—	Secretion (profuse)
Nasopharyngeal glands		—	Secretion
Kidneys	$\alpha_1 \beta_1$	α_1 = ↓ renin release β_1 = ↑ renin release	—
Adrenergic nerve terminals	α_2 (presynaptic)	↓ Release of norepinephrine	
Cholinergic nerve terminals	α_2 (presynaptic)		↓ Release of acetylcholine at ↓some sites

^a *Key to symbols:*

* Where known.

† For far vision.

‡ For near vision.

§ β_2- and α-adrenoceptors are present in the heart also, but they are less important than β_1-receptors.

\# Renal and mesenteric blood vessels have dopamine receptors, which cause dilatation when stimulated. α_2-Adrenoceptors in blood vessels cause contraction when stimulated.

** α_2-Adrenoceptors in the myenteric plexus inhibit acetylcholine release when stimulated.

†† α_1-Adrenoceptor stimulation contracts the uterus during pregnancy.

↑ = increase; ↓ = decrease; Constr = constriction; Dilat = dilatation; Contr = contraction; Relax = relaxation. —— = No effect.

Distribution of Adrenoceptors

This varies from organ to organ, as listed in Table 13-2. The receptor distribution determines the char- acteristic response, because the endogenous release of norepinephrine (and epinephrine) stimulates all adrenoceptors, and the effects in any given organ will depend on the balance between α- and β-receptors and their respective subtypes. (When norepinephrine is administered exogenously as a drug, the effects of α_2 stimulation may not be observed.)

Modulation of Autonomic Nervous System Activity

At least three different levels of control interact to modulate activity in the autonomic nervous system.

Physiological interaction of sympathetic and parasympathetic innervation

At central sites (e.g., the medulla oblongata) cholinergic and adrenergic systems can interact with each other by reflex mechanisms to maintain homeostasis. A drug-induced elevation of mean arterial pressure causes a baroreceptor-mediated negative feedback response that results in marked bradycardia. This is due to increased acetylcholine release at the sinoatrial node, causing a compensatory decrease in heart rate. Bradycardia occurs even when the pressor drug is a potent myocardial stimulant that normally increases the heart rate (e.g., norepinephrine, Chapter 16). In this way the parasympathetic nervous system becomes dominant and overrides sympathomimetic effects on both the sinoatrial and atrioventricular nodes.

Control of transmitter release

This is another mechanism by which one system may be inhibited (or enhanced) relative to the other. Presynaptic α_2-adrenoceptors, when stimulated by released norepinephrine, exert a negative-feedback control that diminishes further norepinephrine release from nerve endings. Conversely, norepinephrine release can be enhanced by stimulation of β_2-adrenoceptors. However, this latter mechanism may be more sensitive to circulating epinephrine.

Presynaptic α_2-adrenoceptors located on parasympathetic nerve endings can also reduce the amount of acetylcholine released at certain sites. In the mesenteric plexus, for example, the release of acetylcholine is decreased to an extent that causes relaxation and reduced motility of the intestine.

Other endogenous substances, e.g., prostaglandins and enkephalins, also inhibit norepinephrine release by interacting with specific presynaptic receptors. Contrasting with this is the effect of angiotensin II (see Chapter 32), which enhances the release of catecholamines.

Changes in postsynaptic receptors

At postsynaptic adrenoceptor sites in target organs, the response of an organ to neurotransmitters may be altered by changes in receptor numbers, e.g., desensitization due to down-regulation of receptors following periods of excessive stimulation. Up-regulation (i.e., increased receptor numbers) may occur in other circumstances, e.g., when a drug acts on neurons to inhibit transmitter release.

SUGGESTED READING

Arunlakshana O, Schild HO. Some quantitative uses of drug antagonists. Br J Pharmacol 1959; 14:48–58.

Burnstock G, Hoyle CHV. Autonomic neuroeffector mechanisms. Chur: Harwood Academic, 1992.

Bylund DB, Eikenberg DC, Heible JP, et al. International Union of Pharmacology nomenclature of adrenoceptors. Pharmacol Rev 1994; 46:121–136.

Gaddum JH. The quantitative effects of antagonist drugs. J Physiol (Lond) 1937; 89:7–9P.

Limbird LE. The alpha-2 adrenergic receptors. Clifton, NJ: Humana Press, 1988.

Ruffolo RR. The alpha-1 adrenergic receptors. Clifton, NJ: Humana Press, 1987.

Schild HO. pA$_2$ and competitive drug antagonism. Br J Pharmacol 1949; 4:277–280.

Starke K. Presynaptic receptors. Annu Rev Pharmacol Toxicol 1981; 21:7–30.

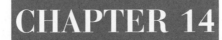

CHAPTER 14

Autonomic Cholinergic Agonists

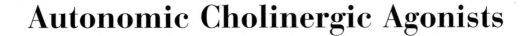

L. SPERO

CASE HISTORY

A 55-year-old man who owned a small nursery and flower shop was found unconscious by his wife in the greenhouse behind his home. During the past week he had been complaining of abdominal discomfort and frequent stools. Since he was usually of robust health, she suspected that he may have poisoned himself with chemicals he used in the garden. She had him taken to the hospital at once.

On arrival at the hospital emergency room the patient was unconscious, he was salivating profusely, and his breathing was shallow. His skin was warm and moist. Blood pressure was 140/90 mmHg, pulse was 45/min and regular, respiration rate was 30/min, and temperature was normal. There was no evidence of trauma. Both pupils were constricted and did not respond to light. Auscultation of the chest revealed moderate wheezing and numerous rhonchi. The heart was normal. Palpitation of the abdomen revealed no abnormalities, but hyperactive bowel sounds were heard. The rectal examination revealed nothing remarkable, and an occult blood test of the stool was negative. The extremities showed subcutaneous muscle fasciculations at the time of admission. These disappeared during the course of the examination, but muscle tone decreased and breathing became shallower during this time. The neurological examination revealed no response to painful stimuli, no localizing signs, and no abnormal reflexes.

During this examination, the wife reported that her husband had mild hypertension controlled by salt restriction (about 5 years' duration), and non–insulin-dependent diabetes controlled by diet (about 10 years' duration). He had no history of mental illness, he did not smoke or drink, and he was not taking medication.

The signs and symptoms of excessive cholinergic activity, together with the patient's occupation, allowed a provisional diagnosis of poisoning by organic phosphorus insecticide to be made. When questioned directly, the wife confirmed that her husband had recently experimented with such chemicals.

An airway and intravenous line were inserted, followed at once by intravenous injections of 2 mg atropine sulfate, repeated every 10 minutes until signs of atropinization appeared, shown by dry, flushed skin and tachycardia of 140 beats/min. Atropinization was continued for 24 hours with intramuscular injections of 2 mg of atropine sulfate every 4 hours.

At the same time the patient was given a slow intravenous infusion of pralidoxime (Protopam chloride), 1 g in 250 mL saline, over a 30-minute period. This dose was repeated 1 hour later because of persisting muscle weakness, which then disappeared, and respiration strengthened. No further treatment with pralidoxime was indicated.

The patient slowly began to recognize his surroundings and regained consciousness about 6 hours after being admitted to hospital. He felt very weak and confused. His respiration and the effects of atropinization continued to be monitored for the next 24 hours, and he remained under observation for an additional 3 days. He was discharged with the admonition to avoid strenuous activity and with instructions in the handling of organophosphate insecticides and the early recognition of signs of poisoning.

ACETYLCHOLINE

As described in Chapter 13, acetylcholine acts as a neurotransmitter at four distinct types of cholinergic site. These are ganglionic synapses, postganglionic parasympathetic (and some sympathetic) terminals, central cholinergic synapses, and neuromuscular junctions.

The synthesis and release of acetylcholine and the characteristics of the receptor systems on which it acts (two types of nicotinic receptor and the muscarinic receptor system, which is also of more than one type) are described in Chapters 13 and 19. Many molecular species of these receptors have been identified. These will be referred to only briefly, since the physiological roles of these subtypes have yet to be clearly defined.

Muscarinic receptors are G protein–linked receptors with a structure that includes seven transmembrane domains. Neuronal muscarinic receptors are of the M_1 and M_2 subtypes, smooth muscle has M_2 and M_3 subtypes, the heart contains the M_2 (also known as $M_{2\alpha}$ cardiac) subtype, and endocrine glands contain the M_3 (also known as $M_{2\beta}$ glandular) subtype. Other muscarinic receptors have been cloned from CNS material but have not been identified with respect to specific physiological sites. The M_1 and M_3 subtypes have been demonstrated to use both the inositol trisphosphate (IP_3) and diacylglycerol (DAG) cascades as second messengers. The M_2 subtype activates potassium channels and inhibits cAMP production.

Principal Actions of Acetylcholine

Muscarinic actions

These are postganglionic parasympathetic actions on exocrine glands and smooth muscle, and they have the following effects.

1. Secretion by exocrine glands, such as sweat, salivary, mucous, and lacrimal glands, is stimulated. Gastric, intestinal, and pancreatic secretions are also increased, although they depend only partly on parasympathetic innervation. Where both sympathetic and parasympathetic innervation are involved, parasympathetic (muscarinic) stimulation produces a watery secretion, while sympathetic stimulation produces a more concentrated one. Both may be required for copious production of a "quality" secretion.

2. Sphincters in the gastrointestinal, biliary, and urinary tracts are relaxed.

3. Stimulation of smooth muscle contraction in bronchi leads to bronchoconstriction and asthmatic symptoms. Stimulation of smooth muscle in the gastrointestinal tract, together with the relaxation of sphincters, results in increased propulsive motility and may cause cramps and diarrhea. In the bile duct and ureters, this action causes increased intraluminal pressure and may result in colicky pain. The gallbladder and urinary bladder are stimulated to contract and expel their contents.

4. The circular muscles of the iris and the muscles of accommodation are stimulated to contract so that the pupil is constricted and the lens of the eye is accommodated for near vision.

5. The heart is slowed.

Nicotinic actions

1. Stimulation of sympathetic and parasympathetic ganglia, i.e., stimulation of postsynaptic neurons within the ganglia so that the postganglionic fibers release their respective transmitters at their peripheral endings.
2. Stimulation of the adrenal medulla to release epinephrine and norepinephrine.
3. Contraction of skeletal muscles.

Acetylcholine as a Drug

Acetylcholine is poorly absorbed following oral or subcutaneous administration. When it is given intravenously, very high doses are required to produce an effect because it is rapidly hydrolyzed by plasma cholinesterase that is found in both the blood and the liver.

The pharmacological effects of intravenous administration of acetylcholine include a transient fall in blood pressure; bradycardia; partial or complete heart block or cardiac arrest; flushing, sweating, salivation, lacrimation, and increased bronchial mucus secretion; and, as secondary consequences, nausea, coughing, and dyspnea. These are all due to muscarinic actions; no nicotinic actions are noted. The effects on skeletal muscle can be observed only after intra-arterial injection. Exogenously administered acetylcholine will not produce effects on the CNS, since the molecule is a quaternary ammonium compound that cannot cross the blood–brain barrier (Fig. 14-1).

Acetylcholine can dilate blood vessels by releasing endothelium-derived relaxing factor (EDRF). This in turn activates guanylyl cyclase and thereby increases cGMP, which relaxes smooth muscle. There is no cholinergic innervation of these blood vessels.

CHOLINERGIC DRUGS

Because acetylcholine is so unsuitable as a drug, substitutes are used if parasympathetic effects need to be produced for diagnosis or therapy.

The contraindications are essentially the same for all the cholinergic drugs. They are contraindicated in patients with intestinal or urinary obstruction, because the increased peristaltic contraction would exacerbate the effects of the obstruction. These agents should be used cautiously in patients with bronchial asthma for similar reasons.

Cholinergic drugs mimic the effects of stimulation of cholinergic nerves. They may do so either by direct action, in the same way as acetylcholine, or by

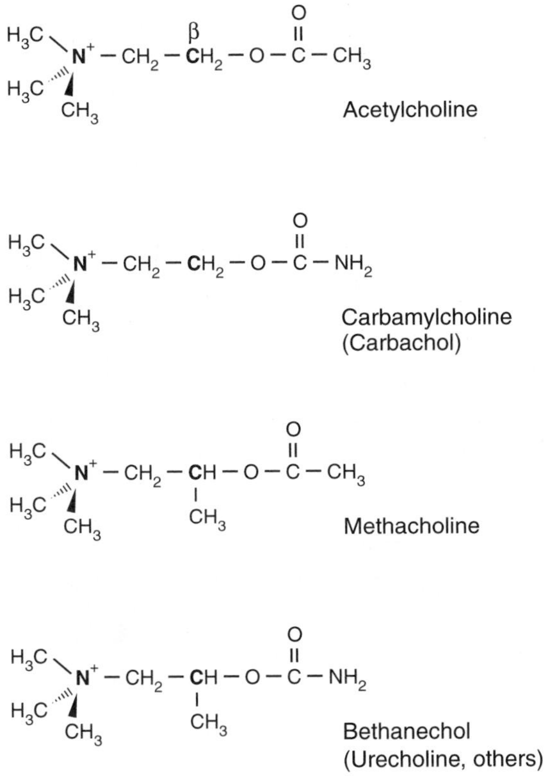

Figure 14-1. Structural formulae of acetylcholine and analogs.

inhibition of acetylcholinesterase, thereby preventing the destruction of endogenous acetylcholine. Stimulation of the mechanism for release of endogenous acetylcholine is not used therapeutically.

Directly Acting Cholinergic Agonists

Naturally occurring alkaloids with direct cholinergic activities

Muscarine is found in the mushroom *Amanita muscaria* (Fly agaric) and related species. It was the agent used to characterize the muscarinic receptor. Its actions are solely muscarinic. Specific muscarinic antagonists (e.g., atropine) are used to treat the poisoning caused frequently by this alkaloid in uninformed mushroom pickers.

Pilocarpine is found in the leaves of *Pilocarpus*, a South American shrub. It has both muscarinic and nicotinic actions. The effects of pilocarpine upon glands, such as the sweat and salivary glands, are particularly pronounced; therefore it has been used to increase salivation and to induce sweating. Pilocarpine is now used mainly in ophthalmology to treat glaucoma (by opening the drainage canals for the ocular fluid and thereby reducing the intraocular pressure), to produce miosis, and to counteract the mydriatic and cycloplegic actions of drugs such as atropine and the ganglion-blocking agents.

Arecoline is derived from a seed commonly known as the betel nut. Its peripheral actions are similar to those of the synthetic agent methacholine (see below). Arecoline has no therapeutic use in humans, but it is of interest because the betel nut is habitually chewed by a large part of the world's population. From Africa to the East Indies, in many countries bordering the Indian and Pacific oceans, millions of people who do not smoke tobacco show an equivalent addiction to chewing the betel nut. Presumably, arecoline has central effects that are analogous to those of nicotine.

Synthetic analogs of acetylcholine

If the acetyl group in acetylcholine is replaced by a carbamyl group, the resulting compound (carbamylcholine) is much more resistant to cholinesterase hydrolysis. Substitution of a methyl group at the β-carbon results in analogs, e.g., methacholine and bethanechol, which have a greater selectivity for muscarinic receptors, and also somewhat reduces the susceptibility to cholinesterase hydrolysis (see. Fig. 14-1).

Carbamylcholine (carbachol) has both muscarinic and nicotinic properties. It selectively stimulates the urinary and gastrointestinal tracts, but it is not used for this purpose because of its concomitant ganglion stimulant effects. It is available for use in ocular surgery to produce miosis and thus reduce intraocular pressure, and it may also be used in the treatment of glaucoma.

Methacholine has a resistance to hydrolysis similar to that of carbachol. It is used to increase gastrointestinal motility and to overcome urinary retention consequent to anesthesia or vagotomy.

Bethanechol (carbamyl-β-methylcholine) may be used to test pancreatic function since it increases secretion but constricts the sphincter of Oddi. This should cause an increase in plasma amylase, because the secreted amylase cannot reach the intestine and is reabsorbed into the blood. Pancreatic function can thus be correlated with plasma amylase levels.

Indirectly Acting Cholinergic Drugs: Cholinesterase Inhibitors

All clinically used cholinesterase blockers inhibit both acetylcholinesterase and plasma cholinesterase, although not always to the same extent. The main pharmacological effects are due to inhibition of acetylcholinesterase.

Following a lethal overdose of most acetylcholinesterase inhibitors, a characteristic sequence of reactions results from the rapid buildup of acetylcholine at the various receptor sites. Restlessness usually develops early and reflects the central actions of acetylcholine. This is accompanied by increasing abdominal distress, with more and more severe pain due to intestinal spasm. There is frequent, involuntary defecation and urination. The pupils of the eyes become constricted (miosis). The skeletal muscles show fasciculation; i.e., small groups of muscle fibers twitch but produce no coordinated movement, so there is virtual paralysis. There is also increased glandular activity with salivation, lacrimation, sweating, and increased bronchial secretion. At the same time there is a bronchiolar constriction that, with the accumulation of bronchial secretions, results in stertorous, difficult breathing. Later there are usually convulsions, during which the breathing ceases. The heart, although slowed, continues to beat for some time after breathing stops. Ultimately, death is due to respiratory failure.

In denervated organs in which no acetylcholine is released, inhibition of acetylcholinesterase is without pharmacological effect. By contrast, directly acting cholinergic drugs often elicit an exaggerated response in such organs because of denervation supersensitivity of the receptors.

Chemically, there are two main classes of compounds that inhibit acetylcholinesterase: carbamate derivatives, which are reversible inhibitors, and organophosphates, which inhibit acetylcholinesterase irreversibly by forming stable complexes with it.

Acetylcholinesterase Structure

The active site of acetylcholinesterase consists of an anionic site, which interacts with the quaternary nitrogen on the choline moiety of acetylcholine, and an esteratic site, which interacts with and hydrolyzes the ester grouping of acetylcholine (Fig. 14-2). A serine hydroxyl group at the esteratic site accepts the acetyl group and becomes acetylated but is subsequently regenerated by interaction with water.

Plasma cholinesterase shows genetic variation, and some individuals have an atypical variant that has very low hydrolytic activity. This will influence the pharmacokinetics of many drugs with ester linkages (see Chapter 12). Acetylcholinesterase variants have not been observed, probably because "atypical" acetylcholinesterase would be lethal in the first hours of life.

Reversible cholinesterase inhibitors

These agents are competitive inhibitors of the cholinesterases (Fig. 14-3). They have carbamyl ester linkages that are slowly hydrolyzed by the enzyme, resulting in carbamylation of the enzyme. Water can then release a carbamic acid molecule from the enzyme. These agents have mainly muscarinic side effects that can be blocked by atropine.

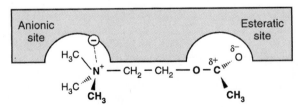

Figure 14-2. Interaction of acetylcholine and acetylcholinesterase.

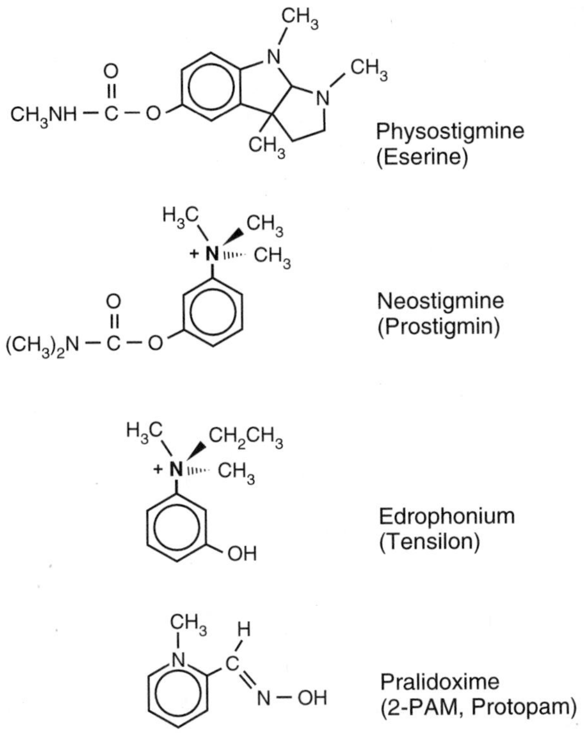

Physostigmine
(Eserine)

Neostigmine
(Prostigmin)

Edrophonium
(Tensilon)

Pralidoxime
(2-PAM, Protopam)

Figure 14-3. Structural formulae of reversible cholinesterase inhibitors, and pralidoxime, a dephosphorylation agent.

Physostigmine (eserine). This is an alkaloid extracted from the Calabar bean; its effects were utilized in many African "trial-by-ordeal" ceremonies. It is lipid-soluble and can therefore cross the blood–brain barrier and produce CNS side effects. Its main use is in the treatment of glaucoma. It is readily absorbed locally from eye drops and, by increasing the availability of acetylcholine, reduces intraocular pressure, mainly by facilitating the outflow of aqueous humor.

Neostigmine, pyridostigmine, ambenonium. These anticholinesterases are all quaternary ammonium compounds and therefore do not readily cross the blood–brain barrier. They also have some direct nicotinic agonist actions in skeletal muscle, which renders them very suitable for the treatment of myasthenia gravis (see Chapter 19). Ambenonium has the longest duration of action; neostigmine, the shortest. They are taken orally in myasthenia gravis. Some CNS side effects are observed with ambenonium, because it does appear to cross the blood–brain barrier, although slowly.

In addition to the common muscarinic side effects

found with cholinesterase inhibitors, all of the reversible inhibitors described above can produce a "cholinergic crisis" as a consequence of excess acetylcholine desensitizing the nicotinic receptors at both the ganglia and, more importantly, the neuromuscular junctions. The major symptom is muscle paralysis resembling myasthenia gravis, the disease these agents are being used to treat.

Edrophonium. This is a short-acting reversible cholinesterase inhibitor that is used by intravenous injection to diagnose myasthenia gravis and to differentiate between it and a cholinergic crisis. It has a brief duration of action (3–4 minutes); the myasthenic patient will experience transient improvement. A patient in a cholinergic crisis will become transiently worse.

Irreversible cholinesterase inhibitors

This class of cholinesterase inhibitors, which consists of hundreds of active organophosphorus chemicals, is important more for toxicological than for therapeutic reasons. These agents include "nerve gases" for biological warfare, and insecticides (Fig. 14-4). They produce phosphonylation or phosphorylation of the esteratic site of acetylcholinesterase, and once this covalent interaction is complete it cannot be reversed. The reaction takes place in three stages, as shown in Figure 14-5.

1. A reversible phase in which the irreversible inhibitor competes with acetylcholine for binding to

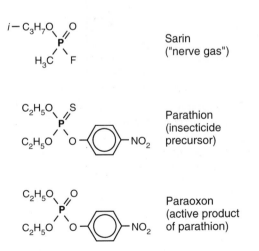

Sarin
("nerve gas")

Parathion
(insecticide precursor)

Paraoxon
(active product of parathion)

Figure 14-4. Structural formulae of irreversible cholinesterase inhibitors.

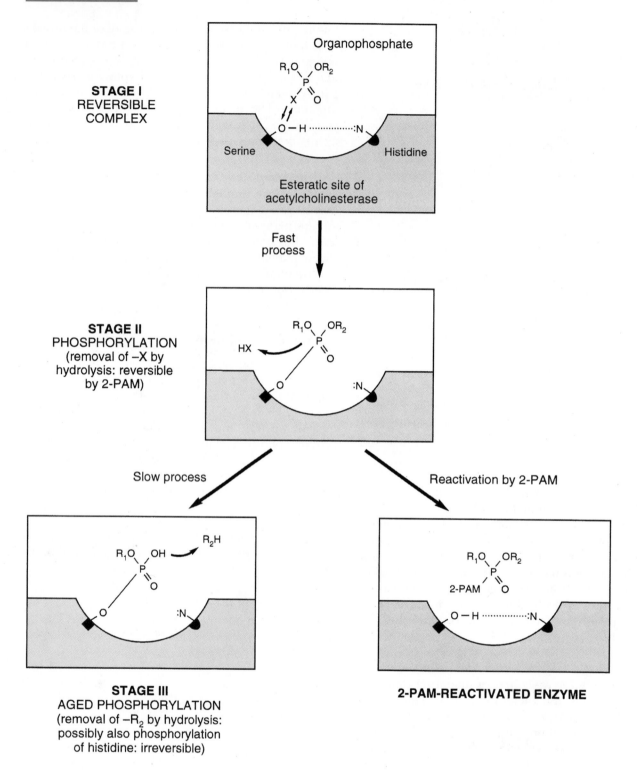

Figure 14-5. The steps of acetylcholinesterase inhibition by organophosphorus compounds, and enzyme reactivation with pralidoxime (pyridine-2-aldoxime, 2-PAM).

the acetylcholinesterase. This stage may be symptom-free.

2. Phosphorylation of the serine residue in the esteratic site. At this stage the acetylcholinesterase can be reactivated by pralidoxime (2-PAM, Fig. 14-3), which binds close to the esteratic site and has a hydroxyl side-chain that can lead to dephosphorylation at a higher rate than the free water present.

3. An "aging" process in which there is loss of an alkyl group or migration of the phosphoryl group to a histidine. The enzyme is now irreversibly inhibited, and restoration of cholinesterase activity requires de novo synthesis of acetylcholinesterase.

Therapeutic use. **Echothiophate** (Phospholine Iodide) is one of the few organophosphates used clinically. It is a thiocholine analog that is fairly stable and has a long duration of action. It is the only one of these compounds used in the treatment of glaucoma. It causes a reduction in the total body content of acetylcholinesterase and should therefore not be used within 4–6 weeks of surgery because of possible complications with muscle relaxants. Muscarinic side effects can be overcome with atropine, or they may be reversed with 2-PAM (see below). Other organophosphate cholinesterases are used in veterinary medicine.

Nerve gases. These inhibitors are volatile liquids that have been studied since World War II as potential chemical weapons to be used as sprays or aerosols. Being very highly lipid-soluble, they rapidly penetrate intact skin and mucous membranes, enter the circulation, and quickly reach all central and peripheral cholinergic synapses. Accidental contact with these agents has occurred through incautious handling in laboratories, storage depots, etc., and during poorly controlled testing in the field. Incidents of deliberate use as chemical weapons during armed conflicts in various parts of the world have occurred in recent years. High concentrations kill almost instantaneously; low concentrations are more insidious because symptoms may develop slowly and resemble mental or neurological illness. The fluorine-containing organophosphate cholinesterase inhibitors, such as sarin, have also been shown to induce a delayed neurotoxicity even when present in trace amounts. Reactivation of the enzyme with 2-PAM can be achieved only within the first few minutes following exposure.

Insecticides. These are organophosphate cholinesterase inhibitors that have been designed to be more toxic to insects than to mammals. They are all thiophosphates that must be converted to phosphates to become activated. This occurs very rapidly in insects but more slowly in humans. They are all designed to be readily inactivated by mammalian metabolism.

However, these compounds cause human toxicity through cumulation from repeated exposure of persons handling them in their daily work. Mild poisoning may produce only nausea, headache, and weakness. This may lead to unusual neurological symptoms that may not be recognized as being due to "intoxication." Since these agents are also very lipid-soluble, they may concentrate in body fat, which will form a reservoir from which the insecticide may leak slowly back into the circulation where it can be activated. Atropine can be used to block muscarinic side effects, and unless the level of inhibitor is very high, careful support of the patient and the use of artificial respiration may allow survival until de novo synthesis of acetylcholinesterase returns the patient to normal.

Cholinesterase reactivators. The phosphorylated acetylcholinesterase can be reactivated before the "aging" process occurs (see Fig. 14-5). The drug used for this purpose is **pralidoxime** (pyridine-2-aldoxime, **2-PAM**, see Fig. 14-3).

The ability of 2-PAM to reactivate the enzyme is a function of the phosphoryl group and the rate at which the "aging" process occurs, which is also a function of the organophosphate structure. 2-PAM does not influence carbamylation of acetylcholinesterase, and because it has some anticholinesterase activity of its own, it is contraindicated in the presence of overdose of reversible cholinesterase inhibitor. It has been suggested that "Gulf War syndrome" (a poorly defined condition that includes fatigue, depression, cognitive problems, rashes, diarrhea, and other symptoms) is due in part to the use of 2-PAM by the United Nations troops as prophylaxis against possible nerve gas attacks by their Iraqi opponents. However, this suggestion has not been proven to be true.

Indirectly Acting Cholinergic Drugs: Dopamine Antagonists

Incompetence of the gastroesophageal sphincter can lead to reflux of acidic gastric contents into the lower esophagus, producing irritation of the esophageal mucosa and reflux esophagitis. Directly acting cholinergic drugs can increase sphincter tone, but they also increase gastric secretion. Indirectly acting agents such as metoclopramide are therefore preferred.

Metoclopramide (Fig. 14-6) increases gastroesophageal sphincter pressure, increases the force of esophageal peristalsis, increases the rate of gastric emptying without influencing the rate of acid secretion, and increases small intestinal motility. It has been shown to markedly reduce reflux esophagitis, but it has not proven to be effective in the treatment of gastric ulcer (see Chapter 45).

Metoclopramide (Maxeran, others) is a dopamine D_2-receptor antagonist with some neuroleptic properties; it is used extensively as a centrally acting antiemetic. Its effects on gastrointestinal motility are employed to speed up the absorption of drugs that are taken up in the lower intestine or to hasten the passage of barium contrast medium through the small intestine. It is also used to facilitate gastrointestinal intubation.

Its mode of action is not clearly understood. It may work by reducing the dopaminergic inhibitory tone on the cholinergic ganglia of the myenteric plexus. This is analogous to the dopaminergic/cholinergic interaction in the basal ganglia (see Chapters 20 and 21) and is consistent with the fact that parkinsonian side effects occur in some patients receiving metoclopramide. It has also been reported to increase the sensitivity of intestinal smooth muscle to acetylcholine. Anticholinergic drugs diminish the effects of metoclopramide.

In spite of its structural resemblance to procainamide, metoclopramide is only a poor local anesthetic.

NICOTINE AND LOBELINE

Nicotine (Fig. 14-7) is not used as a therapeutic agent but there are, nevertheless, three reasons for studying it. First, it is the drug that was initially used to characterize nicotinic pharmacological responses. Second, nicotine is pharmacologically the most active

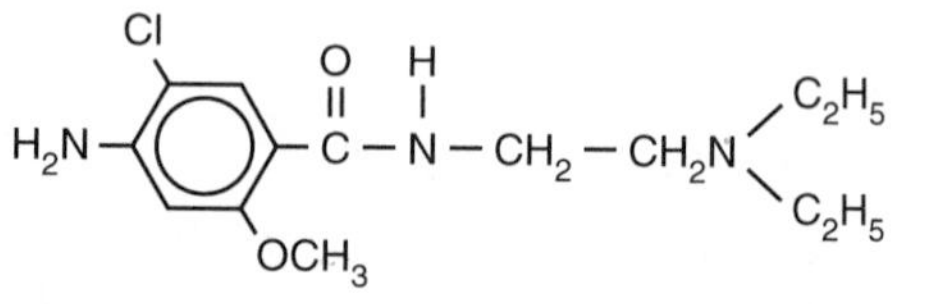

Figure 14-6. Structural formula of metoclopramide.

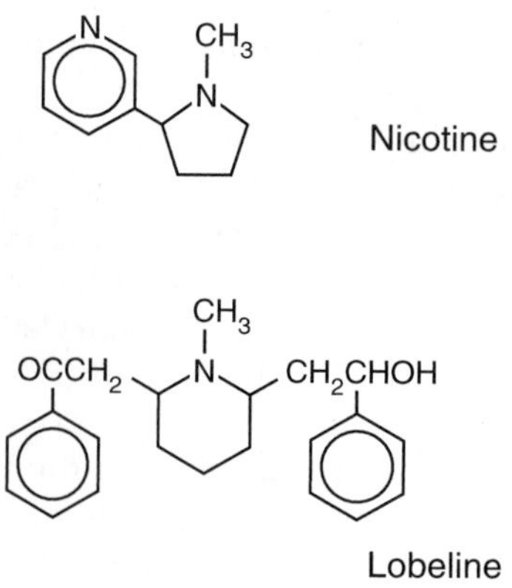

Figure 14-7. Structural formulae of nicotine and lobeline.

ingredient of tobacco smoke, and the use of a nicotine transdermal patch to reduce tobacco use is now widespread. Third, nicotine is a potent and rapidly acting poison that, when used as an insecticide, occasionally takes human life.

Nicotine is an alkaloid; it is a brown liquid that is volatile and, therefore, is easily inhaled with tobacco smoke. It penetrates not only mucous membranes but also intact skin. In the body, most of it is inactivated fairly rapidly (within 2–4 hours) by multiple pathways in the liver and lung, but some is excreted unchanged. The major metabolite is cotinine, formed by the sequential action of a P450 enzyme and an aldehyde oxidase. The other primary metabolite is nicotine N'-oxide.

Nicotine intake, in a dose equivalent to the smoking of one or two cigarettes (roughly 0.3–1 mg), usually causes a slight increase in heart rate, some rise of blood pressure, and a modest increase in respiratory rate. These effects are comparable to those of mild exercise. Skin temperature and cutaneous blood flow decrease. Secretion of vasopressin (antidiuretic hormone, ADH) is stimulated, with consequent suppression of diuresis, and thus smoking tests have been proposed for diagnostic distinction between pituitary and other forms of diabetes insipidus. Nicotine-induced release of epinephrine from the adrenal medulla leads to an increase in blood sugar. Effects on the mood are difficult to measure; some persons feel stimulated, others sedated. All these effects tend to be qualitatively similar whether the person is a smoker or a nonsmoker. In the latter, there may be in addition nausea and vomiting, an urge to defecate, and sometimes tremor.

The effects of small amounts of nicotine are due to the following actions. The smallest doses stimulate the chemoreceptors in the carotid and aortic bodies. This accounts primarily for the effects on respiration. The first circulatory effects are mostly due to norepinephrine release from sympathetic fibers within vascular walls and within the heart muscle. Furthermore, the adrenal medulla is stimulated to release epinephrine, and the supraoptic nucleus is stimulated to release antidiuretic hormone.

Somewhat higher doses of nicotine are necessary to act upon autonomic ganglia. With increasing dosage there is the following sequence: stimulation of sympathetic ganglia, stimulation of parasympathetic ganglia, blockade of parasympathetic ganglia. These actions account for the gastrointestinal effects and the increasing disturbance of circulation and respiration. Blockade of sympathetic ganglia usually requires very high doses and is seen only during the final stages of intoxication. Tremor and nausea are due to separate actions in the CNS. Radioreceptor assays have demonstrated the presence of nicotinic receptors in the CNS, and nicotine can cross the blood–brain barrier rapidly.

After inadvertent intake of toxic amounts, e.g., an insecticide containing 40% nicotine (Black Leaf 40), dyspnea develops rapidly. Gradually, the blood pressure rises exceedingly high (250–300 mmHg) while the pulse is very slow. There is diarrhea. Twitching and fasciculation of skeletal muscles are soon followed by paralysis. Death is due to failure of the respiratory muscles and usually occurs within 15–30 minutes of nicotine intake. This is so because, in a very high dose, nicotine behaves like a depolarizing relaxant of skeletal muscle, and paralysis is the usual cause of death in fatal poisoning (see Chapter 19). The emergency treatment of acute poisoning, therefore, is artificial respiration to tide the patient over the critical period.

Chronic intoxication is possible. The repeated liberation of norepinephrine in the walls of blood vessels, over long periods of time, leads to vasoconstriction and interference with circulation in susceptible vascular beds. Thus, gangrene and loss of limbs or blindness may occur in predisposed persons. Women who smoke during pregnancy often have smaller-than-average babies. It is not entirely clear whether this represents a retardation of growth or premature delivery, but animal data support the idea of growth inhibition due to nicotine, as well as due to high carbon monoxide levels in the blood and tissues.

The effects of tobacco smoke and nicotine are not completely identical. Production of cancer, allergic reactions, and smoking-related impairment of pulmonary function are probably not due to nicotine. More than 260 different chemicals have been identified in tobacco smoke, and there is enough carbon monoxide, cyanide, and oxide of nitrogen for any one of these to kill if a person were to breathe tobacco smoke instead of air. However, the intermittent "puffing" and the dilution of smoke upon inhalation seem to reduce their acute toxicity. (Note, however, that ingestion of a whole or part of a cigarette would involve a toxic dose of nicotine—up to 22 mg. This is an additional reason for keeping cigarettes away from children.)

Nicotine self-administration is an important aspect of smoking. Nicotine has reinforcing effects (see Chapter 72) and is the component of tobacco that causes dependence in the tobacco user. Craving for nicotine, and the withdrawal symptoms associated with it, make it difficult to quit smoking "cold turkey." The symptoms of nicotine withdrawal can be reduced by administering nicotine; this is best accomplished with the transdermal nicotine patch. The nicotine patch, by slowly releasing low concentrations of nicotine, can reduce the craving for a cigarette without producing other pharmacological effects. The dose must be adjusted to the individual user. Many reported failures of the nicotine patch result from the side effects of patches that release too much nicotine. A similar principle applies to nicotine-containing chewing gum (Nicorette) used as a smoking-cessation aid.

The alkaloid **lobeline** (Fig. 14-7) is a nicotinic agonist that has been used to ameliorate nicotine withdrawal symptoms during cessation of smoking. It also increases respiration by stimulating the carotid body, and it was at one time used as a drug for resuscitation.

SUGGESTED READING

Bertrand D. Nicotinic receptor: an allosteric protein specialised for intercellular communications. Semin Neurosci 1995; 7:75–90.

Eglen RM. Muscarinic acetylcholine receptor subtypes in smooth muscle. TIPS 1994; 15:114–119.

Felder CC. Muscarinic acetylcholine receptors: signal transduction through multiple effectors. FASEB J 1995; 9:619–625.

Fryxell KJ. The evolutionary divergence of neurotransmitter receptors and 2nd messenger pathways. J Mol Evol 1995; 41:85–97.

Kaneda M. Neuronal nicotinic receptors: molecular organization and regulation. Neuropharmacol 1995; 34:563–582.

Levitan IB. Modulation of ion channels in neurons and other cells. Annu Rev Neurosci 1988; 11:119–136.

McGehee DS. Physiological diversity of nicotinic acetylcholine receptors expressed by vertebrate neurons. Annu Rev Physiol 1995; 57:521–546.

Rotenberg M. Differentiation between organophosphate and carbamate poisoning. Clin Chim Acta 1995; 234:11–21.

Rubin LL, Anthony DT, Englander LL, et al. Neural regulation of properties of the nicotinic acetylcholine receptor. J Recept Res 1988; 8:161–181.

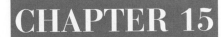

CHAPTER 15

Autonomic Cholinergic Antagonists

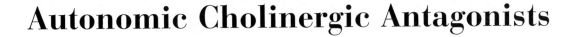

L. SPERO

CASE HISTORY

A thin, 27-year-old woman traveling on the subway fainted when she stood up to leave the train. She was helped to a seat, and her heavy overcoat was removed. Within 5 minutes she appeared to have recovered, but she still looked very pale. She was taken to a nearby hospital where she was found to have a blood pressure of 65/42 mmHg and a heart rate of 42 bpm. Blood glucose was normal. Her eyes were very light-sensitive and her skin was warm and dry. She had difficulty in talking, but during the examination she told of having frequently used her father's "old blood pressure medicine" because it reduced her appetite.

The patient was given an intravenous infusion of 300 mL saline to reverse probable volume depletion. She was given intravenous atropine 0.5 mg, which was repeated every 3–5 minutes up to a total dose of 0.04 mg/kg. Still, her heart rate remained below 50 bpm, and an intravenous dopamine infusion was started at 5 μg/kg/min. This produced some improvement. However, since her systolic blood pressure was still below 70 mmHg, she was given intravenous norepinephrine 5 μg/min. An immediate improvement in blood pressure and heart rate was observed. The norepinephrine was terminated and she was maintained on dopamine 2.5 μg/kg for the next 48 hours.

On review of her history she acknowledged having had difficulty concentrating. Also, she had been in a mental fog since she started taking her father's pills.

Within 10 days of her subway episode, the patient had returned to normal with none of the symptoms remaining or recurring. It was concluded that the pills she had taken were ganglion blockers. She was advised to seek counsel for her self-perceived "appetite" problem and not use medications of unknown origin.

MUSCARINIC RECEPTOR ANTAGONISTS

These antagonists selectively block muscarinic receptors at parasympathetic postganglionic sites and, if they can cross the blood–brain barrier, in the CNS. They are frequently misnamed "cholinergic antagonists" or "anticholinergics" without specific reference to their selectivity for muscarinic receptors.

Principles of Action

As described in Chapter 13, muscarinic agonists appear to bind to receptor sites with three different levels of affinity. However, the antagonists that have been examined appear to bind with equal affinity to all three types (or states?) of the receptor.

Table 15-1 shows the interactions of a number of muscarinic antagonists with radioactive ligands that label muscarinic receptors (see Chapter 9). This table demonstrates that muscarinic antagonists have a similar affinity for the receptor regardless of whether it is labeled with an agonist (^{3}H-oxotremorine) or an antagonist (^{3}H-propylbenzilylcholine). The antagonist binding site is clearly different from the agonist site, but it includes the agonist site within

Table 15-1 Muscarinic Receptor Binding. IC_{50} Values for Various Cholinergic Agonists and Antagonists Against Ligands That Label Muscarinic Cholinergic Receptors

Competing Cold Ligand	^3H Ligand		
	^3H-Propyl-benzilylcholine* (Antagonist)	^3H-Oxotremorine* (Agonist)	^3H-Quinuclidinyl Benzilate† (Antagonist)
Muscarinic agonists			
Acetylcholine	3,300 nM	240 nM	3,000 nM
Oxotremorine	460 nM	38 nM	700 nM
Methacholine	2,000 nM	350 nM	2,500 nM
Muscarine	8,300 nM	> —	> —
Carbachol	15,000 nM	240 nM	25,000 nM
Muscarinic antagonists			
Atropine	0.59 nM	3.0 nM	3.0 nM
Benzhexol	7.10 nM	25.0 nM	> —
Methylatropine	0.35 nM	0.7 nM	0.2 nM
Nicotinic agonists and antagonists			
Nicotine d-Tubocurarine Hexamethonium	> 100,000 nM	> 100,000 nM	> 100,000 nM

Sources: *Birdsal NJM, Burgen ASV, Hume EC. *Mol Pharmacol* 1978; 14:723–736.
†Yamamura HI, Snyder SH. *Mol Pharmacol* 1974; 10:861–867.

its binding domain. These antagonist affinities are much higher (i.e., the IC_{50} values are much lower) than those of agonists (e.g., acetylcholine), even when the radiolabeled compound is an agonist. It is also apparent that nicotinic agonists and antagonists have a very low affinity for the muscarinic receptor, as shown by the very high IC_{50} values.

The radioreceptor assay may thus be used as a predictive indicator of the pharmacological effects of muscarinic antagonists. The higher their affinity in a radioreceptor experiment, the more potent they are clinically. Pirenzepine, a muscarinic antagonist, was predicted (and found) to be a more selective inhibitor of gastric secretion than of gastric motility, on the basis of its unusual relative selectivity for the "high-affinity" (M_1) agonist site over the "low-affinity" (M_2) agonist site.

The blockade of muscarinic receptors by these antagonists is competitive and depends on the relative concentrations of the antagonist and acetylcholine and their relative affinities for the receptors. As is the case with most families of antagonists, they are slightly more effective against exogenously applied agonist than against acetylcholine released endogenously as a neurotransmitter. Preganglionic cholinergic nerve stimulation in the presence of a muscarinic antagonist still stimulates autonomic nicotinic ganglia, but only sympathetic effects are elicited.

Pharmacological Effects

The effects of the prototypical muscarinic antagonist, atropine (Fig. 15-1), will be described.

Exocrine glands

Salivary secretion is impaired even after very small doses of atropine. The subject experiences a dry mouth and swallowing may be very difficult.

Gastric secretion is diminished, although gastric pH is unchanged. Therefore, the main contribution of atropine in the treatment of peptic ulcer is relief of spasm; see below.

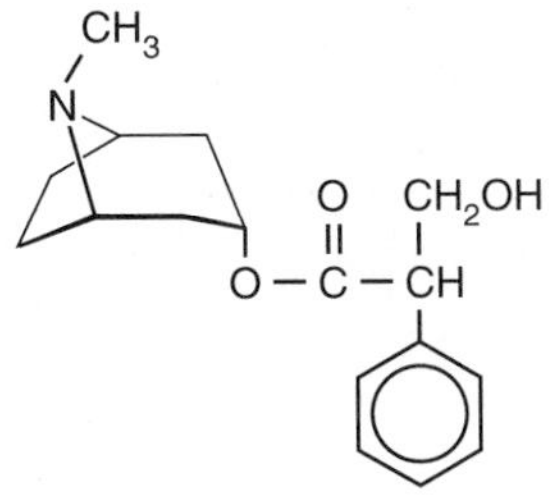

Figure 15-1. Structural formulae of natural muscarinic antagonists.

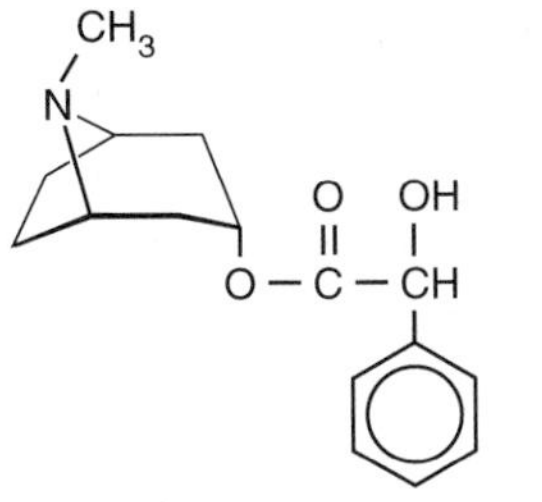

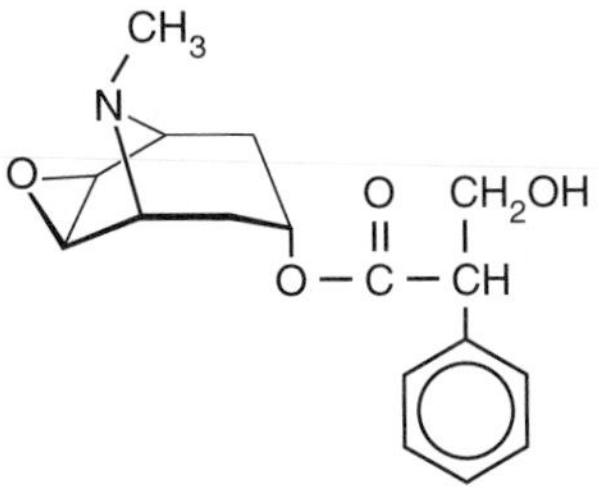

Bronchial secretions are suppressed. This action renders atropine useful for preanesthetic medication.

Sweating is impaired. The inability to perspire may interfere with heat regulation, which can be fatal in very hot weather.

Smooth muscle

Gastrointestinal tract. Atropine abolishes any excessive tone and motility of the intestinal tract, but it has relatively little effect on normal motility. It is therefore spasmolytic but not constipating. Atropine is particularly effective in relieving spasms of the cardiac sphincter of the stomach, whereas effects on the pyloric sphincter are less reliable.

Biliary tract. Atropine has some relaxing action and is moderately effective in relieving biliary colic. It does not influence the formation of bile.

Urinary tract. In therapeutic doses, atropine diminishes the tone of the fundus of the bladder but increases the tone of the vesical sphincter. This may cause retention of urine, which can be a serious side effect in patients after surgery and in elderly men with prostatic hypertrophy. The effect is utilized, however, to suppress the frequency and urgency of micturition in cystitis. This effect is also exploited in the control of nocturnal enuresis.

Atropine also reduces tone and motility of the ureter and thus relieves attacks of renal colic.

Circulation

Large doses of atropine (2 mg) have the expected effect on the heart rate, which increases by 40–50 bpm as a result of vagal blockade. Small doses of atropine (0.2 mg) decrease the heart rate by 10–15 bpm. This is due to stimulation of the medullary centers including the vagal nucleus. Atropine in therapeutic doses of 0.5–1 mg in the adult has usually a dual effect—namely, first a decrease and then an increase of the heart rate. The bradycardia is due to stimulation of the cardioinhibitory center of the medulla, while the tachycardia is in response to the muscarinic antagonist effects of atropine in the S-A node of the heart.

There is no major effect on blood vessels, so blood pressure is not affected. High doses of atropine cause selective vasodilatation, including flushing of the face.

The eye

Atropine has two primary effects on the eye—namely, mydriasis (dilatation of the pupil) and cycloplegia (paralysis of accommodation)—which it causes by antagonizing acetylcholine, as shown in Figure 15-2. Both effects can be produced by systemic application of atropine, but they are most prominent after local application, because local application of concentrated solutions produces much higher intraocular concentrations of atropine than is achieved by systemically tolerable oral or parenteral doses.

This combination of effects makes atropine an important drug in ophthalmology because it permits precise measurements of refraction. The mydriatic effect is utilized in cases of iritis. In eyes with a narrow chamber angle (i.e., the angle between iris and cornea), dilatation of the pupil may cause the iris muscle to block the canal of Schlemm and thereby interfere with the drainage of aqueous humor; in this way atropine may produce an attack of glaucoma in predisposed persons, which may cause them to lose

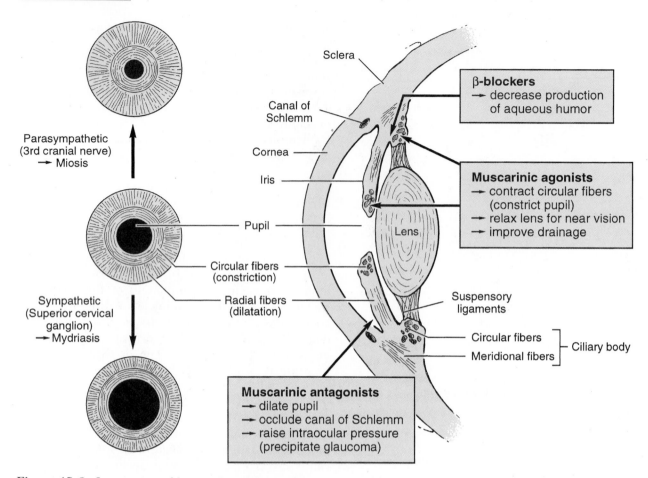

Figure 15-2. Innervation of lens and iris of the eye.

their eyesight. The effects of atropine applied as eye drops may be noticeable for as long as a week.

Central nervous system

Atropine in the usual therapeutic doses has no significant effects upon the central nervous system. It has no uses in this area, except for its beneficial effects in Parkinson's disease, in which it suppresses tremor and rigidity. This is due primarily to a central action (see Chapter 21), but some action upon muscle spindles may also contribute to the effect.

In high doses, atropine has complicated effects on the brain that have been broadly classified as stimulatory, but disorientation is the most characteristic feature (see Chapter 30). After drug intake, the subject first becomes restless and quarrelsome. A state of excitation may be followed by delirium. Usually there is recovery without recollection; only rarely will the delirium progress into coma with respiratory failure and death.

The central effects of atropine-containing plant extracts differ slightly from those of the pure alkaloid because of the admixture of scopolamine (see below). Belladonna alkaloids were used as medicines for many centuries, but they also found much disreputable use in witchcraft and quackery. Remnants of these nonmedicinal medieval uses are found in the mnemonic jingle on atropine poisoning:

> *Dry as a Bone,*
> *Red as a Beet,*
> *Mad as a Hen.*

Drugs in Clinical Use

Naturally occurring plant alkaloids

Atropine (Fig. 15-1). Atropine is *dl*-hyoscyamine extracted from belladonna (deadly nightshade), hyoscyamus (henbane), or stramonium (jimsonweed) plants, all of which belong to the potato family. *l*-Hyoscyamine is more potent than the racemic mixture atropine, but it is less stable.

Atropine is usually given as the sulfate, subcutaneously in doses of 0.5–1 mg. The effects of oral doses are less intense and occur more slowly. In the treatment of anticholinesterase poisoning, atropine may need to be given intravenously. For ophthalmic purposes, atropine is applied directly to the eye in solution or ointment. Narrow-angle glaucoma is a contraindication to its use.

The duration of action varies depending on the dose, route of administration, and respective organ. The systemic effects of atropine, whether it is administered orally or subcutaneously, last only a few hours, so the dose must be repeated every 4–6 hours. Following local application of atropine to the eye, however, impairment of accommodation may persist for 3 or 4 days, and dilation of the pupil even for 6 or 7 days. Reversible cholinesterase inhibitors are sometimes used to overcome this problem. However, the half-life of the inhibitors is shorter than that of atropine, and the visual impairment can reappear unexpectedly.

Insofar as the cardiac and ocular effects of atropine are concerned, little or no tolerance develops. However, repeated doses of the drug produce diminishing effects upon the digestive tract and secretions. Appreciable tolerance can develop in patients receiving relatively large doses of atropine, as in the treatment of parkinsonism, so very high doses in the order of 50 mg per day may become necessary to maintain effectiveness. These changes may occur due to up-regulation (or increase in the number) of muscarinic receptors or because of a change in the conformation of the receptors. Chronic use also tends to cause urinary retention.

Homatropine hydrobromide, homatropine methylbromide. Homatropine, an analog of atropine (Fig. 15-1), has a more rapid onset and a shorter duration of action. However, it is less potent than atropine. The hydrobromide salt of homatropine is used solely by topical application for ophthalmic purposes; since it has a tertiary N, it would be able to enter the CNS if given systemically. The quaternary methyl analogs of homatropine (e.g., homatropine methylbromide) and atropine (methylatropine) are unable to cross the blood–brain barrier and therefore do not have the CNS effects of the parent compounds. Their main use is in the treatment of gastrointestinal disorders.

Scopolamine (Fig. 15-1). Scopolamine, which has the same peripheral actions as atropine, centrally has a pronounced sedative action. For a long time it was the only drug used to subdue highly agitated mentally ill patients. However, some people get excited after taking scopolamine, rather than sedated.

"Twilight sleep," resulting from a combination of scopolamine and morphine, at one time was very popular in surgery and obstetrics because the anticholinergic action of scopolamine produced amnesia for the events surrounding the surgery or childbirth. Its modern counterpart is neuroleptanalgesia by a combination of opioid and neuroleptic (see Chapter 24). In most persons, scopolamine tends to counteract the respiratory depression produced by morphine. For obscure reasons, however, this combination produces in some subjects a pronounced, and potentially fatal, respiratory depression.

Scopolamine is used prophylactically to prevent motion sickness. It is not recommended for nausea and vomiting due to nonvestibular causes.

Synthetic muscarinic antagonists

There are many synthetic substitutes for atropine (Fig. 15-3). They were developed to maximize specific actions of atropine.

Suppression of gastric secretion. These agents are described in Chapter 45. They are all quaternary ammonium compounds and they exist as two types: those with mixed muscarinic and ganglion-blocking properties (e.g., **propantheline** and oxyphenonium), and **pirenzepine,** which is a purely muscarinic antagonist.

These antagonists all reduce gastric secretions, but the mixed antagonists reduce motility as well. The selectivity of pirenzepine for secretion makes it the muscarinic antagonist of choice in ulcer therapy. It is used only in combination with histamine H_2-receptor blockers (e.g., ranitidine), antacids, or "cytoprotective" agents (carbenoxolone).

Suppression of smooth muscle spasm in gastrointestinal tract, biliary tract, and ureter. The drugs advocated for this purpose, e.g., dicyclomine (Bentylol), cause relaxation through their muscarinic antagonist actions as well as through a nonspecific relaxant effect on smooth muscle. They are little used in clinical practice, atropine being preferred.

Ophthalmic use. For this purpose, use is made of short-acting muscarinic antagonists that are well absorbed from eye drops instilled in the conjunctival sacs (e.g., homatropine). However, they are tertiary amines and, therefore, can have CNS side effects including convulsions, psychotic disorders, and behavioral disturbances.

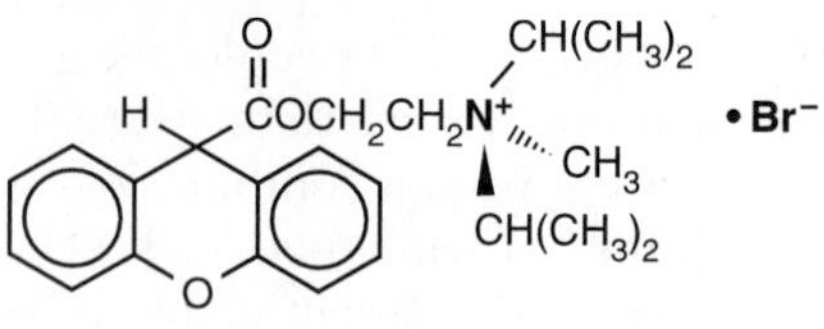

Propantheline
(Pro-Banthine)

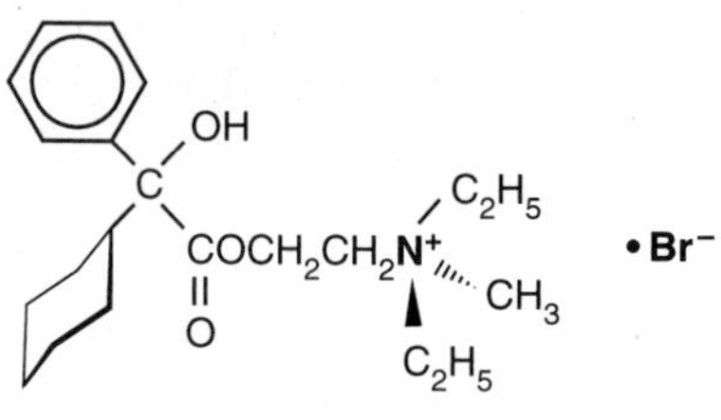

Oxyphenonium
(Spasmophen)

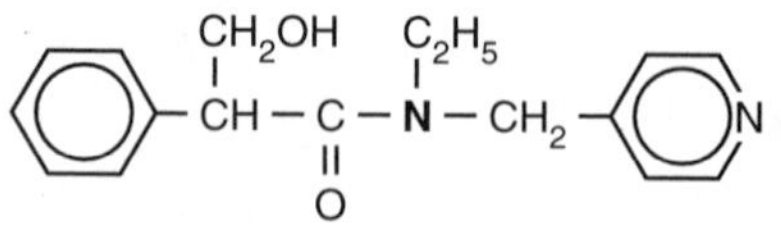

Tropicamide
(Mydriacyl, others)

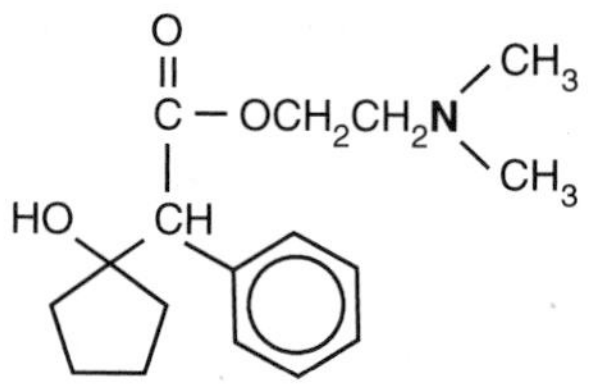

Cyclopentolate
(Cyclogyl, others)

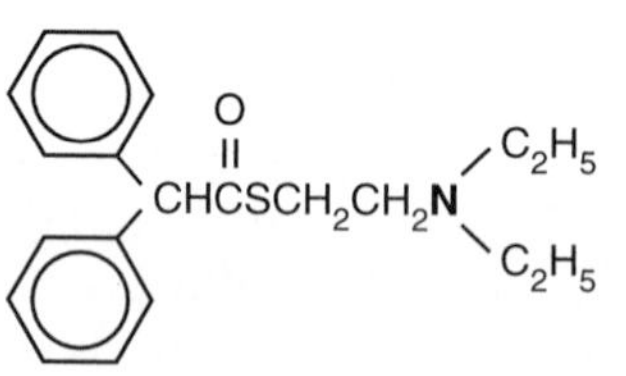

Thiphenamil
(Thiphen)

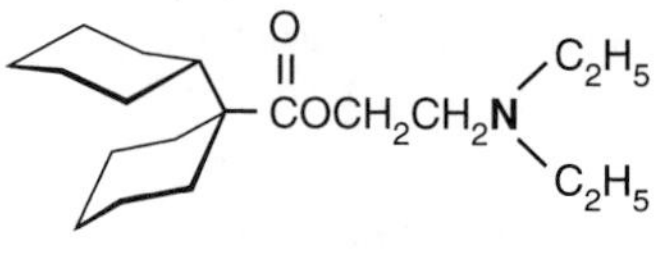

Dicyclomine
(Bentylol)

Figure 15-3. Structural formulae of some synthetic muscarinic antagonists.

Antiparkinsonian drugs. Parkinson's disease, described in Chapter 21, is due to an imbalance between cholinergic activity and chronically declining dopaminergic activity in the basal ganglia. The drug of choice is L-dopa, which can restore dopamine levels, but unfortunately it does not affect the chronically declining numbers of dopaminergic neurons. Muscarinic antagonists, such as **trihexyphenidyl** (Artane) and **benztropine** (Cogentin), can also restore the balance, and they may be useful adjuncts to L-dopa therapy. They are sometimes used in patients unresponsive to L-dopa.

The central effects of these synthetic drugs are relatively stronger than their peripheral cholinergic blocking actions, although the latter exist and cannot be disregarded. However, urinary retention and interference with reading ability (caused by cycloplegia) are usually less bothersome than with atropine.

These drugs are used for symptomatic treatment irrespective of the origin of symptoms. Thus, they are not restricted to parkinsonism but are used also in similar disorders induced by phenothiazine antipsychotics and other drugs. The appearance of mental confusion and urinary retention usually indicates that the muscarinic antagonist has reached its limits of usefulness and should be withdrawn.

In addition to the few muscarinic antagonists mentioned above, or that are shown in Figure 15-3, at least 15 other synthetic compounds have been used for this purpose.

NICOTINIC RECEPTOR ANTAGONISTS; GANGLION BLOCKERS

These are drugs that competitively inhibit the actions of acetylcholine at autonomic ganglia. Nicotine (an agonist) in high doses can also block these receptors through a desensitization mechanism similar to that described for succinylcholine (see Chapter 19). There is no difference between the nicotinic receptors in sympathetic ganglia and those in parasympathetic ganglia. Any apparent selectivity in the blockade of sympathetic pathways as distinct from parasympathetic pathways results from the relative importance of the two pathways in controlling the function of a specific organ. Some differences in selectivity may be related to the anatomical location of the sympathetic ganglia a distance away from the innervated organ involved, whereas the parasympathetic ganglia are generally located within that organ. The blood flow through these two locations, and hence the delivery of drug to them, may be quite different.

The nicotinic receptors in autonomic ganglia are not identical to those at the neuromuscular junction. This is illustrated in Figure 15-4, which shows that the optimum carbon-chain length of a compound for ganglion blockade is not the same as for neuromuscular junction blockade. Nevertheless, drugs chosen for clinical use in neuromuscular blockade will have

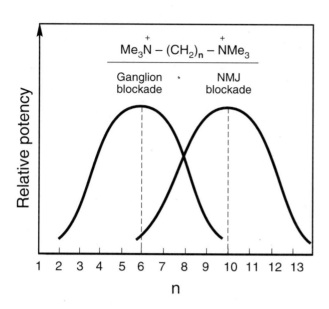

Figure 15-4. Relative nicotinic receptor blockade as a function of optimum chain length of the onium compound for blockade of autonomic ganglia and of neuromuscular junctions (NMJ).

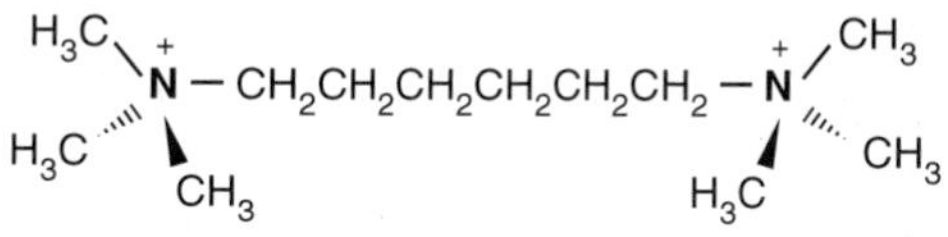

Hexamethonium

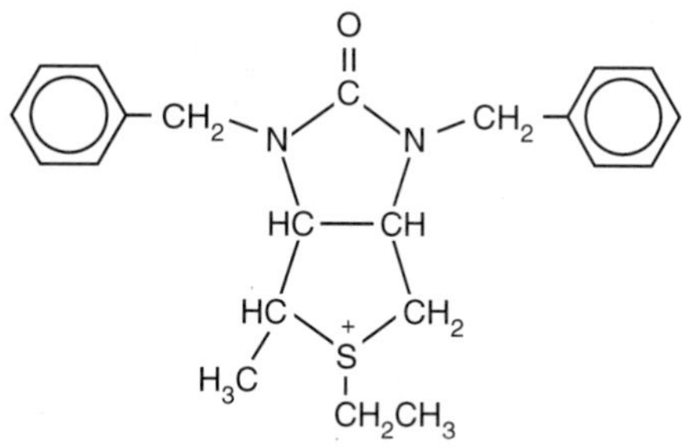

Trimethaphan

Figure 15-5. Structural formulae of the ganglionic blockers hexamethonium and trimethaphan.

some ganglion-blocking side effects. Historically, ganglion blockers were important in the treatment of chronic hypertension because they lowered vascular sympathetic tone. They are no longer used for this purpose. The reasons become apparent from the description given below of the effects of **hexamethonium** (Fig. 15-5), a prototype of this family. The physiology of each organ determines its response to ganglion blockade. The wide spectrum of side effects has led to the withdrawal of these drugs from general use.

Pharmacological Effects

What will happen to a person constantly treated with hexamethonium is illustrated by Paton's tongue-in-cheek description of the "**hexamethonium man**":

He is a pink complexioned person, except when he has stood in a queue for a long time, when he may get pale and faint. His handshake is warm and dry. He is a placid and relaxed companion; for instance he may laugh, but he can't cry because the tears cannot come. Your rudest story will not make him blush, and the most unpleasant circumstances will fail to make him turn pale. His collars and socks stay very clean and sweet. He wears corsets and may, if you meet him out, be rather fidgety (corsets to compress his splanchnic vascular pool, fidgety to keep the venous return going from his legs). He dislikes speaking much unless helped with something to moisten his dry mouth and throat. He is long-sighted and easily blinded by bright light. The redness of his eyeballs may suggest irregular habits and in fact his head is rather weak. But he always behaves like a gentleman and never belches nor hiccups. He tends to get cold and keeps well wrapped up. But his health is good; he does not have chilblains and those diseases of modern civilization, hypertension and peptic ulcer, pass him by. He is thin because his appetite is modest; he never feels hunger pains and his stomach never rumbles. He gets rather constipated so that his intake of liquid paraffin is high. As old age comes on, he will suffer from retention of urine and impotence, but frequency, precipitancy, and strangury will not worry him. One is uncertain how he will end, but perhaps if he is not careful, by eating less and less and getting colder and colder, he will sink into a symptomless, hypoglycemic coma and die, as was proposed for the universe, a sort of entropy death.

The effects of ganglion blockade upon the function of the various systems depend upon the dominant tone, parasympathetic or sympathetic, for each organ. Thus, sympathetic tone predominates in the vasomotor system, and the usual response to hexamethonium is a reduction in blood pressure, particularly in hypertensive subjects. However, the most important feature is the failure of the regulating interplay of vasoconstriction and vasodilatation, which keeps the blood properly distributed in response to exertion or mere changes in posture. After hexamethonium, blood distribution becomes principally determined by gravity. The "hexamethonium man" faints when the blood accumulates in his legs after he has been standing for a while. If the person is lying down and an arm or leg is held up, the limb becomes almost bloodless. Ganglionic blockers are therefore used as an aid in special surgical procedures. The same principle is used if ganglionic blockers are employed to combat pulmonary edema. While furosemide is the generally accepted drug of choice in pulmonary edema, ganglionic blockers have the advantage of decidedly faster action.

The iris is predominantly under parasympathetic control, so the response to ganglionic blockade is mydriasis. The gastrointestinal tract responds with partial or complete inhibition of gastric motility, some inhibition of salivary and gastric secretion, and disturbances of intestinal motility, usually constipation. In the respiratory tract, there is sometimes a decrease in nasopharyngeal secretion and some bronchodilatation. The skin becomes dry and flushed because of sympathetic blockade. There are no significant effects upon the central nervous system.

Ganglionic Blockers in Current Clinical Use

Trimethaphan camsylate (Arfonad, Fig. 15-5) is given only by continuous intravenous infusion. It acts very rapidly and briefly, so the reduction of blood pressure can be controlled by varying the rate of infusion. Its main use is to treat acute hypertensive crises, to reduce blood pressure during surgery so as to minimize bleeding, and to reduce the circulating blood volume in the emergency treatment of pulmonary edema. The drug releases histamine and should be avoided if there is a history of allergy.

SUGGESTED READING

Cutler NR. Muscarinic M1 receptor antagonists: potential in the treatment of Alzheimer's disease. CNS Drugs 1995; 3:467–481.

Fishman PH, Perkins, JP. Receptor desensitization. Adv Second Messenger Phosphoprotein Res 1988; 21:25–32.

Kaneda M. Neuronal nicotinic acetylcholine receptors of ganglion cells in the rat retina. Jpn J Physiol 1995; 45:491–508.

Nathanson NM. Binding of antagonists by muscarinic acetylcholine receptors in intact cultured heart cells. J Neurochem 1983; 41:1545–1550.

Olmez E, Guc MO, Ilhan M. Inhibitory muscarinic cholinoceptors on postganglionic parasympathetic nerves in the guinea pig isolated atrium are of the M3 subtype. Pharmacology 1995; 51:112–117.

Paton WDM. The principles of ganglionic block. In: Scientific basis of medicine, vol. 2. London: Athlone Press, 1954.

Wamsley JK, Gehlert DR, Roeske WR, Yamamura HI. Muscarinic antagonist binding site heterogeneity as evidenced by autoradiography and direct labelling with QNB and pirenzepine. Life Sci 1984; 34:1395–1402.

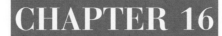

CHAPTER 16

Adrenoceptor Agonists

C. FORSTER

CASE HISTORY

A 6-year-old boy with a history of mild hay fever, which was treated successfully with over-the-counter medications, had an anaphylactic reaction as a result of a bee sting. In this emergency, epinephrine 0.3 mg in sterile water was ordered, to be given subcutaneously. By error, however, the epinephrine was given intravenously by a young attending nurse in the emergency room. It resulted in dangerously high blood pressure (180/125 mmHg) and heart rate (125 bpm). The boy was clearly distressed, tense, and frightened. He had fine tremor of the hands; cold, clammy skin; and appeared to have respiratory difficulty.

He was immediately given intravenous sodium nitroprusside by continuous infusion at a rate of 0.5 μg/kg/min, as well as propranolol by slow intravenous infusion at a rate of a little more than 1.0 mg/min. Careful monitoring of the blood pressure, ECG, and cardiac function accompanied these interventions. Atropine was available, to be used if bradycardia should become a problem.

The hypertension and tachycardia were successfully controlled by these measures. The child's condition stabilized in a couple of hours without any significant rebound hypertension, and he was able to return home. On the recommendation of the family physician, he was given a prescription for a kit containing subcutaneous epinephrine, and his parents were advised to carry it in case he suffered any subsequent attacks.

CLASSIFICATION

The sympathetic nervous system regulates a wide variety of dissimilar biological functions, disorders of which result in a great diversity of clinical problems. It is not surprising, therefore, that agents that mimic or alter sympathetic nervous system activity have made a huge impact on the therapeutic management of such disorders. Moreover, such agents are among the most extensively studied in pharmacological research. The effects of stimulation of the sympathetic nervous system can be reproduced in whole, or in part, by the administration of drugs that mimic the effects of endogenous catecholamines (dopamine, norepinephrine, and epinephrine) on effector organs. The widest spectrum of sympathomimetic activity is exhibited by the catecholamines themselves, which directly stimulate adrenoceptors when administered as drugs. However, since direct stimulation of adrenoceptors is not the only mechanism by which the action of endogenous catecholamines may be mimicked, it is essential to classify the sympathomimetic agents as follows.

1. Drugs that stimulate all α- and/or all β-adrenoceptors, as well as dopamine receptors (e.g., catecholamines, as well as agents that selectively activate specific subtypes of these receptors)
2. Drugs that increase the release of norepinephrine from sympathetic nerves, sometimes with additional direct stimulation of adrenoceptors (e.g., ephedrine, amphetamine)

3. Drugs that block the reuptake ("uptake 1") of norepinephrine (e.g., cocaine, imipramine)

Catecholamine structure

CATECHOLAMINES

Chemical Structures and Structure–Activity Relationships

Phenylethylamine, the parent compound of the catecholamines, consists of a benzene ring and an aliphatic two-carbon side-chain with an amine group on the α-carbon (Fig. 16-1). Substitutions can be made on the aromatic ring, the α- and β-carbons, and on the terminal amino group. These various substitutions yield many compounds with a wide variety of sympathomimetic and sympatholytic activities (Figs. 16-1 and 16-2).

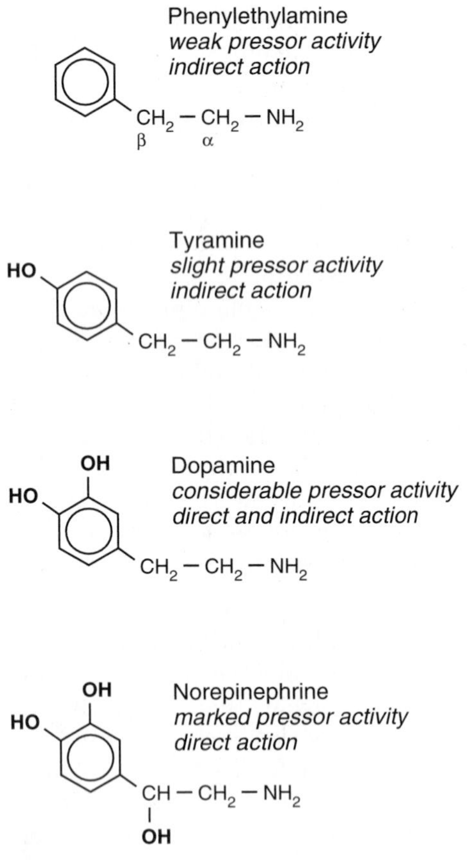

Figure 16-1. Effects of substituting –OH groups in the phenylethylamine molecule. Increasing the number of substitutions increases the pressor activity and introduces direct adrenoceptor-stimulant action.

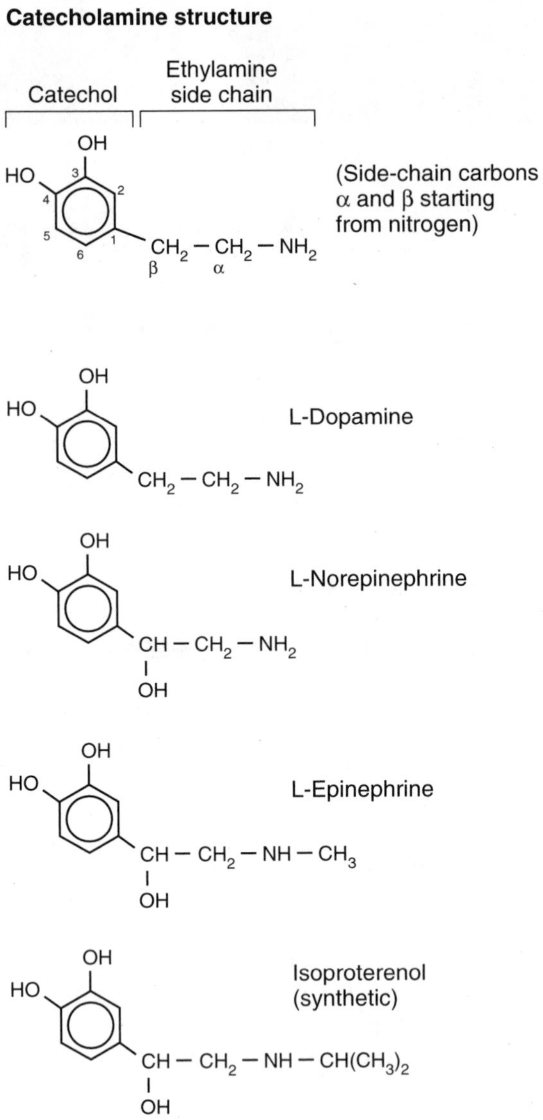

Figure 16-2. Chemical structures of the catecholamines.

A phenol ring with two adjacent hydroxyl groups is called catechol. Therefore phenylethylamine derivatives having hydroxyl groups at C-3 and C-4 on the phenyl ring, such as the endogenous sympathetic neurotransmitters and isoproterenol, are termed catecholamines (Fig. 16-2). Many directly acting sympathomimetics have both α- and β-adrenoceptor activity (Table 16-1), but the ratio of α:β activity varies tremendously from an almost pure α-adrenoceptor agonist (e.g., phenylephrine) to an almost pure β-adrenoceptor agonist (e.g., isoproterenol). Hydroxyls in the C-3 and C-4 positions are required for maximal adrenergic activity. Absence of these hydroxyl groups decreases the overall potency of an agent,

Table 16-1 Classification of Adrenoceptors with their Respective Agonists, Antagonists, and Effector Pathways*

Pharmacologically Defined Receptors	Agonists	Antagonists	Effector Pathway	Clone
α_{1A}	Norepinephrine Epinephrine Dopamine Phenylephrine Methoxamine	Prazosin Phentolamine, WB 4101 Phenoxybenzamine Labetalol *Niguldipine* *5-Methylurapidil*	IP_3/DAG Ca^{2+} influx	α_{1a}
α_{1B}	Norepinephrine Epinephrine Dopamine Phenylephrine	Prazosin Phentolamine Phenoxybenzamine *Chlorethylclonidine* *Spiperone*	IP_3/DAG	α_{1b}
α_{1D}	Epinephrine Norepinephrine Phenylephrine	Prazosin Phentolamine WB 4101 *BMY 7378*	IP_3/DAG	α_{1d}
α_{2A}	Norepinephrine Epinephrine Phenylephrine Clonidine BHT 920 *Oxymetazoline*	Phentolamine Phenoxybenzamine Rauwolscine Yohimbine	$\downarrow$cAMP	α_{2a}
α_{2B}	Norepinephrine Epinephrine Phenylephrine Clonidine BHT 920	Phentolamine Phenoxybenzamine Rauwolscine Yohimbine Prazosin†	$\downarrow$cAMP	α_{2b}
α_{2C}	Epinephrine Norepinephrine	Phentolamine Rauwolscine Prazosin†	$\downarrow$cAMP	α_{2c}
β_1	Norepinephrine Epinephrine Dopamine Isoproterenol *d-Dobutamine*	Phentolamine Labetalol *Atenolol* *Metoprolol*	$\uparrow$cAMP	β_1
β_2	Epinephrine Norepinephrine Isoproterenol *Albuterol (Salbutamol)* *Terbutaline*	Propranolol Labetalol *ICI 118551* *Butoxamine*	$\uparrow$cAMP	β_2
β_3	Norepinephrine Epinephrine Isoproterenol *BRL 37344*	—	$\uparrow$cAMP	β_3

*Italics denote the most selective agents. Propranolol is ineffective at β_3-adrenoceptors. Oxymetazoline is a partial agonist but may show high affinity as an antagonist against α_{1A}; it also has been shown to have high agonist affinity at α_{2A}.

†Prazosin is approximately 100 times less potent at α_{2B}- and α_{2C}- than at α_1-adrenoceptors.

and in particular reduces β-adrenoceptor activity. Phenylephrine, for example, differs chemically from epinephrine in that it has no C-4-hydroxyl group (see Fig. 16-6). It is a strong stimulator of α-adrenoceptors but is, nevertheless, less potent than norepinephrine and epinephrine. However, it has negligible activity on β-adrenoceptors. Hydroxyl groups at C-3 and C-5 positions appear to confer β_2-adrenoceptor selectivity (e.g., terbutaline, metaproterenol). Albuterol (salbutamol) is an important exception to this general rule: Although it lacks a C-5 substituent, and has a –CH_2–OH substituent on position C-3, it has a hydroxyl substituent on C-4, which permits it to exert strong β_2-agonist activity. It is interesting to speculate that C-4-hydroxyl also may confer some properties of α_2-adrenoceptor activation.

Drugs that lack both aromatic hydroxyl groups can produce greater CNS stimulation than epinephrine does (e.g., amphetamine, methamphetamine, ephedrine). Also, the absence of one or both of the hydroxyl groups renders the drug more effective following oral administration and prolongs the duration of action.

Side-chain substitutions also alter the activity of the catecholamines. Substitution on the α-carbon blocks oxidation by monoamine oxidase and therefore increases the duration of action of the noncatecholamines. Substitution on the β-carbon decreases CNS stimulation and increases both α- and β-adrenoceptor activity.

Substitution on either the α- or β-carbon provides optical isomers. Levorotatory substitution on the β-carbon confers greater peripheral activity, so that the naturally occurring *l*-epinephrine and *l*-norepinephrine are 10 times as potent as their unnatural *d*-isomers. Dextrorotatory substitution on the α-carbon results in greater CNS activity compared to the *l*-isomer. Thus *d*-amphetamine is more potent centrally than *l*-amphetamine, but peripherally the *d*- and *l*-isomers are equipotent.

Mechanism of Action

The events following adrenoceptor activation by an agonist to produce a biological response are described in Chapter 13. All adrenoceptors when stimulated by an agonist are coupled to G proteins. G protein–linked receptors include the receptors for a wide variety of hormones and neurotransmitters (see Chapters 9 and 10). Figure 16-3 provides a simplified overview of the events of signal transduction specific for adrenoceptor agonists.

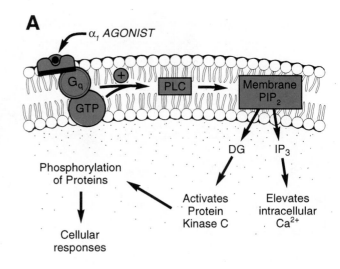

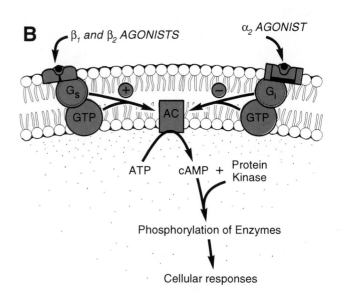

Figure 16-3. Molecular effects of (A) α_1-adrenoceptor agonists and (B) α_2-, β_1-, and β_2-adrenoceptor agonists. PLC = phospholipase C; PIP_2 = phosphatidylinositol bisphosphate; IP_3 = inositol trisphosphate; DG = diacylglycerol; G_i = inhibitory G protein for adenylyl cyclase; G_q = stimulatory G protein for phospholipase C; G_s = stimulatory G protein for adenylyl cyclase; GTP = guanosine triphosphate; AC = adenylyl cyclase; ATP = adenosine triphosphate; cAMP = cyclic adenosine monophosphate; + = stimulates; − = inhibits.

Classification of Adrenoceptors

Adrenoceptors are located ubiquitously throughout the central and autonomic nervous systems, as well as in peripheral tissues (Table 13-2). Adrenoceptors have a wide range of different affinities for many

Table 16-2 Effects of α- and β-Adrenoceptor Agonists on the Cardiovascular System*

Receptor	Drugs	Effects	
α_1	Norepinephrine Epinephrine Dopamine (higher doses) Phenylephrine Metaraminol	Large arteries: ↑tone	
		Arterioles:	↑ tone ↑ peripheral resistance ↑ diastolic pressure ↑ afterload ↑ heart rate (reflex)
		Large veins:	↑ tone ↑ venous return ↑ preload (↑ ventricular volume)
α_2	Norepinephrine Epinephrine	↑ tone in large arteries ↑ peripheral resistance (postsynaptic α_2- receptors in some vascular smooth muscle) ↑ EDRF (nitric oxide) ↑ coronary vasodilatation ↑ coronary transmitter release	
β_1	Norepinephrine Epinephrine Isoproterenol Dopamine Dobutamine	↑ heart rate ↑ automaticity of all pacemaker cells ↑ (arrhythmias can occur) ↑ conduction velocity in atria, A-V node, ↑ and ventricles ↑ velocity of contraction ↑ force of contraction ↑ stroke volume ↑ cardiac output ↑ oxygen consumption ↓ diastolic time for coronary perfusion and ↓ ↓ ventricular filling (with marked ↓ tachycardia) ↓ residual (end-systolic) volume ↑ coronary vasodilatation	

β_2	Albuterol (Salbutamol)
	Terbutaline
	Epinephrine
	Isoproterenol
		↓ arteriolar tone
		↓ peripheral resistance
		↓ diastolic pressure
		↓ afterload
		↓ heart rate: (1) reflex
		               (2) β_1 stimulation with epinephrine
		                    and isoproterenol, and high doses
		                    of selective β_1-agonists	

*No functional distinction between α_{1A}- and α_{1B}-receptors has been identified as yet.

synthetic agents and, as a result, the adrenoceptors have been subdivided into distinct receptor subtypes, as described in Chapter 13. With the development of potent and highly selective α- and β-adrenoceptor antagonists and molecular biological research methods, a series of subtypes have been identified, as listed in Table 16-1.

α_1-Adrenoceptor subtypes

The first suggestion that there are different α_1-adrenoceptor subtypes was based on differences in response to prazosin (an α_1-adrenoceptor antagonist) in functional in vitro assays: This remains an active area of investigation. Radioligand binding and molecular studies identified a number of distinct sites with similar high affinity for prazosin, but different affinities for other compounds. The α_{1A}- and α_{1B}-adrenoceptors were subclassified on the basis of their differential affinity for WB 4101 and chloroethylclonidine. This classification was further supported by the much greater affinity of the α_{1A}-adrenoceptor for 5-methylurapidil and niguldipine. In the rat, tissues with a high population of α_{1A}-adrenoceptors include vas deferens, anococcygeus muscle, and submaxillary gland, whereas spleen and liver have predominantly α_{1B}-adrenoceptors.

Various studies have found blood vessels to contain either α_{1A} or α_{1B} or both, but other reports have suggested that blood vessels have α_1-adrenoceptors with distinctly different properties, including widely differing affinities for prazosin. Such studies led to the identification of further subtypes designated α_{1H}, α_{1L}, and α_{1N}. Finally, the cloning of α_1-receptors, structural analysis of their protein subunits, and formation of recombinant α_1-adrenoceptors gave rise to a different system of nomenclature in which α_{1a}, α_{1b}, and α_{1d} have so far been named. The α_{1a} subtype may correspond to the pharmacologically identified α_{1A}-receptor. The functional significance of these various subtypes in human pharmacology is currently under study.

α_2-Adrenoceptor subtypes

Subclassification of α_2-adrenoceptors was originally based on the ability of prazosin to inhibit $[^3H]$-yohimbine or $[3H]$-rauwolscine binding. Prazosin has high affinity for the α_{2B}- and α_{2C}-adrenoceptor (found in rat lung) but has low affinity for the α_{2A}-adrenoceptor (in platelets). By correlation of antagonist potencies, two additional sites were identified and designated as the α_{2C}- and α_{2D}-adrenoceptor.

All known α_2-adrenoceptors can be activated by norepinephrine and epinephrine and blocked by rauwolscine and yohimbine. Oxymetazoline shows preferential potency at the α_{2A}-adrenoceptor. The α_{2C}-adrenoceptor shares certain similarities with the α_{2B}-adrenoceptor but has higher affinity for rauwolscine; it has been identified in opossum kidney and human retinoblastoma cell lines. The α_{1D}-adrenoceptor has been found in bovine pineal and rat submaxillary glands and has much lower affinity for rauwolscine, as well as low affinity for prazosin. It now appears that the α_{2D}-adrenoceptor is the rat homolog of the human α_{2A}-adrenoceptor.

As in the case of the α_1-adrenoceptors, the α_2 subtypes have now been cloned, and their related genes have been identified and mapped (see Table 16-1). There is a high degree of structural homology and pharmacological similarity among the corresponding subtypes of α_2-adrenoceptor in humans, rats, and mice.

β-Adrenoceptor subtypes

The existence of two distinct β-adrenoceptor subtypes has been well established since 1967. More recently a β-adrenoceptor was found that was insensitive to all of the classical β antagonists. Originally this was referred to as "atypical β-adrenoceptor," but with the identification of selective agonists and expression of a recombinant receptor it is appropriate to call this a β_3-adrenoceptor.

All three β-adrenoceptors can be activated by norepinephrine and epinephrine, but a primary distinction between β_1 and β_2-adrenoceptors can be made in terms of the relative potencies of these two catecholamines. Norepinephrine is slightly more potent than epinephrine at the β_1-adrenoceptor, but at the β_2-adrenoceptor, epinephrine is some 100-fold more potent than norepinephrine. Norepinephrine is more potent than epinephrine at the β_3-adrenoceptor. Isoproterenol is equipotent at all three β-adrenoceptors. All three β-adrenoceptors can be labeled with iodocyanopindolol, and all use adenylyl cyclase as their mechanism for signal transduction.

Selective antagonists for the β-adrenoceptor subtypes will be discussed in Chapter 17. Synthetic agonists with high selectivity for the β_2-adrenoceptor are available and clinically useful (see below), but selective agonists for the β_1-adrenoceptor have limited usefulness because of low selectivity and efficacy. β_1-Adrenoceptors mediate inotropic and chronotropic effects on the myocardium, and relaxation of coronary arteries, whereas β_2-adrenoceptors mediate relaxation of bronchiolar, uterine, and vascular smooth muscle. In addition, the presynaptic β-adrenoceptor (which facilitates transmitter release) shares many characteristics with the β_2-adrenoceptor. Although no selective antagonist for the β_3-adrenoceptor has been discovered, a number of selective agonists have been shown to exist, most notably BRL 37344. The primary actions mediated by β_3-adrenoceptors are lipolysis in white adipose tissue, thermogenesis in brown adipose tissue, and inhibition of gastrointestinal smooth muscle contraction.

All three subtypes of β-adrenoceptor have now been cloned and characterized by their respective pharmacological properties. There is only about 50% structural homology among the three types.

Effects of Catecholamines

Heart

Norepinephrine, epinephrine, and isoproterenol stimulate β_1-adrenoceptors in the heart and produce the following effects.

Tachycardia results from an increased rate of discharge of pacemaker cells in the S-A node. This increases the slope of phase 4 in the action potential (i.e., the rate of diastolic depolarization) because of altered permeability of the cell membrane, allowing a faster influx of Na^+ (and Ca^{2+}). The increase in heart rate is referred to as a *positive chronotropic effect.*

Norepinephrine (and epinephrine in large doses) may **increase the blood pressure** to such an extent that reflex slowing of the heart may occur, mediated by baroreceptor stimulation that causes increased amounts of acetylcholine to be released at the S-A node. Because of reflex slowing, the cardiac output may be unchanged or decreased. The stroke volume, however, is always increased.

Automaticity of latent pacemaker cells is increased, and this may lead to arrhythmias.

Shortening of the refractory period of the A-V node gives rise to acceleration of impulse conduction between atria and ventricles.

The force of contraction of the heart is increased; i.e., there is a *positive inotropic effect.*

Increase in stroke volume and cardiac output is accompanied by **increased oxygen consumption**. There is a decrease in efficiency of the heart; i.e., less work is done relative to the amount of oxygen consumed.

The β_1 effects of norepinephrine on the heart may be observed after administration of atropine or in isolated heart preparations.

Dopamine has a dose-dependent positive inotropic effect on the heart through stimulation of β_1-adrenoceptors. At infusion rates of 5–20 μg/kg/min, cardiac output and rate increase. Dopamine receptors in the periphery (renal and mesenteric vessels) are stimulated at doses of 1–5 μg/kg/min. High doses stimulate α-adrenoceptors.

Although β_1-adrenoceptors are of major importance in modulating cardiac responses, there are also β_2 and α_1 present in the heart. β_2-Adrenoceptors are probably stimulated by circulating epinephrine, resulting in synergism with β_1-receptor stimulation with respect to increasing the heart rate. α_1-Adrenoceptors have a moderate positive inotropic effect and may be an important compensatory mechanism when β-adrenoceptors are down-regulated, as seen in congestive heart failure.

Blood vessels

The basic difference among the catecholamines is that norepinephrine constricts all blood vessels, whereas epinephrine has mixed effects (i.e., it causes vasoconstriction in some vascular beds while dilating blood vessels in skeletal muscle), and isoproterenol is a pure vasodilator. This difference is reflected in the effects of the individual drugs on heart rate.

Norepinephrine causes constriction of arterioles in the skin, skeletal muscle, mucous membranes, and kidneys. In vivo, this is evidenced by an increase in total peripheral resistance, which results in elevation of diastolic blood pressure. Systolic pressure is also increased. Constriction of large veins (capacitance vessels) and larger arteries (conductance vessels) also occurs. These vascular responses to norepinephrine are mediated predominantly through α_1-adrenoceptor stimulation, although in some vascular beds there may be an α_2-adrenoceptor component. The coronary vascular bed is unique in that the predominant adrenoceptor on the smooth muscle cell is believed to be a β_1-adrenoceptor. Furthermore, in some instances, the endothelial cells of coronary blood vessels possess α_2-adrenoceptors which, when activated, cause the release of an endothelium-derived relaxing factor (EDRF, also known to be nitric oxide). Therefore, the net effect of norepinephrine on the coronary bed is vasodilatation, because the vasoconstriction effects of α_1-adrenoceptors are overcome by the vasodilatation effects of β_1- and endothelial α_2-adrenoceptors and of EDRF.

As mentioned earlier, the large increase in blood

pressure produced by norepinephrine slows the heart by a reflex increase in vagal tone, thus masking the β_1-adrenoceptor effects on heart rate. The β_1-adrenoceptor-mediated inotropic action is maintained (Fig. 16-4).

Epinephrine causes vasoconstriction of most blood vessels in the skin, mucous membranes, and kidneys. Dilatation occurs in skeletal muscle vascular beds, which contain β_2- and α_1-adrenoceptors. These β_2-adrenoceptors are sensitive to much lower doses of epinephrine than are the α_1-adrenoceptors. Moreover, epinephrine is much more potent than norepinephrine on the β_2-adrenoceptor than the β_1-adrenoceptor. This dilatation response results in a slight decrease in resistance, causing a small decrease in diastolic pressure, and therefore reflex tachycardia may occur rather than reflex slowing of the heart (Fig. 16-4). Larger doses of epinephrine, however, do stimulate α_1-adrenoceptors, and the actions of epinephrine become similar to those of norepinephrine, and reflex bradycardia occurs.

Isoproterenol lowers peripheral vascular resistance (β_2-adrenoceptor stimulation) in renal and mesenteric blood vessels and in skeletal muscle beds, causing a fall in diastolic pressure. Cardiac output is raised because of an increase in venous return. The increase in cardiac output is enhanced by an increased force of contraction (positive inotropic action) and tachycardia (positive chronotropic effect). Systolic pressure may remain unchanged or rise slightly. Nevertheless, mean arterial pressure typically falls (Fig. 16-4).

Dopamine effects are mediated by several distinct types of receptor (see Chapter 28). At low concentration, dopamine stimulates only dopamine receptors, resulting in dilatation of renal and mesenteric vessels, as well as the coronary bed. Low doses also cause an increase in glomerular filtration rate, renal blood flow, and Na^+ excretion. At higher concentrations, dopamine interacts with α_1-adrenoceptors, causing increased peripheral vascular resistance and vasoconstriction. When dopamine is used for

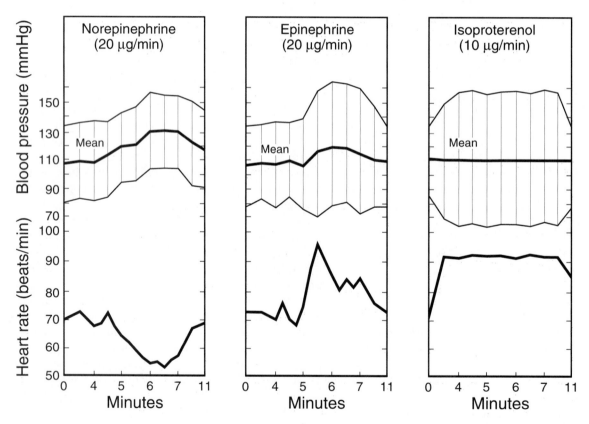

Figure 16-4. Effects of norepinephrine, epinephrine, and isoproterenol infusions on blood pressure and heart rate in humans. Note the increased mean pressure and decreased heart rate following infusion of norepinephrine; the essentially unchanged mean pressure, increased pulse pressure, and elevated heart rate following infusion of epinephrine; and the unchanged mean pressure, increased pulse pressure, and sustained elevated heart rate following infusion of isoproterenol.

treatment of shock, blood pressure and renal function must be carefully monitored.

The effects of catecholamines on the cardiovascular system are summarized in Table 16-2.

Respiratory system

Activation of β_2-adrenoceptors causes relaxation of bronchiolar smooth muscle and decreased airway resistance. Antigen-induced release of asthma mediators is also inhibited. (See Selective β_2-Adrenoceptor Agonists, below).

Activation of α_1-adrenoceptors causes vasoconstriction in the upper respiratory tract mucosa. This decongestant effect in nasal and bronchiolar mucosa is clinically useful. (See Selective α_1-Adrenoceptor Agonists, below).

Epinephrine primarily relaxes bronchial smooth muscle. It has a powerful bronchodilatory action, most evident when bronchial muscle is contracted, as in bronchial asthma. The beneficial effects may also arise from a decrease in antigen-induced release of inflammatory mediators from mast cells and, to a lesser extent, from diminished bronchial secretions and congestion within the mucosa. Similarly, isoproterenol relaxes bronchial smooth muscle, and prevents or relieves bronchoconstriction, but tolerance to this action develops. Isoproterenol also inhibits antigen-induced release of asthma mediators.

Gastrointestinal tract

Stimulation of α- and β-adrenoceptors causes relaxation of gastrointestinal smooth muscle by different mechanisms:

- Norepinephrine, by stimulating presynaptic α_2-adrenoceptors on cholinergic neurons, inhibits the release of acetylcholine, causing decreased smooth muscle tone and reduced amplitude of contractions.
- Stimulation of β_2-adrenoceptors elevates cAMP, resulting in Ca^{2+} sequestration, which reduces the strength of muscle contraction.
- α_1-Adrenoceptor activation causes an increase in K^+ conductance and hyperpolarization, thus reducing muscle cell excitability.

Uterus

The effects of the catecholamines on the uterine tract are dependent on the status of the uterus. Norepinephrine has been observed to increase the frequency of contraction in the human pregnant uterus. Epinephrine inhibits uterine tone and contractions during the last month of pregnancy and at parturition. On the basis of the latter finding, selective β_2-agonists are commonly used to delay premature labor.

Eye

The radial muscle in the iris contains α_1-adrenoceptors that, when stimulated, cause mydriasis (pupil dilatation). In theory, this should tend to raise the intraocular pressure by blocking the outflow of aqueous humor. However, α_1-mediated vasoconstriction decreases the formation of aqueous humor, and this effect usually predominates, lowering the intraocular pressure. Intraocular pressure is influenced by both α- and β-adrenoceptors. Some β-adrenoceptor antagonists (e.g., timolol) are commonly used in the treatment of glaucoma.

Metabolic effects

The important effects of catecholamines on intermediary metabolism include lipolysis, glycogenolysis, and gluconeogenesis.

Lipolysis is associated with β_1 stimulation (and the more recently characterized β_3-adrenoceptor). Receptor-mediated elevation of cAMP levels causes activation of lipase, and the breakdown of triglycerides to glycerol and free fatty acids is enhanced.

Glycogenolysis in the liver is increased by β_2 stimulation, which causes increased glucose release into the circulation and hyperglycemia. α-Adrenoceptors may also play a role.

Gluconeogenesis from lactate and amino acids is also stimulated. Oxygen consumption is increased by both epinephrine and norepinephrine (calorigenic effect).

Epinephrine increases plasma levels of K^+ transiently; this is followed by a more prolonged fall in K^+ plasma levels. This is a β_2-mediated effect. Adrenoceptor agonists of the β_2 type have been used in the management of hyperkalemic familial periodic paralysis because of the ability of the drugs to increase uptake of K^+ into muscle cells.

Endocrine glands

The release of insulin is increased by β_2-adrenoceptor stimulation and inhibited by α-adrenoceptor activation (see Chapter 50). Glucagon secretion from α cells in the pancreas is also increased. Renin release from the juxtaglomerular cells in the kidney is increased by β_1-adrenoceptor activation and inhibited by α-adrenoceptor stimulation.

Central nervous system

Catecholamines are potent stimulants of the central nervous system (Fig. 16-5). The concentration of free catecholamines in the brain is increased by cocaine (via blockade of reuptake of catecholamine neurotransmitters, and possibly enhanced release). A mood-elevating (euphoriant) effect is the basis for the abuse of these drugs. They also enhance alertness and prolong the ability to perform repetitive tasks.

Skeletal muscle

Epinephrine and other β_2-agonists facilitate the release of acetylcholine from cholinergic motor axon terminals, probably by elevating cAMP levels at presynaptic sites. Stimulation of α_2-adrenoceptors on cholinergic neurons in skeletal muscle increases the release of acetylcholine, presumably by increasing Ca^{2+} influx into the neurons. This contrasts with α_2-adrenoceptor stimulation on cholinergic neurons at other sites, e.g., the gastrointestinal tract (see above), where it inhibits the release of acetylcholine. Motor power in myasthenia gravis can be increased by ephedrine and amphetamine, which increase the release of catecholamines in addition to being direct adrenoceptor agonists. β_2-Adrenoceptor agonists (e.g., epinephrine, albuterol) cause muscle tremor

that can be prevented by propranolol. The mechanism responsible for tremor induction is associated with β_2-adrenoceptor-mediated enhancement of muscle spindle discharge.

SELECTIVE ADRENOCEPTOR AGONISTS

α_1-Adrenoceptor Agonists (Fig. 16-6)

Phenylephrine (Neo-Synephrine)

This agent is closely related chemically to epinephrine. It is a powerful, selective, and direct-acting α_1-adrenoceptor agonist that activates β-adrenoceptors only at high concentrations. The pharmacological effects are essentially similar to those of norepinephrine, but it is less potent and has a much longer duration of action. The predominant actions are on the cardiovascular system. Intravenous, subcutaneous, and oral administration all cause a rise in systolic and diastolic pressure in humans and other species. Phenylephrine is useful as a vasoconstrictor, decongestant, mydriatic, and anti-allergy agent. It is also used to treat paroxysmal atrial tachycardia by indirectly causing reflex bradycardia.

Methoxamine (Vasoxyl)

This is another relatively selective α_1-adrenoceptor agent. It does not stimulate β-adrenoceptors, nor

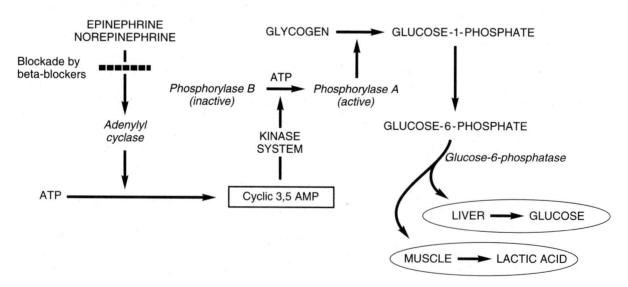

Figure 16-5. Metabolic pathways by which catecholamines stimulate glycogenolysis.

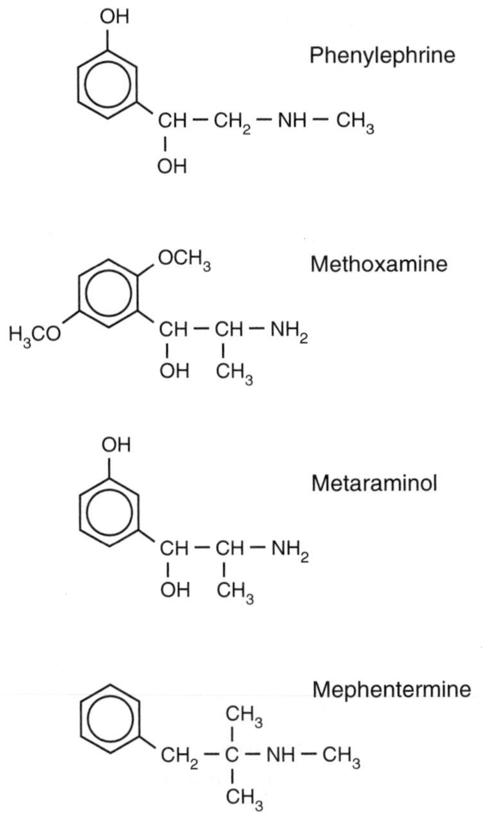

OH

Phenylephrine

$CH-CH_2-NH-CH_3$

OH

OCH_3

Methoxamine

H_3CO

$CH-CH-NH_2$

OH CH$_3$

OH

Metaraminol

$CH-CH-NH_2$

OH CH$_3$

Mephentermine

CH$_3$

$CH_2-C-NH-CH_3$

CH$_3$

Figure 16-6. Structural formulae of α_1-adrenoceptor agonists.

does it stimulate the CNS. Its major action on the cardiovascular system is to raise blood pressure; this effect is associated with reflex bradycardia. Like phenylephrine, methoxamine is used to treat hypotensive states and to relieve paroxysmal atrial tachycardia.

Metaraminol (Aramine)

This agent is both a direct (α_1-adrenoceptor-stimulating) and an indirect sympathomimetic. It causes an increase in both systolic and diastolic pressure that is due to peripheral vasoconstriction and is accompanied by reflex vagal bradycardia. Its effects, like those of methoxamine, are long-lasting. Metaraminol can also release norepinephrine from sympathetic nerves and is a weak β_1-adrenoceptor agonist.

Other selective α_1-adrenoceptor agonists include mephentermine, naphazoline, and cirazoline.

Selective α_2-Adrenoceptor Agonists

Clonidine (Catapres)

When clonidine was first synthesized, it was found to produce vasoconstriction mediated by α-adrenoceptors. However, during trials as a nasal decongestant, it was found to cause hypotension, sedation, and bradycardia. These different responses represent actions on pre- versus postsynaptic α_2-adrenoceptors.

When clonidine is given intravenously, it produces an acute rise in blood pressure because of activation of postjunctional α_1- and α_2-adrenoceptors. This rise in pressure is usually not seen when the drug is given orally. It is followed by a prolonged hypotensive response resulting from decreased central outflow in the sympathetic nervous system. This is due to activation of presynaptic α_2-adrenoceptors in the lower brainstem, possibly in the nucleus of the tractus solitarius.

A withdrawal reaction occurs after abrupt discontinuation of therapy with clonidine.

α-**Methyldopa, guanfacine, and guanabenz** are α_2-adrenoceptor agonists that function in a similar manner to clonidine, and will not be discussed further. The compounds BHT 920 and BHT 933 are useful experimental pharmacological tools for studying α_2-adrenoceptor mechanisms.

Selective β_1-Adrenoceptor Agonist

Dobutamine (Dobutrex)

This agent is a synthetic derivative of dopamine with the catechol group in its structure (Fig. 16-7). It is known as a selective stimulant of β_1-adrenoceptors. Its action on the heart is unique in that it produces more inotropic than chronotropic effects. The precise reason for this is unclear, but may be due to the distinct properties of the *d*- and *l*-isomers. While *d*-dobutamine is a pure β_1-adrenoceptor agonist, the *l*-isomer has some α_1-adrenoceptor-stimulant effects, which may contribute to the overall increase in inotropy.

Selective β_2-Adrenoceptor Agonists

The main problems encountered with β-adrenoceptor agonists used for the treatment of asthma are caused

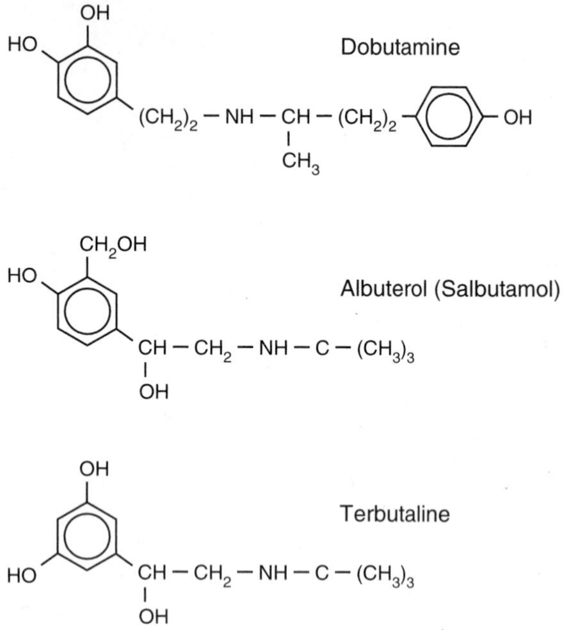

Figure 16-7. Structural formulae of selective β_1- and β_2-adrenoceptor agonists.

by β_1-adrenoceptor stimulation. Therefore there has been much effort put into the development of drugs with selectivity toward β_2-adrenoceptors. **Albuterol** (salbutamol; Ventolin) and other related drugs are effective bronchodilators because of their action on β_2-adrenoceptors in bronchiolar smooth muscle. Because they stimulate β_2-receptors preferentially, these agents lack the myocardial stimulating properties of isoproterenol. High doses of albuterol, however, will cause β_1-receptor-mediated myocardial stimulation. Albuterol also stimulates β_2-receptors in the smooth muscle of vessels supplying skeletal muscle, leading to a decrease in peripheral vascular resistance. Since the uterus reacts to β_2-agonists with relaxation, albuterol can be used to delay delivery in premature labor.

Other selective β_2-adrenoceptor agonists are **terbutaline** (Bricanyl) and **orciprenaline** (Alupent).

Selective β_3-Adrenoceptor Agonists

BRL 37344 is an experimental compound that regulates fat metabolism and gastrointestinal function. Recent research indicates that such agents may have a use in treatment of obesity.

Nonselective β-Adrenoceptor Agonist

Isoproterenol (Isuprel) is the most potent β_1- and β_2-adrenergic agent in use. Peripheral vasodilatation,

tachycardia, myocardial stimulation, and bronchial relaxation are the most important effects produced. Isoproterenol is more potent than epinephrine as a bronchial dilator, but it is not a decongestant. The side effects of isoproterenol, which frequently are very severe, are due primarily to its cardiac action. The tachycardia and myocardial stimulation produce signs of coronary insufficiency by increasing the amount of oxygen required by the heart.

Isoproterenol is metabolized by COMT, just as the endogenous catecholamines are, but it is unaffected by MAO. (For further details, see earlier in this chapter.)

DRUGS THAT RELEASE NOREPINEPHRINE FROM SYMPATHETIC NERVES

These drugs are transported across the adrenergic neuronal membrane and displace norepinephrine from storage sites within the neuron. The released norepinephrine interacts with adrenoceptors to produce characteristic responses in the effector organs, e.g., increase in heart rate and elevation of blood pressure. Most of these drugs (e.g., ephedrine) produce additional sympathomimetic effects by stimulating adrenoceptors directly. Since such drugs have both indirect (norepinephrine-releasing) and direct (adrenoceptor-stimulating) actions, they are frequently classified as drugs with "mixed" actions. However, the direct stimulation of peripheral adrenoceptors by amphetamine is minimal when compared with its norepinephrine-releasing action.

Ephedrine

Ephedrine (Fig. 16-8) is an alkaloid obtained from Ma Huang (*Ephedra equisetina*) and has been used in Chinese medicine from early times. Both carbon atoms on the aliphatic side-chain are asymmetric, resulting in four isomers: (+)- and (−)-ephedrine,

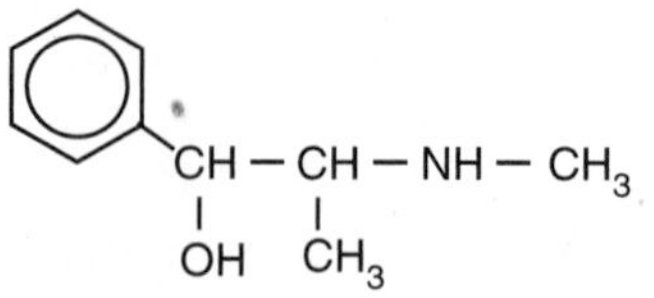

Figure 16-8. Structural formula of ephedrine.

and (+)- and (−)-pseudoephedrine. The most potent form in relation to sympathomimetic activity is (−)-ephedrine, which is used clinically.

Pharmacologically, ephedrine belongs to a special category. Its sympathomimetic effects are due to norepinephrine release from sympathetic nerves (Fig. 16-9, Table 16-3), combined with direct action on α_1-, β_1-, and β_2-adrenoceptors. Tachyphylaxis may occur during chronic administration, because of depletion of the intraneuronal pool of norepinephrine.

The change from the phenolic structure of epinephrine to the phenyl structure of ephedrine results in a marked difference in action. Unlike epinephrine, ephedrine is effective orally, has a prolonged action, is a potent central simulant, but gives rise to tachyphylaxis. Intravenous injection of ephedrine produces a prompt rise in blood pressure. As a vasopressor agent, ephedrine is only 1/1000–1/100 as potent as epinephrine, but its duration of action is seven to 10 times longer. It dilates the coronary vessels, increases the heart rate, and may elevate the arterial blood pressure.

Ephedrine dilates the bronchioles. Although its effect on asthma is not as prompt or pronounced as that of epinephrine, it has the advantage of being active upon oral administration and is longer acting.

Ephedrine increases the tone of skeletal muscle, and for this reason it may be used as an adjuvant drug in the treatment of myasthenia gravis.

Pseudoephedrine (Sudafed) is an active stereoisomer of ephedrine with similar actions and uses.

Amphetamine and Related Drugs

These agents are potent stimulants of the central nervous system; they are described in detail in Chapter 30. The peripheral cardiovascular effects caused by amphetamine are, however, an inherent part of its toxicity.

Amphetamine has a euphoriant (mood-elevating) effect which often causes this substance to be abused (see Chapter 72).

Methamphetamine has a higher ratio of central-to-peripheral effects than amphetamine.

Methylphenidate is used in the treatment of narcolepsy in adults and the hyperkinetic syndrome (attention deficit disorder with hyperactivity) in children. Its abuse potential is similar to that of amphetamine.

Other drugs of this type are **phenmetrazine** and **phentermine.** They are used occasionally as appetite suppressants, although phenmetrazine was withdrawn from the market in Canada because of the risk of abuse, similar to that of amphetamine.

Tyramine

This compound has no direct adrenoceptor-agonist activity; its effects are solely due to release of norepinephrine. Therefore the prior administration of a drug that depletes intraneuronal stores of norepinephrine (e.g., reserpine) will abolish its effects. Tyramine is never used clinically, but it is important as a research drug and in drug interactions when tyramine-containing food is consumed by patients receiving MAO inhibitors.

DRUGS THAT BLOCK THE REUPTAKE OF NOREPINEPHRINE

Cocaine, imipramine, and **amitriptyline** belong to this class of drugs. They interfere with the presynaptic uptake process of a number of neurotransmitters. This causes the concentration of norepinephrine to be elevated at adrenoceptor sites and the responses of effector organs to be exaggerated (see Fig. 16-9). These drugs also prevent the uptake of certain other drugs into the adrenergic neuron; thus, they diminish the responses to ephedrine and block the effects of tyramine.

CLINICAL USES OF α- AND β-ADRENOCEPTOR AGONISTS

Nasal Decongestants

Decongestion of nasal mucous membranes may be achieved by vasoconstriction resulting from local application of α_1-adrenoceptor agonists. Drugs commonly used for this purpose include phenylephrine (Neo-Synephrine), mephentermine (Wyamine), pseudoephedrine (Sudafed), and xylometazoline (Otriven, Otrivin). The beneficial decongestant effects of these drugs may be followed by rebound congestion.

Pressor Agents

Phenylephrine, metaraminol (Aramine), methoxamine (Vasoxyl), and mephentermine may be used parenterally to elevate the blood pressure (e.g., in hypotension associated with spinal anesthesia). The

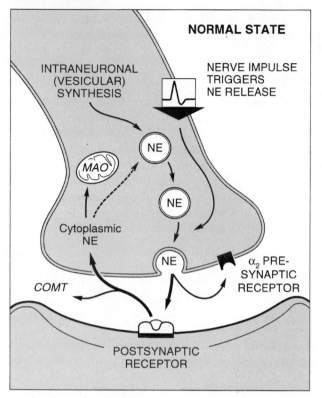

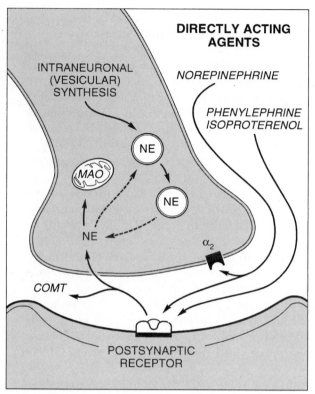

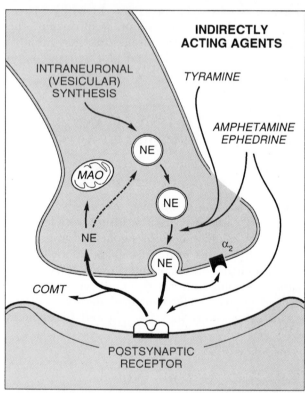

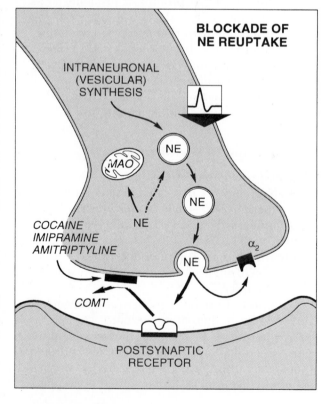

Figure 16-9. Schematic representations of various mechanisms of action of drugs on sympathetic nerve activity. NE = norepinephrine; MAO = monoamine oxidase; COMT = catechol-*O*-methyltransferase; α-CH₃-DOPA = α-methyldopa; α-CH₃-NE = α-methylnorepinephrine.

Although not shown in the diagrams, there is a constant resting release of norepinephrine from adrenergic terminals. (This figure and Table 16-3 are summaries of drug effects on adrenergic nerve activity, as variously discussed in Chapters 16–18).

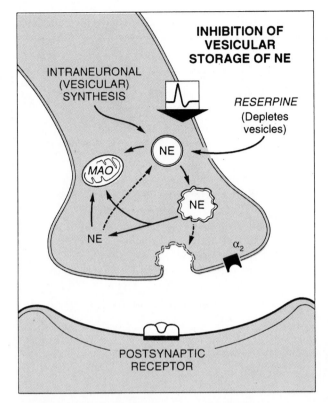

INHIBITION OF VESICULAR STORAGE OF NE

INTRANEURONAL (VESICULAR) SYNTHESIS

RESERPINE (Depletes vesicles)

NE

MAO

NE

NE

α_2

POSTSYNAPTIC RECEPTOR

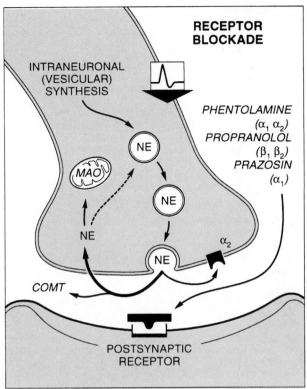

RECEPTOR BLOCKADE

INTRANEURONAL (VESICULAR) SYNTHESIS

PHENTOLAMINE (α_1 α_2)
PROPRANOLOL (β_1 β_2)
PRAZOSIN (α_1)

NE

MAO

NE

NE

NE

α_2

COMT

POSTSYNAPTIC RECEPTOR

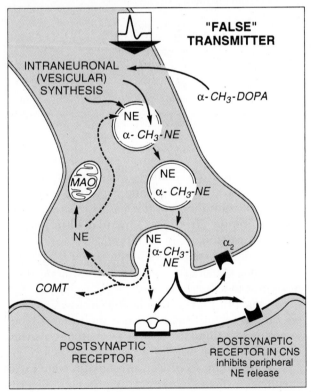

"FALSE" TRANSMITTER

INTRANEURONAL (VESICULAR) SYNTHESIS

α-CH_3-DOPA

NE
α-CH_3-NE

MAO

NE
α-CH_3-NE

NE

NE
α-CH_3-NE

α_2

COMT

POSTSYNAPTIC RECEPTOR

POSTSYNAPTIC RECEPTOR IN CNS inhibits peripheral NE release

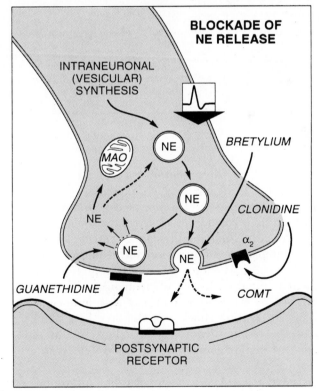

BLOCKADE OF NE RELEASE

INTRANEURONAL (VESICULAR) SYNTHESIS

BRETYLIUM

CLONIDINE

NE

MAO

NE

NE

NE

NE

α_2

GUANETHIDINE

COMT

POSTSYNAPTIC RECEPTOR

Table 16-3 Types of Action of Representative Drugs at Adrenergic Neurons, Synapses, and Neuroeffector Junctions

Mechanism of Action	Drugs	Effects
Interference with synthesis of transmitter	α-Methyl-p-tyrosine Disulfiram	Depletion of norepinephrine
Metabolic transformation by the same pathway as precursor of transmitter	α-Methyldopa	Displacement of norepinephrine by false transmitter (α-methyl-norepinephrine); blockade of release of norepinephrine
Blockade of transport system of axonal membrane, i.e., uptake of norepinephrine	Imipramine Amitriptyline Cocaine	Accumulation of norepinephrine at extra-cellular sites; potentiation of sympathetic response
Blockade of transport system of storage granule membrane	Reserpine	Destruction of norepinephrine by intraneuro-nal MAO, and depletion of adrenergic terminals; super-sensitivity to directly acting amines; subsensitivity to indirectly acting amines
Displacement of transmitter from axonal terminal	Amphetamine Tyramine Ephedrine	Sympathomimetic (indirect)
Prevention of release of transmitter	Guanethidine Bretylium Clonidine	Antiadrenergic; decreased release of norepi-nephrine
Mimicry of transmitter at post-synaptic receptor	Phenylephrine Isoproterenol	Sympathomimetic (direct)
Blockade of endogenous transmitter at postsynaptic receptor	Phenoxybenzamine Propranolol Prazosin	α-Adrenoceptor antagonism β-Adrenoceptor antagonism Selective α_1-adrenoceptor antagonism
Inhibition of enzymatic break-down of transmitter	MAO inhibitors (Pargyline, Tranylcypromine)	Accumulation of norepinephrine at certain sites; potentiation of tyramine

stimulation of α_1-adrenoceptors leads to an increase in peripheral resistance, which increases diastolic (and systolic) pressure. The use of α_1-adrenoceptor agonists in hypovolemic shock is controversial, since there is already a maximal release of catecholamines causing intense vasoconstriction and resulting in decreased tissue perfusion. The microcirculation may be further impaired by use of α_1-agonists. This was the rationale for the proposed use of α_1-adrenoceptor blockers in treating shock (see Chapter 17). Elevation of the blood pressure is of value only in the absence of hypovolemia and/or electrolyte disturbances.

In **cardiogenic shock** (myocardial infarction), norepinephrine (levarterenol, Levophed), dopamine (Intropin), and dobutamine (Dobutrex) may be used. Dopamine, in contrast to norepinephrine, has a va-sodilating action on splanchnic and renal vascular beds, mediated through specific dopamine receptors. The force of contraction of the heart is also increased (β_1-adrenoceptor effects). Glomerular filtration rate and urine production are enhanced.

Dobutamine is relatively selective as a β_1-adreno-ceptor agonist that increases stroke volume at doses that do not increase heart rate.

Norepinephrine is administered intravenously in moderate doses sufficient to raise the arterial blood pressure and stimulate the heart without causing serious vasoconstriction.

Anaphylactic shock is traditionally treated with epinephrine, which counteracts the bronchoconstric-tor and vasodilator actions of histamine. Epinephrine is also used in urticaria, hay fever, and angioneurotic edema.

Bronchodilators

Selective β_2-adrenoceptor agonists are effective in the treatment of reversible airway obstruction associated with bronchial asthma and chronic bronchitis. They cause fewer cardiovascular side effects, such as tachycardia, than do the nonselective β-adrenoceptor agonists, such as epinephrine and isoproterenol. However, with increased dosage of β_2-selective agonists, cardiovascular side effects can occur. These drugs should be used with caution in patients who have thyrotoxicosis or cardiovascular disorders.

Albuterol (salbutamol) is the most widely used β_2-adrenoceptor agonist. It can be used orally or by inhalation from aerosol containers. Terbutaline (Bricanyl) and orciprenaline (Alupent) are similar in action.

Isoproterenol is a potent nonselective bronchodilator with the disadvantage of causing excessive myocardial stimulation.

Epinephrine, used in treating acute attacks of allergy-induced asthma, stimulates not only β_2-adrenoceptors, but also α_1-adrenoceptors, which constrict bronchial mucosal vessels and thereby enhance the reduction in airway resistance.

All β_2-adrenoceptor agonists increase cAMP in bronchial muscle cells, resulting in Ca^{2+} sequestration and relaxation of the bronchiolar smooth muscle.

Cardiac Arrest and Heart Block

Isoproterenol or epinephrine may be administered intravenously or directly into the heart in asystole. These agents may also be used in complete heart block with slow ventricular response or asystole. The long-term maintenance treatment of heart block may also require isoproterenol.

Ophthalmic Applications

Phenylephrine and ephedrine are sometimes applied topically to the eye to dilate the pupil (mydriasis), usually to permit examination of the fundus. They have the advantage of not causing paralysis of accommodation (cycloplegia) as atropine-like drugs do. In glaucoma, phenylephrine or epinephrine may be used to decrease the intraocular pressure by their local vasoconstrictor action, which decreases the production of aqueous humor. All effects described in the eye are mediated by α_1-adrenoceptor stimulation.

SUGGESTED READING

Berridge MJ. The molecular basis of communication within the cell. Sci Am 1985; 254(4):142–152.

Brodde OE. The functional importance of β_1 and β_2 adrenoceptors in the human heart. Am J Cardiol 1988; 62:24C–29C.

Eggleston PA, Beasley PP. Bronchodilatation and inhibition of induced asthma by adrenergic agonists. Clin Pharmacol Ther 1981; 29:505–510.

Emorine L, Blin N, Strosberg AD. The human β_3-adrenoceptor: the search for a physiological function. TIPS 1994; 15:3–6.

Flavahan NA, McGrath JC. Alpha$_1$-adrenoceptor activation can increase heart rate directly or decrease it indirectly through parasympathetic activation. Br J Pharmacol 1982; 77:319–328.

Ford APDW, Williams TJ, Blue DR, Clarke DE. α_1-Adrenoceptor classification: sharpening Occam's razor. TIPS 1994; 15:167–170.

Hicks PE, Barras M, Herman G, Mauduit P, Armstrong AM, Rossignol B. α_1-Adrenoceptor subtypes in dog saphenous vein that mediate contraction and inositol phosphate production. Br J Pharmacol 1991; 102:151–161.

Hon C, Abel PW, Minneman KP. α_1-Adrenoceptor subtypes linked to different mechanisms for increasing intracellular Ca^{++} in smooth muscle. Nature 1987; 329:24–27.

Lafontan M, Berlan M, Prud'hon M. Beta-adrenergic agonists. Mechanism of action; lipid mobilization and anabolism. Reprod Nutr Dev 1988; 28:61–84.

Lulich KM, Goldie RG, Paterson JW. Beta-adrenoceptor function in asthmatic bronchial smooth muscle. Gen Pharmacol 1988; 19:307–311.

Seale JP. Whither beta-adrenoceptor agonists in the treatment of asthma. Prog Clin Biol Res 1988; 263:367–377.

Starke K. Alpha-adrenoceptor subclassification. Rev Physiol Biochem Pharmacol 1981; 88:199–236.

van Zwieten PA, Timmermans PB. Alpha-adrenoceptor stimulation and calcium movements. Recent advances in sympathetic neurotransmission. 6th meeting on adrenergic mechanisms. Porto, Portugal, 1986. Blood Vessels 1987; 24:271–280.

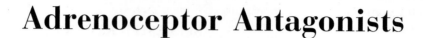

CHAPTER 17

Adrenoceptor Antagonists

C. FORSTER

CASE HISTORY

A healthy 60-year-old man presented for a routine eye examination. He complained of progressive weakening of vision, and his intraocular pressure was found to be 23 mmHg. His arterial blood pressure was found to be mildly elevated (135/98 mmHg) but was not treated at this stage. Since intraocular pressures of greater than 20 mmHg usually indicate a need for drug therapy, the patient was asked to return to the ophthalmology department for a diagnostic test for glaucoma. The patient's brother (aged 65) and father had also been diagnosed as having glaucoma. After an overnight fast and immediately before the test, the patient was asked to consume 1 liter of water. This caused the intraocular pressure to increase by 12 mmHg. The patient had no evidence of trauma, inflammation, or diabetes, nor was he taking any medication. Timolol 0.25% ophthalmic solution was prescribed, to be self-administered at a dose of 1 drop of the solution in each eye, twice daily. On this treatment the intraocular pressure remained elevated at 22 mmHg, and the concentration of the solution was therefore increased to 0.5%. Following regular treatment for 3 weeks, his intraocular pressure appeared to be controlled, and was stable at 15 mmHg (i.e., within the normal range). However, on continuing this regimen, he became significantly hypotensive (85/50 mmHg). Timolol was discontinued and acetazolamide 250 mg/day was introduced. The intraocular pressure was maintained at the previous level and his blood pressure returned to the normal range (118/76 mmHg).

INTRODUCTORY CONCEPT

The characteristic responses of effector organs to endogenous catecholamines and sympathomimetic drugs can be selectively blocked by α- or β-adrenoceptor antagonists. The extent of the blockade obtained is related to (1) the relative concentrations of the agonist and the antagonist present at the adrenoceptor sites in the effector organ cells and (2) their relative affinities for these sites. Selectivity of the antagonist drug for α- or β-adrenoceptors is further enhanced by differing affinities of the drugs for the α-adrenoceptor subtypes (α_1 and α_2) and for β-adrenoceptor subtypes (β_1 and β_2).

Selective inhibition of some of the physiological effects of catecholamines was first reported in 1906 by Dale, who demonstrated that the pressor effects of large doses of epinephrine could be reversed, to cause a fall in blood pressure, by certain ergot derivatives now known to possess α-adrenoceptor-blocking properties. Later work led to the synthesis of a large number of drugs with the ability to antagonize the effects of α-adrenoceptor stimulation. More recently, the development of selective antagonists for α_{1A}-, α_{1B}-, and α_{1D}-adrenoceptors has helped provide functional evidence for the existence of these distinct subtypes. Selective antagonists for α_{1A}-receptors include 5-methylurapidil and niguldipine. Selective antagonists for the α_{1B}- and α_{1D}-adrenoceptors are the irreversible inhibitor **chloroethylclonidine** and **BMY 7378** respectively.

MEASUREMENT OF ANTAGONIST POTENCY

Drug antagonism is quantified by the use of the pA scale, which is an empirical measure of the activity of an antagonist that is not dependent on its mechanism of action. The pA_2 is defined as the negative logarithm (base 10) of the molar concentration of antagonist which reduces the effect of a double dose of agonist to that of a single dose or, in other words, causes a parallel displacement of the concentration–effect curve of a given agonist two-fold to the right without changing the maximum response.

The pA_2 can be determined by measuring the value of the concentration ratio at three or more antagonist concentrations. A graph of log [concentration ratio minus 1] against log [concentration of antagonist] yields a line with a slope of unity, and the x-intercept equals the pA_2 for true competitive antagonism (Schild plot).

Antagonists are never completely receptor-specific. The pA scale can also be used to assess the degree of specificity. A general principle of receptor theory is that drugs acting upon the same receptor can be expected to be antagonized by the same concentration of a particular antagonist and to produce the same dose ratios and the same pA_2 values.

α-ADRENOCEPTOR ANTAGONISTS

These are classified as follows:

1. *Irreversible antagonists* (e.g., phenoxybenzamine). This antagonism outlasts the presence of phenoxybenzamine, and is insurmountable, i.e., its effects are not overcome by agonists such as norepinephrine.
2. *Reversible, competitive antagonists* that produce equilibrium blockade, i.e., the free drug and the drug–receptor complex are in equilibrium, and the blockade disappears as the free drug is destroyed. Phentolamine and prazosin belong to this class.

A further classification distinguishes between selective and nonselective α-adrenoceptor antagonists; e.g., phentolamine and phenoxybenzamine block both α_1- and α_2-adrenoceptors whereas prazosin selectively blocks α_1-adrenoceptors. Rauwolscine, a plant alkaloid with prominent CNS effects, is a selective α_2-adrenoceptor antagonist and 5-methylura-

pidil and chloroethylclonidine are selective for α_{1A}- and α_{1B}-adrenoceptors, respectively.

Irreversible α-Adrenoceptor Antagonists

Phenoxybenzamine (Dibenzyline)

The haloalkylamine phenoxybenzamine (Fig. 17-1) is closely related chemically to the nitrogen mustards. It contains a tertiary amine which cyclizes to form a reactive ethylenimonium intermediate. The molecular configuration directly responsible for blockade is a highly reactive carbonium ion formed when the three-membered ring breaks. The persistence and completeness of the blockade produced appear to be dependent upon covalent bonding to the receptor, which is difficult to reverse. After a single dose of phenoxybenzamine, a progressively decreasing but still significant blockade persists for at least 3 days. With increasing doses of the blocking agent, the dose–response curve for an agonist is shifted progressively to the right and the maximum possible response is reduced as the number of available receptors becomes decreased. Phenoxybenzamine also blocks the reuptake of norepinephrine and enhances its release from sympathetic neurons by blockade of presynaptic α_2-adrenoceptors. This drug also provides a useful pharmacological tool with which to study receptor reserve (spare receptor) characteristics.

In the **cardiovascular system**, a fall in diastolic blood pressure occurs because of decreased peripheral resistance. Systolic blood pressure drops sharply when the patient assumes an upright posture (postural hypotension). Reflex tachycardia is induced when peripheral resistance is decreased, and following decreased venous return to the heart. Tachycardia is also caused by blockade of presynaptic α_2-adrenoceptors, which exert inhibitory feedback control over norepinephrine release.

Metabolic effects consist of an increase in insulin secretion, and sometimes increased lipolysis. The

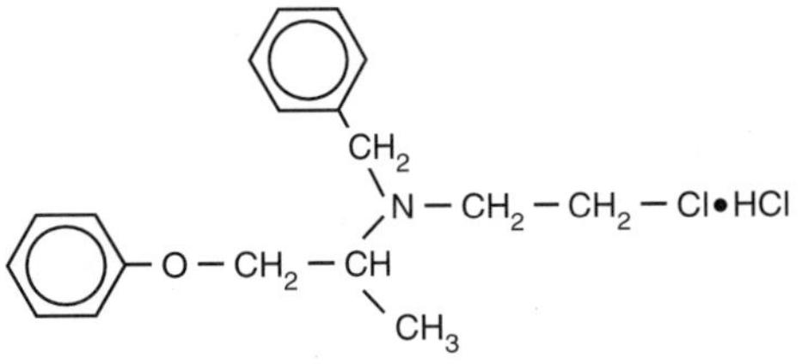

Figure 17-1. Structural formula of phenoxybenzamine HCl.

increase in insulin secretion is due both to α-adrenoceptor blockade, which prevents the inhibitory effects of endogenous catecholamines on insulin secretion, and to the unmasking of the β_2-adrenoceptor activity of endogenous epinephrine, which further enhances the release of insulin.

Reversible α-Adrenoceptor Antagonists

Tolazoline (Priscoline), **phentolamine** (Regitine, Rogitine)

These drugs (Fig. 17-2) have a wide range of pharmacological actions. At high concentrations, they are weak partial agonists at several types of receptor, and they also have some inhibitory effect on neurotransmitter reuptake and inactivation. They produce effective competitive α-adrenoceptor blockade, with a pA_2 value in the range of 8.5–9.0.

Quantitative aspects are of prime importance in discussing drug antagonism. For example, phentolamine in high concentrations not only competitively inhibits norepinephrine action but also blocks that of serotonin. It may, therefore, be assumed that phentolamine has affinity for serotonin (5-HT) receptors but has some 1000-times-higher affinity for the α-adrenoceptor than for the 5-HT receptor.

The cardiovascular effects of phentolamine are similar to those of phenoxybenzamine but are more transient. The cardiostimulating properties of nonselective α-adrenoceptor antagonists, resulting from blockade of presynaptic α_2-adrenoceptors (causing an increased release of norepinephrine from sympathetic nerve endings), can be blocked by atenolol, which is a selective antagonist of β_1-adrenoceptors in the heart.

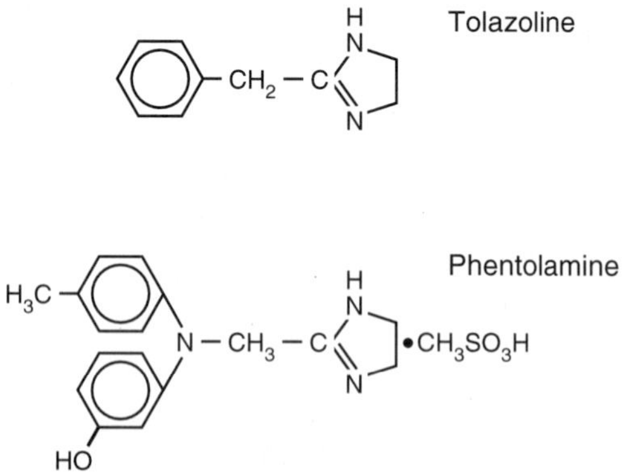

Figure 17-2. Structural formulae of tolazoline and phentolamine mesylate.

Prazosin (Minipress)

This selective α_1-adrenoceptor antagonist (Fig. 17-3) is an effective drug used clinically for the treatment of hypertension. The affinity of prazosin for the α_1-adrenoceptor is some 1000-fold greater than that for the α_2-adrenoceptor. Thus, the pA_2 value for the α_1-adrenoceptor is 9.0 and that against the α_{2B}-adrenoceptor is 7.4; the α_{2A}-adrenoceptor is relatively resistant to blockade by prazosin. The adverse effects that are characteristically observed with nonselective α-adrenoceptor antagonists (e.g., tachycardia, positive inotropy, and renin release) are uncommon with prazosin treatment.

The selectivity of prazosin for α_1-adrenoceptors allows the negative-feedback loop for norepinephrine to be retained. This may prevent the tachycardia observed with the nonselective adrenoceptor antagonists. However, tachycardia mediated by reflex baroreceptor mechanisms may occur occasionally.

Diastolic pressure falls as a result of decreased venous return, caused by decreased peripheral resistance and reduction of circulating blood volume (due to venous pooling in the large veins). Orthostatic hypotension occurs because of α_1-adrenoceptor blockade in the large veins. Dizziness or syncope may occur as a "first-dose phenomenon" and lead to loss of consciousness. This effect may be circumvented by starting with a low dose and increasing it slowly.

The drug is well absorbed following oral administration. The plasma half-life is 3–4 hours. There is extensive protein binding (approximately 97% at therapeutic concentrations). Elimination is by biotransformation in the liver and excretion in the bile.

Other selective α_1-adrenoceptor antagonists in this family include terazosin, doxazosin, and trimazosin. These drugs are pharmacodynamically similar to prazosin, but differ from it in pharmacokinetic profiles.

Indoramin

Indoramin (Fig. 17-4) is a selective competitive α_1-adrenoceptor antagonist that also has been used for

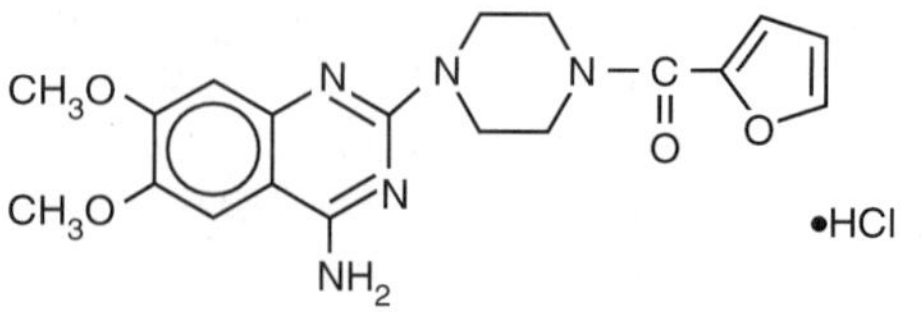

Figure 17-3. Structural formula of prazosin HCl.

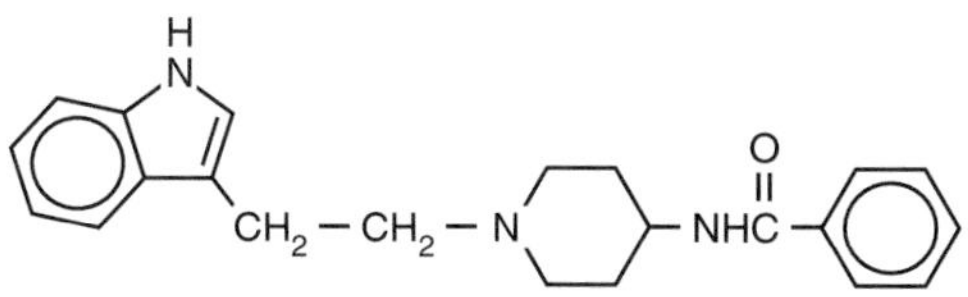

Figure 17-4. Structural formula of indoramin.

the treatment of hypertension. Competitive antagonism of histamine and 5-HT is also evident. Like prazosin, it is selective and therefore lowers blood pressure without producing tachycardia. It also has been used for the treatment of Raynaud's disease.

Yohimbine and rauwolscine

The indolealkylamines yohimbine (Fig. 17-5) and rauwolscine are competitive antagonists at the α_2-adrenoceptor. They are relatively selective in only a narrow dose range, and pA$_2$ values are in the range of 7.5–8.0. Thus, at low doses, yohimbine readily enters the CNS, where it blocks presynaptic α_2-receptors and therefore increases norepinephrine release. As a result, it increases blood pressure and heart rate, and causes behavioral excitation, tremor, and increased release of antidiuretic hormone. In contrast, at higher doses it also blocks peripheral α_1-adrenoceptors and produces a short-lasting fall in blood pressure. Yohimbine has been used to treat impotence, although its benefit in the treatment of sexual dysfunction is not clearly understood.

Other Agents With α-Adrenoceptor-Blocking Properties

5-Methylurapidil and niguldipine are selective competitive inhibitors at the α_{1A}-adrenoceptor. Chloroethylclonidine is an irreversible α_{1B}-adrenoceptor inhibitor.

Other drugs with α-adrenoceptor-blocking activity include neuroleptics (e.g., haloperidol, chlorprom-

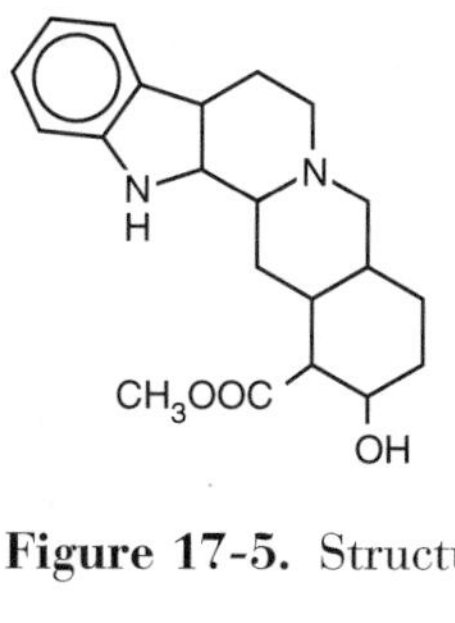

Figure 17-5. Structural formula of yohimbine.

azine), tricyclic antidepressants (e.g., desipramine), and 5-HT-receptor antagonists (e.g., ketanserin).

Therapeutic Uses of α-Adrenoceptor Antagonists

α-Adrenoceptor antagonism has been employed or suggested as therapy in a wide variety of conditions, but as yet it has few established uses.

Although expected to be useful in the treatment of essential hypertension, α-adrenoceptor antagonists other than prazosin have given disappointing results. An important factor in relation to nonselective α-adrenoceptor blockade is that tachycardia and palpitations are added to the other side effects associated with inhibition of sympathetic vasoconstriction. These and other unpleasant side effects prohibit the use of such drugs in therapy for hypertension.

Prazosin also has been suggested as an effective treatment for congestive heart failure, on the grounds that there is excessive activity of the sympathetic nervous system in this condition. Unfortunately, once more, results of some significant clinical trials with prazosin have shown no benefit over placebo.

Formerly, an important use of adrenoceptor antagonists was in the diagnosis of pheochromocytoma, a catecholamine-secreting tumor of the chromaffin tissue of the adrenals. Several agents have been used for this purpose, but phentolamine was most commonly employed. A significant fall in blood pressure within 2 minutes of administering the drug was considered to be a positive response. With the advent of sensitive chemical methods for the determination of catecholamines and their metabolites in urine and plasma, however, the phentolamine test has declined in importance. α-Adrenoceptor antagonists are useful in the preoperative management of cases of pheochromocytoma, for the prolonged treatment of cases not amenable to surgery, and to prevent paroxysmal hypertension during operative manipulation of the tumor.

The use of α-adrenoceptor-blocking drugs is occasionally recommended in the treatment of shock, since vasoconstriction is an important feature, with resultant decrease in tissue perfusion. Some α-adrenoceptor-blocking drugs may be clinically effective in the treatment of Raynaud's disease, a condition characterized by vasoconstriction due to increased sympathetic-nerve activity.

Prazosin is used routinely in the treatment of hypertension, sometimes in conjunction with other drugs such as propranolol and hydrochlorothiazide.

The side effects of prazosin consist of the "first-dose phenomenon" (i.e., a rapid and profound fall in blood pressure, faintness, and palpitations shortly after the first dose, or after a significant increase in dose), orthostatic hypotension, edema, and aggravation of preexisting angina. Other occasional adverse effects are vertigo, headache, depression, vomiting, diarrhea, and constipation.

β-ADRENOCEPTOR ANTAGONISTS ("β-BLOCKERS")

The β-adrenoceptors are classified as β_1, β_2, and β_3 on the basis of the finding that different drugs selectively stimulate or block each of the subtypes of β-adrenoceptor. However, no antagonist for the β_3-adrenoceptor exists to date; this subtype will not be discussed further in this chapter. A subclassification of β-adrenoceptor antagonists into nonselective and selective became necessary because drugs such as propranolol block both β_1- and β_2-adrenoceptors, while other drugs such as metoprolol selectively block β_1-adrenoceptors with only minor effects on β_2-adrenoceptors.

Some examples of β-adrenoceptor antagonists are shown structurally in Figure 17-6. These agents are used extensively in the treatment of cardiovascular diseases, including hypertension, angina pectoris, cardiac arrhythmias, and in the secondary prevention of myocardial infarction and sudden death in patients with coronary thrombosis. The β-adrenoceptor antagonists differ in their profiles of activity, pharmacokinetics, and adverse effects, and some show greater selectivity for β_1-adrenoceptors in the heart. These "cardioselective" β_1-adrenoceptor antagonists are less likely to cause the adverse effects of bronchospasm, intermittent claudication, and cold extremities. They do not block the potentiation of insulin-induced hypoglycemia. However, high doses of cardioselective antagonists can cause some degree of β_2-adrenoceptor blockade and precipitate asthma in some patients.

The membrane-stabilizing (local anesthetic) and intrinsic sympathomimetic (i.e., partial agonist) activity of these compounds should increase their antidysrhythmic effects and reduce the cardiodepressant effects. When patients are dependent on sympathetic drive because of poor cardiac reserve, a partial agonist of β_1-adrenoceptors is preferred (e.g., pindolol, acebutolol), because it is less likely to cause serious impairment of cardiac output. Conversely, a partial

agonist would be less suitable in thyrotoxicosis, which is associated with excessive activity of the sympathetic nervous system.

Propranolol (Inderal)

The development of the class of compounds known as *β-blockers* has drawn enormous clinical attention, and this group of drugs is one of the most widely prescribed throughout the world. The first compound to be developed was dichloroisoprenaline, but this was discovered to be a partial agonist and, therefore, was considered "unsafe." James Black, in the late 1950s and 1960s, initiated the development of additional agents of this class at the laboratories of Imperial Chemical Industries in England. The first compound developed was pronethalol, but this compound was shown to produce thymic tumors in mice. Propranolol and practolol soon followed from the same laboratory. Both the latter compounds were devoid of agonist properties, and practolol was the first cardioselective agent. Practolol was withdrawn from clinical practice in the 1970s because it caused ophthalmic problems. However, propranolol remained, and it is the prototype for developing newer agents with more selective properties.

Propranolol (Fig. 17-6) is a racemic mixture of levorotatory and dextrorotatory forms. The *l*-isomer is some 100 times more potent than the *d*-isomer in blocking β_1- and β_2-adrenoceptors. The two isomers are equally effective as membrane stabilizers, but this action is usually seen only at high concentrations of the drug. Propranolol is a competitive antagonist of endogenous norepinephrine and epinephrine, and of all sympathomimetic drugs acting on β_1- and β_2-adrenoceptors. The effects of propranolol antagonism on endogenously released catecholamines are dependent upon the extent of the sympathetic tone in a given organ.

Pharmacological effects (Table 17-1)

Cardiovascular. Propranolol exerts a negative chronotropic action on the heart, i.e., bradycardia, particularly when sympathetic discharge to the heart is high, as in exercise.

It also produces a decrease in the force of contraction. The rate of rise of tension in the heart (*dp/dt*) and the peak force attained are also decreased. Consequently, cardiac output is reduced; i.e., the amount of blood ejected from the heart per minute is reduced. Oxygen consumption is also decreased, because of the decreased work of the heart. Atrioven-

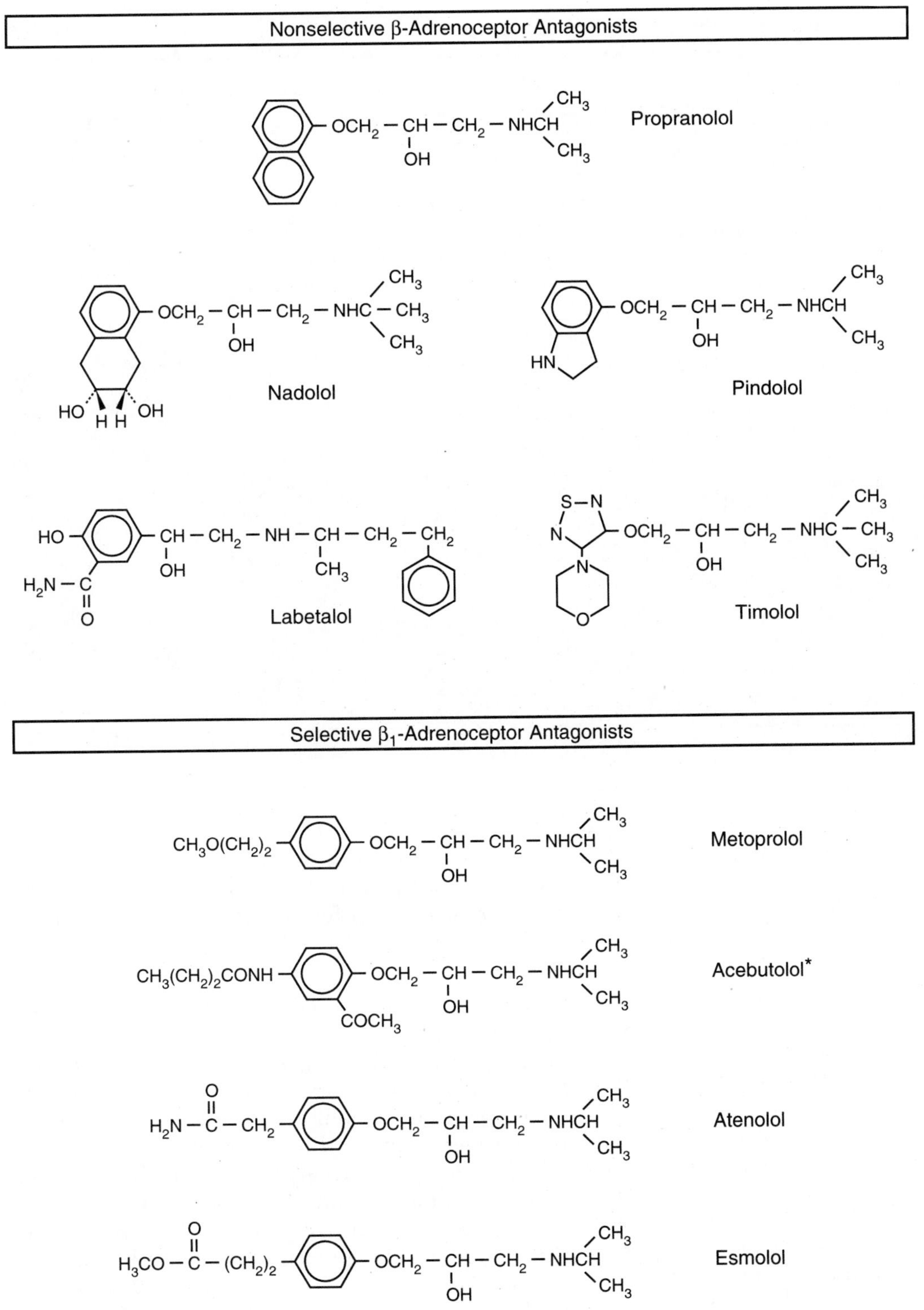

Nonselective β-Adrenoceptor Antagonists

Propranolol

Nadolol

Pindolol

Labetalol

Timolol

Selective β₁-Adrenoceptor Antagonists

Metoprolol

Acebutolol*

Atenolol

Esmolol

Figure 17-6. Structural formulae of β-adrenoceptor antagonists. (*Acebutolol is a selective antagonist, and partial agonist, that is metabolized to a nonselective antagonist.)

Table 17-1 Effects of β-Adrenoceptor Antagonists

β₁-Adrenoceptor Blockade	β₂-Adrenoceptor Blockade
Cardiovascular Effects (effects on cardiac function are more prominent during exercise)	Vasoconstriction in some arterioles, *e.g.*, those supplying skeletal muscle*
Reduced heart rate	Increased airway resistance and precipitation of asthma
Delayed conduction velocity at the A-V node	Decreased glycogenolysis and gluconeogenesis
Decreased rate of diastolic depolarization in all pacemaker cells (the basis for antiarrhythmic action)	Inhibition of insulin release
Decreased force of contraction (negative inotropy) leading to:	Antagonism of catecholamine-induced tremor
reduced stroke volume;	
increased residual (end-systolic) volume; and	
decreased cardiac output (decreased heart rate and stroke volume)	
Reduced velocity of contraction	
Decreased cardiac O₂ consumption (decreased rate and ventricular systolic pressure and contractility)	
Reduced blood pressure	
Inhibition of renin release from kidneys, causing subsequent lowering of angiotensin II	
Edema formation due to sodium retention caused by decreased cardiac output	
Other Effects	
Decreased lipolysis	

*In coronary blood vessels, vasoconstriction would be the predominant effect of β₁-adrenoceptor blockade.

tricular (A-V) conduction velocity is decreased, since vagal action on the A-V node becomes dominant. Automaticity of pacemaker cells is decreased; this is the basis for the use of propranolol in suppressing ectopic foci.

Peripheral vascular resistance is increased as a result of vasoconstriction caused by reflex increase in sympathetic tone and by unopposed α-adrenoceptor stimulation by endogenous norepinephrine in small arteries and arterioles which contain both α₁- and β₂-adrenoceptors (e.g., vessels to skeletal muscles). Nevertheless, hypotension occurs after chronic administration of propranolol, probably because of the decrease in cardiac output, possible central actions, and blockade of renin release from the juxtaglomerular cells in the kidneys, which results in a decreased rate of angiotensin II formation and decreased aldosterone release from the adrenal cortex (Fig. 17-7).

Bronchiolar smooth muscle. Propranolol blocks the bronchodilatation mediated by β₂-adrenoceptor stimulation and potentiates bronchospasm induced by acetylcholine and histamine. Airway resistance is always increased to at least a minor extent by this drug. Bronchospasm following propranolol administration is extremely hazardous in asthmatics.

Metabolic effects. The stimulant effects of endogenous catecholamines and sympathomimetic drugs on carbohydrate and fat metabolism are believed to be mediated via β-adrenoceptors. In humans, propranolol inhibits the increase in plasma free fatty acids induced by catecholamines.

The effects on carbohydrate metabolism are less clear. Propranolol inhibits the secretion of insulin from the pancreas in response to β₂-adrenoceptor stimulants but also prevents the hyperglycemic response to the action of epinephrine on β₂-receptors in the liver. Resting plasma glucose concentrations in nondiabetics are usually normal during treatment with propranolol. However, the rate of recovery of blood glucose levels following insulin administration or muscular exercise may be delayed, resulting in hypoglycemia. Propranolol must be used cautiously

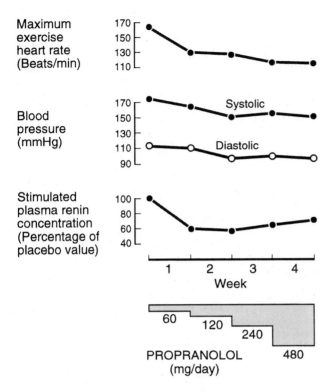

Figure 17-7. Dose–response relationships between the fall in blood pressure, the degree of cardiac blockade, and plasma renin concentration produced by propranolol. Dose increments at weekly intervals.

in diabetics. A cardioselective β_1-adrenoceptor antagonist (e.g., metoprolol) may be less hazardous, since metabolic effects appear to be more closely associated with β_2-adrenoceptors.

Central effects. Propranolol readily crosses the blood–brain barrier and therefore affects central β-adrenoceptors. It is used for the prophylaxis of migraine, although the relevance of β-adrenoceptor blockade in treating this condition is questionable, and drugs with intrinsic sympathomimetic properties are clearly not recommended. The exact mechanism underlying the prevention of migraine by propranolol is not known, but it may be associated with inhibition of β_2-adrenoceptor-mediated vasodilatation in the brain or with blockade of uptake of serotonin by platelets. This would enhance the vasotonic effects of serotonin on cerebral blood flow. The use of propranolol in the treatment of anxiety is no longer recommended.

Tremor due to hyperthyroidism, alcohol withdrawal, or nervousness responds successfully to propranolol.

The antihypertensive effect of propranolol may also be related in part to a central sympatholytic action that results in enhanced vagal tone in the heart.

Pharmacokinetics

Propranolol, because of its lipid solubility, is quickly and completely absorbed from the gastrointestinal tract. Following absorption, it undergoes extensive first-pass metabolism in the liver. Because of rapid hepatic extraction of the drug from the blood, systemic bioavailability of an oral dose is less than 30%. Since the hepatic extraction mechanisms are saturable (and vary between individuals), increasing the dose of propranolol may result in disproportionate increases in plasma levels. Hydroxylation of propranolol in the liver produces an active metabolite, 4-hydroxypropranolol, which has a shorter half-life than the parent compound. A large proportion of circulating propranolol is protein bound, and the plasma half-life is approximately 4 hours. However, the clinical effect may last longer than the reported half-life because of the additive effect of the active metabolite (Table 17-2).

Adverse effects and toxicity

These are predictable on the basis of the action of propranolol in producing β-adrenoceptor blockade. Adverse effects are also widespread because of the diffuse distribution of sympathetic nerves and adrenergic receptors. Serious reactions include:

- Severe bradycardia.
- Congestive heart failure.
- Depression of A-V conduction leading to A-V dissociation, especially in patients with conduction defects, or in those who are receiving digitalis.
- Bronchoconstriction.
- Hypoglycemia, particularly following insulin administration.
- Aggravation of peripheral vascular disease, because of unopposed α_1-adrenoceptor-mediated vasoconstriction by endogenous norepinephrine.
- Fatal disturbances of cardiac rhythm or severe anginal attacks as a result of abrupt withdrawal. The dosage should therefore be reduced gradually over 1 or 2 weeks. The effects of propranolol withdrawal may be associated with rapid reinstallation of sympathetic drive to the heart, or with increased β-adrenoceptor sensitivity.

Table 17-2 Pharmacokinetics of Some β-Adrenoceptor Antagonists

	Atenolol	Metoprolol	Pindolol	Propranolol	Timolol
Extent of absorption (%)	~50	>95	>90	>90	>90
Extent of bioavailability (% of dose)	~40	~50	~90	~30	75
Interpatient variations in plasma levels	4-fold	10-fold	4-fold	20-fold	7-fold
β-Blocking plasma concentration (ng/mL)	200–500	50–100	50–100	50–100	5–10
Protein binding (%)	<5	12	57	93	~10
Lipophilicity	Low	Moderate	Moderate	High	Low
Elimination half-life (hours)	6–9	3–4	3–4	3–5	3–4
Predominant route of elimination	Renal excretion (mostly unchanged)	Hepatic biotransformation	Renal excretion (~40% unchanged) and hepatic biotransformation	Hepatic biotransformation	Renal excretion (~20% unchanged) and hepatic biotransformation
Active metabolites	No	No	No	Yes	No

Other Nonselective β-Adrenoceptor Antagonists (Fig. 17-6)

Nadolol (Corgard) is one of the longest-acting β-blockers, with a half-life of 14–24 hours; therefore, it can be administered on a once-daily basis.

Pindolol (Visken) and **acebutolol** (Monitan) have some sympathomimetic activity. Because of this property, they cause less reduction in heart rate than propranolol does.

Timolol (Blocadren) has a half-life similar to that of propranolol but is less potent. However, it is only moderately biotransformed in the liver.

Selective β_1-Adrenoceptor Antagonists (Fig. 17-6)

Metoprolol (Betaloc, Lopresor) and **atenolol** (Tenormin) are similar in potency to propranolol in blocking β_1-adrenoceptors but much less active in blocking β_2-adrenoceptors. Metoprolol is used in the prophylaxis of angina pectoris and in the treatment of hypertension. Metoprolol also may be useful in some types of heart failure.

Esmolol (Brevibloc) is a short-acting β_1-antagonist for intravenous use. It is rapidly hydrolyzed by esterases in erythrocytes. The drug causes a rapid dose-related reduction in blood pressure and heart rate. It is used in the treatment of supraventricular tachyarrhythmias.

Other Agents

Labetalol (Trandate, Fig. 17-6) is an antagonist at both α_1- and β_2-adrenoceptors. Its β-blocking effects are predominant, with a 3:1 ratio of β:α antagonism. The drug decreases blood pressure without reflex increase in heart rate and cardiac output. For this reason it is useful in controlling elevated blood pressure associated with pheochromocytoma or hypertensive emergency.

Bucindolol and **carvedilol** are antagonists at both α- and β-adrenoceptors. These drugs reduce systemic vascular resistance and can improve left ventricular ejection fraction. Because of these properties, the effects of carvedilol on mild to severe heart failure are at present being evaluated in multicenter trials and, if successful, carvedilol will likely be introduced for the treatment of heart failure.

Therapeutic Uses of β-Adrenoceptor-Blocking Drugs

β-Adrenoceptor antagonists are widely used in disorders of the cardiovascular system (hypertension, angina pectoris, cardiac dysrhythmias) and in thyrotoxicosis. The properties and relative potencies of some of the drugs are shown in Table 17-3.

Timolol, propranolol, and metoprolol are used in the prevention of myocardial reinfarction. The drugs are beneficial and consistently effective regardless of

Table 17-3 Properties and Approximate Relative Potencies of Some β-Adrenoceptor Antagonists*

Drug	Solubility	Membrane-Stabilizing Effects	Intrinsic Sympatho-mimetic Activity	Approximate Cardiac Potency Relative to Propranolol	Hypotensive Doses Used (mg/day)
Propranolol	Lipid	+ +	0	1	160–480
Metoprolol	Aqueous	0	0	1	100–400
Pindolol	Lipid	±	+ +	10	15–45
Timolol	Aqueous	0	±	10	30–60
Atenolol	Aqueous	0	0	1	100–200

* ±, +, + + = relative degrees of activity; 0 = no activity.

age, sex, and site of infarction. Drug therapy is initiated between 5 and 28 days after the infarct. Propranolol is also used in the prophylaxis of migraine, and timolol in the treatment of glaucoma.

Drug Interactions

Cimetidine inhibits the hepatic enzymes associated with the first-pass metabolism of propranolol, metoprolol, and labetalol, and thus confers enhanced bioavailability on these agents. Verapamil may act synergistically to decrease conduction velocity at the A-V node and to enhance the negative inotropic effects of propranolol and other β-adrenoceptor antagonists. Digoxin interacts in a similar manner. Indomethacin and salicylates may decrease the antihypertensive effects of β_1-adrenoceptor antagonists by inhibiting the synthesis of vasodilating prostaglandins. The hypoglycemic effect of insulin may be enhanced or prolonged by the nonselective β-adrenoceptor antagonists.

SUGGESTED READING

Bowery NG, Ruffino RR, eds. Pharmacology of adrenoceptors. Pharmacol Comm 1995; 6:1–280.

Cohn JN, Archibald DG, Ziesche S, et al. The effect of vasodilator therapy on mortality in chronic congestive heart failure: results of a Veterans Administration cooperative study. N Engl J Med 1986; 314:1547–1552.

Cubeddu LX. New α_1-adrenergic receptor antagonists for the treatment of hypertension; role of vascular α receptors in the control of peripheral resistance. Am Heart J 1988; 116:133–162.

Das Gupta P, Broadhurst P, Lahiri A. The effects of intravenous carvedilol, a new multiple action vasodilating β-blocker, in congestive heart failure. J Cardiovasc Pharmacol 1991; 18:S12.

Fitzgerald JD. Introduction to focused section on new developments in beta blockade. Cardiovasc Drugs Ther 1991; 5:545–547.

Fitzgerald JD. The applied pharmacology of beta adrenoceptor antagonists (beta blockers) in relation to clinical outcomes. Cardiovasc Drugs Ther 1991; 5:561–576.

Frishman WH. Beta-adrenergic receptor blockers. Adverse effects and drug interactions. Hypertension 1988; 11(II):21–29.

Kenakin TP. Drug antagonism. In: Kenakin TP, ed. Pharmacologic analysis of drug-receptor interaction. New York: Raven Press, 1993.

Van Zwieten PA. Alpha-adrenoceptor blocking agents in the treatment of hypertension. In: Laragh JH, Brenner BM, eds. Hypertension: pathophysiology, diagnosis and management. New York: Raven Press, 1990: 2233–2249.

Walle T, Webb JG, Bagwell EE, et al. Stereoselective delivery and actions of beta receptor antagonists. Biochem Pharmacol 1988; 37:115–124.

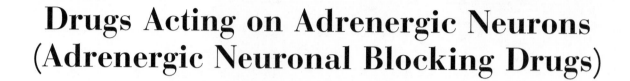

CHAPTER 18

Drugs Acting on Adrenergic Neurons (Adrenergic Neuronal Blocking Drugs)

C. FORSTER

CASE HISTORY

A 45-year-old normotensive (115/72 mmHg) woman had a 3-year history of major depression and suicidal tendencies that were not controlled by standard tricyclic antidepressants (amitriptyline and desipramine) or by fluoxetine. Electroconvulsive therapy was considered inappropriate in this patient. Phenelzine 15 mg/day was prescribed and she was advised that any beneficial effects of the drug could take up to 2 weeks to become evident. She was also provided with a list of foods and drinks to avoid.

After 4 weeks of treatment, her behavioral and mental status began to show some improvement. She was eating regularly, had less insomnia, and had started to go out socially.

One evening, in her fifth month of this treatment, she went to a friend's house for dinner. The main course of the meal included a rich cheese sauce (the patient had forgotten [deliberately?] the contents of the list of foods to avoid and had not informed her friend of the list). During the meal she had an immediate and severe throbbing headache. She was rushed to the hospital where her blood pressure was found to be 180/135 mmHg. She was treated with intravenous phentolamine 2 mg, and her blood pressure returned to normal within 10 minutes. However, she remained in the hospital for further psychiatric assessment.

CLASSIFICATION

The sympathetic nervous system participates in the regulation of arterial blood pressure in both normal and hypertensive individuals. Arteries, arterioles, and veins have direct sympathetic innervation that, by releasing catecholamines, causes vasoconstriction. Also, the rate and force of cardiac contraction and, therefore, the cardiac output are increased by the activity of the sympathetic nervous system. The cardiovascular abnormalities found consistently in sustained hypertension are an increase in peripheral resistance and/or an increase in cardiac output. Historically, it is interesting to note that surgical sympathectomy was used to treat severe hypertension. Early pharmacological treatment was with ganglionic blocking drugs. Subsequently, other antihypertensive drugs were developed, many of which act either on adrenergic neurons or on α- or β-adrenoceptors.

Drugs acting on adrenergic neurons do so by a variety of mechanisms, which include:

- Inhibition of synthesis of catecholamines (e.g., α-methyl-p-tyrosine)
- Interference with catecholamine storage in intraneuronal vesicles, resulting in depletion of catecholamines (e.g., reserpine)
- Blockade of release of norepinephrine (e.g., guanethidine)
- Stimulation of negative feedback by activation of prejunctional α_2-adrenoceptors (e.g., clonidine)

- Inhibition of catecholamine metabolism (e.g., pargyline)
- Destruction of sympathetic terminals (e.g., 6-hydroxydopamine)

Most, but not all, of these drugs act at both central and peripheral sites and cause distinctive, undesirable side effects, many of which are predictable on the basis of the mechanism and site of action of the individual drug.

DRUGS

Reserpine

Reserpine (Serpasil, Fig. 18-1) is one of the alkaloids obtained from *Rauwolfia serpentina* (Indian snake root), which grows in India, where it has been used extensively for the treatment of anxiety, insomnia, psychoses, and hypertension. It is an important tool in pharmacological experimentation because of its action in reducing the concentration of biogenic amines at both central and peripheral sites. Clinically, reserpine is used only occasionally in the treatment of hypertension, usually in conjunction with other drugs such as hydrochlorothiazide. Related alkaloids are deserpidine and rescinnamine. Syrosingopine is a semisynthetic derivative with less effect on the central nervous system, but it remains a useful pharmacological tool with which to study the effects of biogenic amines.

Mechanism of action

Reserpine depletes central and peripheral stores of norepinephrine, 5-hydroxytryptamine, and dopamine. Chromaffin cells in the adrenal medulla are also depleted, but at a lower rate and to a lesser extent than the neurons. Reserpine is a potent inhibitor of the active transport system by which norepinephrine is taken up from the neuronal cell cytoplasm into the storage vesicles within sympathetic nerve endings (Fig. 18-2). The capacity of the storage granules to retain high concentrations of norepinephrine within the vesicles against a concentration gradient is also abolished. This allows leakage of norepinephrine into the cytoplasm and from there to the mitochondria, where it is deaminated by monoamine oxidase, resulting in depletion of norepinephrine stores. The uptake of dopamine from the cytoplasm to the storage vesicle is also impaired, and synthesis of the transmitter is therefore decreased. Noradrenergic and dopaminergic neurons in the periphery and the brain are affected. The concentration of 5-hydroxytryptamine (5-HT, serotonin) is also significantly lowered in central serotonergic neurons, mast cells, platelets, and in the gastrointestinal tract.

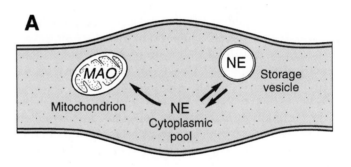

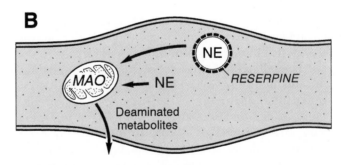

Figure 18-2. Proposed mechanism of norepinephrine depletion from a sympathetic terminal varicosity by reserpine. A. In the normal state norepinephrine (NE) is in equilibrium between the cytoplasm and the storage vesicles, controlled by mitochondrial monoamine oxidase (MAO). B. In the presence of reserpine the norepinephrine uptake into storage vesicles is prevented and norepinephrine from both cytoplasm and storage vesicles is gradually depleted by MAO metabolism.

Figure 18-1. Structural formula of reserpine.

Decrease in catecholamine concentration occurs within an hour of reserpine administration and is maximal by 24 hours.

Pharmacokinetics

Reserpine is well absorbed from the gastrointestinal tract, with a bioavailability of over 80%. At therapeutic levels, about 95% of the drug in plasma is protein-bound. It is highly lipophilic and therefore crosses capillary walls readily, including those in the CNS; and it appears in breast milk. It tends to accumulate in body fat as well as in catecholaminergic and serotonergic terminals. Reserpine is extensively demethylated in the liver and undergoes considerable first-pass biotransformation. However, the slow release from fatty tissues and the high protein binding result in a long half-life of 46–168 hours.

Effects on the cardiovascular system

The antihypertensive actions of reserpine are probably a consequence of the reduced norepinephrine levels in peripheral sympathetic nerve endings, although a central action cannot be excluded. The peripheral depletion causes an impairment of responses to sympathetic stimulation. In the vascular system, therefore, there is less transmitter available for stimulation of adrenoceptors and, in particular, the α_1-adrenoceptor. As a result, there is a reduction of tone in arterioles and large veins, resulting in a fall in diastolic blood pressure and venous pooling of blood. Similarly, in the heart, the β_1-adrenoceptor-mediated excitatory effects of norepinephrine are reduced or abolished, allowing acetylcholine to become the dominant transmitter. This results in bradycardia and decreased cardiac output, which also contribute to the reduction in blood pressure.

The fall in blood pressure is progressive and dose-dependent. Pressure begins to fall 3–6 days after initial administration of the drug and remains depressed for some time after withdrawal of reserpine. The dose should be as low as possible to avoid suicidal or depressive states. The effects of reserpine are additive with those of other antihypertensive agents including angiotensin-converting-enzyme (ACE) inhibitors. Since only small doses are administered in the treatment of hypertension (resulting in less depletion of norepinephrine), the side effects of severe orthostatic hypotension (decreased venous return and reduced cardiac output) are not frequently observed.

During chronic treatment with reserpine, super-sensitivity to the catecholamines (as well as to drugs with direct sympathomimetic effects) occurs. The increased sensitivity is associated with up-regulation of the receptors. In contrast, responses to indirectly acting sympathomimetics (which normally increase the amount of norepinephrine released, e.g., ephedrine, amphetamine, and the experimental drug tyramine) are either decreased or abolished with chronic reserpine treatment, since there is little or no norepinephrine to be released.

Adverse effects

In the presence of reserpine, parasympathetic activity becomes more pronounced because of loss of opposing sympathetic tone. This applies to all organs with dual innervation by both sympathetic and parasympathetic systems. Most side effects can be attributed to the unopposed activity of the parasympathetic system in many organs.

Cardiovascular. Excessive bradycardia may occur in some patients, as do nasal congestion and flushing of the skin, as well as postural hypotension with larger doses. Nasal congestion in the newborns of mothers treated with reserpine may cause serious respiratory problems. Sodium retention and edema may occur because of decreased perfusion pressure in renal blood vessels. Rapid parenteral injection can release norepinephrine initially and cause a transient rise in blood pressure.

The most unpleasant untoward responses to reserpine (and the most important from the point of view of toxicity) are related to the CNS and the gastrointestinal tract.

Central nervous system. Decreased concentrations of dopamine in the brain may cause parkinsonism. Lethargy, sedation, nightmares, and depression (occasionally leading to suicide) also may occur. The depression of mood closely resembles the clinical condition of endogenous depression. Hence, reserpine has been used experimentally to induce depression as a model for testing the efficacy of drugs with antidepressant potential.

Gastrointestinal tract. Increase in tone and motility gives rise to abdominal cramps and diarrhea. Gastric HCl is increased, leading to reactivation or aggravation of peptic ulcer. Release of gastrin via a central vagal action may be responsible for the increased gastric acid secretion induced by reserpine.

Other effects. It has been claimed that long-term treatment with reserpine increases the incidence of breast carcinoma in women, but this is uncertain. The secretion of prolactin is also enhanced, probably because of decreased dopamine concentrations in the brain (see Chapter 28). Galactorrhea may occur occasionally.

Guanethidine

Guanethidine (Ismelin, Fig. 18-3) is actively transported into peripheral sympathetic nerve endings by the uptake system for norepinephrine, with which it competes, and accumulates in storage vesicles. As a result, it reduces norepinephrine concentration in the sympathetic nerve endings and produces a characteristic, prolonged decrease of norepinephrine release, which interrupts transmission of impulses between sympathetic neurons and effector organs.

Other drugs that block the neuronal uptake of norepinephrine, such as cocaine and tricyclic antidepressants, also interfere competitively with the uptake of guanethidine. This competitive interference may prevent the onset of action or reverse the neuronal blocking effects of guanethidine.

Blockade of norepinephrine uptake by guanethidine causes partial depletion of norepinephrine stores, but chronic administration leads to receptor supersensitivity and therefore potentiates the actions of exogenous norepinephrine. Responses to indirectly acting sympathomimetic drugs (e.g., tyramine and amphetamine) are reduced in magnitude or blocked.

Mechanism of action

Following intraneuronal accumulation of guanethidine, norepinephrine release (which normally occurs in response to action potentials) is impaired. This effect is associated with a membrane-stabilizing (local anesthetic) action of guanethidine. Action potentials still occur, but exocytosis is blocked at neuronal membrane sites.

Subsequent and gradual depletion of norepinephrine occurs *selectively* in peripheral sympathetic nerve endings and is attributable to the blockade of

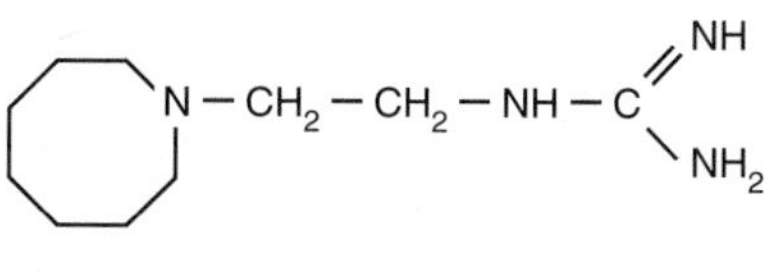

Figure 18-3. Structural formula of guanethidine.

amine uptake coupled with intraneuronal vesicular norepinephrine release and deamination by monoamine oxidase (MAO). The effects of guanethidine on intraneuronal concentration and release of norepinephrine have been described as "drug-induced sympathectomy."

Guanethidine may also act as a false transmitter, since it is released after nerve stimulation but does not act on the receptors.

Pharmacokinetics

Orally administered guanethidine is absorbed to varying degree, in a range from 5 to 30%, with wide interindividual variations in dose requirements for reliable antihypertensive effects. However, the individually effective dose remains relatively constant in a given patient. The peak effect occurs in 6–8 hours, with a duration of action of about 24 hours. Guanethidine is rapidly transported to its intraneuronal sites of action. It is cleared by the kidney, both in unchanged form and as two partly inactive metabolites, with an elimination half-life of about 5 days.

Effects on the cardiovascular system

The primary mechanism by which guanethidine lowers blood pressure is decreased release of norepinephrine, causing a reduction in sympathetic excitatory effects on the heart and vascular smooth muscle. Guanethidine causes a prolonged fall in blood pressure, particularly in hypertensive patients. The response to the drug is greater in the erect than in the supine position, so the drug may cause postural hypotension. This is a characteristic response to drugs that block the sympathetic nervous system. The hypotension is presumably due to a reduction in the capacity of vasoconstrictor fibers to bring about the usual reflex compensations when the erect posture is assumed. This reduces venous return and cardiac output and results in hypotension. The rapid intravenous administration of a large dose of guanethidine can cause a transient, but marked, increase in blood pressure attributable to an initial displacement of norepinephrine from the sympathetic nerves. This is then followed by a prolonged fall in blood pressure, which is due to blockade of release of norepinephrine, followed by subsequent depletion.

Guanethidine has little effect on the catecholamine content of the adrenal medulla and the CNS; in the latter case this is probably because the drug does not readily cross the blood–brain barrier.

The most important aspects of the general pharmacology of guanethidine are attributable to inhibition of responses to sympathetic nerve activity. Guanethidine is used in patients with severe hypertension. It has a very prolonged action, and the effects of a constant daily dose may actually continue to increase for several weeks.

Adverse effects

Orthostatic hypotension (postural hypotension, see above) is aggravated by alcohol, warm weather, and exercise.

Sodium and fluid retention may occur and lead to edema and resistance to the therapeutic effect of the drug if a diuretic is not administered concurrently.

Bradycardia, due to vagal predominance in the heart, may be a decided disadvantage, especially in older patients.

Diarrhea from unopposed activity of the vagus nerve in the gastrointestinal tract is common. Failure of ejaculation may also occur.

Severe hypertensive reactions have been reported in patients with pheochromocytoma and are caused by supersensitivity of the adrenoceptors to catecholamines released from the tumor.

Drug interactions

Uptake of guanethidine into sympathetic neurons is blocked by tricyclic antidepressants, cocaine, and amphetamine (Fig. 18-4). The antihypertensive action of guanethidine can thus be prevented by these drugs. Chronic administration of guanethidine also sensitizes the effector cells to catecholamines as much as 100-fold. The fact that responses are much reduced or absent in the presence of such sensitization indicates that the amount of transmitter released must be very small indeed. The supersensitivity of adrenoceptors reaches a maximum in 10–14 days.

Other Drugs of This Class

Bethanidine, debrisoquin, and **guanadrel** are from the same family as guanethidine, with similar mechanism of action, side effects, and interactions. The half-life of bethanidine is much shorter than that of guanethidine (7–11 hours versus 43 hours, respectively). Bethanidine is excreted unchanged in the urine, while guanethidine is both biotransformed (40%) and excreted unchanged. The biotransformation of debrisoquin shows marked individual differences that are due to genetic variations in the cyto-

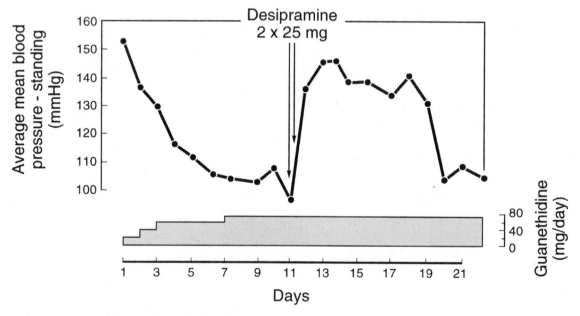

Figure 18-4. Antagonism of the antihypertensive action of guanethidine by desipramine in a hypertensive patient. The dose of guanethidine was adjusted in increments of 20 mg per day, producing a lowering of mean arterial pressure to below 100 mm Hg. Administration of 50 mg of desipramine totally reversed the guanethidine effect for approximately 1 week.

chrome P450 species involved; this is discussed in Chapter 12.

α-Methyldopa

α-Methyldopa (Aldomet, Dopamet) is closely related chemically to L-dopa, which is a precursor in the synthesis of dopamine, norepinephrine, and epinephrine (see Chapter 13).

Mechanism of action

α-Methyldopa becomes a substrate for dopa decarboxylase (aromatic amino acid decarboxylase) within the brain and in the periphery. It is converted to α-methyldopamine, which is in turn converted to α-methylnorepinephrine by dopamine-β-hydroxylase within the vesicles. α-Methylnorepinephrine acts as a "false" transmitter, which is responsible for the reduction of blood pressure in hypertensive patients (Fig. 18-5).

α-Methylnorepinephrine (formed from α-methyldopa) stimulates presynaptic α_2-adrenoceptors, for which it has a high affinity, in the nucleus of the tractus solitarius in the medulla oblongata. Stimulation of these α_2-adrenoceptors inhibits synaptic release of norepinephrine and thus blocks central sympathetic outflow, which in turn decreases the peripheral release of norepinephrine at sympathetic terminals on blood vessels.

In the peripheral nerves, α-methylnorepinephrine is stored in the vesicles and is released by nerve stimulation. It has only weak α_1-adrenoceptor-agonist properties. The central action of α-methylnorepinephrine prevents the peripheral release of both the false transmitter and norepinephrine.

Pharmacokinetics

α-Methyldopa is poorly and somewhat irregularly absorbed from the gastrointestinal tract, and absorption is decreased by food. Oral bioavailability ranges from 10 to 60% (mean value 25%), due in part to first-pass biotransformation. The peak concentration in plasma is reached in about 2 hours. There is rapid distribution to all organs, especially the kidneys, heart, and brain. The elimination half-life is 1.5–2 hours in normal subjects, but it is increased in those with impaired renal function. About 50% of a dose is excreted unchanged in the urine, and 50% is biotransformed to α-methylnorepinephrine and other metabolites.

Cardiovascular effects

α-Methyldopa produces progressive reductions in blood pressure and heart rate that are maximal in 4–6 hours. The fall in blood pressure is greater in hypertensive than in normotensive subjects; it is due to decreases in both cardiac output and peripheral resistance. α-Methyldopa does not produce any major changes in distribution of blood flow. Renal blood flow and glomerular filtration are well maintained in both normotensive and hypertensive subjects.

Adverse effects

Adverse reactions to α-methyldopa include drowsiness, psychic depression, parkinsonism, dryness of the mouth, nasal stuffiness, nausea, and gastrointestinal disturbances. Hypersensitivity reactions include jaundice, pyrexia, and rashes; occasionally hemolytic anemia may occur. Prolonged treatment may cause a positive Coombs test. Liver damage may occur in the occasional patient.

Clonidine

Clonidine (Catapres, Fig. 18-6) is an imidazoline derivative chemically related to the α-adrenoceptor antagonist tolazoline. Clonidine was originally devel-

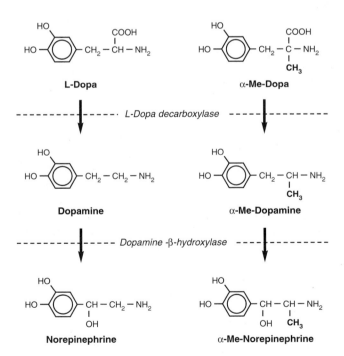

Figure 18-5. Formation of α-methylnorepinephrine from α-methyldopa.

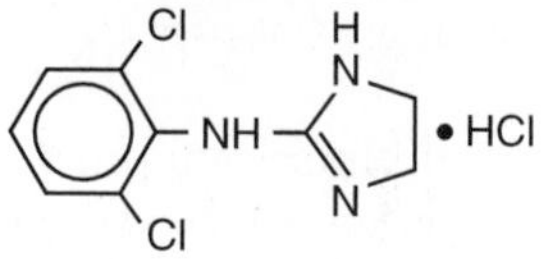

Figure 18-6. Structural formula of clonidine HCl.

oped as a nasal decongestant because of its local vasoconstrictor effects, but when tested for this purpose in humans it produced a marked reduction of blood pressure and heart rate. The fall in blood pressure is due to the α_2-adrenoceptor-stimulant properties of clonidine. Its actions in many respects resemble those of α-methyldopa. Both drugs allow vasopressor centers in the brain to retain some degree of sensitivity to baroreceptor control, thus lowering the incidence of postural hypotension.

Other drugs related to clonidine are **guanfacine** and **guanabenz.**

Mechanism of action

Clonidine has a marked presynaptic α_2-adrenoceptor-stimulant action, which interferes with the neuronal release of norepinephrine at both central and peripheral sites. The central site of action is in the medulla. Stimulation of α_2-adrenoceptors in this area (and possibly of α_1-receptors on inhibitory interneurons) causes a reduction of efferent sympathetic nerve activity that results in a fall in blood pressure and heart rate. At peripheral sites, stimulation of presynaptic α_2-receptors causes a reduction in the release of norepinephrine from the terminal varicosities. The inhibitory effect of the vagus nerve on the heart is augmented, probably both by increased sensitivity of the baroreceptors and by central actions.

Pharmacokinetics

Oral absorption of clonidine is essentially complete but rather slow, peak plasma levels being reached in about 4 hours. Plasma half-life is about 12 hours, but is greatly increased by severe renal disease. About 50% of the absorbed drug is excreted unchanged in the urine, the other half undergoing biotransformation in the liver.

Pharmacological effects

Intravenous administration of clonidine in humans produces an initial brief increase in blood pressure

followed by a fall in blood pressure associated with bradycardia. The initial increase in blood pressure is caused not only by a transient stimulation of α_1-adrenoceptors but also by stimulation of postjunctional α_2-adrenoceptors in blood vessels.

After oral administration, a decrease in blood pressure is evident within 30–60 minutes. The hemodynamic effects of clonidine include bradycardia and a reduced cardiac output, which both contribute to the fall in blood pressure.

Following chronic administration of clonidine, peripheral resistance is also decreased. Clonidine has minor effects on reflex control of blood pressure; therefore, postural hypotension is not a common side effect. A potentially dangerous side effect of clonidine is "rebound" hypertension in patients in whom the drug has been suddenly withdrawn. Prior administration of α-adrenoceptor antagonists (e.g., phentolamine) will prevent this rebound effect. Renin release is also inhibited by clonidine.

Other uses of clonidine

Small doses of clonidine are effective in the prophylactic treatment of migraine by reducing the frequency and severity of attacks. The drug has been used successfully in alleviating opiate withdrawal symptoms and also has been reported to reduce some of the symptoms of alcohol withdrawal that are attributable to adrenergic overactivity (see Chapter 23).

Adverse effects

Sedation, dry mouth, and constipation occur frequently in the therapeutic dose range and limit the use of clonidine. It is possible that clonidine stimulation of α_2-adrenoceptors found on cholinergic fibers innervating salivary glands and intestine may be responsible. Central mechanisms also may be involved.

The rebound hypertensive overshoot described earlier occurs only on sudden withdrawal of the drug; it is associated with overactivity of the sympathetic nervous system, as indicated by elevated plasma and urinary catecholamines. Clonidine can also potentiate insulin-induced hypoglycemia.

Drug interactions

Desmethylimipramine interferes with the antihypertensive action of clonidine, which may be due to the α-adrenoceptor-blocking activity possessed by the antidepressant. Other tricyclic antidepressants and phenothiazine antipsychotics also may block the cardiovascular responses to clonidine administration and should be used with caution.

Monoamine Oxidase Inhibitors (MAOIs)

These drugs were introduced as antidepressants (see Chapter 29), which is their sole remaining use. Because of their important pharmacological effect of inhibiting monoamine oxidase (MAO), which is involved in the intraneuronal catabolism of catecholamines, and therefore in the regulation of cytoplasmic norepinephrine concentrations in sympathetic nerve terminals, the MAOI **pargyline** had formerly been advocated for the treatment of hypertension. The adverse effects and drug interactions of MAOIs (described in Chapter 29), and the development of more modern antihypertensive therapy, rendered these drugs obsolete as antihypertensives.

Bretylium

Bretylium tosylate (Bretylate, Fig. 18-7) was first described in 1959. Like guanethidine, the drug causes inhibition of responses to adrenergic nerve stimulation and to indirectly acting sympathomimetic amines; it decreases the amount of norepinephrine released per stimulus. However, in contrast to guanethidine, a single dose of bretylium produces no detectable reduction in tissue catecholamine levels.

The major cardiovascular effects of bretylium are very similar to those of guanethidine, and at one time bretylium was used quite extensively in the treatment of hypertension. However, tolerance to its effects develops quite rapidly. It is used occasionally in the treatment of ventricular dysrhythmias.

α-Methyltyrosine (Metyrosine)

The biosynthesis of the catecholamines is inhibited by α-methyltyrosine at both central and peripheral sites, including chromaffin cells in the medulla of

the adrenal gland. α-Methyltyrosine is a competitive inhibitor of tyrosine hydroxylase, which catalyzes the formation of L-dopa from L-tyrosine, the rate-limiting step in catecholamine synthesis. As a result, the activity of the sympathetic nervous system is reduced. α-Methyltyrosine is sometimes used to treat hypertension associated with pheochromocytoma, a tumor of chromaffin cells found most commonly in the adrenal medulla. When this tumor occurs at extra-adrenal sites, it may be surgically less accessible and, therefore, drug therapy may be necessary. Surgery may also be contraindicated in some patients. The effectiveness of α-methyltyrosine can be determined by measurement of blood and urinary catecholamines.

Adverse effects include sedation, extrapyramidal symptoms, and psychic disturbances. Severe diarrhea may also occur. The drug is largely excreted in the urine but is not very soluble at urinary pH. Therefore, there is a risk of urinary crystal formation, and increased water intake is required to prevent this.

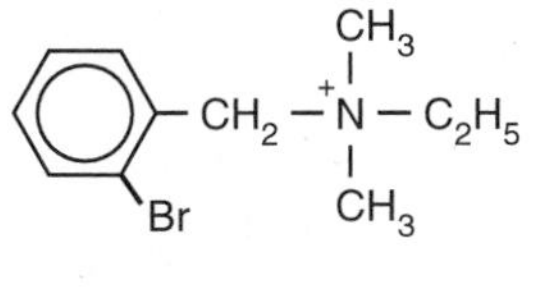

6-Hydroxydopamine

6-Hydroxydopamine is a useful research drug that has a destructive effect on sympathetic nerve endings. It does not penetrate the blood-brain barrier but can be administered intraventricularly. 6-Hydroxydopamine accumulates within the neurons following its uptake by the amine pump and causes a dramatic reduction in catecholamines. This can result in a permanent "functional" sympathectomy and in the loss of approximately 80% of all functional adrenergic neurons. 6-Hydroxydopamine is also a neurotoxin for dopaminergic fibers and has been used extensively for this purpose in order to trace the patterns of such innervation within distinct areas of the brain.

SUGGESTED READING

Curzon G. How reserpine and chlorpromazine act: the impact of key discoveries on the history of psychopharmacology. TIPS 1990; 11:61–63.

Beers MH, Passman LJ. Antihypertensive medications and depression. Drugs 1990; 40:792–799.

Magarian GJ. Reserpine: a relic from the past or a neglected drug of the present for achieving cost containment in treating hypertension? J Gen Intern Med 1991; 6:561–572.

Lederle FA, Applegate WB, Grimm RJ Jr. Reserpine and the medical marketplace. Arch Intern Med 1993; 153:705–706.

Figure 18-7. Structural formula of bretylium.

Mathias CJ. Management of hypertension by reduction in sympathetic activity. Hypertension 1991; 17(4 Suppl):69–74.

Oster JR, Epstein M. Use of centrally acting sympatholytic agents in the management of hypertension. Arch Intern Med 1991; 151:1638–1644.

Weber MA. Clinical pharmacology of centrally acting antihypertensive agents. J Clin Pharmacol 1989; 29:598–602.

Yasuda JM, Schroeder DJ. Guanethidine for reflex sympathetic dystrophy. Ann Pharmacother 1994; 28(3):338–341.

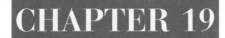

CHAPTER 19

Neuromuscular Transmission and Drugs (Muscle Relaxants)

L. SPERO

L. SPERO

CASE HISTORY

A 25-year-old fashion model saw her physician with complaints of diplopia (double vision), dysphagia (problems swallowing), and what she believed to be a mild cold with generalized fatigue. This fatigue was relieved by rest. She had had these problems for a few weeks and was only now seeking medical assistance because of her increasingly hoarse voice and the apparent inability to fully open her eyes, which interfered with on-camera work for TV commercials.

On examination, the patient had normal deep tendon reflexes and no muscle wasting. She had a poor gag reflex and selective weakness of her neck extensor muscles. She had marked bilateral ptosis (drooping of the eyelids) and bilateral ocular paresis that was elicited by sustained lateral gaze. Her thymus gland was swollen and of a tough consistency.

Myasthenia gravis was suspected, and an edrophonium test was ordered. An initial dose of 2 mg of edrophonium was administered intravenously without effect. An additional 8 mg of edrophonium was administered, and within 2 minutes her muscle strength became normal and was sustained at a normal level for about 5 minutes. There was some salivation and flushing, and a low dose of atropine was administered to reduce the risk of bradycardia.

Her serum IgG antibodies to acetylcholine receptors were measured using a test involving competition with ^{125}I-α-bungarotoxin binding to human acetylcholine receptors. The test was positive. She was also tested with repetitive nerve stimulation, which showed a 20% decline in compound muscle action potential when the nerve was stimulated with surface electrodes six to 10 times at 2–3 Hz.

The neurologist decided that the patient's acute symptoms should be treated with pyridostigmine 60 mg three times a day. She also received prednisone 20 mg/day, which was increased to 40 mg/day in increments of 5 mg every 2 or 3 days.

The symptoms of myasthenia improved over the next 6 months but then began to get worse again. Increasing the dose of pyridostigmine appeared to make the symptoms worse, and another edrophonium test was performed. After an intravenous injection of 2 mg of edrophonium the patient had difficulty breathing, and she lost all muscle tone for a period of about 8 minutes. She subsequently recovered. Her dose of pyridostigmine was then lowered to 40 mg three times a day. This relieved the symptoms and she remained stable for a further 6 months. At this time her serum IgG antibodies to acetylcholine receptors started to climb, and it was decided to remove her thymus gland. Over a 6-month period after the surgery her symptoms gradually abated, and she has remained stable since then.

CELLULAR EVENTS IN NERVE–MUSCLE TRANSMISSION

The motor nerve fibers coming from the anterior horn cells of the spinal cord are myelinated up to the point where the fibers enter the muscle. Each nerve fiber then divides into as many as 200 nonmyelinated branches that are covered by a Schwann cell. Each nerve terminal branch forms a single endplate region on a single muscle fiber (Fig. 19-1). The portion of the muscle cell membrane (sarcolemma) immediately underlying the nerve terminal forms a specialized structure called the muscle soleplate, characterized by infoldings of the sarcolemma. These are known as junctional folds.

The synaptic vesicles within the nerve terminal are clustered immediately opposite the junctional folds of the sarcolemma. The acetylcholine receptors of the sarcolemma are located at the mouths of the junctional folds and constitute at least 90% of the soleplate membrane.

Impulse Invasion of the Nerve Terminal

The nerve action potential travels along the motor nerve fiber by saltatory conduction between nodes of

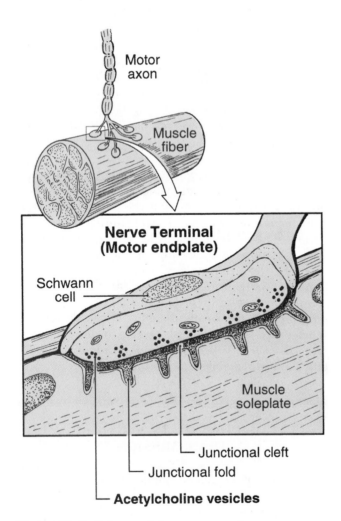

Figure 19-1. Schema of the nerve–muscle junction.

Ranvier until it arrives at the point where the motor fiber enters the muscle. After this point, the action potential propagates into the terminals in the same fashion as it would in any unmyelinated fiber.

Release of Acetylcholine

The events related to the release of acetylcholine constitute a cycle that is illustrated in Figure 19-2. (For synthesis of acetylcholine see Chapter 13). The discrete steps in this cycle are as follows.

1. As with regular action potentials, there is a small influx of Ca^{2+} associated with the action potential of the nerve terminal. This takes place through voltage-gated N-type channels, which have a low sensitivity to the therapeutically used calcium-channel blockers.

2. Since the surfaces of the membranes of the vesicles (and of the cell) are negatively charged, the entering Ca^{2+} neutralizes the charges and causes vesicles to approach the prejunctional membrane.

3. The vesicle then spontaneously fuses with the presynaptic membrane, releasing the enclosed acetylcholine by exocytosis.

4. The membrane of the vesicle, now incorporated into the presynaptic membrane, is pulled back into the cytoplasm by contractile filaments, which form a basket around the empty vesicle.

5. The basket vesicles lose their baskets and form a cistern. Within this cistern, acetylcholine is made by the action of choline acetyltransferase on choline and acetyl-CoA (coenzyme A).

6. Vesicles containing acetylcholine then bud off from this cistern.

The entire cycle from (1) to (6) is very fast, taking place in seconds or minutes at most.

Production of Endplate Potentials

Within 0.1 msec the released acetylcholine diffuses across the 200-Å junctional cleft and interacts with the acetylcholine receptors in the specialized endplate region of sarcolemma.

Each vesicle releases about 10,000 molecules of acetylcholine, which act on the nicotinic cholinergic receptors on the outside of the endplate. (Acetylcholine injected inside the muscle has no effect.)

The stimulated receptors then almost simultaneously open up channels for Ca^{2+}, Na^+, and K^+ in the endplate. The net result is an endplate potential. If only one (a "quantum" of acetylcholine), two, or three vesicles are released, as occurs spontaneously at a rate of about two pulses per second, only a

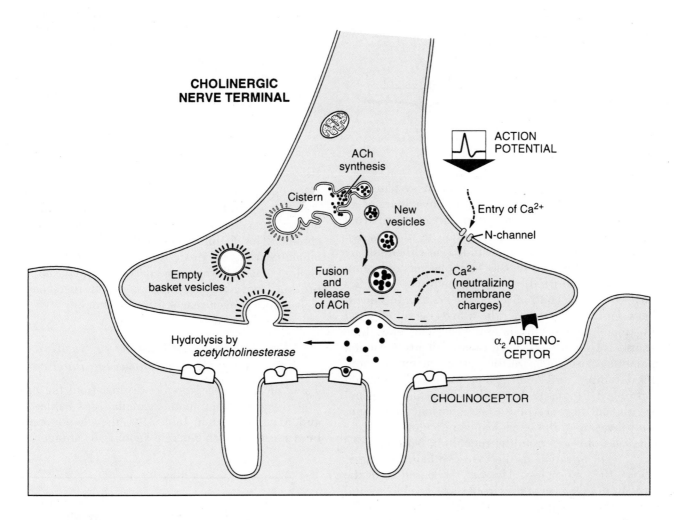

Figure 19-2. Cellular events in nerve–muscle impulse transmission.

miniature endplate potential (MEPP) develops, as shown in Figure 19-3. When a nerve impulse invades the nerve terminal, however, about 200 vesicles are released simultaneously, producing a normal endplate potential of 10–15 mV.

The endplate potential is a graded event and depends on the number of vesicles of acetylcholine released and the number of acetylcholine molecules interacting with the receptors. The amplitude of the endplate potential becomes greater with repeated stimulation of the nerve; this is called post-tetanic potentiation or PTP. It is due to an increased concentration of K^+ within the synapse, which depolarizes the nerve terminal so that an increased amount of acetylcholine is released. If the endplate potential exceeds 15 mV, the sarcolemmal membrane surrounding the endplate is raised above its threshold and an action potential is produced (Fig. 19-4). All-or-none action potentials do not originate within the endplate.

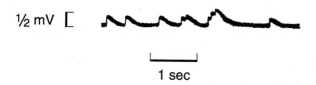

½ mV

1 sec

Figure 19-3. Miniature endplate potentials from the release of single vesicles, or very small numbers of vesicles, of acetylcholine.

Excitation-Contraction Coupling in Muscle

The action potential travels along the surface membrane and is carried into the central portion of the

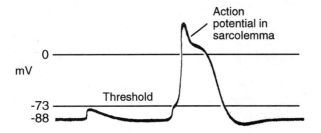

Figure 19-4. Action potential.

muscle fiber by the transverse tubular system. The transverse tubules (T-tubules) are invaginations of the plasma membrane and form part of the internal membrane system (also referred to as the triads). Each transverse tubule is bounded on either side by the lateral cisternae of the sarcoplasmic reticulum (thus the name triad). Electron microscopic studies have revealed a continuity (it appears as a fuzziness) between the membrane of the transverse tubules and the membrane of the lateral cisternae, and these channels have recently been isolated. Thus the action potential can depolarize the plasma membrane and the T-tubules, and it can also pass across the junction between T-tubules and lateral cisternae and depolarize the membranes of the sarcoplasmic reticulum. This invasion of the sarcoplasmic reticulum produces a release of Ca^{2+} from the reticulum. Normally, the Ca^{2+} concentration in the cytosol of the muscle is about 10^{-7} M or less. The Ca^{2+} released from the reticulum may bring the cytosol Ca^{2+} level to around 10^{-6} M or so, thus triggering the troponin-actin-myosin interactions (discussed in Chapter 35) that result in shortening (contraction) of the fiber.

The sarcoplasmic reticulum continuously pumps Ca^{2+} out of the cytosol, and this pump becomes more active during a contraction. Within a few milliseconds the Ca^{2+} concentration in the cytosol is reduced below 10^{-7} M and the muscle relaxes.

The tension developed during the contraction is a function of the intracellular Ca^{2+} concentration, which in turn depends on the rate of release of Ca^{2+} from the sarcoplasmic reticulum and the rate of its reabsorption into the sarcoplasmic reticulum. As the frequency of stimulation of the muscle increases, the sarcoplasmic reticulum is unable to lower the Ca^{2+} concentration below 10^{-7} M between stimuli, so the baseline tension is elevated and there is incomplete relaxation between twitches; this state is called clonus. When the rate of stimulation is increased further there is no significant reduction in Ca^{2+} concentration between stimuli, and a sustained tetanic contrac-

tion results. Once this frequency is reached, further increases in frequency can produce graded increases in the tetanic tension (Fig. 19-5). Tetanic stimulation, and not a single twitch, is the physiological state of muscle contraction, and different types of muscle have different intrinsic frequencies at which they are physiologically stimulated, i.e., become tetanic.

Acetylcholine Breakdown and Reuptake of Choline

When it dissociates from the nicotinic cholinergic receptor and diffuses away, acetylcholine is broken down by acetylcholinesterase into acetic acid and choline. The choline reenters the nerve terminal by an active transport process. Up to 90% of the acetylcholine released from the nerve terminal may be broken down by acetylcholinesterase in the synaptic cleft before it even reaches the receptors.

Characterization of Cholinergic Nicotinic Receptors at the Neuromuscular Junction

These nicotinic receptors are distinct from the nicotinic receptors in autonomic ganglia (see Chapter 13) and, as can be seen in Table 19-1, they do not readily bind muscarinic cholinergic agonists or antagonists.

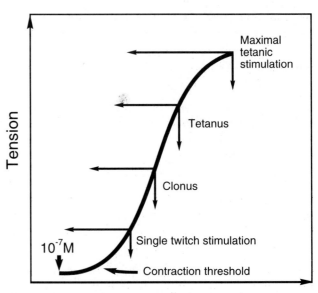

Figure 19-5. Various forms of muscle contraction dependent on baseline tension and intracellular calcium concentration.

Table 19-1 Nicotinic Receptor Binding*

Competing Cold Ligand	Electroplax Receptors†	Rat Brain Receptors‡	Rat Diaphragm Receptors§
Nicotinic agonists			
Nicotine	18.0 μM	3.1 μM	—
Acetylcholine	1.5 μM	30.0 μM	0.47 μM
Carbachol	40.0 μM	90.0 μM	3.5 μM
Nicotinic "depolarizing"-type antagonists			
Decamethonium	0.8 μM	500 μM	2.1 μM
Succinylcholine	—	1,500 μM	1.33 μM
Nicotinic "competitive"-type antagonists			
d-Tubocurarine	0.17 μM	1.9 μM	0.24 μM
Gallamine	0.44 μM	3.5 μM	1.7 μM
Nicotinic ganglion blocker			
Hexamethonium	61 μM	900 μM	118 μM
Muscarinic agonists			
Muscarine	—	10,000 μM	—
Oxotremorine	—	2,000 μM	—
Muscarinic antagonist			
Atropine	—	1,600 μM	—
Cholinesterase inhibitor			
Physostigmine	—	2,000 μM	—

*IC_{50} values for various cholinergic agonists and antagonists against [131]I α-bungarotoxin, a specific nicotinic antagonist at the neuromuscular junction, which labels nicotinic cholinergic receptors at nicotinic sites from various sources. α-Bungarotoxin is a very slowly reversible ligand. These IC_{50} values are therefore obtained from protection experiments and not from competition experiments. They are probably underestimates. The electroplax of the electric eel is a modified nerve–muscle junction, in which the response to the binding of acetylcholine leads to energy discharge as an electric shock, rather than energy utilization for contraction.

Sources:
†Weber M, Changeux JP. *Mol Pharmacol* 1974: 10:15–35.
‡Schmidt J. *Mol Pharmacol* 1977: 13:283–290.
§Colquhoun D, Rang HP. *Mol Pharmacol* 1976: 12:519–535.

This type of nicotinic receptor also has been found in the brain and in the electric organs (electroplax) of certain fish (torpedo) and the electric eel.

From Table 19-1 it is clear that agonists and antagonists bind to the receptor with similar affinities. This receptor does not appear to have separate subsites for agonists and antagonists. The receptor has been isolated and purified and even reconstituted into artificial membranes. The availability of antibodies to the pure receptor has been most useful in determining the level of receptors in a number of skeletal muscle diseases and in identifying the genetic determinants of receptor subtypes.

The radioreceptor binding assay, e.g., with [131]I α-bungarotoxin, can also be used to predict the potency of new nicotinic antagonists as neuromuscular blockers.

Binding of acetylcholine to this receptor leads to the influx of anions and cations through an ionophore that appears not to be ion-specific. The more receptors are occupied, the greater the number of ionophores that are "open" and the larger the ion fluxes down their electrochemical gradients. This is the basis for the graded endplate potential (Fig. 19-6).

Desensitization of Acetylcholine Receptors

The interaction of acetylcholine with the nicotinic receptor first leads to an "activated" state of the receptor, which goes to an inactive (desensitized) state when the acetylcholine dissociates from it. This then slowly reverts to the ground state.

Under physiological conditions, because of the high efficacy of acetylcholine, a response can be elicited by occupying only 20–30% of the receptors; the rest constitutes a receptor reserve ("spare receptors"). This means that at any time as many as 10–20% of the receptors may be in the inactive state. A

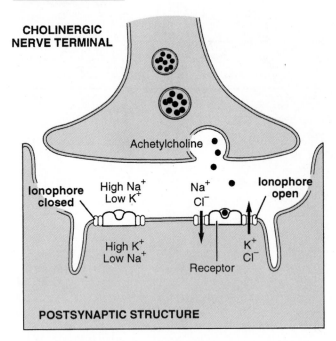

Figure 19-6. The function of ionophores in allowing ion fluxes in relation to receptor occupation by acetylcholine.

situation that would lead to a greater increase in the number of receptors in the inactive state can lead to blockade of the neuromuscular junction.

SUBSTANCES AFFECTING ACETYLCHOLINE RELEASE

Local and general anesthetics have varying degrees of blocking action on the prejunctional nerve terminals, thus preventing nerve impulses from triggering the acetylcholine release sequence (see Chapter 25).

Ethanol. Ethanol at low concentrations (5–20 mM) enhances the fusion of acetylcholine vesicle membranes to the prejunctional membrane. Hence, ethanol increases the amount of acetylcholine released by an action potential. This also occurs in the spinal cord and possibly in the CNS. Higher concentrations (40–80 mM) of ethanol inhibit the release of acetylcholine.

Black widow spider venom. This substance causes a dramatic and almost complete release of all acetylcholine vesicles from the nerve ending. This explains why the victim of such a spider bite initially presents with signs of muscle and abdominal cramps followed by relaxation. The vesicles are not subse-

quently refilled, and de novo synthesis of vesicles is required.

Botulinum toxin. This toxin from the bacterial spores of *Clostridium botulinum* blocks the release of acetylcholine from the vesicles. It kills in very low concentrations by causing paralysis of all muscles, including the respiratory muscles.

Calcium. Ca^{2+} increases the release of acetylcholine, as might be reasoned.

Magnesium. Mg^{2+} decreases the release of acetylcholine, probably by modifying the calcium channels.

NICOTINIC ANTAGONISTS AT THE NEUROMUSCULAR JUNCTION: MUSCLE RELAXANTS

These antagonists selectively block the nicotinic receptors at the neuromuscular junction. They do not affect motor nerves, nor do they block direct stimulation of the muscle. Side effects due to ganglion blockade are occasionally observed. These drugs are used in surgery as muscle relaxants because, while all general anesthetics are able to cause muscle relaxation, this state is reached only during deep general anesthesia when most other nervous functions are also severely depressed. By combining muscle relaxants and anesthetics, one can obtain a surgically adequate skeletal muscle relaxation at relatively moderate levels of CNS depression.

Some degree of muscle relaxation can also be achieved by the blockade of interneurons with drugs of the benzodiazepine and propanediol carbamate classes. These act at the level of the spinal cord. However, the muscle relaxants of this class lack some of the clinically desirable selectivity. Their use is limited to treatment of acute muscle spasms associated with trauma and inflammation and to certain orthopedic manipulations (benzodiazepines are described in Chapter 27).

Nondepolarizing Competitive Blockers

d-Tubocurarine

The classical example of drugs acting in this manner is curare (the generic term for various South American arrow poisons). Claude Bernard demonstrated in 1856 that the site of paralytic action of curare is the synapse between motor nerve and skeletal muscle. The crude agent remained a pharmacological curiosity until the 1940s, when one of the pure alkaloids, *d*-tubocurarine, became available for use as a muscle relaxant in general anesthesia. The designation "tubo-" indicates that the crude material was used by Indian tribes who carried their arrow poison in hollow bamboo tubes.

The competitive nondepolarizing neuromuscular blocking agents are relatively bulky, rigid molecules with two nitrogen groups held apart at a distance of approximately 12–14 Å (Fig. 19-7). These drugs compete with acetylcholine for its receptor sites at the endplate. They have zero efficacy; there is therefore no agonist action and no depolarization, and their actions are purely competitive.

The paralytic effects of *d*-tubocurarine can be reversed by increasing the concentrations of acetylcholine at the neuromuscular junction through inhibition of acetylcholinesterase. The drugs used for this purpose are **neostigmine** and **edrophonium**. The characteristics of their interactions with the neuromuscular junction are illustrated in Figure 19-8.

Tubocurarine (Tubarine) is inactive by mouth and is always administered intravenously. A typical dose is 0.3 mg/kg. It is distributed widely in body tissues but is concentrated in the neuromuscular junctions. It does not enter the CNS and does not pass the placenta. About one-third of the dose is excreted in the urine over several hours. However, the action on the neuromuscular junctions begins to wear off after about 20 minutes because of redistribution of the drug.

Curare causes progressive paralysis, starting with the muscles of the face, then the limbs, and finally the respiratory musculature. Cardiac and smooth muscles are not affected, but very high doses will block autonomic ganglia. Rapid intravenous administration of curare causes release of histamine, resulting in transient hypotension. The drug has no analgesic properties, nor does it affect consciousness.

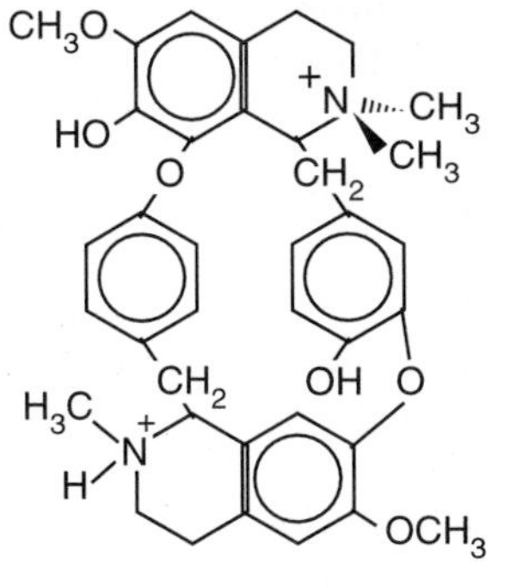

Since clinically useful muscle relaxation requires doses that impair or paralyze respiratory muscles, artificial respiration is necessary and must be available whenever curariform drugs are used. With artificial respiration it is possible to survive without harm doses of tubocurarine that would otherwise be fatal.

Some antibiotics (e.g., aminoglycosides) potentiate curare action, and different general anesthetics require reduction of the optimal dose of curare to different extents.

d-Tubocurarine is used in conjunction with general anesthesia when prolonged or profound muscle relaxation is required for the purposes of surgery. The drug is also used in the treatment of tetanus (i.e., the disease caused by the tetanus bacillus, not the physiological type of muscle contraction) and may have to be applied for days or weeks in some cases.

Pancuronium

Pancuronium (Pavulon; Fig. 19-9) is now widely used in place of *d*-tubocurarine. It is five times as potent as tubocurarine, and has a faster onset and a shorter duration of action. It does not release histamine, and in most patients it has no circulatory effects. It is used with caution in patients with impaired cardiovascular function because it can increase the blood pressure, possibly by ganglionic stimulation.

Atracurium

Atracurium (Tracrium) is a nondepolarizing skeletal neuromuscular blocking agent that has a rapid onset and short duration of action. It is degraded nonenzymatically at pH 7.4 as well as being excreted unchanged by the kidneys. It is of particular usefulness in patients with renal failure. Atracurium, and other neuromuscular blockers such as **vecuronium** (Norcuron), **pipecuronium** (Arduan), and **doxacuronium** (Nuromax), have fewer cardiovascular side effects than other competitive nicotinic receptor antagonists.

Desensitizing (Depolarizing) Blockers

These nicotinic receptor antagonists are noncompetitive and produce their effects by desensitizing the receptors in the neuromuscular junction. They act to produce effects similar to those of an excess of acetylcholine (either added exogenously or accumu-

Figure 19-7. Structural formula of *d*-tubocurarine.

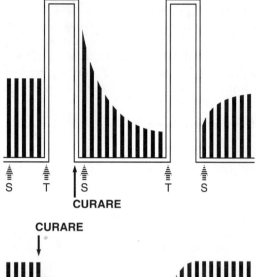

Curare competes with released acetylcholine: single twitch (S) is more sensitive to curare action than is tetanic stimulation (T).

Tetanic stimulation causes release of much acetylcholine: curare is less effective.

Acetylcholine released by tetanus tends to overcome the block and facilitates subsequent single twitch responses.

Curare action is reversed by neostigmine, since more acetylcholine is available because of inhibition of acetylcholinesterase.

Figure 19-8. The effects of curare on skeletal muscle contraction, and their reversal by neostigmine.

lated endogenously after cholinesterase inhibition). In vitro there is an initial stimulation of the endplate, which becomes depolarized, and the muscle contracts. Subsequently the endplate remains depolarized (for about 2–3 minutes) while the muscle relaxes. Within a further few minutes the endplate repolarizes, but the muscle is still relaxed and the endplate is unresponsive to normal acetylcholine release.

These phenomena can be explained in terms of desensitization of receptors. The depolarization occurs because these "antagonists" have both affinity and efficacy, and the receptors are therefore activated. As an excess of receptors become activated, a large fraction of the receptors are converted to the inactive state. Since the endplate membrane is made up very largely of receptor protein, the inactivation leads to a change in the membrane properties, and the endplate potential no longer propagates into the sarcolemmal membrane. There are no further action potentials and the muscle relaxes. At this stage there are still sufficient "spare receptors" for the endplate potential to be maintained. As more receptors are desensitized (inactivated), the endplate potential drops and the endplate repolarizes, but it is now insensitive to acetylcholine or nerve stimulation. The characteristics of the interactions of desensitizing (depolarizing) blockers in the neuromuscular junction are illustrated in (Figure 19-10).

Succinylcholine

This drug (Fig. 19-11) is hydrolyzed by plasma cholinesterase but not by acetylcholinesterase; it acts like an excess of acetylcholine once it reaches the neuromuscular synaptic cleft. It cannot cross the blood–brain barrier or placenta and does not release histamine.

Special features of succinylcholine (Anectine) are

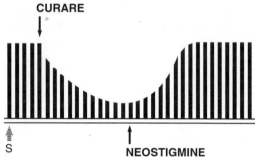

Figure 19-9. Structural formula of pancuronium.

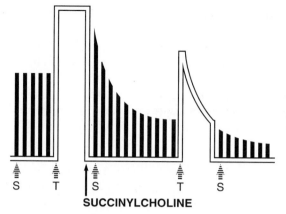

Succinylcholine summates with released acetylcholine during tetanus: tetanus is more sensitive to succinylcholine than to curare blockade, and tetanus (T) is poorly maintained.

Subsequent single twitch (S) stimulation is blocked more strongly.

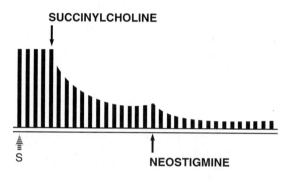

Succinylcholine blockade of neuromuscular junctions is enhanced by neostigmine because of summation of succinylcholine with acetylcholine.

Figure 19-10. The effects of succinylcholine on skeletal muscle contraction (compare with Fig. 19-8).

its rapid onset of action (approximately one circulation time) and short duration of action (2–3 minutes). The latter is a function of the rapid hydrolysis of the drug by plasma cholinesterase. There are rare genetic variants of this cholinesterase that do not readily hydrolyze succinylcholine, as described in Chapter 12. The duration of action may then be greatly prolonged. Therefore, succinylcholine should be used only when facilities are available for giving artificial respiration.

The depolarizing blockade produced by succinylcholine is clinically different from nondepolarizing blockade:

1. Depolarizing blockade is preceded by muscle stimulation that takes the form of an initial, irregular, and uncoordinated contraction of muscle fibers. This state is referred to as fasciculation, it is generally of short duration (5–30 seconds), and its intensity

depends somewhat on the speed of intravenous injection of the drug. Some patients have sore muscles after succinylcholine, much as an untrained subject does after strenuous exercise.

2. Since depolarizing blockade is akin to having an excess of acetylcholine at the neuromuscular junction, it cannot be reversed by cholinesterase inhibitors, and may actually be made worse by them.

3. It is an integral feature of depolarizing blockade that the potassium channels in the muscle membrane around the muscle soleplate remain open so that serum potassium rises. This increase is often minimal and usually of no clinical significance. However, it can lead to symptoms of severe hyperkalemia with consequent cardiac arrest in patients with many freshly denervated muscles (as after spinal injury), with extensive burns, or with uremia.

The clinical use of succinylcholine takes advantage of its rapid and short action. The two main uses are, therefore, to facilitate tracheal intubation for artificial ventilation during general anesthesia and to paralyze skeletal muscles during electroconvulsive (shock) therapy of mental disorders.

Succinylcholine is metabolized by butyrylcholinesterase to succinylmonocholine. This metabolite is

$$H_3C\diagdown \atop H_3C - \overset{+}{N}CH_2CH_2OCCH_2CH_2COCH_2CH_2\overset{+}{N} \diagup CH_3 \atop \diagdown CH_3$$

Figure 19-11. Structural formula of succinylcholine.

a *competitive* cholinergic nicotinic antagonist. It may accumulate during prolonged use of succinylcholine, and its effect may persist following the termination of succinylcholine administration. Competitive blockade by this metabolite can be reversed by cholinesterase inhibitors.

The neuromuscular effects of toxic (lethal) doses of nicotine and of anticholinesterases are similar to those of succinylcholine in principle, although not usually in the rate of development. The action of these drugs on the neuromuscular junction is also of the depolarizing type and, therefore, cannot be antagonized by pharmacological means; survival may depend on prompt artificial ventilation.

DRUGS ACTING ON EXCITATION–CONTRACTION COUPLING IN MUSCLE

Caffeine

Normally a muscle does not begin to contract until the membrane potential has been reduced to about -50 mV. But in the presence of caffeine (in vitro) the muscle begins to contract at about -65 mV.

It is thought that caffeine produces this muscle "sensitization" by releasing Ca^{2+} either from the sarcoplasmic reticulum or from the sarcolemmal membrane.

In the concentration range of 1–5 mM, caffeine (in vitro) produces contracture of muscle, and this may occur without depolarization of the cell membranes.

Caffeine, like theophylline, blocks the phosphodiesterase of tissues, thus enhancing the action of cyclic AMP. It may also inhibit the binding of adenosine to the adenosine receptor, which is involved in the desensitization of the nicotinic receptor in muscle. Thus, caffeine-induced contraction of muscle fibers may result from blockade of this action of adenosine.

Dantrolene in Malignant Hyperthermia

General anesthetics such as halothane and other uncharged anesthetic molecules can make the muscle reticulum "leaky" to Ca^{2+}, particularly in genetically vulnerable subjects (approximately one person in 200,000). Such patients exhibit the life-threatening syndrome of malignant hyperthermia (see Chapter 12). Ca^{2+} stimulates the ATP-dependent contractile mechanism and increases the respiratory quotient of the muscle mitochondria. As a result, the muscles go into contracture and enormous amounts of heat are produced.

The outcome of an attack of malignant hyperthermia is greatly improved if the patient is cooled quickly and given dantrolene (Dantrium), a drug that increases the binding of Ca^{2+} to the sarcolemma and sarcoplasmic reticulum and can restore normal calcium movements across the membranes.

Local Anesthetics

Procainamide and other procaine-like local anesthetics also block the release of Ca^{2+} from muscle reticulum, inhibiting muscle contracture states. These positively charged drugs may simply stop the exit of Ca^{2+} from reticulum by "coating" the reticulum membrane with their positive charges.

DRUGS ACTING ON CHOLINESTERASE

If cholinesterase is inhibited, the effective concentration of acetylcholine in the synaptic cleft is increased. This is the essential mechanism of action of cholinesterase inhibitors. After administration of one of these compounds, the depolarization response to applied acetylcholine is increased.

As described in Chapter 14, cholinesterase inhibitors can be divided into two categories, reversible and irreversible. The reversible inhibitors include physostigmine, neostigmine, and edrophonium. They are used clinically for the termination of curare-induced block and in the treatment of myasthenia gravis. Clinical use of irreversible cholinesterase inhibitors (organophosphates) is rare, although their prolonged action is occasionally useful in the treatment of glaucoma. However, these compounds are used widely as insecticides and occasionally give rise to accidental poisoning. They have occasionally been employed as chemical warfare agents (the so-called "nerve gases").

MYASTHENIA GRAVIS

Myasthenia gravis is a chronic disease characterized by muscular weakness of fluctuating intensity. It is aggravated by physical activity and improved by rest. The weakness is not associated with any significant atrophy of the muscles, at least in the earlier stages of the disease.

Myasthenia gravis was recognized in 1879 by Erb and in 1893 by Goldflam, whose clinical characterization of the disorder is still valid. The symptoms are primarily due to dysfunction of the motor system. The muscles of the eyes, of the larynx, and of mastication are often affected first and most seriously. Later the muscles of the trunk and extremities may become involved (less often, the symptoms of myasthenia gravis first appear in these muscles). Characteristically, an involved muscle rapidly becomes progressively weaker upon exercise. Most patients are better in the morning than in the afternoon. Remissions and relapses occur. Paralysis of the respiratory muscles may cause the death of some patients.

Noting the similarity between the symptoms shown by laboratory animals treated with curare and those of patients suffering from myasthenia gravis, Mary Walker in 1934 treated a myasthenic patient with physostigmine and observed a therapeutic effect. It became generally accepted that the clinically observed muscular weakness was caused by neuromuscular blockade; this concept was confirmed by the supersensitivity of myasthenia gravis patients to tubocurarine (which can be used as a diagnostic test).

It is now known that myasthenia gravis is an autoimmune disease in which antibodies to nicotinic receptors are produced in the thymus. The antibodies reduce the number of available receptors at the neuromuscular junction. The antibody–receptor interaction also leads to structural damage in the synaptic cleft, the postjunctional membrane loses its characteristic folds, and the cleft itself widens. The consequence of all these changes is that less acetylcholine reaches a smaller number of receptors.

Some patients respond to thymectomy, and treatment with immunosuppressant drugs is now used for long-term management. However, pyridostigmine (Mestinon), a physostigmine analog, is used as a supplement (30–180 mg p.o.), often in combination with atropine (to reduce cardiovascular complications). This will increase the concentration of acetylcholine reaching the receptors. The action begins within 1–2 hours, lasting approximately 5 hours. For diagnostic purposes (myasthenic crisis versus neostigmine excess) a short-acting anticholinesterase such as edrophonium (Tensilon) can be used; remission of symptoms during the test indicates a myasthenic crisis.

NERVE–MUSCLE EVENTS FOLLOWING NERVE SECTION OR LESION

In denervated muscles, the acetylcholine receptors are found all along the muscle membrane, not only at the endplate. This gives rise to denervation supersensitivity and the muscle, having more receptors, is now more sensitive to exogenous acetylcholine. Inhibitors of protein synthesis can prevent the development of this supersensitivity, indicating that synthesis of receptors may be involved. Some forms of muscular dystrophy are thought to be associated with partial denervation of the muscles. Nerve fibers contain some trophic factor, not as yet isolated or identified, that acts to keep acetylcholine receptors localized to the endplate region, and that keeps the muscle fully developed. Loss of this trophic factor permits the acetylcholine receptors to spread over the whole surface of the fiber. The spread of nicotinic receptors is accompanied by a spread of acetylcholinesterase. This is illustrated in Figure 19-12. The reverse phenomenon is observed during the embryonic development of neuromuscular junctions. Here the muscle myotube is first covered with receptors, but as a nerve terminal makes contact with it, the receptors concentrate in the endplate region.

In the supersensitive muscle the nature of the action potentials is also changed, as shown by the fact

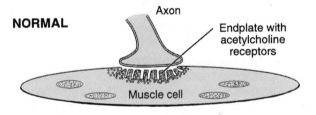

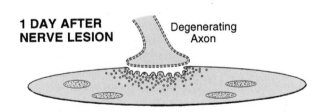

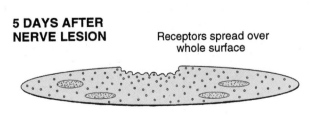

Figure 19-12. Effects of nerve lesion on acetylcholine receptor distribution. Sensitivity to acetylcholine is determined by the spread and distribution of receptors.

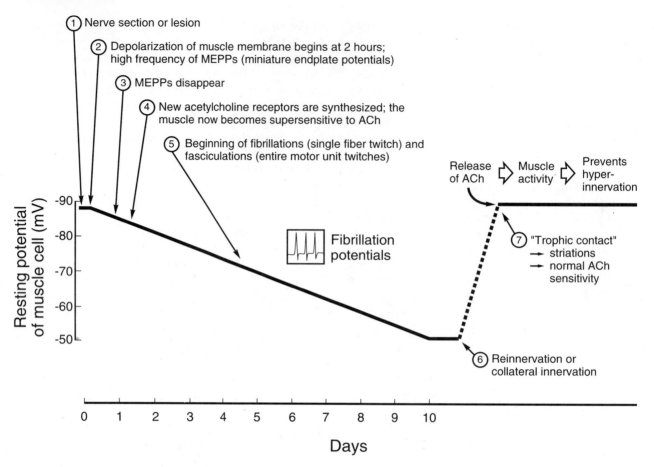

Figure 19-13. Concepts of denervation sensitivity.

that they can no longer be blocked by tetrodotoxin. It is as if all of the properties of the endplate (the graded response of which is not blocked by tetrodotoxin) have spread out. The physiology of denervation supersensitivity is illustrated in Figure 19-13.

SUGGESTED READING

Brehm P, Henderson L. Regulation of acetylcholine receptor channel function during development of skeletal muscle. Dev Biol 1988; 129:1–11.

Fawcelt WJ. Train-of-4 recovery after pharmacological antagonism of pancuronium-induced, pipecuronium-induced and doxacurium-induced NMJ blockade in anaesthetised humans. Acta Anaesthesiol Scand 1995; 39:288–293.

McCoy EP. Comparison of the effects of neostigmine and edrophonium on the duration of action of succinylcholine. Acta Anaesthesiol Scand 1995; 39:744–747.

Myasthenia Gravis. Ann Thorac Surg 1995; 60:223–224.

Stanley EF, Drachman DB. Rapid degradation of new acetylcholine receptors at the neuromuscular junction. Science 1983; 222:67–69.

Torda TA. The neuromuscular blocking drugs. Med J Aust 1988; 149:316–319.

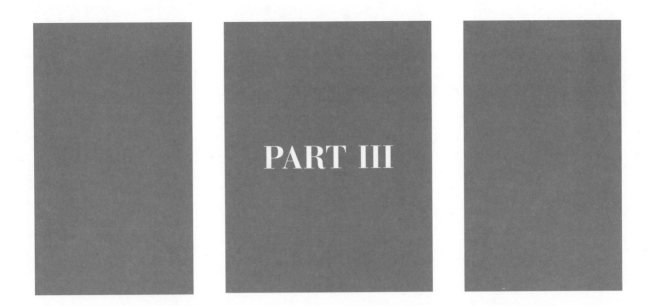

PART III

CENTRAL NERVOUS SYSTEM

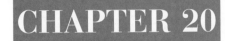

CHAPTER 20

Functional Organization of the Central Nervous System

A.J. LANÇA

In the course of its evolution, the nervous system has developed a highly complex functional and anatomical organization that subserves three main processes: (1) gathering external information (i.e., sensory function or input), (2) storing and processing the information (i.e., integrative function), and (3) triggering an adaptation or response (i.e., motor or secretory function or output).

ANATOMICAL AND MACROFUNCTIONAL ORGANIZATION OF THE CENTRAL NERVOUS SYSTEM

The anatomical organization of the adult human central nervous system (CNS) reflects the basic organization seen in the embryo. By the fourth week of embryonic development, the caudal portion of the neural tube gives rise to the spinal cord, while the anterior portion gives rise to the three primary brain vesicles: the forebrain (prosencephalon), midbrain (mesencephalon), and hindbrain (rhombencephalon) (Fig. 20-1). The relationship between these structures and their main derivatives in the mature brain is summarized in Table 20-1.

The cerebellum is responsible for the coordination of voluntary movements, maintenance of body posture, and coordination of head and eye movements.

The brainstem (pons and medulla oblongata) and midbrain constitute the primary centers for the coordination of vital functions (such as regulation of

respiratory and cardiovascular functions) and reflexes (such as vomiting and swallowing). The reticular formation (which regulates the sleep–arousal cycle and coordination of eye movements) and the most important monoamine-producing neuronal groups are also located in the midbrain and brainstem.

The functional organization of the forebrain is more complex. In the thalamus, motor, general and special sensory, and visceral information is integrated. The hypothalamus receives important ascending input from the spinal cord and brainstem, as well as input from the cortical regions (primarily from the limbic system) and thalamus. The hypothalamus also has sensors that respond to the properties of the circulating blood, such as temperature, osmolarity, and concentrations of different metabolites and hormones. The hypothalamus is responsible for the crucial integration of neural and endocrine functions.

In the telencephalon the final processing and integration of information takes place. The cerebral cortex, the convoluted surface layer of the cerebral hemispheres, is divided into different areas or lobes delimited by well-defined grooves, the sulci. Each cortical region is classified according to its anatomical location (e.g., frontal, temporal, occipital), or type of information processed (e.g., motor, sensory, visual). The cerebral cortex has a characteristic histological organization, with neuronal cell bodies and fibers arranged in layers. The number and characteristics of the different layers are distinctive in each cortical area.

217

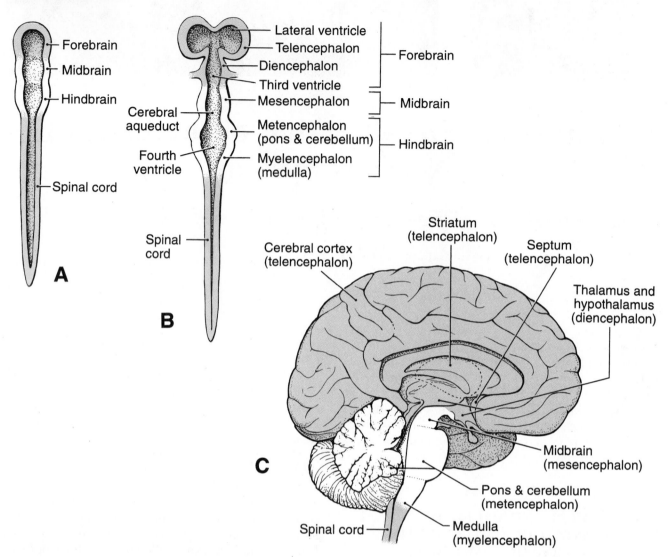

Figure 20-1. The embryonic neural tube forms the brain vesicles and the spinal cord. A. Three-vesicle stage of the neural tube (fourth week of embryonic development). B. Five-vesicle stage of the neural tube (fifth week). C. Mid- sagittal view of the mature central nervous system. (The relationships between developing and mature structures are summarized in Table 20-1.)

The components of the **basal ganglia** are the **caudate nucleus** and the **putamen** (together known as the **corpus striatum**) and the **globus pallidus**. The basal ganglia play an important role in the initiation, control, and modulation of movement (see Chapter 21) and are also involved in cognition.

The **hippocampus** and **septum** are involved in learning and memory, while the **amygdala** is involved in the integration of autonomic and endocrine functions. The hippocampus, septum, and amygdala are parts of the **limbic system,** which also includes portions of the hypothalamus, thalamus, and cerebral cortex. The limbic system is involved in the

mechanisms of motivation, regulation of mood, emotions, and basic behaviors involving survival of the individual and the species.

CELLULAR ORGANIZATION OF THE CENTRAL NERVOUS SYSTEM

Neurons

The morphological and functional unit of the nervous system is the nerve cell, or **neuron,** consisting of a

Table 20-1 Organization of the Embryonic Brain Vesicles and Their Mature Counterparts

Primary Brain Vesicles	Secondary Brain Vesicles	Mature Brain
1. Forebrain (prosencephalon)	1a. Telencephalon (cerebral hemispheres)	Cerebral cortex Basal ganglia Hippocampus Amygdala Septum Olfactory system
	1b. Diencephalon	Thalamus Hypothalamus Retinae Optic nerves Optic tract
2. Midbrain (mesencephalon)	2. Midbrain	Midbrain
3. Hindbrain (rhombencephalon)	3a. Metencephalon	Pons Cerebellum
	3b. Myelencephalon	Medulla oblongata

cell body (**soma**) and its processes. The soma contains a nucleus and surrounding cytoplasm (**perikaryon**), which is packed with **rough endoplasmic reticulum** (Nissl bodies), a network of **smooth endoplasmic reticulum**, a prominent **Golgi complex**, and abundant **secretory vesicles**. These are characteristics of cells active in protein synthesis and secretion.

Neurons have two types of cytoplasmic processes that emerge from the cell body: dendrites and axons. **Dendrites** are usually short, can have highly complex branching patterns, and typically carry signals *toward* the soma (inputs). The **axon** is a long slender process, usually does not have many branchings, and carries signals *away from* the cell body (output) toward the axon terminals.

The neuron has a conspicuous **cytoskeleton**, with abundant microtubules, neurofilaments, and microfilaments, that maintains the cell shape. In addition, the microtubules contain contractile proteins (functionally analogous to myosin) that are responsible for the movement of vesicles and organelles along the axon, both toward the terminal (anterograde transport) and toward the soma (retrograde transport).

In the CNS, neurons are arranged in groups that are connected with each other according to definite patterns. These connective patterns, or **neuronal circuits**, have two types of neurons. (1) Large neurons with long axons, that establish synaptic contacts with other neurons located at some distance elsewhere in the nervous system, are known as **projection neurons** or **Golgi type I neurons**. (2) **Local circuit neurons** or **Golgi type II neurons** are usually small and have short axons that establish synaptic contacts with other neurons located in the same structure or region.

Synapses

Synaptic contacts between neurons are of two types, electrical and chemical. In **electrical synapses**, the apposed membranes of the two neurons contain large transmembrane proteins (**connexins**; see also Chapter 2, Fig. 2-13) made of six identical subunits arranged hexagonally around a central pore. The connexin in the presynaptic membrane is perfectly aligned with its postsynaptic counterpart, so their central pores form a continuous hydrophilic channel through which direct flow of ionic current can occur between the two neurons. Electrical synapses often connect groups of many neurons, synchronizing their activity. Such synapses are also established between neurons and glial cells. Signal transmission between neurons is faster in electrical synapses than in chemical synapses, and can occur in both directions. Electrical synapses are frequent in the nonmammalian brain but are less frequent in the mammalian brain, though they have been found in the retina and in cerebellum, hippocampus, and other structures.

Chemical synapses are the typical synapses found in the mammalian brain and are the major target of pharmacological interventions. These synapses are usually unidirectional and a single synapse establishes connection between only two cells. However, a single presynaptic cell can establish separate synaptic contacts with as many as 100,000 other neurons. This enormous degree of interconnection makes possible the complex circuitry and functional adaptability of the human nervous system.

In chemical synapses there is no cytoplasmic continuity between the adjacent cells, and the release of a chemical messenger is required to pass the information from one cell to the other. The presynaptic axon ends in an expanded terminal that contains in its cytoplasm a large number of **synaptic vesicles** (with diameters ranging from 40 to 200 nm) clustered near the presynaptic membrane and mitochondria.

The arrival of a nerve impulse causes the voltage-dependent ion channels of the presynaptic terminal to open, allowing extracellular Ca^{2+} to enter the terminal. This calcium entry causes the vesicles to "dock" with the presynaptic membrane, fuse with it, and open to discharge their neurotransmitter content into the **synaptic cleft**, the 20–30-nm gap between the pre- and postsynaptic neurons. The functional association of the action potential and exocytosis is known as **action-secretion coupling**. The released neurochemical messenger diffuses across the cleft and binds to specialized receptor structures on the postsynaptic membrane, initiating the postsynaptic response that completes the process of **synaptic transmission**.

The continuous presence of the neurotransmitter in the synaptic cleft would prevent new signals from getting through and render the synapse nonfunctional. It is therefore essential for the neurotransmitter to be removed from the synaptic cleft shortly after release. This occurs by three different mechanisms (diffusion, enzymatic degradation, and reuptake) that together remove the transmitter from the cleft in about 1 msec after its release.

In the CNS, conventional synapses can be established between a presynaptic terminal and different parts of the postsynaptic neuron. They can be between an axon and a dendrite (**axodendritic**), an axon and a soma (**axosomatic**), or even between axons (**axoaxonic**). Axodendritic synapses are often excitatory, while the axosomatic are usually inhibitory. Axoaxonic synapses regulate the amount of neurotransmitter released by the postsynaptic axon.

There are also other less common types of synapses, such as **dendrodendritic**, **dendrosomatic**, and **dendroaxonic**. The physiological properties and relevance of these unconventional synapses are still incompletely understood, but they may take part in intricate local feedback circuits.

Neuroglia

The central nervous system contains a large population of small cells that outnumber the neurons. These cells, known collectively as **glial cells** or **neuroglia** (meaning "nerve glue"), are of two types, the larger-sized or **macroglial cells** and the smaller-sized or **microglial cells**.

There are two main types of macroglial cells: astrocytes and oligodendrocytes. **Astrocytes** are star-shaped cells with cytoplasmic processes rich in thin filaments (made of glial fibrillary acidic protein) and glycogen. Some of their long, slender cytoplasmic processes, known as **pedicels** or **perivascular end feet**, surround the blood vessels and contribute to the formation of the blood–brain barrier (see Chapter 2). Astrocytes act as structural support for neurons and are also involved in the responses to injury and to immunological challenge as well as in regulation of the extracellular concentrations of potassium ions and small molecules such as γ-aminobutyric acid (GABA) and glutamate.

Oligodendrocytes are present in both white and gray matter, they have a smaller and denser nucleus than the astrocytes, and their cytoplasm displays an abundant rough endoplasmic reticulum and polyribosomes, which accounts for their conspicuous electron density. These cells typically have large amounts of myelin basic proteins (MBP), which can be easily identified by immunocytochemistry. Their main function is the production of myelin in the white matter of the CNS (equivalent to the role of the Schwann cells in the peripheral nervous system). They also produce and release growth factors and guide the growth of axons during development and regeneration.

Other macroglial cell types include the **ependymocytes** that form the simple columnar epithelium lining the ventricles and the **epithelial cells of the choroid plexus** that secrete the cerebrospinal fluid (see Chapter 2).

Microglial cells are relatively inactive under normal conditions. They display a moderate phagocytic activity, eliminating cellular debris resulting from neuronal and glial degeneration. Following tissue injury, the microglial cells show greatly increased phagocytic activity. Little is known of their pharmacological responses.

NEUROCHEMICAL MESSENGERS

Concept

The neuron is a secretory cell specialized in the production of **neurochemical messengers**. These are molecules that (1) are synthesized by a neuron, (2) are present in the presynaptic terminal and released into a synapse, (3) exert an action on a postsynaptic neuron or effector cell, (4) are removed from the synaptic cleft by a specific mechanism, and (5) when administered exogenously in physiological concentrations, replicate the actions of the endogenously occurring substance.

There are three types of neurochemical messengers: (1) neurotransmitters, (2) neuromodulators, and (3) neurohormones.

1. Neurotransmitters are released into the synaptic cleft and cause an electrophysiological change (**postsynaptic potential**) in the postsynaptic cell. This change can facilitate the entry of cations such as Na^+ or Ca^{2+} that depolarize the postsynaptic cell membrane, thus producing an **excitatory postsynaptic potential (EPSP)**. Alternatively, it can facilitate the entry of anions such as Cl^- that hyperpolarize the membrane, producing an **inhibitory postsynaptic potential (IPSP)**.

2. Neuromodulators act upon postsynaptic cells but do not themselves produce action potentials. Instead, they change the responsiveness of the postsynaptic cell to the generation of action potentials by neurotransmitters.

3. Neurohormones are synthesized in neurons but are released into perivascular spaces rather than into a synaptic cleft. After entering the bloodstream, these substances are carried to remote sites of action either inside or outside the CNS.

The same neurochemical messenger can act as a neurotransmitter, a neurohormone, or a neuromodulator in different brain sites. For example, the neuropeptide vasopressin is synthesized by neurons in the supraoptic and paraventricular nuclei of the hypothalamus, transported to the neurohypophysis, and released there into the circulation to act as a hormone. The same hypothalamic neurons also send axonal projections to other brain regions (such as the septum and the spinal cord), where vasopressin is released into synaptic clefts and acts as a classical neurotransmitter.

Mechanisms of Synthesis and Functional Implications

Two main groups of neurochemical messengers are used in the nervous system: small-molecule neurotransmitters and large-sized neuropeptides (Table 20-2).

Small-molecule neurotransmitters are formed in short metabolic pathways, from simple and readily available precursors. The pathways of synthesis of the major small-molecule transmitters are summarized in Figure 20-2. Neurotransmitter synthesis occurs in the neuronal cell body, as well as in the presynaptic terminals.

The precursor molecules required for the synthesis of the neurotransmitter are readily transported across the cell membrane, both in the soma and in the presynaptic terminal. The neurotransmitter locally synthesized in the presynaptic terminal is actively transported into small (40–60 nm) synaptic vesicles (**vesicular pool**), where it is stored until released by exocytosis. Enzymes that degrade small-molecule transmitters are also present in the cytosol or mitochondria of the presynaptic terminal, and in some cases also in the synaptic cleft. The amount of transmitter present in the cytosol (**cytoplasmic pool**) is the result of the balance between synthesis and degradation. Pharmacological agents that inhibit the degradative enzymes disturb this equilibrium and increase the amount of neurotransmitter in the cytoplasmic pool.

The synthesis of **neuropeptides** is a more elabo-

Table 20-2 Small- and Large-Molecule Neurotransmitters in the Central Nervous System

Neurochemical Messenger	Molecular Weight (Da)
Classical neurotransmitters:	
Acetylcholine	146
Serotonin	176
Histamine	111
Dopamine	190
Norepinephrine	169
Epinephrine	183
Amino acid neurotransmitters:	
Glutamate	147
Aspartate	133
GABA	103
Glycine	75
Neuropeptides:	
α-Endorphin	1746
β-Endorphin	3438
Dynorphin A	2147
Dynorphin B	1571
Leu-enkephalin	555
Met-enkephalin	573
Vasopressin	1084
Oxytocin	1007
Cholecystokinin 8S	1143
Angiotensin II	1046
Neurotensin	1672
Substance P	1347
Neuropeptide Y	4271
CGRP	3789

Acetylcholine

$$\text{Acetyl-CoA + Choline} \underset{AChE}{\overset{CAT}{\rightleftharpoons}} \text{ACh + CoA}$$

Serotonin

$$\text{Tryptophan} \xrightarrow{TryH} \text{5-OH-tryptophan} \xrightarrow{AAA\ Dec} \text{5-HT} \xrightarrow{MAO + ALDH} \text{5-HIAA}$$

Histamine

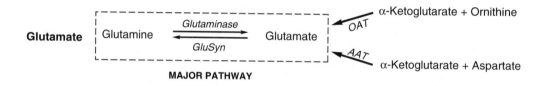

Catecholamines

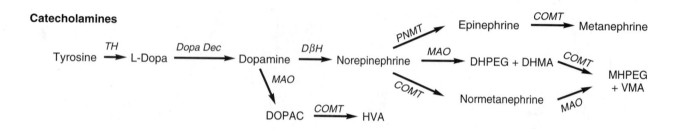

Glutamate

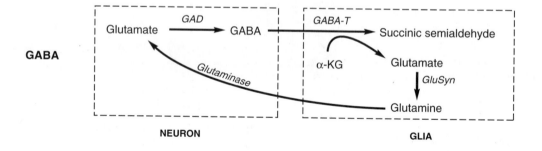

GABA

Glycine Serine $\xrightarrow{SHMT}$ Glycine

Figure 20-2. Principal metabolic pathways of biosynthesis and degradation of the main small-molecule neurotransmitters in the mammalian brain. Abbreviations: AAA Dec = aromatic amino acid decarboxylase; AAT = aspartate aminotransferase; AChE = acetylcholinesterase; ALDH = aldehyde dehydrogenase; CAT = choline acetyltransferase; CoA = coenzyme A; COMT = catechol-*O*-methyltransferase; DβH = dopamine-β-hydroxylase; DHMA = 3,4-dihydroxymandelic acid; DHPEG = 3,4-dihydroxyphenylethylene glycol; DO = diamine oxidase; DOPAC = dihydroxyphenylacetic acid; Dopa Dec = dopa decarboxylase; GABA-T = GABA transaminase; GAD = glutamic acid decarboxylase; GluSyn = glutamine synthetase; 5-HIAA = 5-hydroxyindoleacetic acid; Hist Dec = histidine decarboxylase; HMT = histamine methyltransferase; HVA = homovanillic acid; KG = α-ketoglutarate; MAO = monoamine oxidase; MHPEG = 3-methoxy-4-hydroxyphenylethylene glycol; OAT = ornithine aminotransferase; PNMT = phenylethanolamine-*N*-methyltransferase; SHMT = serine hydroxymethyltransferase; TH = tyrosine hydroxylase; TryH = tryptophan hydroxylase; VMA = vanilmandelic acid.

rate process. Initially, **large precursor molecules** (with molecular weights of up to several thousand daltons) are synthesized by mRNAs associated with the rough endoplasmic reticulum (RER). The molecule is transported into the lumen of the RER together with specific **proteolytic enzymes.** The large peptide molecules and proteolytic enzymes are "packaged" in the same secretory vesicles and carried by anterograde transport to the presynaptic terminals. During transport, the proteases cleave the large precursor into smaller physiologically active peptides. The same large precursor molecules can be formed in many different parts of the CNS but undergo cleavage by different proteolytic enzymes at different sites to release different active peptide products.

The calcium-dependent patterns of release for small-molecule and large-sized messengers differ significantly. First, neuropeptide-containing vesicles are more sensitive to calcium influx than those containing small-molecule neurotransmitters. Second, after stimulation of the neuron, small-molecule neurotransmitters can be rapidly synthesized in the presynaptic terminals and replenish the cytoplasmic and vesicular pools, thus permitting a steady release of the transmitter. Replenishment of the large-sized peptides in a synaptic terminal takes much longer, as a new supply of the peptide has to be synthesized in the cell body and transported to the terminal.

Most, if not all, mature neurons contain more than one chemical messenger. A classical small-molecule transmitter is usually present in association with one or more large-sized neuropeptides in the same neuron. This situation is known as **colocalization** of neurochemical messengers (see examples in Table 20-3). The colocalized chemical messengers are also coreleased, and they interact functionally with each other, the peptide acting to modulate the response of the postsynaptic cell to the classical transmitter; this is known as **cotransmission.** Consequently, any given neuronal population is defined not by the existence of a single messenger but, rather, by a combination of chemical messengers.

Receptors: Concept and Classifications

After release into the synaptic cleft, the neurochemical messenger binds to specific molecules known as **receptors.** The basic criteria for identifying a given molecule as a receptor are discussed in Chapters 9 and 10. In addition, exogenous administration of physiological amounts of the naturally occurring transmitter should produce the same physiological

Table 20-3 Colocalization of Small-Molecule Neurotransmitters with Neuroactive Peptides*

Neurotransmitter	Peptide
Acetylcholine	CGRP
	VIP
	Substance P
	Enkephalin
	Neurotensin
Serotonin	Substance P
	CCK
	Enkephalin
Dopamine	CCK
	Neurotensin
	Enkephalin
Norepinephrine	Neuropeptide Y
	Enkephalin
	Somatostatin
Epinephrine	Neuropeptide Y
	Enkephalin
	Neurotensin
Glutamate	Substance P
GABA	Somatostatin
	CCK
	Enkephalin
	Substance P
Glycine	Neurotensin

*Abbreviations: CCK = cholecystokinin; CGRP = calcitonin-gene-related peptide; VIP = vasoactive intestinal peptide.

response at that receptor and should be blocked by treatment with an antagonist. Receptors should show a selective neuroanatomical distribution in well-defined neuroanatomical pathways and brain structures where the transmitter in question is also found.

Recent advances in molecular techniques have already allowed the isolation and reconstitution of functional receptor molecules as well as the mapping, isolation, and cloning of **receptor genes.**

Receptor proteins are synthesized in the rough endoplasmic reticulum, transported to different parts of the cell, and inserted into the cell membrane of the soma, dendrites, and axons. Binding of a selective ligand to a **presynaptic receptor** regulates the release of neurotransmitter from the presynaptic cell, while binding to a **postsynaptic receptor** produces a response in the postsynaptic cell. Receptors have also been classified as **autoreceptors** or as **heteroreceptors** according to whether they are sensitive to a transmitter released by that same neuron or by another neuron.

Receptors are divided into two classes, ionotropic and metabotropic, according to their mechanism of linkage to ion channels.

1. Ionotropic receptors are directly linked to ion channels. These large molecules (250,000–300,000 Da) consist of four or five subunits embedded in the cell membrane (Fig. 20-3), each subunit containing four membrane-spanning elements. At least one of the receptor subunits has a high-affinity binding site that selectively recognizes the transmitter molecule. The other subunits have low-affinity binding sites and are primarily involved in regulating the opening and closing of the channel (Fig. 20-4A).

These receptors mediate fast responses (on the order of milliseconds). When activated by the transmitter, they undergo conformational changes that allow ions to pass through the channel. The nicotinic acetylcholine receptor (linked to a Na^+ channel) and the $GABA_A$ receptor (linked to a Cl^- channel) are classical examples of ionotropic receptors. Other important examples, including most glutamate receptors, glycine receptors, and the $5\text{-}HT_3$ (serotonin subtype) receptor, are described later in this chapter.

The distribution of ionotropic receptors in different parts of the neuron is not homogeneous. For example, receptors gating Na^+ and K^+ channels are particularly abundant in the soma and cell processes, whereas receptors linked to Ca^{2+} channels are sparse in those structures but particularly abundant in the presynaptic terminals. Accordingly, inactivation of the Na^+ and K^+ channels by tetrodotoxin and tetraethylammonium, respectively, prevents the propagation of an action potential along the axon but does not prevent the release of neurotransmitter by the presynaptic terminal. Conversely, inactivation of the calcium channels prevents the release of neurotransmitter by the terminal but does not significantly disrupt the axonal propagation of an action potential.

Ionotropic receptors can mediate either excitatory or inhibitory activity. In the soma and dendritic processes, the transmitter-induced opening of Na^+ channels causes an influx of positive charges that depolarizes the membrane and produces an **excitatory postsynaptic potential (EPSP)**. Conversely, binding of a transmitter to a receptor that opens a Cl^- channel and allows the influx of Cl^- ions causes hyperpolarization and an **inhibitory postsynaptic potential (IPSP)**.

Each neuron receives a large number of synaptic contacts; EPSPs are generated in some synapses, IPSPs in others. The changes in net polarity of the neuron are therefore determined by summation of all the EPSPs and IPSPs occurring on the surface of that neuron. If enough EPSPs occur to cancel out the IPSPs, then an action potential will be generated. The inhibitory or excitatory effects of a particular type of transmitter are not determined by the intrinsic properties of the transmitter per se but depend on the type of receptor to which the transmitter molecule binds.

2. Metabotropic receptors are *indirectly* linked to ion channels (Fig. 20-4B). The binding of the transmitter to the receptor is followed by coupling of the receptor to a GTP-binding protein (**G protein**). In turn, the G protein will interact with the ion channel either directly, or indirectly through second-messenger systems. The structural features of metabotropic receptors, and the nature of their second-messenger systems are described in Chapter 10. Functionally, metabotropic receptors mediate slow synaptic actions that last seconds or even minutes. The effects on the neuron can be either excitatory or inhibitory, depending on the characteristics of the ion channel activated.

One of the most important functional aspects of second-messenger-mediated transmission is that it induces phosphorylation of regulatory proteins and

A

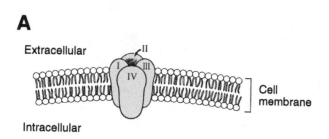

B

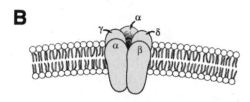

Figure 20-3. Ionotropic receptors (receptor-gated channels) are found in chemical synapses. These receptors have four (A) or five (B) transmembrane subunits.

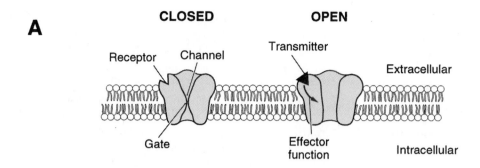

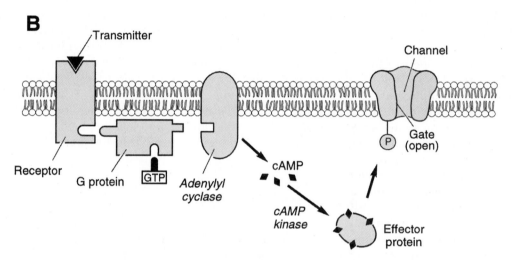

Figure 20-4. A. In ionotropic receptors the high-affinity binding site (receptor site), the effector site, and the gating site are all part of the same molecular structure. B. In metabotropic receptors the high-affinity binding site (receptor site) and the ion-gating channel are two separate molecules. In this case the gating of the ion channel is indirectly mediated through the G protein/second-messenger (cAMP) pathway.

alters gene expression. These mechanisms are likely to constitute the basis for long-term cellular changes, as seen in neuronal development and long-term memory.

BLOOD–BRAIN BARRIER: STRUCTURE AND PHARMACOLOGICAL IMPLICATIONS

Although the CNS is highly vascularized, the histological and functional properties of its capillary network create a barrier, known as the **blood–brain barrier** (BBB), that severely restricts the passage of most molecules between the bloodstream and the parenchyma of the CNS. The histological basis of the BBB is described in Chapter 2; it consists of continuous tight junctions between the capillary endothelial cells, absence of fenestrations, and marked scarcity of pinocytotic vesicles. Brain capillaries are also sur-

rounded by a prominent basement membrane, limited on the outside by a continuous layer of cellular processes belonging to neurons and glial cells (astrocytes and oligodendrocytes). Consequently, in the CNS, the transport of a molecule from the bloodstream to the perivascular space cannot occur by simple diffusion but requires that the molecule either (1) be sufficiently small and lipid-soluble to cross the cell membrane and the cytoplasm of the endothelial cell or (2) bind to a selective carrier and undergo active (i.e., energy-consuming) transport.

In a few structures surrounding the third and fourth ventricles, such as the area postrema, subfornical organ, and the median eminence, the BBB is weak, or leaky, so these parts of the brain are functionally "outside" the BBB. This fact allows them to act as sensors of the chemical and osmotic properties of the blood. The gathered information is then transferred by neuronal impulses to other brain regions inside the BBB, triggering the appropriate responses. In the case of the median eminence, the existence of a weak BBB permits the hormones and releasing factors produced by hypothalamic neurons to pass readily from the perivascular space into the bloodstream.

The very low permeability of the BBB reduces drastically the number of drugs that can effectively cross from the blood into the CNS. With the exception of molecules for which there are specific transport systems (e.g., glucose, amino acids, transferrin, and insulin), only small lipophilic molecules enter the brain. The oil–water partition coefficient of a given molecule can be used as an indicator of its ability to enter the brain.

Several strategies have been developed to facilitate the entry of drugs into the CNS. Molecular changes aimed at increasing liposolubility are the most common approach. Direct delivery of the drug into the brain ventricles or the subarachnoid space is used experimentally to bypass the BBB but is too hazardous for frequent therapeutic use in humans, except for lumbar spinal subarachnoid injection. One of the most elegant and potentially effective strategies is to bind the drug to a **carrier**, such as an antibody against receptors of molecules known to be actively transported into the CNS (e.g., antibodies against transferrin receptors). The drug–antibody complex binds to the receptor, initiating the active transport mechanisms.

NEUROTRANSMITTER SYSTEMS IN THE CENTRAL NERVOUS SYSTEM

Acetylcholine

Cholinergic (AChergic) synapses are found both in the periphery (neuromuscular junction, autonomic ganglia, and parasympathetic postganglionic synapses) and in the brain and spinal cord.

Synthesis and degradation

Choline is taken up into neurons by two different transport processes. In the CNS, a carrier-mediated and Na^+-dependent high-affinity transport exists only in cholinergic terminals, and 50–85% of the choline transported by this mechanism is utilized in ACh synthesis. A low-affinity transport (Na^+-independent passive diffusion) is present in cell bod-

ies of cholinergic neurons. **Choline acetyltransferase** is the rate-limiting enzyme in the synthesis of ACh (Fig. 20-2) and, in the CNS, it is present only in ACh-producing neurons.

After its release, ACh is readily hydrolyzed to acetyl-CoA and choline by cholinesterases in the synaptic cleft. Half of this choline is immediately reutilized in the production of new ACh molecules. There are two types of cholinesterases in the CNS: (1) **butyrylcholinesterase** (also known as nonspecific or "pseudo" cholinesterase) and (2) **acetylcholinesterase** (AChE, also called specific or "true" cholinesterase). AChE is by far the more abundant in the mammalian brain. AChE activity can be decreased by inhibitors that compete with ACh for binding to the anionic and esteratic sites of the enzyme. The types of inhibitor are described in Chapters 14 and 19. By increasing the availability of ACh in the synaptic cleft, these inhibitors cause increased binding of ACh to the postsynaptic cholinergic receptors and thus facilitate cholinergic transmission.

Acetylcholine receptors

There are two classes of cholinergic receptors, muscarinic and nicotinic. **Muscarinic receptors** are metabotropic; they are coupled to G proteins and linked to a variety of ion channels. They have a slow response time (100–250 msec). Five different types of muscarinic receptors (M_1–M_5) have already been identified (Table 20-4) and all are present in the CNS. Autoradiographic studies reveal the highest densities of M_1-receptors (those with high affinity for pirenzepine) in the hippocampus, basal ganglia, substantia nigra, and superficial layers of the neocortex; M_2 and other subtypes are particularly abundant in the septum, superior colliculus, cerebellum, and brainstem.

Nicotinic receptors are ionotropic; they have a faster response than muscarinic receptors (less than 100 msec). In the CNS, high concentrations of nicotinic receptors are found in the periaqueductal gray, cerebellum, dentate gyrus of the hippocampus, and occipital cortex, as well as the perikarya and terminal fields of the nigrostriatal and mesolimbic dopaminergic systems. Cholinergic receptors on spinal Renshaw cells are also nicotinic.

Both muscarinic and nicotinic receptors, when activated by their respective agonists, cause depolarization and excitation of the target neurons. Antagonists of central muscarinic receptors have long-established therapeutic use, but central nicotinic receptor

Table 20-4 Receptor Types and Subtypes for CNS Neurotransmitters: Ligands and Major Effects

Transmitter	Receptor Subtypes	Agonists	Antagonists	Cellular Effects
Classical: Acetylcholine	Muscarinic (M_{1-5})	M_{1-5}: Muscarine	M_1: Pirenzepine, Telenzepine M_2: Methoctramine, Gallamine	$M_{1,3,5}$: $\uparrow IP_3/DG$ (excitatory)
		M_1: Oxotremorine M	M_3: 4-DAMP M_4: Tropicamide	$M_{1,3,5}$: $\uparrow IP_3/DG$ (excitatory) $M_{2,4}$: $\downarrow cAMP$; $\uparrow K^+$ conductance (inhibitory)
	Nicotinic	Nicotine	α-Bungarotoxin	$\uparrow Ca^{2+}$, $\uparrow Na^+$, $\uparrow K^+$ conductance (excitatory)
Serotonin	$5\text{-}HT_{1A,1B,1D}$	$5\text{-}HT_{1A}$: 8-OH-DPAT	$5\text{-}HT_{1A}$: p-MPPI	$\downarrow cAMP$, $\uparrow K^+$ conductance (inhibitory)
		$5\text{-}HT_{1B}$: Anpirtoline	—	$\downarrow cAMP$, $\uparrow K^+$ conductance (inhibitory)
		$5\text{-}HT_{1D}$: L 694247	$5\text{-}HT_{1D}$: GR 127935	$\downarrow cAMP$, $\uparrow K^+$ conductance (inhibitory)
	$5\text{-}HT_{1C}$	—	$5\text{-}HT_{1C}$: Norclozapine	$\uparrow IP_3/DG$ (excitatory)
	$5\text{-}HT_2$	—	$5\text{-}HT_2$: Ketanserin, Ritanserin	$\uparrow IP_3/DG$ (excitatory)
	$5\text{-}HT_3$	$5\text{-}HT_3$: 2-Methylserotonin	$5\text{-}HT_3$: ICS 205930 (Tropanyl)	$\uparrow Ca^{2+}$, $\uparrow Na^+$ and $\uparrow K^+$ conductance (excitatory)
	$5\text{-}HT_4$	SC 53116	—	$\uparrow cAMP$ (excitatory)
Histamine	H_1	2($m\text{-}F$-Phenylhistamine)	Mepyramine	$\uparrow IP_3/DG$ (excitatory)
	H_2	Dimaprit	Cimetidine	$\uparrow cAMP$ (excitatory)
	H_3	Imetit	Thioperamide	$\downarrow cAMP$ (inhibitory) (auto-receptor)
Dopamine	$D_{1,5}$	D_1: SKF 38393 D_5: High affinity for dopamine	D_1: SCH 23390 —	$\uparrow cAMP$ (excitatory) $\uparrow cAMP$ (excitatory)
	$D_{2,3,4}$	D_2: TNPA	$D_2 > D_3$: Raclopride	$\downarrow cAMP$, $\downarrow Ca^{2+}$, $\uparrow K^+$ conductance (inhibitory)
		D_3: 7-OH-DPAT	$D_4 > D_{2,3}$: Clozapine	$\downarrow cAMP$, $\downarrow Ca^{2+}$, $\uparrow K^+$ conductance (inhibitory)
Epinephrine and Norepinephrine	$\alpha_{1A,1B,1C}$	α_1: Methoxamine	α_1: Prazosin α_{1A}: S-Methyl-urapidil	α_{1A}: $\uparrow Ca^{2+}$ conductance (excitatory) $\alpha_{1B,1C}$: $\uparrow IP_3/DG$ (excitatory)
	$\alpha_{2A,2B,2C}$	α_2: Clonidine	α_2: Yohimbine	α_2: $\downarrow cAMP$, $\downarrow Ca^{2+}$ conductance (inhibitory)
	$\beta_{1,2,3}$	β_1: Isoproterenol $>>$ NE $=$ E β_2: Isoproterenol $>$ E $>>$ NE β_3: Isoproterenol $=$ NE $>$ E	$\beta_{1,2,3}$: Pindolol β_1: Atenolol β_2: ICI 118551 β_3: BRL 37344	$\uparrow cAMP$ (excitatory) $\uparrow cAMP$ (excitatory) $\uparrow cAMP$ (excitatory) $\uparrow cAMP$ (excitatory)

antagonists have so far been used only for experimental purposes.

Central cholinergic pathways

Local circuit cholinergic neurons are excitatory interneurons in the caudate-putamen (involved in motor coordination) and in the nucleus accumbens and olfactory tubercle (involved in motivational processes) (see Fig. 20-5). The **cholinergic projection neurons** are organized into two groups, the basal forebrain (BF) and the pontomesencephalotegmental (PMT) cholinergic complexes (Fig. 20-6A). (1) BF neuron cell bodies are located in the medial septum and related areas with axons that project to the hippocampus, olfactory bulb, and nonstriatal fore-

Table 20-4 *Continued*

Transmitter	Receptor Subtypes	Agonists	Antagonists	Cellular Effects
Amino Acids:				
Glutamate and Aspartate	NMDA	*cis*-ACDA	Dizocilpine (MK 801), Kynurenate	$\uparrow Na^+$, $\uparrow K^+$, and $\uparrow Ca^{2+}$ conductance (excitatory)
	Non-NMDA:			
	Kainate	Kainic acid	GAMS	$\uparrow Na^+$, $\uparrow K^+$ conductance (excitatory)
	Quisqualate/AMPA	Quisqualate	CNQX	$\uparrow Na^+$, $\uparrow K^+$ conductance (excitatory)
	L-AP4	—	L-AP4	$\downarrow cAMP$ (inhibitory) (autoreceptor?)
	ACPD	ACPD	AP3	$\uparrow IP_3/DG$ (excitatory)
GABA	GABA$_A$	Muscimol	Bicuculline	$\uparrow Cl^-$ conductance (inhibitory)
	GABA$_B$	Baclofen	Phaclofen	$\uparrow K^+$ and $\downarrow Ca^{2+}$ conductance (inhibitory)
Glycine	Glycine receptor	β-Alanine	Strychnine	$\uparrow Cl^-$ conductance (inhibitory)
Peptides:				
Opioids	μ	DAMGO	CTOP	$\downarrow cAMP$, $\downarrow Ca^{2+}$ and $\uparrow K^+$ conductance (inhibitory)
	δ	DPDPE	ICI 174864	$\downarrow cAMP$, $\downarrow Ca^{2+}$ and $\uparrow K^+$ conductance (inhibitory)
	κ	U 62066	Binaltorphimine	$\downarrow cAMP$, $\downarrow Ca^{2+}$ and $\uparrow K^+$ conductance (inhibitory)
Vasopressin	V$_1$	DGAVP	Manning compound	$\uparrow IP_3/DG$ (excitatory)
	V$_2$	dVDAVP	DDIAAVP	$\uparrow cAMP$ (excitatory)
Oxytocin	—	Oxytocin	Vasotocin	$\uparrow IP_3/DG$ (excitatory)
Cholecystokinin	CCK$_A$	CCK-8: CCK$_A$ > CCK$_B$	Devazepide	$\uparrow IP_3/DG$ (excitatory)
	CCK$_B$	Pentagastrin	CI 988	$\uparrow IP_3/DG$ (excitatory)
Angiotensin	AII$_\alpha$	Angiotensin II	AII$_{\alpha,\beta}$: Saralasin AII$_\alpha$: DuP 753	$\uparrow cAMP$, $\uparrow cGMP$ (excitatory)
	AII$_\beta$	Angiotensin II	AII$_\beta$: PD 123177	$\uparrow cAMP$, $\uparrow cGMP$ (excitatory)

ACDA = 1-Aminocyclobutane-*cis*-1,3-decarboxylic acid; ACPD = (±)-1-Amino-1,3-cyclopentanedicarboxylic acid; AMPA = (±)-α-Amino-3-hydroxy-5-methylisoxazole-4-propionic acid; AP3 = (±)-2-Amino-3-phosphonopropionic acid; cAMP = cyclic adenosine monophosphate; cGMP = cyclic guanosine monophosphate; CNQX = 6-Cyano-7-nitroquinoxaline-2,3-dione; CTOP = D-Phe-Cys-Tyr-D-Trp-Orn-Thr-Pen-Thr amide; DAMGO = [D-Ala^2,N-Me-Phe^4,Gly-ol^5]-Enkephalin; 4-DAMP = 4-Diphenylacetoxy-N-methylpiperidine; DDIAAVP = [d(CH$_2$)$_5$^{1},D-Ile^4,Ile^4,Arg^8,Ala^9]-Vasopressin; DG = Diacylglycerol; DGAVP = [Des-Glycinamide^9,Arg^8]-Vasopressin; DPDPE = [D-Pen^{2,5}]-Enkephalin; dVDAVP = [deamino-Cys^1, Val^4, D-Arg^8]-Vasopressin; E = Epinephrine; GAMS = D-γ-Glutamylaminomethanesulfonic acid; IP$_3$ = Inositol trisphosphate; L-AP4 = L(+)-2-Amino-4-phosphonobutyric acid; Manning Compound = [d(CH$_2$)$_5$^{1}O-Me-Tyr^2,Arg^8]-Vasopressin; NE = Norepinephrine; NMDA = N-Methyl-D-aspartic acid; 7-OH-DPAT = 7-Hydroxy-dipropylaminotetralin; 8-OH-DPAT = 8-Hydroxy-dipropylaminotetralin; TNPA = (±)2,10,11-Trihydroxy-N-propylnoraporphine.

Other abbreviations (e.g., ICI 118551) refer to proprietary codes with the letters standing for abbreviation of the pharmaceutical company and the number referring to the product number.

brain, and are believed to be involved in mechanisms of learning and memory. (2) PMT neuron cell bodies are located in the ventral midbrain, sending ascending projections to the thalamus and remaining diencephalic and mesencephalic areas and descending projections to the pons and medulla, cerebellum, and vestibular nuclei. These projections are involved in mechanisms of arousal and homeostasis.

Serotonin

Synthesis and degradation

Serotonin (5-hydroxytryptamine, 5-HT) is formed by hydroxylation of the neutral amino acid trypto-

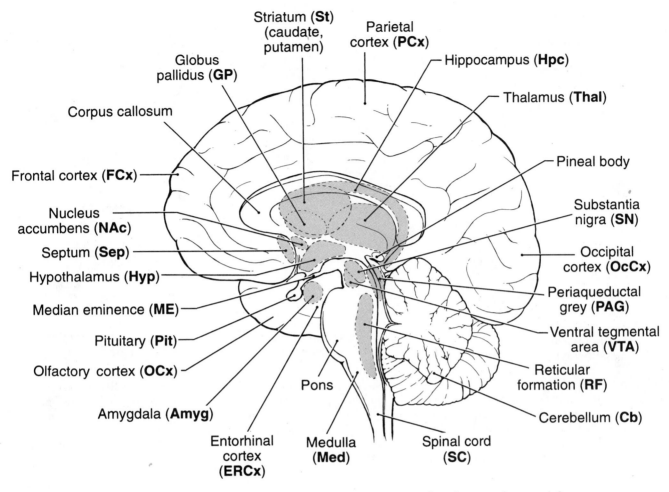

Figure 20-5. Approximate locations of major brain nuclei and structures referred to in subsequent figures.

phan (Fig. 20-2). Tryptophan, the rate-limiting factor in the synthesis of 5-HT, does not cross the BBB and must be actively transported by a carrier that is also responsible for the transport of other amino acids (e.g., tyrosine, phenylalanine, histidine). Cytoplasmic and membrane-bound pools of tryptophan hydroxylase are present in the cell bodies and terminals of 5-HT-producing neurons. Serotonin production can be selectively blocked by inhibitors of tryptophan hydroxylase, such as *p*-chlorophenylalanine; 5-HT produced in the periphery has no central actions, since it does not cross the BBB.

Serotonin is deaminated by **monoamine oxidase** (MAO) to form 5-hydroxyindoleacetaldehyde, which is then oxidized by **aldehyde dehydrogenase** to form **5-hydroxyindoleacetic acid (5-HIAA)**. MAO is widely distributed in both nervous and non-nervous tissues. Two types (MAO-A and MAO-B) have been identified on the basis of their substrate affinities, specificity of inhibition by certain MAO inhibi-

tors, and brain distribution in different species. MAO-A has a higher affinity for 5-HT than MAO-B does, and is mainly localized intracellularly, while MAO-B concentrations are higher extracellularly. In human brain MAO-B is the predominant form. Some drugs, such as pargyline, are irreversible inhibitors of both forms of the enzyme, while other compounds selectively inhibit only one MAO subtype (e.g., MAO-A inhibitor clorgyline, and MAO-B inhibitor deprenyl). However, MAO also participates in the degradation of dopamine and norepinephrine, and inhibition of MAO affects the dopaminergic and noradrenergic systems as well as the serotonergic system (see Chapter 13).

5-HIAA is the most important serotonin metabolite, and its concentration in the CSF is used as a measure of serotonergic activity in the brain. Low CSF concentrations of 5-HIAA have been observed in depressed patients. Drugs that increase the availability of serotonin in the synaptic cleft are used as

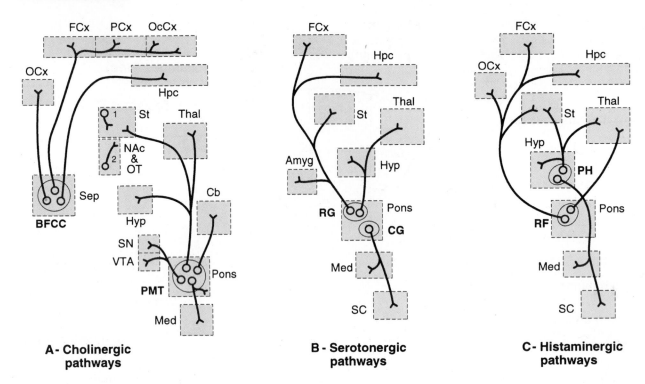

A - Cholinergic pathways

B - Serotonergic pathways

C - Histaminergic pathways

Figure 20-6. Schematic representation of major cholinergic, serotonergic, and histaminergic pathways in the brain. A. **Cholinergic:** 1 = local-circuit neurons in striatum; 2 = local-circuit neurons in nucleus accumbens; BFCC = basal forebrain cholinergic complex; PMT = pontomesencephalotegmental cholinergic complex; OT = olfactory tubercle. B. **Serotonergic:** RG = rostral group of 5-HT perikarya, including the dorsal and medial raphe nuclei; CG = caudal group, including the nucleus raphe magnus. C. **Histaminergic:** PH = posterior hypothalamic cell group; RF = reticular formation cell group. For other abbreviations, see Figure 20-5.

antidepressants (see Chapter 29). Tricyclics (e.g., imipramine) and nontricyclic antidepressants (e.g., fluoxetine) act by blocking the reuptake of 5-HT, while MAO inhibitors prevent its degradation.

Serotonin receptors

There are three main types of serotonin receptors, two of which exist in more than one form. The main subtypes of serotonin receptors, defined by their genetic, pharmacological, and electrophysiological properties, are 5-HT$_{1A,B,C,D}$; 5-HT$_{2A,B}$; and 5-HT$_3$. Their features are summarized in Table 20-4.

Central serotonergic pathways

The classical serotonergic cell nuclei are located in the midline of the pons and upper brainstem (see Fig. 20-5). The more rostral group (RG, mainly the **dorsal and medial raphe nuclei**) send extensive diffuse ascending innervation to the thalamus, hypo-

thalamus, striatal complex, and cortical areas. Limbic brain structures, such as the hippocampus, septum, amygdala, and limbic frontal cortex, receive a very rich serotonergic innervation (Fig. 20-6B). Typically, the 5-HT innervation of each area originates in more than one raphe group. The widespread distribution of ascending serotonergic innervation of the cortical areas contrasts with the well-defined patterns of regional and laminar distribution of the dopaminergic and noradrenergic innervation in the cortex. These findings support the view that the ascending serotonergic innervation exerts a global, yet not necessarily uniform, influence upon cortical functions.

A caudal serotonergic cell group (CG) located in the caudal pons and medulla oblongata sends **descending innervation** to the medulla and spinal cord, where serotonin is involved in mechanisms of cardiovascular control and pain perception.

Serotonergic cell groups have also been identified in other structures such as the **area postrema** and functionally related areas, where they are involved in the integration of information concerning gastrointestinal function and respiratory control.

The **pineal gland** contains high concentrations of serotonin, which is locally produced in secretory cells (pinealocytes) and is the precursor in the synthesis of melatonin, a hormone that inhibits sexual development and maturation. High concentrations of serotonin inhibit melatonin activity.

In addition to its role in homeostasis and pain modulation, the serotonergic system also plays a central role in the mechanisms of sleep, feeding, and sexual behavior. Serotonergic activity is higher in the waking state, decreases during slow-wave sleep, and is almost nonexistent during "rapid eye movement" sleep. Finally, hyperactivity of the serotonergic system is involved in the pathogenesis of anxiety, whereas hypoactivity has been implicated in the etiology of depression.

Histamine

Synthesis and degradation

Histamine is synthesized by decarboxylation of the amino acid **histidine** (Fig. 20-2), which is actively transported into the CNS. Pyridoxal phosphate is required as a cofactor for the decarboxylase. Histamine synthesis can therefore be blocked by pyridoxal phosphate antagonists, or by α-fluoromethylhistidine, a selective and irreversible inhibitor of histidine decarboxylase.

Histamine can be metabolized either by histamine-*N*-methyltransferase to form methylhistamine or by diamine oxidase to form imidazole acetic acid. Histamine concentrations in the brain are relatively low (except in the hypothalamus) but there is a rapid turnover.

Histamine receptors

The major types of histamine receptors in the brain are shown in Table 20-4. They are all present in the periphery as well as in the CNS. H_1-receptors are the site of action of the classical antihistaminic drugs. In the CNS, H_1-receptors mediate excitatory activity and are abundant in the hypothalamus, whereas H_2-receptors mediate inhibitory activity and are found in the hippocampus and cortex. H_3-receptors have the pharmacological profile of autoreceptors, are almost exclusively present in the hypothalamus, and

regulate the synthesis and release of histamine in histamine-producing neurons.

Central histaminergic pathways

The two main histaminergic cell groups are located in the brainstem **reticular formation** (RF) and the ventral **posterior hypothalamus** (PH) (see Fig. 20-5). The hypothalamus is the CNS region with the highest concentrations of histamine and histamine receptors, because many of the PH histaminergic neurons are local interneurons. **Ascending projection fibers** from both the RF and PH join the **medial forebrain bundle** and diffusely innervate the cerebral cortex, hippocampus, basal ganglia, olfactory tubercle, and thalamus. The PH group also sends **descending fibers** to the brainstem and spinal cord (Fig. 20-6C).

Functionally, the central histaminergic system has been implicated in the mechanisms of arousal (RF-mediated), and of PH-mediated regulation of food and water intake. These central actions have long been suspected, since it is well known that systemic administration of antihistaminic drugs also causes sedation and loss of appetite.

Catecholamines: Dopamine, Norepinephine, and Epinephrine

Synthesis and degradation

The metabolic routes of synthesis and degradation of **dopamine** (DA), **norepinephrine** (NE), and **epinephrine** (E) are the same in the CNS as in the peripheral autonomic system. They are summarized in Figure 20-2 and described in detail in Chapter 13. The production of DA can be increased by the administration of L-dopa, which readily crosses the blood–brain barrier and thus bypasses the tyrosine hydroxylase reaction.

The catecholamine neurotransmitters are removed from the synaptic cleft by a combination of degradative reactions and high-affinity binding to membrane-bound **transporters** that carry undegraded transmitters back into the cytoplasm. These uptake mechanisms are blocked by various drugs with strong psychoactive properties, such as amphetamine and cocaine (which block the uptake of DA and NE), and tricyclic and other antidepressants such as imipramine and citalopram, that block the reuptake of NE and 5-HT, respectively.

The concentrations of DA and its metabolites homovanillic acid (HVA) and dihydroxyphenylacetic acid (DOPAc) have been used as indicators of the level of central dopaminergic activity. Stimulation of the DA cells, either by electrical stimuli or by pharmacological means (such as chronic administration of antipsychotic drugs), increases the levels of these metabolites in plasma and CSF. Hypoactivity of the DA system, as in parkinsonism, has an opposite effect.

Similarly, concentrations of NE, E, and their metabolites can be measured in the CSF, plasma, and urine and provide useful biochemical information for the diagnosis of neuropsychiatric disorders (e.g., mania and depression) and endocrine disorders (e.g., pheochromocytoma).

Dopamine receptors

Classically, two types of DA receptors are recognized, D_1-like (D_1 and D_5; they activate adenylyl cyclase) and D_2-like (D_2, D_3, and D_4; they inhibit adenylyl cyclase). Molecular biology techniques have so far identified six different subtypes of DA receptors (D_1, $D_{2(short)}$, $D_{2(long)}$, D_3, D_4, and D_5) that have been pharmacologically characterized. All the known subtypes of dopamine receptors are members of the G protein–coupled receptor family (see Chapter 9).

DA excitatory activity is mediated by the D_1 and D_5 subtypes. The D_5-receptor subtype has an affinity for DA 10-fold higher than that of D_1, is found only in nervous tissue, and is particularly abundant in limbic structures (such as the olfactory tubercle and ventral striatum, including the nucleus accumbens). The D_1-receptor is abundant in the predominantly motor-related dorsal striatum, i.e., the caudate-putamen (see Chapter 21). Smaller numbers of D_1-receptors are present in other limbic structures (e.g., amygdala, frontal cortex, and hypothalamus). In the pituitary gland, D_1 binding is restricted to the neural lobe. All D_1-receptors appear to be located postsynaptically.

The inhibitory activity of DA is mediated by the D_2-receptor. The $D_{2(short)}$ and $D_{2(long)}$ forms have the same pharmacological properties and originate through alternative splicing of the same gene. In the pituitary gland, D_2 binding is very dense in the intermediate lobe, light in the anterior lobe, and absent from the neural lobe. D_2-receptors predominate in areas where most of the DA-producing cell bodies are located; they are probably newly synthe-

sized receptors awaiting transport to the axon terminals where they will become autoreceptors.

Unlike the D_2-receptor, the D_3- and D_4-receptors are present in very high amounts in limbic but not in motor structures. This is consistent with the fact that atypical neuroleptics such as clozapine, which have a much higher affinity for the D_3- and D_4- than for the D_2-receptors, have a very low incidence of extrapyramidal (i.e., motor) side effects, yet retain their antipsychotic properties. The D_3-receptor subtype is characterized by its high affinity for the dopamine agonist quinpirol, and for dopamine autoreceptor inhibitors (such as (+)-AJ76). Very recent evidence suggests that D_4-receptors are located mainly on GABA-containing interneurons, which they inhibit.

Central dopaminergic pathways

There are three types of DA-containing neuronal systems in the CNS. **Ultrashort DAergic** interneurons are found in the retina and the olfactory bulb. **Intermediate-length DAergic** neurons in the hypothalamus project to the hypophysis, where they participate in regulation of the secretion of prolactin and other hormones. The third and largest DAergic system is the **ventral mesencephalic system,** with perikarya located in the substantia nigra pars compacta (SNc) and the ventral tegmental area (VTA) (see Fig. 20-5).

The ascending fibers originating in the SNc constitute the **nigrostriatal system,** projecting mainly to the dorsal striatum. They are involved in motor coordination. Massive degeneration of the DA neurons of the substantia nigra, with severe depletion of DA, is the primary lesion in Parkinson's disease (see Chapter 21). The **mesolimbic system** includes primarily the DA neurons of the VTA that project to limbic areas such as the ventral striatum (including the nucleus accumbens), septum, olfactory tubercle, amygdala, and frontal cortex (Fig. 20-7A). This system is involved in the neural mechanisms of motivation and reward (see Chapters 71 and 72). Disturbed activity in this system seems to play an important role in the etiology of schizophrenia (see Chapter 28).

Adrenergic receptors

Adrenergic receptors are divided into two types: α (antagonized by phentolamine) and β (antagonized by propranolol). NE and E act on both types. Six

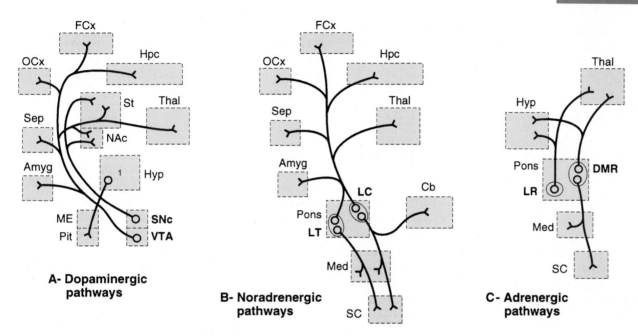

A- Dopaminergic pathways

B- Noradrenergic pathways

C- Adrenergic pathways

Figure 20-7. Schematic representation of major catecholaminergic pathways in the brain. A. Dopaminergic: 1 = hypothalamohypophysial system; SNc = substantia nigra, pars compacta; VTA = ventral tegmental area. B.

Noradrenergic: LC = locus coeruleus; LT = lateral tegmental group. C. Adrenergic: LR = lateral reticular group; DMR = dorsomedial reticular group. For other abbreviations, see Figure 20-5.

subtypes of α-adrenergic (α_{1A}, α_{1B}, α_{1C}, α_{2A}, α_{2B}, and α_{2C}) and three subtypes of β-adrenergic (β_1, β_2, and β_3) receptor have been cloned so far. The α_1-receptors are located postsynaptically. Stimulation of the α_{1A}-receptor activates a calcium channel and causes increased intracellular concentration of Ca^{2+} and excitation of the postsynaptic cell. The α_{1B}- and α_{1C}-receptors activate the diacylglycerol/inositol trisphosphate second messenger system. α_2-Receptors are located both pre- and postsynaptically. They inhibit the adenylyl cyclase/cyclic AMP second-messenger system, and stimulation of postsynaptic α_2-receptors causes hyperpolarization (i.e., inhibition) of the postsynaptic neuron. Drugs that are agonists at presynaptic α_2-receptors (e.g., clonidine) decrease NE turnover in the adrenergic axon terminal, whereas antagonists (e.g., yohimbine) increase the NE turnover.

The α_1-adrenoceptors are distributed in thalamus and neocortex as well as in the dorsal motor nucleus of the vagus nerve (a region involved in blood pressure regulation); the selective α_1-antagonist prazosin is an effective centrally acting antihypertensive agent. The α_2-receptor concentration is highest in the amygdala, locus coeruleus, and temporal cortex. In human brain, both α_1 and α_2 subtypes are also abundant in other cortical areas and hippocampus and moderately abundant in the basal ganglia and substantia nigra. The α_{2A} type is present in all the regions mentioned above, whereas the α_{2B} type is seen only in the basal ganglia.

The β-adrenergic receptors are members of the G protein–coupled receptor family and share the typical structural properties of this family (see Chapter 9). All three subtypes of β-adrenergic receptors (β_1, β_2, and β_3) stimulate adenylyl cyclase and cause excitation of the postsynaptic cell. Some of the main features of these receptor types are summarized in Table 20-4.

The concentration of β-receptors in human CNS is highest in the hippocampus and cerebellum, followed by the thalamic nuclei, basal ganglia, and mesencephalon.

The central noradrenergic and adrenergic systems are involved in the regulation of food and water intake. Stimulation of the α-receptors induces feeding, while stimulation of the β-receptors suppresses feeding. Effects opposite to these have been reported in the regulation of water intake. Hypoactivity of noradrenergic and adrenergic systems has also been implicated in the etiology of depression. Chronic treatment with inhibitors of NE and 5-HT uptake, such as desipramine and fluoxetine, causes alterations in central adrenergic and serotonergic activity that are believed to be responsible for the antidepressant effect of these agents (see Chapter 29).

Central noradrenergic and adrenergic pathways

Noradrenergic. There are two large groups of NE neurons in the CNS (Fig. 20-7B). The locus coeruleus (LC) is a large nucleus in the lateral central gray of the pons. The lateral tegmental group of NE neurons is diffusely distributed in the caudal brainstem, ventral to the LC. Large-sized NE neurons in both groups have long axons that branch profusely and send widespread innervation to many brain regions. The NEergic ascending projections profusely innervate the brainstem, cerebellum, and most forebrain structures. The descending projections innervate the lower brainstem and the spinal cord.

The NEergic projections have a predominantly inhibitory effect on postsynaptic neurons in the cortex, thalamus, cerebellum, and spinal cord. In the hippocampus, however, the effects of the rich NEergic innervation are more complex, and they vary in different subregions.

Adrenergic. Adrenergic neurons are organized into two main groups located in the reticular formation of the brainstem, the lateral reticular group, and the dorsomedial reticular group (Fig. 20-7C). These groups send ascending projections to the hypothalamus (where they are involved in neuroendocrine regulation), thalamus (pain modulation), dorsal motor nucleus of the vagus nerve and nucleus of the solitary tract (respiratory and cardiovascular control), and locus coeruleus. Descending projections are sent to the central gray matter of the spinal cord. The existence of a rich adrenergic innervation of the locus coeruleus raises the possibility that adrenergic neurons regulate the activity of NE-producing neurons in this region.

Amino Acid Neurotransmitters

The role of glutamate, aspartate, γ-aminobutyrate, and glycine as neurotransmitters is now well established. However, the amino acid (AA) neurotransmitter systems differ from the classical neurotransmitter systems in many respects. Some of the major differences are (1) the high content and ubiquitous distribution of AA neurotransmitters in the nervous system, (2) their extensive role in peripheral and central synapses at all phylogenetic levels, and (3) their involvement in multiple metabolic pathways. Glutamate and aspartate are excitatory neurotransmitters while γ-aminobutyric acid (GABA) and glycine (in most instances) are inhibitory.

Excitatory amino acid neurotransmitters: Synthesis and degradation

The negatively charged amino acid L-glutamate (and also L-aspartate) is abundant in the adult mammalian CNS. Glutamate does not cross the blood–brain barrier but is synthesized locally in the CNS, mainly from glutamine but also from a variety of other precursors (Fig. 20-2).

The calcium-dependent release of aspartate and glutamate into the synaptic cleft is followed by inactivation through the reuptake of the neurotransmitter molecules by a high-affinity sodium-dependent transport system, similar to those mediating the reuptake of the catecholamines and serotonin. Aspartate and glutamate share the same reuptake system, located in the terminals of aspartate- and glutamate-producing neurons, as well as in the adjacent glial cells. The glutamate taken up by glial cells is transformed into glutamine, by the action of glutamine synthetase, which is found only in glial cells. However, the glutamine can diffuse back into glutamate neurons and be reconverted to glutamate by the enzyme glutaminase.

Excitatory amino acid receptors

The excitatory AA receptors have been classified into two main types: the NMDA (*N*-methyl-D-aspartate) *receptor*, and the non-NMDA receptors, of which there are four subtypes, named for their selective agonists—kainate, quisqualate/AMPA (α-amino-3-hydroxy-5-methyl-isoxazole-4-propionic acid), L-AP4 (L-2-amino-4-phosphonobutyrate, L-APB) and ACPD (1-amino-cyclopentane-1,3-dicarboxylic acid) (see Table 20-4).

The NMDA receptor is an ionotropic receptor linked to a channel that is permeable to monovalent cations and highly permeable to calcium. The NMDA receptor responds rather slowly to glutamate, which is more effective in opening the ion channel when the cell is already depolarized. The increase in intracellular calcium concentration in the postsynaptic cell may lead to the activation of various Ca^{2+}-dependent enzymes that mediate the cell responses (e.g., protein kinase C, calcium/calmodulin-dependent protein kinase II, and nitric oxide synthase).

The NMDA receptor complex consists of four different subunits bearing five distinct binding sites. (1) The **glutamate binding site** and (2) the **glycine binding site**, both located near the extracellular end of the channel, act as co-agonists to open the channel. (3) The **phencyclidine (PCP) binding site**, located inside the channel, (4) the **voltage-dependent magnesium binding site**, located at the intracellular end of the channel, and (5) the **zinc binding site**, located at the extracellular end of the channel, are all inhibitory sites. **Dizocilpine** (MK-801) and **ketamine** act similarly to phencyclidine as channel blockers. The glycine-binding site is selectively blocked by kynurenate and (+)HA-966 and stimulated by D-serine. The NMDA receptor is widely distributed in the CNS, but particularly in the cerebral cortex and hippocampus.

The non-NMDA **kainate** receptor is an ionotropic receptor that regulates a channel permeable to sodium and potassium. This receptor is particularly abundant in the hippocampus.

The **quisqualate/AMPA** receptor also is an ionotropic receptor that regulates sodium and potassium exchange. Its distribution in the CNS is ubiquitous, and similar to that of the NMDA receptor.

Activation of the L-AP4 receptor subtype inhibits the presynaptic release of glutamate. Further pharmacological characterization and study of the neuroanatomical distribution of the L-AP4-receptor are still required.

Finally, the **ACPD** subtype is a metabotropic receptor that activates phospholipase C and the diacylglycerol/inositol trisphosphate second-messenger system.

The excitatory effects of glutamate and structurally related compounds can, if carried beyond physiological limits, give rise to seizure activity and convulsions (see Chapter 22). These substances can also produce neurotoxic effects. For example, kainic acid and ibotenic acid are used experimentally by intracerebral injection to induce selective degeneration and death of neuronal cell bodies at the injection site, while sparing the axons terminating in, or passing through, that area. The neurotoxic effects of glutamate and its analogs are due to prolonged and exacerbated excitation and calcium influx that irreversibly damages the metabolic and functional activity of the neuron. Glycine binding site blockers, and other NMDA receptor antagonists, are currently being assessed for their therapeutic potential as antiepileptic agents and as drugs that might prevent ischemic brain damage after stroke or trauma. Glutamate receptors (especially the NMDA type) are involved in processes of neuronal plasticity that are the cellular basis of learning (e.g., long-term potentiation or LTP).

Central pathways containing aspartate and glutamate

These amino acid neurotransmitters are ubiquitously present in the CNS, but glutamate is particularly abundant in certain structures and pathways (Fig. 20-8A). Large populations of glutamate-containing neurons are seen in the **cerebral cortex**, where they provide the major excitatory cortical output, directed heavily to the hippocampus, basal ganglia (caudate-putamen and nucleus accumbens), thalamus, olfactory tubercle, and amygdala.

The **hippocampus** also contains many glutamatergic neurons (i.e., pyramidal and granular cells) that project to **limbic structures**, such as the lateral septum and nucleus accumbens. These pathways are thought to be involved in learning.

In the **retina**, glutamate is the major excitatory neurotransmitter, and it is found in the photoreceptors and in the bipolar cells.

Inhibitory Amino Acid Neurotransmitters

GABA

Synthesis and degradation. γ-Aminobutyric acid (GABA) is the main inhibitory neurotransmitter in the mammalian CNS and is found in concentrations 1000 times higher than those of classical monoamine neurotransmitters. It is synthesized locally by decarboxylation of glutamate (Fig. 20-2).

After its release into the synaptic cleft, its activity at postsynaptic receptors is terminated through selective reuptake by a glycoprotein, the GABA transporter, located in the presynaptic terminals and surrounding glia. The recaptured transmitter is reused in the nerve terminal or metabolized by GABA transaminase in glial cells.

GABA receptors. There are two subtypes of GABA receptors, designated $GABA_A$ and $GABA_B$ (see Table 20-4). The $GABA_A$ receptor, the more abundant type in the mammalian CNS, is an ionotropic receptor. Its stimulation by GABA results in the opening of a chloride channel, influx of Cl^-, and hyperpolarization (i.e., inhibition) of the postsynaptic cell. The $GABA_A$ receptor is a tetramer with five separate binding sites. (1) The **GABA binding site** and (2)

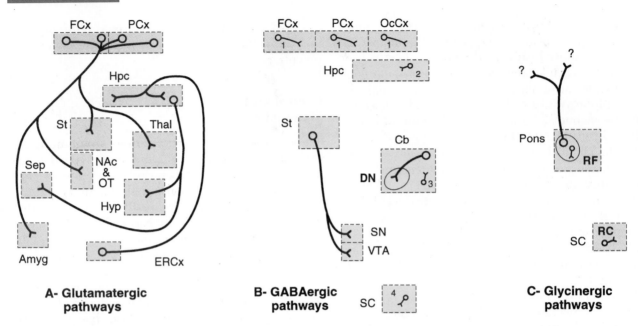

A- Glutamatergic
pathways

B- GABAergic
pathways

C- Glycinergic
pathways

Figure 20-8. Schematic representation of major amino acid neurotransmitter pathways in the brain. A. **Glutamatergic:** OT = olfactory tubercle. B. **GABAergic:** 1 = cortical local-circuit neurons; 2 = hippocampal local-circuit neurons; 3 = cerebellar local-circuit neurons; 4 = spinal local-circuit neurons; DN = deep nuclei of cerebellum. C. **Glycinergic:** RF = reticular formation cell group; RC = Renshaw cells, spinal interneurons. For other abbreviations, see Figure 20-5.

the **benzodiazepine binding site** are located at the extracellular end of the channel. (3) The **barbiturate,** (4) the **steroid,** and (5) the **picrotoxinin binding sites** are all located inside the Cl⁻ channel.

The hyperpolarizing action of GABA exerts an anticonvulsant effect, and specific $GABA_A$ agonists, such as muscimol and tetrahydroxyisoxazolopyridinone (THIP), have anticonvulsant properties, while specific $GABA_A$ antagonists (e.g., bicuculline) produce vigorous convulsions. Binding of benzodiazepines to their selective binding site on the $GABA_A$ receptor facilitates GABA activity by *increasing the frequency* of channel opening. Clinically, benzodiazepines are depressant drugs with anticonvulsant, sedative, and anxiolytic properties (see Chapter 26). Some drugs, such as the β-carbolines, which bind to the benzodiazepine binding site but *decrease* GABA activity, are known as **inverse agonists.** It has also been suggested that the depressant effects of ethanol may be exerted through the $GABA_A$ receptor, and there is a positive correlation betweeen the potencies of anesthetic agents and their ability to increase GABA-mediated chloride uptake.

Barbiturates (e.g., phenobarbital and pentobarbital) act by *increasing the opening time* of the chloride channel, and are also anticonvulsants. Neuroactive steroids, such as alphaxalone, facilitate the binding of agonists to the GABA site and modulate benzodiazepine binding, and in high concentrations they can activate the $GABA_A$ receptor. Picrotoxin and pentylenetetrazol (metrazol) *decrease* the opening time of the Cl⁻ channel and thus are convulsants.

The **$GABA_B$ receptor** was first identified by its lack of affinity for muscimol and bicuculline and its selective affinity for the agonist baclofen and the antagonist phaclofen. $GABA_B$ receptors are located presynaptically and act through G proteins to inhibit cyclic AMP production, open a K⁺ channel (causing hyperpolarization), and decrease Ca²⁺ influx, thus reducing the presynaptic release of neurotransmitters.

Central GABAergic pathways. Most GABA-containing neurons are inhibitory local **interneurons** located in the retina, cerebral cortex, hippocampus, cerebellum, and spinal cord (Fig. 20-8B). To date, two main inhibitory **GABAergic pathways** have been identified in the CNS: (1) the projections from the **Purkinje cells** to the cerebellar nuclei, and (2) the **striatonigral pathway,** the descending component of the loop involved in the regulation of motor activity and limbic functions (see Chapters 21 and 71).

Glycine

Synthesis and degradation. Glycine, the smallest amino acid [$CH_2(NH_2)COOH$], is a potent inhibitory neurotransmitter in the mammalian CNS. It is formed from serine by the enzyme **serine hydroxymethyltransferase** (SHMT) (Fig. 20-2). The brain metabolism of glycine is still unclear. After release into the synaptic cleft and binding to the active sites, glycine is removed by a selective reuptake mechanism.

Glycine receptors. The glycine receptor, like the $GABA_A$ receptor, is an ionotropic receptor linked to a Cl^- channel in the postsynaptic membrane. It is selectively blocked by the natural alkaloid strychnine and by RU 5135. Several other amino acids (serine, proline, taurine, and β-alanine) activate the glycine receptor (see Table 20-4). This receptor is distinct from the accessory glycine binding site on the NMDA receptor, which is excitatory in effect and is not blocked by strychnine.

Central pathways containing glycine. The neuroanatomical distribution of glycine in the mammalian CNS is rather restricted (Fig. 20-8C). In the **ventral spinal cord** glycine is found in interneurons (Renshaw cells) that exert an inhibitory action on the motor neurons; this action is blocked by strychnine. At supraspinal levels, glycine is found in only a few structures, including the **brainstem, reticular formation,** and **amacrine cells of the retina.**

Neuropeptides

In recent years, more than 50 neuropeptides have been identified in the mammalian CNS. An exhaustive presentation of the different peptides is beyond the scope of this chapter. Those for which physiological roles have been best established are the opioid peptides, vasopressin, oxytocin, cholecystokinin, and angiotensin.

Opioid peptides

Three different groups or families of opioid peptides are found in the CNS, originating from three different precursors encoded by three different genes. These precursors are **proopiomelanocortin** (POMC, with 267 amino acids [a.a.]), **proenkephalin** (Pro-Enk, 267 a.a.), and **prodynorphin** (Pro-Dyn, 256 a.a.).

The fragments derived from POMC include the nonopioid peptides α-, β-, and γ-melanocyte-stimulating hormone (MSH) and adrenocorticotropic hormone (ACTH), as well as β-lipoptropin (β-LPH, 91 a.a.). β-LPH is the immediate precursor of the opioid fragments β-endorphin (31 a.a.), γ-endorphin (17 a.a.), and α-endorphin (16 a.a.). Most neurons expressing POMC-derived peptides, and β-endorphin in particular, are located in the **arcuate nucleus** of the hypothalamus, intermediate and anterior lobes of the **pituitary,** and nucleus of the solitary tract.

The most important Pro-Enk-derived opioid fragments are the pentapeptides methionine-enkephalin (Met-Enk) and leucine-enkephalin (Leu-Enk). Each molecule of Pro-Enk contains six copies of Met-Enk and one copy of Leu-Enk. A heptapeptide, an octapeptide, and two larger fragments (peptide E and peptide F) are also derived from Pro-Enk. The smaller fragments Met-Enk and Leu-Enk are more abundant in nervous tissue, while the larger fragments predominate in the adrenal medulla. Enkephalins are present in interneurons, as well as in projection neurons. A large population of Enk-producing neurons in the striatum sends projections to the globus pallidus, the brain area with the highest concentration of enkephalins. Enkephalinergic neurons are also present in the hypothalamus, ventral mesencephalon, pons, and cerebellum.

Pro-Dyn contains three copies of Leu-Enk. C-terminal extensions of Leu-Enk form the four peptide fragments α- and β-neoendorphin, dynorphin A, and dynorphin B. The general distribution of Pro-Dyn-derived peptides in the brain overlaps with the distribution of enkephalins. Additionally, high concentrations of dynorphins are also present in the amygdala, septum, and spinal cord (see Fig. 20-9).

These peptides bind selectively to the three major groups of opioid receptors, μ, δ, and κ (see Table 20-4 and Chapter 23), all of which are metabotropic receptors linked to ion channels via the adenylyl cyclase/cyclic AMP second-messenger system. Binding of opioid peptides to these receptors inhibits adenylyl cyclase activity via an inhibitory G protein. Ultimately, activation of the μ- and δ-receptors results in opening of a K^+ channel, while binding to the κ receptor leads to the closing of a Ca^{2+} channel, and both actions have inhibitory effects on the neuron. The endogenous opioids have different receptor affinities: β-endorphin binds to the μ-receptor, the enkephalins have higher affinity for the δ-receptor, and dynorphin binds selectively to the κ-receptor.

The μ-receptor subtype is most abundant in the cerebral cortex, hippocampus, and various sites in the thalamus, hypothalamus, brainstem, and dorsal horn of the spinal cord. This distribution of μ-recep-

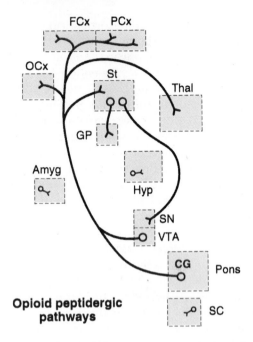

Figure 20-9. Schematic representation of major opioid peptidergic pathways in the brain. CG = central gray. In this diagram, St also includes the NAc.

tors is consistent with their involvement in pain regulation and sensorimotor integration. The δ-opioid receptors are particularly concentrated in the olfactory system, neocortex, and various limbic structures, where they may play an important role in olfaction, motor integration, reward (see Chapter 71), and cognitive functions. Finally, the κ-receptors are also very abundant in the caudate-putamen, various limbic and hypothalamic sites, and the neural lobe of the pituitary, where they have been implicated in the regulation of food intake and water balance, pain perception, and neuroendocrine function.

Vasopressin and oxytocin

The octapeptides arginine vasopressin (AVP) and oxytocin originate from large peptide precursors, the neurophysins, that are normally synthesized in separate populations of hypothalamic neurons located in the supraoptic (SON), paraventricular (PVN), and suprachiasmatic (SCN) nuclei of the hypothalamus (Fig. 20-10). Large axons from the SON and PVN travel through the median eminence and terminate near blood vessels in the neurohypophysis, where the AVP and oxytocin are released into the bloodstream to be carried to their peripheral targets. Other small-sized AVP- and oxytocin-producing neurons send

axonal projections to other regions of the CNS. AVP-containing projections are scarce in the cerebral cortex but are abundant in the mediodorsal thalamus and limbic system (including limbic-related cortical areas, septum, and parts of the amygdala). Caudal projections are also present in the brainstem and dorsal horn of the spinal cord. In general, oxytocin-containing fibers have a fairly similar distribution. In the spinal cord, many oxytocin fibers are found in the dorsal horn and central gray.

To date, two different types of vasopressin receptors have been identified: V_1 and V_2 (Table 20-4). Both types are metabotropic and G protein–linked. V_1 activation leads to cell stimulation via the inositol trisphosphate (IP_3) second-messenger system. In the CNS, AVP binding sites are most abundant in the extrahypothalamic limbic structures (septum, amygdala, and ventral hippocampus), but they are also numerous in the hypothalamus, pons, and medulla. The central AVP system has been implicated in mechanisms of learning and memory, including long-term potentiation.

Oxytocin binding occurs predominantly in various limbic structures and ventral hippocampus. The functional role of oxytocin as a central neurotransmitter is still not clear, but recent studies have suggested that it might play an important role in the initiation of maternal behaviors and in the etiology of obsessive-compulsive disorder and related behaviors.

Cholecystokinin

Pharmacological, behavioral, and neuroanatomical studies have shown that the octapeptide cholecystokinin (CCK) is synthesized in the CNS and acts as a neurotransmitter. CCK-producing neurons have been identified in limbic cortical areas, hypothalamus, amygdala, and ventral mesencephalon (Fig. 20-10C), and are particularly numerous in the nucleus accumbens and median eminence. CCK is colocalized with dopamine and neurotensin in the substantia nigra and ventral tegmental area and with oxytocin in the paraventricular and supraoptic hypothalamic nuclei.

Two types of CCK receptors (CCK_A and CCK_B) have so far been identified (Table 20-4). Both types are found in many parts of the CNS. Abundant CCK_A and CCK_B receptors are found together, and may have opposing actions, in the caudate-putamen, nucleus accumbens, and ventral mesencephalon. For example, in the nucleus accumbens, stimulation of the CCK_A receptor facilitates the release of dopamine while stimulation of the CCK_B receptor inhibits it.

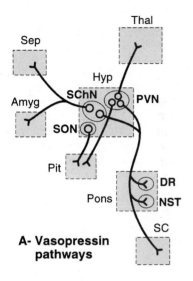

A- Vasopressin pathways

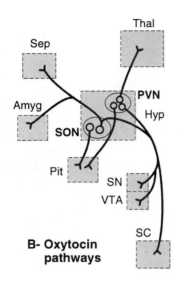

B- Oxytocin pathways

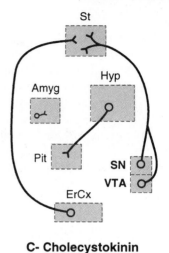

C- Cholecystokinin pathways

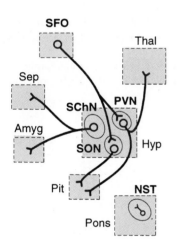

D- Angiotensin II pathways

Figure 20-10. Schematic representation of other peptidergic pathways in the brain. A. **Vasopressin:** Hypothalamic nuclei containing vasopressin-synthesizing cells; SON = supraoptic nucleus; PVN = paraventricular nucleus; SChN = suprachiasmatic nucleus; DR = dorsal raphe; NST = nucleus of solitary tract. B. **Oxytocin:** SON and PVN as above. C. **Cholecystokinin.** D. **Angiotensin II:** PVN, SON, SChN, and NST as above; SFO = subfornical organ. For other abbreviations, see Figure 20-5.

The central CCKergic system appears to be involved in the regulation of food intake and in the etiology of anxiety.

Angiotensin

The octapeptide **angiotensin II** (AII) is well known for its effects on water intake and on blood pressure.

Its metabolism and physiological role in the periphery are described in Chapters 32 and 38. In the brain, AII is produced in neurons that are able to synthesize all the required substrates and enzymes. The larger precursor, **angiotensinogen** (14 a.a.), is converted to the immediate precursor, the decapeptide **angiotensin I.** This is converted to AII by cleavage of the last two amino acids of the carboxylic terminal by **angiotensin-converting enzyme** (ACE). In the diencephalon, the AII-producing neurons are located in the subfornical organ, and in the PVN, SON, and SChN of the hypothalamus (Fig. 20-10D). AII-containing perikarya are also found in various sites in the thalamus and brainstem, while angiotensinergic innervation is abundant in limbic forebrain regions and median eminence. In the hypothalamus, AII is colocalized with vasopressin (but not with oxytocin), dynorphin, Leu-enkephalin, and cholecystokinin.

The brain renin–angiotensin system, which is separate from that of the periphery, is involved in the regulation of water and electrolyte balance and neuroendocrine control (stimulation of prolactin, ACTH, and LH release).

There are two types of AII receptors (Table 20-4). The AII_{α} subtype predominates in the areas involved in regulation of water intake and of cardiovascular and endocrine function. The AII_{β} receptor is abundant in areas involved in the modulation of sensory input.

SUGGESTED READING

Angevine JB. The nervous tissue. In: Bloom W, Fawcett DW, eds. A textbook of histology. 12th ed. New York: Chapman & Hall, 1994:309–367.

Barr ML, Kiernan JA. The human nervous system: an anatomical viewpoint. 6th ed. Philadelphia: Lippincott, 1993.

Chiu AT, Herblin WF, McCall DE, et al. Identification of angiotensin II receptor subtypes. Biochem Biophys Res Commun 1989; 165:196–203.

Cooper JR, Bloom FE, Roth RH. The biochemical basis of neuropharmacology. 7th ed. New York: Oxford, 1996.

Davson H, Zloković B, Rakić L, Segal MB. An introduction to the blood-brain barrier. London: Macmillan, 1993.

Hall ZC, ed. An introduction to molecular neurobiology. Sunderland, MA: Sinauer, 1992. See especially Chap 2, electrical signalling; Chap 3, ion channels; Chap 4, chemical messengers at synapses.

Harrington MA, Zhong P, Garlow SJ, Cianarello RD. Molecular biology of serotonin receptors. J Clin Psychiatry 1992; 53(Suppl 10):8–27.

Kandel ER, Schwartz JH, Jessell TM. Elementary interactions between neurons: synaptic transmission. In: Principles of neural science. 3rd ed, Part III. New York: Elsevier, 1991:120–269.

Larsen WJ. Development of the brain and cranial nerves. In: Human embryology, Chap 13. New York: Churchill Livingston, 1993:375–418.

Siegel GJ, Agranoff BW, Albers RW, Molinoff PB. Basic neurochemistry. Molecular, cellular and medical aspects. 5th ed. New York: Raven Press, 1994.

Woodruff GN, Hill DR, Boden P, et al. Functional role of brain CCK receptors. Neuropeptides 1991; 19(Suppl):45–56.

CHAPTER 21

Agents Modifying Movement Control

W.M. BURNHAM

CASE HISTORY

Amanda C., a prominent 58-year-old ophthalmologist, began to experience motor difficulties. Her movements became slow and her posture stiff and rigid. She found it increasingly hard to get up from chairs and sofas or to keep up with friends when walking. She also noticed an irritating tremor in her hands. Recognizing the early signs of Parkinson's disease, she consulted her physician, who prescribed a trial of L-dopa. This was unsuccessful because she was unable to tolerate the persistent nausea and occasional vomiting. She did well, however, on a lower dose of L-dopa combined with carbidopa and was able to continue work, although she did experience temporary dizziness on standing up from a sitting or lying position. Gradually, however, she began to display abnormal, involuntary movements (dyskinesia) during the time when the drug was effective, and also a sudden loss of mobility as the effects of the drug began wearing off ("on/off syndrome"). Bromocriptine was added at a starting dose of 2.5 mg daily and gradually increased to 40 mg. This somewhat alleviated the problem, but at the high dosage she began to experience brightly colored visual hallucinations and confusion, which disappeared when the dose was reduced. Over the next 2 years she began to complain of gradually deteriorating memory, and at age 65 she retired and withdrew from professional and public activities.

In mammals, the control of conscious ("voluntary") movement depends on a large number of CNS structures. The highest of these is the motor cortex. Closely allied to the motor cortex is a group of subcortical structures called the basal ganglia. While the exact function of the basal ganglia is not yet clear, pathology of these structures is known to cause a loss of control over voluntary movements. In some cases, voluntary movement slows or stops (progressively greater degrees of impairment are called bradykinesia, hypokinesia, and akinesia), and the individual freezes into immobility. In other cases, seemingly voluntary-type movements begin to occur even when they are not wanted (dyskinesia, hyperkinesia). In both cases, reflex function remains normal.

Traditionally, the prognosis for patients afflicted with the hypo- or hyperkinetic syndromes was poor. During the past 30 years, however, the biochemical basis of basal-ganglion dysfunction has become better understood, and drugs have been developed that can alleviate (though not cure) two of the most common syndromes: Parkinson's disease and Huntington's chorea.

BASAL GANGLIA

Definitions

The term "basal ganglia" is applied to a group of subcortical forebrain structures which includes the caudate-putamen (striatum) and the globus pallidus (the pallidum) (Fig. 21-1). The caudate and putamen are structurally distinct in the human, but they are joined as a single structure in lower mammals,

POSTERIOR (OBLIQUE) VIEW

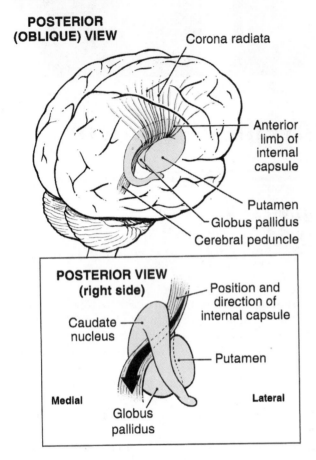

Figure 21-1. The caudate-putamen and the globus pallidus. Substantia nigra and subthalamus are not shown.

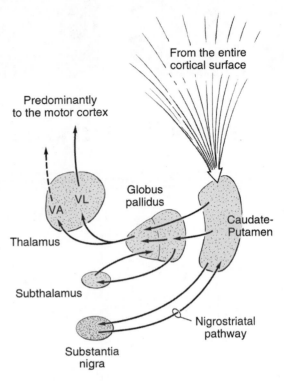

Figure 21-2. Schematic, simplified representation of major connections of the basal ganglia. VA = thalamus ventralis anterior; VL = thalamus ventralis lateralis.

and they are generally considered to function as a unit. Closely associated with the basal ganglia are two small brainstem nuclei, the substantia nigra and the subthalamus.

Neural Connections

The complete connections of the basal ganglia are complex and not fully understood. Major pathways, however, are as shown in Figure 21-2 (see also Chapter 20).

Through-put pathway

All parts of the neocortex project to the caudate-putamen. The caudate-putamen projects to the globus pallidus, which in turn projects to areas in the thalamus (VA, VL in Fig. 21-2). These project back to the cortex, including the frontal and especially the motor areas. Thus, the major "through-put" pathway seems to be a progression from the cortex as a whole to the basal ganglia and then back to the motor cortex.

Side pathways

In addition to the through-put pathway, there are two side pathways that play important roles in basal-ganglia dysfunction. One of these runs from the caudate-putamen to the substantia nigra and back. The connections from the substantia nigra to caudate-putamen are called the **nigrostriatal pathway.** This loop is crucially involved in Parkinson's disease, a disorder involving bradykinesia and akinesia. The second side path connects the outer (lateral) segment of the globus pallidus to its inner (medial) segment via the subthalamic nucleus. This is now considered an alternate or indirect part of the through-put pathway and is believed to inhibit movement, whereas the direct pathway promotes it. Damage to the subthalamus—a part of this pathway—causes a rare hyperkinetic syndrome called **hemiballismus,** a condition in which the contralateral limbs make large, uncontrolled swinging motions.

Neurotransmitters

The caudate-putamen contains a number of putative neurotransmitter substances, including norepinephrine (NE), serotonin (5-HT), glutamate (Glu), γ-aminobutyric acid (GABA), dopamine (DA), and acetylcholine (ACh). Figure 21-3 indicates the postulated relationship of three of the most important, GABA, ACh, and DA. Output pathways of the caudate-putamen, including the fibers that go to the substantia nigra, are postulated to be GABAergic. Activity in these pathways is modulated by ACh interneurons and by dopaminergic input from the substantia nigra. (The connections shown in Fig. 21-3 are schematic. The actual connections are more complex.) Normal function of the caudate-putamen depends on the balance of these transmitters, and particularly on the balance between DA and ACh. In terms of the behavioral output, DA seems to be the "go" system, while ACh seems to be the "no-go" system. An excess of DA, therefore, produces an excess of movement, while an excess of ACh produces

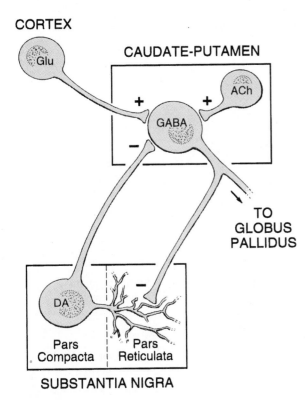

Figure 21-3. Possible (hypothetical) interrelation between transmitters in the caudate-putamen and substantia nigra (see text.) Glu = glutamate; ACh = acetylcholine; DA = dopamine; GABA = γ-aminobutyric acid; (+) = excitatory; (−) = inhibitory.

immobility. The effects of DA are mediated both by D_1 dopamine receptors, which excite neurons in the direct (movement-excitatory) pathway from striatum to medial globus pallidus, and by D_2 dopamine receptors, which inhibit neurons in the indirect (movement-inhibitory) pathway from the striatum to the lateral globus pallidus and subthalamus.

PARKINSON'S DISEASE

Clinical Syndrome

Parkinson's disease is the most common of the basal-ganglia disorders, with a lifetime prevalence of one in 400. Its cardinal symptoms are:

- Bradykinesia and akinesia (slowness or inability to initiate voluntary movements)
- Rigidity (stiffness in the skeletal muscles)
- Tremor at rest (shaking, which ceases when the affected limb is moved, but which returns when the movement comes to an end)

Parkinson's disease is a syndrome rather than a specific disease, and its causes are varied. The most common of the identified pathological causes are atherosclerosis and encephalitis lethargica. Most cases, however, are idiopathic (i.e., they have no known cause). The onset of idiopathic Parkinson's disease usually occurs late in life (age 50–65). The syndrome gradually worsens over a period of about 10 years until the patient becomes helpless.

Neuropathology

A number of abnormalities are found in parkinsonian brains. The crucial anatomical change, however, seems to be a progressive loss of the pigmented cells in the substantia nigra, the cells that give rise to the nigrostriatal tract. In most cases, 80% or more of these are gone before symptoms appear. Since these cells release DA from axon terminals in the caudate-putamen, their loss causes a secondary biochemical change, a reduction of DA content in the caudate-putamen, eventually to 10% or less of normal. This results in a DA/ACh imbalance, which is the actual cause of the parkinsonian syndrome. Since ACh ("no-go") predominates, immobility results.

A drug-induced parkinsonian syndrome occurs frequently as a reversible side effect of the antipsychotic drugs, which block D_2 dopamine receptors (see Chapter 28). A permanent and irreversible parkinsonian syndrome is induced by 1-methyl-4-phenyl-1,2,5,6-tetrahydropyridine (MPTP), a compound originally discovered as a toxic byproduct of the illicit synthesis of meperidine in the United States. MPTP selectively destroys dopaminergic neurons in the substantia nigra. It is biotransformed to two toxic metabolites, MPDP$^+$ and MPP$^+$, which cause an overflow of DA from these neurons. The free DA undergoes a nonenzymatic oxidation to a quinone-semiquinone derivative and free hydroxyl radicals, which cause peroxidation of membrane lipids. This in turn increases membrane permeability to calcium, causing a massive influx of Ca^{2+} that is responsible for the cell death. Currently, much research is directed toward a possible role for similar changes in the production of idiopathic parkinsonism.

Nondrug Therapies

Two surgical approaches are sometimes used in the treatment of Parkinson's disease: (1) surgical lesions of the thalamus or globus pallidus and (2) cellular transplants. Lesioning of the thalamus or globus pallidus has been done for some years; it is effective in relieving rigidity and tremor but less effective in controlling hypokinesia. More recently, transplantation of catecholamine-rich tissue containing dopaminergic neurons (sometimes derived from aborted fetuses) into the striatum has been attempted. Transplants have had some success but remain controversial and are not widely practiced. Most patients with Parkinson's disease are treated with drug therapy.

Drug Therapy

All of the drugs used in the treatment of Parkinson's disease are intended to correct the DA/ACh imbalance in the striatum.

L-Dopa

When it was discovered that Parkinson's disease was associated with decreased DA in the caudate-putamen, attempts were made to raise DA levels. Dopamine itself does not cross the blood–brain barrier, but its precursor, L-dopa (3,4-dihydroxyphenylalanine, Fig. 21-4), crosses via active transport and is taken up by catecholaminergic neurons. In the presence of excess precursor, the surviving DA neurons increase their output of DA, and most parkinsonian patients quickly return to normal mobility. L-dopa is the mainstay therapy for Parkinson's disease.

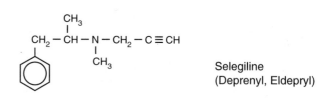

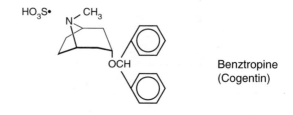

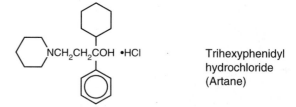

Figure 21-4. Drugs used in the treatment of Parkinson's disease. (See Fig. 58-2 for amantadine hydrochloride.)

Pharmacokinetics

L-dopa is well absorbed from the gastrointestinal tract and reaches maximum plasma levels 1–2 hours

Table 21-1 Pharmacokinetic Parameters of Drugs Acting on the Basal Ganglia

Name	Half-life (hours)	Bioavail-ability (oral %)	Urinary Excretion (%)	Bound in Plasma (%)	Volume of Distribution (L/kg)	Effective Plasma Concentration
Amantadine	16 ± 3.4	50–100	50–90	67	6.6 ± 1.5	300 ng/mL
Bromocriptine	7 ± 5	3–6	2	93	2 ± 1	
L-Dopa	1.4 ± 0.4	41 ± 16	<1		1.7 ± 0.4	8 ± 3 nmoles/L
Selegiline	1.9 ± 0.1	?	45	94	1.9	

after an oral dose. Most of the drug is rapidly decarboxylated by dopa decarboxylase in the periphery, but a small amount is converted by catechol-*O*-methyltransferase (COMT) to 3-*O*-methyldopa, which has a longer serum half-life than the original compound. Other important pharmacokinetic parameters of L-dopa are shown in Table 21-1.

Limitations of therapy

While the introduction of L-dopa (Larodopa, Dopar, and others) has greatly improved the status of parkinsonian patients, the drug has major drawbacks.

Relief is symptomatic. L-Dopa does not replace lost neurons; it just allows the surviving cells to work with greater efficiency. Thus, relief is symptomatic and lasts only while the compound (which has a short half-life) remains in the blood. The patient must take L-dopa several times a day.

Duration of relief is limited. Most researchers believe that substantia nigra cells continue to die even in the presence of L-dopa. Eventually, perhaps due to continued cell loss, L-dopa loses its potency in many patients.

Side effects

L-dopa has serious side effects, many of them related to the fact that L-dopa raises DA levels in blood and in brain areas outside the caudate-putamen. In the first few months of therapy, nausea is a problem in about 80% of the patients; it is due to the effect of DA in the blood on the chemoreceptor trigger zone. Cardiac arrhythmias appear in about 30% of patients, as a result of the effect of circulating DA on β_1-adrenoceptors of the heart. Orthostatic hypotension is also seen; the mechanism is unknown. Tolerance to these early effects gradually develops. After 2–4 months, however, another set of side effects

begin to develop. Paradoxically, these late side effects seem to relate to the development of DA hypersensitivity. They consist of hyperkinesias (seen in 80% of patients after 1 year) and psychiatric abnormalities, such as anxiety, agitation, or psychosis (seen in 15% of patients). Tolerance to these late side effects does not develop, although they disappear when L-dopa is discontinued.

Carbidopa and Benserazide

When L-dopa is administered orally, more than 90% of each dose is decarboxylated to DA in the periphery and less than 5% enters the brain. The systemic DA circulating in the blood causes side effects but has no therapeutic action since it cannot enter the brain. Carbidopa (Fig. 21-4) is a peripheral decarboxylase inhibitor that prevents the peripheral conversion of L-dopa to DA. Benserazide (available in Canada but not in the United States) has a closely similar action. By increasing the level of L-dopa in the blood, these agents increase the rate of entry of L-dopa into the brain. Neither carbidopa nor benserazide itself enters the brain, since these are polar compounds. When carbidopa and L-dopa are given in combination, a much smaller dose of L-dopa is required, and the early side effects (nausea, cardiac arrhythmia) are lessened. A combination of carbidopa and L-dopa, in a ratio of 1:10, is marketed as a standard commercial preparation (Sinemet). A similar mixture of benserazide and L-dopa, in a ratio of 1:4, is marketed in Canada (Prolopa).

Pharmacokinetics

Both carbidopa and benserazide are incompletely absorbed from the gastrointestinal tract; their oral bioavailabilities are 40–70%. The maximum plasma concentration of carbidopa is reached at 2–3 hours after a dose, and absorption may be somewhat delayed by food, particularly by dietary protein. The elimination $t^{1/2}$ of carbidopa is about 2 hours, and 30% is excreted unchanged in the urine. There are numerous metabolites, all of them pharmacologically inactive. Both carbidopa and benserazide tend to slow the absorption of L-dopa, probably by competing for mucosal transport systems. As a result, they reduce the C_{max} of L-dopa after each dose, but prolong the effect and smooth out the plasma peaks and troughs.

Amantadine

Amantadine (Symmetrel) was originally developed as a synthetic antiviral agent (see Chapter 58). Its usefulness in Parkinson's disease was discovered by chance. Amantadine appears to work by increasing DA release from the surviving nigral neurons. Amantadine alone is less effective than L-dopa, but it also has fewer side effects. Insomnia and hallucinations may occur, but only at toxic levels. Unfortunately, tolerance to its therapeutic action develops after 6–8 months.

Pharmacokinetics

Amantadine absorption from the gastrointestinal tract is essentially complete but slow; maximum plasma levels are reached in 2–4 hours after a single dose. It distributes throughout the body, including the brain. The plasma $t^{1/2}$ is about 12–18 hours but is markedly influenced by the state of renal function, because over 90% is eliminated unmetabolized in the urine by a combination of glomerular filtration and tubular secretion. Adverse effects are therefore more common in elderly patients with reduced renal function.

Dopamine Agonists

Recently, two new strategies to enhance DA activity have been based on the use of DA receptor agonists and MAO-B blockers.

Dopamine receptor agonists

A number of DA receptor agonists are able to cross the blood–brain barrier and act directly on DA receptors (e.g., bromocriptine, pergolide, lisuride). The advantage of these agents is that, at least in theory, they should be able to act directly on postsynaptic DA receptors even if the presynaptic DA-releasing

neurons have died. **Bromocriptine** (Parlodel, Fig. 21-4) is now available for use as an adjunct to L-dopa in the therapy of Parkinson's disease. Side effects are similar to those of L-dopa.

MAO-B inhibitors

Another way to raise DA levels is by blocking monoamine oxidase (MAO), the enzyme that breaks down DA. Nonspecific MAO inhibitors (MAOI) have been used for some time in the treatment of depression (see Chapter 29). They must be used with great care, because a hypertensive crisis may occur if the patient eats certain foods or takes a drug with pressor effects. Recently, drugs have been developed that specifically block MAO-B, the enzyme responsible for most of the DA metabolism in brain. One of these is **selegiline** (Fig. 21-4), also called deprenyl (Eldepryl). It is an irreversible inhibitor with a much greater affinity for MAO-B than for MAO-A. Selegiline elevates DA levels in the brain at doses that do not have the dangerous side effects associated with the traditional MAO inhibitors. It has only a mild therapeutic effect when given alone, but it significantly enhances the effects of L-dopa when the two drugs are given in combination. It has been claimed that selegiline, in addition to its immediate therapeutic effects, may slow the progression of Parkinson's disease, possibly by an antioxidant effect independent of its MAO-inhibitory action. (This is based on the experimental finding that selegiline can block the DA cell death caused by MPTP.) To date, however, clinical trials have not provided unambiguous support for this claim.

Selegiline is rapidly absorbed from the gastrointestinal tract and widely distributed into the tissues. The elimination $t^{1/2}$ is only about 10 minutes, but the action of selegiline is much longer because it binds irreversibly to MAO-B in the striatum, hippocampus, thalamus, and substantia nigra. In the liver, it is biotransformed by the cytochrome P450 system to yield three metabolites: N-desmethylselegiline (which is also an irreversible inhibitor of MAO-B) and minor amounts of amphetamine and methamphetamine (which have DA-releasing action of their own). Therefore it is possible that the metabolites contribute to the therapeutic effect of selegiline. The metabolites are excreted mainly in the urine.

Anticholinergics (Muscarinic Blockers)

An alternate way to correct the DA/ACh imbalance in Parkinson's disease is to lower ACh activity. This can be achieved with muscarinic blockers (see Chapter 15), atropine-like drugs such as **benztropine** (Cogentin) and **trihexyphenidyl** (Artane) (Fig. 21-4). Anticholinergic therapy was actually the *first* pharmacological treatment for Parkinson's disease, having been used (without theoretical basis) for more than a century. The muscarinic blockers, however, are less effective than L-dopa, and they produce unpleasant side effects, including blurred vision, dryness of the mouth, constipation, urinary retention, and ataxia (see Chapter 15). Since the introduction of L-dopa, anticholinergics have been relegated to secondary status. However, they may be useful as supplementary agents. Since they work by a different mechanism than L-dopa, combination with L-dopa will increase the maximum therapeutic effect obtained.

Therapeutic Approaches

The drugs available for Parkinson's disease may be administered in a number of different ways. In each case, L-dopa is the major drug, and the other agents are used as adjuncts. One approach is to start with muscarinic blockers when the syndrome is mild and to add L-dopa and finally carbidopa as the syndrome worsens. Other physicians prefer to use L-dopa from the start. Amantadine may be administered for short periods to help the patient over "flare-ups," and dopamine receptor agonists or selegiline may be used as adjunct therapy.

Whatever the approach, a crucial aspect of therapy is to balance the therapeutic effects of L-dopa against its side effects (e.g., nausea). A good plan is to start with a low initial dose of L-dopa and to increase the level gradually as tolerance develops to the early side effects of the drug.

Prognosis for Drug Therapy

While impressive results can be achieved in the short term, the long-term prognosis for control of Parkinson's disease is still not good. Studies suggest that the average patient obtains relief for up to 5 years and then reverts to pretreatment conditions, perhaps because of the continued loss of cells in the substantia nigra. Since the disease often occurs late in life, the addition of 5 "good" years may be highly significant. Nevertheless, the present drugs are far from ideal, and the search for new ones continues.

HUNTINGTON'S CHOREA

Clinical Syndrome

Huntington's chorea occurs with a frequency of one in 10,000 people. The predominant symptom is not akinesia but hyperkinesia. The patient makes uncontrolled, repetitive movements, which get worse during excitement and cease only during sleep. Since the movements are well coordinated and *appear* to be voluntary, they give a dance-like impression (hence the name "chorea"). A separate, unrelated feature is the development of mental deterioration, which progresses to outright dementia. Huntington's chorea is an inherited disorder, transmitted by an autosomal dominant gene. Its onset is gradual, occurring in early middle age (age 30–50).

Neuropathology

Examination of the brains of Huntington's chorea patients reveals widespread alterations, including degeneration of the neocortex and of the caudate-putamen. The caudate-putamen is drastically affected, often being reduced to less than half of its normal mass. The missing neurons are predominantly ACh and GABA neurons. As a result of this degeneration, ACh levels are often low in the patient's caudate-putamen, and GABA levels are *invariably* low. DA levels are normal. The mechanism responsible for the neuron loss is unknown, but one current hypothesis attributes it to a defect in mitochondrial energy metabolism.

Drug Therapy

Barbiturates

The traditional treatment (without theoretical basis) for Huntington's chorea was barbiturate therapy. This simply served to keep the patient quiet.

Phenothiazines and butyrophenones

The antipsychotics are DA-blockers that are usually used in the treatment of schizophrenia (see Chapter 28). More recently, they have also been administered to Huntington's chorea patients, on the premise that if ACh is low, DA must be predominant. In line with expectations, antipsychotics such as **fluphenazine, bromperidol,** and **clozapine** have proven to be successful at suppressing choretic movements, and neuroleptic therapy is now standard. Unfortunately, these agents do nothing to relieve the dementia that accompanies the chorea. This dementia is believed to result from degeneration of structures other than the basal ganglia, perhaps from loss of neurons in the cortex.

New Directions in Research

Acetylcholine enhancers

One approach to therapy has been to attempt to raise ACh levels by dietary choline supplements or by use of physostigmine. So far the results have been equivocal. It seems possible that the GABA neurons normally controlled by the ACh interneurons (Fig. 21-3) have also degenerated. If so, raising ACh levels would not be effective.

γ-Aminobutyric acid agonists

Another approach has been to raise GABA activity by means of GABA-agonist drugs. Several compounds, including imidazole acetic acid and muscimol, have been tried with ambiguous results. Alternatively, benzodiazepines, which enhance the effect of GABA at the GABA$_A$ receptor, have been reported to decrease the choretic movement in a dose-dependent manner, but their long-term therapeutic value is not yet clear.

AMYOTROPHIC LATERAL SCLEROSIS

Amyotrophic lateral sclerosis ("Lou Gehrig's disease") is a degenerative disease characterized by progressive wasting and weakness of skeletal muscles that is eventually fatal because of paralysis of the respiratory muscles. It is believed to be due to excitotoxic damage to upper and lower motor neurons, i.e., cell death caused by massive calcium influx as a result of excessive action of glutamate at postsynaptic receptors. There is some evidence to suggest that the problem is partly due to defective reuptake of glutamate at presynaptic excitatory terminals. No effective treatment for it has been available, but **riluzole** has recently been approved for this purpose.

Riluzole (2-amino-6-trifluoromethoxybenzothiazole; Rilutek) is believed to inhibit presynaptic release of glutamate, possibly by blocking voltage-activated sodium channels. Recent controlled studies have indicated that riluzole produces a dose-depen-

dent prolongation of the mean survival time of patients with this disease, but the effect is of relatively short duration (less than 18 months). However, the drug is well tolerated; the main adverse effects are weakness, dizziness, nausea, and increased serum levels of aminotransferases. Therefore, the drug offers a possibility of some prolongation of life with an acceptably low risk of toxicity.

SUGGESTED READING

Agid Y. Parkinson's disease. Pathophysiology. Lancet 1991; 337:1321–1327.

Albin RL, Young AB, Penney JB. The functional anatomy of basal ganglia disorders. Trend Neurosci 1989; 10:366–375.

Bergman H, Wichmann T, DeLong MR. Reversal of experimental Parkinsonism by lesions of the subthalamic nucleus. Science 1990; 249:1436–1438.

Cedarbaum JM. Clinical pharmacokinetics of anti-parkinsonian drugs. Clin Pharmacokinet 1987; 13:141–178.

Cesura AM, Pletscher A. The new generation of monoamine oxidase inhibitors. Prog Drug Res 1992; 38:171–297.

Chiueh CC, Wu R-M, Mohanakumar KP, et al. In vivo generation of hydroxyl radicals and MPTP-induced dopaminergic toxicity in the basal ganglia. Ann NY Acad Sci 1994; 738:25–36.

Gerlach M, Youdim MB, Riederer P. Is selegiline neuroprotective in Parkinson's disease? J Neural Transm 1994; 41(Suppl):177–188.

Heinonen EH, Lammintausta R. A review of the pharmacology of selegiline. Acta Neurol Scand 1991; 136(Suppl):44–59.

Juncos JL. Levodopa: pharmacology, pharmacokinetics and pharmacodynamics. Neurol Clin 1992; 10(2):487–509.

Kopin IJ. The pharmacology of Parkinson's disease therapy: an update. Annu Rev Pharmacol Toxicol 1993; 32:467–495.

Lacomblez L, Bensimon G, Leigh PN, et al. Dose-ranging study of riluzole in amyotrophic lateral sclerosis. Amyotrophic Lateral Sclerosis/Riluzole Study Group II. Lancet 1996; 347:1425–1431.

Lewitt PA. Treatment strategies for extension of levodopa effect. Neurol Clin 1992; 10(2):511–526.

Lewitt PA. Levodopa therapeutics: new treatment strategies. Neurology 1993; 43(12 Suppl 6):S31–37.

Montastruc JL, Rascol O, Senard JM. Current status of dopamine agonists in Parkinson's disease management. Drugs 1993; 46(3):384–393.

Pletscher A, DaPrada M. Pharmacotherapy of Parkinson's disease: research from 1960 to 1991. Acta Neurol Scand 1993; 146(Suppl):26–31.

Ransmayr G, Kunig G, Gerstenbrand F. Modern therapy of Parkinson's disease. J Neural Transm 1992; 38(Suppl): 129–140.

Ross RT. Drug-induced parkinsonism and other movement disorders. Can J Neurol Sci 1990; 17:155–162.

Rothstein JD. Excitotoxic mechanisms in the pathogenesis of amyotrophic lateral sclerosis. [Review] Adv Neurol 1995; 68:7–20.

Saint-Cyr JA, Taylor AE, Lang AE. Neuropsychological and psychiatric side effects in the treatment of Parkinson's disease. Neurology 1993; 43(12 Suppl 6):S47–52.

Standaert DG, Young AB. Treatment of central nervous system degenerative disorders. In: Hardman JG, Limbird LE, Molinoff PB, Ruddon RW, Gilman AG, eds. Goodman & Gilman's the pharmacological basis of therapeutics. 9th ed. New York: McGraw-Hill, 1996: 503–520.

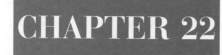

CHAPTER 22

Antiseizure Drugs

W.M. BURNHAM

Michael F., an active youngster, was an avid skier and first in his class at a school in rural Manitoba. At age 12, he started to report "visions" and often seemed moody and confused. He began to do poorly in school. A tentative diagnosis of early onset schizophrenia was made, and he was started on a trial of haloperidol. He began to show tremor and muscular stiffness, and his physician added benztropine to the medication. On this treatment he became somnolent, nonresponsive, and confused, and he was hospitalized for investigation. After 12 days, Michael had a tonic-clonic seizure. His condition was rediagnosed as complex partial epilepsy, and he was started on carbamazepine. At first, he reacted to this with dizziness and diplopia about 2 hours after each dose. He was therefore changed to a slow-release oral preparation and these symptoms disappeared. Carbamazepine has prevented further tonic-clonic attacks, but he still experiences occasional complex partial seizures, in which he has visual or auditory hallucinations similar to those with which his illness began. He has been able to continue with his schooling, but requires very careful monitoring of his drug dosage.

EPILEPSY

Definitions

Epilepsy is a disorder of the central nervous system that is characterized by spontaneous, recurring seizures. It is one of the most common of the CNS disorders, occurring in one of every 100 people. Onset is often in childhood, although it may occur at any time during life. In many patients, epilepsy is a permanent condition.

Seizures are self-sustaining (but self-limiting) episodes of neural hyperactivity. During a seizure, the neurons of the brain cease their normal activities and begin to fire in massive, synchronized bursts. Such synchronized activity produces characteristic "spike" or "spike and wave" patterns in the electroencephalogram (EEG) (Fig. 22-1). After a few seconds or minutes, the inhibitory mechanisms of the brain regain control, the seizure stops, and the person returns to normal.

Seizures by themselves do not equal epilepsy. Every brain contains the circuitry necessary to produce seizures, and every brain will do so if subjected to the proper stimuli, such as electric current or convulsant drugs. The essence of epilepsy is a **chronic low seizure threshold,** which leads to the production of **spontaneous attacks.**

Causes

Pathology versus biochemistry

In some cases of epilepsy, low seizure threshold is associated with some sort of obvious pathology (e.g.,

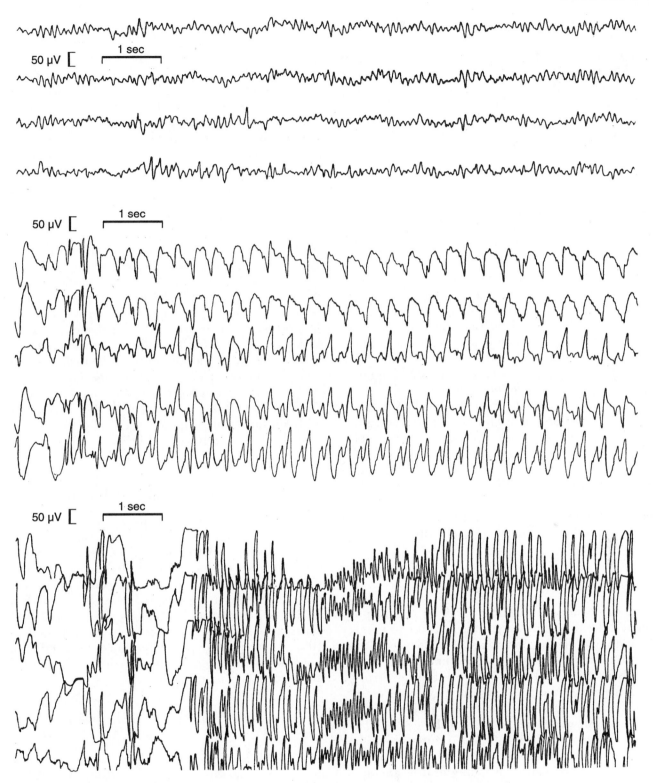

Figure 22-1. EEG patterns during seizures. Top: Normal during seizure-free interval. Middle: 3/sec spike and wave (absence). Bottom: "Spikes" (tonic-clonic).

an infection; a tumor; a scar due to a wound, stroke, or birth injury). In other cases, the brain of an epileptic patient appears to be entirely normal. This suggests that the basic problem in epilepsy may be biochemical in nature—perhaps a subtle mismatch between excitatory and inhibitory transmitters. Such a mismatch might be caused by structural pathology in some patients and by genetic factors in others.

Biochemical hypotheses

Over the years, there have been a number of hypotheses concerning the biochemical flaw in epilepsy. Currently, the most popular hypotheses relate to the amino acid transmitters GABA and glutamate. Normal brain function depends upon a balance of excitation and inhibition. If excitation exceeds inhibition, brain tissue becomes hyperexcitable (= low seizure threshold). If the imbalance is sufficiently large, a seizure occurs. Researchers are currently investigating the hypotheses that chronic low threshold results either from too much activity in the excitatory glutamatergic system (the *glutamate hypothesis*) or from too little activity in the inhibitory GABA system (the *GABA hypothesis*). There is pharmacological evidence to support both hypotheses: Drugs that enhance glutamatergic activity cause seizures, as do drugs that decrease GABAergic activity. Currently, researchers are searching for evidence of either too much glutamatergic activity or too little GABAergic activity in human epileptic brain tissue. As yet, neither hypothesis has been conclusively proven.

Seizure Types

There are a number of different types of epileptic seizures. Because of this, some theorists prefer to talk of "the epilepsies" rather than of "epilepsy." It is important to distinguish among the seizure types because they respond differently to antiseizure drugs. The wrong drug may be useless, or may even exacerbate a seizure condition. Four types of seizures commonly seen in adults are described in Table 22-1. The names and characteristics of these seizures should be learned, since misdiagnosis of seizure type is one of the most common causes of failure in drug therapy. In particular, mild complex partial seizures tend to be confused with absence attacks.

In addition to the adult seizure types, there are a number of seizure syndromes seen primarily in childhood. These are not discussed in this chapter.

Status Epilepticus

Very-long-lasting or constantly repeating seizures of any type are called "status epilepticus." This syndrome is rare, but it is life-threatening when the seizures are of the tonic-clonic variety. Tonic-clonic status is a medical emergency that requires immediate treatment in a hospital setting. An ambulance should be called if any tonic-clonic seizure continues for more than 5 minutes.

THERAPY FOR EPILEPSY

Most people with seizures are perfectly normal between attacks, and seizures themselves are usually brief and relatively harmless. The question arises, "Why treat epilepsy?" The answer is that seizures have an impact on human life which is far out of proportion to their medical significance. Seizures look strange, even frightening, and the public reacts badly to them. People with uncontrolled seizures may face the loss of friends, jobs, and housing. In addition, they are not permitted to drive motor vehicles. Drivers' licenses are canceled with the first seizure and reinstated only if the seizures are perfectly controlled. Thus, seizure control becomes a major issue in patients' lives.

Drug Versus Nondrug Therapy

A number of nondrug therapies are available for epilepsy, including diet, biofeedback, vagal stimulation, and surgery. Of these, only surgery has gained widespread acceptance. For selected patients, neurosurgery offers a chance to reduce seizures or eliminate them altogether. It is attempted, however, only when attacks arise from a clear-cut focal area, and only when they are frequent and drug resistant. Less than 10% of the epileptic population meet these criteria. Thus, for most epileptic patients, the major therapy for seizures is drug therapy.

General Principles of Drug Therapy

A large number of drugs suppress seizures (e.g., most hypnotics, sedatives, and anesthetics). A small number of the safest and least toxic are used in therapy. These are called antiseizure drugs or, more commonly, anticonvulsants. (Anticonvulsant is not an ideal term, since many seizures do not involve convulsions.) Before individual drugs are discussed, a number of general statements can be made about

Table 22-1 Common Seizure Types*

Generalized (appears to involve the whole brain from the outset):

Absence ("petit mal")	Attack	Brief period of unconsciousness; patient stares blankly, eyelids may flutter
	Duration	<30 seconds
	EEG	3/second spike and wave, whole brain
Tonic-clonic ("grand mal")	Attack	Unconsciousness with dramatic tonic-clonic convulsions; may be preceded by an aura;† may involve an "epileptic cry," profuse salivation, tongue-biting, and incontinence
	Duration	<5 minutes
	EEG	Constant spiking, whole brain

Partial (at least initially, involves only part of the brain):

Simple partial ("focal cortical")	Attack	Sensory, motor, or perceptual/emotional signs; patient is conscious (will respond to questions)
	Duration	Varies
	EEG	Localized spiking in a neocortical or limbic area
Complex partial ("psychomotor", "temporal lobe")	Attack	Patient is out of contact with the environment (will not respond to questions) and may perform automatic movements ("automatisms"); no subsequent memory of the attack; often follows a simple partial attack of temporal-lobe origin, e.g., an olfactory aura,† a perceptual aura† (déjà vu, distortion of perspective), or an emotional aura†
	Duration	Varies
	EEG	Spiking in both temporal lobes

*Traditional names in parentheses.
†Simple partial seizures may generalize to produce complex partial or tonic-clonic attacks. The simple partial seizure is then called an "aura."

these drugs, their mechanisms of action, and the way in which they are used.

Characteristics of antiseizure drugs

- Antiseizure drugs do not cure epilepsy; they simply suppress seizures on a temporary basis. Patients must take them once, twice, or three times a day, often for life.
- Antiseizure drugs are fairly safe, but most of them can cause rare, life-threatening, non–dose-related adverse drug reactions (ADRs), such as liver toxicity or suppression of bone marrow. These rare ADRs, which probably relate to genetic abnormalities in the patient, usually occur within the first few months of therapy. All patients should be closely monitored during this period.
- Most antiseizure drugs also cause dose-related ADRs, such as stomach upsets and/or, at higher doses, sedation. Sedation is a particular problem with the older drugs, which are chemically relat-

ed to the barbiturates. Thus, the antiseizure drugs are often perceived as unpleasant to take. Compliance is a problem; abuse is not.

Mechanisms of antiseizure drug action

In the past decade, we have begun to understand the mechanisms of action of the antiseizure drugs. Three major mechanisms are now proposed:

Drugs that bind to the voltage-dependent sodium channel. Three important antiseizure drugs—phenytoin, carbamazepine, and lamotrigine—are believed to bind to the voltage-dependent sodium channel which initiates neuronal action potentials. Each time the neuron fires, the sodium channel cycles through its "active," "inactive," and "resting" states. It is believed that these three drugs hold the channel a little longer in its inactive state. This means that the neuron can fire at moderate rates (e.g., those involved in thinking) but not at very rapid rates (those involved in seizures).

Drugs that enhance activity in the GABA$_A$ system. The barbiturates, the benzodiazepines, valproate, and vigabatrin are thought to increase activation in the GABA$_A$ receptor system. This enhances GABA$_A$-mediated Cl$^-$ influx, which stabilizes the membrane near its resting potential and results in decreased neuronal excitability (see Chapter 27).

Drugs that bind to T-type voltage-dependent calcium channels. Two drugs active against absence seizures—trimethadione and ethosuximide—are thought to bind to T-type voltage-dependent calcium channels. These channels are particularly important in the thalamus, where they are thought to contribute to the genesis of absence attacks. Trimethadione and ethosuximide decrease activity in T-type calcium channels.

Principles of clinical therapy

Whom to treat. Before starting therapy, it is important to rule out pseudo-seizures (not uncommon), poisoning, or active pathology. If active pathology is present (e.g., a growing tumor, an infection), attention should be directed primarily to treatment of the pathology, not the seizures. Also, before initiating therapy, it is important to make sure that the seizure problem is chronic. Occasionally people have a single seizure that is never repeated.

Choice of drug. Before therapy is started, the type of seizure must be carefully established. Different seizure types require different drugs.

Monotherapy, not polypharmacy. Treatment is initiated with a single drug. If the first drug is not effective, another single drug is tried. Eventually, if the seizures are drug resistant, polypharmacy is attempted. (Note: The recent advent of new compounds with few side effects or drug interactions has reawakened an interest in "rational" polypharmacy.)

Drug interactions. Antiseizure drugs interact with each other and also with the drugs used for a variety of other disorders. These interactions, which tend to be pharmacokinetic involving increases or decreases in blood levels, are too numerous to discuss. (Some of them are discussed in Chapter 64.) A general rule of thumb is that valproate tends to increase blood levels of other drugs by inhibiting

hepatic enzymes, while phenobarbital, phenytoin, and carbamazepine tend to decrease blood levels of other drugs by inducing hepatic enzymes. Several of the antiseizure drugs, including phenytoin and carbamazepine, decrease the blood levels (and effectiveness) of oral contraceptive drugs by inducing enzymes of the cytochrome P450 system in the liver.

Use of blood levels to regulate therapy. Therapeutic blood concentrations are now known for all of the older antiseizure drugs (see Table 22-3), and the monitoring of anticonvulsant blood concentrations has become standard practice. At the start of therapy, or whenever dosage is adjusted, blood samples are taken to determine whether concentrations are in the therapeutic range. The same blood samples are used to check for the occurrence of adverse drug reactions (ADRs) involving liver, kidney, or blood toxicity.

Compliance. Noncompliance is an important cause of failure in antiseizure drug therapy (see Chapter 62). It is typically revealed by blood samples, which indicate that the patient is not taking the medication. Compliance can be improved by programs that provide the patient with information about seizure disorders and the ways in which antiseizure drugs control them.

Withdrawal of drugs. If a patient has no seizures or EEG abnormalities for several years, the drugs may be slowly withdrawn. Children outgrow a number of types of childhood seizure (e.g., absence seizures), and even adults occasionally outgrow their attacks. Note: Except in hospital, antiseizure drugs should never be withdrawn quickly. Rebound seizures, and even status epilepticus, may occur. This is particularly true with the barbiturates (phenobarbital) and the benzodiazepines (clonazepam, clobazam).

Drug therapy during pregnancy. Most women taking antiseizure drugs remain well controlled during pregnancy. There is a slightly increased incidence of fetal malformations in the children of epileptic mothers, however, and this relates in part to the drugs they take. In the general population, the incidence of serious fetal malformations is about 2%. In women with seizures, it is slightly higher at about 3%. It remains at 3% in women taking only one antiseizure drug, but rises to 5% in women taking two antiseizure drugs, to 10% in women taking three, and to over 20% in women taking four antiseizure drugs.

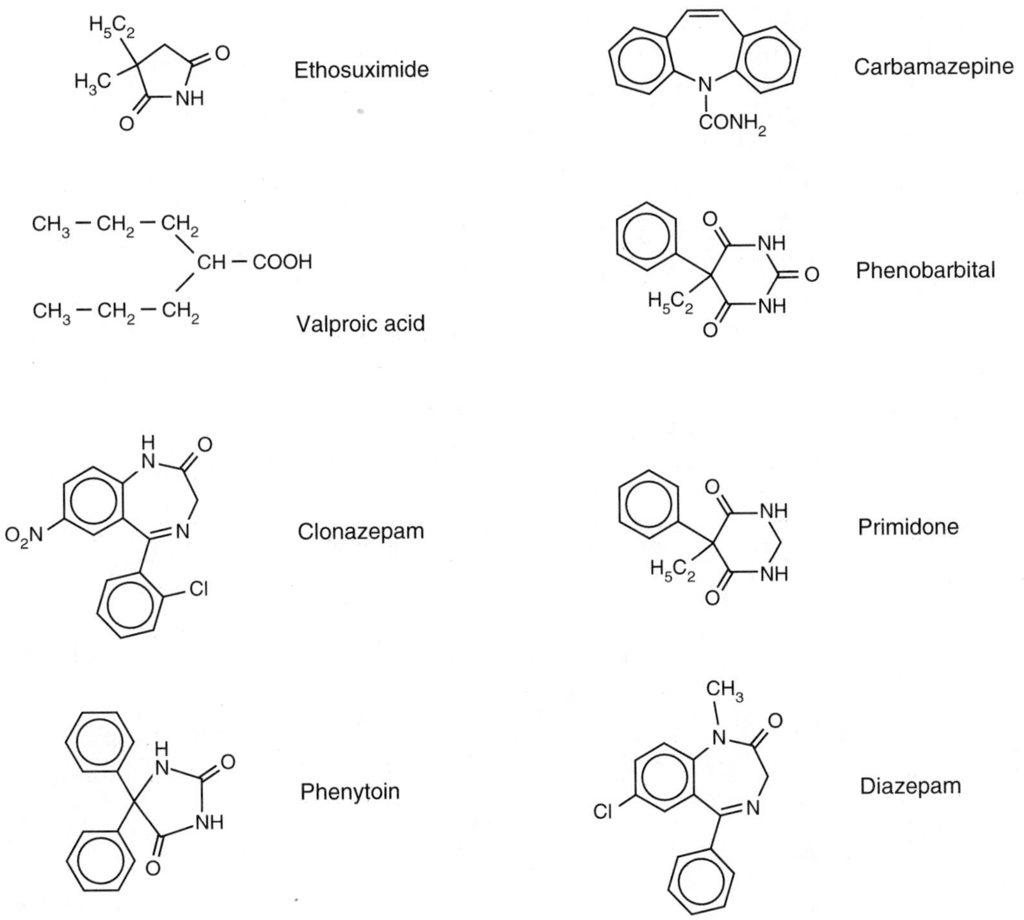

Figure 22-2. Structural formulae of antiseizure drugs.

SPECIFIC DRUGS

The drugs most commonly used in North America are discussed below, grouped in terms of their therapeutic applications. Their chemical structures (Fig. 22-2) and main side effects are summarized in Table 22-2, and their pharmacokinetic features in Table 22-3. Discussions of the less common agents, such as the older succinimides and hydantoins, may be found in medical handbooks.

Drugs Used Only for Absence Seizures

Ethosuximide

Ethosuximide (Zarontin) is the current drug of choice for absence seizures. It has replaced trimethadione (Tridione), a more toxic and less effective drug that has been withdrawn from the market. Ethosuximide is used *only* in the treatment of absence epilepsy. It is not effective against tonic-clonic or partial seizures.

Mechanism of action (probable). Ethosuximide binds to and inhibits the T-type voltage-dependent calcium channel.

Advantages. Ethosuximide is relatively effective, safe, and nonsedating. It has a long half-life, providing sustained control with a single daily dose.

Disadvantages. Ethosuximide may cause gastrointestinal disturbances, fatigue, photophobia, and other side effects. Less common but more serious adverse effects include liver and kidney damage, lupus erythematosus, and blood dyscrasias.

Table 22-2 Commonly Used Antiseizure Drugs

Name (Trade Name)	Chemical Structure (see also Fig. 22-2)	Common Side Effects (at Therapeutic Blood Levels)
Drugs for absence seizures:		
Ethosuximide (Zarontin)	Resembles phenobarbital	GI disturbances, sedation, photophobia
Drugs for tonic-clonic and partial seizures:		
Carbamazepine (Tegretol)	Resembles tricyclic anti-depressants	Diplopia, dizziness, GI disturbances, sedation, transient mild depression of leukocyte count
Gabapentin (Neurontin)	Resembles GABA	Sedation
Phenobarbital (Luminal)	A barbiturate	Sedation, paradoxical excitement in children (abrupt withdrawal is dangerous)
Phenytoin (Dilantin, others)	Resembles phenobarbital	GI disturbances, hirsutism, gingival hyperplasia, acne, sedation (at toxic doses: nystagmus, ataxia)
Primidone (Mysoline)	Resembles phenobarbital	Sedation, psychiatric disturbances, decreased libido
Vigabatrin (Sabril)	Resembles GABA	GI disturbances, sedation, transient psychotic states
Broad-spectrum drugs:		
Clonazepam (Rivotril)	A benzodiazepine	Sedation, personality change, and/or paradoxical excitement in children (abrupt withdrawal is dangerous)
Clobazam (Frisium)	A benzodiazepine	Similar to clonazepam (though milder)
Lamotrigine (Lamictal)	Novel	GI upsets, sedation, rash
Valproate (Depakene)	Branched-chain fatty acid	Tremor, weight gain, GI disturbances, bruising, hair loss
Drugs for status epilepticus:		
Diazepam (Valium) 10–20 mg i.v., at 2 mg/min	A benzodiazepine	Not used in chronic therapy
Lorazepam (Ativan)	A benzodiazepine	Not used in chronic therapy

Drugs Used Only for Tonic-Clonic and Partial Attacks

Phenytoin

Phenytoin (Dilantin) is an older drug (formerly called diphenylhydantoin) that is still widely used for tonic-clonic and partial attacks. It is not effective against absence attacks. Phenytoin replaced phenobarbital as drug of choice just before World War II because it was less sedating. It was for many years the mainstay of antiseizure therapy.

Mechanism of action. Phenytoin binds to and inhibits the voltage-dependent sodium channel, thus preventing the high-frequency discharge typical of seizure activity.

Advantages. Phenytoin has a long half-life and is relatively nonsedating.

Table 22-3 Pharmacokinetic Parameters of Commonly Used Antiseizure Drugs

Drug	Absorption	Half-Life (hours)	Availability (oral) (%)	Urinary Excretion (%)	Bound in Plasma (%)	Volume of Distribution (L/kg)	Effective Concentration in Plasma
For absence seizures:							
Ethosuximide	Rapid	45 ± 8	?	25 ± 15	0	0.72 ± 0.16	40–100 µg/mL
For tonic-clonic and partial seizures:							
Carbamazepine	Slow–moderate	15 ± 5	>70	<1	74 ± 3	1.4 ± 0.4	4–10 µg/mL
Gabapentin	Rapid	6.5 ± 1.0	60	100	0	0.80 ± 0.09	>2 µg/mL
Phenobarbital	Slow–moderate	99 ± 18	100 ± 11	24 ± 5	51 ± 3	0.54 ± 0.03	10–25 µg/mL
Phenytoin	Slow	6–24	90 ± 3	2 ± 8	89 ± 23	0.64 ± 0.04	>10 µg/mL
Primidone	Slow–moderate	15 ± 4	92 ± 18	46 ± 16	19	0.69 ± 0.18	8–12 µg/mL
Vigabatrin	Rapid	4–9	?	60–70	0	0.8	?
Broad-spectrum drugs:							
Valproic acid	Rapid	14–30	100 ± 10	1.8 ± 2.4	93 ± 1	0.22 ± 0.07	30–100 µg/mL
Clobazam	Rapid	10–30	100	<1	85	"Large"	50–300 ng/mL
Clonazepam	Rapid	23 ± 5	98 ± 31	<1	86 ± 0.5	3.2 ± 1.1	5–70 ng/mL
Lamotrigine	Rapid	12–60	98	70	50	1.1–1.3	1.6 ± 1.3 µg/mL

Disadvantages. Phenytoin has a number of annoying side effects, which sometimes occur at therapeutic dose levels. These include gastrointestinal disturbances, acne, gingival hyperplasia (excess growth of gum tissue, seen in over 30% of patients), and hirsutism (excess growth of body hair). Sedation is the most frequent nervous system side effect. At toxic doses, ataxia, nystagmus, and impaired motor coordination may occur. A rare non–dose-related ADR is the "anticonvulsant hypersensitivity syndrome," often indicated by a rash and fever. This ADR necessitates immediate withdrawal of the drug.

Phenytoin also has an unusual metabolism, which complicates dosing. Somewhere within the therapeutic concentration range (10–20 µg/mL, 40–80 µmoles/L), phenytoin tends to saturate the degradative enzymes in the liver. When this happens, phenytoin switches from a normal first-order metabolism to a "pseudo–zero-order" metabolism, which means that elimination begins to take place much more slowly. The physician who has been gradually raising dose levels may find that the patient suddenly begins to show toxic effects. Phenytoin toxicity (usually nystagmus and ataxia) occasionally presents in idiosyncratic forms that are hard to recognize (pseudo-psychosis, increased seizure frequency). Monitoring of blood levels is particularly important, therefore, when phenytoin dosage is being adjusted.

Phenytoin is a substrate for the hepatic cytochrome P450 system, for which it can also act as an inhibitor acutely and an inducer during chronic administration. Therefore it can interact with many other drugs by reciprocal effects on biotransformation and consequent effects on the plasma levels and pharmacological activities, both of phenytoin and of the other drugs involved (see Chapters 4 and 64).

Carbamazepine

Carbamazepine (Tegretol), which has fewer side effects than phenytoin, is now widely used for the treatment of tonic-clonic and partial seizures. It is not effective against absence attacks. The compound is also available in a slow-release formulation (Tegretol CR).

Mechanism of action. Carbamazepine binds to and inhibits the voltage-dependent sodium channel.

Advantages. Carbamazepine is as effective as phenytoin, and even less sedating for most patients.

It does not cause acne, gingival hyperplasia, or hirsutism.

Disadvantages. Gastrointestinal disturbances and double vision sometimes occur at therapeutic dose levels. Occasionally patients show sedation. A mild depression in leukocyte count is often seen early in treatment, but this usually disappears without discontinuation of therapy. Rare non–dose-related ADRs (anticonvulsant hypersensitivity syndrome, severe anemias) occasionally occur and do require withdrawal of the drug. The half-life of carbamazepine varies from 35 hours (at the start of therapy) to 10–12 hours (after prolonged therapy) due to autoinduction of liver enzymes. It is therefore wise to start patients on a low dose and gradually increase the dose as the liver enzymes are induced. After induction has occurred, the short half-life of carbamazepine may make it hard to maintain stable blood levels. Many patients do better on the new controlled-release formulation.

Phenobarbital

Phenobarbital, introduced in 1911, was the first modern antiseizure drug. It is effective against tonic-clonic and some partial seizures, but not against absence attacks. Recently the use of phenobarbital has declined because of the excessive sedation it causes. It is still used in very young children due to its safety, and in patients who are allergic to the other drugs.

Mechanism of action. Phenobarbital enhances GABA-mediated inhibition by binding to the barbiturate receptor site on the ligand-gated chloride channel associated with the $GABA_A$ receptor (see Chapter 27).

Advantages. Phenobarbital is one of the cheapest and safest anticonvulsants. Its long half-life simplifies dosing.

Disadvantages. Phenobarbital causes serious sedation in many patients at therapeutic dose levels. Its original use, before the discovery of its anticonvulsant effects, was as a daytime sedative. In some patients, particularly the very old or very young, phenobarbital causes "paradoxical excitement." In these cases the patient becomes restless and agitated, rather than calm and sleepy. Like phenytoin, phenobarbital also interacts with many drugs through inhi-

bition or induction of the hepatic cytochrome P450 system.

Primidone

Primidone (Mysoline) is a slight variant of phenobarbital. In the body it is biotransformed into phenobarbital, and most of its therapeutic effects probably depend on this active metabolite.

Mechanism of action. Primarily, primidone converts into phenobarbital.

Advantages. Primidone is long-acting and fairly safe.

Disadvantages. Like phenobarbital, primidone is sedating. For this reason, it has also declined in popularity.

Broad-Spectrum Drugs (Active Against Absence, Tonic-Clonic, and Partial Seizures)

Valproate and the benzodiazepines were first used for the treatment of absence seizures. It was later realized that they were also effective in tonic-clonic and partial seizures. They are also used in several forms of drug-resistant childhood epilepsy. The newly released drug, lamotrigine (below), is also a broad-spectrum agent.

Valproate (valproic acid)

Valproate (Depakene) is used for absence attacks, particularly when they are combined with tonic-clonic attacks. Recently, it has also been used for tonic-clonic seizures, partial seizures, and for drug-resistant childhood seizures. It has now joined phenytoin and carbamazepine as one of the "big three" drugs in antiseizure therapy. A slightly different version of the compound, divalproex sodium (Epival), has similar therapeutic effects and is said to cause less gastrointestinal distress.

Mechanism of action. Valproate enhances GABA-mediated inhibition. The exact mechanism of enhancement is unknown.

Advantages. Valproate is one of the least sedating of the antiseizure drugs. Because of its broad-spectrum activity it can be used for patients with mixed seizure types. Traditionally, these patients were given separate drugs for each type, but valproate alone may be sufficient.

Disadvantages. Valproate has a short half-life, which necessitates two or more doses every day. Side effects are still being discovered. Known side effects include gastrointestinal disturbances (frequent in the early stage of therapy), tremor, hair loss, weight gain, and bruising and bleeding. Hepatitis is a rare, but potentially fatal (especially in very young children), non–dose-related ADR.

Clonazepam

Clonazepam (Rivotril), a benzodiazepine, is effective against a broad spectrum of seizure disorders. Its usefulness, however, is limited by the sedation and ataxia it often causes. It may be used in absence epilepsy, but, because of its side effects, it is often reserved for other, drug-resistant forms of childhood epilepsy. Tolerance to the CNS depressant effects, as well as to the antiseizure effect, may develop when the drug is used chronically to control convulsive seizures.

Mechanism of action. Clonazepam enhances GABA-mediated inhibition by binding to the benzodiazepine receptor site on the ligand-gated chloride channel associated with the $GABA_A$ receptor (see Chapter 27).

Advantages. Clonazepam is safe, has a long half-life, and is *not* associated with prominent gastrointestinal disturbances or life-threatening ADRs.

Disadvantages. Clonazepam causes sedation or personality change (paradoxical excitement) in up to 50% of the patients who take it. In children, the paradoxical excitement may take the form of impatience, rudeness, or overt aggression. Like other benzodiazepines, its CNS depressant effects are enhanced by alcohol, opioids, and a variety of sedative and hypnotic drugs.

Clobazam

Clobazam (Frisium) is also a benzodiazepine, recently introduced in Canada and not yet available in the United States. Most benzodiazepines have a nitrogen atom at positions 1 and 4 (1,4-benzodiazepines), but clobazam is a 1,5-benzodiazepine. This difference is said to maximize its therapeutic antiseizure effects and to minimize its sedative side effects.

In some patients, tolerance to the therapeutic effects develops, often within a year after starting the drug.

Mechanism of action. Clobazam, like clonazepam, enhances GABA-mediated inhibition by binding to the benzodiazepine receptor site on the ligand-gated chloride channel associated with the $GABA_A$ receptor.

Advantages. Clobazam has the same advantages as clonazepam, and is believed to have fewer side effects. Like clonazepam, it has a fairly long half-life, and it has active metabolites that probably prolong its duration of action.

Disadvantages. Though side effects may be less than with clonazepam, some patients taking clobazam clearly show sedation or personality changes. Its CNS depressant effects, like those of clonazepam, are also potentiated by alcohol and other CNS depressants.

New Drugs Recently Introduced in North America

Since 1993, three new antiseizure drugs have been introduced in North America—vigabatrin, gabapentin, and lamotrigine. As a group, these compounds are fairly broad-spectrum, have relatively mild side effects, and are associated with few drug interactions. Blood-level testing is not yet available.

The final role of these new compounds in antiseizure therapy is not yet clear. It is already known that they are not "wonder drugs" that could replace all of our present compounds. It is also known, however, that they are effective in some patients whose seizures have long resisted control, including patients with complex partial seizures and with certain types of drug-resistant childhood epilepsy. At present, physicians are using the new compounds cautiously, often as adjunct medications in poorly controlled patients. If a patient is well controlled on the standard drugs, there is no particular need to change over to the newer compounds. If a patient is poorly controlled on the standard drugs, however, the newer compounds should certainly be tried.

Vigabatrin

Vigabatrin (Sabril) has recently been introduced into North America after having been used in Europe for some years. It is effective against tonic-clonic and partial seizures plus several types of drug-resistant childhood seizures. The drug was formerly known as γ-vinyl-GABA.

Mechanism of action. Vigabatrin enhances GABAergic activity by covalently binding to, and irreversibly inactivating, the catabolic enzyme for GABA, GABA transaminase.

Advantages. Vigabatrin has relatively mild side effects and is not associated with any life-threatening ADRs. It is unlikely to be involved in drug interactions. It is effective in some cases of drug-resistant epilepsy in which all other drugs have failed, and it may eventually find a major use in the control of complex partial attacks. It has a short half-life, but this is not important, since it binds covalently to an enzyme. When drugs bind covalently, their therapeutic effects continue after the blood levels have declined.

Disadvantages. Vigabatrin is expensive. It sometimes causes stomach upsets and sedation. Up to 6% of patients are reported to experience transient psychotic episodes, which clear when the drug is withdrawn.

Gabapentin

Gabapentin (Neurontin) was originally designed to act as an agonist at the $GABA_A$ receptor. It has proved not to be a $GABA_A$ agonist, but it is still a useful antiseizure drug, effective against tonic-clonic and partial seizures.

Mechanism of action. The mechanism of action of gabapentin is not yet clear.

Advantages. Gabapentin has relatively mild side effects (below) and is not associated with any life-threatening ADRs. It has *no* known drug interactions. Because of its mild side effects and lack of drug interactions, gabapentin is an ideal "add on" drug. It may eventually find an important role in adjunct therapy.

Disadvantages. Gabapentin is expensive. Some patients experience somnolence, dizziness, ataxia, and fatigue; these side effects are dose-related.

Lamotrigine

Lamotrigine (Lamictal) is a true broad-spectrum drug, effective against absence seizures, tonic-clonic seizures, and partial seizures. It has succeeded in some cases of drug-resistant epilepsy where all other drugs have failed.

Mechanism of action. Lamotrigine, like phenytoin and carbamazepine, is believed to bind to the voltage-dependent sodium channel. It must have other actions as well, since drugs that act on the sodium channel do not usually antagonize absence seizures.

Advantages. Lamotrigine has a broad spectrum of action, has mild side effects, and is not associated with any life-threatening ADRs. It has few known drug interactions.

Disadvantages. Lamotrigine is expensive and has a short half-life. A rash has been reported in up to 6% of patients. This occurs more frequently in children, particularly if they are also taking valproate, and it is less likely to occur if patients are started on low doses that are increased gradually. The rash may abate without discontinuation of the drug.

Drugs for Status Epilepticus

Drugs for status epilepticus are administered intravenously. High doses are used, and it is important that the drugs be infused slowly to avoid bolus effects.

Benzodiazepines

Two benzodiazepines, diazepam (Valium) and lorazepam (Ativan), are the mainstay treatment for all varieties of status epilepticus. Diazepam was the drug of choice for many years. The adult i.v. dose is 10–20 mg, and the infusion rate should not exceed 2 mg/min. If necessary, this dose may be repeated after 20–30 minutes. While diazepam stops status attacks quickly, its effect wears off in time, possibly because of drug redistribution in the body, and status may restart. To prevent this, the patient may be given a secondary i.v. infusion of phenytoin or phenobarbital. Alternatively, lorazepam may be used instead of diazepam. Lorazepam has a slower onset but a longer duration of action. Because of its long duration, it is preferred by many hospitals.

Table 22-4 Success Rate of Antiseizure Drug Therapy (First 2 Years)

Seizure Type	Patients Showing	
	Total Seizure Suppression %	Significant Improvement %
Absence	50	25
Tonic-clonic	60–65	20
Simple partial	Figures unknown—probably like tonic-clonic	
Complex partial	<30	<50

Other drugs

If tonic-clonic status resists the benzodiazepines, i.v. phenytoin or phenobarbital may be tried. If these fail, paraldehyde (i.m.) or lidocaine (i.v.) may be administered. If none of these works, general anesthesia will be required.

PROGNOSIS FOR SEIZURE CONTROL AND QUALITY OF LIFE

First Two Years

Table 22-4 indicates the percentages of seizure suppression that can be achieved early in therapy, assuming proper diagnosis and patient compliance. As indicated, many patients are greatly helped by the antiseizure drugs. These drug-responsive patients are usually well controlled by low doses, and they lead entirely normal lives, experiencing few side effects. Other patients are less responsive to drugs. These drug-resistant patients continue to have some, or many, seizures even when they take high drug doses that are associated with serious side effects. Drug-resistant patients (about 20% of seizure patients, or one in 500 in the general population) find it very hard to live with epilepsy.

Patients with complex partial seizures are especially likely to be drug resistant. This is unfortunate, since complex partial epilepsy is the most common type of epilepsy in adults. Patients with uncontrolled complex partial seizures are frequent candidates for seizure surgery.

Long-Term Therapy

The figures given in Table 22-4 apply only to the first 2 years of therapy. A large-scale study done in the 1960s indicated some tendency for seizures to reappear as time passes.

Summary

Although the present drugs represent a great advance in the therapy of epilepsy, more and better drugs are needed. Most urgently needed are drugs that are effective against complex partial attacks. Agents with fewer side effects would also be welcome. It is possible that new drugs that have been recently introduced may, in part, fill these needs. A long-term goal in therapy is to discover drugs that *cure* epilepsy, rather than simply suppress seizures.

SUGGESTED READING

Brodie MJ, Dichter MA. Antiepileptic drugs. N Engl J Med 1996; 334:168–175.

Macdonald RL, Kelly KM. Mechanisms of action of currently prescribed and newly developed antiepileptic drugs. Epilepsia 1994; 35(Suppl 4):S41–50.

McNamara JO. Drugs effective in the therapy of the epilepsies. In: Hardman JG, Limbird LE, Molinoff PB, Ruddon RW, Gilman AG, eds. Goodman & Gilman's the pharmacological basis of therapeutics. 9th ed. New York: McGraw-Hill, 1996:461–486.

CHAPTER 23

Opioid Analgesics and Antagonists

H. KALANT

CASE HISTORY

A frail 78-year-old woman, looking older than her stated age, was admitted to hospital with a history of severe lower back pain of 3 weeks' duration. Her family physician had made a diagnosis of degenerative arthritis of the lumbar spine and prescribed nonsteroidal anti-inflammatory drugs (NSAIDs) for the pain and diazepam as a muscle relaxant and sedative. The pain persisted, however, and radiological examination revealed a compression fracture of the L-4 vertebra.

On admission, the patient was 5'4" (162 cm) in height and weighed 98 lb (44.5 kg). An order was written for morphine sulfate, 7.5 mg intramuscularly, every 6 hours. The first injection produced a very marked reduction in her pain. However, she felt somewhat nauseated and had no appetite for the meals that were served to her. By the second day on this treatment, she was very drowsy and mentally clouded. Her urine volume fell to 270 mL in 24 hours, and she had no bowel movement. Her color became grayish, and her respiratory rate fell to 5–6/min, with shallow and somewhat irregular breathing.

At this point, an injection of naloxone, 100 μg (0.1 mg), was given, and her breathing and color recovered almost immediately, although her pain also returned. One hour later she was again very drowsy, with depressed respiration. The order for i.m. morphine was cancelled and consideration was given to the initiation of patient-controlled analgesia (PCA) with intravenous morphine, 1–2 mg per injection,

and a maximum permissible delivery of 7 mg in any one hour. Supplementary therapy with oral low-dose NSAIDs was also considered, but was held in reserve while the effect of PCA was assessed.

OPIATES, OPIOIDS, AND NARCOTICS

The opium poppy (*Papaver somniferum*) has been known and used in Asia Minor and southeastern Europe for over 2000 years. Its juice was known to contain an agent that relieved pain (=analgesic), produced sleep or drowsiness (*somniferum* = bringing sleep), relieved diarrhea, and in low doses produced a blissful or euphoric state. Only crude preparations were available for medical use until the isolation and purification of morphine by Sertürner in 1805. Other alkaloids with similar properties were isolated from crude opium over the next decades, and by the mid-19th century these pure compounds (opiates) began to replace opium in medical use. Morphine was named after Morpheus, the Greek god of sleep. The Greek word *narkē* means stupor. Therefore these compounds, which produced drowsiness, analgesia, and a dreamy stuporous state, were called **narcotics.**

In legal terminology, however, a narcotic is any drug included under the Harrison Act in the United States, the Narcotic Control Act in Canada, or equivalent legislation in other countries. Most of these drugs are morphine-like analgesics or synthetic substitutes. However, these Acts generally also cover cocaine and cannabis, which have pharmacological properties quite different from those of the opiate analgesics (see Chapter 30). Therefore the term "narcotic" is no longer used in pharmacology.

In recent years, the term "opioid" was introduced to include not only the opiates with morphine-like action but also substances that are not derived from opium (hence, are not "opiates") and do not have a morphine-like chemical structure but do have morphine-like pharmacological properties. The whole group, including the opiates, is now known as **opioid analgesics**. In 1973, stereospecific receptors for opioid drugs were proven to exist in the central nervous system. Since it seemed improbable that the animal brain would have evolved receptors for plant alkaloids to which it was never exposed, researchers postulated that these receptors must normally take up endogenous material produced in the brain itself. In 1975, the first such materials were isolated and were found to be short peptides with morphine-like properties, which were named **enkephalins**. Soon afterward, longer peptides with similar properties (**endorphins, dynorphin**) were discovered. These are known collectively as **endogenous opioids**.

OPIUM ALKALOIDS

Opium is the dry residue of juice from the seedpod of *Papaver somniferum*. It contains a mixture of alkaloids of two main types (Fig. 23-1).

Benzylisoquinoline Alkaloids

The main example is **papaverine**. This is a smooth muscle depressant that causes relaxation of peripheral arterioles (and therefore lowers blood pressure), coronary arteries, and gastrointestinal and other smooth muscle and has a direct quinidine-like effect on the myocardium. Although it is an opiate (i.e., derived from opium), it has no analgesic effect and does not bind to opioid receptors. Papaverine HCl is marketed for the relief of cerebral and peripheral ischemia due to arterial spasm, but its therapeutic value in these conditions has been questioned.

Phenanthrene Alkaloids

These are mainly **morphine, codeine,** and **thebaine**. Morphine is a potent analgesic, but it also has strong excitatory effects in some tissues and some species; **thebaine** has predominantly excitatory rather than analgesic effects and can cause convulsions.

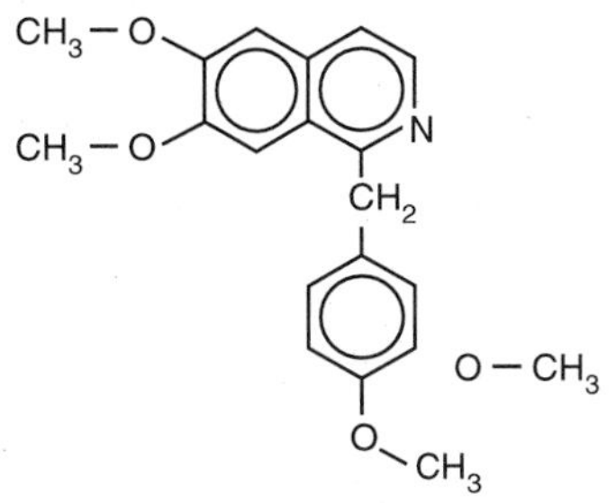

Papaverine - *a benzylisoquinoline alkaloid*

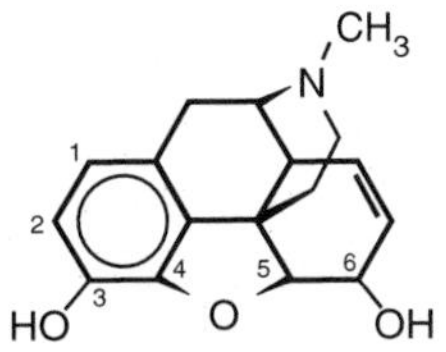

Morphine - *a phenanthrene alkaloid*

Figure 23-1. Structural formulae of the two major classes of opium alkaloid. For codeine, CH_3O- replaces $HO-$ at C-3 of morphine. Thebaine has CH_3O- groups at both C-3 and C-6 of morphine. Heroin is the 3,6-diacetate of morphine.

There are **asymmetric C atoms** in the opiates. Hence, all opiates can exist in either the levo-form (*l-* or levorotatory form) or the dextro-form (*d-* or dextrorotatory form).

All morphine synthesized by opium poppy enzymes is the levorotatory or (−) isomer. The dextro- or (+) isomers of the opiates have no analgesic action, except for d-propoxyphene, a weak synthetic codeine-like analgesic.

PHARMACOLOGICAL ACTIONS OF OPIOIDS

Opioids have a large number of actions, both centrally and peripherally. Although most opioids produce analgesia, they may differ a great deal in their other effects. Morphine, for example, produces euphoria in many people, whereas the opioid ketocyclazocine produces marked dysphoria. The discovery of different classes of opioid receptor has helped to explain this dissociation of effects and the different spectra of effects shown by some of the newer synthetic opioids.

Opioid Receptors and Endogenous Opioids

Properties of opioid–receptor binding

Binding studies (see Chapter 9) have revealed the following properties of the opioid–receptor binding process:

1. Structural specificity, such that small modifications of the drug molecule cause large changes in drug binding (and in drug effect in vivo).
2. Stereospecificity; the $l(-)$ isomer has much higher binding affinity than the $d(+)$ isomer; and only the $l(-)$ isomer is active as an analgesic (with the exception of d-propoxyphene).
3. Competition between agonists and antagonists; drugs of partially similar structure, but lacking certain molecular features essential for opioid action, can bind to the receptor and block the binding of agonists such as morphine. Antagonists must also be $l(-)$ isomers; $d(+)$ isomers do not bind to the receptor.
4. Reversibility; bound drug can be displaced from the receptors by an excess of other molecules with binding ability.
5. A good correlation between the affinity of binding to the receptors and the potency of agonist or antagonist effects in vivo or on isolated tissues (Fig. 23-2).

Subtypes of opioid receptors and ligands

The major clinical use of opioids is in the relief of pain, but all of them have numerous other effects. When they are administered in doses that produce the same degree of analgesia (equianalgesic doses), the drugs differ with respect to the relative degrees of other effects that they produce. This observation led to the current concept of multiple receptor types mediating different effects of the opioids (Table 23-1). The opioids could then be classified according to their relative affinities at the different types of receptor. None of the drugs appear to have absolute specificity for a single receptor type; rather, each drug has a major affinity for one type, with lesser degrees of affinity for the other types (Table 23-2).

Three major classes of opioid receptor are recognized, which have different patterns of affinity for the various opioid agonists and antagonists. The prototypic agonist at the μ-receptor is morphine, at the κ-receptor it is ketocyclazocine, and for the δ-receptor it is the enkephalins. However, the synthesis of highly selective opioid agonists and antagonists has permitted the recognition of subtypes with differ-

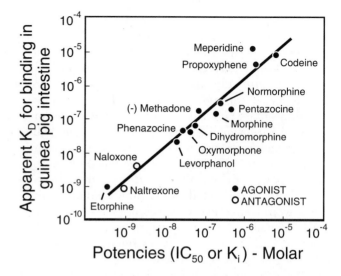

Figure 23-2. Correlation of pharmacological potencies of opiate agonists and antagonists with their affinities for receptor binding in the guinea pig intestine. Potencies refer to IC_{50} for inhibition of electrically induced contraction of isolated gut by agonists, or to K_i for inhibition of opioid activity by antagonists. These compounds show the same rank order of potencies for inhibition of contraction of the isolated gut as for in vivo analgesia.

ent affinities for various ligands. At present, seven subtypes of opioid receptor have been characterized: μ_1 and μ_2; κ_1, κ_2, and κ_3; and δ_1 and δ_2. A fourth class was formerly believed to exist, the σ-receptor, but this is no longer considered to be an opioid receptor.

Of the various types mentioned above, a μ-, a δ-, and κ_1- and κ_2-receptors have been cloned from the corresponding cDNAs and their amino acid structures have been determined. They have the structure characteristic of G protein–linked receptors, with seven membrane-spanning regions. These transmembrane regions and the intracellular loops connecting them are closely similar in the different opioid receptors, but the extracellular connecting loops and the –NH$_2$ and –COOH terminals are different in the different types and presumably account for the different ligand affinities and effects. The receptors are linked through G proteins to their second messengers and act to inhibit adenylyl cyclase activity, decrease voltage-gated Ca^{2+} currents, and increase a receptor-gated K^+ current. The end result is hyperpolarization of the neuron bearing the receptor, with a reduction in its activity and its transmitter release.

Opioid ligands can act at these receptors in four different ways:

- If they activate the receptor and its linked response system, they are **agonists.**

Table 23-1 Types of Opioid Receptors, Their Prototypic Ligands, and Their Most Important Physiological Effects

Receptor Type	Ligands		Major Effects
	Endogenous	*Exogenous*	
Mu			
μ_1	β-Endorphin	Morphine	Supraspinal analgesia
		Hydromorphone	Euphoria
		Etonitazene	Prolactin release
			Miosis
μ_2	β-Endorphin	Morphine	Spinal analgesia
	(dynorphin?)		Inhibition of intestinal motility
			Respiratory depression
Kappa			
κ_1	Dynorphin	Ethylketocyclazocine	Hypothermia?
		Pentazocine	Miosis (weak)
		Tifluadom	Sedation
			Spinal analgesia
κ_2 and κ_3		Nalorphine	Supraspinal analgesia
		Ethylketocyclazocine	Dysphoria
		Bremazocine	Hallucinations
Delta			
δ_1	met-Enkephalin	Etorphine	Spinal analgesia
		D-Pen^2-D-Pen^5-enkephalin	Inhibition of smooth muscle
δ_2		D-Ala^2-Glu^4-deltorphin	Supraspinal analgesia
		D-Ser^2,Leu^5-enkephalin-Thr^6	

- If they occupy the receptor but do not activate it, they are **antagonists,** and can block the activity of agonists.
- If they activate the receptor incompletely, producing a lower maximum response, they are **partial agonists.**
- If they have substantial affinity for more than one receptor type, and act as an agonist at one type and as an antagonist at another, they are **mixed agonist/antagonists.**

Types of endogenous opioid peptides

A possible explanation for the lack of strict specificity of the opiates and synthetic opioids was that the different receptor types had evolved as binding sites for various endogenous ligands, not for exogenous drugs. To date, three groups of peptides have been discovered in the central nervous system, with properties similar to those of the opioid analgesics.

Endorphins are large peptides that are split off enzymatically from known protein hormones of the pituitary and hypothalamus. For example, β-endorphin consists of amino acids 61–91 of β-lipotropin (β-LPH).

Enkephalins are pentapeptides, and met-enkephalin (Tyr-Gly-Gly-Phe-Met) consists of amino acids 61–65 of β-LPH, i.e., 1 through 5 of β-endorphin (Fig. 23-3). Leu-enkephalin is the same as met-enkephalin except that it has a leucine in place of methionine.

Dynorphin is an intermediate-length peptide (17 amino acids), of which the first five amino acids are the same as those constituting leu-enkephalin.

These peptides are synthesized within the brain itself as large precursor proteins, which contain the opioid peptides and other neuroendocrine peptides as parts of their amino acid sequences. The same precursor may occur at several sites in the brain but be split by different enzymes, thus giving rise to different products at different sites. For example, the precursor protein proopiomelanocortin contains within itself the sequences of eight different peptide hormones or neuromodulators (see Fig. 23-3). How-

Table 23-2 Opioid Receptor Selectivity: Agonist, Partial Agonist, and Antagonist Actions at Different Classes of Opioid Receptor*

Compound	Receptor Types					
	μ_1	μ_2	κ_1	κ_3	δ_1	δ_2
Morphine	++++	+++	+	+	0/+	0/+
Buprenorphine	P		−		−	
Nalorphine	−	−	P	P?	0	0
Nalbuphine	−	−	++	+	−?	
Pentazocine	−/P	−	+(P)	0/+		
Ethylketocyclazocine	+	+	+++	++	+	
met-Enkephalin	+	+	0	0	+++	+++
Naloxone	−−−	−−−	−−	−−	−	−
Naloxonazine	−−−	0/−				
β-Funaltrexamine	−−−	−−−				
Naltrindole						−−−
Naltriben						−−−
7-Benzylidene naltrexone (BNTX)					−−−	
Norbinaltorphimine			−−−	−−−		
Quadazocine			−−− (κ_2)			
Naloxone benzoylhydrazone				−−−		

*+++ = strong agonist; + = weak agonist; 0/−, 0/+ = dubious effect.
−−− = strong antagonist; − = weak antagonist; 0 = no effect.
P = partial agonist.

ever, enzymatic activity splits it primarily to β-lipotropin and ACTH in the anterior pituitary, but to β-endorphin and β-MSH in the intermediate lobe of the rat pituitary (see also Chapter 51).

Unfortunately, these peptides have not proven to be specific for individual types of opioid receptors. β-Endorphin, for example, is almost equally active at μ- and δ-receptors, and somewhat less so at κ_3-receptors. Therefore, the biological significance of the various categories of receptors and peptides is still under investigation.

Regional distribution in the nervous system

The distribution of opioid receptors and opioid peptides is not uniform throughout the nervous system. Autoradiographic and binding data, together with studies of the effects of microinjection of opioids into specific loci in the nervous system, have shown that (1) receptors mediating analgesia are concentrated mainly in the dorsal horn of the spinal cord, the periaqueductal gray matter, and the thalamus; (2) those mediating effects on respiration, cough, vomiting, and pupillary diameter are concentrated in the ventral brainstem; (3) those affecting neuroendocrine secretion are mainly in the hypothalamus; and (4) those producing effects on mood and behavior are mainly in the limbic structures (hippocampus, amygdala, etc.).

Within the brain, enkephalins are found in highest concentration in the striatum and nucleus accumbens; β-endorphin in the hypothalamus, pituitary, and periaqueductal gray; and dynorphin in anterior hypothalamus and substantia nigra. Lesser concentrations of all three are found in many other structures. β-Endorphin and ACTH appear to be released together from the anterior pituitary in response to stress, while dynorphin and vasopressin are coreleased from the posterior pituitary by dehydration.

Opioid receptors are also found in the myenteric plexus of small intestine, the vas deferens, and possibly other peripheral tissues where opiates act. Enkephalins are found in the adrenal medulla and in axon terminals from various parts of the spinal cord, especially in areas with high concentrations of opiate

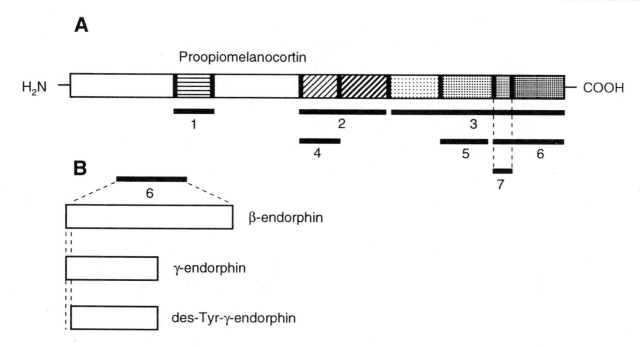

Figure 23-3. Schematic diagram of relationships among the neuropeptides derived from proopiomelanocortin (POMC). A. POMC contains the amino acid sequences of γ-MSH (1), ACTH (2), and β-LPH (3); ACTH contains the sequence of α-MSH (4); β-LPH contains the sequences of β-MSH (5) and β-endorphin (6); β-endorphin contains the sequence of met-enkephalin (7). All of these are marked off by pairs of basic amino acids (black bars), which theoretically can serve as points of cleavage by various peptidases. B. β-Endorphin also contains the sequences of γ-endorphin and des-tyrosine-γ-endorphin, but these are not marked off by cleavage points and are probably not formed from β-endorphin (see also Fig. 51-3, Chapter 51).

receptors. They appear to be the natural transmitter that binds to the receptors inhibiting transmission of pain stimuli. Met-enkephalin is also found in the myenteric plexus, where it binds to the receptors that inhibit gut contractility by inhibiting release of acetylcholine.

Afferent pain stimuli arriving in the dorsal horn appear to activate ascending neurons of the spinothalamic tract by the release of excitatory amino acids, substance P, and other transmitters. Descending modulatory fibers from the central gray, the locus coeruleus, the nucleus raphe magnus, and other brain loci inhibit the transmission of afferent pain stimuli in the dorsal horn by the release of endogenous opioids, serotonin, norepinephrine, and other transmitters. The complex picture of interactions of the endogenous opioids with each other and with other neurotransmitters and modulators is still being filled in. However, enough is already known to provide a rational basis for the use of exogenous opioids, serotonin reuptake inhibitors, and other agents in the treatment of various types of pain (see also Chapter 29).

Major Central Effects of the Opioids

Neuronal activity

Opioids appear to act essentially as inhibitors of neuronal electrical activity, both spontaneous and evoked, and of neurotransmitter release. For example, single-unit recordings from the neocortex show that firing rates, both spontaneous and evoked by the excitatory transmitter glutamate, are reduced after local application of met-enkephalin, β-endorphin, or morphine. The decrease is promptly abolished by naloxone, an opioid-receptor blocker. Hippocampal pyramidal cells show *increased* activity under the influence of morphine, but this is because morphine blocks the inhibitory interneurons that are activated by recurrent collaterals from the pyramidal cell axons (Fig. 23-4). A similar process occurs at the axon terminals of sensory primary afferents entering the spinal cord, where morphine may block transmitter release and thus contribute to the analgesic effect. This locus of action is exploited in the

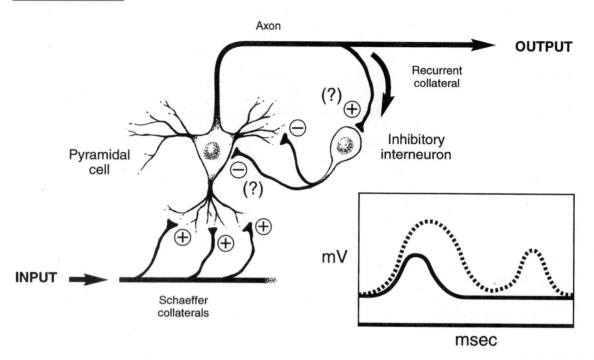

Figure 23-4. Action of morphine on hippocampal pyramidal cell activity. Inhibition of synapse activity occurs either (?) at the excitatory synapse (+) of the recurrent collateral on the interneuron or at the inhibitory synapse (−) on the pyramidal cell. *Inset:* As a result, the compound action potential (pyramidal cell output) evoked by excitatory stimulation of the Schaeffer collaterals is increased after morphine (-----), compared to control conditions (———), and repetitive firing may occur.

technique of continuous epidural or intrathecal infusion of opioids that is used to maintain smooth, prolonged analgesia in patients while minimizing effects on the brain.

Analgesia

Morphine relieves pain both by raising the threshold for pain perception and by diminishing the discomfort even if the pain is perceived, i.e., *increasing the pain tolerance.* Increase in pain threshold is readily measured experimentally (radiant heat, mechanical pressure, etc.), but pain tolerance is greatly affected by individual temperament, setting, and other factors. Narcotic analgesics have a greater effect on pain tolerance (which probably reflects action in the limbic system) than on pain threshold (which probably reflects action in the spinal cord and periaqueductal gray), so a patient can still be aware of the presence of pain but not be bothered or distressed by it.

There is evidence that spinal and supraspinal mechanisms of opioid-induced analgesia interact synergistically. Thus, simultaneous administration of morphine by both systemic and spinal routes produces a very marked increase in analgesic effect. Such synergism can also be shown between the actions of morphine at different sites in the brain, such as the periaqueductal gray and the nucleus raphe magnus. The mechanisms underlying these synergistic effects are not yet well understood.

Morphine relieves all types of pain—visceral, somatic, and cutaneous. It is more effective against dull, constant pains than against sharp, severe, intermittent ones.

Respiratory depression

μ-Receptor agonists have pronounced respiratory depressant activity. They cause a decreased sensitivity of the respiratory center to CO_2. The major acute toxicity from morphine and other μ-agonists is death from respiratory failure. In patients with chronic respiratory disease (e.g., emphysema) morphine may be fatal. In all subjects, increased P_{CO_2} tends to cause cerebral vasodilatation; this leads to an increase in CSF pressure, which may be exaggerated in the presence of head injury. The respiratory depressant effect of opioids is additive with that of alcohol, barbiturates, and other CNS depressants.

Respiratory depression has so far not been separable from analgesic action. The two effects increase with dose in parallel fashion, and equianalgesic doses of different μ-agonists produce equal degrees of respiratory depression. This appears to be true even of the partial agonists and mixed agonist-antagonists.

Change in mood

Part of the analgesic effect is due to a foggy, unreal feeling of being "detached" from things. For some people this is alarming or unpleasant; for others, it is a pleasant, relaxed, dreamy state (euphoria). Euphoria is a poor term because it means different things in relation to different drugs; e.g., with amphetamines and cocaine it means a sense of energy, power, and exhilaration; with the opioids it means the dreamy, pleasant state just mentioned; with heroin and some other opioids taken intravenously it includes, in addition, an intense visceral sensation of warmth and thrill that may be related to the peripheral actions. Not all opioids produce euphoria in all subjects, but they all produce the clouded state.

Sedation

Not all opioids produce the same degree of sedation with equianalgesic doses, but most (especially κ-agonists) produce some, and it appears to be part of the basic neurophysiological effect. The lesser sedative effect of methadone may possibly be due to protein binding, with slower onset of action; with repeated dosage, it causes marked sedation. Even opioids with marked excitatory action may cause convulsions alternating with periods of sedation. The sedative effect of opioids is *at least* additive with that of alcohol and other CNS depressants.

Separate Central Effects

There are other actions that are not intimately related to the analgesic action. These effects may be produced to varying degrees by nonanalgesic opiates such as papaverine or thebaine.

Excitation

In cats, horses, pigs, cows, and a number of other species, and *in some humans, relatively low doses of morphine cause restlessness*, fright, hyperactivity, and fever. Higher doses may cause convulsions.

Miosis

Miosis is seen in humans and in most species in which morphine is sedative. In species in which excitation occurs, mydriasis is noted. However, in the monkey, which is sedated by morphine, the pupils nevertheless dilate. Miosis is blocked by atropine and by decortication; therefore it is thought to be due to removal of cortical inhibitory action on the third cranial nerve nucleus. (**Meperidine**, a synthetic opioid analgesic, is an exception in not causing pupil constriction.)

Nausea and vomiting

Nausea and vomiting are due to stimulation of the chemoreceptor trigger zone and are aggravated by vestibular stimulation (e.g., turning the head suddenly) and by delayed gastric emptying, which is also produced by opioids. **Apomorphine**, *a nonanalgesic derivative of opium, which is an agonist at dopamine receptors and not at opioid receptors, causes a much greater emetic effect than morphine does*, and is sometimes used deliberately to produce vomiting in some types of poisoning (see Chapter 74).

Antitussive action

Direct depression of the cough center is not related to respiratory depression. *Nonanalgesic nonopioid derivatives* (e.g., **dextromethorphan**) *can have antitussive action.*

Endocrine effects

Endocrine effects are produced by actions of the opioids in the thalamus and hypothalamus. These agents inhibit the release of luteinizing-hormone-releasing hormone (LHRH; see Chapter 49) so the pituitary output of luteotropin (LH) and follicle-stimulating hormone (FSH) is diminished. This in turn decreases the secretion of testosterone by the testis and results in decreased libido, reduced volume of ejaculate, and decreased motility of sperm in males; in females, anovulatory cycles or amenorrhea occur. In contrast, serum prolactin level is raised, because the opioids inhibit the release of dopamine by hypothalamic neurons, which normally exert a tonic inhibitory influence on the prolactin secretory cells. In the past it was thought that morphine stimulates release of vasopressin from the posterior lobe of the pituitary. Recent investigations, however, indicate that the direct effect is to inhibit vasopressin secretion; the antidiuresis caused by morphine apparently results from a peripheral action on the kidney.

Poikilothermia

Most opioids inhibit the thermoregulatory mechanism centered in the preoptic anterior hypothalamic region. As a result, the ability to maintain a constant body temperature is impaired, and the direction and degree of change in body temperature depend on the ambient temperature. At normal or low room temperature, excessive heat loss to the environment occurs as a result of opioid action, and the body temperature falls.

Peripheral Effects

Histamine release

Most opioids provoke the release of histamine, causing peripheral arteriolar and venous dilatation. This results in postural hypotension, cutaneous flushing, and increased loss of body heat.

Venous dilatation results partly from histamine release but mainly through neuronal action on vascular smooth muscle. It increases the capacity of the venous bed and decreases the venous return to the heart. This effect of morphine can be very helpful in the emergency treatment of acute left ventricular failure, although it is used less frequently since the advent of potent loop diuretics such as furosemide (see Chapter 41).

Contraction of smooth muscle

Contraction of smooth muscle in the biliary and bladder sphincters is stimulated by morphine and other μ-agonists. The tone of the gastrointestinal and biliary tracts and of the ureter is increased, so the intraluminal pressure in these structures increases and there may be spasm. At the same time, inhibition of acetylcholine release from the myenteric plexus causes a marked reduction in propulsive peristaltic movement, resulting in constipation. This is the basis of the antidiarrheal effect of opioids (see Chapter 46).

Contact dermatitis and urticaria

Contact dermatitis and urticaria occur occasionally among nurses and pharmacists who handle the drugs frequently.

Therapeutic Versus Adverse Effects

Most of the effects of opioids noted above can be regarded as therapeutically desirable under some circumstances and adverse under others. For example, the analgesic action is therapeutic when the drug is given for the relief of pathological or postoperative pain, but it may be an adverse effect if it masks the pain of an acute abdominal emergency such as a ruptured appendix or diverticulitis. Similarly, the inhibition of gastrointestinal motility is therapeutic when opioids are given to relieve a severe diarrhea, but it is an adverse effect when an opioid, given for the relief of pain, results in constipation and abdominal distension. Sedation contributes to the therapeutic effect when morphine is given for the relief of immediate postoperative pain, but is an adverse effect at a somewhat later stage if it interferes with depth of breathing or with early ambulation.

In general, however, the effects most commonly used therapeutically are analgesia, sedation, antidiarrheal effect, and cough suppression. The effects most often regarded as adverse or undesirable are respiratory depression, nausea and vomiting, hypothermia, constipation, and the effects of histamine release. A troublesome but very infrequent adverse effect is a muscular rigidity resembling that of parkinsonism, apparently resulting from opioid inhibition of dopamine release in the striatum (see Chapters 20 and 21). Some opioids, especially meperidine (see below), produce serious interactions with monoamine oxidase inhibitors; this is described in greater detail under Meperidine.

THERAPEUTIC USES

The major therapeutic uses of opioids are consistent with the actions described above. They include the following:

- Relief of pain, both acute (e.g., obstetrical, traumatic, myocardial infarction, postsurgical, etc.) and chronic (musculoskeletal pain of various types, palliative care in cancer with metastases, etc.)
- Preoperative sedation, neuroleptanalgesia, epidural analgesia, and other special procedures
- Severe dyspnea, as in acute left ventricular failure
- Symptomatic treatment of diarrhea
- Suppression of the cough reflex
- Detoxication or maintenance therapy of opioid addiction

Further details of choice of agents and manner of

use are given below in the description of individual opioids.

FATE IN THE BODY

Absorption

Opioids are generally well absorbed from the gastrointestinal tract, especially the more lipid-soluble ones such as heroin, which was formerly given by mouth as a cough suppressant. Methadone is normally given by mouth in methadone maintenance therapy of opioid addicts, and codeine, *d*-propoxyphene, and others are given by mouth for the relief of mild or moderate pain. However, there is a significant first-pass metabolism in the gastrointestinal tract and liver, so bioavailability is appreciably less after oral administration than after parenteral injection. For example, after a single oral dose of morphine only 15–30% reaches the systemic circulation. As a result, the oral dose required for analgesia is initially about six times as large as the intravenous or intramuscular dose. In contrast, the ratio for codeine is only 1.5:1 (oral:parenteral). During chronic oral administration of morphine, however, the ratio falls to 3:1 or 2:1. This increase in oral potency may be due to the accumulation of an active metabolite of morphine (see Metabolism below).

The advantages of oral administration are avoidance of the discomfort of injections and a more prolonged and smooth effect; the disadvantage is slowness of onset. When opioids are being given chronically, however, as for continuous relief of chronic pain in cancer patients, slowness of onset is not really relevant because doses are given frequently enough to produce continuous analgesia. This is facilitated by the use of sustained-release oral tablets which, combined with the increase in oral potency mentioned above, frequently permit effective analgesia with twice-a-day oral dosage.

Distribution

Morphine enters all tissues. In adults relatively little enters the brain because the N is ionized at normal plasma pH. In infants, whose **blood–brain barrier** is less effective, morphine enters more readily, so infants are more susceptible to its action. Morphine also diffuses across the **gastric mucosa** into the lumen of the stomach, where the acidity converts it into the ionized form, which cannot diffuse back across the mucosa into the blood. As a result, morphine accumulates in the lumen, a process known as "ion trapping." For this reason, gastric lavage used to be employed in the emergency treatment of morphine overdose (before naloxone became available), even when the drug had been given parenterally.

Morphine and other opioids also diffuse readily across the **placenta** into the fetal circulation. For example, after administration of meperidine to pregnant women in labor, equilibrium of drug concentration in the maternal and fetal circulations is reached in 6 minutes. Since hepatic drug-metabolizing enzyme activity is very low in the fetus and newborn, the major route of elimination of opioids from the fetus is back-diffusion across the placenta into the maternal circulation. Therefore, if the infant is born too soon after the mother has received meperidine, the drug cannot be eliminated rapidly enough, and severe respiratory depression can occur in the infant.

Onset of analgesic action is usually quite rapid after subcutaneous or intramuscular injection, especially with the more lipid-soluble opioids. The time may range from 5 to 15 minutes, depending on the drug, dose, and route. After intravenous injection, the effect begins almost immediately. Continuous subcutaneous or intravenous infusion by means of a portable pump is being tested for the relief of chronic pain, especially in cancer patients.

Protein binding of opioids in the plasma varies quite markedly from drug to drug. At therapeutic concentrations, morphine is about 30% bound, meperidine about 60%, and methadone about 85%. This difference probably contributes to the disparity of apparent half-life: e.g., 2–3 hours for morphine and 15–22 hours for methadone. However, the dosages for the various opioids are adjusted accordingly, so the usual duration of analgesic effect is about 4 hours for most of them.

Metabolism

Metabolism also varies with the drug. For morphine, biotransformation is fairly rapid and consists mostly of glucuronic acid conjugation of the 3- and 6-hydroxyl groups by the hepatic smooth endoplasmic reticulum. About 90% of a dose is found as glucuronide in the urine, and 7–10% in the feces (via the bile).

The major product is morphine-3-glucuronide, but morphine-6β-glucuronide constitutes a significant fraction of the total. The 6β-glucuronide has a high affinity for the μ-receptor and is just as potent an analgesic as morphine itself. Moreover, it has a considerably longer half-life than morphine, so the area under the concentration–time curve is 11 times as great for morphine-6β-glucuronide as for morphine itself, and much of the total analgesic action of a dose of morphine may be due to the 6β-glucuronide. Since it is more polar than morphine, it crosses the blood–brain barrier into the central nervous system more slowly than morphine but also leaves more slowly. Therefore, it tends to accumulate gradually, both centrally and peripherally, during chronic morphine treatment, and this is probably the major factor in the increase in oral potency of morphine during chronic administration. Enterohepatic circulation may also play a small role: The glucuronides are excreted in the bile but are partially broken down by bacterial enzymes in the large bowel, releasing free morphine which can be reabsorbed into the circulation.

With other opioids, *N*-demethylation, hydrolysis, cyclization, and other reactions are quantitatively important, depending on the individual drug. Heroin (diacetylmorphine), for example, is rapidly hydrolyzed to monoacetylmorphine and morphine. Liver disease may reduce the rate of elimination of various opioids and lead to overdose as a result of accumulation of active drug. Renal disease can lead to accumulation of normeperidine, a toxic metabolite of meperidine.

ROUTES OF ADMINISTRATION

The most common routes by which opioids are administered to patients by physicians or nurses are the intravenous, intramuscular and subcutaneous routes; oral administration may also be used by medical or nursing attendants, or by the patient or family members. The advantages and disadvantages of these routes have been mentioned above. In recent years, however, three additional routes or methods of administration have gained considerable prominence: epidural or intrathecal administration, patient-controlled analgesia, and percutaneous absorption.

Epidural or Intrathecal Administration

Injection and infusion of opioids into the spinal epidural space through which the sensory nerve roots pass, or (much less frequently) directly into the spinal subarachnoid space, is now used in many centers to produce localized analgesia with a reduced risk of respiratory depression, drowsiness, and the other undesired effects. These methods make use of the existence of spinal mechanisms of analgesia noted above. They provide excellent postoperative pain relief, but

a small percentage of patients do suffer serious respiratory depression from opioids used in this way.

In the case of intrathecal injection, respiratory depression is usually the result of an overdose. It is more likely to occur if supplementary systemic opioids are given as well. The estimated frequency of this complication is as high as 5% after intrathecal administration but not more than 0.3% after epidural administration. Redistribution of opioid from the injection site toward the brainstem is well demonstrated with morphine but is much less likely with more lipid-soluble opioids that can diffuse more readily into the blood vessels and be carried away from the central nervous system.

Patient-Controlled Analgesia (PCA)

Recently, a number of devices have been marketed that consist essentially of a pump for injecting opioid solution, a switch that the patient can operate to activate the pump, and control equipment by which the physician or nurse can preset the size of the dose, the minimum interval between doses, and the maximum number of doses in a defined period of time. Such equipment can be used for intravenous, subcutaneous, or epidural administration of the drug. It is simple enough that it can be used in children as well as adults. PCA can be used as the sole method of administration of opioid, or it can be used to provide supplementary analgesia on top of a basal level provided in the conventional manner.

The main advantage claimed for PCA is a more even and continuous analgesia that avoids the wide fluctuations between maximum and minimum plasma levels that can occur when successive doses are given at fixed time intervals. Patient satisfaction is correspondingly greater. However, several studies have indicated that the total amount of opioid required may not differ in PCA versus conventional administration, and the frequency of adverse effects does not appear to differ greatly. Indeed, some types of complication, such as adynamic ileus (intestinal paralysis) or urinary retention due to bladder paralysis by opioids, are more common in patients treated with PCA than with conventional opioid therapy. This probably reflects the more constant level of opioid-induced suppression of acetylcholine release, without intervals in which recovery can occur.

Percutaneous Absorption

Transdermal patches (see Chapter 2) of fentanyl (Duragesic) provide effective delivery of amounts that are sufficient for sustained analgesia in patients with chronic cancer pain. Patches containing different doses of fentanyl permit gradation of the opioid effects.

TOLERANCE AND PHYSICAL DEPENDENCE

Tolerance to the effects of morphine develops rapidly on repeated administration, and larger and larger doses are required for the same effect (see Chapter 72). In animal experiments, continuous slow intravenous infusion of morphine for as little as 4 hours can produce some tolerance. Human addicts can stand many times the normal acute lethal dose without getting respiratory arrest.

The development of tolerance is usually accompanied by the development of physical dependence. Compensatory changes in the cell are unmasked by removal of opiates and a picture of hyperexcitability is seen: restlessness, extreme anxiety, vomiting and diarrhea, runny nose, muscle twitching, chills, fever and sweating, pupillary dilation, and sometimes circulatory collapse. This picture varies in time of onset and in severity after withdrawal of different opiates, but *can be precipitated almost immediately by opiate antagonists. It can be abolished by giving more narcotic analgesic.* (The ability of a new opiate to abolish morphine withdrawal symptoms in human volunteers is used as a method of assessing dependence liability of the new drug; see Chapter 72.)

A number of **hypothetical mechanisms** have been proposed to explain the development of opiate tolerance and physical dependence.

1. If the drug blocks release of a neurotransmitter, postsynaptic receptors for that transmitter might be induced, or their sensitivity might be increased, thereby compensating for the drug effect (i.e., tolerance). Withdrawal of the drug would allow normal release of transmitter, but increased receptor numbers and sensitivity would cause excessive postsynaptic effects (i.e., withdrawal reaction). So far, no good evidence of supersensitivity to acetylcholine, catecholamines, or serotonin has been found in opiate-dependent subjects. However, increased sensitivity to norepinephrine following opioid withdrawal appears to be responsible for some of the more obvious and uncomfortable withdrawal symptoms, such as anxiety, gooseflesh (the source of the term "cold turkey"), intestinal cramps, and disturbances in body temperature. These symptoms can be relieved by administration of **clonidine,** an α_2-adrenoceptor agonist (see Chapters 16 and 18) that decreases the release of catecholamines from presynaptic terminals.

2. An enzyme that is inhibited by the opiates acutely might undergo compensatory induction. As noted above, opioid agonists inhibit adenylyl cyclase activity acutely and reduce cAMP levels in brain cells. In tolerant animals the adenylyl cyclase increases and cAMP levels return to normal; in the withdrawal reaction they are both above normal. However, there is so far no proof that changes in adenylyl cyclase and cAMP *cause* the tolerance, rather than *reflect* it.

3. If the drug blocks release of a neurotransmitter, the transmitter might theoretically accumulate intracellularly until its concentration is high enough to overcome the block (tolerance). Withdrawal of the drug would allow massive release of the accumulated transmitter. However, there is no evidence for such a mechanism.

4. More than one neuronal pathway might serve the same physiological function ("redundancy"). If the major one is inhibited by opiates and the minor one is not, the minor one might hypertrophy and compensate for the drug effect. When the drug is withdrawn, both pathways would function, causing excessive activity. Again, there is no evidence to demonstrate the importance of such a mechanism.

5. High doses of exogenous opioids would lead to a loss ("down-regulation") of their receptors, causing tolerance. At the same time, the excessive presence of the drug would cause a feedback inhibition of the biosynthesis and release of endogenous opioid peptides. Withdrawal of the exogenous opioids would leave a deficiency of the endogenous peptides and their receptors (withdrawal reaction) until readaptation occurred. A decreased rate of synthesis of β-endorphin has recently been reported in morphine-tolerant rats, but there is no evidence of change in receptors during tolerance, although there is cross-tolerance between morphine and the opioid peptides.

Tolerance and physical dependence are not the same as addiction. A normal subject can be made physically dependent, and after going through a withdrawal reaction will not resume drug-taking. Addiction also involves a compulsion to take the drug again after going through withdrawal, i.e., a strong psychological dependence on it. Drug dependence is covered in detail in Chapter 72.

MORPHINE CONGENERS

Codeine is a relatively weak analgesic, having one-tenth the potency of morphine, and consequently shows little respiratory depression and relatively little addiction liability. About 10–15% of a codeine dose is metabolically converted into morphine in the human body, and this fraction accounts for the analgesic activity; however, most of the antitussive effect is thought to be due to codeine itself. It is used widely in combination with nonopioid analgesics such as acetaminophen and ASA, and as a cough suppressant in doses of 10–15 mg. Codeine undergoes relatively little first-pass metabolism in the liver, so it is about 60% as potent by mouth as by parenteral injection.

Hydrocodone (Hycodan and others), a derivative of codeine, is particularly effective as an analgesic, being as potent as morphine, and it is also commonly used as an antitussive.

Most of the **semisynthetic morphine derivatives** are fairly old. Of these, **heroin** is twice as potent as morphine in terms of its initial effects. The addict likes heroin because its high lipid solubility enables it to enter the brain much more rapidly than morphine, and its initial action is more intense. However, the later effects are the same as those of morphine, because it is converted to morphine in the body. Because of narcotic control regulations, heroin is no longer available for clinical use in the United States. In Canada, its use is limited to the control of chronic intractable pain in terminal cancer.

Hydromorphone (Dilaudid) has strong analgesic and antitussive activity; it is more potent than morphine and codeine, respectively, on a weight basis. It is better absorbed than morphine following oral administration, with an onset of analgesic action in about 15 minutes and a duration of action of more than 5 hours. This drug can therefore be given by mouth as well as by subcutaneous or intramuscular injection, and as rectal suppositories.

Levorphanol (Levo-Dromoran) is one of the more potent **synthetic analgesics** presently in wide use; it is four to five times as potent as morphine. It is less constipating than morphine and is longer-acting. This drug has a levo-rotatory structure; its dextro-rotatory isomer, **dextrorphan**, has no analgesic activity but is an effective antitussive. Similarly, **levomethorphan** is an analgesic, whereas **dextromethorphan** is not, but it is widely used in cough mixtures, in adult doses of 10–30 mg.

Meperidine (pethidine; Demerol and others) is the first and perhaps still most widely used *synthetic* congener. It is a relatively old preparation and has many trade names. The chemical structure resembles that of atropine as well as that of morphine, and it was originally believed to be an antispasmodic rather than a constrictor of smooth muscle like morphine. However, this is now known to be false; it does cause spasm. Its action is shorter than that of morphine,

and it is less potent by a factor of about 10. In equianalgesic doses it causes at least as much respiratory depression as morphine. Meperidine does not produce miosis and is, therefore, a favorite of addicted nurses and doctors (it is less likely to be detected). It is quite effective when given by mouth. Normeperidine, a metabolite of meperidine, causes CNS excitatory effects and can produce seizures.

Meperidine is especially likely to interact adversely with monoamine oxidase inhibitors (MAOIs; see Chapter 29) to produce a severe and potentially fatal syndrome characterized by coma, hyperpyrexia, and hypotension. This interaction appears to have two components: (1) the MAOIs inhibit meperidine *N*-demethylase and thus potentiate the action of meperidine, and (2) meperidine inhibits the neuronal uptake of serotonin and thus potentiates the effect of the MAOIs. The excessive concentration of free 5-HT is probably responsible for the hyperpyrexia. Morphine is much less likely than meperidine to interact with MAOIs in this way.

Methadone (Dolophine; Fig. 23-5) has about the same analgesic potency as morphine but differs from it essentially in two respects. It has a much longer duration of action because it is more slowly eliminated from the body, and in single doses it causes little sedation. The lack of sedative effect did detract from its original popularity. However, because of its much slower clearance from the body, its withdrawal effects are much milder than those of morphine. The main current use of methadone is, therefore, to substitute for morphine in addicts prior to withdrawal.

In the 1960s, V. Dole and M. Nyswander began testing the use of **long-term methadone maintenance for the management of opiate addiction.** The purpose is to maintain a sufficiently high level of tolerance that the addict's usual dose of heroin or other opioid produces little or no "high," so there is no inducement to continue taking it. The patients are kept on methadone for months or years while undergoing psychological and social rehabilitation.

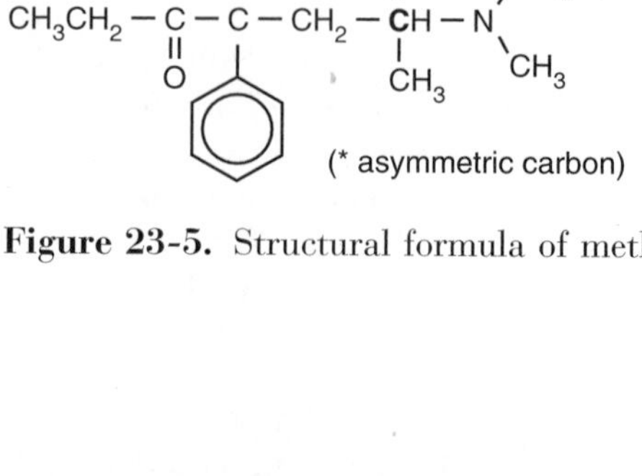

$$CH_3CH_2 - \overset{\overset{\textstyle O}{\|}}{C} - C - CH_2 - \overset{*}{CH} - N \overset{CH_3}{\underset{CH_3}{\diagdown}}$$

(* asymmetric carbon)

Figure 23-5. Structural formula of methadone.

Between 50% and 80% of patients in well-run methadone maintenance programs continue in treatment and show significant improvement in social and work performance. In the most successful cases, methadone dosage can be gradually reduced and eventually withdrawn, replaced in some cases by naltrexone (see below) to prevent a return to heroin.

Propoxyphene (Darvon) is a commonly used analgesic structurally related to methadone but 12–15 times less potent. In equianalgesic doses it has properties similar to those of the other opioid analgesics.

Fentanyl (Sublimaze), **sufentanil** (Sufenta), and **alfentanil** (Alfenta) are chemically related to meperidine. They are all strong analgesics, with potency ratios (relative to morphine) of about 80:1, 800:1, and 20:1 respectively. They produce all the other effects that morphine does, in about the same ratio as the analgesia. The main advantages of fentanyl are that, when given intravenously, it has almost immediate onset of action and a short duration, the half-life of the redistribution phase being only 12.5 minutes. Therefore it lends itself very well for **neuroleptanalgesia** (see Chapter 24). It is injected intravenously in a dose of 1 μg/kg mixed with droperidol or a similar neuroleptic, and supplementary doses of 50–100 μg are given intravenously every 30–45 minutes during surgery. An important advantage is that fentanyl causes very little depression of left ventricular function, so it carries little risk of hypotension during surgery. However, there is some danger of drug accumulation if doses are repeated too frequently. Because of the short half-life, the patient can wake up rapidly when the surgery is over and has little difficulty with respiratory depression and constipation postoperatively. Sufentanil and alfentanil are used for the same purpose. These drugs are also now used frequently for continuous epidural analgesia in PCA regimens, and in transdermal delivery systems.

High doses of fentanyl tend to produce muscular rigidity, perhaps by action at enkephalin receptors in the striatum, which may inhibit dopamine release there. The effect can be overcome by muscle relaxants or by naloxone (see below).

OPIOID ANTAGONISTS

In the morphine molecule (see Fig. 23-1), the methyl group attached to the N is of critical dimensions for agonist activity when the molecule has combined with its receptor. If the CH_3 is changed to an allyl group, or if a cyclopropyl or cyclobutyl group is attached to the methyl, the molecule still binds to the receptor, but no longer initiates a typical morphine response. It therefore functions as a receptor blocker, or opioid antagonist (Fig. 23-6). Replacement of the –OH at carbon 6 by a ketonic oxygen results in a highly specific and powerful blocking action.

Naloxone (Narcan) is said to be a pure opioid antagonist since it has no analgesic activity of its own but has the ability to reverse or block the actions of opioid analgesic agonists. It has the greatest affinity for μ-receptors, where it prevents or reverses the activity not only of morphine and its congeners but also of β-endorphin and enkephalins. It is less effective as a blocker of κ-receptors.

Naltrexone (Trexan) is a related compound that is also a pure blocker, but it has a much longer half-life than naloxone and is well absorbed when given by mouth.

When given together with morphine, these drugs antagonize many of its important actions, including analgesia, respiratory depression, euphoria, increase in CSF pressure, miosis, smooth muscle spasm, and hypotension. Their **clinical uses** are (1) to reverse the respiratory depression caused by morphine-like drugs; (2) for diagnostic tests in opioid addicts, in whom they precipitate an acute withdrawal reaction; and (3) in the treatment of addicts, after they have been withdrawn from opioids, to prevent the "high" from self-administered heroin or morphine, and thus to decrease the risk of relapse. They are also used as supplementary therapy to help prevent relapse in alcoholism (see Chapter 26).

MIXED AGONIST-ANTAGONISTS AND PARTIAL AGONISTS

Opioids with allyl or 4- or 5-carbon substituents on the N, but that retain the –OH group at C-6, display

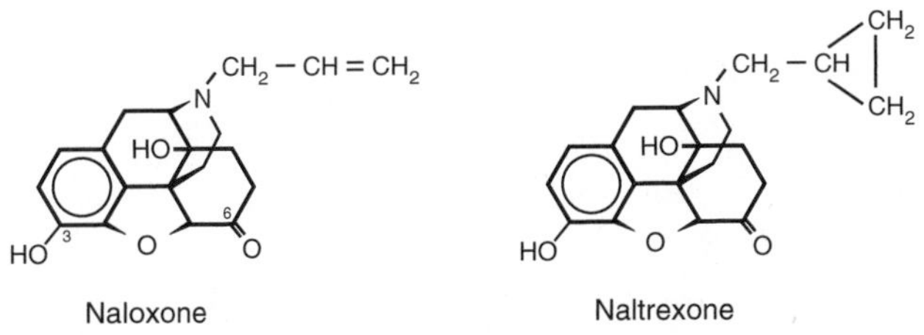

Figure 23-6. Structural formulae of two potent opioid antagonists. Compare these with Figure 23-1. Numbers designate the C-3 and C-6 positions mentioned in the text.

a mixture of agonist and antagonist properties. Examples include nalorphine and nalbuphine (Fig. 23-7). Pentazocine is a synthetic analog with similar properties.

Nalorphine (Nalline) and **levallorphan** (Lorfan) act as μ-receptor blockers, preventing the analgesic, respiratory depressant, and euphoriant actions of morphine. However, they are weak agonists at κ-receptors and therefore have some analgesic and sedating effects when given by themselves. When given in larger doses they cause agitation, dysphoria, and hallucinations. Therefore, they carry a lower risk of abuse and dependence than μ-agonists do.

Pentazocine (Talwin), **cyclazocine,** and **nalbuphine** (Nubain) are also mixed agonist-antagonists that have some morphine-antagonist (μ-blocking) effect but exert reasonably good analgesic action through κ-receptors. Their mental effects seem to be intermediate between those of morphine and nalorphine. They do not cause severe mental disturbance as nalorphine does, but they are less likely than morphine to produce euphoria (see Table 23-2).

Buprenorphine has a cyclopropylmethyl substituent on the N, the same as that of naltrexone, and a $-OCH_3$ group like that of codeine in place of the $-OH$ on C-6. These offset each other to some extent, so, instead of being a μ-receptor blocker, it is a partial μ-agonist. That means that it has some morphine-like action, but the maximum response attainable is considerably less than that of morphine, no matter how much the dose is increased. Thus, when it competes with morphine or heroin for μ-receptors, it can reduce their maximum effect. It has been suggested that this makes it less attractive to addicts and less likely to be abused.

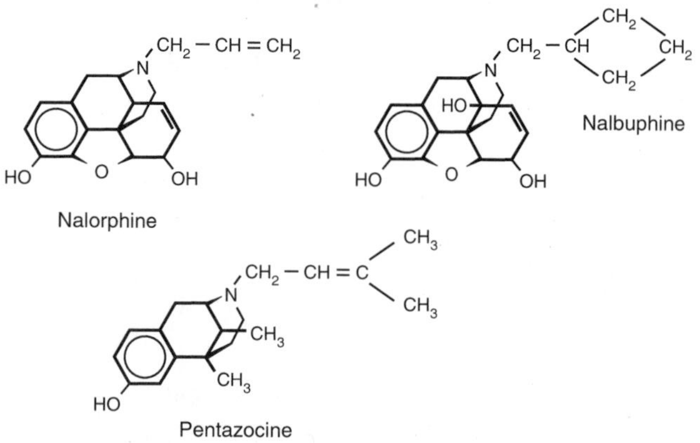

Tramadol (Ultram) is an orally administered analgesic, newly approved in the United States and Canada though used in Europe for over 20 years. It has some structural resemblances both to the opioids and to various nonsteroidal anti-inflammatory agents. Both tramadol and its active metabolite O-desmethyltramadol bind weakly to the μ-receptor, but their analgesic effect is only partially reversible by naloxone. It is not yet clear whether tramadol should be regarded primarily as a partial opioid agonist, or whether its analgesic effect is largely due to its ability to block reuptake of serotonin and norepinephrine at their central synapses. At the recommended dose of 50–100 mg (daily maximum, 400 mg), the analgesic effect of tramadol is comparable to that of codeine-aspirin or codeine-acetaminophen therapy. Adverse effects include dizziness, sedation, constipation, and synergism with alcohol and hypnotics; at higher doses it can give rise to seizures, hallucinations, and confusion.

FINAL COMMENT

The field of opioid peptides, opioid receptors, and synthetic opioids is undergoing rapid change as a result of recent research. Over the next few years there will probably be major developments permitting better separation of analgesic, euphoriant, endocrine, and other effects, and therefore better therapeutic specificity.

SUGGESTED READING

Adler MW, Geller EB, Rogers TJ et al. Opioids, receptors, and immunity. Adv Exp Med Biol 1993; 335:13–20.

Bushnell TG, Justins DM. Choosing the right analgesic. A guide to selection. Drugs 1993; 46:394–408.

Costa E, Trabucchi M, eds. Regulatory peptides from molecular biology to function. Adv Biochem Psychopharmacol 1983; 33:1–561.

Cross SA. Pathophysiology of pain. Mayo Clin Proc 1994; 69:375–383.

Etches RC, Sandler AN, Daley MD. Respiratory depression and spinal opioids. Can J Anaesth 1989; 36:165–185.

Fowler CJ, Fraser GL. Mu-, delta-, kappa-opioid receptors and their subtypes. A critical review with emphasis on radioligand binding experiments. Neurochem Int 1994; 24:401–426.

Knapp RJ, Malatynska E, Collins N et al. Molecular biology and pharmacology of cloned opioid receptors. FASEB J 1995; 9:516–525.

Martin WR. Pharmacology of opioids. Pharmacol Rev 1983; 35:283–323.

Figure 23-7. Structural formulae of some mixed agonist-antagonist opioids that act as μ-receptor blockers, but as agonists at κ- and/or σ-receptors.

Pasternak GW. Pharmacological mechanisms of opioid analgesics. Clin Neuropharmacol 1993; 16:1–18.

Payne R. Role of epidural and intrathecal narcotics and peptides in the management of cancer pain. Med Clin North Am 1987; 71(2):313–327.

Schug SA, Zech D, Grond S. Adverse effects of systemic opioid analgesics. Drug Saf 1992; 7:200–213.

Special issue: Mixed agonist-antagonist analgesics. Drug Alcohol Depend 1985; 14(3–4):221–431.

Symposium: Update on opioids, hypnotics and muscle relaxants. Anaesth Intensive Care 1987; 15(1):7–96.

Takemori AE, Portoghese PS. Selective naltrexone-derived opioid receptor antagonists. Annu Rev Pharmacol Toxicol 1992; 32:239–269.

CHAPTER 24

General Anesthetics

F.J. CARMICHAEL AND D.A. HAAS

CASE HISTORY

A 19-year-old woman was having an operation to remove four impacted wisdom teeth under general anesthesia. She was fit and healthy, as were her parents and siblings. She had no allergies and was taking no medication.

The patient was given an intravenous injection of fentanyl (50 μg) and a precurarizing dose of *d*-tubocurarine (3 mg). Propofol had not yet been adopted as an inducing agent in that hospital, and induction was therefore carried out with an intravenous injection of thiopental (5 mg/kg). Following the administration of thiopental, her blood pressure fell to 80/50 mmHg and her heart rate rose to 115 bpm. When fully unconscious, she was paralyzed with succinylcholine (1.5 mg/kg intravenously) and about 45 seconds later her heart rate was noted to be 44 bpm. When fully relaxed, she had a nasal endotracheal tube inserted to protect her airway and maintain mechanical ventilation. At this point her blood pressure was 125/75 mmHg and her heart rate was 82 bpm. She was given atracurium, an intermediate-acting muscle relaxant, to facilitate ventilation during the dental extraction. Nitrous oxide and isoflurane were started for maintenance of anesthesia and gradually over 4–5 minutes her blood pressure fell to 92/60 mmHg and her heart rate remained at about 80 bpm.

At the time of surgical incision, her blood pressure jumped to 150/95 mmHg and her heart rate increased to 135 bpm. This was treated with an additional injection of fentanyl (100 μg), and the inspired concentration of isoflurane was increased temporarily. The surgery then proceeded without further incident. At the completion of the procedure, the inhalational agents were discontinued and neostigmine (2.5 mg) and atropine (0.6 mg) were given intravenously in order to reverse the muscle relaxation. In about 5 minutes the patient was awake and responding to commands, the endotracheal tube was removed, and the patient was transfered to the postanesthetic recovery unit. During recovery, the only problem was that the patient experienced nausea and vomited once.

Anesthesia can be defined as a reversible, drug-induced loss of sensation in the entire body or in a part of it. In *general* anesthesia, this definition must be extended to include the blocking of sensory responses to painful stimuli; blocking of cardiovascular, respiratory, and gastrointestinal reflexes; blocking of motor functions; and the production of amnesia and unconsciousness.

The proper use of anesthesia in surgery began in the 1840s, following Morton's successful demonstration of the effectiveness of ether anesthesia in dentistry. Since that time new anesthetic agents have been developed and introduced into clinical practice, and methods for administering these drugs have been improved. The newer agents are safer for the patient in that they are nonexplosive. Improved methods for delivering anesthetic drugs and monitoring their effects have allowed the anesthesiologist to give safer anesthesia to patients with compromised cardiovascular, respiratory, or central nervous system function.

Also, these newer agents and methods have contributed immensely to the expansion of the scope of surgery from short operative procedures limited to the extremities or abdomen to the major surgical accomplishments of the present.

DESIRABLE ACTIONS OF GENERAL ANESTHETICS

Hypnosis (loss of consciousness). Although some surgery is conducted on the awake patient, many operative procedures are better carried out with the patient asleep. Many present-day surgical procedures are done with the patient intubated and perhaps mechanically ventilated. These latter procedures require that the patient be "asleep" or unconscious.

Analgesia (loss of pain). Surgical procedures, by their nature, are painful, and it is incumbent upon the anesthetist to alleviate this pain whether the patient is asleep or awake.

Amnesia (loss of recall). Since surgery can be a frightening ordeal for the patient, it is desirable that there be little or no memory of the event.

Muscle relaxation. Many surgical procedures are made considerably easier when there is reduced muscle tone. Also, when a patient is to be intubated and ventilated there is a need for relaxation of laryngeal and respiratory muscles.

There is, therefore, a spectrum of separate pharmacological actions required to achieve the various goals of anesthesia. During anesthetic administration, one must deal with each of these components and determine the level of these effects separately. The depth of anesthesia relates to the degree of reduction of these parameters during surgery, and consequently the degree of unconsciousness, analgesia, amnesia, and muscle relaxation.

No single anesthetic agent has yet been developed in which these properties are combined in optimal proportions. It is unlikely that any single agent could provide optimal anesthesia for all patients and all types of procedures. A combination of different anesthetic agents allows better control of the individual components of the anesthetic spectrum. Full loss of consciousness and loss of pain-induced reflexes, with good muscular relaxation but minimal disturbance of circulation, are usually obtained with a combination of light anesthesia together with specific opioid analgesic and muscle-relaxant drugs, a procedure known as *balanced anesthesia.*

THEORIES OF ANESTHESIA

The mechanism by which general anesthetics exert their effects remains uncertain, although various theories have enjoyed scientific popularity at different times. Any theory of general anesthesia must attempt to identify a common basis for a reversible interaction between nerve cells and drugs of quite varied physical and chemical properties to explain how such diverse substances can produce closely similar patterns of general anesthetic effects.

Metabolic Theories

Early theories attributed the phenomenon of anesthesia to interference with nerve-cell function by the anesthetic agent through depression of neuronal respiration or metabolism. Most investigators now feel that the metabolic disturbances are the result, rather than the cause, of decreased nerve-cell activity.

Membrane Theories

Most theories of anesthesia have been based on the concept that the drug interferes with alterations in cell membranes that normally occur during neuronal excitation, impulse conduction, and synaptic transmitter release.

Lipid solubility theory

The lipid solubility theory was based on the direct correlation between the lipid/water partition coefficients of different substances and their general anesthetic potencies. This correlation, described by Meyer in 1899 and Overton in 1901, led to the view that the degree of anesthesia is proportional to the concentration of anesthetic dissolved in the lipid or lipophilic phase of the cell membrane.

Thermodynamic activity theory

In 1939, Ferguson proposed this theory to account for exceptions to the Meyer-Overton correlation. He multiplied the concentration of dissolved anesthetic by its thermodynamic activity coefficient (TAC), which is a correction factor reflecting the degree of physicochemical interaction between the molecules of anesthetic and those of the phase in which it is located: Thermodynamic activity = molar concentration × TAC. Ferguson claimed that equal thermodynamic activity of different anesthetics in the cell membrane produced equal degrees of anesthesia.

Membrane occupancy theory

Since there were still exceptions that did not fit Ferguson's theory, Mullins (1954) introduced a further correction to take account of the molecular size of the anesthetic agent. At the same thermodynamic activity, a larger molecule would occupy a larger space within the membrane. Mullins proposed that the degree of anesthesia is proportional to the fractional volume of the cell membrane occupied by the anesthetic.

Membrane expansion theory

The membrane expansion theory (Eyring; Seeman; K.W. Miller) extends Mullins' theory by proposing a mechanism of action. According to this hypothesis, the anesthetic molecules enter hydrophobic regions of the membrane (i.e., in the interstices of membrane proteins and between lipid molecules), expanding and distorting the membrane, as well as the proteins associated with the sodium-conductance channel (Fig. 24-1). This expansion would compress ion channels and thus prevent the ion flux associated with the action potential. The effect of this impairment on Na^+ influx is seen in a slower rise of the action potential and a correspondingly higher threshold of depolarization before the neuron responds with an action potential. All neurons would be affected in a similar way, but some are much more sensitive than others. Clinically usable anesthesia and analgesia, without fatal cardiorespiratory depression, depends upon this difference in sensitivity of different neurons to the same drug. To block the excitability of small neurons in the brain, and thus produce general anesthesia, it has been calculated that the anesthetic agent must reach a concentration of 500 μmoles/100 mL of membrane volume.

Various investigators showed that all lipid-soluble anesthetics at effective anesthetic concentration expand cell membranes by about 1%. If anesthetized small laboratory animals, single nerve cells, or axons are subjected to 100–200 atmospheres of pressure so that the membranes are recompressed by about 1%, the animals wake up, or nerve function returns, even though the anesthetic is still present. This phenomenon is called *pressure reversal of anesthesia*, and it has been cited as evidence supporting the membrane expansion effects of anesthetic agents.

The site of interaction between anesthetic agent and cell membrane likely includes hydrophobic areas of membrane protein molecules or protein–lipid interfaces. These interactions could interfere with synthesis or release of neurotransmitters from presynaptic cells, with the removal or reuptake of neurotransmitters from the synaptic cleft, with the binding of neurotransmitters to postsynaptic receptors, and with electrochemical changes in the postsynaptic neural membrane. At present there is substantial evidence that the primary target for general anesthesia is a membrane protein with a site that has both polar and nonpolar regions that bind anesthetic molecules of widely varying sizes and shapes.

There are known specific drug–receptor interactions for certain intravenous agents used in anesthesia, such as central nervous system opioid receptors for opioid analgesics, the nicotinic receptors at the neuromuscular junction for muscle relaxants, the central dopaminergic receptors for neuroleptic drugs, and the central GABA receptors for benzodiazepines.

There is now a considerable body of evidence that a number of intravenous and possibly inhalational anesthetics exert at least part of their anesthetic actions in the central nervous system through interactions at the $GABA_A$-receptor/chloride-channel complex. These agents appear to enhance the binding of the GABA molecule to its receptor. GABA is the most common inhibitory neurotransmitter that increases chloride influx into nerve cells, resulting in CNS depression. Barbiturates, benzodiazepines, and propofol have been suggested to bind to specific sites in the $GABA_A$/chloride-channel complex and activate GABA binding to the $GABA_A$ receptor.

PREMEDICATION

Before a patient undergoes a procedure requiring general anesthesia, premedication may be required. There are a number of indications for premedication, such as relief of anxiety, induction of sedation, analgesia, amnesia, vagal blockade, reduction of secretions in the upper respiratory tract, lessening of postoperative nausea and vomiting, increase in pH and decrease in volume of gastric contents, and potential reduction of the dose of general anesthetic agent required for induction. A most effective and simple means to reduce anxiety is the time-honored preoperative visit to the patient by the anesthesiologist to provide information and answer questions. The following classes of drugs are routinely employed by many physicians.

Opioids. Opioid analgesics such as morphine or

NORMAL MEMBRANE

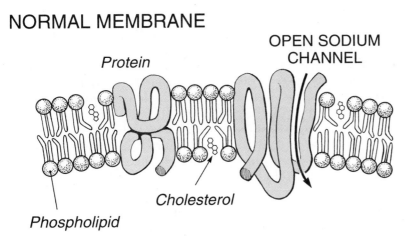

EXPANDED MEMBRANE

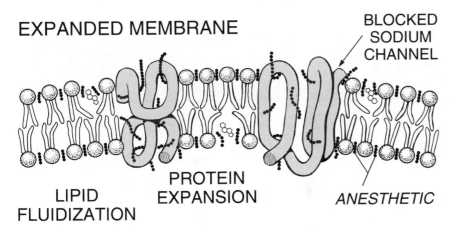

Figure 24-1. Blockade of sodium channels in excitable membranes through expansion of the membrane in the presence of anesthetic molecules.

its synthetic analogs offer analgesia, euphoria, and sedation. Complicating problems can be respiratory depression, nausea and vomiting, gastric retention, and reduced sympathetic tone. (For further details, see Chapter 23.)

Benzodiazepines. These anxiolytics, most notably diazepam, midazolam, and lorazepam, provide a reduction in anxiety without significant effects on respiration or cardiovascular function (see Chapter 27). They are also effective in providing some amnesia and sedation.

Antimuscarinics. Atropine, glycopyrrolate, and scopolamine may be used as premedicants to block vagal reflexes and inhibit salivary and respiratory tract secretions (see Chapter 15). The resulting dry mouth can be unpleasant for the patient, and therefore these drugs may be better used during induction rather than as premedication. Scopolamine also has

central effects leading to sedation and amnesia. Glycopyrrolate does not cross the blood–brain barrier and is also less likely to induce tachycardia than is atropine.

Antihistamines. Both H_1 and H_2 antagonists may be given for premedication. H_1 antagonists such as hydroxyzine and promethazine offer antiemetic effects as well as some sedation. H_2 antagonists such as cimetidine and ranitidine will decrease gastric acidity and reduce the volume of stomach contents. This is important in some patients because general anesthesia eliminates the usual protective reflexes that prevent aspiration following regurgitation of stomach contents. The dopaminergic antagonist metoclopramide is sometimes administered in order to increase the rate of gastric emptying.

Antiemetics. Postoperative nausea and vomiting are common adverse events following general anesthesia. In order to minimize these, patients who are predisposed to nausea and vomiting may be given one of a variety of agents which include the phenothiazines droperidol, prochlorperazine, and promethazine; the antihistamines, such as dimenhydrinate and hydroxyzine; and selective serotonin 5-HT$_3$-receptor antagonists such as ondansetron (Zofran).

SIGNS AND STAGES OF GENERAL ANESTHESIA

The classical signs of general anesthesia with diethyl ether were described by Guedel, who divided the process into stages and planes (Fig. 24-2). These classical signs, while still essentially correct because

they reflect physiological events in response to CNS-depressant agents, are no longer useful with the modern anesthetic agents and techniques in current use. Now, depth of anesthesia is judged by the presence or absence of a response to verbal commands, of the eyelash reflex, of rhythmic respiration, and of the response of heart rate and blood pressure to surgical stimulation. However, the classical signs are given here because they draw attention to some important principles and physiological mechanisms of general anesthesia.

Stage I

This is the period from the beginning of anesthetic administration to the loss of consciousness. The pa-

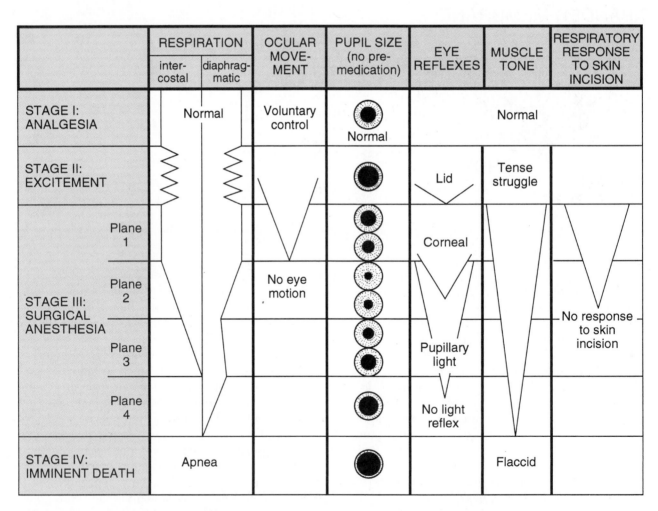

Figure 24-2. Signs and reflex reactions characterizing the stages and planes of anesthesia (after Guedel, who devised this scheme with diethyl ether anesthesia for the training of inexperienced medical personnel during World War I). The wedges indicate the progressive disappearance of signs and reflexes, which may vary somewhat from person to person.

tient progressively loses pain sensation, but motor activity and reflexes remain normal. *Analgesia* in this stage is primarily the relief of pain from cutaneous receptors.

Stage II

This period extends from the loss of consciousness, through a *stage of irregular and spasmodic breathing*, to the reestablishment of regular breathing. The eyes still move in roving motion; the pupils are often dilated but still react to light; the eyelid reflex still occurs; and the patient may swallow, retch, vomit, or struggle intensely. It is a stage of general excitement, not without danger to the patient.

Excitement is thought to occur as a result of anesthetic blockade of small inhibitory cells of the Golgi type II category, unmasking excitatory effects such as gross motor movements.

Stage III

This is the stage of anesthesia during which surgery may be performed. In Guedel's scheme it is subdivided into four planes of increasing anesthetic depth. The movements of the eyes gradually stop; the pupils first constrict and then dilate progressively; the eyelid and then the corneal and pupillary reflexes are extinguished; swallowing, retching, and vomiting stop; skeletal muscles relax; the response of increased respiration at the time of surgical stimulation gradually fades. Respiration, which at first is deep and regular, becomes more shallow and in the deeper planes more diaphragmatic.

This stage of *surgical anesthesia* is associated with progressive depression of the brainstem reticular systems (both activating and inhibiting pathways).

Stage IV

In this stage of *imminent death* the pupils are completely dilated and breathing stops. It is the stage of anesthetic overdose, which is reversible if anesthetic administration is discontinued and artificial respiration is applied.

The spontaneous rhythmicity of the two (bilateral) respiratory centers in the medulla oblongata is reduced. Cardioregulatory centers in the medulla are also depressed. Monosynaptic reflexes are completely abolished.

Beyond stage IV (medullary paralysis), respiratory arrest is followed by circulatory failure (paralysis of vasomotor center) and death.

INHALATIONAL ANESTHESIA

Technique

Anesthetic gases (such as nitrous oxide) and vapors (of volatile liquids such as halothane) are administered to patients at appropriate inspired concentrations, which are achieved by the use of accurate flow meters and other ancillary machinery.

The gases are supplied in compressed form and are passed through pressure reduction valves prior to the delivery of the gas through a flow meter to the patient. The gas is then administered to the patient through a mask fitted over the mouth and nose or larynx (laryngeal mask), or through a tube inserted past the larynx directly into the trachea (endotracheal tube).

The volatile anesthetics (or vapors) are supplied as liquids at room temperature and atmospheric pressure and are delivered in gaseous form from thermocompensated wick vaporizers designed to deliver a precise amount (concentration) of vapor, usually as a percentage of total gas flow.

General Pharmacokinetics

Anesthesia results when appropriate concentrations or partial pressures of the anesthetic agent are present in brain tissue. Between the anesthetic machine and the brain there are a series of diffusion sites as the gas or vapor moves from the machine to the alveoli, into the blood, and finally into body tissues including the brain. At each of these interfaces there is a partial-pressure gradient that depends on the physicochemical properties of the anesthetic agent and the body compartments involved.

Uptake

The rate of rise of anesthetic concentration in the blood, and therefore in the tissues, is dependent upon a series of clearly defined factors:

1. The *concentration* of the agent in the inspired air.

2. The *pulmonary ventilation*, i.e., delivery of the agent to the alveoli. The subsequent transfer from the alveoli to the blood depends upon the solubility of the agent in blood. The more soluble the anesthetic agent is in the blood, the more important is pulmonary ventilation rate as a limiting factor (Fig. 24-3).

3. *Solubility,* measured as the partition coefficient of the agent between blood and gas phase ($P_{b/g}$). As the concentration in the inspired air rises, the tensions or partial pressures of the anesthetic agents in the blood rise more rapidly with the less soluble agents such as nitrous oxide than with the more soluble ones such as methoxyflurane (Fig. 24-3). Therefore the less soluble inhalational agents reach equilibrium more quickly. Yet, even though the tension of the less soluble agents such as nitrous oxide or sevoflurane rises more quickly, less of the agent is transferred and dissolved in blood and tissue when compared to the more soluble agents (Table 24-1). The **lipid solubility,** measured as the partition coefficient of the agent between oil and gas ($P_{o/g}$) at equilibrium, correlates with anesthetic potency. As the lipid solubility increases, the anesthetic potency increases (MAC [minimum alveolar concentration] decreases), as predicted by the membrane theories of anesthesia. Note: There is virtually no barrier to the movement of anesthetic agents between the alveoli and blood.

4. *Cardiac output,* which delivers the agent to the tissues. Alterations in cardiac output have opposing effects on uptake. Increases in pulmonary blood flow will result in more rapid transport of anesthetics from the alveoli; therefore rate of uptake is increased but the equilibration between the alveolar and arterial partial pressures is delayed. However, increases in cardiac output will increase the delivery of anesthetic to the brain, increasing the rate of tissue equilibration, and thereby hastening the onset of anesthe-

sia. Except for extreme conditions of drug solubility or changes in cardiac output, this factor has a minor overall effect.

5. *Transfer of anesthetic from blood into tissues,* which depends upon the solubility of the agent in tissue and the concentration gradient between blood and tissue. The blood flow, i.e., the rate of delivery, to the tissues is also important. Brain, heart, kidneys, gut, and endocrine glands receive the highest blood flow. This is the vessel-rich group of tissues, and they reach peak concentrations of anesthetic agent faster than tissues such as muscle or fat (Fig. 24-4).

Distribution

All anesthetic agents have some degree of lipid solubility, and they will therefore cross cell membranes and distribute into the total body water. They readily cross the blood–brain barrier; otherwise they would not be able to act as general anesthetics.

Biotransformation

Although initially it was thought that the volatile anesthetics were chemically inert, it is now known that all are biotransformed to some degree in the

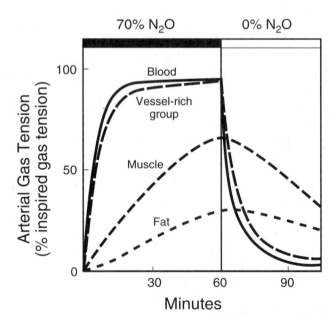

Figure 24-4. Idealized tensions of inhaled anesthetic in blood, tissues, and fat during 60 minutes of inhaling nitrous oxide and 45 minutes of its elimination. (Modified from Cowles AL, Borgstedt HH, Gillies AJ. *Anesth Analg* 1968; 47:404–414.)

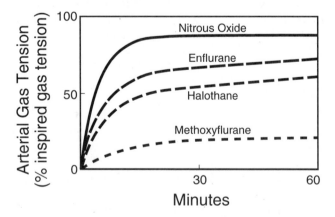

Figure 24-3. Idealized tensions of inhalational anesthetics in blood expressed as a percent of the inspired gas tension with time. (Adapted from Eger EI. *Anesthetic Uptake and Action.* Baltimore: Williams & Wilkins, 1974.)

Table 24-1 Partition Coefficients and Minimum Alveolar Concentrations for Some Anesthetic Gases and Vapors

Agent	$P_{b/g}$*	$P_{br/b}$†	$P_{o/g}$‡	MAC§
Desflurane	0.42	1.3	18.7	6.0
Nitrous oxide	0.47	1.1	1.4	104.0
Sevoflurane	0.60	1.7	53.4	1.71
Isoflurane	1.4	2.6	90.8	1.16
Enflurane	1.9	1.4	98.5	1.68
Halothane	2.3	2.9	224.0	0.76
Methoxyflurane	12.0	2.0	970.0	0.16

*Blood/gas partition coefficient at equilibrium.

†Brain/blood partition coefficient at equilibrium.

‡Oil/gas partition coefficient.

§Minimum alveolar concentration (μmoles/100 mL) required to prevent movement of 50% of patients in response to a surgical stimulus.

Data from Barash PG, Cullen BF, Stoelting RK. *Clinical Anesthesia*, 1992.

liver. The proportion of anesthetic agent taken into the body that is biotransformed ranges from as much as 50% for methoxyflurane and 20% for halothane to 3% for sevoflurane, 2% for enflurane, 0.2% for isoflurane, and 0.02% for desflurane. Biotransformation may continue for a period of 4–5 days following the administration of an anesthetic, as the remaining drug is mobilized from muscle and fat stores back into the circulation.

Elimination

Recovery from a volatile anesthetic occurs once the administration is stopped and the drug diffuses from the blood into the alveolar gas space and is exhaled. The rate of elimination from the body is dependent upon:

1. Transfer of anesthetic from tissue into blood. This can be slow for highly lipid-soluble agents, such as methoxyflurane, coming out of muscle and adipose tissue. This accounts for the prolonged biotransformation of some drugs over 4–5 days. Transfer is, however, more rapid from the brain, so a patient is usually awake from the inhalational agents 5–10 minutes after administration of the anesthetic is stopped.

2. Cardiac output, which affects the rate of delivery of the agent to the lungs.

3. Relative solubilities of the anesthetic in blood and in alveolar gas ($P_{b/g}$). As with uptake, elimination of an inhaled anesthetic from the blood into alveolar air in the lung is more rapid for the less

blood-soluble agents such as N_2O, desflurane, and sevoflurane.

4. Rate of alveolar ventilation.

Figure 24-4 shows uptake and elimination phases of a relatively water-insoluble inhalational anesthetic such as N_2O.

Minimum alveolar concentration

In order to compare the potencies of the various inhalational anesthetic agents as well as to give a quantitative basis for their administration, the concept of the "minimum alveolar concentration" (MAC) was developed. This is the minimal concentration of the inhalational anesthetic agent (expressed as percent of total gas mixture) in the alveolus that will inhibit purposeful movement of 50% of patients following surgical stimulation, such as a skin incision. Since this is measured at or near steady-state conditions, the concentration of anesthetic agent in the brain tissue will be about 500 μmoles/100 mL of membrane volume for any inhalational anesthetic agent used. To achieve this concentration in the neuronal membranes, and thus inhibit purposeful movement by the patient, for halothane the inspired concentration must be about 0.76% (v/v), while the more lipid-soluble agent methoxyflurane will require only 0.16% (v/v).

Note that MAC is the alveolar concentration at equilibrium and is independent of the time required to reach this. However, the time for induction of anesthesia and the time required to reach equilibrium depend upon the blood/gas solubility of the agent, being more rapid for the less soluble agents (see above).

ANESTHETIC GASES

The three best-known anesthetic gases are nitrous oxide (N_2O), ethylene, and cyclopropane. Of these, only N_2O is in current use. The other agents, which have explosion potential, are of historical interest and can be read about in older textbooks.

Nitrous Oxide

N_2O is a nonirritating, colorless gas with a mildly sweet odor. Its boiling point is $-89°C$, and its critical temperature is $36.5°C$. It is furnished in tanks under pressure, as a liquid in equilibrium with its gas phase. It is nonflammable and nonexplosive but does support combustion. Its relevant partition coefficients are shown in Table 24-1.

Pharmacokinetics

N_2O is characterized by its low solubility in blood ($P_{b/g} = 0.47$) and tissue. It therefore readily reaches its limiting concentration in blood and tissues, leading to rapid uptake and rapid elimination. It is not biotransformed and is excreted unchanged. In the blood N_2O is 34 times more soluble than nitrogen. Because of this, N_2O can enter a closed space such as an obstructed bowel, pneumothorax, or middle ear at a faster rate than nitrogen can be removed, and the volume of gas contained within that closed space can significantly expand.

Pharmacological effects

N_2O has a MAC of 104%, consistent with it being a very weak general anesthetic and being unable to provide general anesthesia when administered as the sole agent. It does, however, provide analgesia and sedation even in lower concentrations.

N_2O is used clinically in concentrations up to 70% in combination with oxygen as a supplement to other inhalational or intravenous anesthetics. Its major advantage is that it will reduce the MAC of volatile agents such as halothane when administered concurrently. This, in turn, allows for a reduction in the dose of volatile agents, with a consequent reduction in their dose-dependent adverse effects.

N_2O on its own has minor effects on respiration, but it will potentiate the respiratory depression produced by other agents such as thiopental, opioids, or other inhalational agents. Its effects on the cardiovascular system include mild myocardial depression, but this is counteracted by a mild sympathomimetic effect.

Short-term administration of N_2O for a few hours is not associated with toxicity, but prolonged exposure may have toxic sequelae. N_2O can oxidize and inactivate vitamin B_{12}, the coenzyme for methionine synthase. This can potentially lead to reversible hematopoietic changes such as megaloblastic anemia, leukopenia, and thrombocytopenia, as well as a myeloneuropathy similar to that found in pernicious anemia (see Chapter 43). These changes may assume clinical significance if N_2O is administered continuously for more than 6 hours, or is self-administered repeatedly, as occurs when it is used as a drug of abuse. Occupational exposure is of concern for health professionals, because chronic, low-dose exposure may cause these toxic effects. (Scavenging of waste gases in operating rooms, which is now applied routinely, has greatly reduced the concerns of occupational exposure.)

Oxygen

Although not an anesthetic agent, oxygen is always included as part of the anesthetic gas mixture and must be considered a drug. It is a clear, colorless, odorless gas, with a boiling point of $-182.5°C$ and critical temperature of $-118°C$. It supports combustion.

O_2 is normally present at a partial pressure of 159 mmHg or 21.2 kPa in the atmosphere. Clinically it is generally used in elevated concentrations during anesthesia and in patients in intensive care units.

When inhaled continuously for 24 hours or more in concentrations greater than 50%, O_2 is toxic to lung tissue. In premature infants it is also toxic to the retina.

VOLATILE ANESTHETICS

Diethyl Ether

This agent, once the most widely used, is now only of historical interest in the western world; it is rarely used anywhere. Diethyl ether is a potent anesthetic agent that maintains good respiration during light anesthesia. It maintains a stable blood pressure by releasing endogenous catecholamines. However, this same action may give rise to cardiac arrhythmias. Unfortunately this agent is explosive, making it a great hazard in modern-day operating rooms.

Halothane

This volatile agent was introduced into anesthetic practice in the late 1950s and was for many years the most common agent of its class in use in North America.

Halothane (see Fig. 24-5 and Table 24-1) is a pleasant-smelling, nonirritating and nonexplosive liquid with a boiling point of 50.2°C and a vapor pressure of 243 torr (mmHg) at 20°C. It is soluble

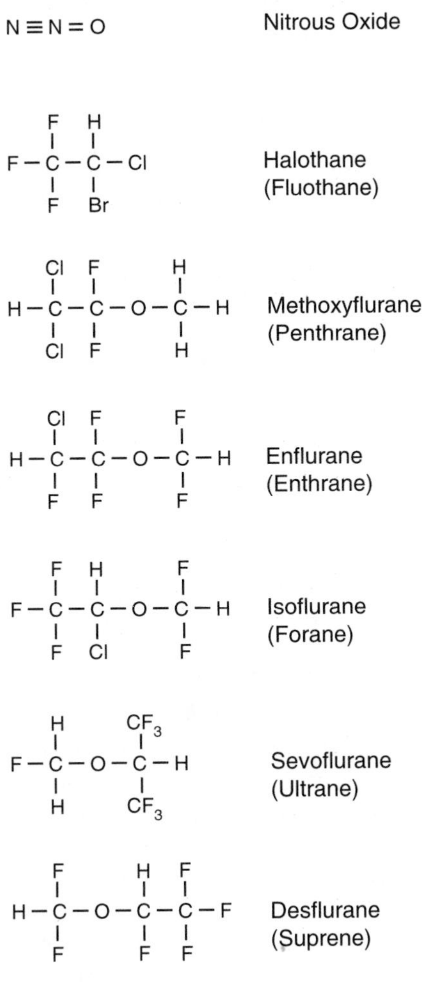

Figure 24-5. Structural formulae of some inhalational anesthetics.

in rubber and is therefore taken up by the tubing in anesthetic equipment.

Pharmacokinetics

The uptake of halothane from the lung is moderately rapid (see Fig. 24-3), so it can be used for inhalational induction of anesthesia in concentrations up to about 4% (v/v). It is used for the maintenance of anesthesia at 0.5–2% (v/v). About 20% of the inhaled dose is biotransformed in the liver; the remainder is rapidly eliminated via the respiratory tract after administration is discontinued.

Pharmacological effects

CNS. Halothane is a potent anesthetic agent, with MAC of 0.76%. It has only a mild, clinically unsatisfactory analgesic effect, usually requiring the addition of an analgesic agent such as N_2O or an opioid.

Respiratory. Halothane vapor does not irritate the respiratory mucosa. It produces a dose-dependent depression of ventilation, with increased rate of respiration but a greater reduction in tidal volume, resulting in a characteristic pattern of short, rapid breaths during anesthesia. There is a reduced respiratory response to raised CO_2 and a greatly depressed response to decreased O_2 (hypoxia).

Cardiovascular. Halothane causes a dose-dependent depression of the myocardium coupled with a relaxation of vascular smooth muscle, resulting in a *fall in blood pressure. The drug sensitizes the myocardium to catecholamines*, so exogenous administration of these agents can produce arrhythmias.

Other. It causes dose-dependent relaxation of uterine contractility that can lead to bleeding in obstetrical surgery such as caesarean sections. It also depresses motility and tone of the gut. Halothane is a poor skeletal muscle relaxant, but it will potentiate neuromuscular blocking agents, allowing for the use of less neuromuscular blocker to achieve the same degree of muscle relaxation.

Toxicity

Although halothane has the lowest mortality risk of any general anesthetic, postoperative hepatitis has been described as a rare complication in about one in 35,000 cases of halothane anesthesia (see Chapter 46). However, a cause-effect relationship is difficult to establish.

In genetically susceptible subjects, halothane (and other volatile general anesthetics) may precipitate a malignant hyperthermia crisis (see Chapter 12).

Methoxyflurane

This volatile anesthetic agent was specifically designed to have high solubility in blood (see Table 24-1), resulting in a slow induction and emergence. These properties were chosen deliberately because they were thought to provide more safety because of better control during induction, even though they also meant slower recovery from anesthesia. Methoxyflurane (see Fig. 24-5) gained some popularity in the late 1960s. However, approximately 50% of the inhaled dose is biotransformed, releasing free fluoride, which is toxic to the kidney. Therefore this agent is rarely used in North America today. It is a good analgesic and has been used for pain relief during labor or during short procedures such as wound dressing changes.

Isoflurane

Along with its isomer enflurane, this drug is the most popular volatile anesthetic in use today in North America. Isoflurane (see Fig. 24-5 and Table 24-1) is a pleasant-smelling, nonirritating, nonexplosive vapor. Its boiling point is 48.5°C and its vapor pressure is 238 torr (mmHg) at 20°C.

Pharmacokinetics

The uptake of isoflurane is similar to that of halothane. The concentration used for induction of anesthesia is usually 2–4% (v/v), and for maintenance 1–2% (v/v) in an O_2:N_2O mixture. Only about 0.2% of the inhaled dose is biotransformed.

Pharmacological effects

CNS. This potent inhalational anesthetic has mild analgesic properties. It produces CNS depression, reducing cerebral metabolic rate. The MAC for isoflurane is 1.16% (v/v).

Respiratory. A concentration-dependent depression of minute ventilation occurs, resulting in in-

creasing arterial P_{CO_2} concentrations. There is a reduced ventilatory response to CO_2 and a greatly depressed response to hypoxia. Isoflurane inhalation results in bronchodilatation.

Cardiovascular. Isoflurane produces concentration-dependent depression of the myocardium, with a resulting fall in blood pressure. However, this agent does *not* sensitize the myocardium to catecholamines, which is one of its advantages over halothane. One of the advantages of isoflurane is that it tends to maintain cardiac output by dilating peripheral vascular beds and thus reducing blood pressure or afterload.

Other. It produces only a mild degree of muscle relaxation, but it will potentiate neuromuscular blocking agents.

This agent will also precipitate malignant hyperthermia in genetically susceptible individuals.

Enflurane

This isomer of isoflurane (see Fig. 24-5 and Table 24-1) is a potent inhalational anesthetic with a MAC of 1.68%. It has physical and pharmacological properties that offer some advantages when compared to isoflurane. However, enflurane produces excitation at higher doses, resulting in seizure-like activity in the EEG that may be manifested as twitching of muscles. Like isoflurane and halothane, it causes bronchodilatation. For surgical cases lasting more than 8 hours the administration of this agent results in elevated circulating fluoride concentrations, since about 2% of the inhaled dose is biotransformed. Enflurane can precipitate a malignant hyperthermia crisis in susceptible individuals.

Sevoflurane

This volatile anesthetic (see Fig. 24-5 and Table 24-1) was first used in humans in 1971. It has low solubility in blood ($P_{b/g}$ = 0.6), similar to that of nitrous oxide, and therefore the induction of anesthesia is rapid, limited primarily by the adequacy of alveolar ventilation and the rate of increase in the inspired concentration. Elimination of the agent from the body is likewise rapid, so patients wake up and recover relatively quickly. Sevoflurane is a potent anesthetic agent with a MAC value of 1.71% of the inspired gas. Like isoflurane and enflurane, sevoflurane causes a decrease in blood pressure and cardiac output, and it does *not* sensitize the myocardium to catecholamines. It produces a concentration-dependent decrease in alveolar ventilation. About 3% of the inspired dose of sevoflurane is metabolized to release fluoride. As with all currently used inhalational anesthetic agents, sevoflurane can trigger malignant hyperthermia.

Desflurane

This volatile anesthetic (see Fig. 24-5 and Table 24-1) was first used in humans in 1987. Like sevoflurane and nitrous oxide, it has low blood solubility ($P_{b/g}$ = 0.42); therefore induction and recovery from anesthesia are relatively rapid. Unfortunately, desflurane has a pungent odor which limits its use for inhalational induction. Like other volatile anesthetics, it causes concentration-dependent reductions in blood pressure and respiration, and it does *not* sensitize the myocardium to catecholamines. Desflurane is resistant to biodegradation; only about 0.02% of the inspired dose is metabolized. Its MAC is 6.0% in adults. The agent can also trigger malignant hyperthermia in susceptible individuals.

INTRAVENOUS ANESTHETICS

Rapidly acting and short-acting intravenous agents are commonly used today for the induction of anesthesia. The most commonly used drug is thiopental. Other agents used for the same purpose include methohexital, propofol, and ketamine. High doses of opioid analgesics, such as fentanyl, can also be used intravenously for the induction and maintenance of anesthesia. The disadvantages attached to all of these are the irrevocability of intravenous administration of a potent drug and the consequent dangers of overdosing the patient.

Furthermore, while quite safe in the hands of specialists who are prepared to deal with side effects and anesthesia accidents, the intravenous anesthetics are very dangerous when used on an occasional basis by the inexperienced practitioner who falls prey to the temptations of convenience!

Thiopental Sodium

This thiobarbiturate is available as a pale yellow powder. It is a weak acid, pK_a 7.6 and is therefore readily soluble in alkaline medium. It is usually prepared as a 2.5% aqueous solution at pH 10.5.

Pharmacokinetics

Thiopental is highly lipid-soluble, having a $P_{o/w}$ = 35 in the unionized form. Thus it can readily cross cell membranes and rapidly enter brain tissue.

With rapid intravenous administration there is prompt distribution into the vessel-rich group of tissues (brain, heart, lung, kidney, liver, intestine, endocrine glands) which induces unconsciousness in 10–15 seconds. The onset of action, therefore, is partly a function of the speed of injection.

The termination of action, however, is due to redistribution of the drug out of the brain and other vessel-rich tissues into less well-perfused tissues including skeletal muscle, and then into adipose tissue, where peak levels are not reached until more than 2 hours later (Fig. 24-6).

Thiopental is biotransformed in the liver by the cytochrome P450–dependent mixed-function oxidase system, resulting in side-chain oxidation and demethylation. This process, with a half-life of 6.5 hours, is much slower than the redistribution process. Because of the long half-life, with repeated doses of thiopental the various body stores begin to fill up and the drug accumulates in the body. As a result, patients with such accumulation may be asleep for a very long period (days). This is why thiopental is not used as the sole anesthetic agent except for procedures of very short duration. Renal excretion of the parent compound is negligible.

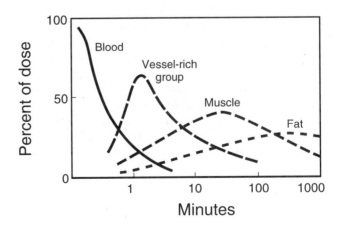

Figure 24-6. Distribution of anesthetic agent in various compartments following intravenous administration. Note the log-scale for time.

Thiopental crosses the placenta readily, and peak fetal blood levels occur in about 3 minutes.

Pharmacological Effects

CNS. The rapid injection of 3–5 mg/kg will produce loss of consciousness in one arm–brain circulation time. The duration of sleep is approximately 5 minutes, depending on the dose given.

However, thiopental lowers the threshold for pain, resulting in an increased sensitivity to pain or hyperalgesia. It is also a poor muscle relaxant.

It reduces brain metabolic rate and consequently brain blood flow. This will reduce intracranial pressure. Therefore, under controlled conditions, thiopental is very effective for the acute treatment of raised intracranial pressure.

Respiratory. It is a potent respiratory depressant, so there is usually a period of apnea during induction of anesthesia. This effect is enhanced by premedication with other depressant drugs. Thiopental causes a dose-dependent decrease in the response of the respiratory center to changes in P_{CO_2} and P_{O_2}.

Cardiovascular. Thiopental is a direct myocardial depressant and vascular smooth muscle relaxant, producing a dose-dependent fall in blood pressure. Accidental intra-arterial injection of concentrations greater than 2.5% causes vascular spasm, primarily due to the alkalinity of thiopental solutions. The vasospasm can result in tissue damage and loss of part of the limb.

Other. Clinically, thiopental is used in doses of 3–5 mg/kg in a normal patient. This agent would be relatively contraindicated in patients with hypovolemic shock, and the dose must be greatly reduced in the elderly and in patients with myxedema. The use of all barbiturates, including thiopental, is contraindicated in patients with the relatively rare defect in heme synthesis seen in the porphyrias. Because barbiturate administration results in a marked increase in the porphyrin synthetic pathway, resulting in an overproduction of intermediate products of heme synthesis, an exacerbation of the disease process can occur.

Methohexital

This is an ultrashort-acting oxybarbiturate with pharmacological properties similar to those of thiopental. It is about three times as potent as thiopental, the usual induction dose being about 1 mg/kg i.v.

Propofol

Propofol, 2,6-diisopropylphenol, belongs to a new class of anesthetic agent. It is practically insoluble in water, so its clinical use requires it to be formulated as a 1% aqueous emulsion containing soybean oil, glycerol, and egg phosphatide.

Pharmacokinetics

Intravenous administration of propofol, like that of thiopental, results in a distribution of the drug into the vessel-rich group of tissues, including brain. Unconsciousness is induced in 15–30 seconds, depending on the speed of injection. Propofol can be irritating to the blood vessel at the site of injection, necessitating a somewhat slower rate of injection and thus a slow onset of anesthesia. The termination of action is due to the redistribution of the drug out of the brain into less well perfused tissues such as muscle and fat, such that the patient will wake up in 5–10 minutes. The redistribution $t_{1/2\alpha}$ is about 5 minutes.

As well, propofol is rapidly and extensively metabolized in the liver. About 98% is excreted in the urine: 40% is found as propofol-glucuronide or -sulfate, while approximately 60% is metabolized by the cytochrome P450–dependent mixed-function oxidase system to 2,6-diisopropyl-1,4-quinol, which is then conjugated to glucuronide or sulfate. This elimination process has a half-life of about 2–3 hours. Because of rapid biotransformation and elimination, this drug does not accumulate in the body to any great extent and therefore, unlike thiopental, it can be used to maintain anesthesia with continuous infusion. At subhypnotic doses propofol can be used for sedation.

Pharmacological effects

CNS. Propofol induces unconsciousness following a dose of 1–2 mg/kg i.v. The duration of sleep is about 5–10 minutes, depending on the dose used.

Unlike thiopental, propofol does not cause hyperalgesia, so it is useful for intravenous sedation and for the maintenance of anesthesia during surgery.

Respiratory. Induction of anesthesia with propofol is frequently accompanied by a period of apnea that may last for more than 1 minute depending on the dose administered. The maintenance of anesthesia with propofol results in a dose-dependent decrease in ventilation and a rise in blood CO_2 levels. This respiratory depression is increased when propofol is administered with other anesthetic adjuvants such as opioids and benzodiazepines.

Cardiovascular. Propofol administration results in a reduction in both systolic and diastolic blood pressure and is associated with reduced cardiac output and vascular resistance. This effect is potentiated by prior opioid analgesic administration. When propofol is used for the maintenance of anesthesia, the blood pressure is reduced by about 20%.

Other. As with most other induction agents, propofol must be used with great caution in patients with hypovolemia or shock, and in the elderly. Propofol does not trigger malignant hyperthermia crises; it can be used to induce and maintain anesthesia in susceptible individuals.

Etomidate

Etomidate is a methylbenzyl-imidazole derivative that is structurally unlike the other intravenous anesthetics. It is a weak base, pK_a 3.0, that is dissolved in propylene glycol for use as an intravenous anesthetic. At a dose of 0.3 mg/kg, it produces a rapid induction of anesthesia much as thiopental does. Consciousness is regained in 5–10 minutes, but full recovery may take longer than with thiopental. The drug is biotransformed in the liver with a half-life of 2.9 hours. The major advantage of etomidate is its minimal effect on the cardiovascular system. It produces a dose-related depression of respiration.

The drug depresses adrenal steroidogenesis and therefore cannot be used for long-term administration. Although available in Europe and the United States (as of 1992), this drug has not been licensed for use in Canada.

Midazolam

Midazolam is a water-soluble benzodiazepine that is most commonly used for sedation or as an adjunct to anesthesia. It can also be used for the induction and maintenance of anesthesia. In a dose of 0.15–0.4 mg/kg administered over 4–5 seconds, it induces unconsciousness in about 60 seconds and patients remain asleep for 7–15 minutes, which is longer than with thiopental or propofol. The induction of anesthesia with midazolam is generally preceded by administration of an opioid such as fentanyl, which will prolong the sleep time. Midazolam provides a smooth induction of anesthesia with minimal effects on the cardiovascular system.

Midazolam is biotransformed in the liver. It has a half-life of elimination of about 2.7 hours, which is considerably shorter than the 24–36 hours for diazepam (see Chapter 27).

Ketamine

Ketamine is a phenylcyclohexylamine derivative that can be used for rapid induction of anesthesia by the intravenous (1–2 mg/kg) or intramuscular (5–10 mg/kg) route. In lower doses it induces sedation, analgesia, and amnesia. As with other intravenous anesthetics, it is initially distributed to highly perfused tissues and is then redistributed to less well perfused tissues. The redistribution results in termination of its action. The redistribution half-life is about 10–15 minutes. Ketamine is biotransformed in the liver into multiple metabolites, including norketamine, which has an anesthetic potency approximately one-third that of ketamine. Its elimination half-life is 2–3 hours.

Ketamine appears to exert its anesthetic and analgesic actions by blocking the cation channels that are activated by the *N*-methyl-D-aspartate (NMDA) subtype of receptor for the excitatory neurotransmitter glutamate.

Ketamine produces a unique state that has been described as *dissociative anesthesia*, which is characterized by profound analgesia, amnesia, and catalepsy. The dissociation component refers to a functional and electrophysiological separation of the normal communications between the sensory cortex and the association areas in the brain. The result resembles catalepsy, in which the eyes may remain open with slow nystagmus and intact corneal reflexes. Patients are generally noncommunicative, although they appear to be awake. Varying degrees of skeletal muscle hypertonus may be present, along with nonpurposeful skeletal muscle movements that are independent of surgical stimulation.

Ketamine differs from most anesthetic agents in that it *stimulates the cardiovascular system*, producing increases in heart rate, cardiac output, and blood pressure. Its ability to maintain arterial blood pressure is particularly useful in hypovolemic patients and those in cardiogenic shock. Conversely, ketamine is contraindicated when an elevation of blood pressure should be avoided, as in patients with a history of significant coronary artery disease, hypertension, or cerebrovascular disease. Furthermore, ketamine potentially increases cerebral blood flow and is therefore contraindicated in patients with raised intracranial pressure.

Ketamine can maintain normal lung volumes and can induce bronchodilatation. It is therefore useful in patients with asthma. It is a potent stimulator of salivary and tracheobronchial secretions; therefore antimuscarinics such as atropine are often administered concurrently. Emergence phenomena, described as vivid dreams, hallucinations, and delirium, have been reported. They appear to be related to the dose and rate of drug administration. The incidence of these phenomena is reduced when benzodiazepines are administered concurrently.

High-Dose Opioid Anesthesia

This procedure has proven to be highly effective in cardiovascular surgery. Although morphine was used initially, the commonly preferred drug today is fentanyl (see Chapter 23) at doses of up to 150 μg/kg (the usual analgesic dose is only 1 μg/kg). The high dose of fentanyl is combined with a muscle relaxant, endotracheal intubation, and ventilation with 100% O_2. This technique of anesthesia provides a high degree of stability of blood pressure and cardiac output, but because of the very large dose of fentanyl used, ventilatory support is required postoperatively while the opioid is biotransformed and excreted.

Neuroleptanalgesia/Anesthesia

This has been described as a state of drug-induced depression of activity, lack of initiative, and reduced response to external stimuli. The patient has good analgesia and is sedated, yet is able to respond to simple commands.

For example, neuroleptanalgesia in a 60–70-kg

individual is usually produced by means of intravenous injection of a combination of a potent, short-acting opioid such as fentanyl (50–100 μg) and a short-acting benzodiazepine such as midazolam (0.5–1.0 mg). To this may be added a small dose of the butyrophenone droperidol (0.5–1.25 mg), or propofol (10–20 mg), as required for adequate sedation.

This neuroleptanalgesic state can be readily converted into unconsciousness (neuroleptanesthesia) by the addition of small doses of an induction agent such as thiopental or propofol or by the addition of a mixture of O_2:N_2O or N_2O:O_2:halothane.

Intravenous Sedation

Intravenous sedation is commonly used in conjunction with local infiltration or regional anesthesia to help the patient relax and perhaps experience amnesia for the period of the surgical procedure. Commonly used agents include fentanyl, midazolam, and propofol. These patients must be monitored closely because of the severe consequences of an overdose and of respiratory depression.

SUGGESTED READING

Barash PG, Cullen BF, Stoelting RK. Clinical Anesthesia. 2nd ed. Philadelphia: JB Lippincott, 1992.

Dripps RD, Eckenhoff JE, Vandam CD. Introduction to anesthesia: the principles of safe practice. Philadelphia: WB Saunders, 1982.

Franks NP, Lieb WR. Mechanisms of general anesthesia. Environ Health Perspect 1990; 87:199–205.

Miller RD. ed. Anesthesia. 3rd ed. New York: Churchill Livingstone, 1990.

Tanelian DL, Kosek E, Mody I, MacIver MB. The role of the GABA$_A$ receptor/chloride channel complex in anesthesia. Anesthesiology 1993; 78:757–776.

Ueda I, Kamaya H. Molecular mechanisms of anesthesia. Anesth Analg 1984; 63:929–945.

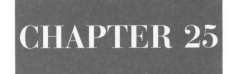

CHAPTER 25

Local Anesthetics

D.A. HAAS AND F.J. CARMICHAEL

CASE HISTORY

A 58-year-old male patient required local anesthesia for the surgical removal of an abscessed tooth, a procedure that was estimated to require 30 minutes of surgical time. The patient's medical history included mild hypertension, which was well controlled with daily administrations of a diuretic; his blood pressure on examination was 124/80 mmHg. His history also included a pseudocholinesterase deficiency that had been discovered some years earlier in relation to surgery under general anesthesia and succinylcholine, and he reported that he had a "bad reaction" to the administration of a local anesthetic in the past. When questioned on this last point, he recalled that he once fainted following an injection of local anesthetic for a dental procedure many years ago but since that time has had local anesthetic administered uneventfully.

The presence of infection necessitated administration of local anesthetic in a site away from the abscess, and a regional nerve block was chosen instead of infiltration directly adjacent to the tooth. The estimated length of time for the surgical procedure indicated the use of an intermediate-acting local anesthetic with vasoconstrictor. The history of pseudocholinesterase deficiency ruled out the use of an ester-type anesthetic. Because of the patient's cardiovascular history, a relatively low concentration of vasoconstrictor was advised as a cautionary measure. The combination of drugs was therefore 1.5 mL of lidocaine 2% with 5 μg/mL (1:200,000) epinephrine for this regional nerve block.

Within 2 minutes of injection the patient felt faint. He was placed in a supine position with his legs elevated, which quickly relieved his symptoms. This reaction was quite likely psychogenic in nature, unrelated to the selection of drugs. Addressing the patient's anxiety would have helped to lessen the likelihood of this reaction.

Once the patient reported feeling well, the signs and symptoms of a successful nerve block were noted, and the surgery was carried out successfully.

Local anesthetics are drugs that can reversibly block the generation and propagation of nerve impulses. They are capable of depressing conduction in all excitable cells and therefore potentially interfere with the function of tissues in which impulse transmission occurs. This includes both sensory and motor peripheral nerves, autonomic ganglia, the central nervous system, neuromuscular junction, cardiac muscle, and smooth muscle. Their primary indications are to temporarily eliminate sensation at a specific site in order to permit surgical treatment or to relieve pain. A number of these agents can also be used as antiarrhythmics, as discussed in more detail in Chapter 37. Overall, local anesthetics rank among the most widely used drugs.

The history of local anesthetics began with cocaine, which had been isolated in 1860. It was the active ingredient of the extracts of the leaves of the Andean shrub *Erythroxylon coca*, which were known to confer insensitivity to delicate tissues. In 1884 Koller demonstrated the local anesthetic effects of cocaine on the conjunctiva of animals, and Hall used cocaine in dentistry. It was used by Halstead in 1885 for nerve blocks and by Bier in 1898 for the first spinal anesthesia in man. In 1904 Einhorn synthesized procaine, and in subsequent years many new local anesthetic agents have been synthesized and used clinically.

CHEMISTRY

Local anesthetics have in common specific fundamental structural features, as illustrated in Figure 25-1. The first of the three characteristic features is a lipophilic portion composed of an aromatic nucleus derived from para-aminobenzoic acid (PABA) as in procaine, or from aniline as in lidocaine. This portion is then joined by an amide or ester linkage to an intermediate alkyl chain, the second characteristic feature. The third feature is a hydrophilic secondary or tertiary amino terminus. The lipophilicity of the aromatic group facilitates penetration into the nerve sheath and subsequently into the nerve membrane itself. Both the hydrophilic and lipophilic groups are necessary for drug action. Because of the amino terminus, local anesthetics are weak bases that can exist as either charged or uncharged molecules. The free base form is only slightly soluble in water and local anesthetics are therefore usually formulated as the water-soluble hydrochloride salts. The properties of local anesthetics are summarized in Table 25-1.

MECHANISM OF ACTION

Nerve Membrane and Action Potentials

The function of the nerve cell is to convey information from one part of the body to another. This information is passed along the nerve fiber, or axon, in the form of electrical action potentials or impulses. Peripheral nerves are generally a mixed population of nerve fibers with different diameters and rates of impulse conduction. These nerve fibers are arranged in a series of bundles, or fascicles, that are surrounded by layers of connective tissue. A single axon is a long cylinder of neural cytoplasm, the axoplasm, surrounded by the nerve membrane, which is further encased in either a thin sheath in the case of nonmyelinated nerves, or multiple layers of myelin in the case of myelinated nerves. The nerve membrane itself consists of a double layer of phospholipid molecules, with their polar head-groups oriented toward the two surfaces and their nonpolar carbon chains oriented

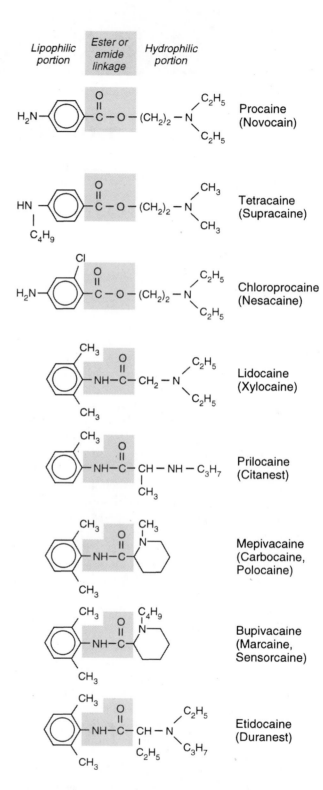

Figure 25-1. Structural formulae of local anesthetics, illustrating common structural features (see text).

Table 25-1 Properties of Representative Local Anesthetics

Drug	Pk_a	Ionized/Unionized at pH 7.4	Partition Coefficient*	Plasma Protein Binding (%)	Onset	Duration	Relative Toxicity† (Nonvascular Administration)
						of Action	
Procaine	8.9	32/1	0.02	6	Slow	Short	0.5
Tetracaine	8.2	6/1	4.1	85	Slow	Long	5
Chloroprocaine	9.0	40/1	0.14	?	Rapid	Short	0.3
Lidocaine	7.9	3/1	2.9	64	Rapid	Intermediate	1
Prilocaine	7.9	3/1	0.9	55	Rapid	Intermediate	0.9
Mepivacaine	7.6	1.6/1	0.8	78	Rapid	Intermediate	1
Bupivacaine	8.1	5/1	27.5	96	Slow	Long	4
Etidocaine	7.7	2/1	141	94	Rapid	Long	2

*Heptane/buffer (pH 7.4).
†Toxicity relative to lidocaine = 1.

toward the middle of the membrane (see Fig. 2-4, Chapter 2). Interspaced among the lipids are protein molecules which constitute the various ion channels, also known as ionophores, as well as structural proteins and enzymes. The ionophores are very selective for specific ions, including Na^+ and K^+, and are regulated, or *gated*, by a membrane potential that is measured in terms of its voltage differential. Therefore these are known as *voltage-gated channels*. There are also passive ion channels for Na^+, K^+, and Cl^-, which contribute to the resting membrane potential and the leakage of ions into and out of the nerve cell (see Fig. 24-1, Chapter 24).

The electrophysiological properties of the nerve membrane are dependent on the concentration of electrolytes on either side of the nerve membrane as well as its permeability to Na^+ and K^+. The resting neural membrane is relatively impermeable to Na^+ and selectively permeable to K^+. In the resting state there is a voltage gradient across the nerve membrane of approximately -70 mV, with the interior negative relative to the exterior. This potential difference is maintained by the $(Na^+ + K^+)$-ATPase pump through the constant extrusion of Na^+ from inside the cell in exchange for K^+, with resultant high intracellular K^+ and high extracellular Na^+ concentrations.

Action potentials are transient depolarizations of these excitable nerve cells. The reversal of the membrane potential during the generation or conduction of an action potential has been shown to be due to an increased permeability of the membrane for Na^+.

This leads to the membrane potential becoming less negative, which in turn is followed by a rapid influx of Na^+ into the cell, thereby further accelerating depolarization. The Na^+ channels then close, and this is followed by the more slowly developing outflow of K^+ of a similar magnitude, which repolarizes the membrane. Figure 25-2 shows the changes in membrane potential and the corresponding ionic currents during an action potential.

Ionophores can be present in three configurations. In the resting nerve most Na^+ channels are in a *closed* state, such that the nerve cell is relatively impermeable. Depolarization causes these channels to be in the *open or activated* conformation, which allows Na^+ influx. Rapidly after this, however, the channels change to an impermeable *inactivated* conformation. This latter state is refractory to further stimulation until it returns to the resting, or *closed*, state. The *inactivated* state results in nerve conduction being unidirectional. The impulse is propagated along the axon by a local electrotonic current created by the potential difference between the depolarized section and the adjacent nondepolarized membrane.

Site and Mode of Action of Local Anesthetics

Local anesthetics exert their effect on impulse conduction through an action directly on the nerve membrane. They induce a reversible and dose-dependent reduction in the rate of rise and height of the action potential, progressing to the point of total inhibition. There is also an elevation of the firing threshold and

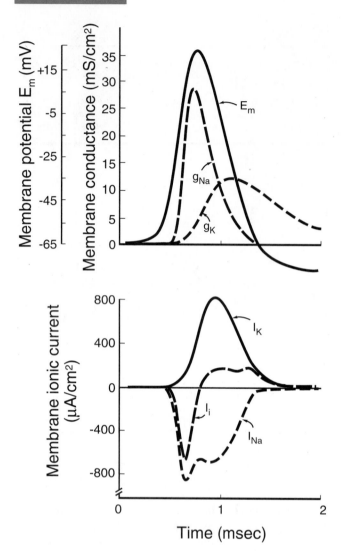

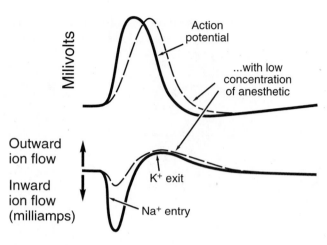

Figure 25-3. Voltage clamp experiments show that the local anesthetics primarily block the entry of Na^+ without affecting the exit of K^+.

Figure 25-2. The course of changes in membrane potential (E_m), membrane conductances of Na^+ (g_{Na}) and K^+ (g_K) (top), and the related Na^+ currents (I_{Na}), K^+ currents (I_K), and total membrane ionic current (I_i) (bottom), during propagation of an action potential in squid giant axon. The early, inward I_{Na} drives the regenerative depolarizing phase of the impulse, whereas the more slowly developing I_K underlies the rapid phase of repolarization. (Adapted from Butterworth JF and Strichartz GR. *Anesthesiology* 1990; 72:711–734.)

a slowing of the spread of conduction down the length of the axon. In myelinated nerves these phenomena occur only at the nodes of Ranvier.

As shown in Figure 25-3, voltage clamp experiments have demonstrated that local anesthetics exert their effects primarily by blocking the entry of Na^+ into the cell, thereby preventing the expected transient increase in its permeability. It is believed that

this is accomplished by binding of the ionized drug either to a site directly in the Na^+ channel itself, at the membrane–protein interface, or within the protein subunits of the channel. This prevents opening by inhibiting conformational changes of the protein and preventing the normal cycling process. The effect of local anesthetics on K^+ conduction is less than that on Na^+ conduction. Local anesthetics share this property of blocking Na^+ entry with the highly specific channel blockers tetrodotoxin and saxitoxin, which have been used to advance our understanding of the mechanism of action of local anesthetics.

That the charged cationic form of the local anesthetic molecule blocks neuronal conduction more effectively than the uncharged free base can be demonstrated by altering the pH of the bathing solution in an isolated nerve preparation. The effect of pH on the ability of local anesthetics to block action potentials is illustrated in Figure 25-4. The local anesthetic is more effective at pH 7.0 when more of it is in the form of the charged cation, than at pH 8.0 when more is present as uncharged free base.

Once the necessary minimum number of channels are blocked over a length of the axon, the action potential can not be propagated. This is illustrated in Figure 25-5, which represents a small- and large-diameter axon, each having approximately the same density of Na^+ channels per unit of surface area. Following generation of the nerve impulse, depolarization spreads electrotonically further and more rapidly down the large axon than down the smaller axon. These local currents trigger the opening of the Na^+ channels, drawn as empty circles in Figure 25-5. The spread is unidirectional as the open channels

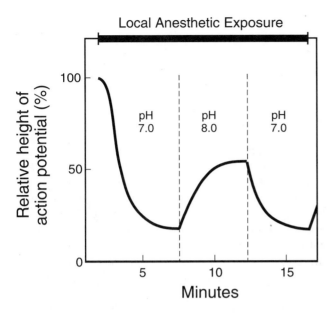

Figure 25-4. Effect of changing the pH of the internal bathing solution on the height of the action potential in the isolated giant axon of the squid while exposed to local anesthetic action. (Adapted from Narahashi T, Frazier DT, Yamada M. *J Pharmacol Exp Ther* 1970; 171:32–51.)

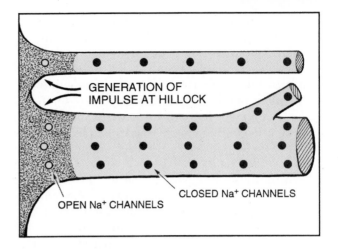

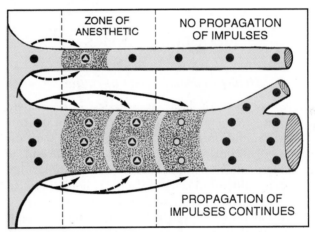

Figure 25-5. Blockade of impulse propagation in small- and large-diameter axons (see text).

then cycle into the refractory closed state. The large axon will have more excited channels than the small axon. When the anesthetic is applied in a fixed concentration to a limited area of each axon, the small axon becomes completely blocked because its few excited channels are prevented from opening by the anesthetic. The larger axon escapes blockade because more Na^+ channels are being excited and the limited amount of anesthetic blocks only a portion of them. This property leads to a differential sensitivity of nerve fibers, such that the smaller fibers are more susceptible to blockade than larger fibers. As a result, there may be differential sensory and motor blockade. There are no intrinsic differences between sensory and motor nerves; however, there are differences in fiber size and myelination that account for this phenomenon.

Anesthetic action can be increased by repeated stimulation of the nerve fiber. This is known as a *frequency-dependent or phasic block* and appears to be due to local anesthetic gaining access more readily to the binding site, as well as having a greater affinity for the binding site, when the channel is open. The result is that noxious stimuli, which can cause repeated bursts of depolarization, may be blocked preferentially to motor activity due to the relative differences in frequencies of stimulation.

TYPES OF LOCAL ANESTHETIC BLOCK

Topical. Local anesthetic is applied to the surface of the skin, wounds, burns, or mucous membranes.

Infiltration. Local anesthetic is injected directly into or around an area to be treated. This type of block is used for minor surgical procedures.

Regional nerve block. To obtain regional anesthesia, local anesthetic is injected in close proximity to the nerve supplying the area to be anesthetized. This block is used for surgical and dental procedures as well as pain relief.

Spinal. Local anesthetic is injected into the lumbar subarachnoid space to reach the roots of the spinal nerves that supply the site of operation. Spinal block is used in surgery on the lower limbs and pelvis, as well as in obstetrics.

Epidural, peridural, or extradural. Local anesthetic is injected into the extradural space through which the nerve roots pass. Uses are the same as for spinal anesthesia, but the advantage is that the anesthetic agent cannot accidentally rise to a higher segment of the spinal cord than was intended.

Intravenous. Local anesthetic is injected into the venous system of a limb, distal to the point at which the circulation in that limb is interrupted by a tourniquet. Intravenous block is used for surgery on that limb.

Sympathetic. Sympathetic nerve blocks can be used in the treatment of pain caused by reflex sympathetic dystrophies such as causalgia and the shoulder–hand syndrome, or for the intractable pain of carcinoma of the pancreas or the upper abdomen.

PHARMACOKINETICS

Absorption and Onset of Action

The *absorption* of local anesthetics is dependent upon the site of administration, dose, vasodilating properties, and presence of vasoconstrictor. With the exception of intravenous block, it is important to understand that local anesthetic action, unlike that of systemically administered drugs, is not dependent on absorption into the circulation. On the contrary, absorption into the systemic circulation is a major factor in terminating the action. The *onset* of action of local anesthetics depends on the following factors.

Dose

To a limited extent, increases in the administered dose will result in a more rapid onset of action. This is due to the greater number of molecules available to reach the site of action.

Lipid solubility

Uptake by the nerve is facilitated by an increase in lipid solubility of the agents, as this allows more rapid penetration through the nerve sheath. As listed in Table 25-1, relative lipid solubility is reflected in the lipid:water partition coefficient, which is also often related to the potency of the drug.

Site of injection

Diffusion to the site of action is a factor; the further the drug is deposited away from the nerve fiber, the longer it will take to act. Thus, the onset for the in-

filtration technique is quite rapid, whereas that for brachial plexus block may be prolonged. The speed of diffusion is influenced by tissue binding, removal by the circulation, and, in the case of esters, local hydrolysis.

Nerve morphology

The morphology of the nerve bundle must be taken into account when considering the onset of action, as each nerve fiber has a differential sensitivity to the conduction-blocking effects of the agent, as stated earlier. The small, slowly conducting A-δ and C fibers, which conduct pain sensation, are blocked with lower concentrations of local anesthetics than the larger A-α motor fibers. The result of this is a *differential sequence of onset of anesthesia, with pain sensation most susceptible, followed by temperature, touch, proprioception, and finally motor function.*

pH of the tissue

This will determine the ratio of ionized to unionized drug. Although local anesthetics are usually formulated as the hydrochloride salt, and therefore acidic, the strong buffering ability of extracellular fluid rapidly brings the pH of the solution to physiological levels. Carbonation of the local anesthetic may improve the depth of neuronal blockade because the diffusion of carbon dioxide through the nerve membrane will decrease axoplasmic pH. This, in turn, promotes the formation of the charged form of the anesthetic molecule. Carbonated local anesthetics are formulated by the manufacturer by adding CO_2 and sealing the vial under pressure. The clinical advantage of carbonation is equivocal with respect to speed of onset, but it does appear to improve depth of blockade when the local anesthetic is administered epidurally.

pK_a of the drug

The ratio of ionized to unionized drug is also dependent on the pK_a of the drug. The relative degree of ionization has an important influence on rate of onset, duration, and pharmacodynamics. The uncharged base penetrates the membrane and has some activity of its own; therefore a higher ratio of uncharged-to-charged species will increase the speed of onset of action. Some local anesthetic solutions are prepared in buffered alkaline media with the intention of promoting a faster onset attributable to the higher proportion of uncharged molecules. Again, the strong buffering ability of the tissue minimizes this effect. Furthermore, there is a limit to the amount that the pH can be raised because of the need to avoid causing local tissue necrosis.

The ionization of local anesthetics depends on the hydrogen ion concentration of their environment and their pK_a. For example:

$$R - N \underset{CH_3}{\overset{CH_3}{<}} + H^+ \rightleftharpoons R - \overset{\oplus}{\underset{H}{N}} \underset{CH_3}{\overset{CH_3}{<}}$$

These effects may be represented in the following:

$$\underset{\text{Aqueous phases}}{BH^+ \rightleftharpoons H^+ + B} \rightleftharpoons \underset{\substack{\text{Nerve} \\ \text{sheath}}}{\| B \|} \rightleftharpoons \underset{\text{Membrane phase}}{B + H^+ \rightleftharpoons BH^+}$$

Let B represent the local anesthetic base (unionized), and BH^+ the ionized form. The anesthetic has been administered by injection in an aqueous solution in which the ionized and unionized forms exist at equilibrium. Only the unionized form *(B)* can effectively penetrate through the nerve sheath into the nerve membrane, where it once again establishes an equilibrium with the ionized molecule. Once inside the nerve membrane, it is the ionized form that is necessary for effective blockade of Na^+ influx. The less ionized, the greater the uptake into the nerve; but the more ionized, the greater the effect at the membrane itself.

The relative ratios are determined by the pK_a of the agents. This relationship is described by the Henderson-Hasselbalch equation:

$$pK_a - pH = \log [\text{ionized/unionized}]$$

The pK_a of most anesthetics ranges from 7.6 to 9.0. At physiological pH 7.4, most of the local anesthetic will therefore be in the ionized state, as a charged base. An example is lidocaine, which has a pK_a of 7.9. At physiological pH it exists in a ratio of 3:1 ionized to unionized, based on this formula. Another example is procaine with a pK_a of 8.9. The higher pK_a value means that at physiological pH procaine exists in a ratio of approximately 32:1 ionized to unionized. Comparison of these two anesthetics shows that lidocaine has a relatively greater proportion of the unionized form and would be expected to have a more rapid onset of action, which is confirmed clinically. In general, all other factors being equal, the most rapid onset would be expected from agents with the lowest pK_a values (see Table 25-1).

The pH of the tissue may become more acidic during a localized infection and cause a greater proportion of ionized anesthetic, thereby delaying or preventing the onset of action. For example, if lidocaine (pK_a 7.9) is administered into a site of infection in which the local pH is 5.9, there would be a resulting ratio of 100 times as many ionized as unionized forms. Greatly reduced penetration into the nerve tissue would be expected, and this is confirmed clinically.

Duration of Action

The duration of action of local anesthetics depends primarily on the redistribution of the drug away from the site of action. These drugs can often be categorized as short-acting, such as procaine and chloroprocaine; intermediate-acting, such as lidocaine, mepivacaine, and prilocaine; and long-acting, such as bupivacaine, etidocaine, and tetracaine. The duration of action can be altered by the following factors, some of which also influence onset.

Dose

Increases in the administered dose can increase the duration of action. Doubling the dose prolongs duration by about one half-life.

Lipid solubility

Within limits, increases in lipid solubility increase the potency and duration of action. This is due to the greater ease with which the drug penetrates the connective tissue layers and nerve sheath into the hydrophobic portion of the nerve membrane. Since it penetrates more readily, more molecules are now present at the site of action, thus allowing for a longer duration. The relative potencies of local anesthetics, as well as their protein binding, correlate reasonably well in rank order with their lipid solubilities, as measured by their partition coefficients.

Diffusion away from the site

This is the major factor in determining duration of action. It is dependent in part on the vascularity of the tissue surrounding the nerve. Removal from the site is highest with intercostal nerve blocks, followed by lumbar epidural blocks and brachial plexus blocks; slowest removal occurs in poorly vascularized subcutaneous sites. Vasodilating properties differ among the agents, with procaine and lidocaine having strong dilating properties and agents such as bupivacaine having less. Except for cocaine, all local anesthetics are inherently vasodilating to the extent that administration alone in vascular tissues can result in an inappropriately short duration of action.

Diffusion away can be reduced by the addition of a vasoconstrictor. This causes a local reduction of blood flow which in turn reduces the rate of uptake and removal of the drug into the circulation, thereby allowing a longer exposure of the nerve to the local anesthetic. In addition, this reduces the likelihood of systemic toxicity by decreasing the rate of systemic uptake, and it provides localized hemostasis during infiltration for surgery. Epinephrine is most commonly used for this purpose, being supplied as an accompanying agent in a range of concentrations from 5 μg/mL(1:200,000) to 20 μg/mL(1:50,000). Other vasoconstrictors that have been used include phenylephrine, norepinephrine, and levonordefrin.

Protein binding

Highly protein-bound agents such as bupivacaine, etidocaine, and tetracaine have an extended duration of action. It is assumed that the degree of plasma protein binding of local anesthetics correlates with the degree of binding to the nerve membrane proteins that constitute the ion channels. Greater affinity at this latter site would be expected to prolong action. Binding to tissue proteins may also contribute to the duration of action by preventing the free form from diffusing away from the site. Furthermore, increased protein binding of the more lipid-soluble compounds tends to reduce their toxicity and reduce transfer across the placenta.

Distribution, Biotransformation, and Elimination

The distribution of local anesthetics when absorbed into the circulation can be described by a two- or three-compartment model. They distribute widely, with highly perfused tissues having greater concentration, as expected. There is rapid extraction by lung tissue.

Biotransformation is dependent on whether the drug is an ester or amide. Esters are hydrolyzed by plasma cholinesterase or by liver esterases, in most cases releasing free para-aminobenzoic acid (PABA), which is known to be allergenic. As discussed in Chapter 12, patients with atypical plasma cholinesterase would be expected to metabolize procaine at a much lower rate. Clinically, however, this is of little consequence unless potentially toxic levels of anesthetic are employed. Half-lives of elimination of ester-type agents are less than 1 minute.

Amides are biotransformed exclusively by the liver, with the exception of prilocaine, which is also metabolized in plasma and kidneys. Lidocaine, mepivacaine, bupivacaine, and etidocaine are N-dealkylated followed by hydrolysis. One of the active metabolites of lidocaine is monoethylglycine xylidide, which is approximately 80% as potent as lidocaine and may be responsible for the toxicity or adverse effects, such as sedation, when excessive doses are used. One of the metabolites of prilocaine is ortho-toluidine, which reduces hemoglobin to methemoglobin, which may lead to methemoglobinemia if produced in excess. Half-lives of elimination of amide-type agents range from 90 to 160 minutes.

The pharmacokinetic characteristics may be altered depending upon the health of the patient. If hepatic function or blood flow is significantly altered, changes in the plasma levels of the amide anesthetics would be expected. Reduced hepatic function would predispose to toxicity (see below) but, unlike its effect on systemically administered drugs, it would not be expected to cause a significant increase in the duration of action of locally administered anesthetics. Progesterone-induced alterations during pregnancy may possibly lead to increased sensitivity to local anesthetics.

ADVERSE REACTIONS AND TOXICITY

Adverse reactions may be a result of toxicity, allergy, or an anxiety-induced psychogenic reaction. Toxic effects are a function of systemic absorption. High blood levels may be secondary to excessive amounts injected extravascularly, or they could be the result of a single inadvertent intravascular administration into a major vessel. Many factors modify toxicity, such as a raised CO_2 or H^+ level in the patient, which will increase the amount of the more active ionized form. In general, toxicity manifests itself in the central nervous system and cardiovascular system. The nervous system effects include both excitatory and inhibitory phenomena. With increasing doses, central nervous system effects are characterized progressively by mild sedation, lightheadedness, dizziness, sensory disturbances, disorientation, tremors, muscle twitching, tonic-clonic seizures, cardiovascular instability, and ultimately respiratory arrest, cardiovascular collapse, and coma. The ability to cause central excitation is correlated with the intrinsic anesthetic potency.

Local anesthetics have significant cardiovascular effects both on the myocardium and on peripheral vascular smooth muscle. The direct effect on the myocardium is also correlated with anesthetic potency and is reflected in a depression of excitability, rate of conduction, and force of contraction, resulting in decreased cardiac output, hypotension, and eventually cardiovascular system collapse. The effects on myocardial conduction are related to those of some of the antiarrhythmic agents (see Chapter 37).

The drugs are believed to be devoid of direct toxicity to nerves, and nerve function recovers completely following a nerve block or spinal anesthesia. Local skeletal muscle damage may occur, but this effect is reversible.

In general, the incidence of toxicity of local anesthetics is very low. This is largely due to the administration of these drugs into a restricted area of the body, from which systemic absorption occurs only gradually. Recommendations for maximum doses are often given, but these must be assessed critically. Toxicity is dependent upon numerous factors, such as site of administration, speed of injection, and presence of vasoconstrictor. Given this caveat, the maximum recommended doses for infiltration or regional nerve block anesthesia in healthy adults are summarized in Table 25-2.

A true allergy to an amide local anesthetic is rare, whereas esters are somewhat more allergenic because of the metabolite PABA. Allergies to other ingredients in the drug formulation are possible. These include the preservative methylparaben or the antioxidant metabisulfite.

Anxiety-induced psychogenic events are relatively common adverse reactions associated with local anesthetic administration. They may manifest as syncope, nausea, vomiting, or alterations in heart rate or blood pressure, or they may mimic an allergic reaction. Adverse events may also be the result of inadvertent intravascular administration of vasoconstrictor, which would produce the expected cardiovascular signs of sympathetic stimulation.

COMMONLY USED LOCAL ANESTHETICS

Local anesthetics are usually classified by structure on the basis of intermediate linkage of ester or amide type (see Fig. 25-1).

Esters

Cocaine is primarily of historical interest for regional block techniques; this drug is too toxic for other than topical use. Cocaine is unique among local anesthetics in that it induces vasoconstriction and has addiction potential. It may be used for topical application to mucous membranes, including oropharyngeal and nasal cavities, prior to local surgical procedures, bronchoscopy, or nasal intubation.

Procaine was the first synthetic local anesthetic. It has a slow onset, short duration of action, and weak potency. Although procaine has low systemic toxicity, esters in general, as noted above, are more allergenic than the amides. Procaine is most effective when used for infiltration anesthesia or nerve blocks. Although used widely in the past, it has been superseded by amides.

Tetracaine is approximately 10 times as potent as procaine with respect to its anesthetic action and systemic toxicity. It has a long duration of action but a slow onset, due to its relatively high pK_a. Its major clinical application is spinal anesthesia, where it has a more rapid onset due to the reduction in barriers to diffusion. Tetracaine is effective topically, but this use is limited by its significant toxicity, which may occur following absorption through mucous membranes.

Chloroprocaine has a rapid onset of action, short duration, and relatively low systemic toxicity. Its rapid onset of action occurs in spite of its high pK_a because it is formulated in relatively high concentrations, which is feasible because of its low toxic-

Table 25-2 Maximum Recommended Doses of Local Anesthetics*

Drug	Plain Solution (mg/kg)	With Vasoconstrictor (mg/kg)
Procaine	5	8
Tetracaine	1.4	2.8
Chloroprocaine	11	14
Lidocaine	4	7
Prilocaine	7	8
Mepivacaine	4	7
Bupivacaine	2.5	3
Etidocaine	4	6

*Toxicity depends on numerous factors, of which the total administered dose is only one (see text).

ity. It is used for infiltration, nerve block, intravenous, and epidural techniques. Potential local neurotoxicity was shown to be due to the antioxidant metabisulfite, which is no longer contained in the formulation.

Benzocaine is poorly soluble and therefore available for topical use only. Excessive absorption may lead to methemoglobinemia.

Propoxycaine is formulated in combination with procaine and a vasoconstrictor, which provides a prolonged duration of action.

Amides

Lidocaine is the most commonly used local anesthetic agent. This xylidine derivative is the prototype for the amide group; it has a rapid onset with an intermediate duration of action. It has prominent vasodilating properties and therefore specific formulations include epinephrine. It is effective for most types of local anesthetic blocks.

Prilocaine is a toluidine derivative similar to lidocaine in properties and uses, except that it is less inherently vasodilating. It provides a similar duration of action and has similar indications to those of lidocaine. It is reported to be the least toxic of the amides in use, but it is associated with risk of methemoglobinemia.

Mepivacaine is a xylidine derivative similar to lidocaine; it may be used for infiltration, nerve block, and epidural procedures. It is not effective as a topical agent, and it is not used in obstetric anesthesia because its biotransformation is prolonged in the fetus.

Bupivacaine is a xylidine derivative characterized by a long duration of action. Its onset of action is slower than that of lidocaine, but it is very potent and has good separation of sensory and motor blockade. Bupivacaine has a greater relative toxicity than lidocaine—in particular, a greater potential for cardiotoxicity. There is a smaller difference between the doses that lead to cardiovascular collapse and those with central-nervous-system effects. It can be used for infiltration, nerve block, epidural, and spinal procedures.

Etidocaine is a xylidine derivative similar to bupivacaine in that it is characterized by a long duration of action, strong potency, and relatively high cardiotoxicity. However, it differs in that it has a rapid onset of action and little separation of sensory and motor blockade. It is used for infiltration and nerve block.

Articaine is a thiophene derivative that appears to be similar to lidocaine.

SUGGESTED READING

Butterworth JF, Strichartz GR. Molecular mechanism of local anesthesia: a review. Anesthesiology 1990; 72:711–734.

Covino BG. Pharmacology of local anaesthetic agents. Br J Anaesth 1986; 58:701–716.

Strichartz GR, ed. Local Anesthetics. Handbook of experimental pharmacology, vol 81. Berlin: Springer-Verlag, 1987.

Strichartz GR, Covino BG. Local Anesthetics. In: Miller RD, ed. Anesthesia. 3rd ed. New York: Churchill Livingstone, 1990.

Seeman P. The membrane actions of anesthetics and tranquilizers. Pharmacol Rev 1972; 24:583–655.

CHAPTER 26

The Alcohols

H. KALANT AND J.M. KHANNA

CASE HISTORY

J. N., a 56-year-old vice-president of a brokerage firm, was required to undergo a thorough medical examination in connection with a large company-sponsored insurance policy. He denied any current illness, but laboratory test results indicated mildly elevated levels of aspartate transaminase (79 mU/mL), γ-glutamyl transpeptidase (62 mU/mL) and carbohydrate-deficient transferrin (41 mg/L). His physical examination had also revealed a slightly enlarged liver, but of normal consistency and not tender. The physician therefore took a more detailed history and functional enquiry, and learned that J.N. had been under gradually increasing pressure at work for the past 6 or 7 years. He had previously used alcohol socially without apparent problems, but had started to increase his intake and now drank an average of five or six drinks a day, and as much as eight drinks on occasion.

His blood pressure had increased in the last few years and was now 185/100 mmHg, despite the initiation of therapy with enalapril by his own family physician. He had also been using diazepam more frequently for relief of tension, and used flunitrazepam two or three times a week for relief of insomnia. Some years earlier he had consulted a gastroenterologist because of epigastric pain, which was diagnosed as being due to a duodenal ulcer, and he was started on therapy with ranitidine, which he continued up to the present. However, the gastric discomfort had recurred twice in the past 2 years, during therapy with naproxen, a nonsteroidal anti-inflammatory agent that he took during flare-ups of osteoarthritis in his knees.

Finally, J.N. admitted to the physician that three years ago he had been arrested for impaired driving when coming home from a party. A breath test had indicated a blood alcohol concentration of 154 mg/dL, and he had pleaded guilty. He was fined and his license was suspended for 1 year. This had been a major inconvenience to him, as well as an emotional jolt, and he claimed that since his license had been restored he never drove after drinking, but his wife hinted that this might not be entirely true.

The use of ethyl alcohol dates from prehistoric times and occurs in almost all parts of the world. Probably this is because the requirements for production of alcohol are extremely simple: some plant material containing starch or sugar, some moisture, yeast (even wild strains from the air), and a temperature high enough to permit fermentation. The earliest technological "improvement" (still used in some primitive societies) was to chew grain or tubers to crush them and mix them with yeasts from the chewer's mouth, then spit them back into a container with water, and leave them to ferment. In ancient times, this crude method gradually evolved into fairly sophisticated methods for producing wines and beers of relatively low alcohol content. Distillation was invented by Arabic chemists, from whom it spread to Europe in the Middle Ages; this permitted the production of much more potent beverages.

In view of the very long association of alcohol with human life and culture, it is not surprising that alcohol has many religious, symbolic, social, economic, and legal roles. These are reviewed in Chapter 72. The present chapter deals primarily with pharmacological, biochemical, and clinical aspects.

CHEMISTRY, METABOLISM, AND METABOLIC EFFECTS

Physical Chemistry

The aliphatic alcohols form a homologous series beginning with methanol:

CH_3-OH	Methanol (wood alcohol)
CH_3-CH_2-OH	Ethanol (grain alcohol)
$CH_3-CH_2-CH_2-OH$	n-Propanol
$CH_3-CH-CH_3$	Isopropanol
$\quad\ \ $ OH	
$CH_3-CH_2-CH_2-CH_2-OH$	n-Butanol

etc.

The first two are completely miscible with water and have very low lipid/water partition coefficients, but water solubility decreases as chain length increases, so octanol is virtually insoluble in water. Within the series of straight-chain alcohols, potency is proportional to the chain length, increasing by a factor of two to three with each additional carbon. However, because of the decrease in water solubility it is hard to achieve a toxic concentration in the body with longer-chain alcohols than pentanol or hexanol. All of the lower alcohols are used as solvents, but only ethanol is sufficiently nontoxic to be used as a beverage, though trace amounts of other alcohols are found in many alcoholic beverages. The amount of alcohol contained in 1.5 oz. (43 ml) of distilled spirits (40% v/v), 12 oz. of most regular beers (4–5% v/v), or 5 oz. of an average table wine (12% v/v), is approximately the same (13.6 g). This is referred to as a standard drink.

Absorption and Distribution

Ethanol is readily absorbed through any mucosal surface by simple diffusion. This can occur in the stomach, but is faster in the intestine, so a delay in gastric emptying, as by food or strenuous physical activity, slows the absorption. The rate of ethanol absorption is highest with 20–30% ethanol; with very dilute solutions it is slower because of a lower diffusion gradient. More concentrated alcohol may slow absorption by causing gastric irritation and pylorospasm. Ethanol vapor can also be absorbed readily through the lung, and rats and mice can easily be made deeply intoxicated by this route.

After absorption from the GI tract, ethanol is carried to the liver and then to the systemic circulation, diffusing into all tissues and body fluids including the CSF, sweat, urine, and breath. The equilibrium partition coefficient for ethanol between blood and alveolar air in humans is approximately 2200:1. Therefore the ethanol concentration in end-expiratory air can be measured and multiplied by this partition coefficient (e.g., by Breathalyzer or Intoxilyzer machines) to provide a fairly accurate estimate of the ethanol concentration in the blood.

Since ethanol is highly water-soluble and its molecular weight is only 46, it moves easily through aqueous channels in cell membranes. *Therefore it distributes and equilibrates quickly throughout the entire body water*, and its V_d equals the volume of total body water. Alcohol dilution can therefore be used to measure total body water (see next section and Fig. 26-3). The blood alcohol concentration (BAC) produced by a given number of standard drinks varies from one person to another as a function of individual differences in volume of total body water. This volume is greater in persons with greater height and weight. However, as a percentage of total body weight it is inversely related to the percentage of body fat, so that it tends to decrease with age, to be lower in women than in men, and to be lower in obese individuals than in lean, muscular ones of the same body weight.

Though alcohol passes rapidly across capillary walls, differences in blood flow to different tissues result in differences in the rates at which alcohol concentrations in the various tissues and fluids come into equilibrium with the concentration in the blood. This is most marked during the phase of rapid rise of blood alcohol level. During this phase, the rapid diffusion of ethanol from capillary blood into tissue fluid causes the ethanol concentration to be lower in the venous blood leaving the tissue than in the arterial blood entering it. The smaller the volume of blood flow per gram of tissue per minute, the larger is this early arterial–venous (A–V) difference in ethanol concentration. During this time, therefore, the concentration in a sample of blood from a hand or forearm vein is misleadingly low in comparison to the concentration reaching the brain (Fig. 26-1). Once distribution is complete, the A–V difference disappears.

Since diffusion is a first-order process, the rate

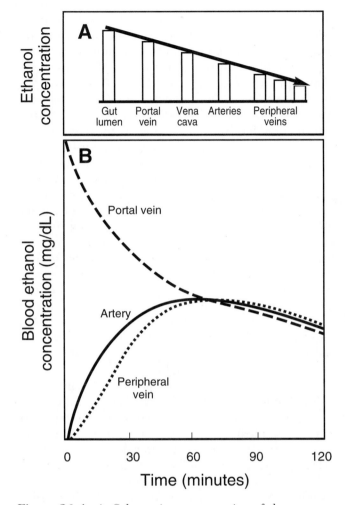

Figure 26-1. A. Schematic representation of the concentration gradient of ethanol from jejunal lumen to peripheral veins during the early stage of absorption and distribution. B. Time course of arterial–venous (A–V) differences in ethanol concentration during absorption and distribution.

etaldehyde and then to acetate, primarily in the liver (Fig. 26-2).

The three principal enzymatic mechanisms that can oxidize ethanol to acetaldehyde are **alcohol dehydrogenase (ADH), catalase,** and a **microsomal ethanol-oxidizing system (MEOS),** which is essentially part of the cytochrome P450 system. All evidence favors the view that normally *ADH is by far the most important hepatic enzyme responsible for the in vivo oxidation of ethanol.* Small amounts of ADH are also present in the gastrointestinal mucosa, renal tubular epithelium, lung, and brain, and may be responsible for the small amount of extrahepatic oxidation of ethanol.

Chronic ingestion of substantial amounts of ethanol leads to induction of the cytochrome P450 system, especially CYP2E1, which has a high substrate specificity for ethanol. This induction may be an important factor in the increased rate of alcohol oxidation seen in regular heavy drinkers. It is also related to the ability of chronic heavy drinking to induce the metabolism of a number of other drugs that are substrates of the P450 system.

Most of the acetaldehyde formed from ethanol is oxidized to acetate by the mitochondrial acetaldehyde dehydrogenase in the liver. Small amounts of acetaldehyde that escape into the circulation are oxidized rapidly in other tissues. Acetaldehyde is a highly reactive substance, and even transient elevation of levels in the blood can result in formation of permanent (covalently bonded) complexes with hemoglobin and plasma proteins. These complexes act as antigens, which can be measured by appro-

at which ethanol is lost from the body in the urine, breath, and sweat is proportional to the plasma concentration of ethanol. Over the range of concentrations produced by light to very heavy drinking, between 2% and 10% of the ingested dose can be lost in this way.

Biotransformation

Minute amounts of ethanol are conjugated with glucuronic or sulfuric acid (see Chapter 4) and excreted in the urine. By far the most important biotransformation reaction, however, is oxidation to ac-

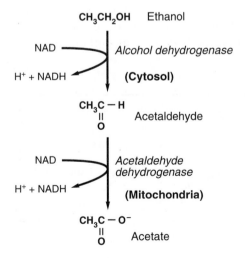

Figure 26-2. The two initial steps of ethanol metabolism in the liver.

priate antibodies. Alcoholics have significantly raised plasma levels of such antigens, and this finding may give rise to a useful diagnostic or screening test for heavy drinking.

Some of the acetate is converted to acetyl-CoA in the liver and oxidized to CO_2 and H_2O, or converted to amino acids, fatty acids, or glycogen in the same way as acetyl-CoA from other sources. However, large amounts of acetate pass into the systemic circulation and are taken up in other tissues, converted to acetyl-CoA, and oxidized in those tissues.

The rate-limiting step in the whole process is the alcohol dehydrogenase (ADH) step. The rate of this reaction in vivo, in normal well-nourished individuals, is determined both by the concentration of the ADH enzyme and by the NAD concentration or NAD:NADH ratio, which in turn depend on the rate of reoxidation of NADH.

There are differences between individuals, and within the same person from time to time, but *on average a 70-kg human can oxidize about 10 g of ethanol per hour*. This means that the typical blood alcohol curve, after oral ingestion in the fasting state, rises to a peak level in 30–90 minutes depending on the dose and then falls steadily at a rate of 15–20 mg/100 mL/hr until the concentration reaches about 25 mg/dL; below this point it falls exponentially (Fig. 26-3). However, ADH actually exhibits Michaelis-Menten kinetics, so the apparently linear portion of the curve is really a very shallow curve, and its slope is affected by the starting concentration. Therefore the initial rate of descent is greater if the maximum concentration is higher.

If the apparently linear portion of the curve is projected back to t_0 (see Fig. 26-3), the intercept on the vertical axis is C_0, i.e., the theoretical concentration that would have been found if all the administered dose of ethanol had been instantaneously ab-

sorbed and uniformly distributed throughout its V_d. Since ethanol is distributed almost entirely in the body water, and blood contains about 80% water, C_0 in the blood corresponds to 80% of the C_0 in the water phase, or $C_{0 \text{ water}} = 1.25 \times C_{0 \text{ blood}}$. $C_{0 \text{ water}}$ = dose/volume of body water. Therefore, if dose and $C_{0 \text{ water}}$ are known, total body water can be estimated; this method has been used clinically for that purpose.

It has been suggested that a sex difference in gastric mucosal ADH activity (lower in women than in men) may cause a difference in gastric first-pass metabolism and thus be responsible for higher BACs in women than in men after the same dose of ethanol per unit of body weight. However, it is doubtful that gastric first-pass metabolism of ethanol plays any significant role in humans, because estimates of total body water by the ethanol dilution method are identical whether the ethanol is given by mouth or intravenously. This means that bioavailability of alcohol by mouth must be essentially complete. Moreover, BACs in men and women are identical if they are given the same dose of alcohol per unit of body water rather than per unit of body weight.

Since the oxidation of ethanol requires simultaneous reduction of NAD to NADH, anything that makes NAD more available by reoxidizing NADH more rapidly will help to keep the rate of alcohol metabolism at the maximum permitted by the amount of ADH present. Fructose, insulin plus glucose, and other sources of pyruvate may do this. However, it is not possible to speed the process past its normal maximum by this means. Dinitrophenol can increase the rate of NADH reoxidation (and hence of ethanol oxidation) beyond the normal limit by uncoupling oxidation from phosphorylation, but it is too toxic to use clinically.

Metabolic Effects of Ethanol

The change of NAD to NADH, resulting from the metabolism of ethanol and acetaldehyde, affects other NAD-linked metabolic processes. Some of the better-studied examples are listed below (Fig 26-4).

1. Pyruvate is reduced to lactate by lactate dehydrogenase (simultaneously oxidizing NADH to NAD), causing varying degrees of *elevation of serum lactate and metabolic acidosis*. The raised lactate inhibits renal secretion of urate and thus can *precipitate attacks of gout*.

2. Increased hepatic NADH also favors reduction of glyceraldehyde-3-phosphate to glycerol-3-phos-

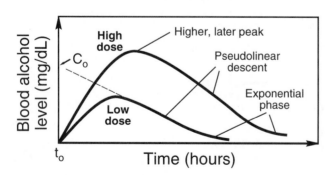

Figure 26-3. Dose dependence of peak blood alcohol levels and rate of descent from the peak.

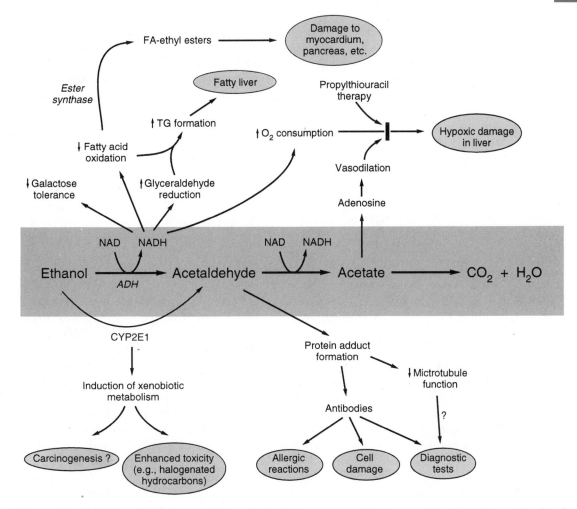

Figure 26-4. Evolving concepts of the relation between ethanol metabolism and alcohol-related organic damage. The pre-1960 vision of ethanol metabolism is shown in the central shaded area. Discoveries since 1960 have added everything else shown in the figure. The end-results, in terms of organ damage or its detection, are circled. (Reproduced by permission of the editor and publishers of the *Keio Journal of Medicine.*)

phate and inhibits glycerophosphate dehydrogenate, leading to an elevated glycerol-3-phosphate level.

3. At the same time, the excess production of acetate from acetaldehyde, together with the raised NADH level, stimulates the synthesis of fatty acids in the liver while their oxidation via the tricarboxylic acid cycle is blocked.

4. The excess of glycerol-3-phosphate and of fatty acids leads to increased esterification and accumulation of neutral triglycerides in the liver.

5. The increase in NADH and decrease in pyruvate result in a reduced rate of gluconeogenesis. Therefore, if hepatic glycogen supplies are depleted by lack of adequate food intake, ethanol causes hypoglycemia.

6. The raised NADH level also inhibits the en-

zyme systems that convert galactose to glucose and that conjugate glycine and benzoate to form hippuric acid (see Chapter 4), so the liver function tests based on these enzymes are disturbed.

These changes are all reversible when alcohol oxidation is finished.

7. However, chronic heavy ingestion of alcohol increases not only the rate of alcohol oxidation but also the rate of O_2 consumption. Consequently the risk of hypoxia in the liver is increased, especially at the hepatic venous end of the sinusoid where the Po_2 is normally lowest anyway (see Chapter 46). This may explain why liver cell necrosis in heavy drinkers is chiefly around the collecting veins ("central veins").

8. In the brain, ethanol can be oxidized to acetaldehyde by the very small amount of alcohol dehydrogenase present there, as well as by catalase and possibly by other neuronal or glial enzymes. Even though the amount of acetaldehyde formed is probably quite small, its high reactivity causes it to form condensation products with dopamine, serotonin, and other neuroamines, or with the aldehydes produced by the action of MAO on these amines (Fig. 26-5). The possible roles of such condensation products in the actions of ethanol on the brain are not yet clear.

Numerous other metabolic effects of ethanol are produced in other tissues, but their pharmacological or pathological significance is not well established.

ETHANOL ACTIONS AND INTOXICATION

Membrane and Cellular Effects of Ethanol

All tissues and cells can be affected by high-enough concentrations of ethanol, but they differ greatly in sensitivity. At bactericidal concentrations (about 70% or more) denaturation and precipitation of protein occurs, as in fixation of tissues for histology. At much lower concentrations (e.g., less than 0.1%) the actions are quite different and involve a modification of various cell membrane functions.

Although ethanol is much more water-soluble than the major anesthetic agents, its membrane actions are similar in many respects to those of other anesthetics on excitable cell membranes (see Chapters 24 and 25). In very high concentrations that

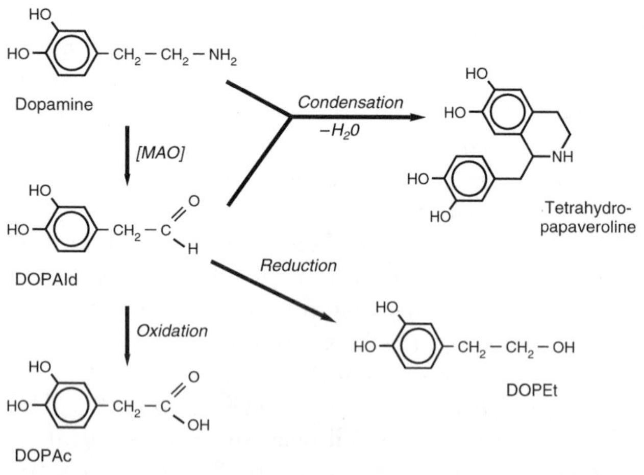

Figure 26-5. Formation of biogenic aldehyde condensation products through the action of alcohol in the brain.

cause profound general anesthesia or death, ethanol causes expansion and fluidization of the membranes, just as other general anesthetics do. This disordering effect on membrane lipids also affects the interactions between the lipids and protein inclusions in the membranes, such as receptors, membrane-bound enzymes, and ion channels. As a result, almost every membrane function is altered, in ways that produce or reflect altered excitability.

At much lower concentrations, however, such as those resulting from moderate social use of alcohol, the membrane effects are much less diffuse and more selective. This may reflect a more specific interaction of ethanol at the lipid–protein interfaces of particular protein inclusions in the cell membrane.

Among these alterations are the following:

1. Acute exposure to relatively low concentrations of ethanol (20 mM or higher) produces a concentration-dependent inhibition of the NMDA subtype of glutamate receptor. Glutamate is the major excitatory neurotransmitter in the brain and activation of NMDA receptors opens a receptor-linked cation channel, leading to influx of Ca^{2+} and Na^+ into the neuron. This influx activates processes involved in learning and memory, but more massive influx can cause epileptic seizures and neuronal death. Inhibition of NMDA receptors may explain the impairment of learning and memory formation during alcohol intoxication as well as the elevation of stimulus intensity needed to elicit seizures. The other subtypes of glutamate receptor (kainate and AMPA receptors) are also inhibited by ethanol, but the functional consequences are not yet clear.

When the brain is exposed chronically to ethanol, however, the number of NMDA receptors is increased. This up-regulation may result in neuronal hyperexcitability, contributing both to tolerance to the neuronal depressant actions of ethanol and to the major signs of ethanol withdrawal, such as tremor, exaggerated tendon reflexes, and seizures. Overactivity of glutamate receptors, and the consequent increase in Ca^{2+} influx, may also be one factor in the production of alcohol brain damage.

2. Low concentrations of ethanol have also been reported to enhance the effects of GABA on the GABA-benzodiazepine-receptor/Cl^--ionophore complex (see Chapters 21 and 26). Under normal conditions, GABA increases Cl^- influx into the cell body and increases Cl^- efflux from axon terminals, in both cases lowering the excitability of the membrane. Enhancement of this action by ethanol is most clearly and consistently demonstrable at very high (anesthe-

tizing) concentrations, and can be blocked by Ro 15-4513, a benzodiazepine receptor "inverse agonist" that also reverses some of the behavioral and physiological signs of ethanol intoxication.

3. At somewhat higher concentrations, ethanol reduces the excitation-dependent influx of Ca^{2+}, thus diminishing Ca^{2+}-dependent cell responses such as neurotransmitter release.

4. Receptor-activated second-messenger systems are also affected by ethanol. Norepinephrine-activated adenylyl cyclase activity is increased by ethanol in some types of neuron, whereas norepinephrine- and acetylcholine-activated phosphoinositol turnover is inhibited. However, the pattern of changes in different parts of the nervous system is complex, and it is not yet clear what role they play in mediating the actions of ethanol.

5. At higher concentrations, ethanol inhibits the active reuptake of adenosine, thus increasing the free adenosine concentration at adenosine receptors.

6. At quite high ethanol concentrations, Na^+ channel opening is impaired. Therefore the rate of rise of action potentials is reduced, so their maximum height is diminished. Nerve conduction and muscle contraction, including myocardial contraction, are thus impaired. At the same time, active transport of Na^+, K^+, and amino acids by the cell membrane $(Na^+ + K^+)$-ATPase is impaired. This may affect the resting potential of the membrane, on which maintenance of excitability depends.

7. Ethanol increases both the spontaneous and the impulse-triggered release of acetylcholine at cholinergic nerve terminals at the nerve–muscle junction and the anterior-horn-cell recurrent collateral. In brain slices, however, alcohol inhibits the synaptic release of acetylcholine more than that of other neurotransmitters. It is not known if the effect is exerted on the membrane of the cholinergic synapse itself or on the axons that carry electrical impulses to the synapse. In the living organism, the overall effect of alcohol on acetylcholine release is complex, but intoxication generally reduces it in parallel with the onset of drowsiness.

While these membrane effects are most prominent in excitable tissues such as brain and muscle, they probably apply to all tissues but at different alcohol concentrations. Even in the central nervous system, some cells are more sensitive than others, and complex polysynaptic pathways are generally more sensitive than simple spinal reflex arcs. In general, ethanol causes a dose-dependent reduction of both spontaneous and evoked firing rates of single units in the cerebral cortex, hippocampus, and other parts of the brain. However, depending on differences in sensitivity of small interneurons, large pyramidal or Purkinje cells, myelinated versus unmyelinated fibers, etc., some units may show increased activity (disinhibition) at concentrations that decrease activity in others. Death occurs by depression of the respiratory control mechanism at blood alcohol concentrations too low to produce serious *direct* effects on most other tissues.

Effects of Ethanol on Integrated Functions of the Nervous System

Relatively low concentrations of ethanol affect the hippocampus, the hypothalamus, and the ascending reticular formation, which is an important arousal mechanism for the forebrain. One of the earliest effects produced by small doses of ethanol (10–20 g, equivalent to 1–2 oz. of distilled spirits given to an adult) is cutaneous vasodilatation of central origin. This appears to be due to disturbed functioning of the thermoregulatory center in the preoptic area and anterior hypothalamus. The skin is flushed and warm, and there is sweating and increased heat loss from the skin. As a result, in a cool environment there may be a fall in body temperature. The vasodilatation also contributes to a fall in peripheral arteriolar resistance, tachycardia, and increased amplitude of pulse pressure.

Hypothalamic actions of ethanol also lead to increased gastric secretion of HCl and increased gastrointestinal motility.

Subjectively, low doses usually produce relaxation and mild sedation in an individual at rest. If alcohol is infused slowly intravenously, the progressive increase in total dosage leads to increasing sedation, sleep, and ultimately to anesthesia and coma.

In the usual social setting in which alcohol is drunk, the picture is modified. At first the sedation is accompanied by loss of inhibitory control of emotions and the *subjects become talkative and emotionally labile*. This is not a unique effect of alcohol; it can be caused by many sedatives in appropriate doses, but these are not normally taken in a social setting. *Small doses* do not impair complex intellectual ability and may even improve it slightly in tense, nervous people. Even after *higher doses*, the impairment stems principally from slowing (increased reaction time) and inability to concentrate, rather than from loss of actual intellectual ability. However, *high alcohol levels* do produce marked impairment of mental functioning, including impaired judgement, increased risk-taking, confusion, and disruption of rational thought. Impaired memory formation may lead to blackouts, i.e., inability to recall in the sober state events that occurred during the intoxicated state. The impairment of the reticular activating system results in decreased ability to attend to incoming sensory information from several sources simultaneously, so complex tasks requiring alertness and rapid decision-making are more readily disrupted than those in which time is not a critical factor. Visual and other sensory acuity is impaired, and at higher blood alcohol concentrations anesthesia is produced.

Electroencephalographic (EEG) changes are not specific for ethanol, but are reflections of the state of arousal or depression. At low blood alcohol levels, during the stage of excitation and talkativeness, there is a desynchronized (aroused) EEG with an increase in the mean frequency of β activity. At higher levels, with increasing drowsiness, there is a progressive shift toward EEG synchronization with increased amplitude and steady fall in dominant frequency toward the 1–3-Hz range. Cortical and hippocampal evoked responses at first show increased amplitude, but as severe depression develops the amplitude falls. The latency is also increased, not only in the cortex but also in the afferent paths in the brainstem; this is indicative of a fall in conduction velocity and of a delay in synaptic transmission.

The action of ethanol on the midbrain and medullary reticular formation, and on the input to cerebellar Purkinje cells, also affects descending fibers that modulate the responses of sensory organs and spinal motor synapses. Loss of descending inhibitory control at synapses in the motor pathways, together with impaired proprioceptor sensation, results in *motor ataxia*, *positive Romberg sign*, and *slurred speech*. Changes in reflexes vary with the complexity of the pathways. Loss of descending inhibitory influences may facilitate simple reflexes, such as tendon jerks, at low or moderate alcohol levels. In contrast, *complex polysynaptic reflexes* are impaired easily. At very high alcohol levels, even monosynaptic reflexes are blocked.

Endocrine Effects

Numerous endocrine effects, mediated via the hypothalamus, have been shown.

1. Pituitary **antidiuretic hormone secretion is inhibited** by rising blood ethanol levels, causing *diuresis* of low specific gravity and of variable intensity and duration. This can be *abolished by the action of nicotine* on the hypothalamus. This led to the suggestion that the effect of ethanol might result from decreased excitatory input to the supraoptic and paraventricular nuclei, rather than from direct suppression of secretory cells in the neurohypophysis. However, low concentrations of ethanol have also been shown to inhibit Ca^{2+} channels and enhance K^+ currents in the secretory cells, so inhibition of AVP release may be due to direct action of ethanol.

2. Secretion of oxytocin is inhibited, and intravenous infusion of dilute ethanol was, for a time, used clinically to stop uterine contractions and prevent premature labor. This practice has been abandoned because of the risk of damage to the fetus.

3. Release of β-endorphin from the intermediate lobe and probably the anterior lobe of the hypophysis is *increased*. The possible role of increased endorphin release in the effects of ethanol is not yet clear.

4. Increased secretion of epinephrine, norepinephrine, and adrenal corticosteroids occurs during severe intoxication with respiratory and circulatory depression. However, small doses of ethanol diminish stress responses to a variety of stressors. This antistress effect includes reduction or prevention of the elevations in plasma corticosteroid and catecholamine levels. The blood ethanol level at which stress reduction is replaced by ethanol-induced stress probably varies with the person and the circumstances.

5. Secretion of luteinizing hormone (LH) is impaired and, as a result, serum **testosterone levels tend to fall**. Another factor contributing to the reduction in testosterone output is the inhibition of steroid hydroxylation in the testis as a result of NADH accumulation caused by alcohol dehydrogenase activity in the testis itself.

Ethanol Intoxication

Signs of intoxication appear at different blood levels, depending on individual differences in tolerance and also on the speed of drinking and thus on the rate of rise of the blood ethanol level.

Mild signs appear in most people at levels below 500 mg/L (0.05%, or slightly over 10 mmol/L). Frank intoxication with psychomotor impairment is present in many subjects at levels below 1000 mg/L (0.1% or 21 mmol/L), but in practically everyone at 1500 mg/L (0.15%, just under 33 mmol/L). Profound intoxication, with anesthesia or coma, is likely at 2500 mg/L (0.25%, 54 mmol/L) or higher, although chronic heavy use of ethanol many increase tolerance to such a degree that some individuals are still conscious and active at blood levels of well over 0.35%.

Death occurs, as a result of respiratory depression in most cases, at levels of 5000 mg/L (0.5% or 108 mmol/L) or higher. *Barbiturates and other sedatives, benzodiazepines, phenothiazines (both antipsychotics and antihistamines), opioids, many antidepressants, and many "over-the-counter" cough and cold medications show additive or potentiating effects when taken together with alcohols.* When such drugs are used to quiet someone who is "roaring drunk," great care must be taken to avoid fatal overdosage.

In many countries, it is illegal to drive a motor vehicle at blood levels specified in the traffic criminal codes. In various European countries, this is 0.05% (500 mg/L, about 11 mmol/L). In Canada and some parts of the United States it is 0.08% (800 mg/L, 17 mmol/L). In many parts of the United States, it is 0.1%. These values do not, in most jurisdictions, constitute a legal definition of intoxication, but form the basis of "per se legislation"; i.e., even at 0.1% some individuals with very high tolerance might not be demonstrably intoxicated, but enough drivers are likely to be impaired to varying degrees at the designated blood alcohol levels to justify making it an offense to drive at these levels, whether a given individual is impaired or not.

Treatment of Acute Intoxication

Treatment might theoretically be aimed at either (1) speeding the disappearance of alcohol from the body or (2) counteracting its effects. As already mentioned, metabolic disappearance cannot be speeded up very much. In extreme cases, where death may occur, hemodialysis is undoubtedly rapid and effective in removing the alcohol. Usually, however, such treatment is not needed.

Pharmacological reversal of the effects of ethanol is not usually attempted in mild intoxication. Many compounds have been tested for their claimed **amethystic** (anti-intoxicant) properties; a recent example is the antiparkinsonian agent amantadine (see Chapter 21). However, the results are not very convincing. In serious intoxication with profound coma, central nervous system stimulants (analeptics) are occasionally used, but they are not very helpful because there is a small margin between doses that are ineffective and those that are too large and cause seizures. As noted earlier in this section, the benzodiazepine

receptor inverse agonist Ro 15-4513 can reverse some of the signs of alcohol intoxication, but it does not antagonize the lethal effect of ethanol overdose. The opioid antagonist naloxone has been reported to reverse alcoholic coma, but there are numerous reports that it has failed to work, and in experimental animals it works only at doses that have an analeptic effect of their own. Therefore *supportive therapy (intravenous fluids, artificial respiration if needed, etc.) is the principal approach.* This is kept up until metabolism lowers the blood alcohol level to the point where the danger is past.

ALCOHOLISM AND RELATED PROBLEMS

Alcoholism ("Chronic Alcoholism," Alcohol Dependence, Alcohol Addiction)

Alcoholism constitutes a very complex medical and social problem. The factors involved include such things as the prevalent social attitudes toward drinking and drunkenness, parental attitudes and habits, drinking practices among certain occupational groups, personal emotional conflicts, and perhaps excessively rewarding pharmacological effects of ethanol. There is considerable evidence suggesting a hereditary (genetic) predisposition in many cases. Much research is currently being directed at a search for biochemical markers for detecting those who have a genetic predisposition, and also for biochemical tests for identifying heavy drinkers at an early stage. In almost every case, most of these factors are involved in varying degrees, so there is no single cause of alcoholism. This question is examined in more detail in Chapter 72.

The adverse consequences of alcoholism are also seen in many different aspects of the individual's life, including physical and mental health, family relations, work and economic performance, accidents, legal problems, and others. Most of these are beyond the scope of this chapter. Only a few of the pharmacological problems can be covered here.

Nutritional Problems

Oxidation of ethanol yields 7 cal/g. At an average oxidation rate of 10 g/hr or 240 g daily, one could derive nearly 1700 cal/day from ethanol. In many individual cases, especially in regular heavy drinkers, the amount may be much higher. If the average dietary intake of a man with sedentary occupation is

2500–3000 cal/day, steady drinking can provide well over half of the total. Since alcoholic beverages contain little or no protein, vitamins, or lipotropic factors, a variety of nutritional deficiency diseases can result. **Peripheral neuropathy, Korsakoff's psychosis, Wernicke's disease,** *and* **pellagra** *are examples of B vitamin deficiencies occurring in alcoholics;* they became much less frequent once vitamin supplementation of bread and other foods began. Since nutrition is frequently insufficient during drinking bouts and hepatic glycogen content is reduced, serious hypoglycemia can occur, as explained above under Metabolic Effects of Ethanol.

Organ Damage

Fatty liver is common among alcoholics as a result of the metabolic disturbances described earlier. **Alcoholic hepatitis and cirrhosis,** however, appear to result from different processes than fatty liver. As noted in the section on metabolism, chronic ingestion of large amounts of ethanol leads to increased O_2 consumption by the hepatocytes, and therefore to a much lower Po_2 at the venous end of the sinusoid. Anything that reduces arterial Po_2 can therefore precipitate hypoxia in that zone, resulting in alterations of cell membrane permeability, leakage of various macromolecular constituents, and ultimately hepatocellular necrosis and a local inflammatory cell response (alcoholic hepatitis). Early cell damage that has not yet progressed to necrosis can often be detected by raised levels of hepatocellular enzymes (e.g., various transpeptidases) and carbohydrate-deficient transferrin in the plasma. Ethanol also reduces the hepatic level of reduced glutathione, and this effect may contribute to the production of hepatocellular necrosis (see Chapter 46). Current research is also exploring the possibility that autoantibodies formed against acetaldehyde complexes with hepatocellular proteins may produce liver cell necrosis. Repeated episodes of necrosis lead to fibroblast response, which eventually produces portal cirrhosis (see Chapter 46). Even if the hepatocellular damage is reversible, the cells remain sensitive to ethanol for months after the cessation of heavy drinking; even small doses can produce a prompt rise in serum alanine aminotransferase and γ-glutamyltransferase levels.

Another important type of organic damage in alcoholics is **cerebral cortical atrophy,** with widening of the sulci and enlargement of the ventricles. This can be revealed by computerized tomography (CT) scanning and magnetic resonance imaging (MRI) at a stage before gross neurological or psychological deficits are detectable clinically. This is a different type of lesion from the nutritional-deficiency effects previously noted, and may possibly reflect a direct toxic effect of ethanol itself. Fortunately, it is often reversible if drinking is stopped at an early stage.

Some alcoholics, after years of heavy drinking, show a relatively sudden "break" or loss of tolerance, becoming quite intoxicated by amounts of alcohol that previously produced only mild symptoms. This is usually the result of organic damage to either the liver or the nervous system. Liver damage, resulting in reduced ethanol-oxidizing ability, causes the same amount of ethanol to yield higher and more prolonged blood alcohol levels than previously. Brain damage, with cortical and hippocampal neuron loss, may render the nervous system more sensitive to the same blood alcohol level.

The **fetal alcohol syndrome** (FAS) is a complex picture of *irreversible* damage to the fetus and results from ingestion of alcohol by pregnant women. The complete picture includes small head, widely separated eyes with short palpebral fissures and epicanthic folds, a broad upper lip that lacks the normal midline vertical groove (the philtrum), a short nose, mental and physical retardation, often cardiac valvular defects, and continued retardation of development postnatally. FAS appears to be caused by a direct toxic effect of ethanol and/or acetaldehyde, perhaps in part by impairment of placental circulation, rather than a consequence of maternal malnutrition. The severity appears to be dose-dependent, but the minimum dose required to produce it is not known. Therefore many obstetricians advise total abstinence during pregnancy.

In general, alcoholics have a higher mortality rate than the general population of the same age and sex. The **excess mortality** is due not only to liver cirrhosis but to many different causes including hypertensive heart disease, stroke, cancer of the pharynx and esophagus, and accidents. In contrast, there is considerable epidemiological evidence suggesting that a low or moderate alcohol intake may reduce the risk of fatal myocardial infarction; the mechanism is not yet known. At average daily alcohol intakes in excess of one to two standard drinks, the excess mortality outweighs the cardiac protective effect.

Tolerance and Physical Dependence

With steady intake of alcohol, tolerance develops, i.e., larger amounts of alcohol are required to produce the same degree of effect. This reflects both **metabolic tolerance** produced by faster oxidation in the liver, and **functional tolerance** in the nervous system. Absorption may actually be somewhat faster in tolerant individuals, because they show less alcohol-induced delay of gastric emptying. Distribution of the alcohol is not significantly altered.

Functional tolerance is an actual change in sensitivity of the CNS. Acute tolerance occurs within the course of a single exposure to ethanol, so there is less intoxication at a given blood alcohol level on the descending limb of the blood alcohol curve than there was at the same level on the rising limb (the Mellanby effect). Chronic tolerance is the gradual decrease in degree of intoxication at the same blood alcohol level over the course of repeated alcohol exposures. The relation between acute and chronic tolerance is not yet wholly clear. The maximum degree of tolerance to ethanol is considerably smaller than the maximum tolerance that can develop to opioids or to benzodiazepines.

The mechanism of functional tolerance to ethanol is complex and not yet fully known. Experimental evidence indicates that not only the presence of alcohol itself, but also the genetic background of the individual, the environmental and behavioral circumstances under which alcohol is consumed, and the degree of use of drugs with effects that resemble those of alcohol (such as benzodiazepines and other sedatives) all influence the speed and degree of development of tolerance to alcohol. The neural mechanisms underlying tolerance appear to include serotonin, glutamate (NMDA receptors), acetylcholine, vasopressin, dopamine, and GABA receptors, especially in pathways in the septum and hippocampus that are also involved in learning and memory. Tolerance appears to be related to the development of physical dependence, with which it proceeds more or less in parallel. **Physical dependence** is revealed by the occurrence of physiological disturbances, referred to as **withdrawal symptoms,** when alcohol intake is reduced or stopped (see also Chapter 72).

Ethanol Withdrawal Syndrome

Since ethanol depresses neuronal excitability and spontaneous activity in various parts of the brain, adaptation must involve some type of compensatory hyperactivity to offset the alcohol effect. This is seen as tolerance when the alcohol is present. When the alcohol is withdrawn the hyperactivity gives rise to the withdrawal symptoms. Their severity and dura-

tion depend upon the severity and duration of the preceding period of drinking.

Following a single intoxicating dose of alcohol or a single short period of drinking, e.g., one evening, the only consistent physiological change that can be correlated with "hangover" (and is suggestive of withdrawal effect) is some degree of *neuronal hyperexcitability* (Fig. 26-6).

After longer drinking bouts lasting several days or more, the symptoms include marked hyperirritability, exaggerated reflexes, sleeplessness, tremor, muscular tension, cold sweaty skin, nausea, and marked thirst. In severe cases there may be generalized convulsions.

After chronic drinking for many weeks or months, abrupt cessation or even some reduction of alcohol intake can precipitate a two-stage withdrawal

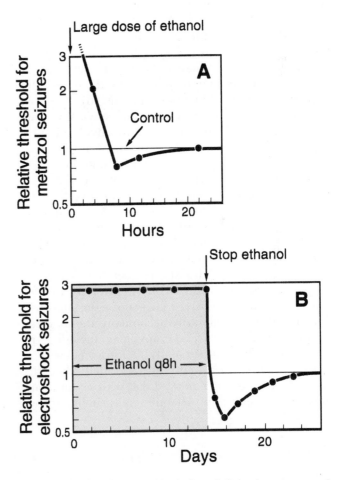

Figure 26-6. Effects of alcohol withdrawal on neuronal excitability by pentylenetetrazol (metrazol) or electric shock. A. After a single large dose of ethanol at zero time. B. After prolonged ingestion of ethanol. Note the difference in the time scales in A and B.

reaction. In addition to the symptoms already described, which begin very soon after withdrawal, there can be a second stage beginning 2 or more days later. This is characterized by severe hyperactivity with delirium, hallucinations, fever, profuse sweating, intense vasodilatation, and severe tachycardia. This stage (delirium tremens) is still sometimes fatal despite the newer treatments. One hypothesis is that this picture results from rebound hypersensitivity of β-adrenergic receptors that have been suppressed during prolonged intoxication and early withdrawal.

Treatment of the withdrawal syndrome depends on its severity. In many mild cases, rest, quiet, and reassurance are all that are required. In more severe cases, long-acting benzodiazepines such as **chlordiazepoxide** or **diazepam** are usually effective in reducing the irritability, tremor, and sleeplessness, and are the drugs of choice. The first dose is sometimes given parenterally for rapid action (see Chapter 27). **Chlormethiazole** is widely used in Europe to treat alcohol withdrawal symptoms but is not yet available in North America. Symptoms due to adrenergic overactivity may be relieved by the α_2-adrenoceptor agonist clonidine (see Chapter 16).

Phenothiazines do not prevent convulsions, and may even increase the risk, so anticonvulsant drugs may also be necessary. The anticonvulsant benzodiazepine carbamazepine may be helpful in such cases. **Barbiturates, paraldehyde,** etc., are useful but less safe and probably somewhat less effective than the drugs mentioned. They are now very seldom used clinically. Ethanol itself is effective, and a tapering-off treatment is preferred in some countries. However, such a regimen is hard to adhere to and is psychologically bad for the patient who wishes to stop drinking, unless the alcohol is given by a different route (intravenously) that is not associated with the stimuli that ordinarily accompany the ingestion of alcohol. Supportive therapy may include large amounts of fluid either orally or intravenously, but some patients are actually overhydrated when first seen. A high-calorie balanced diet with vitamin supplements, especially thiamin, is usually recommended.

Pharmacotherapy of Behavioral Dependence

Physical dependence, though commonly found in alcoholic patients, is not the fundamental feature of alcoholism. Rather, it is "psychological" or behavioral dependence, which is believed to be related to the reinforcing effects of ethanol. These topics are discussed in Chapters 71 and 72. Drug therapies aimed at reducing dependence by blocking or decreasing the reinforcing effects are not specific for alcohol, but are used also in dependence on other drugs. Therefore they are covered in Chapter 72. Disulfiram and other drugs described below are specific for alcoholism but do not act on the reinforcement system. Instead, they interact with the metabolism of alcohol in such a way as to give rise to highly unpleasant effects. The hope is that the patient's desire to drink alcohol will be offset by the fear of these consequences.

Disulfiram and Related Drugs

Tetraethylthiuram disulfide (disulfiram, or TETD) inhibits the hepatic enzymes that oxidize acetaldehyde to acetate. Consumption of ethanol therefore produces accumulation of acetaldehyde in the blood and tissues, causing acetaldehyde poisoning. Within minutes, the subject becomes hot, flushed, and cyanotic. The pulse rate, cardiac output, and respiratory rate rise. These effects are thought to result from excessive release of catecholamines from sympathetic nerve endings under the influence of acetaldehyde. However, disulfiram also inhibits dopamine-β-hydroxylase, so the stores of catecholamines in the nerve endings are low to begin with. Therefore, after 30–60 minutes the sympathetic tone falls abruptly and there is a marked drop in blood pressure, pallor, and nausea. This reaction lasts for up to 2 hours and can be very severe and occasionally fatal. Alcoholics are often given disulfiram so that fear of a reaction will deter them from drinking. *It is not a cure for alcoholism,* merely a deterrent (see Chapter 72).

Disulfiram is absorbed rapidly from the GI tract, begins to act within 2–4 hours, and reaches its maximum effect in 24 hours. It should not be started until 12–24 hours after the last drink of alcohol. The drug is metabolized in the body by splitting the disulfide bond to form diethyldithiocarbamate, which may be the active form. This in turn is broken down to form CS_2, which appears in the breath, and to sulfate, which is excreted slowly in the urine over the next week.

Disulfiram itself has some toxicity apart from the inhibition of dopamine-β-hydroxylase and possibly some other enzymes. Toxic symptoms may include weakness, dizziness, mental disturbances, cardiac arrhythmias, skin reactions, and impotence. It can also inhibit metabolism of other drugs by liver microsomal enzymes, thus altering the effects of these drugs. Patients using disulfiram must be monitored carefully.

Citrated calcium carbimide also inhibits acetaldehyde dehydrogenase. However, it does not inhibit dopamine-β-hydroxylase, and its toxic effects are much less severe than those of disulfiram. It has therefore found clinical use (in Canada and some other countries, but not in the United States). The reaction to alcohol is also less severe than with disulfiram, and possibly not so effective a deterrent to drinking.

Tolbutamide, metronidazole, and **cephalosporins** have similar interactions with alcohol. Patients being treated with these drugs should be warned not to drink alcohol. Conversely, chronic intake of alcohol may cause faster biotransformation of tolbutamide, with correspondingly shorter duration of action (see Chapter 4).

METHANOL INTOXICATION

Methanol is a milder intoxicant than ethanol in that larger doses are necessary to produce the same degree of intoxication. Its serious toxicity is not that of methanol itself, but of its metabolic products. It is oxidized by catalase, as well as by alcohol dehydrogenase, to **formaldehyde,** which is in turn oxidized to **formic acid.** These substances are specifically toxic to the retina and optic nerve and may produce partial or complete permanent blindness. In addition, the formic acid gives rise to severe metabolic acidosis, which may be fatal.

Treatment requires (1) vigorous measures to correct the acidosis with intravenous sodium bicarbonate solution and (2) attempts to eliminate the methanol before it can be oxidized. This is achieved by combining hemodialysis (for removing methanol) with administration of repeated doses of ethanol, which competitively inhibits oxidation of the methanol. Folate is also used, to enhance oxidation of any formate produced.

HIGHER ALCOHOLS

Propyl and isopropyl alcohols are used as antiseptics and for alcohol rubs. The higher alcohols (butyl, pentyl, etc.) are used mainly as solvents for industrial processes. They are of concern pharmacologically for two reasons. (1) Distilled beverages contain small amounts of higher alcohols and aldehydes, referred to as "congeners." There is some slight evidence that they may contribute to the toxicity of the ethanol. (2) They are often consumed by "skid row" alcoholics in the form of antifreeze, cleaning fluid, and numerous other toxic mixtures with gasoline, benzene, etc. The intoxicating effects are similar to those of ethanol but much more severe for the same dose. Organic toxicity, especially to the liver, kidney, and bone marrow, is also more severe with these mixtures.

Certain other higher alcohols, mainly unsaturated tertiary alcohols such as ethchlorvynol (Placidyl), and certain acetaldehyde derivatives (trichloracetaldehyde hydrate or paraldehyde), were formerly used fairly widely as sedatives and hypnotics. They are still used occasionally but have been replaced almost completely by the benzodiazepines. They are therefore no longer described in detail in this text.

SUGGESTED READING

Brewer C, Hardt F, Petersen EN, eds. Antabuse—experiences from 40 years of clinical use and the discovery of an active metabolite. Acta Psychiatr Scand, Suppl 1992; 369:1–72.

Deitrich RA, Dunwiddie TV, Harris RA, Erwin VG. Mechanism of action of ethanol: initial nervous system actions. Pharmacol Rev 1989; 41:498–537.

Gorelick DA. Overview of pharmacologic treatment approaches for alcohol and other drug addiction. Intoxication, withdrawal, and relapse prevention. Psychiatr Clin North Am 1993; 16(1):141–156.

Kalant H. Pharmacokinetics of ethanol: absorption, distribution and elimination. In: Begleiter H, Kissin B, eds. The pharmacology of alcohol and alcohol dependence, vol. 2. New York: Oxford University Press, 1996: 15–58.

Kalant H, Khanna JM. Methods for the study of tolerance. In: Adler MW, Cowan A, eds. Testing and evaluation of drugs of abuse. New York: Wiley-Liss, 1990: 43–66.

Kalant H, Lê AD. Effects of ethanol on thermoregulation. In: Schönbaum E, Lomax P, eds. Thermoregulation: pathology, pharmacology, and therapy. Internat Encycloped Pharmacol Therap, Section 132. Oxford: Pergamon, 1991: 561–617.

Lê AD, Khanna JM. Dispositional mechanisms in drug tolerance and sensitization. In: Goudie AJ, Emmett-Oglesby MW, eds. Psychoactive drugs—tolerance and sensitization. Clifton, NJ: Humana, 1989: 281–351.

Lieber CS. Mechanisms of ethanol-drug-nutrition interactions. J Toxicol Clin Toxicol 1994; 32:631–681.

Lieber CS. Alcohol and the liver: 1994 update. Gastroenterology 1994; 106:1085–1105.

Majchrowicz E, Noble EP, eds. Biochemistry and pharmacology of ethanol (2 volumes). New York: Plenum, 1979.

Tabakoff B, Hoffman PL. Alcohol: neurobiology. In: Lowinson JH, Ruiz P, Millman RB, eds. Substance abuse: a comprehensive textbook. 2nd ed. Baltimore: Williams & Wilkins, 1992: 152–185.

Tabakoff B, Hellevuo K, Hoffman PL. Alcohol. In: Schuster CR, Gust SW, Kuhar MJ, eds. Handbook of experimental pharmacology, vol 118, Pharmacological aspects of drug dependence. New York: Springer-Verlag, 1996: 373–458.

Treistman SN, Bayley H, Lemos JR, et al. Effects of ethanol on calcium channels, potassium channels, and vasopressin release. Ann NY Acad Sci 1991; 625:249–263.

Wallgren H, Barry H, III. Actions of alcohol (2 volumes). Amsterdam: Elsevier, 1970.

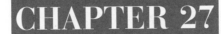

CHAPTER 27

Anxiolytics and Hypnotics

E.M. SELLERS, J.M. KHANNA, AND M.K. ROMACH

CASE HISTORY

Ms. K., 30 years old, was referred by her family doctor for assessment and management of her pattern and amount of alcohol consumption. Since her early teens, she had experienced anxiety accompanied by heart palpitations, lightheadedness, tremulousness, muscle tension, sweating, and difficulty concentrating when she was in any social situation—one-on-one discussions with her teachers, parties, family gatherings. As a result, she frequently avoided such situations. She then discovered that alcohol facilitated her ability to socialize, and she would drink two to three glasses of wine to relax in these situations.

By the time she entered university her anxiety had generalized to other situations, and even to the anticipation of them. As a result she started drinking alcohol before leaving home to attend such events. She found the alcohol to be moderately effective, but noted that as she drank more her anxiety became more persistent throughout the day. Her consumption of alcohol increased over the past 10 years from two to three glasses of wine twice weekly to five or more glasses daily.

Ms. K. was embarrassed by these symptoms, and had not discussed them with anybody until 3 months ago, when she confided to her family doctor the difficulties she was having but did not reveal how much she was drinking. Following a discussion about ways of managing symptoms of anxiety, her doctor prescribed alprazolam 0.5 mg twice a day. There was little discussion about how long the medication would be prescribed.

Within the first week of medication Ms. K. found her anxiety significantly but not entirely reduced. Over the next 3 weeks the dose was titrated to 0.5 mg four times per day. At this dosage she felt able to conduct her daily activities in a calm and competent manner and became engaged in more social interactions. At times she felt somewhat drowsy, but this abated over time. She also decreased her alcohol consumption significantly. Her intention was to stop drinking entirely, but she wished to reduce her intake gradually.

After 3 months, her physician suggested tapering off the alprazolam because he was concerned that she might become "addicted." However, the patient feared that she might find it impossible to stop taking the drug.

Her ambivalence between the doctor's recommendation to stop the medication and her fear of relapse of her anxiety began to generate an anxiety of its own. She related her concerns about a relapse to the physician, as well as her fear that she would resort once again to heavy drinking. Hearing of her past drinking history, the physician became more insistent that she stop the alprazolam and referred her to a treatment center for substance abuse. Ms. K. was not currently using any other drugs, licit or illicit, aside from the prescribed alprazolam and four to six glasses of wine per week.

DEFINITIONS

The terms "sedative" and "hypnotic" are rather old and are not very precise when applied to modern therapy. When alcohol, opioids, and belladonna were the only available psychopharmacological drugs, a wide variety of behavior disorders were managed by sedating the anxious or disturbed patient. A sedative drug decreases activity and agitation and calms the patient. The word "hypnotic," on the other hand, is derived from the Greek word *hypnos* for sleep and was applied to drugs used to promote sleep in any patient, not necessarily an anxious or agitated one. In fact, however, most of the drugs with sedating activity are also hypnotic.

The main use of hypnotics is to promote drowsiness and facilitate the onset or maintenance of sleep, which ideally should have all the characteristics of normal sleep. Hypnotic-induced and -maintained sleep is, however, never identical to normal physiological sleep.

The anxiolytic drugs constitute a large and chemically heterogeneous group (Table 27-1), which includes some drugs covered in other chapters. With the possible exception of benzodiazepines, most modern anxiolytic drugs have sedative action such as that seen with barbiturates. Even benzodiazepines share this property when high doses are given. Benzodiazepines are among the most commonly prescribed or used drugs in the world. About 10% of North Americans use a benzodiazepine at some time in the course

---

Table 27-1 Anxiolytic, Hypnotic Drugs

Alcohols (see Chapter 26)
   Ethchlorvynol*
   Chloral hydrate

Benzodiazepines

Barbiturates*

Piperidinediones
   Glutethimide*
   Methyprylon*

Miscellaneous
   Propanediol carbamates* (e.g., meprobamate)
   Methaqualone*
   Paraldehyde*
   Bromides*
   Monoureides*
   Ethinamate*
   Antihistamines (see Chapter 33)

*Note: These drugs, even though occasionally still used as anxiolytics and hypnotics, are mainly of historical interest. They have been largely replaced by drugs with greater efficacy, lesser abuse and dependence liability, and a wider margin of safety (e.g., benzodiazepines). The same can be said of all barbiturates except thiopental and phenobarbital.

---

of each year. Between 30 and 50% of hospitalized patients receive such drugs.

Sedation

Mild suppression of arousal and behavior, with slight reduction of alertness and responses to stimuli, is called sedation, and the drugs are called sedatives.

The mechanism of sedation produced by drugs is not fully known because of the complexity of their actions. Several features are important: (1) such drugs act on polysynaptic pathways; (2) they usually increase presynaptic inhibition; (3) different parts of the brain have different sensitivity toward them (i.e., regional selectivity and specificity); and (4) the drugs enhance pre- (and occasionally post-) synaptic effects of γ-aminobutyric acid (GABA).

Sleep

Further depression, by larger doses of the same drugs, causes sleep, and the drugs may then be used as hypnotics. The user can normally be roused by strong-enough stimuli (e.g., pain, alarm clock).

Normal sleep consists of at least two phases: (1) slow-wave sleep (SWS, or stages 3 and 4), so-called because the EEG shows predominantly high-voltage synchronous activity, but with sustained tonus of skeletal muscles; and (2) rapid-eye-movement (REM) sleep, in which the EEG shows an arousal pattern, the eyes move rapidly and irregularly, skeletal muscles relax completely, and dreaming is thought to take place. These two phases alternate throughout the total sleep period, REM sleep making up about 25% of the total. This alternation appears to depend upon a balance of serotonin (5-HT) and catecholamine influences on the reticular formation. Hypnotic drugs suppress the reticular formation to different degrees.

The **sleep produced by hypnotics** differs from normal sleep, in that SWS patterns are altered and shortened by the appearance of EEG spindles, REM sleep is suppressed, and total sleep time is prolonged. Most of the benzodiazepines produce similar effects on the patterns of sleep, although to a lesser degree. With chronic use the effects tend to decrease but do not disappear. If after 3–4 weeks the drug is suddenly stopped, the amount and intensity of REM increase to levels greater than in normal sleep ("REM rebound"). This is considered by some investigators to represent a mild degree of physical dependence and withdrawal reaction (see Adverse Effects of Barbiturates, and Chapter 72).

Anesthesia

Deeper depression, such that even intense stimuli do not cause arousal, is called anesthesia (see Chapter 24).

These three divisions are merely differences of degree and give no indication of different mechanisms. For drugs that have general CNS-depressant actions, decreased anxiety, sedation, sleep, and general anesthesia fall along a continuum of increasing CNS depression. However, modern drugs tend to have more selective actions (e.g., benzodiazepines are normally incapable of producing anesthesia).

In addition to sedation, sleep, or anesthesia, CNS-depressant drugs can depress other central states characterized by neuronal excitation. Hence, these drugs may be useful as antiepileptics or muscle relaxants.

BENZODIAZEPINES

Chlordiazepoxide was first marketed in 1960. This was followed by diazepam (1963) and oxazepam (1965), and many others since then. The popularity of these drugs is the result of a combination of their pharmacological actions, their relative safety, and the demand for agents of this type by both physicians and patients. Benzodiazepines can be classified on the basis of their chemical structure, kinetic characteristics, and therapeutic indications.

Structure

All benzodiazepines are variations upon the 5-aryl-1,4-benzodiazepine nucleus (Fig. 27-1). 1,5-Benzodiazepines also exist, but are not different in pharmacological action. Other than the apparent requirement for the 5-aryl group, the structure–activity relationships are not stringent, and many benzodiazepine metabolites are pharmacologically active.

Chlordiazepoxide and diazepam are the prototypical benzodiazepines. Diazepam and many other benzodiazepines are metabolized to the active metabolite *N*-desmethyldiazepam, also called nordiazepam (ND; see Fig. 27-4). ND is marketed as a separate drug in some countries. Chlorazepate and prazepam are quite rapidly converted to ND, one by acid hydrolysis and the other by dealkylation, and owe their clinical effects to the active metabolite (see Fig. 27-1).

The 3-OH substituent of oxazepam and lorazepam determines that the principal metabolic pathway is conjugation rather than production of ND. Triazolobenzodiazepines (e.g., triazolam) undergo rather rapid biotransformation without production of active metabolites.

Mechanism of Benzodiazepine Action

In 1977, specific receptors for the benzodiazepines were discovered in the nervous system. These receptors are characterized by the following properties:

- **Saturability.** The receptors are saturable by ^{3}H-diazepam with a K_D of 3.6 nM, or by ^{3}H-flunitrazepam with a K_D of 1–3 nM.
- **Stereoselectivity.** The (+)-enantiomers of benzodiazepines are about 200 times more active than the (−)-enantiomers in inhibiting the specific binding of ^{3}H-diazepam.
- **Receptor distribution in the CNS.** The receptors are highest in density in the cerebral cortex, as shown in Table 27-2, but are also present in significant numbers in the cerebellum and parts of the limbic system.

  Two subclasses of receptors, designated I and II, have been postulated. Type I receptors predominate in the cerebellum, cerebral cortical layer IV, and the substantia nigra. Type II receptors are found in hippocampus, superior colliculus, and cerebral cortical layers I–III. The prevalent view now is that both anxiolytic and sedative effects are mediated by the type I receptor, and anticonvulsant and muscle relaxation effects are related to type II receptor activation. All the benzodiazepines in current clinical use act on both type I and type II receptors, but a number of experimental compounds have been synthesized that are selective for one or another receptor type. The differences in pharmacological profiles of various benzodiazepines are related to differences in their intrinsic activities. Compounds with low intrinsic activity (partial agonists) at type I receptors display anxiolytic activity and are nonsedating, whereas compounds with high intrinsic activity are primarily sedatives. Amnesic effects are exerted even at a low level of receptor occupancy, and therefore the partial agonists still carry the disadvantage of producing amnesia.
- **Endogenous ligands.** None of the common neurotransmitters compete for binding with ^{3}H-diazepam. Norepinephrine, dopamine, GABA, glutamate, glycine, and histamine have no direct effect on the benzodiazepine receptor. An octapeptide isolated from brain has been claimed to be the

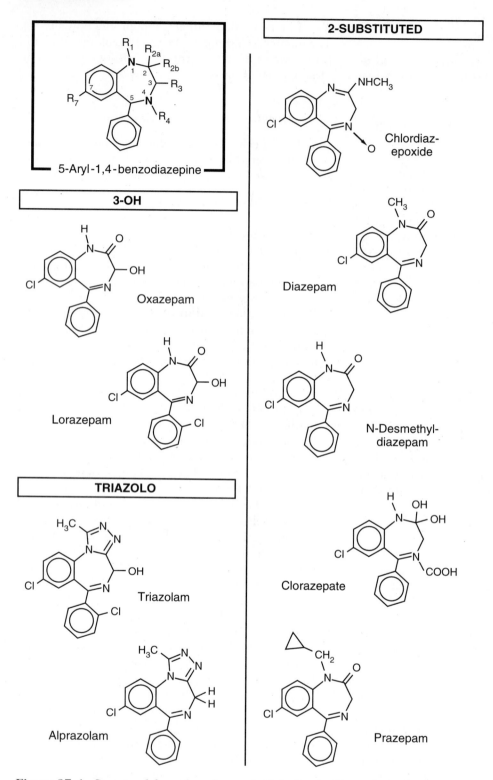

Figure 27-1. Structural formulae of several clinically significant benzodiazepines.

Table 27-2 Density of Benzodiazepine Binding Sites in Different Regions of the Human Brain

Region	^3H-Diazepam B_{max} (fmoles of ^3H-ligand per mg protein)
Cerebral cortex	1200
Cerebellar cortex	730
Amygdala	720
Hippocampus	610
Hypothalamus	520

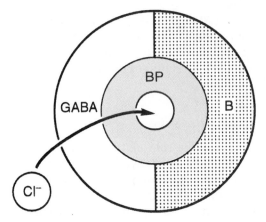

Figure 27-2. Schematic representation of the GABA/chloride-ionophore receptor complex, transected in the plane of the cell membrane. (Note that this is an evolving field of investigation with at times conflicting views. See Chapter 22 for additional interpretations.) GABA = GABA receptor; B = benzodiazepine receptor; BP = barbiturate and picrotoxinin receptor, believed to be closely associated with the chloride ionophore; Cl^- = chloride channel.

endogenous ligand for the benzodiazepine receptor, but there is not yet agreement on this point.

GABA-linked benzodiazepine receptors

Since both GABA (at 1 μM) and the GABA-agonist muscimol (at 100 nM) enhance the binding of ^3H-diazepam to its receptor, it is thought that the benzodiazepine receptor is linked cooperatively to the GABA receptor as described below (see also Chapter 22). Elevated GABA levels in brain are associated with stable, electrically suppressed nervous tissue. Benzodiazepines are thought to produce their anticonvulsant effect by increasing the effect of GABA at its receptor.

Postsynaptic GABA receptors are functionally linked to benzodiazepine receptors, barbiturate receptors, and a Cl^- ion channel that collectively constitute the GABA-receptor/chloride-ionophore complex. This entire complex is involved in the mediation and modulation of GABAergic inhibitory transmission. The physiological effects of GABA are mediated by increases in chloride conductance, but all three receptors contribute to the regulation of the chloride ionophore.

Figure 27-2 is a theoretical model of the GABA-receptor/Cl^--ionophore complex. This transverse two-dimensional view of the receptor complex represents the chloride channel located centrally, surrounded by three distinct receptors: the GABA receptor, the benzodiazepine receptor, and the picrotoxinin-barbiturate receptor. The ion channel may be a separate component or could be a part of one of the proteins bearing the receptors. Neurotransmitters or drugs that open the Cl^- channel are thought to have antiseizure activity, and those that block the Cl^- channel are convulsant in nature.

The GABA-receptor/Cl^--ionophore complex is composed of subunits (designated α, β, and γ), each of which exists in several isoforms (α_1, α_2, β_1, β_2, etc.). The expression of the mRNAs for these subunits varies greatly across brain regions, so the actual set of subunits making up a receptor complex varies in different regions. This diversity may be functionally important, because different combinations of subunits offer the possibility of specificity or selectivity for different drugs. The different benzodiazepine receptor types (I and II) presumably reflect different subunit combinations that may permit the future development of new benzodiazepines with selective actions.

Interaction of the benzodiazepines with their specific binding sites increases chloride conductance in the presence of GABA by increasing the frequency of Cl^- channel openings, and this effect can be blocked by the GABA antagonist bicuculline. These findings indicate that benzodiazepines act to potentiate GABAergic inhibition and that a functional GABA receptor is required for the action of the benzodiazepines. Anticonvulsant barbiturates such as phenobarbital potentiate GABAergic inhibition by prolonging the period during which the Cl^- channels stay open in response to GABA-receptor activation. This effect is inhibited by picrotoxin, a CNS-stimulatory drug that is thought to cause convulsions by blocking the Cl^- channels without affecting the binding of GABA to its receptor site.

So far, work on the linkage between the benzodiazepine receptor and the GABA/Cl⁻-ionophore complex has offered a possible explanation of the anticonvulsant effects of benzodiazepines. It is not yet clear whether this linkage is related to the anxiolytic properties of these drugs.

Benzodiazepine antagonist

The investigation of the role of the benzodiazepine receptor has been advanced by the discovery of a selective and specific antagonist, flumazenil (Ro 15-1788). This substance (Fig. 27-3) blocks or reverses diazepam effects but has no apparent intrinsic activity of its own. When given to monkeys to which diazepam has been administered chronically, the antagonist precipitates a benzodiazepine withdrawal syndrome.

β-Carbolines

Benzodiazepine-antagonistic properties have also been discovered among receptor ligands structurally different from flumazenil. Various β-carboline derivatives bind specifically to the ³H-diazepam receptors but produce effects opposite to those of benzodiazepines; i.e., they show proconvulsant activity and anxiogenic effects. Therefore they have been called inverse agonists rather than antagonists. It has been suggested that β-carbolines produce effects opposite to those of benzodiazepines because these agents reduce the coupling of GABA receptors to the Cl⁻ ionophore, thereby decreasing the frequency of chloride channel opening. Interestingly, flumazenil also blocks the effect of β-carbolines, since it blocks the receptor binding of inverse agonists as well as of agonists.

Pharmacokinetics

Absorption

After oral administration, the absorption of diazepam, alprazolam, and triazolam is very rapid. The

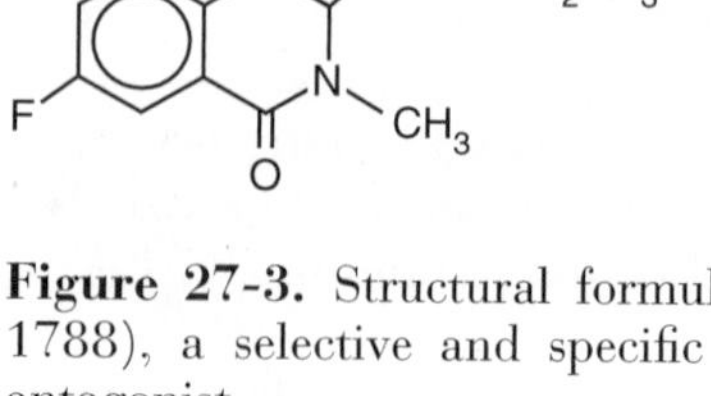

Figure 27-3. Structural formula of flumazenil (Ro 15-1788), a selective and specific benzodiazepine receptor antagonist.

peak plasma concentration occurs about 1 hour after ingestion. Such rapid absorption can account for the acute subjective drowsiness, "spaced-out" feeling, or motor impairment after the drug is ingested. Such effects are also dose-related. Diazepam has a systemic bioavailability of 100%. Oxazepam, lorazepam, and prazepam are absorbed more slowly, maximum plasma concentration occurring 2–3 hours after ingestion; the bioavailability of oxazepam taken orally is about 50–70%. Clorazepate is converted by acid hydrolysis in the stomach to its active form, desmethyldiazepam; antacids reduce the rate of conversion and decrease the drug's peak effects.

After intramuscular injection of diazepam or of chlordiazepoxide in healthy persons or alcoholics in withdrawal, absorption is slow (the plasma concentration peaking at 10–12 hours) and erratic, but eventually complete. As a consequence, clinical effects may be delayed and unpredictable. Therefore, these drugs should generally not be given intramuscularly.

Protein binding

Most benzodiazepines are extensively bound to serum albumin (e.g., diazepam is 98% bound at therapeutic concentrations). The binding decreases the concentration of free active drug in equilibrium with the sites of action and elimination. However, drug can rapidly go off its protein binding sites and become available to the sites of action. Glomerular filtration of many benzodiazepines is low because of their extensive serum protein binding.

Biotransformation and disposition of individual drugs

All benzodiazepines undergo biotransformation in the liver, mainly by cytochrome P450 activity or by conjugation. Rates and patterns of benzodiazepine biotransformation vary considerably among healthy and sick humans.

Figure 27-4 summarizes the typical patterns of biotransformation. Even though there are many benzodiazepines, there are only a few patterns of biotransformation. Metabolites indicated with an asterisk in Figure 27-4 are pharmacologically active. Table 27-3 classifies the benzodiazepines on the basis of their half-lives and patterns of disposition.

Chlordiazepoxide and **diazepam** each have two major active metabolites that contribute to their clinical effects and toxicity: (1) Chlordiazepoxide is converted to desmethylchlordiazepoxide and then to demoxepam; (2) diazepam is converted to desmethyl-

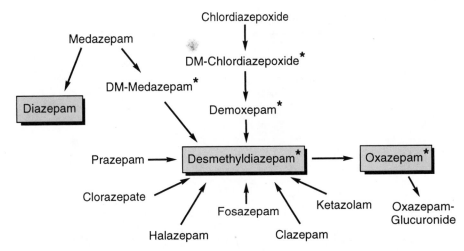

Figure 27-4. Patterns of benzodiazepine biotransformation. DM = desmethyl; * = active metabolites.

diazepam and then to oxazepam, itself a marketed benzodiazepine. Desmethyldiazepam has a longer mean half-life than the parent drug (50.9 ± 6.2 hours versus 32.6 ± 11.3 hours). By coincidence, the half-life of diazepam in hours is about equal to the patient's age in years; however, there are many exceptions to this rule. Little diazepam is excreted in the bile, and enterohepatic recirculation is not responsible for the slow elimination.

These long half-lives and the extent of variation between patients make prediction of the time of maximum clinical effect or toxicity very difficult, but during long-term therapy one can expect cumulative and long-lasting effects of the benzodiazepines with long half-lives. On average, the time for cumulation to peak concentration during long-term oral administration is roughly five times the half-life of the drug, i.e., for chlordiazepoxide it is 3 days, for diazepam 7 days, and desmethyldiazepam 10 days. The slow cumulation of drug means that the full therapeutic effect or toxicity cannot be determined for a considerable time; therefore the dosage should not be adjusted until cumulation is maximal. Conversely, elimination of the drug is slow and the offset of drug effect may be delayed.

Because of the long half-lives of chlordiazepoxide and diazepam, multiple daily doses may in theory be unnecessary. However, if the entire 24-hour dosage is given as a single dose, it may cause extreme sedation. Because of this sedating action, it is best to give most of the daily dose at bedtime.

The biotransformation of chlordiazepoxide, diazepam, and desmethyldiazepam is impaired in patients with severe liver disease, and the half-life may increase up to sixfold. The biotransformation of chlordiazepoxide and diazepam is inhibited by concurrent administration of disulfiram or ethanol.

Lorazepam, a more potent benzodiazepine, is similar to **oxazepam** in structure and in pattern of disposition. Its bioavailability after intramuscular injection is complete. Unlike chlordiazepoxide and diazepam, lorazepam and oxazepam are biotransformed simply by glucuronide conjugation to inactive metabolites. Furthermore, since the mean half-life of oxazepam is 7 hours, cumulation is minor and a full therapeutic response occurs after a few doses. Similarly, excessive sedation rapidly disappears. However, for the therapeutic effect to be maintained the drug should be given three times a day. Neither liver disease nor advanced age alters the half-life of oxazepam or lorazepam. These drugs may be preferable for treating acute anxiety disorder, when dose titration is required and hangover or daytime lethargy are particularly to be avoided. The slower absorption of oxazepam and lorazepam, however, somewhat detracts from their usefulness as hypnotics.

Triazolam is well absorbed, has a rapid onset of action, is rapidly metabolized, and has no active metabolites. It is widely used as a hypnotic agent.

Flurazepam, though marketed as a hypnotic, has few properties to recommend it as such. The cumulation of the slowly eliminated active metabolite, desalkylflurazepam, over 7–10 days results in slow onset of the hypnotic effect and causes drowsiness as a side effect during long-term use. Older patients are particularly likely to experience toxic effects because they are more sensitive to various psychoactive drugs and may have altered biotransformation of the drug.

Table 27-3 Kinetic Classification of Some Benzodiazepines by Half-Life

Drug	Maximum Recommended Daily Dose (mg)	Time to Peak Effect (hours)	Half-Life (hours)	Therapeutic Indications	Active Metabolites (half-life in hours)
Long half-life					
Rapid pro-drug conversion					
Clorazepate* (Tranxene)	60	1–2	1	Anxiety	DM-diazepam (30–200)
Flurazepam* (Dalmane)	30	1	1.5	Insomnia	Desalkylflurazepam (40–250)
Slow pro-drug conversion					
Chlordiazepoxide* (Librium)	100	2–4	130	Anxiety	DM-diazepam (30–200)
Diazepam* (Valium)	40	1–2	20–100	Anxiety	DM-diazepam (30–200) Oxazepam (5–15)
Prazepam* (Centrax)	60	3	3	Anxiety	DM-diazepam (30–200)
Intermediate half-life					
Alprazolam (Xanax)	3	1–2	6–20	Anxiety/pain	
Lorazepam (Ativan)	6	1–6	10–20	Anxiety	
Nitrazepam (Mogadon)	10	2	15–40	Insomnia	
Oxazepam (Serax)	120	1–4	5–15	Anxiety	
Temazepam (Restoril)	30	0.8–1.4	10–20	Insomnia	
Short half-life					
Brotizolam	0.125–0.5	1–2	2–7	Insomnia	
Midazolam (Versed)	7.5–15	0.25–0.5	1.5–5	Sedation	
Triazolam (Halcion)	0.25	1–2	1.5–5	Insomnia	

*Biotransformation results in desmethyl (DM) derivative, which has long half-life as indicated.

Alprazolam has been marketed primarily for the treatment of panic disorders, for which it has become quite popular. It is well absorbed by mouth and reaches its peak concentration in 1–2 hours after a single dose. It has a half-life of about 11 hours, which is increased substantially in the elderly and in patients with liver or kidney disease. One of its primary metabolites, α-hydroxyalprazolam, is further metabolized to desmethylalprazolam, and both of these are active.

Clonazepam is a long-acting benzodiazepine, and the half-life of the parent compound varies from approximately 18 to 50 hours. Although its pharmacological profile is similar to those of other benzodiazepines, it is used primarily for the treatment of epilepsy (petit mal; see Chapter 22).

Midazolam is a short-acting (half-life 1–4 hours) benzodiazepine that is available only as an injectable formulation of its water-soluble hydrochloride salt. It is used for both preoperative sedation and induction of anesthesia. Midazolam itself is highly lipophilic and onset of effect is rapid; offset of effect is also rapid, because of both redistribution and biotransformation. Administration of midazolam is often followed by anterograde amnesia.

Temazepam is a hypnotic agent very similar in pharmacokinetic properties to other intermediate-half-life benzodiazepines. It is useful for short-term management of insomnia.

Zopiclone (Imovane) is structurally not a benzodiazepine, but a cyclopyrrolone derivative. Nevertheless, its pharmacological properties are so similar to those of the intermediate-acting benzodiazepines that it is usually grouped with them. Zopiclone has a half-life of approximately 5 hours. It has a rapid onset of action and peak plasma concentrations are produced within 90 minutes. The drug is marketed as a hypnotic.

Distribution

Benzodiazepines are distributed widely in the body; tissue concentrations in brain, liver, and spleen exceed those of unbound drug in the serum. The volumes of distribution of the benzodiazepines correlate well with in vitro measures of their lipid solubilities. Thus, diazepam is more lipophilic than chlordiazepoxide and has a larger apparent volume of distribution. Similarly, the volumes of distribution of chlordiazepoxide and diazepam are larger in females than in males, and in elderly patients (over 70 years of age) than in younger ones. The larger volume of distribution accounts in part for the prolonged half-life in older patients (see Chapters 5 and 66). Chlordiazepoxide, diazepam, and desmethyldiazepam enter the CNS at rates proportional to their lipid solubilities, while steady-state concentrations in cerebrospinal fluid are determined by the degree of serum protein binding of the drugs. Diazepam and chlordiazepoxide also cross the placenta and appear in small amounts in breast milk.

Pharmacological Actions and Therapeutic Uses

Behavioral effects

Antianxiety action. The effects of the benzodiazepines in the relief of anxiety can be demonstrated readily in experimental animals. In conflict punishment procedures (see Chapter 71), benzodiazepines greatly reduce the behavior-suppressing effects of punishment, so the animals will continue to seek food or water despite the concurrent presence of electrical shock. Other drugs such as barbiturates may show similar effects, but the benzodiazepines produce these effects without sedation or alteration of other animal behaviors. No benzodiazepine has been shown to be superior in efficacy to chlordiazepoxide for the treatment of acute anxiety disorder or chronic anxiety states.

The majority of the benzodiazepines have been approved for use in acute anxiety disorders. Although most of these drugs are also used for chronic anxiety states, their efficacy decreases somewhat after a few weeks. Thus, there is less indication for the drugs to be used for chronic anxiety.

Most benzodiazepines have no antidepressant and no antipsychotic (neuroleptic) actions, but recently alprazolam has been shown to have some activity in depression.

Anticonvulsant activity. Benzodiazepines are potent anticonvulsants (see Chapter 22) and have been shown to prevent or abolish seizures in various animal models of epilepsy. These drugs are very potent in preventing pentylenetetrazole-induced sei-

zures but are less potent in electroshock-induced seizures. Although very effective in the treatment of status epilepticus (e.g., with diazepam), absence attacks, and other types of childhood seizures (e.g., with clonazepam), oral benzodiazepines have only a limited role in the long-term management of seizure disorders because of the development of tolerance to their anticonvulsant effect.

Alcohol withdrawal. Most benzodiazepines are effective in the treatment of alcohol withdrawal syndrome (see Chapter 26). The longer-acting benzodiazepines, such as chlordiazepoxide or diazepam, are more effective than shorter-acting benzodiazepines in the treatment of the alcohol withdrawal syndrome.

Muscle relaxant effects. Benzodiazepines reduce elevated skeletal muscle tone and are effective in various neuromuscular disorders including cerebral palsy, tetanus, and "stiff-man syndrome" (a rare autoimmune disease of the CNS, in which autoantibodies against glutamate decarboxylase interfere with GABA interneuron function in the spinal cord). They are frequently used in a variety of problems for which the efficacy of benzodiazepines is unproven, such as backache and muscle trauma.

Amnesia with sedation. The wide margin of safety of the benzodiazepines permits their use in a variety of clinical situations in which the objective is simply to produce sedation and amnesia (e.g., endoscopy, bronchoscopy, preanesthetic sedation, anesthesia induction, cardioversion, delivery). In these situations, intravenous diazepam is at least as effective as and safer than barbiturates, but it is probably not superior to other parenterally administered benzodiazepines. Midazolam, a benzodiazepine with very rapid elimination, is available for induction of anesthesia or acute sedation, and also produces amnesia in over two-thirds of such cases.

These drugs should be chosen with consideration of the desired duration of action (see Table 27-3).

Insomnia. Insomnia is a symptom or sign and is not a diagnosis or disease. Except for a very rare patient who may have a primary chronic sleep disorder, insomnia is always due to some other primary event or process.

Transient insomnia is short term (less than 2 weeks) and typically due to factors that are readily understood as being disruptive of sleep (e.g., jet lag, situational anxiety, shift-work, physical factors such as noise and cold, bereavement, pain). Medications are often not needed since simple "sleep hygiene" and common sense measures are sufficient. If a hypnotic is prescribed, the shorter-acting medications (e.g., oxazepam, temazepam, triazolam, zopiclone) are preferred, to minimize morning "hangover." Since triazolam rapidly enters the brain, it produces an early onset of sleep. However, this property also contributes to the anterograde amnesia seen particularly at higher doses. Other marketed hypnotics have a slower rate of onset.

The initial prescription should be for up to 1 week, with one repeat permitted before a full reassessment. Such short-term use is not associated with physical dependence, (i.e., a clinically important withdrawal syndrome) or abuse. In order to avoid drug side effects, the initial doses should not be "routine," but rather initiated at the lowest effective dose. The elderly are more sensitive to most psychotropic drugs, and therefore initial doses in those over 60 years of age should be 50% of those listed. The most common side effect of hypnotics is feeling sedated or mentally "fuzzy" in the morning. The longer the drug's half-life, the greater the probability of this. No hypnotic should be combined with alcohol, and patients must be warned of this. Some patients may have a mildly disrupted sleep pattern for one or two nights upon abrupt discontinuation.

Experience with triazolam is far more extensive than with most of the other hypnotics, but recently concerns about its safety have been raised. It has received extensive negative publicity because of complaints of confusion, amnesia, bizarre behavior, agitation, or hallucination. This drug has been withdrawn from sale in some countries. In North America, the recommended starting dose has been reduced to 0.125 mg from 0.25 mg, and the recommended maximum dose is now 0.25 mg instead of 0.5 mg. Triazolam has been reported to be associated with paradoxical rage reactions, but these are extremely rare, and it is not clear in most cases that the drug was an important etiological factor.

Chronic insomnia requires a comprehensive medical and psychiatric assessment, since it is associated with such a wide range of etiologies (e.g., alcohol or drug abuse; depression; anxiety disorders; bipolar disorder; adjustment disorder; cardiovascular and CNS disease, including dementia; medication side effects; chronic pain; use of excessive amounts of caffeinated beverages). Hypnotics have no primary role in the management of these types of problems. Patients with primary chronic insomnia should have their management directed by specialists in the field.

In most such cases, it is best not to use hypnotics at all. However, such medications can be very effective in more severely affected individuals, and may give much-needed relief. In that situation they should be used only for short periods of time in transient insomnia, or as adjuncts in the management of clinical problems that can cause insomnia.

Responsiveness

Dose requirements for patients vary greatly. For example, the diazepam concentration required to produce sufficient sedation and relaxation to permit passage of a gastroscope varies 22-fold; hence, there must be such great differences in receptor sensitivity that it is virtually impossible to predict a clinical response at a particular dose in a particular patient. The sensitivity to benzodiazepines increases with age and liver disease and decreases with smoking and with recent use of benzodiazepines, alcohol, or other drugs that produce cross-tolerance to benzodiazepines. As a rule of thumb the initial dose of benzodiazepine should be reduced by 50% in the elderly (over 65 years), patients with liver disease, or those concurrently receiving other CNS depressants.

Relation of drug concentration and effect

Single measurements of the concentration of chlordiazepoxide or diazepam in whole blood or plasma do not correlate closely with the therapeutic or toxic effects because of the presence of active metabolites, the variation between patients in the concentration of free drug, the development of tolerance, and the inaccurate quantitation of the response. (However, *within* patients the drug effect increases with drug concentration.) These drugs are slowly eliminated from the body; hence metabolites may be detected in plasma or urine for weeks after administration of a single dose, even though clinically significant effects are no longer present.

Tolerance, dependence, and withdrawal

Acute, subacute, and chronic tolerance to benzodiazepines have been demonstrated in studies with animals and humans (see also Chapter 72). During long-term administration, tolerance commonly manifests itself as a decrease in side effects.

Tolerance to benzodiazepines appears to be primarily functional rather than metabolic in nature. Tolerance to the sedative, anticonvulsant, and muscle relaxant effects of benzodiazepines has been shown. In general, their anxiolytic effects persist during chronic treatment, although there is some disagreement about this. Physical dependence may develop in patients taking large amounts of diazepam (more than 40 mg/day) or chlordiazepoxide (more than 200 mg/day), and the consequent signs and symptoms of withdrawal may be seen when use of the drug is stopped. However, elimination of diazepam and chlordiazepoxide (and their metabolites) is slow enough that the withdrawal reaction is delayed and often mild, because tissue levels of these benzodiazepines decline slowly and the receptors have more chance to return to a normal state. (This is equivalent to "tapering.") When a reaction occurs, anxiety, tremor, insomnia, disorders of perception, and, rarely, seizures are the clinical features.

More rapidly eliminated benzodiazepines may produce a more severe clinical withdrawal syndrome. The reason for this is that, after termination of treatment with a short-acting benzodiazepine, the tissue levels of drug decline rapidly, causing rapid onset of the withdrawal reaction before there has been any return toward normal sensitivity. Just as with opioids, the precipitated withdrawal reaction induced with benzodiazepine antagonists may not be identical to the withdrawal reaction resulting from cessation of drug administration.

Psychological dependence can occur at any dose, and the resultant signs and symptoms are difficult to distinguish from those of withdrawal reaction and from anxiety. Patients who have taken therapeutic doses of benzodiazepines for a long time frequently experience severe anxiety when an attempt is made to discontinue the drug. Recent reports indicate that some of these patients, in fact, are experiencing drug withdrawal effects. The risk of physical dependence can be minimized by avoiding long-term (more than 6 weeks) therapy. Concern has been expressed that the high-potency, short-half-life benzodiazepines are more prone to produce dependence and have a greater incidence of withdrawal reactions after stopping the drug.

For most conditions for which efficacy of benzodiazepine therapy has been proven, only 2–4 weeks of therapy is required, and such short-term therapy will ordinarily not give rise to clinically important withdrawal symptoms. Sometimes the diagnosis is not clear and a trial of therapy with a benzodiazepine is reasonable. At the commencement of such a trial, the desired therapeutic goal and the duration of therapy should be specified.

Drug Interactions

Benzodiazepines interact with many psychoactive drugs. The combination of ethyl alcohol and benzodiazepines can impair driving skills to a degree greater than that caused by the same amount of either drug alone. This fact is of forensic importance and physicians should warn their patients about the hazards of drinking alcohol when they are taking benzodiazepines. Interactions among benzodiazepines, analgesics, antihistamines, phenothiazines, and tricyclic antidepressants are also well documented. A list of such proven interactions is not helpful, and patients must always be cautioned, when taking other psychoactive agents together with benzodiazepines, against driving a car or engaging in other activities in which there is risk to themselves or others.

Benzodiazepines do not induce the synthesis of drug-biotransforming enzymes, have less risk of interaction with coumarin anticoagulants than barbiturates do, and are safer to use in combination with anticoagulants, antiarrhythmics, antineoplastic agents, and antiepileptic drugs, with which metabolic interactions are most common during barbiturate therapy.

Adverse Reactions

Orally administered benzodiazepines cause side effects, which are not life-threatening, in less than 10% of hospitalized patients who receive them. The common adverse effects of benzodiazepines are direct extensions of their pharmacological actions: drowsiness, ataxia, lethargy, and, rarely, coma. However, paradoxical excitation may on occasion be observed.

Benzodiazepines may interfere with memory acquisition, consolidation, and recall, and all are able to produce an anterograde amnesia.

The frequency of side effects of chlordiazepoxide and diazepam therapy increases with age, dose, duration of therapy, and presence of liver disease and hypoalbuminemia.

Hematological, renal, and hepatic toxicity have seldom been reported for benzodiazepines. Various unusual responses have been observed, including nightmares, paradoxical delirium and confusion, depression, aggression, and hostile behavior. Rarely, patients experience a dry mouth, a metallic taste, or headaches. It is important for the physician to be aware of the sometimes-bizarre effects of these drugs.

Uncommon but important acute adverse effects after **intravenous administration** include respira-

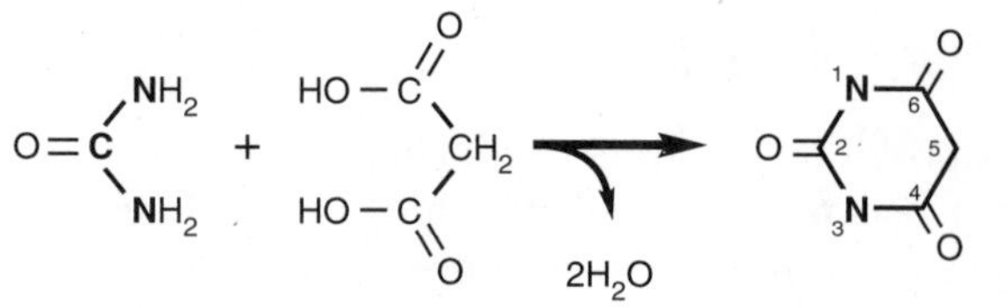

Figure 27-5. Production of barbituric acid, the parent compound of barbiturates, from urea and malonic acid.

tory or cardiac arrest or both, hypotension, and phlebitis at the site of injection. Life-threatening adverse reactions occur with a frequency of about 2% after rapid intravenous administration of diazepam. Patients particularly at risk often have coexisting severe pulmonary or cardiac disease or have concurrently received cardiorespiratory-depressant medications. Whenever possible and practical, the rate of injection should be less than 12.5 mg/min for chlordiazepoxide and less than 2.5 mg/min for diazepam. Phlebitis is most common after repeated injections at the same site and can be minimized by flushing the vein with 50 mL of saline after each injection.

Since the administration of benzodiazepines to pregnant women has not been proven to be safe for the fetus, these drugs should be prescribed during pregnancy only when their use is mandatory, and then for the shortest time possible.

An **overdose** of benzodiazepines alone is never fatal. On the basis of this wide margin of safety alone, benzodiazepines should replace barbiturates. However, since 35% of drug overdoses involve more than one drug, combinations of benzodiazepines and more dangerous drugs, such as alcohol, are common and may cause death.

BARBITURATES

The uses of barbiturates are very limited in modern therapeutics. These drugs have largely been replaced by the benzodiazepines, which are, on balance, safer.

Chemical Structure

A barbiturate results from the condensation of malonic acid and urea, as shown in Figure 27-5. Barbituric acid itself has no sedative effect, but if the two hydrogen atoms on C-5 are replaced by ethyl (C_2H_5) or larger hydrocarbon groups, the resulting products

are pharmacologically active. British pharmacopoeial names for these drugs end in "-itone," the American names in "-ital." Drugs in which the oxygen on C-2 is replaced by sulfur are called thiobarbiturates; e.g., the thio equivalent of pentobarbital is called thiopental. Such compounds are extremely rapid- and short-acting when injected intravenously, and they are used exclusively in this way as general anesthetics (see Chapter 24).

Pharmacokinetics

Factors determining speed of onset and duration of barbiturate action include the following.

Lipid solubility

In general, the speed of onset and duration of action both depend on the relative lipid solubility, as reflected by the membrane/water partition coefficient. As Table 27-4 indicates, the barbiturate derivatives with higher lipid solubility have a more rapid onset but a shorter duration of action. Thiopental and other ultrashort-acting barbiturates are very highly lipid-soluble and enter the brain very quickly, producing anesthesia almost instantaneously. However, within a few minutes they are widely redistributed throughout the body, with the result that the concentration in brain and, therefore, the depth of central depression both decrease (see Chapter 24 and Fig. 27-6).

Barbiturates with lower lipid solubility and a longer duration of action (pentobarbital and secobarbital) enter the brain less readily than thiopental and are therefore less suitable as intravenous anesthetics. Moreover, these agents are usually taken by mouth, so wide distribution in the body does not lag so far behind entry into the central nervous system. Recovery from oral pentobarbital and secobarbital, therefore, depends more on biotransformation of the drug than on redistribution.

Ionization

Barbiturates are weak acids. For some, the pK_a is such that urinary excretion can be increased by alkalinization of the urine. This applies, for example, to phenobarbital, which has a pK_a of 7.2 (see Chapter 7).

Table 27-4 Characteristics of Some Barbiturates

C-5 Substituents	Nonproprietary Name	Duration (half-life—hours)	Membrane/Buffer Partition Coefficient ($P_{m/b}$)
Phenyl and ethyl	Phenobarbital	Long (35–150)	9
Isopentyl and ethyl	Amobarbital	Intermediate (8–42)	11
Methylbutyl and ethyl	Pentobarbital	Intermediate (15–48)	11
Methyl and cyclohexenyl	Hexobarbital	Ultrashort (2.7–7)	36

Biotransformation

Most barbiturates are extensively biotransformed to inactive metabolites by the hepatic drug-hydroxylating system (see Chapter 4). Some barbiturates are biotransformed slowly. In humans, about 20% of a sedative dose of phenobarbital is converted to *p*-hydroxyphenobarbital and excreted in the urine over a 5-day period; 15–20% is eliminated unchanged in the same period. The mean plasma half-life of unchanged phenobarbital is about 86 hours. With barbital, up to 90% is eliminated unchanged.

Recently, other pathways of barbiturate metabolism have been discovered, including *N*-glucosylation. Oriental populations show much more glucosylation relative to hydroxylation of barbiturates than occidental populations do. However, the clinical significance of this difference is not yet clear, and it does not affect the overall elimination half-life of the drug.

Clinical Uses

There are few recommended uses of barbiturates today. Some barbiturates (e.g., phenobarbital) are anticonvulsants and may be employed clinically to reduce the frequency and severity of seizures in epileptics (see Chapter 22).

Other uses are in anesthesia induction (e.g., thiopental) referred to above and in Chapter 24, in special neuropsychiatric investigations, and to reduce cerebral edema (potentially effective).

Barbiturates are no longer considered appropriate for the treatment of anxiety or insomnia. Although they are still used to some extent as hypnotics, they have largely been replaced for this purpose by short-acting benzodiazepines.

Adverse Effects of Barbiturates

1. In very low doses, instead of sedation the barbiturates may occasionally produce uncontrolled **hyperactivity of the cortex.** The patient may be euphoric, excited, restless, agitated, or violent. This resembles early alcohol intoxication, or the early stage of ether anesthesia (see Chapter 24). In chronic users who have developed some tolerance, an otherwise-normal hypnotic dose may produce these effects.

2. With large doses of barbiturate, depression may persist for longer than intended, and the patient feels **groggy and "doped"** the next day. This is the result of the relatively long half-lives of the drugs used as hypnotics (e.g., pentobarbital and secobarbital) with continuation of drug action into the following day.

3. Chronic use of barbiturates, especially as daytime sedatives in repeated doses, may lead to **tolerance, dependence,** and the risk of a **withdrawal syndrome.**

Tolerance is in part metabolic, by induction of the liver cytochrome P450 system. To be effective as an inducer, the drug must be present for a sufficiently long uninterrupted period. Therefore, the long-acting (i.e., slowly eliminated) barbiturates such as barbital and phenobarbital are the best inducers of the biotransformation of other drugs; however, they do not induce their own biotransformation appreciably. Short-acting barbiturates act as inducers only if repeated doses are given at short intervals so as to maintain an appreciable blood level for some time. When induction does occur, the metabolism of a whole range of other drugs can be greatly speeded up (see Chapter 4).

The other major component of tolerance is an

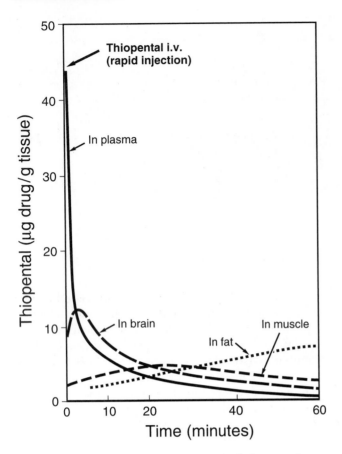

Figure 27-6. Calculated time courses of thiopental concentration in human tissues.

adaptive change in the nervous system itself, which compensates for the drug effect by an increase in neuronal excitability. When the drug is withdrawn, a barbiturate abstinence syndrome occurs that is very similar to the alcohol withdrawal syndrome (see Chapters 26 and 72).

4. In **congenital porphyria**, barbiturates can precipitate or aggravate attacks by increasing the production of porphyrins in the liver.

5. With severe **overdose**, depression extends to the hypothalamus and the medullary centers for cardiovascular and respiratory control. Respiration is slow and shallow, and heart rate and blood pressure are reduced.

6. Death from overdose: Barbiturates are encountered in about 12% of acute drug ingestions (toxic overdoses). Alone or in combination with other drugs such as alcohol they can cause death, usually due to respiratory failure. **Treatment of overdose** consists of support of cardiovascular and respiratory function, removal of drug by gastric lavage, and occasionally forced diuresis and alkalinization of the urine (see Chapter 74).

SUGGESTED READING

Busto U, Kaplan HL, Zawertailo L, Sellers EM. Pharmacological effects and abuse liability of bretazenil, diazepam and alprazolam in humans. Clin Pharmacol Ther 1994; 55(4):451–463.

Busto U, Sellers EM, Naranjo CA, et al. Withdrawal reaction after long-term therapeutic use of benzodiazepines. N Engl J Med 1986; 315:854–859.

Giusti P, Romeo E, Auta J, Guidotti A. Structural variety of GABA$_A$ receptors and specificity of benzodiazepine pharmacological profiles. Adv Biochem Psychopharmacol 1992; 47:163–177.

Greenblatt DJ, Shader RI. Pharmacokinetics of antianxiety agents. In: Meltzer HY, ed. Psychopharmacology: the third generation of progress. New York: Raven Press, 1987:1377–1386.

Hallström C, ed. Benzodiazepine dependence. Oxford: Oxford University Press, 1993.

Mendelson WB. Neuropharmacology of sleep induction by benzodiazepines. Crit Rev Neurobiol 1992; 6:221–232.

Romach MK, Busto U, Somer G, Kaplan HL, Sellers EM. Clinical aspects of chronic alprazolam and lorazepam use. Am J Psychiatry 1995; 152:1161–1167.

Sanger DJ, Benavides J, Perrault G, et al. Recent developments in the behavioral pharmacology of benzodiazepine (omega) receptors: evidence for the functional significance of receptor subtypes. Neurosci Biobehav Rev 1994; 18:355–372.

Sellers EM, Ciraulo DA, DuPont RL, et al. Alprazolam and benzodiazepine withdrawal. J Clin Psychiatry 1993; 54(10, Suppl):64–75.

Shader RI, Greenblatt DJ. Use of benzodiazepines in anxiety disorders. N Engl J Med 1993; 328:1398–1405.

CHAPTER 28

Antipsychotics

S. KAPUR AND P. SEEMAN

W. G. was 19 years old when he enrolled in university. His academic record was good, he won a place on the university rowing team, and he enjoyed his share of late nights throughout first year. When he returned to school for his second year, his roommate observed that W. G. was staying by himself, avoiding the company of friends, and skipping school and athletic training, things he had never done before. Some time later, he was heard speaking to himself as he sat isolated in his room, mumbling and smiling. Soon after, he confided to his roommate that he had uncovered a "grand conspiracy" to rob him of his athletic abilities and that he could hear the conspirators' voices as they made plans to destroy him. Finally, he accused his roommate of being a part of the conspiracy.

At this point, his friends called his parents and he was taken to see a psychiatrist. The psychiatrist diagnosed him as showing early symptoms of schizophrenia, and he was admitted to the hospital. Blood and urine tests were negative for signs of any general medical condition or the presence of any street drugs. He was therefore treated with haloperidol at a starting dose of 10 mg per day. On the second day of his treatment, while a medical student was interviewing him, he seemed to develop a "seizure." His neck was strained backward with his face turned upward toward the ceiling. He was having difficulty speaking but was quite conscious of his surroundings. The attending physician recognized this as an acute dystonic reaction to the medication rather than a seizure.

The doctor immediately ordered an injection of benztropine, which resolved the situation in a matter of minutes. Following this experience, W.G. refused to have anything more to do with haloperidol. However, he agreed to take loxapine instead after it was explained to him that he was less likely to have the dystonic reaction with this drug, especially if it was accompanied by benztropine.

The dose of loxapine was gradually increased to 40 mg/day. He experienced sedation, blurred vision, drying of his eyes that made it difficult for him to wear contact lenses, and dry mouth. However, over the next 3 weeks his delusions and hallucinations disappeared. He developed insight into his problems, and the sedation, the dry mouth, and the dry eyes became much more bearable. He left the hospital a month later, went back to his dormitory, and resumed his academic life.

Over the next few months, W.G. put on about 5 kg of weight and started feeling "low" since he had lost his physical prowess and was experiencing difficulties in concentration at school. About 6 months after discharge, his physician noticed a return of some of the previous delusions and hallucinations. On detailed enquiry it turned out that he had been taking "pep pills," on the recommendation of a fellow athlete, to help him with his problems of feeling low and weight gain. The doctor asked him to bring in one of these pep pills, which were identified as amphetamine in the hospital laboratory. On receiving the report of the analysis, the doctor advised him never to take those pills because they might be responsible for the relapse of his delusions and hallucinations.

Since then, W.G. has continued treatment as an

outpatient. Life hasn't been perfect, but he has been able to lose most of his weight gain through diet and exercise. With some accommodations for the time lost, he was able to achieve a passing grade for that year and, while he missed the university rowing squad, he was allowed to train with them on the B team.

As the name "antipsychotics" suggests, this class of drugs is used to treat psychosis. However, it is important to be clear about the distinctions between some related terms: *antipsychotics* and *neuroleptics, psychosis* and *schizophrenia*. The terms neuroleptic and antipsychotic are commonly used interchangeably. But there is a difference. The word "neuroleptic" has its origin in early animal experiments, when it was noted that these medications caused profound sedation and abnormal motor posturing in animals, almost as if the animal or its nervous system had been "seized" by the drug (*neuro* for nerve, and *lepsis* for seizure). All the early neuroleptics had antipsychotic action and vice versa. Now, however, there are drugs that do not have classical neuroleptic action in animals but nonetheless are potent antipsychotics (e.g., clozapine). Therefore, the broader term antipsychotic will be used here.

The main clinical use of antipsychotics is to treat **psychosis,** which is the name given to a clinical syndrome characterized by the following symptoms.

1. **Delusions,** which are fixed false beliefs (e.g., the patient feels that Martians are tapping his phone lines to control his behavior, and no amount of reasoning can shake the patient's belief in this false assumption).
2. **Hallucinations,** which are the experience of perceptual sensations in the absence of any stimulation (e.g., the patient may report hearing a running commentary by a "voice," or may report having "visions" of holy processions).
3. **Grossly disorganized behavior and speech** (i.e., patients are unable to take care of themselves, may be mute, mumbling incoherently, or smiling to themselves, and may respond in incomprehensible speech to questions or comments).

It is important to distinguish between psychosis and schizophrenia. Schizophrenia is the most common illness in which psychosis is observed. However, psychosis may also be encountered in patients with severe dementia, depression, or severe metabolic disturbances from liver failure or kidney failure. Sometimes prescription medications or illicit street drugs may cause psychosis. Antipsychotics are useful in treating psychosis in any of these circumstances, although the dose, mode of administration, and duration of therapy may vary from condition to condition.

Schizophrenia, however, is more than just psychosis. Most patients with schizophrenia also have difficulties with other cognitive abilities (e.g., memory, concentration, attention, executive function) and have a complex of problems called *negative symptoms* (e.g., apathy, low mood, restricted range of emotion). The current antipsychotics are most helpful with the psychotic component of schizophrenia (the so-called *positive symptoms*).

The story of antipsychotics begins in the early 1950s. Laborit, a surgeon in Paris, was testing various antihistamine drugs, such as promethazine, to prevent postoperative surgical shock. These drugs had a calming effect which was not just sleepiness or sedation but a form of "autonomic stabilization." In 1950, Charpentier synthesized a chemically related compound, chlorpromazine, which, when used in anesthesia, not only reduced the amount of surgical anesthetic required but also reduced the patient's anxiety. Because of the noted calming effects of this drug, Laborit urged psychiatrists to use it for treating psychosis; at the time, little else was available. The first psychotic patients were treated by Delay and Deniker in 1952. (The discovery of antipsychotics has been described by Ayd and Blackwell [1984].)

Since their introduction, these drugs have transformed psychiatric wards. Rarely does one see patients who are unkempt, violent, incontinent, catatonic, or actively hallucinating and requiring physical restraint. Antipsychotics have made it possible for a large number of these patients to leave mental hospitals, to stay out of them, and to lead a reasonably normal life in the community, free of, or with greatly reduced, symptoms (Figs. 28-1 and 28-2). However, the current antipsychotics are not very effective against the cognitive and the negative components of schizophrenia, which cause these patients ongoing social or work-related problems.

MECHANISMS OF ACTION OF ANTIPSYCHOTICS

Molecular Mechanism of Action

Most antipsychotics, at concentrations that elicit clinical effects, act selectively on dopamine receptors

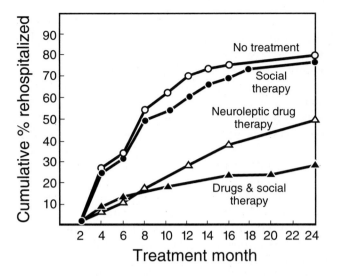

Figure 28-1. Rehospitalization rates of schizophrenic patients. After being discharged from hospital after a 2-month stay, patients taking antipsychotic medication were much less likely to be rehospitalized. (Adapted from Hogarty et al., 1974.)

throughout the brain and the body. The fundamental molecular explanation for the selective blocking of dopamine receptors is that these drugs adopt a conformation in which certain aspects of the molecule are identical to the corresponding features of dopa-

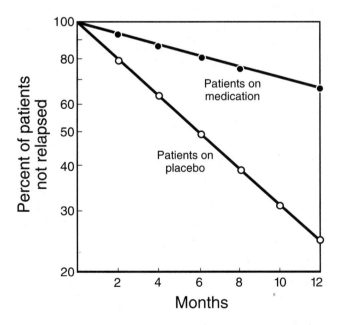

Figure 28-2. Effect of antipsychotic medication on relapse rate of schizophrenic patients. (Adapted from Davis 1976.)

mine. The molecular formulae of **chlorpromazine (a phenothiazine)** and **haloperidol (a butyrophenone)** and their similarity to dopamine are shown in Figure 28-3. One can readily appreciate that the antipsychotic medications share an affinity for the dopamine system which is recognized as a crucial aspect of their clinical effectiveness. Several observations buttress the essential connection between the antipsychotic effect of these drugs and their action on the dopamine system:

1. Reserpine, which depletes the brain of dopamine and norepinephrine, also has an antipsychotic

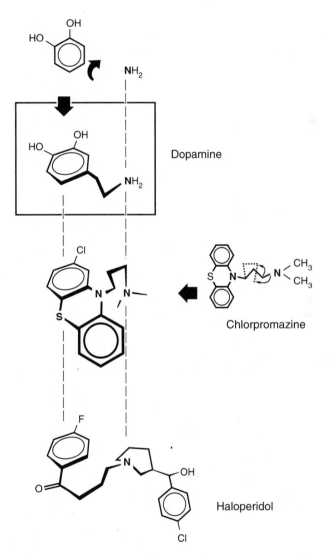

Figure 28-3. Structural overlap (benzene rings and nitrogen atoms; broken lines) of dopamine and the antipsychotics chlorpromazine (a phenothiazine) and haloperidol (a butyrophenone).

effect, although it is no longer used clinically for this purpose.

2. Amphetamine can induce psychosis in humans and in animal models. This is thought to result from a release of dopamine from the vesicles in dopaminergic nerve terminals. Antipsychotics block the psychotomimetic actions of amphetamine.

3. Antipsychotics block the peripheral and central actions of L-dopa, apomorphine, and bromocriptine, which are all dopamine agonists. (For example, motor dyskinesias, which can be caused by L-dopa, are suppressed by typical antipsychotics.)

The Dopamine System

The dopaminergic system arises from groups of cells in the midbrain and the hypothalamus (Fig. 28-4). Of the cells originating in the midbrain, the neurons arising in substantia nigra ascend to the striatum (the nigrostriatal pathway) and are primarily involved in the modulation of motor behavior. This pathway is implicated in Parkinson's disease and in the parkinsonian side effects induced by typical antipsychotics. The other prominent midbrain projections arise from the ventral tegmental area, project to various limbic (nucleus accumbens, olfactory tubercle, septum) and cortical regions (cingulate, entorhinal, prefrontal, and pyriform cortices), and are called the mesolimbic and mesocortical pathways, respectively. These neurons are involved in cognition, modulation of motivation, reward-linked behavior, and emotion. In addition, discrete groups of dopaminergic cells originate in the hypothalamus and project to the pituitary and are involved in the neuroendocrine regulation of prolactin secretion (see also Chapter 20).

It was thought that the effects of dopamine were mediated via two distinct receptor types, the D_1- and D_2-receptors. However, recent developments in molecular genetics have led to the identification of further subtypes, and it is now thought that the dopamine system consists of two *receptor families:* D_1 and D_2. The *D_1-family* contains the original D_1-receptor and the newly cloned D_5-receptor. These receptors share a similar genetic sequence, and both activate adenylyl cyclase and increase the production of the second messenger cAMP. The *D_2-family* contains the original D_2-receptor and the newly distinguished D_3 and D_4 subtypes. These receptors are grouped together because they share a high degree of genetic sequence similarity and have a similar, though not identical, pharmacological profile. The

D_2-receptor subtype is predominantly expressed in the caudate-putamen regions, while the D_3- and D_4-receptors have a higher distribution in the limbic regions of the brain.

The dopamine receptors are localized both presynaptically and postsynaptically. The presynaptic receptors located on the cell bodies are termed somatodendritic autoreceptors, while those on the axonal terminal are called terminal autoreceptors. The somatodendritic autoreceptors modulate the firing of the dopamine neurons, whereas the autoreceptors on the axon terminal modulate the release of dopamine. The postsynaptic dopamine receptors mediate the effect of dopamine on the nondopaminergic cell bodies. D_1-receptors are primarily postsynaptic, while the D_2- and D_3-receptors are found both presynaptically and postsynaptically. To add to this complexity, studies have revealed the existence of high-affinity and low-affinity forms for both D_1- and D_2-receptors, and it is suggested that the high-affinity conformation may be more relevant to the actual signal transduction and may play a special role in psychotic symptoms.

Action of Antipsychotics on Dopamine Receptors

The one feature common to all antipsychotics is their ability to bind to the dopamine receptors and antagonize the action of dopamine. Furthermore, the antipsychotic action seems to be more closely linked to D_2 than to D_1 antagonism. This assertion is backed by the following observations.

1. While most antipsychotics have both D_1- and D_2-blocking abilities when tested in vitro, they are prescribed clinically at doses that have little or no effect on the D_1-receptors but block 60–80% of the D_2-receptors. This has been confirmed by positron emission tomography (PET) in patients (Fig. 28-5).

2. Drugs that act exclusively to block the D_2-receptors (e.g., raclopride) are effective antipsychotics, but those that act only on the D_1-receptors are not effective as antipsychotic agents.

3. There is a high correlation between the D_2 affinity of a drug and the dose at which it is used as an antipsychotic agent (Fig. 28-6). However, no such correlation exists for the D_1-receptors. In fact, recent studies using PET imaging have demonstrated a relationship between the percent of D_2-receptors blocked and the antipsychotic response in patients.

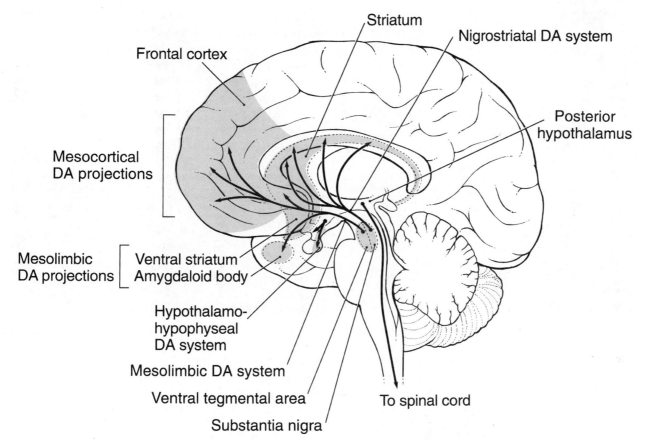

Figure 28-4. Dopaminergic pathways. The nigrostriatal dopamine system originates in the substantia nigra and terminates in the main dorsal part of the striatum. The ventral tegmental area gives rise to the mesolimbic DA system, which terminates in the ventral striatum, amygdaloid body, frontal lobe, and some other basal forebrain areas. The hypothalamohypophyseal system innervates the median eminence as well as the posterior and intermediate lobes of the pituitary, and dopamine neurons in the posterior hypothalamus project to the spinal cord. (Adapted from Heimer L. *The Human Brain and Spinal Cord. Functional Neuroanatomy and Dissection Guide*, 2nd ed., Fig. 133. New York: Springer-Verlag, 1985.) (See also Chapter 20, Figs. 20-5 and 20-7A.)

Antipsychotic Action: Where in the Brain?

As shown in Figure 28-4, the dopamine system is widely distributed throughout the CNS. It is presently held that psychosis is related to a hyperdopaminergic state in the mesolimbic and the mesocortical dopamine tracts. Therefore, it would be ideal if one could block the transmission in these circuits alone without doing so in the rest of the dopamine circuits. At present, this is not possible. Thus, while blocking the mesolimbic and the mesocortical pathways results in antipsychotic action, blocking the other pathways results in the unwanted side effects that accompany treatment with these drugs.

The nigrostriatal pathway is involved in the coordination of movement. Blocking this dopamine pathway, while not essential for the antipsychotic response, results in the parkinsonian side effects of these drugs. Similarly, the hypothalamohypophyseal pathway plays a role in the control of prolactin secretion, and the unintended blockade of dopamine in this pathway results in the endocrine side effects (see below).

Antipsychotic Action: More Than Just Dopamine D_2-Receptors?

While it is possible to achieve an effective antipsychotic response with a drug that affects only the D_2-receptors, two new questions arise. (1) Would it be possible to obtain antipsychotic responses through

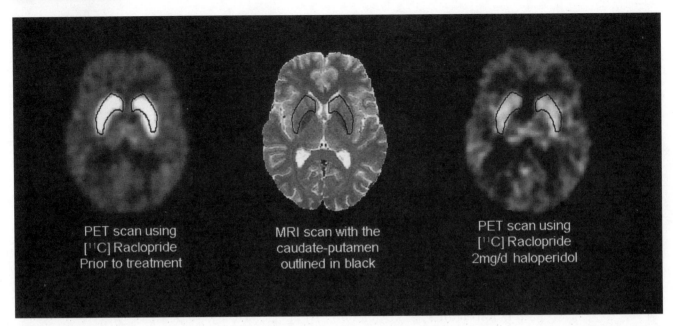

PET scan using
[¹¹C] Raclopride
Prior to treatment

MRI scan with the
caudate-putamen
outlined in black

PET scan using
[¹¹C] Raclopride
2mg/d haloperidol

Figure 28-5. PET scans showing the effect of antipsychotics on the D_2 dopamine receptors. The figure on the left is a PET scan using ^{11}C-raclopride, an agent that binds specifically to D_2 dopamine receptors. The scan shows a high intensity of dopamine receptors, localized in the caudate-putamen. The caudate-putamen can be better appreciated on a corresponding MRI (middle) from the same subject. The subject then received 10 days of treatment with 2 mg haloperidol. Haloperidol occupies D_2 dopamine receptors in the caudate-putamen, and as a result the ligand ^{11}C-raclopride is unable to bind to them. Therefore, as seen on the scan on the right, the signal from the caudate-putamen is much attenuated. Mathematical modeling of the data revealed that in the second scan the number of receptors measured by ^{11}C-raclopride was 30% of the first scan, suggesting that 70% of the receptors were occupied by haloperidol. (Scan courtesy of the author, The PET Centre, Clarke Institute of Psychiatry, University of Toronto.)

some other mechanism? (2) Would combining the receptor blockade of another transmitter system, along with the blockade of dopamine D_2-receptors, result in a better profile of antipsychotic response?

Active research is currently underway to explore these questions. A valuable clue in this search has been an antipsychotic drug called **clozapine** (Fig. 28-7). This drug has certain unique properties. At a pharmacological concentration it has a relatively high affinity for the D_4- as opposed to the D_2-receptor and a higher affinity for the serotonin S_2-receptor than for the dopamine D_2-receptor. At clinical concentrations it is an effective antipsychotic agent without causing parkinsonian side effects (presumably by sparing the nigrostriatal pathway), and also without causing a rise in prolactin (by sparing the hypothalamohypophyseal pathway). For this reason clozapine, which is often referred to as an "atypical neuroleptic," has provided valuable leads toward understanding the mechanism of antipsychotic action beyond the dopamine D_2-receptors. Researchers are now studying the effects of the serotonin S_2- and dopamine D_4-selective agents in greater depth. Results with S_2-only drugs have not been very encouraging, and studies of D_4-only agents are just getting underway.

A more productive line of work has been to study drugs with combined S_2- and D_2-blocking activity. Combining S_2 blockade with adequate D_2 blockade improves the antipsychotic response and also diminishes the parkinsonian side effects. The mechanism of this response may be as follows. The serotonin system inhibits the dopamine system in the nigrostriatal circuit. When patients take antipsychotics, their nigrostriatal circuit is under inhibition from two sources: inhibition from endogenous serotonin and inhibition from the administered D_2-blocking antipsychotic agent. The addition of an S_2-blocking agent then releases the nigrostriatal circuit from the endogenous serotonin inhibition, and this results in the relief of parkinsonian symptoms. This mechanism is being exploited by a new class of antipsy-

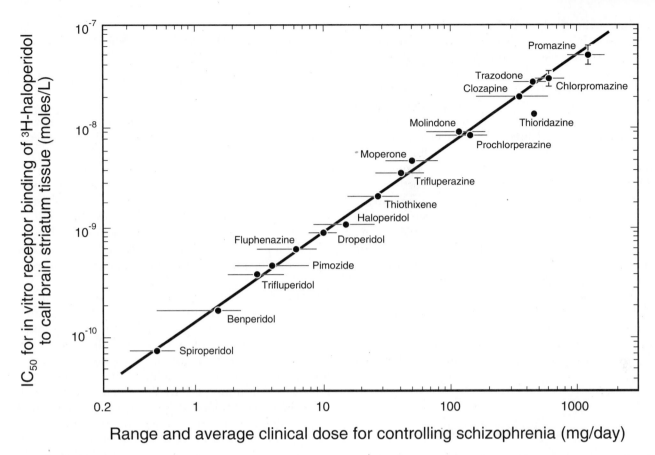

Figure 28-6. Relation between doses of antipsychotics to control schizophrenia and their respective receptor-binding potencies.

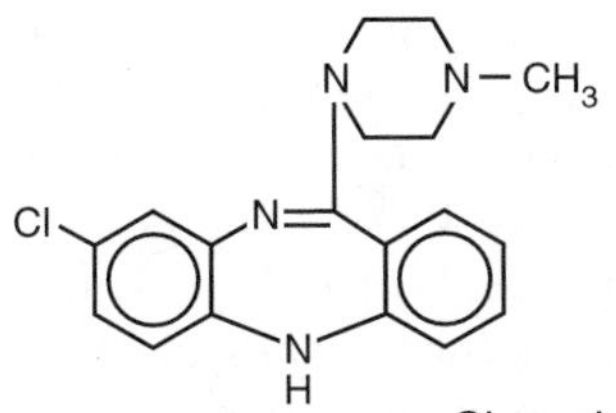

chotic agents, of which **risperidone** (Fig. 28-7) is the first representative, that have been shown to be effective in treating psychotic symptoms with fewer parkinsonian side effects.

At present, it is reasonable to assume that a certain minimum level of dopamine D_2 blockade is essential for antipsychotic response, and that it may be possible to improve the quality of response and achieve it with fewer side effects by combining D_2 blockade with blockade of other receptors, most notably S_2 and D_4.

Clozapine
(Affinity for D_4 and S_2 receptors)

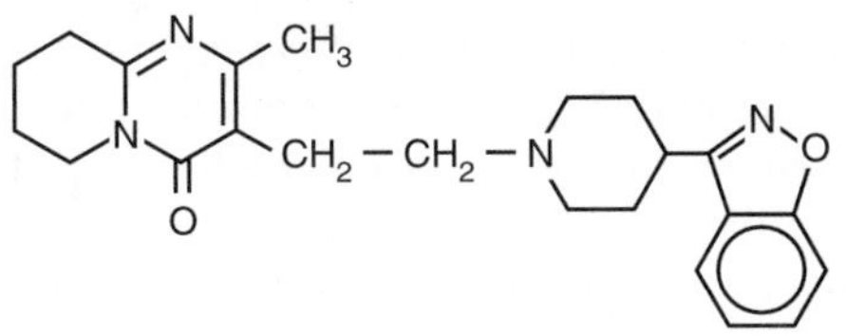

Risperidone
(Affinity for D_2 and S_2 receptors)

Figure 28-7. Structural formulae of the "atypical" antipsychotics clozapine and risperidone, and their dopamine and serotonin receptor-subtype affinities (see text).

FUNCTIONAL EFFECTS OF ANTIPSYCHOTIC AGENTS

Antipsychotic Action

The main use of these agents is to combat psychosis. When given to patients they produce decreases in bizarre behavior, in delusions, and in hallucinations.

These are collectively called "antipsychotic action." The antipsychotics are also effective in decreasing anxiety (or nervousness) and promoting sleepiness or sedation. It should be pointed out that it is not necessary for all of these three effects to be linked. In fact, there are very effective antianxiety agents and sleep-inducing agents that are not effective as antipsychotics (see Chapter 27). Conversely, some of the antipsychotics can achieve antipsychotic effects without prominent sedative effects (e.g., risperidone or other high-potency agents). In other words, sedative effects of these medications are not a prerequisite for antipsychotic effect. However, it is often desirable to use drugs with sedative and sleep-inducing properties in the early stage of psychosis, to help calm the patient and simplify management before the antipsychotic effect (i.e., the effect on delusions and hallucinations) manifests itself completely.

There was a tendency in the past to use antipsychotic agents as antianxiety or sleep agents. However, while they are often effective, there are safer and more specific agents available for this purpose.

Antinausea and Antivomiting Action

The chemoreceptor trigger zone (CTZ) is a region of the reticular formation in the medulla oblongata outside the blood–brain barrier, the stimulation of which leads to nausea and vomiting. The CTZ is rich in D_2-receptors, and the blockade of these D_2-receptors protects from CTZ-induced vomiting. Thus antipsychotic drugs, by virtue of their D_2-blocking activity, effectively reduce nausea produced by other drugs, pregnancy, radiation sickness, cancer, etc. In fact, the location of the CTZ outside the blood–brain barrier makes it possible to achieve this antinausea effect with drugs that do not cross into the brain and hence do not cause other side effects. While most of the antipsychotics are effective against the types of nausea mentioned above, many are not very effective in nausea secondary to bowel obstruction or motion sickness. Only particular phenothiazines (such as promethazine, meclizine, and thiethylperazine) are effective in motion sickness, possibly because these compounds localize in high concentrations in the vestibular nucleus. However, because of side effects, some of them potentially irreversible, antipsychotic agents should not be the indiscriminate first choice when considering the treatment of nausea.

PHARMACOKINETICS AND DOSAGE

Absorption, Biotransformation, and Elimination

The commonly used antipsychotics show quite variable bioavailability, despite their high lipid solubility. This may indicate a large and variable first-pass effect in the gastrointestinal mucosa or the liver. Bioavailability (see Chapter 5) is increased as much as 10-fold by intramuscular injection. Most of these drugs show a high degree of serum protein binding, and they also accumulate in tissues with a large blood supply, such as brain, lung, and kidney. They also cross the placenta into the fetal circulation quite readily.

The kinetics of elimination are complex, because these drugs follow multiple pathways of biotransformation, with different rate and affinity constants. Sulfoxidation, N-dealkylation, ring hydroxylation, and glucuronide conjugation are among the more important reactions, and each parent compound may have a large number of different metabolites, most of them inactive. Prolonged administration may cause some induction of hepatic microsomal enzymes, and the plasma concentrations of the drugs may fall despite a constant level of dosage. Excretion occurs into the urine (the more polar metabolites) and into the bile.

Most of these agents show plasma elimination half-lives in the range of 10–20 hours. However, if body fat has accumulated a large store of drug, traces of the drug and its metabolites may continue to appear in the urine for many weeks or months after the last dose. The long half-life and the lipid accumulation permit one to administer these drugs in once-a-day dosage. These factors may also account for the observation that after chronic treatment of a psychotic patient there may be no relapse for months after the drug is stopped.

Onset of action of antipsychotics is difficult to interpret. The typical physiological effects (e.g., on circulation, arousal, emesis, thermoregulation) appear rapidly, as one would expect from the high lipid solubility. In fact, the anxiolytic and sedative effects also appear almost immediately. In contrast, the antipsychotic effects usually take several weeks to develop, and may not be maximal until after several months of treatment. This suggests that the antipsychotic action is complex and that the change in thinking and behavior is the end result of a cascade of alterations that is started by the drug.

It is now possible to measure the concentrations of most antipsychotics in the plasma of patients receiving these medications. However, it has been very difficult to develop a clear "therapeutic range" that is of clinical utility. Therefore, at present, antipsychotic drug levels are measured only for research and in cases where one suspects pharmacokinetic drug interactions. It is also now possible to measure the effects of an antipsychotic agent on the dopamine D_2-receptors in vivo in patients, using PET imaging. While this remains primarily a research tool, preliminary studies do suggest that adequate antipsychotic response requires a D_2-receptor occupancy in the range of 60–80%.

Lipid Solubility and Drug Dosage

The association between a drug and its receptor is favored by higher lipid solubility of the drug. This is true even if the receptor is on the outside surface of the cell membrane. In other words, drugs with high lipid solubility generally have very low dissociation constants or K_D values. The reason for this is that once the lipid-soluble drug attaches to the receptor, the drug's lipid solubility greatly reduces its dissociation from the receptor; i.e., the drug "sticks" to the receptor. In terms of the oral dose in milligrams, therefore, a more lipid-soluble drug is more potent and a smaller dose of it is required.

Lipid solubility also plays a role in the absorption of orally administered drugs and their ability to cross the blood–brain barrier. It is reasonable to expect that the more lipid-soluble antipsychotics permeate membranes more readily, reach their target tissues more rapidly, and thus may have faster onset of action and require lower doses for equivalent antipsychotic action than do less lipid-soluble drugs.

Domperidone (Fig. 28-8) is a special case since it is not sufficiently lipid-soluble to permeate the blood–brain barrier. Thus, domperidone is not an antipsychotic because it cannot enter the brain. It does, however, block all the actions of dopamine and dopamine-like drugs on the peripheral tissues of the body. For example, when one is using high doses of the dopamine receptor agonist bromocriptine to treat Parkinson's disease (see Chapter 21) or galactorrhea, there are undesirable side effects on the dopamine-sensitive peripheral tissues (vasodilatation, flushing, hypotension). These side effects of bromocriptine are readily blocked by domperidone, so the bromocriptine can be used at a high dose, without incurring peripheral side effects. Typical antipsychotics could not be used for this purpose because of their central actions.

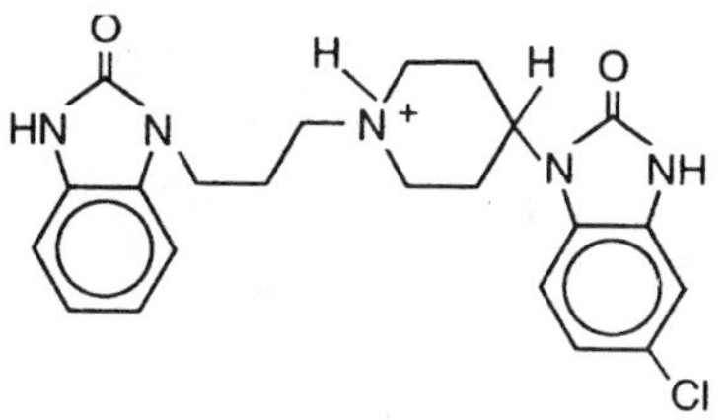

Depot Injections of Antipsychotics

Some antipsychotics, of which **fluphenazine** is perhaps the most common example, have an alcohol substituent (–OH) attached to the end of the molecule, and an ester can be formed by linking it to such fatty acids as enanthic or decanoic acid (Fig. 28-9). When injected intramuscularly, the fatty esters remain as an oil drop within the muscle tissue, diffusing out slowly because the fluphenazine ester is poorly soluble in the tissue and plasma water. When

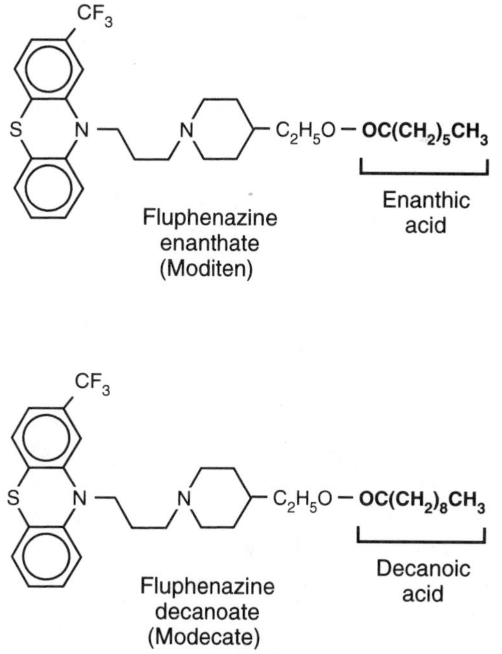

Figure 28-8. Domperidone, a peripheral dopamine receptor blocker, is a positively charged molecule that does not readily enter the brain.

Figure 28-9. Fluphenazine enanthate (Moditen) is slightly less lipid-soluble and is injected intramuscularly at a dose of 25 mg once every 2 weeks. The more lipid-soluble decanoate ester (Modecate) needs to be injected only once every 3 weeks on average.

the fluphenazine ester does diffuse into plasma, the plasma esterases immediately split off the fatty acid, freeing the fluphenazine to act directly on the brain. Decanoic acid contains 10 carbon atoms and is much more lipid-soluble than enanthic acid, which contains only seven carbon atoms; thus, a single injection of the enanthate lasts for only about 2 weeks while the decanoate lasts for about 3 weeks. Depot injections are useful in the clinical management of certain patients as they reduce the inconvenience of having to take a pill every day and also make it possible to ensure compliance with a medication regimen.

FUNCTIONAL CLASSIFICATION OF ANTIPSYCHOTIC AGENTS

All the antipsychotics (with the possible exception of clozapine) are equal in producing antipsychotic effects. Thus, the main reasons for choosing between them usually are their particular side effects. Antipsychotics may be chosen on the grounds that they have few side effects, or they may be chosen when a given side effect is actually desirable (e.g., sedation of an agitated patient). While over three dozen antipsychotic agents are available in markets around the world, they can be functionally divided into different classes, based mainly on their affinity for the dopamine receptors, and hence the dose at which they are given. A few agents, however, have atypical profiles and are therefore classified separately and referred to as "atypicals" (Table 28-1).

Most of the side effects of the drugs originate from their actions on the cholinergic, adrenergic, and histaminergic receptors; their antipsychotic effects originate from the antidopaminergic actions. Thus, drugs with very high affinity and selectivity for the dopamine receptors (high-potency agents) can be administered at lower doses that occupy a requisite number of dopamine receptors without disturbing the other receptor systems to any appreciable degree. However, since they block the dopamine system with great affinity, high-potency agents give rise to dopamine-related side effects much more prominently (e.g., parkinsonian and endocrine side effects).

The low-potency agents have lower affinity for the dopamine system, and they are not very selective. At the doses needed to occupy the requisite number of dopamine receptors, they also block the cholinergic, adrenergic, and histaminergic systems to a substantial degree. This results in a high level of sedation, anticholinergic effects, and hypotension, but the dopamine-related side effects are minimized.

As their classification implies, the midpotency agents lie between the two potency extremes in terms of their affinity for the dopamine system and their functional effects. The atypical agents (clozapine and risperidone) are distinguished pharmacologically by their affinity for the serotonin receptors and the general absence of parkinsonian side effects. In terms of other side effects, clozapine behaves more like a low-potency agent, whereas risperidone is more similar to high-potency agents.

ADVERSE EFFECTS OF ANTIPSYCHOTICS

Side effects or adverse effects of antipsychotic medication occur in practically all patients treated with these drugs. Most of the side effects can be easily understood to result from the pharmacological properties of antipsychotics. First, these drugs act both in the brain and peripherally. All of their peripheral actions are unwanted side effects (e.g., hypotension, constipation, tachycardia). Second, in the brain these drugs act on a variety of receptors other than the dopamine receptor (e.g., histamine, acetylcholine), and these actions create unwanted side effects. Finally, even within the dopamine system the drugs act on all four major pathways. Their actions on the mesolimbic and mesocortical pathways improve psychotic symptoms, but their effects on the nigrostriatal and hypothalamohypophyseal pathways give rise to side effects. In about a third of patients these side effects are minimal. In the rest of the patients, side effects are sufficiently significant that they should be monitored and treated if necessary. Some of these effects (antipsychotic-induced parkinsonism, dyskinesias and dystonias, and akathisia) appear within days or weeks of initiation of therapy, whereas others (e.g., tardive dyskinesia) require months or years to develop.

Antipsychotic-Induced Parkinsonism

In a large proportion of patients the antipsychotics cause extrapyramidal signs that mimic Parkinson's disease. These result from the unwanted effects of the antipsychotics on the nigrostriatal pathways, the mechanism of which is shown schematically in Figure 28-9. The signs include the following:

Akinesia. The patient has shorter steps that appear like a shuffling gait, reduced arm swing, and cramped handwriting called "micrographia." In addition, the patient may show little spontaneous

Table 28-1 Different Antipsychotics Ranked by Functional Class[a]

Drug	Chemical Class	CPZ* Equiv.	DA$_2$† Affinity	Ch-M‡ Affinity	Adr$_1$§ Affinity	Side Effects Extra-pyramidal	Anticholinergic Sedation Hypotension
Low potency							
Chlorpromazine *Largactil*	Aliphatic phenothiazine	100	+	+++	+++		
Thioridazine *Mellaril*	Piperidine phenothiazine	100	+	+++	+++		
Midpotency							
Perphenazine *Trilafon*	Piperazine phenothiazine	8	++	++	++		
Loxapine *Loxapac*	Dibenzoxazepine	10	++	++	++		
High potency							
Haloperidol *Haldol*	Butyrophenone	2	+++	−	+		
Fluphenazine *Moditen*	Piperazine phenothiazine	2	+++	−	+		
Atypical							
Clozapine *Clozaril*	Dibenzodiazepine	80	+	+++	++	Absent	High
Risperidone *Risperdal*		2	++	−	++	Low	Low

[a] *Key to symbols:*

*Functional equivalence with 100 mg of chlorpromazine.

†DA$_2$ dopamine receptor affinity.

‡Cholinergic muscarinic receptor affinity.

§Adrenergic receptor affinity.

Relative antagonist affinities: +++ = highest; ++ = midlevel; + = low; − = negligible.

Relative frequency of side effects indicated by arrows.

---

motion and there is difficulty in initiating motion, such as getting up from a chair.

Rigidity. The patient complains of feeling stiff, and examination reveals a uniform stiffness throughout the range of motion—a "cogwheel" type of rigidity.

Tremor. This tremor is similar to the "pill-rolling" tremor seen in Parkinson's disease and may interfere with the patient's ability to carry out fine manual tasks.

Neuroleptic Malignant Syndrome

This is a rare, but very severe and sometimes fatal side effect. It resembles severe parkinsonism in that one of the cardinal features is extreme rigidity. This is accompanied by fever, marked autonomic disturbances, and muscle destruction that results in very high levels of creatine phosphokinase in the blood, as well as myoglobinemia and myoglobinuria. Although the syndrome is related to dopamine D$_2$ blockade, it is unpredictable and is not directly dose-related. Some individuals seem to have a greater susceptibility to it, although there is not yet any prospective method to identify these individuals.

Antipsychotic-Induced Dyskinesias and Dystonias

Acute dyskinesia may set in within 1–3 days of antipsychotic therapy and consists of involuntary motions of the lips, jaw, and tongue; the patient may grimace, chew, or have difficulty speaking. Acute dystonias consist of involuntary twisting motion of the neck, the pelvis, and the eyes (oculogyric crises). Acute dystonias arise early in the course of treatment, and young muscular men are particularly susceptible.

Antipsychotic-Induced Akathisia

Akathisia or restlessness is a common side effect of antipsychotic therapy. Despite the fact that the patient feels rigid or stiff and has difficulty initiating motion, there is a tremendous urge to keep walking and moving around. This is a particularly difficult side effect to diagnose, as restlessness and anxiety usually accompany psychosis itself. In typical cases of akathisia the onset of the restlessness coincides with the start of the medication, and patients claim that their restlessness has a "physical" component, almost as if the legs themselves were restless. Also, the patients report a marked relief if they move their legs, either on the spot or by pacing.

Treatment of Antipsychotic-Induced Parkinsonism, Dystonias, and Akathisia

As shown in Figure 28-10, and discussed in greater detail in Chapter 21, there is normally a balance between the cholinergic and dopaminergic inputs into the neurons in the striatum (caudate and putamen). When an antipsychotic blocks the dopamine receptors, the cholinergic influence becomes relatively excessive. This relative dominance of the cholinergic system results in parkinsonian signs and acute dystonias. Thus, the treatment of these side effects aims at restoring the cholinergic-dopaminergic balance, which is best done by administering an anticholinergic drug such as **benztropine** or **biperiden.**

In principle, the cholinergic-dopaminergic balance can also be restored with L-dopa. This would, of course, be defeating the purpose of giving the antipsychotic in the first place, since the high doses of L-dopa required to restore the chemical balance would antagonize the action of the antipsychotic, and the patient's psychosis would reappear.

Some physicians routinely prescribe the anticholinergic medication together with antipsychotic therapy. This is good practice when dealing with children who have childhood autism or schizophrenia-like symptoms, because children are particularly predisposed to dystonic reactions. Such reactions can be

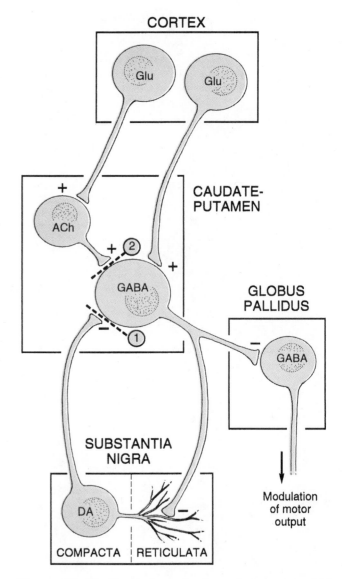

Figure 28-10. Sites of production of extrapyramidal ("parkinsonian") signs by antipsychotics (1), and of "antiparkinsonian" therapeutic effects by benztropine and other anticholinergic agents (2). Glu = glutamate; ACh = acetylcholine; GABA = γ-aminobutyric acid; DA = dopamine. + indicates an excitatory synapse, − an inhibitory synapse.

fatal when the tongue goes into spasm, occluding the respiratory passages. Coadministration of antipsychotic and anticholinergic medications is also good practice in muscular young men and in any patients with a previous history of having responded to antipsychotics with parkinsonian side effects. However, this is not recommended as a routine in all patients, as anticholinergic activity has its own side effects (see below). Therefore, in the majority of adult patients the antipsychotic is administered first, and the anticholinergic drug is added, if needed. After about 1 or 2 months of antipsychotic therapy, most patients develop tolerance to the stiffness-producing side effect of the antipsychotic, and the anticholinergic drug is no longer needed. However, about 25% of patients will continue to require anticholinergic therapy together with the antipsychotic drug for an indefinite period.

Development and Treatment of Tardive Dyskinesia

After many months or years of antipsychotic therapy, the patient may develop tardive dyskinesia (TD). The signs are the same as those sometimes seen in acute dyskinesia—namely, involuntary oral, buccal, and lingual motion, as if the patient were chewing gum. There may also be dystonic motions of the neck, chest, and trunk.

It was formerly thought that TD was caused by an up-regulation of dopamine receptors in response to the prolonged dopamine receptor blockade by the antipsychotic drug. This synthesis of additional receptors was thought to make the cell more sensitive to the small amounts of dopamine still getting through the drug-induced blockade. However, up-regulation occurs rapidly, whereas the dyskinesia develops very slowly and gradually. More recent evidence suggests that the cause of TD also involves dysfunction of the GABAergic neurons in the caudate-putamen.

Two paradoxical aspects of TD are noteworthy. First, it may seem to improve when the dose of the antipsychotic is increased. This increase of dose may intensify the rigidity side effect and thus mask the involuntary movements of TD. However, anticholinergic drugs, which improve parkinsonian side effects, may worsen TD. This may represent cholinergic effects on dopamine and GABA systems, although the exact mechanism is unclear.

Treatment of TD by depleting the brain dopamine content by means of reserpine, or giving cholinergic agonists to stimulate the GABA cells, has not been very successful. However, some clinicians feel that the most effective measure so far is to discontinue antipsychotic therapy for a time, provided the patient's psychotic symptoms are improved enough to permit this. For patients whose TD is made worse by the antipsychotic, but who cannot do without it, the introduction of the atypical agent **clozapine** provides a new treatment option. Most of the patients who can be switched to clozapine notice either a diminution, or at least no further worsening, of TD.

However, clozapine is not used routinely in all patients, because it is a low-potency agent that has attendant side effects of sedation, anticholinergic activity, and hypotension. In addition, it causes agranulocytosis (which may be fatal) in about 1% of patients receiving it and therefore can be given only if the blood is monitored weekly.

Unwanted Sedation

One of the troubling side effects of antipsychotics is sedation, because sedative effects are not essential for the antipsychotic actions and are, in most situations, unwanted. The sedation reflects a complex interaction of antihistaminergic, antiadrenergic, and anticholinergic actions of these agents. As a general rule, the sedation is greatest for the low-potency agents and least for the high-potency agents. It manifests itself as excessive daytime drowsiness, tiredness and fatigue, and difficulty with attention and concentration. Thus, it may be an important disabling side effect that can interfere with the rehabilitation and routine functioning of a patient.

Orthostatic Hypotension

The antipsychotics depress blood pressure by dilating the arterioles via a direct action on the α-adrenoceptors responsible for vasoconstriction. The patients thus show orthostatic hypotension. In addition, the drugs may have a direct effect on the vasomotor center, which may contribute to the hypotension observed with these agents.

Anticholinergic Side Effects

Some antipsychotics have prominent cholinergic blocking activity, which leads to a series of side effects. Cholinergic blockade in the eye produces blurred vision by causing mydriasis and by weakening the ciliary muscles. It may also lead to dry eyes due to decreased tear secretion. Furthermore, mydriasis may decrease the outflow of aqueous humor and thus may precipitate glaucoma in subjects with a tendency toward narrow-angle glaucoma. Dry mouth and constipation result from anticholinergic action in the gastrointestinal tract, while urinary hesitancy results from such action on the bladder. Low-potency agents are highly anticholinergic; high-potency agents are not. (The intrinsic anticholinergic activity of low-potency agents may in fact be partly responsible for the relative absence of extrapyramidal effects of these agents.)

Pseudopregnancy

The dopamine neurons in the hypothalamus (arcuate cells) release dopamine, which then travels via the hypophyseal portal blood vessels down to the pituitary to inhibit the release of prolactin from the mammotroph cells (Fig. 28-11). Antipsychotics will block the dopamine receptors on these mammotrophs, resulting in a release of prolactin. At the same time, the antipsychotics block the release of follicle-stimulating hormone (FSH) and luteinizing hormone (LH). Thus, a woman does not ovulate, does not menstruate, but has hyperprolactinemia with swollen breasts and possibly galactorrhea; the whole picture simulates pregnancy. Breast swelling and galactorrhea can occur in men as well.

Seizures

Since high doses of antipsychotics decrease the seizure threshold, they can produce seizures in susceptible patients who are epileptics or have other predisposing causes. This effect is most prominent with the low-potency agents.

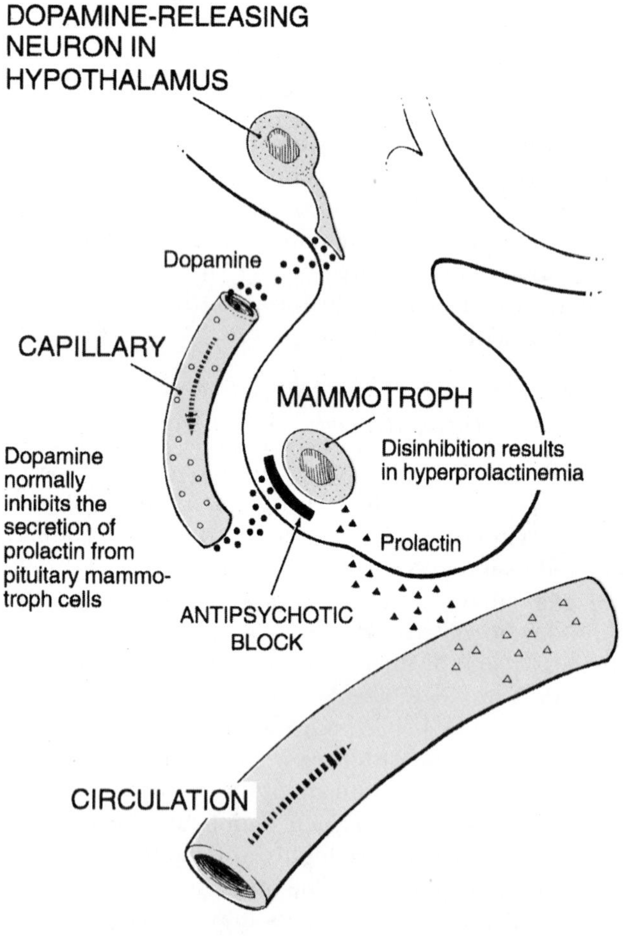

Jaundice

Phenothiazine-induced jaundice occurs in a very small number of patients. It is of the obstructive type with elevated plasma bilirubin, but without fever, liver tenderness, or pruritus. It is thought to be a hypersensitivity reaction since there is eosinophilia, and the severity of the jaundice is not related to the dose of the antipsychotic.

Dermatitis and Photosensitivity

This occurs in a small number of patients, mostly those who are receiving low-potency antipsychotics. These patients become extrasensitive to sunlight, and they develop exaggerated sunburn. Some patients also notice a general hyperpigmentation of the skin, cornea, and the lens.

Figure 28-11. Mechanism of production of hyperprolactinemia by antipsychotics.

SUGGESTED READING

Ayd FJ, Blackwell B, eds. Discoveries in biological psychiatry. Baltimore: Ayd Medical Communications, 1984.

Davis JM. Comparative doses and the costs of antipsychotic medications. Arch Gen Psychiatry 1976; 33:858–861.

Farde L, Nordström AL, Wiesel FA, Pauli S, Halldin C, Sedvall G. Positron emission tomographic analysis of central D_1 and D_2 dopamine receptor occupancy in patients treated with classical neuroleptics and clozapine. Relation to extrapyramidal side effects. Arch Gen Psychiatry 1992; 49:538–544.

Hogarty GE, Goldberg SC, Schooler NR, Ulrich R. Drug and sociotherapy in the aftercare of schizophrenic patients. Arch Gen Psychiatry 1974; 31:603–608.

Meltzer HY. The role of serotonin in schizophrenia and the place of serotonin-dopamine antagonist antipsychotics. J Clin Psychopharmacol 1995; 15:S2–S3.

Nordström AL, Farde L, Wiesel FA, et al. Central D_2-dopamine receptor occupancy in relation to antipsychotic drug effects: a double-blind PET study of schizophrenic patients. Biol Psychiatry 1993; 33:227–235.

Seeman P, Guan HC, Van Tol HHM. Dopamine D_4 receptors elevated in schizophrenia. Nature 1993; 365:441–445.

Seeman P, Lee T, Chau-Wong M, Wong K. Antipsychotic drug doses and neuroleptic/dopamine receptors. Nature 1976; 261:717–719.

Strange PG. Dopamine D_4 receptors: curiouser and curiouser. TIPS 1994; 15:317–319.

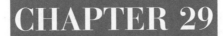

CHAPTER 29

Antidepressant and Mood Stabilizing Agents

J.J. WARSH AND J.M. KHANNA

CASE HISTORY

A 44-year-old man with a history of bipolar affective disorder had his first medical contact for a manic episode 20 years ago, when he was hospitalized and treated with haloperidol in doses of 20–40 mg/day. After a second episode of mania, treatment with lithium carbonate was recommended. Pretreatment hematological, renal, hepatic, and thyroid function indices, as well as ECG, were normal, showing no contraindications to lithium therapy. The patient was placed on lithium carbonate, beginning with 900 mg/day and increasing to 1500 mg/day, with the major portion of the daily dose administered in the evening. Monthly serum lithium levels were in the range of 0.6 to 0.8 mmol/L. The patient remained symptom-free on a maintenance dose of 1500 mg/day.

Two years later he was hospitalized for another manic episode during which he received haloperidol, and the lithium dosage was increased to 2100 mg/day. His mood stabilized over a 3-week period, haloperidol was slowly discontinued, and he was discharged on 2100 mg/day lithium carbonate. This was then slowly reduced to 1800 mg/day, plasma lithium levels stabilized at 0.8–1.0 mmol/L, and over the next 15 years on this maintenance therapy the patient experienced only two depressive episodes of moderate severity, the second of which responded to nortriptyline. Hematological, biochemical, thyroid, and cardiac monitoring performed at 6-month inter-

vals remained normal. In recent years, however, the patient reported increased urinary output and increased consumption of liquids.

About a year ago the patient's serum lithium levels gradually rose to 1.0–1.1 mmol/L, and serum creatinine increased to 110 μmol/L. The lithium carbonate dosage was decreased to 1500 mg/day, and then to 1200 mg/day, to maintain plasma lithium concentrations in the range of 0.8 to 1.0 mmol/L. At a routine visit 6 months later the patient's blood pressure was 160/110 mmHg, serum creatinine was 160 μmol/L, BUN was 7.5 mmol/L, and microhematuria was noted on urinalysis. ECG indicated first-degree heart block. Elevated IgA antibodies, elevated serum creatinine, and 24-hour urine output of 4.5 liters with reduced urine osmolality allowed the diagnosis of IgA nephropathy and lithium-induced nephrogenic diabetes insipidus.

The lithium dosage was gradually reduced and stopped at the end of a 4-week interval. The hypertension was controlled with enalapril 20 mg/day. Because of the absence of recurrences of affective disorder for many years, the patient was allowed a drug-free period of observation. A week after lithium had been stopped, he experienced an abrupt shortening of his usual sleeping time, increased activity, irritability, and expansive mood. He was brought to the hospital in a hypomanic state, which escalated rapidly into a full manic episode within 48 hours. Treatment was instituted with perphenazine 24–32 mg/day, and clonazepam 2.5 mg/day in three to four divided doses, followed by carbamazepine 400 mg/day in divided doses. After 1 week, serum carbamazepine levels were 20 μmol/L, which rose to 24 μmol/L over the next week and then declined to 17 μmol/L. His mania resolved quickly, and after 16 days in hospital he was discharged with maintenance doses of carbamazepine 400 mg/day and perphenazine 12 mg/day.

He soon experienced increasing tiredness and lack of interest, felt "a bit slowed down," and complained of difficulty reading, annoying dryness of the mouth, and some constipation. Therefore the dose of perphenazine was tapered and discontinued and the carbamazepine dosage was increased to 600 mg/day to bring serum levels to 20 μmol/L. Shortly thereafter he began to have feelings of depression, guilt, failure, suicidal thoughts, loss of interest, poor appetite, and marked anxiety and agitation in the morning. He still complained of poor visual accommodation and dry mouth. It was decided to treat this depressive episode with sertraline, starting with 50 mg/day and increasing to 100 mg/day after 1 week because of worsening depression. The concomitant treatment with carbamazepine and sertraline, to which was added clonazepam 2.0 mg/day in divided doses to control anxiety and insomnia, brought this episode under control after 3 weeks. The patient's depression subsided and suicidal thinking ceased. Clonazepam was very slowly tapered and discontinued after a dose of 0.25 mg/day was reached. Further symptomatic improvement occurred gradually between 8 and 12 weeks of therapy, and the patient became symptom-free thereafter. Chronic maintenance therapy consisted of carbamazepine and sertraline at the lowest therapeutic doses or plasma levels.

Antidepressants and mood-stabilizing agents such as lithium salts, carbamazepine, and valproate are used to treat the major affective disorders. These disorders include major depression (depressive episodes without a history of mania) and bipolar affective disorder (manic-depressive illness characterized by episodes of mania and of depression). The cardinal feature of major depression is sustained (at least 2 weeks) depressed mood and/or pervasive loss of interest or pleasure in activities, accompanied by sleep disturbance, changes in appetite and body weight (usually reductions), loss of energy, altered psychomotor activity (retardation or agitation), feelings of self-reproach, and suicidal thoughts. In a manic episode the mood state is marked by abnormal and sustained (at least 1 week) elevation, expansiveness, or irrita-

bility, and the patients show at least three of the following symptoms: inflated self-esteem or grandiosity, decreased sleep, hypertalkativeness, racing thoughts, distractability, increased goal-directed behavior, and excessive involvement in pleasurable activities.

While the etiology of the major affective disorders is still unknown, earlier psychobiological studies and research on antidepressant drugs led to several hypotheses implicating alterations in brain monoamine neurotransmitter function (monoamine hypothesis). It is widely held that manic and depressive symptoms are caused by disturbances in brain neurotransmission mediated by 5-hydroxytryptamine (5-HT) and/or catecholamines (norepinephrine, dopamine). However, these disorders are likely heterogeneous, both diagnostically and pathophysiologically. Furthermore, recent research suggests the involvement of postreceptor signaling disturbances in the pathogenesis of some subtypes of the affective disorders, particularly bipolar affective disorder.

Antidepressant drugs may be categorized into four principal groups: the **tricyclic antidepressants** (TCAs), the **monoamine oxidase inhibitors** (MAOIs), **other cyclic agents,** and the more recently introduced **selective serotonin reuptake inhibitors** (SSRIs). The first two classes of agents were introduced into the clinical therapy of affective disorders in the late 1950s and still have important roles in the treatment of major depressive episodes. Common to all antidepressants is the delayed onset of therapeutic efficacy, generally 2–4 weeks. This phenomenon is thought to reflect the need for development of biochemical and physiological adaptive changes in monoaminergic function for a therapeutic response to occur. Regardless of the class, all antidepressants exhibit side effects. These vary, however, with the specific group of agents and have become increasingly important considerations in the choice of drug for management of depression.

The demand for antidepressant drugs with fewer side effects (especially less anticholinergic and cardiotoxic effects) and faster onset of action, together with the observation that tricyclic antidepressants block the neuronal reuptake of norepinephrine (NE) and/or serotonin (5-HT), led to the synthesis of a large number of new antidepressant compounds, often referred to as "second- and third-generation antidepressants." Some of these antidepressants do not inhibit MAO and have little or no effect on the amine reuptake process. Others, such as the SSRIs, were developed on the basis of their selectivity in blocking neuronal reuptake of 5-HT.

TRICYCLIC ANTIDEPRESSANTS

These drugs, of which there are several types, were developed by modification of the central ring of the phenothiazine molecule, as shown in Figure 29-1. The iminodibenzyl type, including imipramine and related drugs, has a –C–C– bridge in place of the S atom. This is also true of the dibenzocycloheptene type (e.g., amitriptyline), which in addition has the N atom of the phenothiazine ring replaced by a doubly bonded carbon. Additional modifications gave rise to the dibenzoxazepine and dibenzoxepine types (Fig. 29-1). Although many of the original compounds of this class, including imipramine and amitriptyline, were synthesized as potential antipsychotic agents, they were found to be ineffective in quieting agitated psychiatric patients but proved to be effective in treating "endogenous" depression, a depressive subtype now referred to as melancholic.

Pharmacological Properties

Actions on central nervous system and behavior

Tricyclic antidepressants do not elevate mood or the level of arousal in normal persons. In fact, they

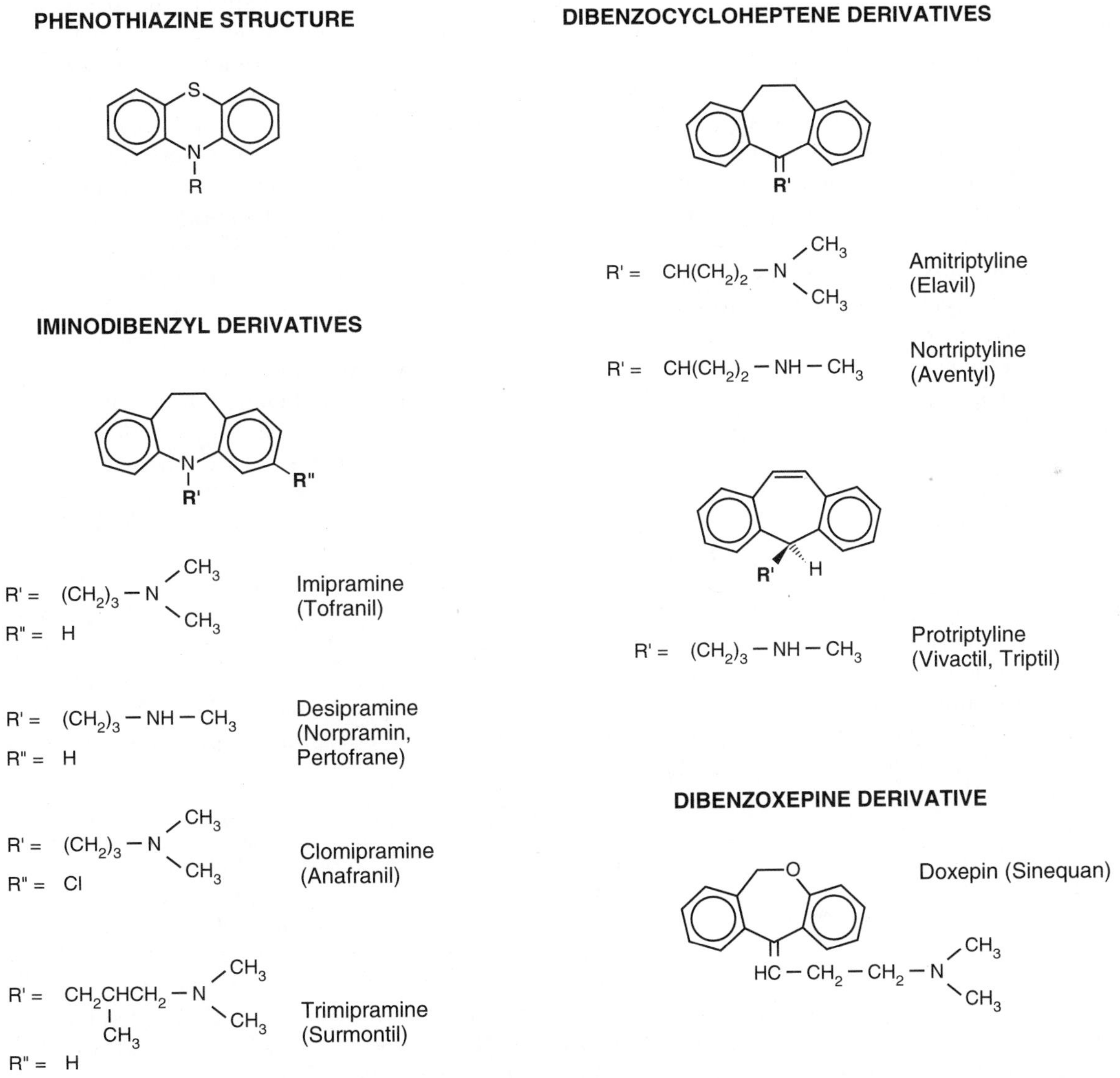

PHENOTHIAZINE STRUCTURE

IMINODIBENZYL DERIVATIVES

DIBENZOCYCLOHEPTENE DERIVATIVES

DIBENZOXEPINE DERIVATIVE

Figure 29-1. Molecular structures of commonly used tricyclic antidepressants.

tend to produce drowsiness and fatigue in healthy subjects. In depressed patients, however, they cause a rise of mood, interest level, and pleasure in activities, which develops gradually over a period of 2–4 weeks.

In laboratory animals, TCAs prolong hexobarbital-induced sleep and impair both learning and performance of various behaviors, such as conditioned avoidance responses. These sedative-like effects are accompanied by slowing and synchronization of the EEG, as seen with barbiturates or other sedatives. Only at high doses do the tricyclics produce EEG signs of stimulation, such as an increase in fast beta-wave activity and seizure activity.

Inhibition of norepinephrine and serotonin reuptake

Tricyclic antidepressants (Table 29-1 and Fig. 29-1) are potent inhibitors of the neuronal reuptake of NE and 5-HT. Generally speaking, tricyclic secondary amines (e.g., desipramine, nortriptyline) are more potent than the corresponding tertiary amines in inhibiting NE reuptake. However, tertiary amine tricyclics (e.g., imipramine, amitriptyline, clomipramine) are more potent inhibitors of 5-HT reuptake than the corresponding secondary amines. In humans, tertiary amine tricyclics are biotransformed by demethylation into the secondary amine tricyclics (e.g., imipramine is converted to desipramine and amitriptyline into nortriptyline).

The mechanism of antidepressant action of these drugs is not clear. Although it was initially believed that their therapeutic effect was related to the inhibitory effects on reuptake of NE and/or 5-HT, this has been questioned for two reasons. First, the effects on monoamine reuptake occur rapidly, whereas the therapeutic benefit develops gradually over several weeks after initiation of therapy. Second, some of the second-generation antidepressant drugs (iprindole and bupropion) do not inhibit the uptake of NE or 5-HT, nor do they inhibit MAO. Recent work seems to implicate two important series of changes in the mechanism of action of antidepressants which occur with a time course that parallels the delayed onset of therapeutic effect. These changes are described below (Fig. 29-2).

Receptor effects

Tricyclic antidepressants have potent antagonist effects at a number of CNS receptors, as listed in Table 29-1. These effects, however, account not for the therapeutic action but for the profile of adverse effects elicited by these agents, which parallel their respective receptor affinities. In general, all tricyclic antidepressants exhibit significant anticholinergic effects, although the tertiary TCAs are more potent in this regard than the demethylated TCAs such as desipramine and nortriptyline. Various TCAs are also potent blockers of H_1 histamine receptors and α_1-adrenoceptors; this action accounts for the sedative and hypotensive effects seen with a number of these agents. The receptor antagonist effects of TCAs also occur rapidly and account for the early onset of side effects seen during treatment. Moreover, these effects occur at lower dosages than those required for therapeutic response.

Two very important receptor changes induced by TCAs may be more directly related to the mechanism of their therapeutic action. These are down-regulation of cerebral cortical β-adrenergic receptors and sensitization of postsynaptic serotonergic receptors leading to enhanced serotonergic neurotransmission. The former effect is produced not only by different types of antidepressant drugs (TCAs, MAOIs, and some second-generation antidepressants) but also by electroconvulsive therapy (ECT), which is a very effective treatment modality for depression.

Initially, the increased intrasynaptic levels of 5-HT activate serotonergic somatodendritic $5-HT_{1A}$-autoreceptors, thus reducing the neuronal firing rate and synaptic release of 5-HT at axon terminals (Fig. 29-2). With time (1–2 weeks), however, the somatodendritic autoreceptors become desensitized, so 5-HT neuronal firing rate progressively recovers and release of 5-HT from presynaptic terminals is enhanced.

These changes, together with the elevated intrasynaptic 5-HT levels at axonal terminals resulting from the continuing blockade of 5-HT reuptake, cause a net increase in serotonergic neurotransmission, an effect hypothesized to be critical to the mechanism of action of all antidepressant agents.

Anticholinergic and antihistaminic effects

The tricyclic antidepressants, like many phenothiazines, possess strong anticholinergic properties. Thus, their side effects include blurred vision, dryness of the mouth, constipation, and urinary retention. As noted above, some are also potent antihistamines. The feelings of sedation and fatigue observed with tricyclic antidepressants are related to their antihistaminergic action.

Table 29-1 Relative Effects of Tricyclic, Second-Generation, and SSRI Antidepressants on Neurotransmitter Reuptake and Receptor Blockade, and Other Pharmacological Actions*

Drug	Reuptake Inhibition			Receptor Blockade							Side Effects		
	NE	5-HT	DA	$5\text{-}HT_1$	$5\text{-}HT_2$	mACh	H_1	$\alpha_1\text{-}AR$	$\alpha_2\text{-}AR$	D_2	Sedation	Anticholinergic	Cardiotoxic
Tricyclics													
Amitriptyline (Elavil)	+ +	+ +	−	+ +	+ + +	+ + + +	+ + + +	+ + + +	+ + +	+	+ + + +	+ + + +	+ + +
Clomipramine (Anafranil)	+ +	+ + + +	−	+	+ + +	+ + + +	+ + + +	+ + + +	+ +	+	+	+ + + +	+ + +
Desipramine (Norpramin)	+ + + +	+	−	+	+ +	+ + +	+ +	+ +	+	±	+	+	+
Doxepin (Sinequan)	+ +	+	−	+ +	+ + +	+ + +	+ + + +	+ + + +	+ +	+ + +	+ + + +	+ + + +	+ + +
Imipramine (Tofranil)	+ +	+ + +	−		+ +	+ + +	+ + +	+ + +	+ +	+ +	+ +	+ + +	+ + +
Nortriptyline (Aventyl)	+ + +	+	−		+ + +	+ +	+ + +	+ + +	+ +	+	+ +	+ +	+
Protriptyline (Triptil)	+ + + +	+	−	+	+	+ + + +	+ + + +	+ +	+	+	+	+	+ + +
Trimipramine (Surmontil)	+	+	−	+	+ +	+ + + +	+ + + +	+ + + +	+ + + +	+ +	+ + + +	+ + + +	+ + +
Other cyclic agents													
Amoxapine (Asendin)	+ + +	+	+ + +	+ +	+ + +	+ +	+ + +	+ + +	+ +	+ + + +	+ +	+ +	±
Maprotiline (Ludiomil)	+ + +	+	+	+	+	+ + +	+ + +	+ + +	+	+ +	+ +	+ +	±
Trazodone (Desyrel)	+	+	−	+ + +	+ + +	−	+	+ + + +	+ + + +	+	+ + + +	±	±
Bupropion (Wellbutrin)	+	−	+ + +	−	−	−	±	+	−	−	+	±	±
SSRIs													
Fluoxetine (Prozac)	+	+ + +	±	+	+ +	+	+	+	±	±	+	−	±
Fluvoxamine (Luvox)	±	+ + +	+	±	+ +	+	±	+	±	±	+	+	−
Sertraline (Zoloft)	±	+ + + +	+ +	−	+	+	±	+ +	+	±	+	±	±
Paroxetine (Paxil)	+	+ + + +	+	−	±	+ +	±	+	±	−	+	+	±

*α-AR = α-adrenoceptors; mACh = muscarinic cholinergic receptors; D_2 = dopamine D_2-receptors; DA = dopamine; H_1 = histamine H_1-receptors; 5-HT = serotonin; NE = norepinephrine.
−, ±, +, + +, + + +, + + + +: absence, or increasing degrees, of reuptake inhibition, receptor blockade, and side effects.

Pharmacokinetics

Absorption of tricyclic antidepressants from the gastrointestinal tract is essentially complete. Patients treated with identical doses show great interindividual differences in their steady-state plasma concentrations. These differences may be related to interindividual variation in hepatic blood flow, resulting in differences in the amount of drug being biotransformed on the first pass through the liver. Clinical improvement has been shown to correlate well with plasma drug levels of some tricyclic antidepressants (nortriptyline, imipramine, desipramine).

The slow onset of antidepressant action may be related, in part, to the time required to achieve adequate steady-state tissue levels for changes in central 5-HT or NE pathways (e.g., receptor desensitization) to take place. The half-life of unchanged tricyclics in humans ranges from 9 to 20 hours (a $t_{1/2}$ of more than 48 hours has been reported in some

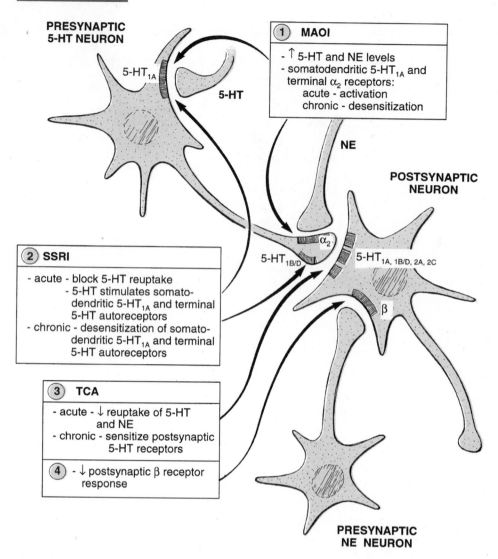

Figure 29-2. Mechanisms and sites of action of mono-amine oxidase inhibitors (1—MAOI), selective serotonin reuptake inhibitors (2—SSRI), and tricyclic antidepressants (3—TCA) in the regulation of 5-HT-mediated neu-rotransmission; α_2 and β refer to noradrenergic receptors. *The overall effect of all three classes of drugs is increased 5-HT synaptic transmission* (see text).

studies), and a steady-state plasma concentration is generally not reached until the second week of treatment. The pharmacokinetics of the many active metabolites have not been thoroughly studied.

In elderly patients, the steady-state levels of tricyclics tend to be higher than in younger subjects on the same dose because of reduced rates of hepatic clearance. This may explain the increased risk of toxicity and the need for lower doses in the elderly.

The biotransformation of tricyclic antidepressants involves demethylation, hydroxylation, and conjugation. Many of the metabolites have antide-pressant action themselves. In patients receiving the tertiary amine tricyclic antidepressants, the ratio between the plasma concentrations of the tertiary amine and its secondary amine metabolite shows great interindividual differences. Much of the variation appears to be genetically determined (see Chapter 12).

Excretion of tricyclic antidepressants is slow (40% in 24 hours, 70% in 72 hours). The greatest portion is excreted as the N-oxide or as the unconju-gated or conjugated 2-OH derivative.

Adverse Effects

Pronounced anticholinergic activity (atropinic effects)

In addition to the regularly observed atropine-like side effects of the tricyclics noted above, there is a danger of acute glaucoma; tricyclic antidepressants must therefore be prescribed with caution to patients with narrow-angle glaucoma or prostatic hypertrophy.

Cardiovascular system

Tricyclic antidepressants have potent and complex effects on the cardiovascular system related to their anticholinergic properties, their inhibition of catecholamine uptake, and their quinidine-like actions. The tricyclic antidepressants also exhibit lidocaine-like effects that can aggravate some preexisting cardiac disorders, yet, almost paradoxically, may be of therapeutic benefit in preventing certain ventricular arrhythmias. Side effects include postural hypotension, tachycardia, hypertension, ECG changes (T-wave abnormalities, arrhythmias, impaired conduction), and congestive heart failure. These reactions are more likely to occur in the presence of existing cardiovascular disease, and with high doses. The risk of cardiotoxic effects of tricyclic antidepressants increases proportionately with plasma concentrations above 1 μg/mL.

CNS effects

Drowsiness is very common with the tertiary tricyclics. A fine rapid tremor, especially in the upper extremities, occurs in about 10% of elderly patients; it may be treated with propranolol, 40 mg twice daily. Tricyclic antidepressants lower the seizure threshold, as do phenothiazines, and may produce tonic-clonic seizures in high doses. Psychotoxic side effects vary from impaired memory to delirium. Although best documented for tricyclics, there is a definite risk with all antidepressants of precipitating a hypomanic or manic episode in depressed patients with a history of bipolar affective disorder.

Withdrawal symptoms

In patients receiving more than 150 mg of imipramine or its equivalent daily for more than 2 months, withdrawal symptoms may start as early as 4 days, but usually between 1 and 2 weeks, following abrupt discontinuation. Symptoms consist of gastrointestinal disturbances, anxiety, and insomnia. Gradually reducing the dose over a period of several weeks can avoid or substantially reduce such symptoms.

Drug Interactions

Hypertension and hyperpyrexia may result when tricyclic antidepressants are given in combination with MAO inhibitors, because both groups of drugs tend to increase the amounts of biogenic amines available to act at postsynaptic receptors. For this reason, practitioners should wait 2 weeks after stopping a MAOI before starting treatment with a tricyclic antidepressant.

Concurrent administration of tricyclic antidepressants and sympathomimetic amines can augment the amine pressor effects to the point of a hypertensive crisis. These antidepressants can also interfere with the therapeutic effects of certain antihypertensive agents (e.g., guanethidine, clonidine, see Chapter 18).

In epileptic patients maintained on anticonvulsant drugs, reduction of the seizure threshold by the tricyclics could be clinically important.

Tricyclic antidepressants tend to enhance the effects of all oral hypoglycemic agents.

Because of the extensive hepatic microsomal metabolism of tricyclic antidepressants, coadministration of drugs that induce (e.g., carbamazepine) or inhibit (e.g., SSRIs) these enzymes can cause up to twofold reductions or elevations, respectively, in plasma tricyclic antidepressant levels, with prominent adverse effects. Thus, considerable attention must be given to such potential metabolic interactions whenever tricyclic antidepressants are coadministered with other medications that affect hepatic drug metabolism.

Overdosage

The clinical picture of overdosage is dominated by marked anticholinergic activity (see above). In severe cases, myoclonic seizures, hyperpyrexia, hypotension, impaired cardiac conduction and contractility, ventricular arrhythmias, and coma may occur.

In addition to routine life-support measures and gastric lavage, anticholinergic toxicity marked by confusion, delirium, agitation, or coma may be managed with physostigmine (1–2 mg by slow intravenous injection, repeated at 30–60-minute intervals as necessary), which counteracts both the central and peripheral anticholinergic effects. Close monitoring of cardiac function is critical in the early stage of tricyclic-antidepressant overdose treatment. Hemodialysis may be required to prevent or treat cardiotoxic complications.

Choice Among Tricyclic Antidepressants

There is no conclusive evidence that any one tricyclic antidepressant or class of antidepressant drugs is superior to another with respect to antidepressant response. The choice in clinical practice depends largely on the individual patient's tolerance of the side effects of a particular antidepressant and the presence of any preexisting medical illness. Certain tricyclic antidepressants may be chosen for their strong sedating properties (e.g., amitriptyline) when insomnia or excitation is present. Nortriptyline produces less hypotension and therefore may be preferred in the treatment of the elderly, who may sustain injuries from falls brought on by unsteadiness and lightheadedness due to orthostatic hypotension. Several new antidepressants such as the SSRIs (see later in this chapter) should be considered for those patients who are particularly predisposed to the cardiotoxic properties of the tricyclics. Although the SSRIs have been widely adopted as the preferred initial drug for treatment of depression, the tricyclics are still frequently used, especially in severe cases.

Other Therapeutic Uses

Tricyclics are also used in two other conditions that are not obviously related to depression. In **chronic pain syndromes**, such as trigeminal neuralgia or posttraumatic pain syndrome, amitriptyline and nortriptyline have an analgesic action at low doses (up to 75 mg/day) that are well below the range required for antidepressant action. The mechanism of the analgesic action is unclear.

MONOAMINE OXIDASE INHIBITORS

Iproniazid (an isopropyl derivative of isoniazid, an antitubercular drug) was synthesized in 1951 in a search for a better chemotherapeutic agent for tuberculosis. When this drug was given to patients, they became cheerful and energetic, and showed marked improvement in their outlook, even though there was no change in their lung pathology. In 1952, Zeller and co-workers discovered that iproniazid inhibits the enzyme monoamine oxidase (MAO). Iproniazid

was introduced for treatment of depression in 1957 but was abandoned because of its hepatotoxicity. However, its effects on mood spurred pharmaceutical chemists to synthesize other monoamine oxidase inhibitors (MAOIs) in a search for less toxic ones. The structures of some of the MAOIs used clinically are shown in Figure 29-3.

Monoamine oxidase exists in two forms—MAO-A, for which 5-HT and NE are preferred substrates, and MAO-B, for which phenylethylamine is the specific substrate. In the human brain MAO-B is the predominant form, but it is localized mostly extracellularly. The intracellular enzyme is mainly the MAO-A subtype. Inhibition of MAO-A may be more important for antidepressant effects, as the selective MAO-B inhibitor deprenyl (selegiline; see Chapter 21) produces little or only weak response in depressed patients.

Pharmacological Properties

Because of their potential to produce a serious hypertensive reaction in patients who inadvertly consumed

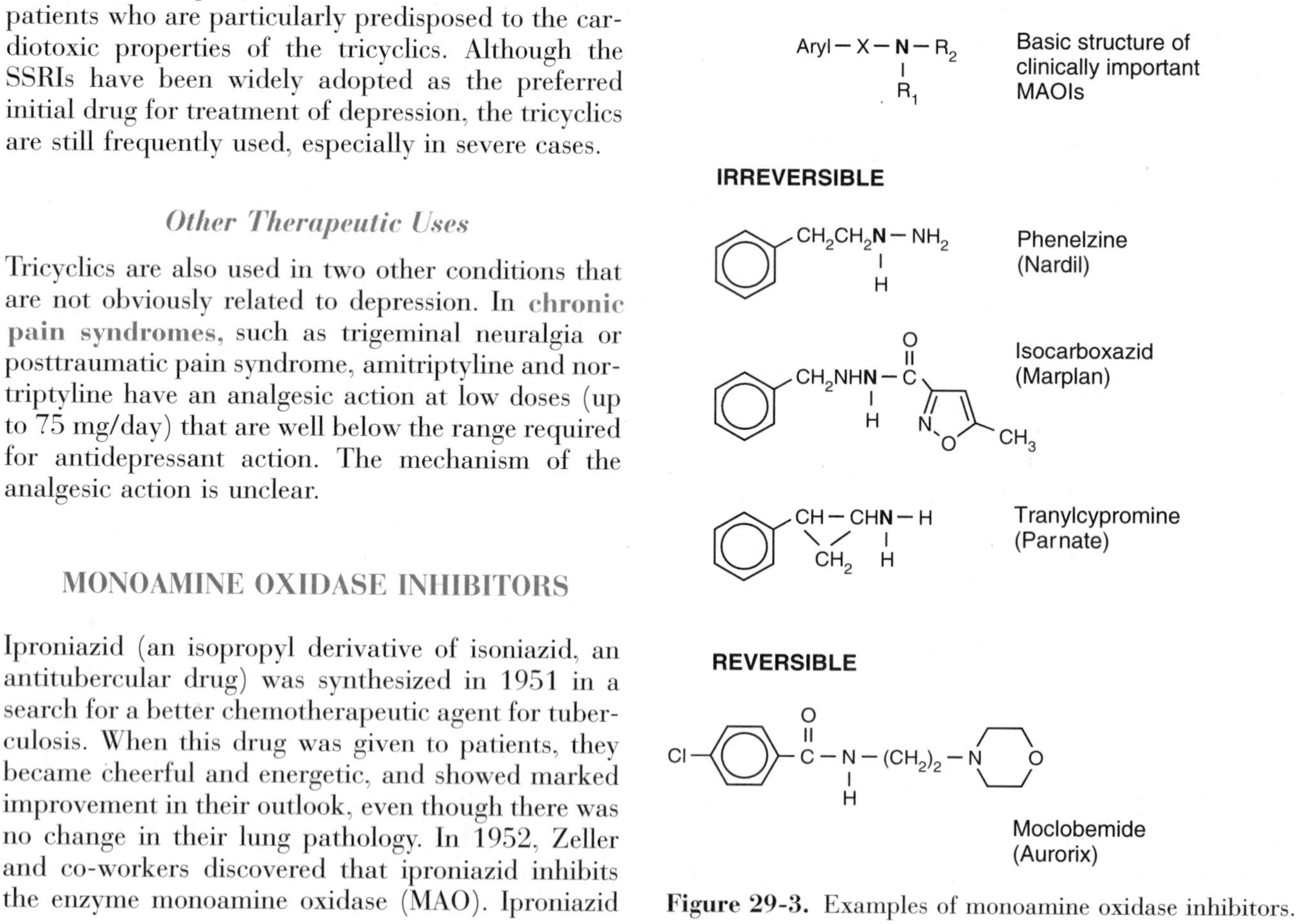

Figure 29-3. Examples of monoamine oxidase inhibitors.

foods high in tyramine, or medications containing pressor amines, the MAOIs were relegated to a secondary role in the treatment of depression for many years. The results of numerous studies, however, now indicate that these agents have therapeutic efficacy comparable to that of other antidepressants.

Following inhibition of MAO, concentrations of 5-HT, DA, and NE are markedly elevated in the body. It has been hypothesized that it is the increased availability of 5-HT in the brain, producing a net increase in serotonergic neurotransmission, and not the inhibition of MAO-A per se, which is particularly important in the mechanism of action of MAOIs. In addition, the simultaneous effect of MAOIs in increasing NE levels may be instrumental in actually enhancing net serotonergic neurotransmission. It has been proposed that the increased levels of NE caused by inhibition of MAO desensitize inhibitory α_2-noradrenergic receptors located presynaptically on 5-HT axon terminals. This results in a release of 5-HT neurons from α_2-noradrenergic receptor-mediated inhibition, and therefore an increased rate of neuronal firing and release of 5-HT. Just as in TCA therapy, a 2–3 week time lag in producing these receptor-desensitization effects following the initiation of MAOI treatment mirrors the delayed onset of therapeutic response to these agents.

MAO inhibitors lower blood pressure, but it is uncertain whether this action is related to MAO inhibition.

Some MAOIs (e.g., phenelzine, tranylcypromine) also have sympathomimetic activity similar to that of amphetamine due to increased release of stored norepinephrine.

The currently available MAOIs are readily absorbed when given by mouth, but excretion is slow. The onset of antidepressant action is slow, but because the drugs inhibit MAO irreversibly, their effects are long-lasting. Termination of drug effects depends upon synthesis of fresh enzyme, a process taking more than a week to reach normal levels.

Adverse Properties

Because MAO is widely distributed throughout the body and is present in many different cell types, diverse pharmacological effects can be expected to occur after the administration of MAOIs.

Unlike some tricyclics, of which the whole dose is sometimes administered at night for its beneficial effect on sleep, MAOIs cause insomnia, and therefore evening and night doses should be avoided. Tranylcypromine may produce stimulant effects in some

individuals, which is thought to be related to its amphetamine-like structure.

Other side effects are similar to those of the tricyclic antidepressants. They may be grouped as (1) signs of excessive central nervous system stimulation, including insomnia, irritability, ataxia, and seizures; (2) peripheral vascular effects, including orthostatic hypotension and dizziness; and (3) atropine-like effects such as dry mouth, impotence, urinary retention, constipation, and other gastrointestinal disturbances that probably reflect imbalance between sympathetic and vagal tone.

As noted, these agents may also precipitate a manic episode in patients with personal or family histories of bipolar depression.

Drug Interactions

Because MAOIs inhibit catecholamine breakdown, coadministration of other substances that contain or release catecholamines may result in marked increase in adrenergic activity, with such consequences as hypertension, tachycardia, agitation, occipital headache, and occasionally intracranial bleeding (secondary to increase in blood pressure, see Chapter 18). Drugs that may interact in this way with MAOIs include tricyclic antidepressants, reserpine, L-dopa, and opioid analgesics. Foods containing large amounts of tyramine, including aged cheeses, bananas, beer, wine, yeast products, yogurt, and meat extracts (e.g., Bovril), can also precipitate a hypertensive reaction. Patients being treated with MAOIs must be warned to consult their physicians before using over-the-counter medications of any kind (especially medicines for coughs and colds, many of which contain sympathomimetic amines), and must receive detailed instructions about their diet. Hypertensive crisis resulting from such interactions can be treated with short-acting α-adrenoceptor blockers (e.g., phentolamine) or calcium channel blockers (e.g., nifedipine).

MAOIs potentiate the effects of numerous other drugs, including alcohol, sedative-hypnotics, general anesthetics, opioids, and other analgesics. This effect is thought to be due mainly to inhibition of biotransformation of these other drugs, but direct CNS interactions cannot be ruled out. After the discontinuation of MAOIs, MAO-inhibiting action will continue for at least a week. If tricyclic antidepressants or another MAOI is to be substituted for an MAOI that is being discontinued, it is recommended that an interval of 2 weeks be allowed before the new drug is started. Treatment with MAOIs should also be discontinued at least 10 days prior to elective surgery in order to avoid possible interactions with the anesthetic or preanesthetic medications. Similarly, a medication-free interval of at least 7 days should be allowed before initiating MAOI treatment in order to avoid interaction with drugs that may have been used previously.

When coadministered with tryptophan (the precursor of serotonin) or SSRI antidepressants, MAOIs may produce a neurological syndrome characterized by confusion, restlessness, elevated body temperature (hyperpyrexia), and muscle spasms (myoclonus). This "serotonin syndrome" is now recognized to be due to the marked elevation of 5-HT levels produced under these conditions.

Overdosage

The clinical picture of MAOI overdosage consists of hyperpyrexia, hypertension, hyperreflexia, involuntary movements, agitation, hallucinations, and coma. These signs and symptoms closely resemble those of major overdosage with amphetamine or atropine-like drugs (see Chapters 15 and 30), which result in excessive central and peripheral catecholaminergic and anticholinergic activity, respectively. Hypotension may sometimes occur, probably as a result of a different type of pharmacological action.

There is an initial asymptomatic period of up to 12 hours after drug ingestion, during which manifestations of overdosage may not be apparent.

Utmost care is recommended in the management of overdosed patients. Many drugs (e.g., sympathomimetics, barbiturates) tend to be potentiated by MAOIs, as noted above, and should be used only under expert guidance.

Indications for MAO Inhibitors

Although a number of earlier studies suggested that MAOIs are more effective for "atypical depressions" characterized by depression with profound feelings of lethargy, mood reactivity, sensitivity to rejection, increased sleep, and increased food intake with carbohydrate craving, more recent investigations have shown these agents to be effective in the treatment of major depressive episodes in general, as well as in panic disorder. Because of their potential to induce serious side effects, however, they continue to be used as a second line of treatment in individuals who

have responded poorly to tricyclic or other antidepressants.

Dosage

Therapeutic doses for phenelzine (Nardil) and tranylcypromine (Parnate) range from 45 to 90 mg/day and 20 to 60 mg/day, respectively. There is no good evidence supporting the use of a lower dosage during maintenance therapy with these agents. Because insomnia is not uncommon during treatment with MAOIs, they are usually given in divided doses early in the day.

Reversible MAOIs

Recently several new MAO inhibitors have been developed that do not block MAO irreversibly. **Moclobemide,** a benzamide derivative chemically distinct from the irreversible MAOIs, which inhibits MAO-A, is a recently introduced member of this subclass. It is rapidly absorbed, is subject to a high first-pass effect, and has a short elimination half-life of 1–2 hours. Treatment with it is initiated in a dose range of 300–450 mg/day in divided doses, and it has a therapeutic range of 300–600 mg/day. The adverse effects of this agent are similar to those of the irreversible MAOIs, with the important exception that it shows a much reduced ability to elevate tyramine levels following ingestion of tyramine-containing foods. Thus there is a much reduced possibility of developing a hypertensive reaction with tyramine-containing foods, although moderation in the use of such foods, and avoidance of over-the-counter drugs, should still be observed as with other MAOIs.

The therapeutic indications for these agents are similar to those for MAOIs in general, i.e., for treatment of major depression.

SECOND-GENERATION ANTIDEPRESSANTS

The introduction of TCAs and MAOIs in the late 1950s revolutionized the treatment of affective disorders. However, both types of drug produced troublesome or potentially dangerous adverse effects, as noted above. Moreover, only about 70–80% of patients responded to treatment with these agents. Therefore, there was a need for new compounds of equal or greater clinical efficacy with fewer and less serious side effects. This led to the development of a number of new antidepressants, the so-called "second/third-generation antidepressants." Many of these are not tricyclic, and they have structures and pharmacological effects quite distinct from those of the typical TCAs (Fig. 29-4), but are as effective as TCAs in treating depression. A brief description of some of the compounds follows (see also Table 29-1).

Amoxapine

In addition to being a strong inhibitor of NE reuptake, amoxapine (Asendin) has strong 5-HT-blocking activity. It has no significant effect on 5-HT reuptake and its anticholinergic activity is weak. Although its antidopaminergic activity is theoretically useful for

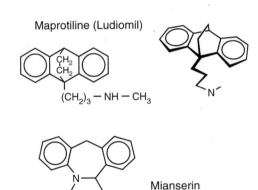

Figure 29-4. Molecular structures of second-generation antidepressants and selective serotonin reuptake inhibitors.

some patients, it has many side effects (orthostatic hypotension) similar to those of TCAs and of antipsychotics (see Chapter 28).

Maprotiline

Maprotiline (Ludiomil) strongly inhibits NE reuptake but only weakly blocks reuptake of 5-HT. It has a strong antihistaminergic and a weak anticholinergic action. There is a lower incidence of cardiovascular complications associated with its use than with that of the TCAs. A higher risk of seizures with this antidepressant has resulted in recommendations for administering lower treatment dosages than originally suggested.

Mianserin

Mianserin has only weak effects in blocking monoamine reuptake, but it blocks presynaptic α_2-receptors, thereby increasing NE turnover. In addition, its independent strong sedative and anxiolytic properties are useful for some patients. Mianserin, like maprotiline, has no significant anticholinergic effects and is much less cardiotoxic than TCAs in therapeutic doses.

Mianserin is not available in the United States and Canada.

Trazodone

A relatively selective but weak inhibitor of 5-HT reuptake, trazodone (Desyrel) also has weak anticholinergic and cardiovascular effects. It does, however, produce sedation. Nefazadone, which is related to trazodone, is much less sedating, and both are beneficial in having minimal adverse effects on sexual function.

Bupropion

Bupropion (Wellbutrin) is an aminoketone related structurally to the phenylethylamines. The mechanism of action of this agent is still poorly understood. While it decreases the density and sensitivity of β-noradrenergic receptors in cerebral cortex of rats receiving chronic dosing, this effect occurs at doses above the therapeutically relevant range. Bupropion exhibits weak dopamine-reuptake-blocking effects. It is rapidly metabolized in humans, and plasma concentrations of the active metabolites such as hydroxybupropion substantially exceed those of the parent compound. Hydroxybupropion shows low but equipotent inhibition of reuptake of dopamine and norepinephrine, which is thought to indicate that this active metabolite may also contribute to the overall therapeutic response. Electrophysiological studies have shown that, acutely, bupropion reduces noradrenergic but not serotonergic neuronal firing rates, whereas suppression of dopaminergic neuronal firing occurs only above therapeutically relevant concentrations. In animal behavioral models used for antidepressant screening, hydroxybupropion appears to account for the major part of this drug's effects. Finally, in clinical biochemical studies, bupropion administration appears to enhance CNS noradrenergic function. Thus, the bulk of evidence implicates noradrenergic processes in the mechanism of therapeutic action of bupropion; some findings suggest the potential for dopaminergic effects, but little evidence supports an action on CNS serotonergic systems as for most other antidepressants.

Bupropion is rapidly absorbed, reaching peak plasma levels in 1–3 hours, and has a mean half-life of about 10 hours. Its three biologically active metabolites, hyroxybupropion, erythrohydrobupropion, and threohydrobupropion, have half-lives of 20–27 hours. Clinically, bupropion has a stimulating effect which may cause agitation, increased motor activity, tremor, and insomnia. Its low anticholinergic potency and lack of effect on cardiac conduction account for its lower potential for cardiotoxicity. It produces a range of gastrointestinal side effects similar to the SSRIs, including nausea, vomiting, and loss of appetite, and it is more likely to be associated with weight loss. A particularly worrisome side effect of bupropion is its propensity to produce seizures at dosages above 450 mg/day, particularly within the time interval between peak plasma levels. For these reasons, it is recommended that bupropion be administered in divided doses not greater than 150 mg/dose, at least 4 hours apart; the maximum total daily dose should not exceed 450 mg.

SELECTIVE SEROTONIN REUPTAKE INHIBITORS (SSRI)

Evidence implicating reduced brain serotonergic function in depression led to the search for potential antidepressant compounds that acted selectively on these systems. It was reasoned that such agents might have enhanced therapeutic effects with fewer troublesome side effects attributable to nonselective actions on other neurotransmitter systems and receptors. At least five SSRIs are now in clinical use throughout the world, the widest experience in North America being with **fluoxetine** (Prozac), **sertraline** (Zoloft), **fluvoxamine** (Luvox), and **paroxetine** (Paxil) (Fig. 29-4). Unlike the tricyclic antidepressants, the SSRIs do not share a common chemical structure but are classified on the basis of their common functional effects. All are potent and very selective inhibitors of neuronal 5-HT reuptake and show little or no inhibition of NE or DA reuptake. They also cause essentially no blockade of α_1-, α_2-, or β_1-adrenoceptors or dopamine D_2-, $5\text{-HT}_{1\&2}$-, or histamine H_1-receptors (Table 29-1).

Pharmacological Effects

As with other antidepressants, the response to SSRIs is delayed for several weeks following institution of treatment. Thus, the mechanism of therapeutic action of SSRIs is also thought to be related to adaptive changes in neuronal function resulting in enhanced brain serotonergic neurotransmission, as already described for TCAs and MAOIs.

Pharmacokinetics

The SSRIs are generally well absorbed from the gastrointestinal tract, reaching peak plasma levels in 4–8 hours. Sertraline tends to be absorbed a little more slowly than the other SSRIs. At therapeutic concentrations, all of these agents show extensive binding to plasma protein (fluoxetine 94%, fluvoxamine 77%, paroxetine 95%, and sertraline 99%). Sertraline and paroxetine have plasma half-lives in the range of 24 hours; fluvoxamine has a shorter $t_{1/2}$ of about 15 hours. In contrast, fluoxetine has a $t_{1/2}$ of 3 days.

The SSRIs undergo extensive hepatic biotransformation. The primary metabolite of sertraline, desmethylsertraline, is only a weak inhibitor of 5-HT reuptake with five to 10 times lower potency, and no active metabolites have been identified for paroxetine or fluvoxamine. The major metabolite of fluoxetine, norfluoxetine, is also a specific and potent inhibitor of 5-HT reuptake, and has a $t1/2$ of 7–15 days. This prolonged half-life for fluoxetine and its major metabolite merits close consideration when this agent is used to treat depression, as it may prolong the duration of intolerable side effects encountered by some patients because of the drug's slow elimination. However, it may have an advantage in individuals who show poor compliance, because occasional missed doses will not result in marked reductions in steady-state plasma levels.

There is little evidence supporting a relationship between plasma levels and response to SSRIs. Fluoxetine and paroxetine show nonlinear pharmacokinetics, because these agents inhibit their own clearance, leading to an increased half-life at higher doses and a disproportionate elevation in plasma concentrations with subsequent dose increases. While some patients require higher levels of certain SSRIs to produce a clinical response, there is no clear explanation for this observation, nor is there yet a means of identifying such individuals in advance of instituting therapy.

Adverse Effects

The lack of effect of SSRIs at various neuroreceptors noted above accounts for the marked reduction in adverse effects reported for these antidepressants compared with the classical tricyclic agents. For example, they do not cause orthostatic hypotension, produce little sedation, and cause little or no dry mouth, constipation, urinary retention, or memory dysfunction. They do, however, produce troublesome side effects, including nausea, increased anxiety, and headache in particular. Some of these adverse effects may be related to the increased stimulation of 5-HT receptor subtypes, such as 5-HT_{1A}, as a result of the 5-HT elevation. This may account for the increased feelings of anxiety and restlessness experienced by as many as 15–20% of patients taking these agents. Paroxetine has a weak blocking effect on muscarinic cholinergic receptors that likely accounts for its ability to cause dry mouth in some patients during treatment.

SSRIs do not produce significant sedation although some patients may experience daytime somnolence, and they do not induce weight gain. The SSRIs appear to have a much greater margin of safety and are less toxic in overdosage than the tricyclics, and they are more suitable for treatment of depression in individuals with coexisting cardiovascular disease. Extrapyramidal side effects have been reported with these agents, possibly mediated by an indirect action on dopaminergic function. Although rare, the possibility of such occurrences should be carefully monitored in long-term maintenance treatment with these agents.

SSRIs cause significant sexual dysfunction, particularly anorgasmia in women and delayed or absent ejaculation in men.

Drug Interactions

Several of the SSRIs are competitive inhibitors of specific hepatic P450 isozymes, and they therefore have the potential for significant drug interactions. Fluoxetine and paroxetine are potent inhibitors of the hepatic P450 isozyme 2D6 in vitro and in vivo, whereas sertraline is much less potent. Thus, fluoxetine and paroxetine can produce marked elevations in the plasma levels (and consequently the side effects) of other drugs that are biotransformed by this hepatic isozyme. For example, plasma tricyclic levels can double during coadministration of fluoxetine, a situation which may occur while switching from a TCA to this SSRI. Fluoxetine also inhibits the hepatic 3A/4 and 2C isozymes, interfering with the clearance of alprazolam and diazepam, respectively; but at the usual minimum effective dose of fluoxetine the effect on 2D6-mediated drug metabolism is much greater than on the 3A/4 and 2C isozymes. Sertraline at usual therapeutic doses of 50–100 mg is much less likely to interfere with the clearance of other drugs.

Because of their high degree of protein binding, SSRIs can increase the plasma levels and toxicity associated with other drugs (e.g., warfarin, digitoxin) that also show extensive plasma protein binding. Ample time must be allowed for the washout of these drugs (2 weeks for sertraline, paroxetine, and fluvoxamine, 5 weeks for fluoxetine) when switching from SSRIs to MAOI treatment to avoid the production of a hypermetabolic state marked by hyperpyrexia, confusion, agitation, muscular rigidity, myoclonus, and autonomic instability. This reaction has considerable similarity to the 5-HT and antipsychotic malignant syndromes and may involve marked augmentation of central serotonergic function.

LITHIUM

Lithium differs from other psychotropic drugs in that it does not produce obvious depressant or euphoriant effects in healthy individuals. Therefore it stabilizes mood in the manic patient without producing drowsiness or motor incoordination. Just as with the antidepressants discussed above, the full effects of lithium are not obtained until 2–3 weeks after initiation of treatment. For this reason, lithium is usually given initially together with an anxiolytic or antipsychotic drug in order to provide immediate relief of symptoms. Once the patient is stabilized, the tranquilizing medication is withdrawn and lithium treatment is maintained.

Mechanisms of Action

It is not clear how lithium works in stabilizing mood, but recent work suggests important actions of lithium on key processes in receptor-stimulated G protein-coupled adenylyl cyclase and phophoinositide (PI) second-messenger systems (Fig. 29-5). Evidence has been obtained that lithium at therapeutic concentrations (0.5–1.0 mmol/L) blocks the enzymatic hydrolysis of inositol monophosphate, resulting in alterations of PI signal transduction by limiting the regeneration of inositol, an essential precursor in PI synthesis. Lithium also inhibits receptor-, guanine nucleotide-, and directly stimulated adenylyl cyclase activity in vitro and in vivo, which suggests that it attenuates receptor-activated adenylyl cyclase signaling at the level of both the G proteins that couple receptors to adenylyl cyclases and the adenylyl cyclases themselves. These effects account for the suppression of hormonal responses in peripheral tissues which underlie important side effects of lithium treatment (e.g., thyrotropin activation of thyroid adenylyl cyclase and antidiuretic hormone activation of renal adenylyl cyclase). They may also be important, however, in the therapeutic mechanism(s) of lithium action in the CNS.

Lithium also appears to interfere with PI-dependent signaling by attenuating protein kinase C (PKC)-mediated responses. This may involve alterations in the intracellular disposition or levels of specific PKC isozymes in certain brain areas such as the hippocampus. Lithium has also been reported to accelerate the uptake of NE by synaptosomes, to enhance brain 5-HT turnover, and to inhibit cell membrane $(Na^+ + K^+)$- and calcium-ATPase activity. The fact that these effects on neuronal signal transduction occur at therapeutically relevant concentrations suggests that they may be the basic mechanism of the therapeutic effects.

Pharmacokinetics and Dosage

Lithium absorption from the gastrointestinal tract is rapid, with peak blood levels occurring about 2–4 hours after a single dose. The serum half-life is approximately 24 hours. However, it has been reported that the half-life of lithium increases with continuous lithium therapy, and a mean $t\frac{1}{2}$ of 57.6

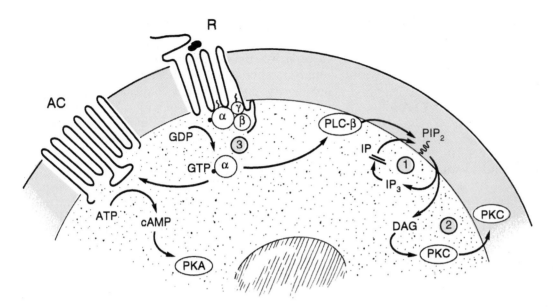

Figure 29-5. Effects of lithium ion on major intracellular signaling mechanisms. (1) Blockade of inositol cycle. (2) Translocation of PKC to membrane. (3) Inhibition of G protein function. *Abbreviations:* α, β, γ = subunits of G proteins; AC = adenylyl cyclase; ATP = adenosine triphosphate; cAMP = cyclic adenosine monophosphate; DAG = diacylglycerol; GDP = guanosine diphosphate; GTP = guanosine triphosphate; IP_3 = inositol-1,4,5-trisphosphate; PIP_2 = phosphatidylinositol-4,5-bisphosphate; PKA = protein kinase A; PKC = protein kinase C; PLC = phospholipase C; R = receptor.

hours has been demonstrated in patients who had been on lithium for more than a year.

Lithium is not protein-bound. The optimal serum lithium concentration for control of manic symptoms is 0.7–1.3 mmoles/L determined 12 hours after the most recent dose. A daily dose of 900–2100 mg, depending on the patient's weight and age, generally provides serum lithium levels within the therapeutic range.

There is a competitive interaction between sodium and lithium ions in the renal tubule. An increase in sodium intake decreases renal reabsorption of lithium and thus lowers the serum lithium level slightly, while reduced sodium intake elevates it. Thus, patients on a sodium-restricted diet or taking drugs that impair sodium reabsorption, such as diuretics and nonsteroidal anti-inflammatory agents, are at risk of lithium intoxication. As lithium is excreted mainly by the kidneys, patients with impaired renal function are also at great risk of lithium accumulation and lithium intoxication. Plasma lithium levels also must be monitored carefully in pregnant women, because renal lithium clearance increases during pregnancy and decreases after childbirth.

Side Effects and Toxicity

Gastrointestinal disturbances, polyuria and polydipsia, fatigue, dizziness, muscle hyperirritability (fasciculation and twitching), and fine tremor of the hands may occur at serum lithium levels within the therapeutic range.

Severe poisoning (serum lithium above 2 mmol/L) primarily affects the central nervous system. Disturbances in higher cortical functions, motor incoordination, slurred speech, and coma may develop.

Endocrine and metabolic effects may occur during lithium therapy. These include hypothyroidism and goiter, alterations in carbohydrate and steroid metabolism, and pitressin-resistant diabetes insipidus-like syndromes.

Some patients show leukocytosis during long-term lithium therapy, which is reversible when therapy is stopped.

ECG changes (especially T-wave depression), arrhythmias, and peripheral circulatory disturbances have been observed.

The key measure to avoid toxicity is the monitoring of serum lithium levels and the avoidance of tissue accumulation. Lithium therapy is generally not recommended for patients with renal and cardio-vascular diseases.

MOOD-STABILIZING ANTICONVULSANT AGENTS

It was observed that some patients with seizure disorders and concomitant mood disturbances often showed improved mood while being treated with the antiseizure agents **carbamazepine** or **valproate** (see Chapter 22). This observation stimulated intensive work in recent years to explore the role of these anticonvulsant drugs in the management of mania and as mood-stabilizing agents. There is now substantial evidence supporting the antimanic actions of these agents and building support for the notion that these agents, valproate in particular, may be more effective in treating manic and hypomanic episodes in certain subtypes of bipolar affective disorder. These include bipolar disorders with rapid cycling (more than four episodes of mania and depression per year), dysphoric mania (mania coexisting with depressive symptoms), and mania secondary to neurological disorders. These agents, however, show only modest antidepressant efficacy at best, and their effectiveness in preventing the recurrence of manic and depressive episodes still remains to be demonstrated unequivocally.

The pharmacology of these agents is described in Chapter 22. Their use in the management of bipolar affective disorder is subject to the same pharmacological and side-effect considerations that apply to their use in seizure disorders. The mechanism of the antimanic and mood-stabilizing action of carbamezepine and valproate is still unknown, but it is thought to be unrelated to their anticonvulsant actions. The onset of anticonvulsant effects of these drugs is relatively rapid (24–48 hours), in contrast to the delay in antimanic response. For this reason, it is unlikely that their effects on voltage-sensitive sodium channels, peripheral-type benzodiazepine receptors, and chloride or other membrane ion channels, to which their anticonvulsant effects are ascribed, are responsible for their effects on mood. Carbamazepine has effects on a number of neurotransmitter systems, some of which may be related to the antimanic action of this drug. Recent research, however, suggests that the effects of mood-stabilizing agents on cellular signal transduction mechanisms may be responsible for their therapeutic action. For example, lithium and valproate modify the disposition of specific protein

kinase C (PKC) isozymes that are key intraneuronal regulatory enzymes in the phosphoinositide signaling cascade. Carbamazepine inhibits cGMP accumulation in lymphocytes, an effect that may be linked to nitric oxide and calcium second-messenger systems.

Side effects encountered with carbamazepine and valproate in the treatment of bipolar disorder are the same as those found when these drugs are used for management of neurological disorders. There is no evidence to support a specific range of doses or plasma concentrations for the antimanic effects of carbamazepine and valproate. Accordingly, therapeutic plasma concentration ranges established for antiseizure activity are also used as a guide in treating mania. Antimanic response to valproate appears to be optimal at levels in the range of 50–100 μg/mL.

OTHER PSYCHIATRIC INDICATIONS FOR ANTIDEPRESSANTS

There is substantial evidence that antidepressants are useful in the management of other psychiatric disorders, particularly a number of the anxiety disorders. For example, patients with **panic disorder** respond to a number of different antidepressants including the tricyclics, MAOIs, and SSRIs. Although comparisons have not been done with all antidepressants, there is no reason to suspect that the antipanic effects are selectively produced by only a few subtypes of antidepressant drugs. Patients with panic disorder are likely to be more sensitive to the adrenergic (stimulating) side effects of these agents, and therefore treatment of panic disorder with antidepressants should be initiated at lower doses and increased much more gradually than in treating depression. The optimal dose range for antipanic activity, however, is similar to that required for the management of depression.

Similarly, clomipramine, a tricyclic antidepressant with more potent 5-HT reuptake blocking action, and the SSRIs have proved useful in the management of **obsessive-compulsive disorder**. Therapeutic doses for treatment of this anxiety disorder are also the same as for treating major depression.

SUGGESTED READING

American Psychiatric Association. Practice guideline for major depressive disorder in adults. Am J Psychiatry 1993; 150:(Suppl) 1–26.
American Psychiatric Association. Practice guideline for the

treatment of patients with bipolar disorder. Am J Psychiatry 1994; 151:(Suppl) 1–36.

Feighner JP, Boyer WF. Selective 5-HT re-uptake inhibitors: the clinical use of citalopram, fluoxetine, fluvoxamine, paroxetine and sertraline. Perspectives in Psychiatry, vol 1. New York: Wiley, 1991.

Manji HK, Potter WZ, Lenox RH. Signal transduction pathways: molecular targets of lithium's actions. Arch Gen Psychiatry 1995; 52:531–543.

McDaniel KD. Clinical pharmacology of monoamine oxidase inhibitors. Clin Neuropharmacol 1986; 9:207–234.

Pinder RM, Wiering JH. Third-generation antidepressants. Med Res Rev 1993; 13:259–325.

Post RM, Weiss SRB, Chuang D-M. Mechanism of action of anticonvulsants in affective disorders: comparisons with lithium. J Clin Psychopharmacol 1992; 12:23S–35S.

Potter WZ, Rudorfer MV, Manji H. The pharmacologic treatment of depression. N Engl J Med 1991; 325:633–642.

Potter WZ, Ketter TA. Pharmacological issues in the treatment of bipolar disorder: focus on mood-stabilizing compounds. Can J Psychiatry 1993; 38:(Suppl 2) S51–S56.

Preskorn SH, Magnus RD. Inhibition of hepatic P-450 isoenzymes by 5-HT selective reuptake inhibitors: in vitro and in vivo findings and their implications for patient care. Psychopharmacol Bull 1994; 30:251–259.

Price LH, Heninger GR. Lithium treatment of mood disorders. N Engl J Med 1994; 331:591–598.

Rudorfer MV. Monoamine oxidase inhibitors: reversible and irreversible. Psychopharmacol Bull 1992; 28:45–57.

van Harten J. Clinical pharmacokinetics of selective 5-HT reuptake inhibitors. Clin Pharmacokinet 1993; 24:203–220.

CHAPTER 30

Hallucinogens and Psychotomimetics

H. KALANT

CASE HISTORY

R.W., a 19-year-old male, was brought to the physician by his roommate, who found him in a very depressed state, his arms covered with scratches, lacerations, and small abscesses.

The history revealed that R.W. was a chronic drug-user who began using alcohol when he was only 11 years old. His absentee father was alcoholic; his mother had to work full-time to support the children. An older brother had personality problems but was not using drugs and had obtained employment in another city. At age 13, R.W. started using cannabis, often together with alcohol. He had a poor academic record and dropped out of school at age 15. His friends introduced him to "crack" cocaine, and he became both a regular user and a small-scale dealer. When using cocaine, he tended to use alcohol, benzodiazepines, or marijuana to "cool off." He tried LSD several times, and although he enjoyed the visual effects he did not like the drug in general because it made him feel rather anxious and strange. He also experimented with the amphetamine derivative MDMA (also known as "Ecstasy") and with something that was sold to him as mescaline.

A year ago worsening personal problems led him to escalate his use of cocaine. It made him feel powerful and euphoric but also made him suspicious of his friends and led to frequent fights with them. If he stopped using the drug, his depression returned in a more acute form. Three weeks ago he markedly raised his daily dosage, taking between 1 and 2 g of cocaine a day, around the clock. He became ex-

tremely hyperactive, with fragmented sleep of not more than 2 hours at a time. He became quite paranoid, heard voices talking to him from the ceiling, and thought people in the next room were pounding drums to annoy him. The pattern on the wallpaper began to move, and he thought he was able to make it move at will. He had sexual fantasies that he sustained for hours, but without orgasm. He had no interest in food, and lost 7 lb in weight. When he began to feel crawling sensations under his skin, he started to dig into his arms with a needle to extract the imaginary worms. Finally he ran out of the drug and went into a deep sleep from which he woke feeling severely depressed, tremulous, and still anorexic.

On examination he was thin and malnourished, restless, and slightly short of breath. He had a moderate tachycardia, cold clammy skin, some tremor, and a very short attention span. The physician began to treat him with desipramine, but referred him immediately to the youth program of a local drug-dependence treatment agency.

A hallucination is defined as the subjective experience of a perception in the absence of a corresponding external reality. Many drugs can produce transient distortions of perception, sometimes giving rise to hallucinations and behavior such as may be seen in psychotic patients. The drugs that are most potent and selective for this action, and that are sometimes used deliberately to produce it, are called **hallucinogens** or **psychotomimetics.** They have also been given a variety of other designations reflecting different points of view. Those who advocate their use as a means of self-discovery call them **psychedelics.** In some people the drug experience may trigger a panic state or a true psychosis, so the drugs are also called **psychodysleptics** and **psychotogens.**

All these names are inappropriate because each emphasizes one effect, rather than the underlying actions. A further problem is that the drugs are not identical in their mechanisms and consequences of action. Amphetamines and cocaine do produce a psychotic state that has frequently been mistaken for paranoid schizophrenia; therefore the term "psychotomimetic" is appropriate. In contrast, the pictures produced by LSD, mescaline, and similar drugs may contain elements reminiscent of true psychoses, but they are seldom mistaken for psychoses, and the user can generally recognize that the symptoms are due to the drug. Therefore, "hallucinogens" is a better term for such drugs.

DRUGS AND METHODS OF STUDY

The two largest groups of drugs considered in this chapter are indolealkylamine derivatives related chemically to serotonin (5-hydroxytryptamine, 5-HT) and phenylethylamine derivatives related chemically to catecholamines. The chemical structures of a number of drugs in each group are shown in Figures 30-1 and 30-2.

In addition to these major groups, dissociative anesthetics such as ketamine, drugs related pharmacologically to atropine, and drugs derived from cannabis can sometimes produce hallucinations when given in high dose or under certain circumstances. Therefore they are also reviewed here in relation to their perceptual and behavioral effects.

Unfortunately, this division into families does not correspond to any clear-cut separation of their pharmacological actions and effects. The mescaline-like drugs shown in the lower half of Figure 30-2 are closely similar in actions and effects to the LSD-like drugs shown in Figure 30-1, even though they are chemically related to amphetamine. Therefore a meaningful classification must be based on a functional approach, and three complementary techniques have been used to generate a functional classification.

The first technique is that of **receptor-binding studies.** LSD (lysergic acid diethylamide) is ex-

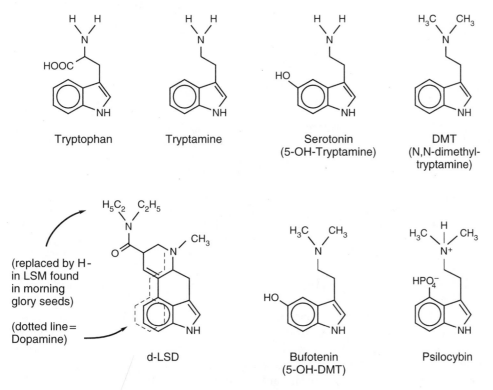

Figure 30-1. Chemical structures of some representative members of the lysergic acid and psilocybin families of hallucinogenic substances.

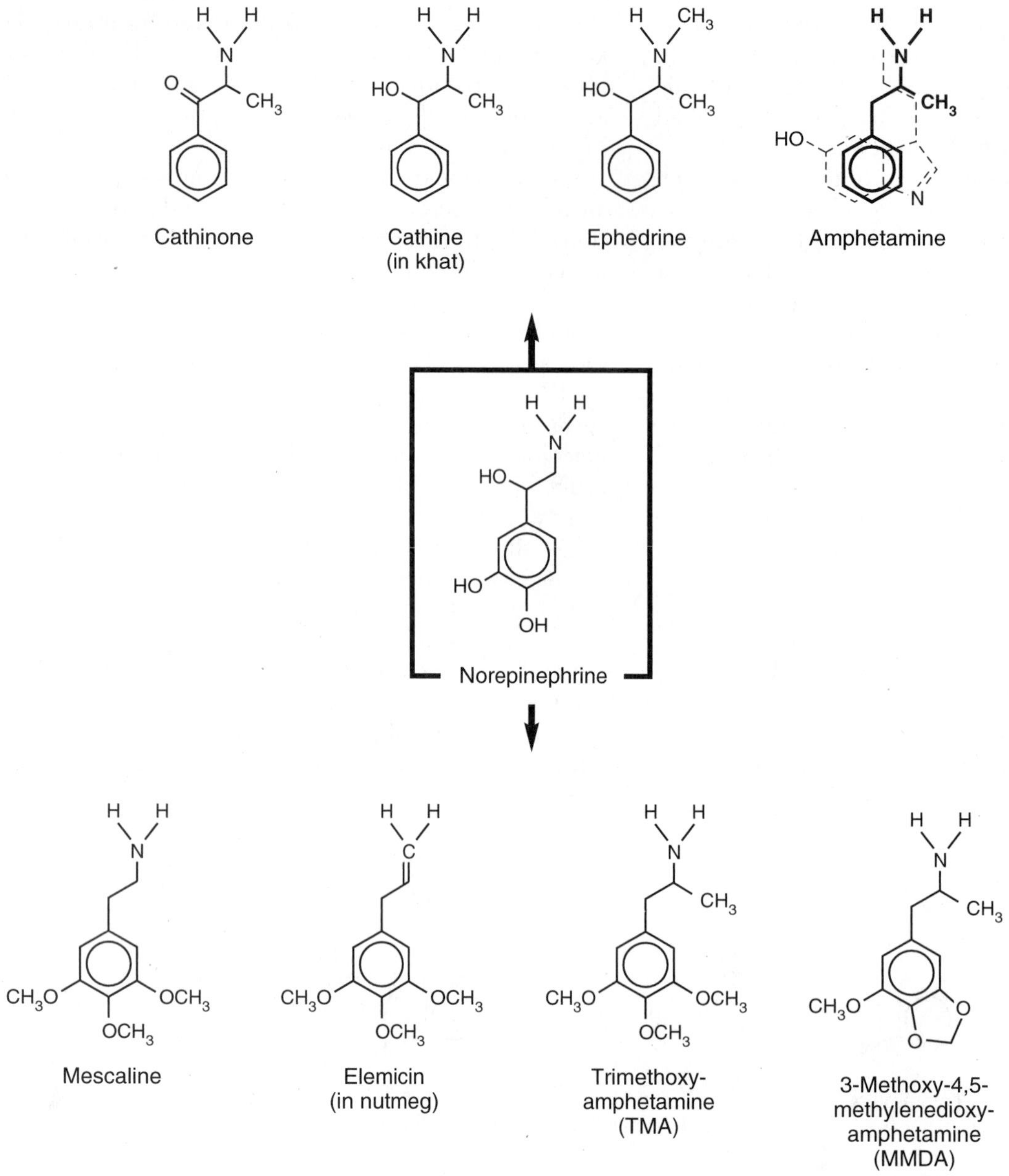

Figure 30-2. Chemical structures of norepinephrine and some representative members of the phenylethylamine group of hallucinogens. Upper row: Members of the amphetamine family. Lower row: Mescaline and related compounds. Superimposed on the amphetamine formula are the main features of the 5-hydroxytryptamine molecule.

tremely potent: A hallucinogenic dose in an adult human can be as little as 2 μg/kg (150-μg total dose). Moreover, it is highly stereospecific; only the *d*-form has activity. These characteristics are consistent with receptor-mediated action, but there has been scientific debate for several decades concerning the identity of the receptors involved in hallucinogen action and the nature of the drug–receptor interaction. The indole nucleus in LSD and related compounds (see Fig. 30-1) is structurally related to 5-HT, and the phenylethylamine structure of the amphetamines and related drugs (Fig. 30-2) is related to dopamine (DA) and norepinephrine (NE). However, the molecular structures of LSD and similar compounds also correspond in part to DA, and the amphetamine and mescaline families also overlap with essential parts of the 5-HT structure. Therefore recent investigations have involved systematic com-

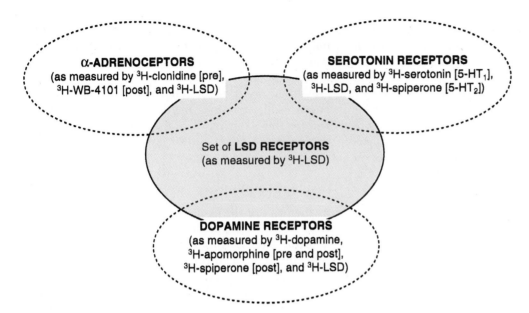

Figure 30-3. Possible receptor interactions of LSD, serotonin, dopamine, and α-adrenoceptor agonists, as revealed by in vitro receptor binding assays: [pre] indicates presynaptic receptors; [post] indicates postsynaptic receptors; [5-HT₁] indicates high-affinity postsynaptic receptors; [5-HT₂] indicates low-affinity (presynaptic?) receptors.

parison of the in vitro binding affinities of all of these compounds at both 5-HT and DA receptors, using the techniques described in Chapter 9.

The results demonstrate an extensive overlap of binding patterns (Fig. 30-3). For example, LSD has about equal affinity for 5-HT_2- and dopamine D_2-receptors, and slightly less for the D_1. Its affinity for the DA receptors is equal to that of lisuride, a potent DA agonist. Conversely, hallucinogenic amphetamine derivatives such as DOM (4-methyl-2,5-dimethoxy-amphetamine) bind strongly to 5-HT_2-receptors. The strongest evidence at present implicates $5\text{-HT}_{2A/2C}$- and D_2-receptors in the hallucinogenic actions of these two major groups of "classical" hallucinogens. For example, ritanserine and spiperone displace LSD from the 5-HT_{2A}-receptors and block many of its subjective and behavioral effects and neurophysiological actions. But it is also antagonized by clozapine, a blocker of D_2- and muscarinic receptors as well as 5-HT_2-receptors, and by sulpiride, which displaces it from D_2-receptors.

The second technique is the in vivo observation of the **patterns of behavioral effects** produced by the drugs in experimental animals. The behaviors that are especially useful in this connection are exploratory activity, stereotypy, food-reinforced operant behavior, and certain motor patterns such as head-twitching, ear-scratching, etc. (see Chapter 71).

The LSD-like hallucinogens produce decreases in exploratory activity, a tendency for the animal to stay close to the walls and corners of the observation chamber, sudden interruptions in food-rewarded bar-pressing activity, stereotypy, and bizarre behaviors such as prolonged staring or visually following the movement of nonexistent objects.

The third technique, also in vivo, is the study of **discriminative stimulus generalization** (see Chapter 71). Rats are trained to press one lever for food reward while under the influence of a drug and a second lever while under placebo. They are then tested under a different drug, and the relative numbers of responses they make on the training drug lever and on the placebo lever indicate whether they perceive the subjective effects of the test drug to be more like those of the training drug or more different from them. Again, the results indicate a considerable overlap of subjective effects. When compared against the training drugs quipazine (predominantly a 5-HT agonist), 5-methoxy-DMT (a pure 5-HT₁ agonist), and amphetamine (predominantly a catecholamine receptor indirect agonist), most of the drugs of both the indoleamine and phenylethylamine groups show varying degrees of cross-generalization.

In general, the results of the receptor-binding studies are in agreement with those of the discriminative stimulus generalization studies and with the behavioral observations. A drug with a very high affinity for 5-HT$_1$-receptors is likely to show high generalization to 5-methoxy-DMT training stimuli and little or none to amphetamine stimuli. A drug with lower receptor specificity will show more cross-generalization. There appears to be a continuum of gradation between the two "pure" pictures. Therefore the spectrum of subjective and objective effects contains similar elements for the two families, but in different proportions. The typical pictures for the various drug groups are described below.

LSD SYNDROME

Typical Sequence

The typical sequence of effects of LSD and similarly acting drugs includes three phases.

Somatic symptoms

The first phase, beginning within minutes of the administration of an effective dose, includes a variety of subjective symptoms such as dizziness, weakness, tremors, nausea, wakefulness, restlessness, and paresthesias, indicative of strong central stimulant action. Muscle tension and hyperreflexia result in some degree of incoordination. Centrally produced sympathomimetic effects include pupillary dilatation, blurred vision, hyperthermia in some species, tachycardia, hyperglycemia, piloerection, and dry mouth. There is also a direct stimulatory effect on uterine muscle, reflecting the relation between LSD and the ergot alkaloids (see Chapter 47).

Perceptual symptoms

These begin about an hour after ingestion of the drug and tend to be mainly visual. The first effect is fluctuation in the perceived brightness of illumination. Shapes become distorted and undulating; colors become brilliant, constantly varying in tone and intensity; and objects appear surrounded by colored halos or rainbows. Distances between objects become confused. The body image becomes distorted, hands and feet may feel enormous, or the whole body may seem to be shrinking away. Sense of hearing is sharpened and, occasionally, senses become fused (synesthesia), e.g., "the noise of water gushing from the faucet was transformed into optical illusions," or colors appear to have specific smells, etc. With mescaline there is a tendency to see geometric pat-terns, even with the eyes closed. The sense of time may become distorted; things seem to hang in sus-pended animation for a long time that, to an observer, is really only a few seconds. During this stage there are often rapid mood changes, the subject being happy, sad, irritable, meditative, or frightened at various times during the same drug experience; some degree of anxiety is almost universal.

Psychic symptoms

At the peak of the experience, about 2 hours or more after ingestion of the drug, there is marked difficulty in expression of thoughts, dream-like feeling, and difficulty in concentration on voluntary thought. At the same time, there is a tendency to fixation on specific stimuli and difficulty in moving the attention away from them. The visual illusions may lead into actual hallucinations. Depersonalization is common; the subject feels that the mind has left the body and is looking down on it from a distance. In this state, the users may feel that they are freed from their bodies and are becoming united with the whole universe, much as in a state of religious ecstasy obtained without drugs. In contrast, the same feeling of drift-ing away from one's concrete self may prove terrify-ing and give rise to panic or an acute psychosis. *The emotional reaction is strongly influenced by the setting and by other people present*, as well as by the user's previous drug experience, expectations, and emotional state at the time of taking the drug.

Psychological Effects

As with all hallucinogenic drugs, the content and nature of the experience depend strongly on the individual user. The neurological and perceptual phe-nomena are probably the same in all subjects, but the way in which these effects are subjectively perceived differs widely. Aesthetically sensitive people place great emphasis on the beauty of the experience, while insensitive people experience mainly the mood changes. Artists refer to the effect of these drugs on creativity, but their artistic skills actually deteriorate badly during the drug effect, so it is the memory or insight retained *after* the drug experience that may be relevant. This memory tends to be selective, most subjects remembering only pleasant or beneficial as-pects of the drug experience, while jitteriness, depres-sion, hostility, auditory hallucinations, and paranoid delusions tend to be forgotten unless they are severe and threatening.

Related Drugs

Despite the many common features, other drugs in the group of phenylalkylamine and indolealkylamine hallucinogens do show some differences from LSD. One of the most widely used is MDMA ("Ecstasy"), an amphetamine derivative (Fig. 30-2). Like both LSD and amphetamine, it increases the release of catecholamines from NE and DA nerve terminals and produces an initial rush of energy and alertness, starting between 20 and 60 minutes after ingestion, but this is later followed by a period of calm, decreased anger and hostility, and increased sensory awareness but without visual distortions; this phase may last for several hours. However, MDMA increases the response to amphetamine, and its major physical risks are like those of amphetamine (see below), including tachycardia, hypertension, and hyperthermia.

Pharmacological Mechanisms

Small doses of LSD, mescaline, etc., cause increased frequency and desynchronization of the EEG, and they reduce the stimulation threshold of the midbrain reticular formation. This hyperarousal state resembles that produced by amphetamines and raises the possibility that sensory overload plays a role in the hallucinogenic effect. With larger doses, the EEG shows intermittent bursts of slow-wave high-voltage activity that appear to coincide with hallucinatory periods. Spontaneous electrical activity of the retina increases and its excitation threshold is lowered, but synaptic transmission in the lateral geniculate nucleus is partially impaired and the cortical evoked potentials after visual stimuli are markedly altered. These findings suggest that the predominantly visual nature of the hallucinations is due to excessive input from the retina, coupled with incomplete transmission to the optic and association cortex. One functional consequence is that afterimages are prolonged, intensified, and fused ("palinopsia"). Possibly this factor contributes to the production of visual hallucinations. Effects on spinal reflexes are variable, but small doses tend to facilitate tendon reflexes and to inhibit polysynaptic reflexes.

Like LSD, MDMA appears to act on serotonergic nerve terminals, but it has a neurotoxic action on these terminals that is preventable by citalopram (a blocker of 5-HT uptake) or by SKF 525A (an inhibitor of cytochrome P450 activity), so the neurotoxicity may be due to a toxic metabolite of MDMA formed after uptake into the nerve terminals. The resulting decrease in 5-HT levels is thought to increase the effects of released DA.

Molecular Mechanisms

As noted earlier, there is considerable evidence that LSD acts primarily at 5-HT receptors but also to some extent at DA and other receptors. However, the nature of the actions at these receptors is not entirely clear. Both the phenylethylamine hallucinogens and the indolealkylamine hallucinogens produce the same electrophysiological effects at the $5-HT_2$-receptors: decreased spontaneous and evoked neuronal activity, prolonged postactivity inhibition, decreased resting K^+ conductance, and increased IP_3 turnover; the net effect is increased excitability. LSD acts as an agonist or partial agonist at both 5-HT and DA receptors, but other evidence appears to support an antagonist action. For example, LSD decreases the turnover of both 5-HT and DA in some parts of the brain and increases it in others, but the nonhallucinogenic analog lisuride has the same effects. Another analog, 2-brom-LSD, inhibits the activity of 5-HT-containing neurons in the midbrain raphe nuclei, and pretreatment with 2-brom-LSD blocks the action of LSD, yet 2-brom-LSD has no hallucinogenic effect of its own. LSD stimulates DA receptors in the striatum, and this effect (as well as the hallucinogenic effect) is blocked by chlorpromazine; yet depletion of brain catecholamines does not block the effect of LSD and may even enhance it. These examples illustrate the complexity of interaction of the 5-HT and DA systems in the brain and underline the fact that the mechanism of action of LSD is not yet fully understood.

Absorption, Distribution, and Biotransformation

All the commonly used drugs in this group are readily absorbed by mouth, except DMT, which must be injected, sniffed, or smoked. Effective doses vary widely; e.g., for LSD 2 μg/kg is usually quite potent in humans, while equivalent doses are 150 μg/kg for psilocybin and 5 mg/kg for mescaline. In part, this difference is due to distribution differences: Mescaline is tightly bound to plasma proteins, and only a small proportion is free to diffuse into the tissues. In contrast, LSD is also largely protein-bound in the plasma, but the binding is loose and the drug passes rapidly into the tissues. This also affects duration of action: the half-life of LSD in humans is about 3 hours while that of mescaline is about 6 hours. With all of these drugs, the bulk of a given dose is found in the liver, spleen, kidneys, and adrenals, and only a minute fraction in the brain. However, LSD enters the brain rapidly, possibly by active transport. Within the brain the highest concentrations are found in the pituitary, pineal gland (possibly in relation to 5-HT uptake sites), hypothalamus, limbic system, and visual and auditory relays. Biotransformation occurs in the liver by routes that differ for each drug. LSD is converted chiefly (almost 90%) to its glucuronide, which is excreted mainly in the bile and a little in the urine; the remainder (10–12%) is oxidized to 2-oxy-LSD and a variety of other oxygenated or hydroxylated derivatives. Mescaline undergoes oxidative deamination to 3,4,5-trimethoxyphenylacetic acid. Psilocybin is dephosphorylated to psilocin, which is also active, but is in turn N-demethylated and oxidized to a hydroxyindole acetic acid.

Relation to Other Drugs

The preferred symptomatic treatment for all these drugs is diazepam. Reserpine enhances the effects of all of them.

Tolerance develops rapidly to LSD on repeated use if the drug is taken at too short intervals. This is apparently due to down-regulation of 5-HT$_2$-receptors, which occurs within 2–3 days of repeated exposure to LSD; no withdrawal reaction has been reported. Cross-tolerance is then found to the other drugs in this group, but not to cannabis or amphetamine.

LSD Toxicity

LSD has a very large margin of safety; no human fatality due to direct toxicity of the drug has been reported. The few known deaths were the result of accidents (falls, jumps, etc.) occurring during the hallucinated state.

The most common ill effects are psychological: "Bad trips" or panic states, arising from the loss of contact with reality, may trigger serious psychotic breakdown in people with chronic emotional problems. "Flashbacks" are spontaneous (and usually frightening) sensations of being under the influence of LSD even though the person has taken none. They occur in regular users and can be triggered by cannabis in former LSD users. It is not known whether they are really a form of drug toxicity or are a conditioned behavioral response to subjective stimuli formerly experienced under the effects of the drug.

Chromosome damage, leukemia, and teratogenic effects have been reported in humans and other species exposed to LSD, but there are many contradictory reports, and the question is not settled. Women using LSD appear to have a higher proportion of spontaneous abortions, and their offspring have more chromosome breaks and more congenital anomalies than nonusers. But the role of LSD is not clear, since other drugs, viral infections, and other incidental factors may have been important causative or contributing factors.

AMPHETAMINES AND COCAINE

Pharmacology of Amphetamines

The amphetamines and related compounds are strong CNS stimulants that are related, both chemically and pharmacologically, to NE (see Fig. 30-2). Amphetamine has an asymmetric carbon, so optical isomers, d- and l-forms, exist (Fig. 30-4). While both forms are active peripherally, only the d-form (Dexedrine) is a central stimulant.

These drugs are sympathomimetics, which act by causing release of NE and DA from their storage sites in catecholaminergic nerve terminals. Amphetamine also appears to have some direct agonist effect on postsynaptic receptors and a weak inhibitory effect on monoamine oxidase. It has peripheral effects on the heart, GI motility, blood vessels, pupil, etc., similar to those of ephedrine and other sympathomimetic drugs (see also Chapter 16). In the central nervous system, d-amphetamine causes a higher turnover rate and a reduced content of catecholamine neurotransmitters. The resulting noradrenergic hyperactivity is probably responsible for the marked increase in wakefulness, alertness, speed of response, hyperreflexia, and amount of voluntary activity. In normal individuals, this often leads to feelings of well-being or even euphoria, and of increased energy and capacity for work. With overdose, however, mental processes are speeded up so much that the subject becomes submerged in a flood of thought associations, and the attention jumps rapidly and ineffectually from one thought to another, as in a manic psychosis.

Dopaminergic hyperactivity is believed to be responsible for the reinforcing effect (see Chapter 71), but also for a different set of effects, including stereotypy (continuously repeated, purposeless movements), paranoid ideas, and hallucinations. All of

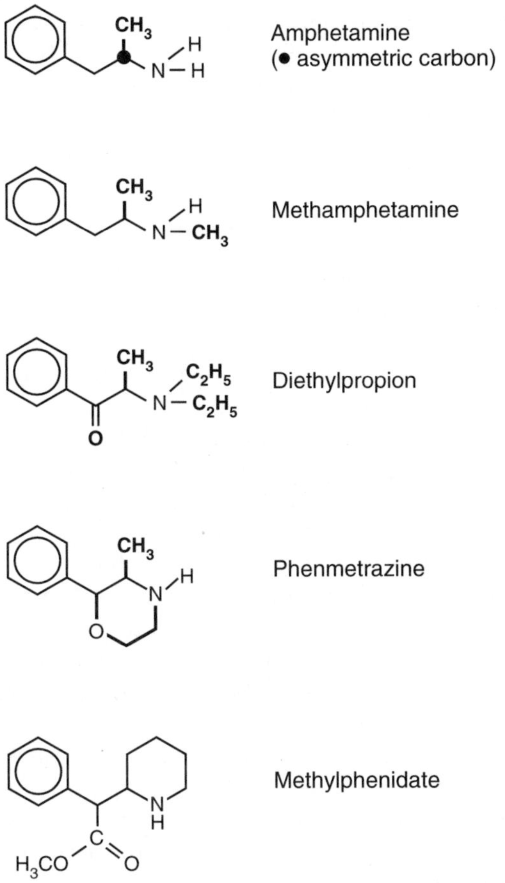

Amphetamine
(● asymmetric carbon)

Methamphetamine

Diethylpropion

Phenmetrazine

Methylphenidate

Figure 30-4. Structural formulae of amphetamines and related compounds.

these effects have been produced experimentally in human volunteers by the administration of large doses of amphetamine, and they were blocked by phenothiazines or butyrophenones. The picture can be mistaken for paranoid schizophrenia.

Medical and Other Uses of Amphetamines

Amphetamine was originally developed as a substitute for ephedrine to raise the blood pressure if hypotension occurred during surgical anesthesia. Its vasoconstrictor properties also led to its use as a nasal decongestant. For both of these uses, it has been replaced by newer sympathomimetics with less central effect.

In many activities, amphetamines will delay the onset of mental and physical fatigue, and they are sometimes used to **enhance performance**—for example, by soldiers on forced marches, by truck drivers on long overnight drives, by students "cramming"

for examinations, by athletes striving for peak performance. In rare situations, such as a temporary emergency, this use may be justified, but in the other cases mentioned it can be very dangerous. *It maintains performance not only by maintaining wakefulness, but also by diminishing the awareness of fatigue,* which normally warns a person that reserve strength is nearly exhausted. Therefore, the subject may push the exertion to the point of serious damage or even death.

In neurology, the main use of the amphetamines is for treatment of **narcolepsy,** a disease of unknown cause characterized by sudden attacks of sleep occurring in completely inappropriate situations. Large doses of amphetamine, as much as 30–200 mg a day, depending on the frequency of attacks, are quite effective. Because of its DA-releasing action, which occurs in the striatum as well as in other locations, amphetamine is also useful as a supplementary therapy in some cases of Parkinson's disease (see Chapter 21).

Amphetamine-type drugs, especially methylphenidate (Ritalin), are also widely used in the treatment of behavioral disorders in children. They reduce the restlessness and hyperactivity in **hyperkinetic children** (attention deficit disorder with hyperactivity). There is no adequate explanation for this apparently paradoxical effect of these drugs. However, barbiturates are also known to produce an opposite effect in these children (i.e., hyperactivity rather than sedation) and further aggravate the condition. It has been reported that all children show sedation with amphetamines, but that the effect is more obvious in hyperkinetic children. There is considerable argument about the long-term value of amphetamine-like drugs in the treatment of hyperkinetic children.

In psychiatry, the drugs are sometimes used to **raise the mood and activity** of certain depressed lethargic patients. However, stimulation of the reticular activating system only guarantees an increase in mental activity, not necessarily a change in mood, and cases have been recorded of depressed inert patients who were roused by amphetamines to the point that, instead of remaining inert, they committed suicide. Atypical reactions are by no means rare: Some patients become acutely anxious and irritable; some become relaxed and drowsy. Therefore these drugs should be used only under close supervision.

By far the most common use was formerly as an aid in losing weight. Amphetamine causes anorexia by some central nervous action that is not fully understood. Thus it helps people to adhere to a reducing diet. Amphetamine itself is no longer permitted to be used for this purpose. It was replaced by newer drugs such as **diethylpropion** (amfepramone; Tenuate, M-Orexic), **phenmetrazine,** and **phenter-mine** (Ionamin, Fentrol, etc.) (see Fig. 30-4). Although these are merely modifications of amphet-amine, they have somewhat less peripheral sympathomimetic action. But they are basically similar and have similar dangers. (For this reason, phenmetrazine was withdrawn from the market, although the closely related phendimetrazine is still sold in the United States.)

Absorption, Distribution, and Elimination

Amphetamines are readily absorbed from the gastro-intestinal tract, so they can be administered orally as well as parenterally. They are sufficiently lipid-soluble (in the non-ionized form) to cross cell membranes readily, including the blood–brain barrier, so they distribute rapidly to all tissues. Biotransformation occurs almost entirely in the liver, and several different pathways are involved: hydroxylation of the phenyl ring, N-demethylation (in the case of methamphetamine and related drugs), deamination, and conjugation reactions. The metabolites, as well as an appreciable fraction of the unchanged drug, are excreted in the urine. Because of the numerous different reactions involved, the half-life of drug in the plasma shows considerable individual variation, but it is usually in the range of 12–18 hours.

Side Effects and Toxicity

When these drugs are given for one purpose, the other usual actions constitute the principal side effects: e.g., when they are given as a mental stimulant, anorexia is a side effect, and vice versa.

When death occurs from poisoning, it is by excessive sympathomimetic activity, resulting in hypertension, severe tachycardia and collapse, hyperpyrexia, delirium, and convulsions.

The two main nonlethal risks are (1) psychic dependence and tolerance, and (2) psychotic episodes. Dependence was much more common than physicians at first realized when the drugs were widely used for treatment of obesity or mild depression. Psychotic episodes usually occur after continued intake of large amounts, and they closely resemble paranoid schizophrenia, for which they are often mistaken. Tolerance may be very marked, some addicts taking hundreds of milligrams daily. (The normal dose is 5 mg of d-amphetamine, two to three times daily.) The drug is largely excreted in the urine

for a day to a week or more after the last ingestion, depending on the amount taken. Disappearance from the body is thus gradual, and withdrawal symptoms are relatively mild, consisting of profound sleepiness and depression and a huge rebound in appetite.

Amphetamine Syndrome

In high doses, amphetamines give rise to an acute psychotic picture with hyperactivity, anxiety, paranoid delusions, and auditory and tactile hallucinations, but with clear consciousness and little or no disorientation. This last point differentiates the picture from that of the delirium produced by atropine-like drugs (described in the following section). The picture is differentiated from that of the LSD group by the prominence of paranoid ideas and the predominance of auditory and tactile rather than visual hallucinations. Moreover, amphetamine-induced hallucinations are more a matter of misinterpretation than of distorted perception. Stereotyped behavior is a common finding, and is probably related to DA release by amphetamine.

Intravenous injection ("speed") greatly increases the rate of onset and intensity of effects. Experiments in human volunteers produced typical amphetamine psychoses in 2–3 days, as compared to weeks or months with oral use.

After the drug is stopped, the psychotic picture usually clears rapidly at a rate that depends directly upon the speed of elimination of the drug from the body. The rate can be increased by acidification of the urine, which increases the degree of ionization of the nitrogen and thus reduces the reabsorption of amphetamine in the renal tubule. However, in some instances, a frank schizophrenic state was precipitated by the drug use in persons already close to clinical breakdown, and in such cases the symptoms may continue even after the drug is totally eliminated.

In addition to the amphetamine toxicity already mentioned, death also may result from opportunistic complications of intravenous injection, such as viral hepatitis, necrotizing angiitis, acquired immune deficiency syndrome (AIDS), or septicemia. However, most deaths in amphetamine users are due to violence: accident, suicide, or murder related to aggressiveness and abnormal behavior while "high."

Cocaine

Cocaine was isolated from coca leaves in the 1850s, but clinical interest in it did not arise until 1884, when both its central stimulant and local anesthetic actions were reported. It was at first recommended for the treatment of depression and of morphine and alcohol dependence, but within a few years it was recognized to give rise to dependence itself. It rapidly became popular among drug addicts (see Chapter 72) and eventually came under strict legal controls in most countries.

The pharmacology of cocaine is discussed in Chapter 24. The main points in the present context are that it is absorbed rapidly through the nasal mucosa, enters the central nervous system rapidly, inhibits the reuptake of NE and DA in catecholaminergic neurons by binding to the transporter in the presynaptic membrane, and thus gives rise to intense central stimulation. Cocaine is *almost identical to amphetamine* in its acute effects and its patterns of toxicity. Double-blind experiments in humans have shown that even experienced cocaine users have great difficulty in distinguishing between the two drugs after intravenous injection. The *main differences* are:

- A shorter duration of effect for cocaine.
- Lower incidence of complications associated with intravenous use, since cocaine is usually sniffed or smoked (as "crack"; see below); instead, rhinitis and perforated nasal septum can occur.
- Ambiguous evidence about tolerance to cocaine; tolerance occurs to some effects, such as anorexia, but it is not clear whether there is any tolerance to the hallucinatory and stereotypy effects, and there may even be sensitization.

Cocaine is biotransformed in several different ways. The major reaction is hydrolysis of the ester linkage by the nonspecific serum esterase, but substantial amounts are also hydroxylated by hepatic cytochrome P450 activity, yielding a reactive metabolite that is thought to be responsible for the small number of cases of serious hepatotoxicity resembling that caused by acetaminophen (see Chapter 46).

In recent years there has been a rapid increase, in North America, of a crudely prepared (and therefore inexpensive) cocaine in the free base form popularly known as "crack." This form, unlike the salts of cocaine, is volatile when heated. It can be volatilized directly by heating it on a piece of aluminum foil, or it can be mixed with tobacco in a cigarette or pipe and, as the tobacco burns, the free cocaine base volatilizes, because of the heat of the combustion zone. The cocaine vapor can be inhaled, and is absorbed rapidly into the pulmonary circulation, so that its central effects are experienced more rapidly. This is entirely analogous to the amphetamine free base that, being volatile, could be used in nasal inhalers and has a very rapid onset of effect, whereas the hydrochloride or sulfate salts are nonvolatile, must be taken orally or by injection, and have much slower onset of action when swallowed.

ATROPINE SYNDROME

The pharmacology of anticholinergic drugs is described in Chapter 15. In the present context, the important point is that antimuscarinic agents that can cross the blood–brain barrier induce a toxic delirium which is deliberately sought by some people as another form of drug "high" and can be mistaken for the effects of LSD-type drugs. The drugs include atropine, scopolamine, benactyzine, piperidyl benzylate esters, and a variety of crude belladonna preparations. The main features of the atropine syndrome are:

- Strong peripheral antimuscarinic effects.
- Much more severe disruption of thought processes than with LSD-type drugs.
- Confusion, disorientation, and memory loss (this was the basis of the former use of these drugs in the so-called "twilight sleep" analgesia in obstetrics).
- Tactile, auditory, and visual hallucinations, including microhallucinations (vivid and brightly colored images of tiny humans, animals, scenery, etc.).
- Somnolence combined with restlessness, incoordination, and hyperreflexia.
- Hyperthermia, with dry hot skin and flushing.

The full-blown drug state may last for well over 24 hours, and residual effects may last for several days. Chlorpromazine does not relieve the symptoms and may even make them worse, because phenothiazines and tricyclic antidepressants have some degree of atropine-like effect of their own. Treatment is usually symptomatic, using diazepam or some other sedative.

PHENYLCYCLOHEXYLAMINE DERIVATIVES

These compounds, of which phencyclidine (PCP) was the first example, produce a mental state similar in some respects to that caused by the atropine group. However, there are some major differences in the clinical picture, and a different basic action. They

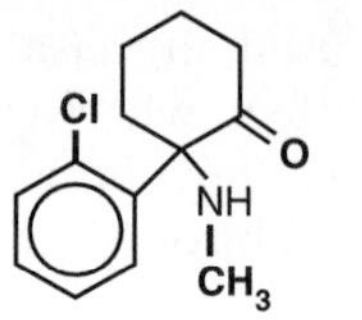

Ketamime

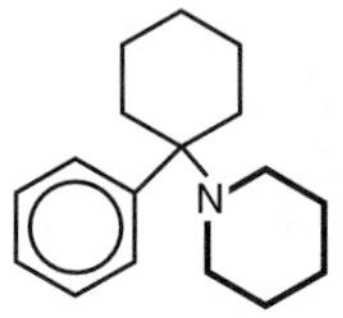

Phenylcyclohexyl-
piperidine
(PCP)
(Phencyclidine)

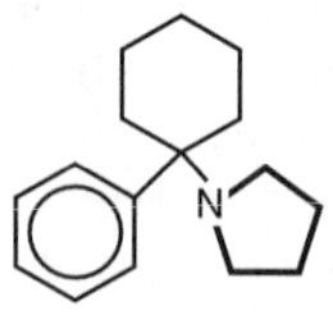

Phenylcyclohexyl-
pyrrolidine
(PHP)

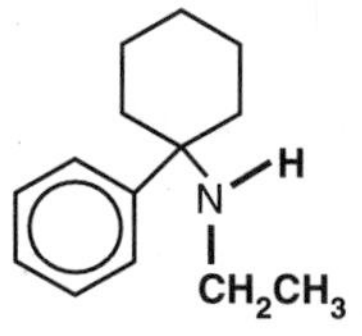

Phenylcyclohexyl-
ethylamine
(PCE)

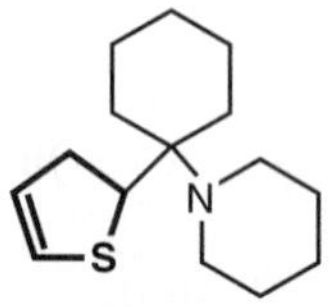

Thienylcyclohexyl-
piperidine
(TCP)

Figure 30-5. Structural formulae of ketamine and its phenylcyclohexylamine analogs. The thienyl ring in TCP is sterically equivalent to a phenyl ring.

are chemically and pharmacologically related to the dissociative anesthetic ketamine (Fig. 30-5).

The peripheral autonomic effects of these drugs differ somewhat in pattern from those of atropine. Although they are predominantly antimuscarinic in type, phencyclidine tends to cause hypersalivation rather than the dryness of the mouth typical of atropine action. In addition, phenylcyclohexylamines have direct sympathomimetic action; e.g., they enhance the effect of NE on isolated gut preparations. They cause tachycardia, hypertension, and hyperthermia, as amphetamine does in high doses, and these effects can be life-threatening. Muscle tone is increased, sometimes to the point of rigidity, and the

resulting heat production may contribute to the hyperthermia. At higher doses, the drugs cause hyperreflexia and seizures. The EEG shows rhythmic spontaneous discharges in the parietal cortex and increased amplitude of sensory evoked responses.

The behavioral effects of PCP and its congeners are characterized by restless, bizarre, repetitive movements (stereotypy), as well as by the analgesia and anesthesia for which the drugs were introduced clinically. Ataxia and dysarthria are common, and the person appears drunk. Excitement, agitation, depression, euphoria, and dysphoria may alternate rapidly or even coexist. After a large dose, the person may not return to normal for up to 2 weeks. In addicts, PCP can cause a schizophrenia-like psychosis characterized by flattened affect, dissociative thought disturbances, depersonalization, catatonia, and long-lasting memory deficits; it can also exacerbate true schizophrenia.

Like the indolealkylamines, the phenylcyclohexylamines interact with multiple neurotransmitters. They are noncompetitive blockers of the Ca^{2+} channel associated with the NMDA type of glutamate receptor (see Chapter 20). This action is important in the hippocampus, resulting in marked impairment of memory and learning. These agents indirectly increase the firing rate of midbrain DA neurons, increase DA output, and inhibit DA uptake in the striatum and NE uptake in the hypothalamus. The increased DA activity causes a secondary increase in neurotensin levels in the striatum that is prevented by D_1-receptor blockers. These drugs are also much more potent inhibitors of 5-HT uptake. The stereotypy and motor hyperactivity are reversed or prevented by DA blockers, but many of the other effects are preventable only by combined blockade of both D_2- and $5-HT_2$-receptors (e.g., by risperidone). It has also been suggested that the PCP receptor is identical to the σ-receptor (see Chapter 23). However, an irreversible blocker for σ-receptors had no effect on PCP–receptor binding. This suggests that PCP receptors are separate from σ-receptors.

PCP undergoes hydroxylation of the cyclohexyl ring in humans, and of all three rings in the rat. The 4-hydroxy derivatives are pharmacologically active. However, the hydroxy derivatives undergo subsequent conjugation reactions that inactivate them and allow them to be excreted in the urine. The biotransformation of other drugs may be affected by the fact that PCP itself suppresses the activity of CYP2C11 and CYP2D in the liver. PCP itself is highly lipid-soluble and accumulates in brain and fat, where it persists for days or weeks. This may account for the slow return to normal after a large dose.

CANNABIS

The hemp plant *(Cannabis sativa)* produces a series of related compounds called "cannabinoids" of which 1-Δ^9-tetrahydrocannabinol (THC) is the main active ingredient. It is a constituent of the resinous material that coats the immature flowering tops and also occurs at lower concentration in the leaves at a certain stage during the life of the plant. The dried leaf material is variously known as "marijuana," "bhang," "ganja," "maconha", etc., in different parts of the world. The resinous material is known as "hashish," "kif," "charas," etc., and is five to 10 times as potent as marijuana in terms of the THC content. In the past two decades, the average content of THC in marijuana sold in North America has increased from about 1% to 3–4% or more, and carefully selected and cloned plants yield as much as 15%.

Pharmacological Effects of Cannabis

At doses normally used by humans, cannabis produces rather trivial physiological effects. The most consistent are a dose-dependent increase in heart rate and congestion of the conjunctival blood vessels. The EEG shows somewhat more persistent alpha rhythm of slightly lower frequency than normal. Cerebral blood flow is decreased by cannabis in inexperienced users; this may be an effect of anxiety rather than a primary pharmacological action of THC. Sensory acuity may be sharpened slightly. However, thinking is slowed and less accurate. Impairment of short-term memory is one of the most consistent findings; free recall is more impaired than recognition. Emotional reactions are more labile; there is usually mild euphoria, talkativeness, laughter, and a subjective feeling of relaxation. These changes are very similar to those found with mild alcohol intoxication.

In experimental animals, THC displaces the dose-response curves for ethanol and PCP to the left (sensitization) in rate and accuracy of performance on complex schedules of food-reinforced responding. Similarly, in humans, driving skills are impaired (decreased alertness, shorter attention span, longer response latency, decreased accuracy of motor responses, etc.) and the effects are at least additive with those of alcohol. In the early stages of cannabis

action there may be synergism with amphetamine, but later there is usually drowsiness and synergism with barbiturates. Part of this effect may be due to cannabidiol (rather than THC itself), which can impair the biotransformation of barbiturates and other drugs by microsomal enzymes in the liver.

After very high doses of THC (e.g., 400 μg/kg or more in humans), there are effects similar in some ways to those of mescaline and LSD, including marked distortion of time and space perception, altered body image, depersonalization, auditory and visual hallucinations, transcendental or panic reactions, and even acute psychotic episodes. Visual hallucinations tend to be more of the reverie or daydream type, rather than abstract forms and colors. Ataxia can occur, with selective impairment of polysynaptic reflexes.

The mechanism of action is not yet fully known but has been greatly clarified in recent years. THC binds stereospecifically to a receptor, designated CB_1, that is found in high density in the cerebral cortex, hippocampus, and striatum and in moderate density in parts of the hypothalamus, amygdala, central gray, and laminae I–III and X of the spinal cord. A second type of receptor, termed CB_2, is found only in the periphery, in splenic macrophages and possibly in cells of the immune system. Both receptors are G protein–linked, decrease adenylyl cyclase activity, inhibit calcium N channels, and disinhibit K^+_A channels. The endogenous ligand for the CB receptors is a lipid material derived from arachidonic acid (cf., prostaglandins, Chapter 31), known as anandamide (see Fig 30-6). A competitive antagonist against THC at the anandamide receptor was recently discovered and should help greatly to elucidate the normal functions of the receptor and the mechanism of action of THC.

Activation of the CB_1-receptor increases the release of DA from DA terminals in the nucleus accumbens in a manner similar to that of nomifensine, a known blocker of DA reuptake. However, it is also possible that the increased release is due to disinhibition, i.e., inhibition of an inhibitory neuron that decreases DA release. The effect on DA release is believed to be linked to the reinforcing effects of cannabis (see Chapter 71). The actions of cannabis are more complex, however, and probably involve several different neurotransmitters. There is evidence, for example, that DA is involved in the effects of cannabis on response latency (see below), whereas 5-HT is involved in its effects on stimulus differentiation. The effects of cannabis are different from those of other hallucinogens: There is neither discrimina-

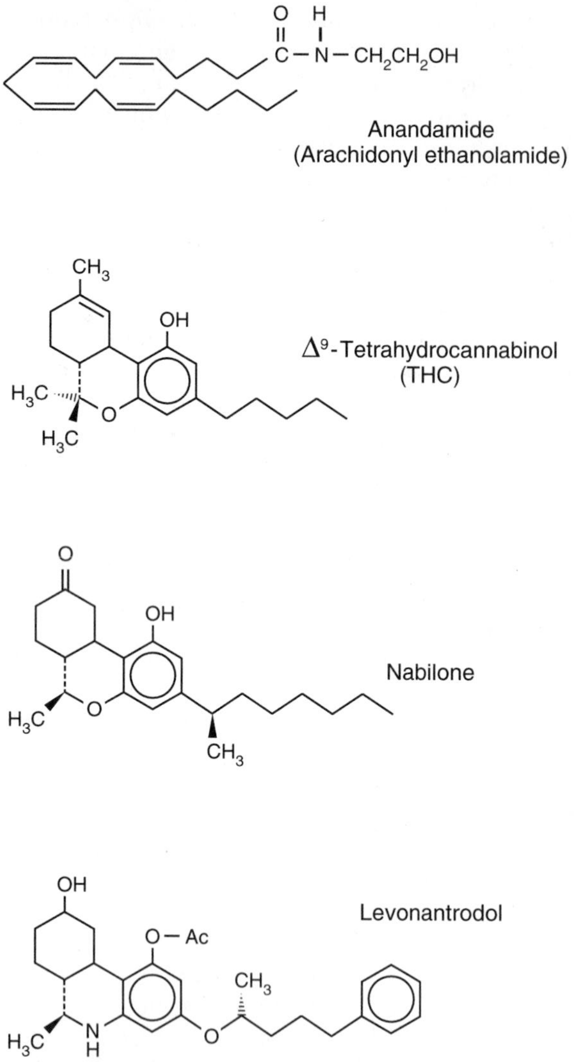

Anandamide
(Arachidonyl ethanolamide)

Δ^9-Tetrahydrocannabinol
(THC)

Nabilone

Levonantrodol

Figure 30-6. Structural formulae of anandamide (the endogenous ligand for the cannabinoid receptor), Δ^9-tetrahydrocannabinol, and two synthetic pharmacologically active analogs, nabilone and levonantrodol.

tive stimulus generalization from, nor cross-tolerance with, either the LSD-like or the amphetamine-like drugs. Some tolerance develops on regular use of high doses of cannabis, but not uniformly to all its effects.

THC is highly lipid-soluble and is absorbed rapidly across the alveolar and capillary membranes when the smoke is inhaled, so the onset of drug action is rapid. It is less well absorbed by mouth, and equivalent effects require about three times as large an oral dose as an inhaled one. THC is converted rapidly to 11-hydroxy-THC, but this is also pharmacologically active, so the drug effect outlasts

measurable THC levels in the blood. Because of the lipid solubility, measurable amounts of THC persist in body fat for days after a single dose. This slow phase of elimination has a half-life of about 56 hours in humans.

Chronic Toxicity of Cannabis

The best-documented adverse effect of chronic heavy use of cannabis by humans is bronchopulmonary irritation caused by the inhalation of cannabis smoke. Cannabis smoke has a much higher tar content than most tobacco smoke, and the tar contains a higher percentage of known irritants and procarcinogens. Chronic heavy smokers of cannabis, therefore, have a high incidence of **chronic bronchitis** with increased airway resistance and impaired gas exchange. Most cannabis users are also tobacco smokers, and the observed effects of cannabis are at least additive with those of tobacco smoke. Precancerous changes have been found in bronchiolar epithelium after only a few years of daily smoking of hashish or marijuana, and several cases of bronchopulmonary cancer have been reported in heavy cannabis smokers at a much earlier age than is usual for tobacco-induced cancer.

Chronic heavy users of cannabis often exhibit a condition of mental slowing, loss of memory, difficulty with abstract thinking, loss of drive, and emotional flatness. This picture has been called the **amotivational syndrome.** It probably represents a chronic intoxication state, and in most cases it clears gradually when use of the drug stops. In some cases, however, the symptoms remain long afterward, and they may be indicative of organic brain damage, analogous to that seen in severe alcoholics. It is possible that malnutrition, injury, infections, or concurrent use of other drugs may contribute to this picture. However, experimental studies in rats have shown that daily administration of cannabis alone, in moderately heavy doses for 3 months, does not impair general health, but does cause long-lasting or permanent impairment of learning of a type resembling that caused by hippocampal damage.

Studies in experimental animals and in humans have shown decreased output of gonadotropic hormones, reduced serum testosterone level, and low sperm count in males, and anovulatory cycles in females, as a result of chronic use of cannabis. However, there are also contradictory reports, and it is also possible that tolerance develops to these effects of cannabis.

Chromosomal damage has been reported in

leukocyte cultures from regular cannabis users. As in the case of LSD, the information is so far inconclusive. This also applies to reports of **impaired immune responses** in cannabis users, although experimental studies in animals have confirmed that cannabis does indeed depress T-lymphocyte function.

Psychiatric problems, other than the "amotivational syndrome," consist mainly of short-duration **psychotic episodes** characterized by severe anxiety or panic provoked by high-dose effects on perception. These usually respond rapidly to reassurance and sedation with benzodiazepines, although they occasionally last for several days or weeks. A more serious problem is the precipitation of a relapse of true endogenous psychosis (schizophrenia) in patients who were previously compensated or borderline.

Newborn infants of mothers who smoke cannabis regularly during pregnancy tend to be small for age and show chronic hyperirritability and poor feeding for several months after birth. By the time they reach school age, their physical development is normal, but they tend to show deficits in verbal learning that may affect subsequent school performance.

Therapeutic Uses of Cannabinoids

Cannabis extracts were used extensively in the 19th and early 20th centuries, on medical prescription, as sedatives, hypnotics, and "tonics," but their variability of composition and their limited shelf life made them unreliable, and they were replaced by pure synthetic drugs of known composition. In recent years there has been a revival of interest in the possible use of pure cannabinoids for a number of other purposes, including nausea and vomiting, anorexia, epilepsy, glaucoma, spasticity, migraine, and Tourette's syndrome. The only one of these applications that has found some measure of medical acceptance is the treatment of nausea and vomiting due to anticancer chemotherapy in a small number of cases that do not respond to conventional medications. **Dronabinol**, a synthetic preparation of THC, is the form usually used for this purpose; it has also been tested as an agent for improving appetite in patients with anorexia caused by AIDS.

When cannabinoids are used for these purposes, most patients find the psychoactive effects undesirable. Therefore there has been interest in developing modified cannabinoids with greater selectivity of action. **Nabilone**, a 9-keto derivative of THC with a modified side-chain (Fig. 30-6), is about 10 times as potent as THC but very similar in its actions, except that it may have slightly less psychoactive effect. **Levonantrodol**, another synthetic modification of THC, is also under study. None of these agents appears to have any major therapeutic role at present, but the recent advances in the pharmacology of the cannabinoids and cannabinoid receptors may lead to more useful drugs in the future.

SUGGESTED READING

Asghar K, De Souza E, eds. Pharmacology and toxicology of amphetamine and related designer drugs. NIDA Res Monogr 94. Rockville MD: NIDA, 1989.

Bock GR, Whelan J, eds. Cocaine: scientific and social dimensions. Ciba Foundation Symposium 166. Chichester: Wiley-Interscience, 1992.

Ellison G. The N-methyl-D-aspartate antagonists phencyclidine, ketamine and dizocilpine as both behavioral and anatomical models of the dementias. Brain Res Rev 1995; 20:250–267.

Fehr KO, Kalant H, eds. Cannabis and health hazards. Toronto: Addiction Research Foundation, 1983.

Hall W, Solowij N, Lemon J. The health and psychological consequences of cannabis use. Nat Drug Strategy Monogr 25. Canberra: Australian Govt Publ Service, 1994.

Hammer RP Jr, ed. The neurobiology of cocaine—cellular and molecular mechanisms. Boca Raton: CRC Press, 1995.

Heym J, Jacobs BL. Serotonergic mechanisms of hallucinogenic drug effects. In: Marwah J, ed. Neurobiology of drug abuse. Mongr Neural Sci, vol 13. Basel: Karger, 1987:55–81.

Kalant OJ. The amphetamines—toxicity and addiction. 2nd ed. Toronto: University of Toronto Press, 1973.

Kalant OJ, ed and translator. *Maier's* Cocaine addiction (Der Kokainismus). Toronto: ARF Books, 1987.

Lin GC, Glennon RA, eds. Hallucinogens: an update. NIDA Research monograph 146. Rockville MD: NIDA, 1994.

Murphy L, Bartke A, eds. Marijuana/cannabinoids—neurobiology and neurophysiology. Boca Raton: CRC Press, 1992.

Pletscher A, Ladewig D, eds. 50 Years of LSD—current status and perspectives of hallucinogens. New York: Parthenon, 1994.

Pertwee R, ed. Cannabinoid receptors. London: Academic Press, 1995.

Schultes RE. Hallucinogens of plant origin. Science 1969; 163:245–254.

Washton AM, Gold MS, eds. Cocaine—a clinician's handbook. Chichester: John Wiley, 1987.

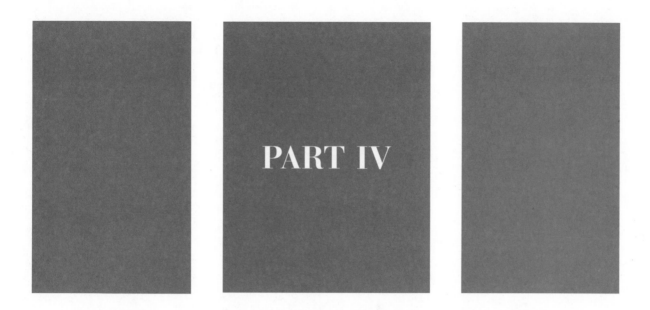

PART IV

MEDIATORS AND MODIFIERS OF TISSUE RESPONSES

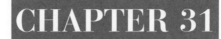

CHAPTER 31

The Eicosanoids

C.R. PACE-ASCIAK AND D. KADAR

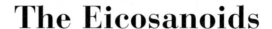

CASE HISTORIES

Case 1

A 26-year-old woman was brought to the Emergency Department with gross edema of both legs and some cyanosis of the feet. She had started using oral contraceptives at the age of 16, but after using them for 9 months she had developed bilateral deep vein thromboses and a small pulmonary embolus. At that time she responded well to anticoagulant therapy and discontinuation of the contraceptive pills. At age 22 she had two spontaneous abortions, one at 9 weeks and one at 8 weeks. A third pregnancy was terminated at 30 weeks because of intrauterine death, shortly before the last admission, and 2 weeks later she developed left iliofemoral venous thrombosis despite being treated with heparin. Four weeks later, while she was still on heparin, a large thrombus was removed surgically from the lower aorta and both iliac and femoral arteries. She developed renal failure as a result of extension of the thrombus into the renal arteries. Intravenous epoprostenol (prostacyclin) was therefore combined with the heparin, and her renal function improved progressively. After 6 weeks, both drugs were discontinued. For the past 2 years she has been maintained on warfarin, aspirin, and dipyridamole and has remained asymptomatic.

Case 2

A 55-year-old woman was brought to hospital with an 8-year history of Raynaud's phenomenon associated with intractable pain and ischemic skin ulcers of the extremities. She had sclerosis of the systemic arteries and nongangrenous digital ulcers. In addition she had borderline hypertension (145/85) and mild angina on effort. In the past, she had been treated with systemic as well as topical antibiotics to care for the ulcers, and nifedipine as a vasodilator, but the results had not been satisfactory.

On this admission, all other medications were discontinued for 24 hours, and she was then given alprostadil (in a solution of 1 mg/mL in 0.9% saline) by constant infusion pump through a central venous line. The initial rate of infusion was 6 ng/kg/min for 12 hours. Since she experienced no adverse effects, the infusion rate was increased to 10 ng/kg/min for 60 hours. The blood pressure, pulse, and respiratory rate were monitored frequently. After 4 weeks there was a remarkable improvement in the pain and increased warmth of the hands. Attacks of vasospasm were much less severe, and four of the five ulcers that she had on admission were healed. The treatment with alprostadil was repeated with the same dosage, and by 2 weeks later the remaining ulcer was healed. After discharge, she was followed up for a period of 18 months, during which the Raynaud's symptoms remained much improved, and the cutaneous ulcers did not recur.

The eicosanoids (*eicosa*, Greek for twenty) constitute families of oxygenated products derived from 20-carbon-atom polyunsaturated fatty acids in which successive double bonds are separated by methylene groups. They are formed via three main oxidative

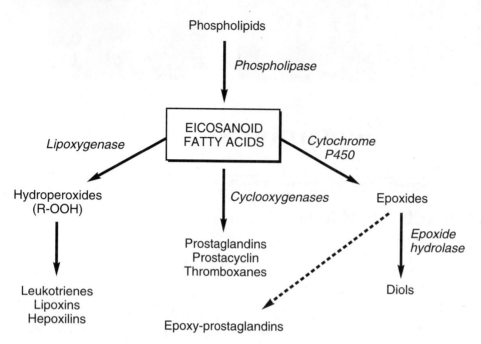

Figure 31-1. Three major pathways for the biological oxidation of eicosanoid fatty acids.

pathways that utilize molecular oxygen as cosubstrate (Fig. 31-1). Products in these pathways possess a variety of biological activities and are believed to act as "local hormones," since they are rapidly inactivated in the circulation.

THE CYCLOOXYGENASE PATHWAY

Since their discovery in the early 1930s and their chemical identification in the early 1960s, considerable effort has been expended on the study of the biological properties and cellular importance of the eicosanoids derived from the cyclooxygenase pathway (Fig. 31-2).

Synthesis

The precursors of the eicosanoids are arachidonic, linoleic, linolenic, eicosapentaenoic, and docosahexaenoic acids, which are obtained from dietary sources.

Prostaglandins (PGs; Table 31-1) were once believed to be the most potent pharmacologically active compounds known; however, the thermolabile prostaglandin endoperoxides (PGG$_2$ and PGH$_2$) ($t_{1/2}$ = 5 minutes) were isolated later and shown to be 50–200 times more potent than the prostaglandins in certain test systems.

Another unstable compound ($t_{1/2}$ = 30 seconds)

derived from the endoperoxides was isolated from human platelets and termed thromboxane A$_2$ (TXA$_2$). This compound possesses 1000-fold greater potency than the prostaglandins in inducing platelet aggregation and contracting the isolated rabbit aorta. Prostacyclin (prostaglandin I$_2$, PGI$_2$) was isolated from the reaction of the rat stomach fundus or the vascular endothelium with the prostaglandin endoperoxides and was found to oppose the actions of TXA$_2$.

The **prostaglandins** constitute a family of naturally occurring cyclopentane-containing straight-chain C-20 carboxylic acids of varying degrees of unsaturation. All "primary" prostaglandins contain the same carbon skeleton, conveniently termed **prostanoic acid,** from which stems the systematic numbering and naming of structures of biological origin and those derived through chemical synthesis. There are ten groups of prostaglandins, designated A through J to indicate the differences in their molecular structures. The E and F classes are named according to whether a keto or a hydroxyl group is present in the cyclopentane ring at the 9-position; the D class is distinguished from the E class in that the former has a keto group at the 11-position instead of the 9-position. The number of double bonds in the alkyl side-chains distinguishes members within each class and is indicated by subscript 1, 2, or 3 (see Fig. 31-2). Three subclasses, A, B, and C, are

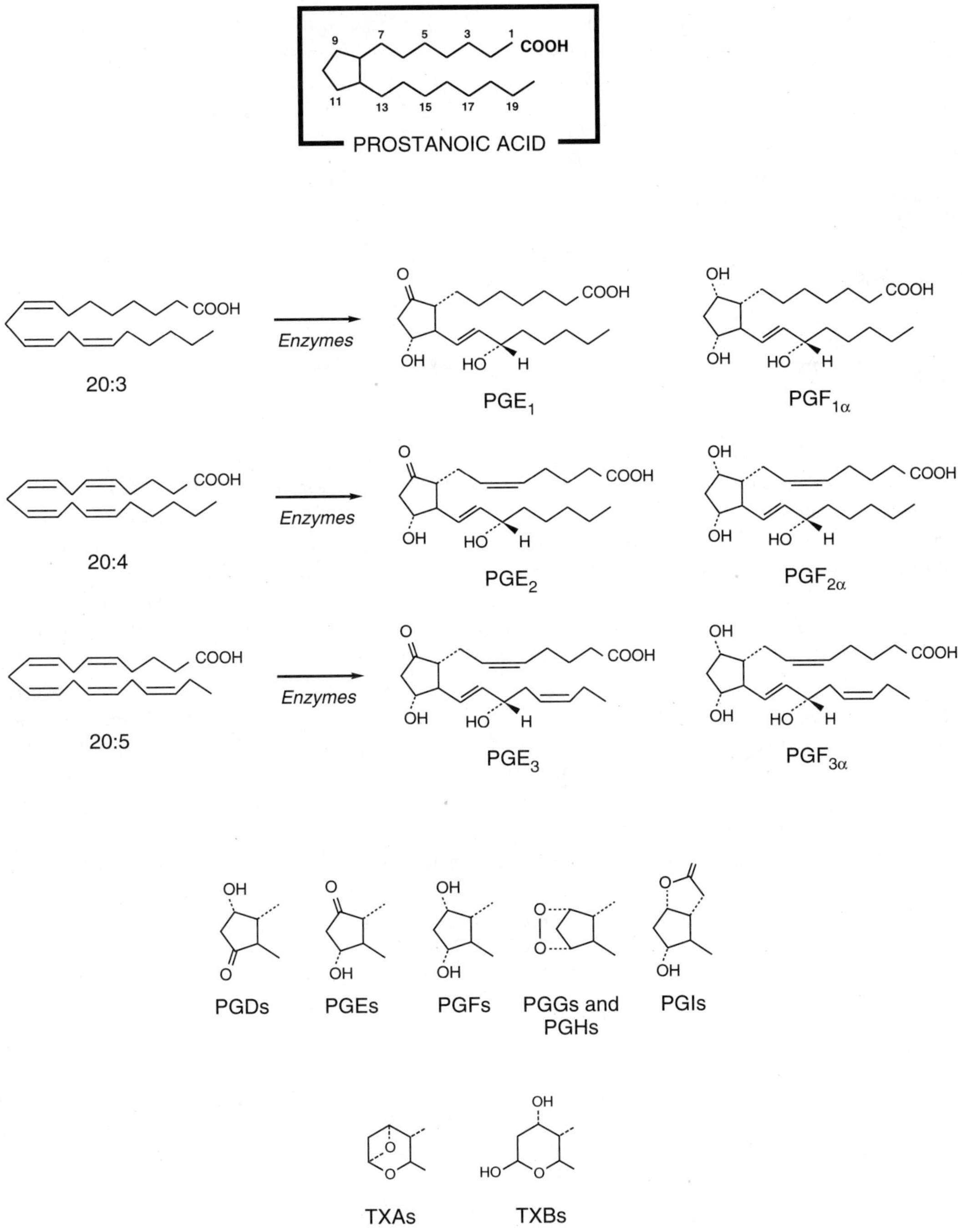

Figure 31-2. General structures of prostaglandins and thromboxanes.

formed chemically from the E compounds by dehydration with either mild mineral acid or alkali.

All of the prostaglandins and related substances can be produced from free eicosatrienoic acid (1-series), arachidonic acid (2-series), and eicosapentaenoic acid (3-series), which are released from tissue glycerophospholipids by the enzyme phospholipase A$_2$ or by a combination of phospholipase C and glyceride lipase.

Thromboxanes are not prostaglandins; they are named after a hypothetical "thrombanoic acid" with a six-membered oxane ring.

The other essential enzymes in the synthesis of prostaglandins, prostacyclin, and thromboxanes are

Table 31-1 Analogs of the Principal Prostaglandins in Clinical Use or Under Development

Prostaglandins	Alprostadil (PGE$_1$)	Dinoprostone (PGE$_2$)	Dinoprost (PGF$_{2\alpha}$)	Epoprostenol (Prostacyclin, PGI$_2$)	Synthetics
Analogs	Enisoprost	Arbaprostil	Carboprost	Beraprost	Nocloprost
	Gemeprost	Enprostil	Cloprostenol	Ciprostene	Rosaprostol
	Limaprost	Meteneprost	Fenprostalene	Iloprost	
	Mexiprostil	Sulprostone	Fluprostenol	OP-41833	
	Misoprostol	Trimprostil	Luprostiol		
	Ornoprostil	Viprostol	Prostalene		
	Rioprostil		Tiaprost		

cyclooxygenases (Cox). CoxI (the predominant form) and CoxII are sensitive to inhibition by steroids and nonsteroidal anti-inflammatory drugs such as acetylsalicylic acid (ASA) or indomethacin. Cyclooxygenases convert arachidonic acid to unstable cyclic **prostaglandin endoperoxides** (PGG$_2$ and PGH$_2$). The enzyme **prostaglandin endoperoxide isomerase** converts the endoperoxides to the prostaglandins PGD$_2$, PGE$_2$, and PGF$_{2\alpha}$. TXA$_2$ and PGI$_2$ are formed by the cytochrome P450 enzymes called **thromboxane synthase** and **prostacyclin synthase**, respectively (Fig. 31-3). All these enzymes together are referred to as the **prostaglandin synthase complex** and are bound to the plasma membrane and/or endoplasmic reticulum of many types of cells.

The synthesis of eicosanoids is stimulated by the release of arachidonic acid, trauma to the cell membrane, antigen–antibody reactions, oxygen deprivation, changes in ion influxes, proteases such as thrombin, and hormones.

Although the prostaglandin synthase complex is ubiquitous, there is a considerable degree of specificity (reasons unknown) for the occurrence of each of the pathways. Human platelets convert the endoperoxides into TXA$_2$, the factor responsible for initiation of the "release reaction" and aggregation of platelets (see Chapter 42). This cytochrome P450 enzyme is also abundant (although not exclusively) in macrophages, lung, spleen, and brain, yet it is almost undetectable in many other organs including heart, stomach, and liver. Prostacyclin synthase, a cytochrome P450 enzyme in the stomach and the smooth muscle and endothelial cells of blood vessels, converts endoperoxide to PGI$_2$, which opposes the action of TXA$_2$; i.e., it inhibits platelet aggregation and is very potent in lowering systemic arterial blood pressure. PGI$_2$ undergoes spontaneous hydration to the inactive 6-keto PGF$_{1\alpha}$ and is excreted in urine.

The kidney appears to contain enzymes that specifically convert the endoperoxides into PGD$_2$, PGE$_2$, and PGF$_{2\alpha}$. It is not yet known what endogenous factors channel the enzymatic activities to favor one pathway or another, but it should be quite possible to manipulate these transformations in the future with drugs that act specifically to block or activate one or several of these related and competing pathways.

The whole prostaglandin sequence is dependent on the availability of the precursor fatty acids in the free form, since phospholipid-bound fatty acid or the ester derivatives are not converted into prostaglandins. At the opposite end of the sequence, PGE$_2$, PGF$_{2\alpha}$, and PGD$_2$ are inactivated by a specific NAD-dependent enzyme, 15-hydroxyprostaglandin dehydrogenase (15-PGDH), that is abundant in all tissues investigated. This inactivation is rapid and extensive; for example, a single passage through the lungs inactivates over 90% of PGE$_2$. The metabolic products are then excreted into the urine.

Sites of Drug Action

There are at least four stages at which drugs can influence the fate of products of the arachidonic acid cascade (Fig. 31-3).

1. Phospholipase step—liberation of arachidonic acid from phospholipids.
2. Cyclooxygenase and lipoxygenase steps—conversion of arachidonic acid into the prostaglandin endoperoxides or precursors of leukotrienes, hepoxilins, and lipoxins.
3. Prostaglandin endoperoxide catabolic step—channeling of the endoperoxides to TXA$_2$, PGE$_2$, PGF$_{2\alpha}$, PGD$_2$, or PGI$_2$.
4. Catabolic step—termination of the biological ac-

tivity of prostaglandins, prostacyclin, thromboxanes, and leukotrienes.

The **corticosteroids** are believed to influence the arachidonic acid cascade by moderating the activity of phospholipase A_2; i.e., they induce synthesis of the inhibitory protein lipocortin-1 (LC-1, annexin-1) and prevent the induction of CoxII by interleukin-1. However, calcium, calmodulin, and vasoactive peptides such as bradykinin and angiotensin II apparently activate the release of fatty acids, resulting in an enhancement of prostaglandin biosynthesis.

The activities of CoxI and CoxII are inhibited by **nonsteroidal anti-inflammatory drugs** (NSAIDs). ASA and indomethacin inhibit both, but act preferentially on CoxI, whereas corticosteroids and flurbiprofen preferentially inhibit CoxII. ASA is known to inactivate the cyclooxygenase by irreversible acetylation of serine in CoxI and CoxII, but the other NSAIDs compete with arachidonic acid for the active center of the enzyme. The excess arachidonic acid may enhance the formation of leukotrienes because NSAIDs do not influence lipoxygenase activity. Imidazole and substituted derivatives inhibit thromboxane synthase. While cyclooxygenase is activated by hydroperoxides, prostacyclin synthase is destroyed by hydroperoxides and inhibited by tranylcypromine (an MAO inhibitor). Phenylbutazone appears to affect cyclooxygenase and prostaglandin endoperoxide isomerases as well. It is quite obvious that drugs with a great deal of specificity for the individual pathways would be of immense benefit to the understanding of the functional importance of each pathway.

Inactivation

Intravenously administered prostaglandins are rapidly inactivated, not only by 15-PGDH, but also by numerous other enzymes present in many tissues. The prostaglandin biotransformation products are finally excreted in the urine. Figure 31-4 illustrates some of these pathways. In humans the major urinary product of PGE_2 is the 16-carbon dicarboxylic acid shown. These pathways are tissue- and species-specific, and the activity of several of these enzymes has been shown to change with age.

THE LIPOXYGENASE PATHWAY

The lipoxygenase pathway involves the addition of molecular oxygen at one or other of the double bonds of the polyunsaturated fatty acid via different site-specific enzymes (see Fig. 31-3). Different lipoxygenases are designated according to the site at which they insert molecular oxygen into the arachidonic acid molecule with the formation of the corresponding hydroperoxyeicosatetraenoic acid (HPETE). The most important products in humans are 5-HPETE, 12-HPETE, and 15-HPETE. These are unstable peroxides that yield their corresponding hydroxy derivatives (HETEs) or are converted to other biologically potent compounds.

Leukotriene (LT) biosynthesis starts with the transformation of 5-HPETE, the precursor, into the unstable triene LTA_4 that is converted into LTB_4 in polymorphonuclear leukocytes and into LTC_4 in mast cells. LTD_4, LTE_4, and LTF_4 are metabolites of LTC_4. Slow-reacting substance of anaphylaxis (SRS-A), first described in 1938 and later found to be released from guinea pig lungs upon antigen–antibody reaction, appears to be a mixture of LTC_4 and LTD_4.

Hepoxilins A and B, with a corresponding hydroxyl group at C-8 or C-10 and epoxide at C-11 and C-12 for both, are derived from 12-HPETE by intramolecular rearrangement to hydroxyepoxides. These products are inactivated via specific epoxide hydrolases to the corresponding inactive trihydroxy derivatives.

Metabolites of the 15-HPETE with biological activity give rise to the lipoxins (LX), products that possess three hydroxyl groups at positions 5, 6, and 15 for LXA and positions 5, 14, and 15 for LXB.

THE EPOXYGENASE PATHWAY

A cytochrome P450 monooxygenase system has been described that epoxidizes the double bonds of the precursor acid to the corresponding mono-epoxide derivatives of the fatty acid (EPETEs; see Fig. 31-3), that may be involved in the maintenance of vascular tone, ion transport, cellular growth, signal transduction, hemostasis, and hematopoiesis. The epoxide products are transformed into the corresponding dihydroxy derivatives through the action of epoxide hydrolases.

MECHANISM OF ACTION OF EICOSANOIDS

The eicosanoids act on distinctive cell membrane-bound G protein-linked receptors that modify adenylyl cyclase activity or that activate phospho-

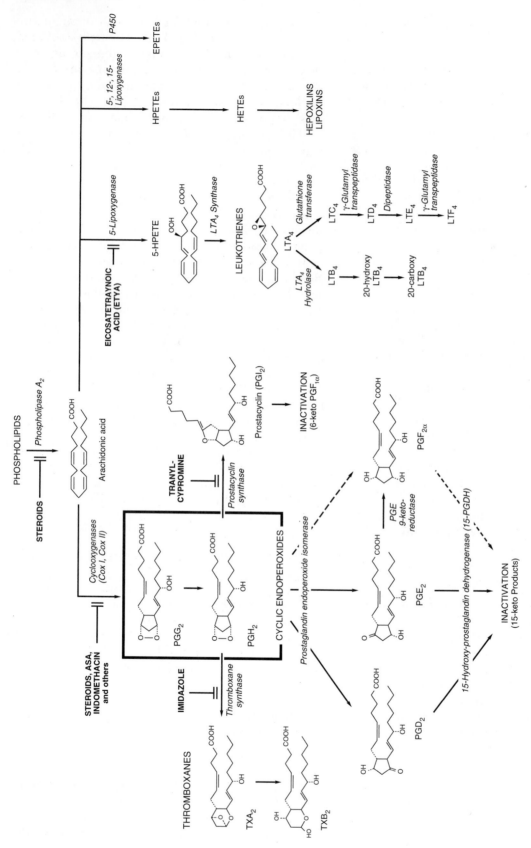

Figure 31-3. Pathways in the eicosanoid fatty acid cascade (simplified). Some sites of inhibition by selected pharmacological agents are indicated by ‖. (Abbreviations are explained in the text.)

lipase C and increase the formation of diacylglycerol and inositol trisphosphate, which brings about increased cytosolic calcium concentration. At the present time, five main types and several subtypes of distinctive eicosanoid receptors are known. They are named after the eicosanoid with the highest affinity, the type of tissue it is found in, and the type of response elicited. PGG_2, PGH_2, and TXA_2 initiate platelet aggregation by increasing calcium concentration, but PGE_1, PGD_2, and PGI_2 inhibit platelet aggregation by increasing cyclic AMP concentration. In general, eicosanoid-induced calcium release causes contraction of smooth muscles, while increased cyclic AMP generation causes relaxation.

BIOLOGICAL EFFECTS

The eicosanoids are formed when the phospholipase or other lipases are activated in a tissue. This activation can result from the action of a physiological stimulus (e.g., angiotensin, bradykinin, norepinephrine) or a pathological stimulus (tissue injury or disease). Once the substrate is released from its esterified stores in the membrane, it is then transformed into the spectrum of products guided by the specific enzymes that it is exposed to. Thus, although the cyclooxygenase and the lipoxygenases in general are ubiquitous, there is considerable tissue specificity in the types of products that are formed. For example, blood platelets contain both a cyclooxygenase and a lipoxygenase, but the main products expressed by this tissue are TXA_2 and 12-HPETE. The main products expressed by the renal papilla are PGE_2 and $PGF_{2\alpha}$. Because prostaglandins and lipoxygenase products are formed in all tissues, and because they exhibit considerable biological potency in test systems, yet are inactivated in one or two passes in the circulation, several physiological roles as local hormones have been proposed, some of which are outlined below.

Prostaglandins, Prostacyclin, and Thromboxane

Cardiovascular system

In most species and vascular beds, **prostaglandins D_2, E_2, and I_2** evoke dilatation of arterioles, precapillary sphincters, and postcapillary vessels and thus increase blood flow; cardiac output is increased; blood pressure generally falls. $PGF_{2\alpha}$ in most species

is a vasoconstrictor of pulmonary arteries and veins, albeit a weak one. **TXA_2,** previously termed rabbit aorta contracting substance, is a potent vasoconstrictor. In certain vessels such as those in the nasal mucosa, prostaglandins evoke a vasoconstrictor effect and have been proposed as nasal decongestants. TXA_2 is a powerful initiator of platelet aggregation; conversely, **PGI_2** opposes the aggregation through elevation of cyclic AMP levels within the platelet. PGI_2 is further capable of deaggregating platelet clumps. It inhibits thrombus formation and is regarded as one of the cooperative factors responsible for the maintenance of hemofluidity (see Chapter 42). The opposing properties of TXA_2 and PGI_2 on platelet function provide a mechanism of regulation of hemostatic function; thus, an imbalance of the TXA_2:PGI_2 ratio might provide an explanation of some pathological states of thrombus formation and inflammation. In experimental models, PGI_2 reduces the size of myocardial infarcts, reduces hypoxic damage in the isolated perfused cat liver, and reduces ischemic damage during kidney transplantation in the dog. PGI_2, PGE_2, and nitric oxide are simultaneously released from endothelial cells. PGE_2 inhibits B-lymphocyte differentiation into antibody-secreting plasma cells, the proliferation of T lymphocytes, and the release of lymphokines.

Smooth muscle

Smooth muscle can be either contracted or relaxed by prostaglandins, depending on the organ studied, the species, and the prostaglandin. **Bronchial muscles** are relaxed in humans and most other species by PGE_1, PGE_2, and PGI_2, although they are contracted by TXA_2, LTC_4, and LTD_4. **Human pregnant uterine muscle** is always contracted in vivo by PGE_1, PGE_2, and $PGF_{2\alpha}$; hence these compounds induce abortion. The nonpregnant uterus is contracted by PGI_2 and TXA_2 but relaxed by PGEs.

Gastrointestinal tract

PGEs and PGI_2 *inhibit the secretion of gastric acid* (see Chapter 44). Also, the volume of secretion and the pepsin content are reduced, but bicarbonate secretion, mucus production, and blood flow are increased. The secretion of pancreatic enzymes and mucus from the small intestine is increased. Prostaglandins also induce the movement of water and electrolytes into the intestinal lumen; therefore they can *produce diarrhea*. While prostaglandins and prostacyclin are cytoprotective, TXA_2 is pro-ulcero-

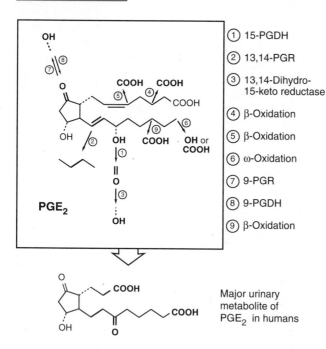

① 15-PGDH

② 13,14-PGR

③ 13,14-Dihydro-15-keto reductase

④ β-Oxidation

⑤ β-Oxidation

⑥ ω-Oxidation

⑦ 9-PGR

⑧ 9-PGDH

⑨ β-Oxidation

Major urinary metabolite of PGE_2 in humans

Figure 31-4. Pathways of prostaglandin catabolism. (See text for explanation of abbreviations.)

genic in the dog and can exert cytolytic effects in myocardial and hepatic tissues.

PGEs cause contraction of intestinal longitudinal muscle and relaxation of the circular muscle, but PGFs, PGG_2, PGH_2, TXA_2, PGI_2, LTB_4, and LTC_4 contract both muscle layers.

Renal system

Prostaglandins increase urine formation, natriuresis, and kaliuresis by altering renal blood flow and renal tubular function. PGD_2, PGE_2, and PGI_2 are active in stimulating renin release. PGEs inhibit the reabsorption of water that is induced by antidiuretic hormone (see also Chapter 47).

Nervous system

After intracerebroventricular injection, prostaglandins cause catatonia and sedation in experimental animals. More importantly, PGE_2 induces a *hyperthermic* response that may be related to pyrogen-induced fever. The antipyretic action of ASA and similar drugs may result from their interference with cyclooxygenase activity. In humans, prostaglandins cause *pain* when injected intradermally and PGEs, PGI_2, and LTB_4 sensitize the nerve endings to the

pain caused by histamine, bradykinin, or mechanical stimuli.

Endocrine systems

Different prostaglandins can stimulate the release of ACTH, growth hormone, prolactin, and gonadotropins, and in addition they have thyrotropin-like and LH-like effects. In several mammals $PGF_{2\alpha}$ can evoke regression of the corpus luteum, which interrupts early pregnancy in these animals; however, this effect has not been observed in human females. 12-HETE increases aldosterone release both directly and through angiotensin II formation.

Possible roles in physiology and pathology

Eicosanoids have been implicated in the function of almost all physiological systems, some of which have been mentioned. One of the roles of eicosanoids is the support of renal perfusion in many diseases associated with decreased effective circulation volume. However, ASA (an inhibitor of CoxI and CoxII) does not influence most of these physiological systems; therefore the role of prostaglandins is questionable. Stronger evidence exists for a role of eicosanoids in tissue inflammation and injury. Prostaglandins act synergistically with agents producing pain, possibly by lowering pain thresholds and sensitizing pain receptors (e.g., potentiating the pain induced by histamine or bradykinin). As PGE_1, PGE_2, and PGI_2 are also potent vasodilatory substances, they potentiate the abilities of histamine, bradykinin, and LTD_4 and LTB_4 to produce edema. The inhibition of cyclooxygenase may be the basis of the analgesic and antiedema actions of nonsteroidal anti-inflammatory compounds (e.g., indomethacin, ibuprofen). Eicosanoids may play a further role in chronic inflammatory joint diseases, which induce destruction of cartilage and resorption of bone (see also Chapters 33, 34).

Leukotrienes

Leukotrienes are now believed to be the biologically active constituents of SRS-A (slow-reacting substance of anaphylaxis). They are formed from arachidonic acid by 5-lipoxygenase. The leukotrienes LTB_4, LTC_4, and LTD_4 can be produced in human, rabbit, and rat polymorphonuclear leukocytes and, upon immunological challenge, they are released from human or guinea pig lungs.

LTC_4, LTD_4, LTE_4, and LTF_4 possess potent vasoconstrictor activity (e.g., in the coronary arteries) and cause constriction of small airways. Tracheal mucus secretion is also increased.

LTB$_4$ is a powerful chemotactic agent and promotes superoxide generation and transendothelial neutrophil migration. Leukotrienes increase vascular wall permeability, evoking leakage from postcapillary venules and thus causing tissue edema. These actions are potentiated by prostaglandins.

Leukotrienes may play an important role in immediate hypersensitivity responses as mediators of allergic bronchoconstriction and increased vascular permeability. The ability of corticosteroids to reduce the production of leukotrienes, by decreasing the release of arachidonic acid and formation of endoperoxides, might explain the antiallergic, anti-inflammatory, and antiasthmatic activity of the corticosteroids. ASA, which does not influence leukotriene production, is devoid of antiallergic and antiasthmatic properties. In fact, ASA-induced asthma might be brought on by the redirection of the substrate, arachidonic acid, into the leukotriene synthesis pathway.

LTB$_4$ can be produced by human polymorphonuclear leukocytes and is a potent chemokinetic, chemotactic, and aggregating agent in many types of cells. It may have a role in inflammation and tissue damage. LTB$_4$ has been found to induce accumulation of polymorphonuclear leukocytes in joint diseases such as gout and arthritis, as well as in skin lesions of patients with psoriasis.

HPETEs and EPETEs

The HPETEs have been shown to possess a variety of biological actions in vitro. These actions lead to such diverse effects as relaxation of vascular smooth muscle of the isolated rat and rabbit stomach, in which contraction has previously been induced with norepinephrine; reversal of the effects of PGI$_2$ on the release of insulin from perfused rat islets of Langerhans; modulation (inhibition) of the effects of PGI$_2$ on the release of renin; and a neuromodulatory role in signal transduction in the sensory neurons of *Aplysia*. The effects could be produced by the HPETEs themselves or, since they are rapidly transformed into other products, their effects may be due to conversion into the leukotrienes, lipoxins, or hepoxilins.

Few studies have concentrated on the biological role of the EPETEs. These products have been shown to possess marginal activity on the release of calcium from liver microsomes and on the release of pituitary hormones from the hypothalamus.

THERAPEUTIC USES

Uterus Stimulation

Prostaglandins induce contractions of the pregnant uterus and, in larger doses, of the nonpregnant uterus. Various preparations are available.

Dinoprostone, PGE$_2$

Prostin E$_2$ vaginal suppositories contain 20 mg of dinoprostone and are used primarily to induce abortion between the 12th and 20th gestational weeks. They are administered every 3–5 hours for not more than 48 hours, until abortion occurs. This product is available only in a limited number of countries.

Prostin E$_2$ oral tablets contain 0.5 mg dinoprostone for elective induction of labor, and for induction made necessary by postmaturity, hypertension, toxemia of pregnancy, premature rupture of amniotic membranes, Rh incompatibility, diabetes mellitus, intrauterine death, or fetal growth retardation. It is administered orally every hour until a satisfactory response is obtained. Single doses should never exceed 1.5 mg, and the duration of treatment should not exceed 18 hours. If oxytocin is to be used, it should not be administered within 1 hour of the last dose. The most frequently observed adverse reactions are nausea, vomiting, diarrhea, fetal heart rate changes, and uterine hypertonus.

Prostin E$_2$ vaginal gel is a semitranslucent viscous vaginal gel supplied in a special applicator syringe that contains 1 or 2 mg of dinoprostone per 3 g of gel. It is used for induction of labor at term or near term. The dose is 1–2 mg intravaginally and may be repeated 6 hours later depending on the patient's initial response. The adverse effects are very similar to those observed with oxytocin, such as fetal heart rate abnormalities, fetal distress, and uterine hypercontractility.

Carboprost, 15-methyl PGF$_{2\alpha}$ (Hemabate, Prostin/15M)

Carboprost tromethamine salt is used only by intramuscular administration, to induce abortion during the 12th to 20th gestational weeks. The dose is 250 μg every 1–3 hours, depending on the uterine response. It is also used for refractory postpartum bleeding due to uterine atony. Carboprost methyl (U-36384) is carboprost methyl ester.

Dinoprost (PGF$_{2\alpha}$; Leutalyse, Prostin F$_2$ Alpha) injectable is for intra-amniotic administration to induce abortion or labor. It is marketed in 5 mg/mL strength. The initial dose is 5 mg, which is repeated as required up to a total of 40 mg. If response is not satisfactory within 24 hours and the membranes are still intact, an additional dose of 10–40 mg can be administered. This product is available in North America but is not advertised or promoted.

Ductus Arteriosus

In premature infants the ductus may remain open, probably because of excessive PGI$_2$ production. In such cases, injectable indomethacin is administered to reduce prostaglandin synthesis and close the ductus.

In neonates with congenital heart defects such as pulmonary atresia or stenosis, tricuspid atresia, coarctation of the aorta, tetralogy of Fallot, interruption of the aortic arch, or transposition of the great vessels, a patent (open) ductus may be essential for survival. In such cases, PGE$_1$ is administered to keep the ductus open until surgical correction can be carried out. The preparation used for this purpose is **alprostadil** (PGE$_1$; Prostin VR), an injectable preparation containing 0.5 mg of PGE$_1$ in anhydrous ethanol. Before administration it must be properly diluted with sterile sodium chloride or dextrose solution. It is administered with the aid of a pump capable of delivering small-volume constant infusions. The initial infusion rate is 0.1 μg/kg body weight/minute until the desired effect is achieved; it is then dropped to 0.05–0.01 μg/kg/min. The drug can be administered into a large vein or through an umbilical artery catheter positioned with its tip at the ductal opening. Numerous precautionary measures must be followed (as listed in the product monograph) before administration is started. The most frequently observed serious side effects are apnea and seizures. The others which are considered to be less serious are flushing, bradycardia, fever, and diarrhea. Long-term use may cause weakening of the walls of the ductus arteriosus and pulmonary arteries; gastric outlet obstruction and cortical proliferation of long bones may occur.

Gastrointestinal Tract

Misoprostol (Cytotec) is a synthetic methyl ester analog of PGE$_1$ used for the prevention of drug-induced gastric ulceration during NSAID, corticosteroid, or anticoagulant administration. In addition, it can be used alone or in combination with antacids for the treatment of duodenal ulcer (see Chapter 44). It is available in oral tablet formulations of 100 and 200 μg. The dosage for the prevention of drug-induced ulcer is 400–800 μg/day, and for duodenal ulcer 800 μg/day in divided doses. Women should be advised not to become pregnant while taking misoprostol. The most frequent side effects are diarrhea, abdominal pain, flatulence, and spotting.

Platelet Aggregation

Epoprostenol (PGI$_2$, prostacyclin; Cyclo-Prostin, Flolan) is used as a replacement for heparin in some hemodialysis patients and for the prevention of platelet aggregation in extracorporeal circulation systems. PGI$_2$ improves the harvest and storage of platelets for therapeutic transfusion. The drug is available in North America on request from the manufacturer, Glaxo-Wellcome Inc.

Impotence

Alprostadil (PGE$_1$; Caverject) is administered into the corpora cavernosa to initiate and maintain complete or partial erection lasting for 1–3 hours. It has been tried in combination with papaverine and with phentolamine to reduce the frequency of adverse reactions. Caverject is available in 10- and 20-μg strengths in the form of a lyophilized powder to be dissolved in normal saline by the patient before administration. In some countries the commercially available Prostin VR is used in institutional pharmacies to prepare a suitable product. The starting dose is 2.5 μg, increased to a total of 40 μg if required. The side effects are pain on injection, priapism, fibrosis, and orthostatic hypotension.

SUGGESTED READING

Bergström S, Carlson LA, and Weeks JR. The prostaglandins: a family of biologically active lipids. Pharmacol Rev 1968; 20:1–48.

Coleman RA, Smith WL, Narumiya S. International Union of Pharmacology classification of prostanoid receptors: properties, distribution and structure of the receptors and their subtypes. Pharmacol Rev 1994; 46:205–229.

Fiddler GI, Lumley P. Preliminary clinical studies with thromboxane synthase inhibitors and thromboxane receptor blockers: a review. Circulation 1990; 81:169–178.

Janssen-Timmen U, Tomic I, Specht E, Beilecke U, Habenicht AJ. The arachidonic acid cascade, eicosanoids, and signal transduction. Ann NY Acad Sci 1994; 733:325–334.

Moncada S, ed. Prostacyclin, thromboxane and leukotrienes. Br Med Bull 1983; 39(3):209–300.

Reilly M, Fitzgerald GA. Cellular activation by thromboxane

A$_2$ and other eicosanoids. Eur Heart J 1993; (14 Suppl)K:88–93.

Samuelsson B, Paoletti R, eds. Advances in prostaglandin and thromboxane research. New York: Raven Press, 1987.

Schror K, Hohlfeld T. Inotropic actions of eicosanoids [Editorial]. Basic Res Cardiol 1992; 87:2–11.

Walt RP. Misoprostol for the treatment of peptic ulcer and anti-inflammatory drug-induced gastroduodenal ulceration. N Engl J Med 1992; 327:1575–1580.

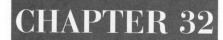

CHAPTER 32

Autacoids

D. KADAR

CASE HISTORY

A 57-year-old male high school teacher with moderate hypertension was adequately treated with atenolol 50 mg daily for several years. In addition, he had suffered from migraine in his youth, but with age it became much less frequent and required no special medication. Recently, he complained that the occasional sexual dysfunction he had experienced since taking atenolol had become more frequent, and he tired easily without any obvious reason. His blood pressure medication was changed to captopril 25 mg twice daily, and was increased to three times daily after 2 weeks. His sexual performance and physical endurance improved somewhat after 3 months, but the previously occasional migraine attacks became more frequent and severe, and he experienced frequent coughing. Prophylactic treatment of his migraine with pizotifen, methysergide, or cyproheptadine was not practical because the pain occurred only in the morning and was unpredictable. A trial with sumatriptan succinate produced significant improvement of his headache, but the transient chest pain and sensation of tightness were intolerable side effects. The antihypertensive medication was changed to losartan 50 mg daily to avoid the coughing spells that occurred with captopril. A combination preparation containing acetaminophen 500 mg, caffeine 15 mg, and codeine phosphate 8 mg was prescribed for the headache, two tablets to be taken every 4 hours when required. Blood and urine chemistry were found to be normal after 3 and 9 months of therapy, and the blood pressure was adequately controlled. Routine follow-up 1 year later showed that this treatment plan was satisfactory.

ANGIOTENSINS AND ANGIOTENSIN-CONVERTING ENZYME (ACE) INHIBITORS

Occurrence and Synthesis of Angiotensins

The angiotensins are peptides of known amino acid composition and structure that are derived from angiotensinogen, a plasma α_2-globulin. Angiotensinogen is converted to the decapeptide angiotensin I by the enzyme renin, which is released by the kidneys. Peptidyl dipeptidase (angiotensin-converting enzyme, ACE), which is found in high concentration in plasma and tissues (glands, kidneys, blood vessels, heart, etc.), converts angiotensin I (inactive) to the octapeptide angiotensin II, the biologically most active form. Angiotensin II circulates in blood and is further catabolized to a less active heptapeptide (angiotensin III) or to inactive fragments (Fig. 32-1).

Angiotensin II has a powerful vasoconstrictor action, 40 times more powerful than that of epinephrine. Angiotensin II stimulates the synthesis and release of aldosterone from the adrenal cortex and the release of antidiuretic hormone (ADH, vasopressin) from the pituitary gland, promoting sodium and water retention. Extremely high concentrations of circulating angiotensin II, as seen in terminal liver failure, directly inhibit sodium reabsorption in the distal tubule. This action is only of academic interest, however, because the intense renal artery constriction

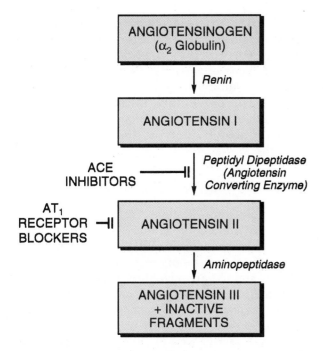

Figure 32-1. Pathway of angiotensin formation and degradation, and classes of drugs acting on it (‖ indicates specific blockade).

markedly reduces renal blood flow and reduces glomerular filtration rate to almost complete renal shutdown.

Renin release can be induced by a decrease in blood pressure or blood volume, by renal ischemia, by depletion of sodium ions, and by stimulation of β_1-adrenoceptors of the juxtaglomerular cells. The induction of renin release by any of these stimuli, and the subsequent production of angiotensin II, increases blood pressure and induces the retention of sodium; this acts as feedback, slowing down the release of renin, bringing about a return to homeostasis.

The vasoconstrictor action of angiotensin II is mediated through direct stimulation of specific angiotensin AT_1-receptors located on pre- and postcapillary vascular smooth muscle cells and indirectly by stimulation of the sympathetic nervous system. Stimulation of AT_1-receptors, which are coupled to G proteins, results in inhibition of adenylyl cyclase and stimulation of phospholipase C activity. Inositol-1,4,5-trisphosphate and diacylglycerol are second messengers. The most strongly affected vessels are those of the skin, splanchnic region, and kidney. Vessels of brain and skeletal muscle are less constricted. Angiotensin II has no important direct effects on the heart; however, due to the elevation of

systemic blood pressure, the work of the heart may increase. Stimulation of AT_1-receptors of the zona glomerulosa cells releases aldosterone.

Angiotensin AT_2-receptors located mainly in the uterus, chromaffin cells, and a number of fetal tissues do not appear to be coupled to G protein.

Angiotensin is used clinically in some parts of the world to raise blood pressure. The preparation employed is angiotensinamide (Hypertensin). This must be given by slow intravenous infusion, during which the blood pressure is monitored continuously. The preparation may be used to restore blood pressure if the hypotension is not due to loss of blood.

More importantly, *antagonists of the renin-angiotensin system have a wide use as antihypertensive agents.* Specific inhibitors of renin release and of renin enzymatic activity are **ditekiren** and **enalkiren**.

Angiotensin II Receptor Blockers

Saralasin, an angiotensin analog, was the first clinically effective angiotensin II receptor blocker, but it was found to have partial agonist activity that caused transient increases in blood pressure. Additional drawbacks were short half-life and the lack of effect from oral administration.

Losartan (Cozaar, Fig. 32-2), a recently introduced nonpeptide imidazole derivative, blocks AT_1-receptors, and it has been approved for the oral treatment of hypertension.

Mechanism of action

Losartan and its 5-carboxylic acid active metabolite lower systolic and diastolic blood pressure by competitive blockade of AT_1-receptors in blood vessels, causing vasodilatation. In addition, it reduces aldosterone release (causing subsequent increase in serum potassium concentration) by blocking AT_1-receptors on zona glomerulosa cells. It blocks the effect of exogenously administered angiotensin II. It does not affect bradykinin or substance P metabolism or the activity of angiotensin-converting enzyme. The plasma half-life of losartan is 1.5–2.5 hours; that of its active metabolite is 6–9 hours.

Therapeutic effects

Several clinical trials have confirmed that losartan lowers the blood pressure in hypertensive patients and that it is as effective as the ACE inhibitor enalapril or the β-blocker atenolol. The antihypertensive

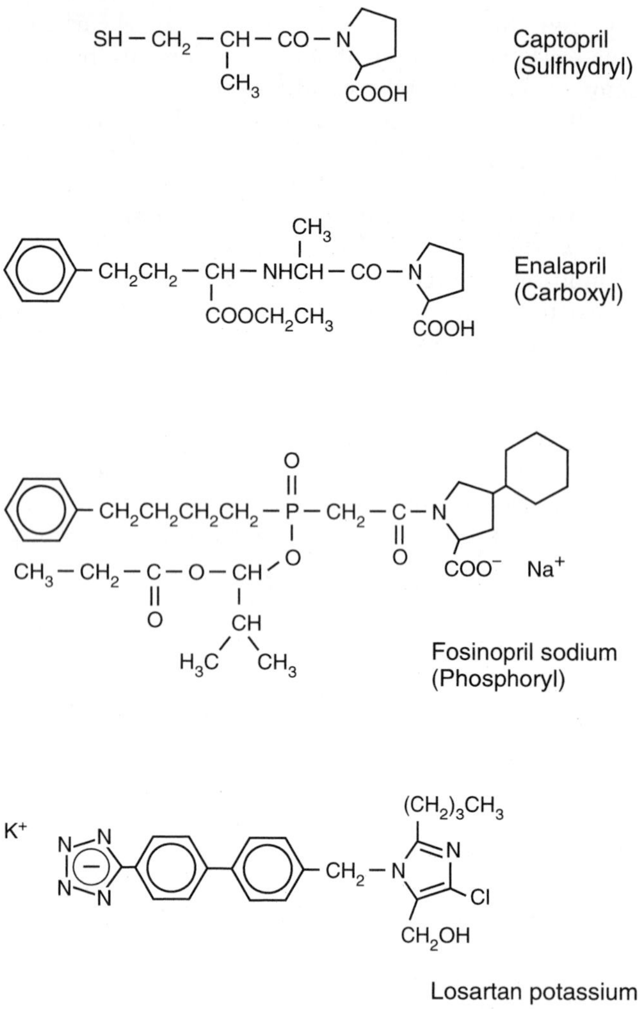

Figure 32-2. Structural formulae of representative ACE inhibitors and the AT_1-receptor-blocker losartan potassium.

effect is enhanced by the coadministration of hydrochlorothiazide. It has less antihypertensive effects in black patients. It has a tendency to raise serum potassium concentration while lowering elevated serum uric acid levels. It does not affect the blood pressure of normotensive individuals. The dose range is 25–200 mg/day. The drug is also marketed in fixed-dose combination of losartan 50 mg and hydrochlorothiazide 12.5 mg. Clinical studies are in progress with a number of other AT_1 receptor blockers (valsartan, irbesartan, candesartan, telmisartan, etc.) that may be released shortly.

Adverse effects

The only side effect attributed to losartan is occasional dizziness. Increased serum potassium concen-

tration observed in some patients was not serious enough to change medication. The safety of losartan during pregnancy or breast feeding has not been established. None of the side effects associated with ACE-inhibitor administration were observed. There is no evidence at present that losartan prolongs survival of patients with heart failure or myocardial infarction or that it prevents the development of nephropathy in diabetes.

ACE Inhibitors

ACE inhibitors were developed during a systematic search for inhibitors of the kininases that break down kinins such as bradykinin and kallidin, and that convert angiotensin I to angiotensin II.

ACE inhibitors are classified according to the chemical nature of their ligand, which binds to the zinc ion at the active site of the enzyme. The inhibitors that are used at present, or that are in their final stages of study, are (1) sulfhydryl compounds (alacepril, captopril, moveltipril, zofenopril); (2) carboxyl compounds (benazepril, cilazapril, enalapril, delapril, lisinopril, pentopril, perindopril, quinapril, ramipril, spirapril, trandolapril); and (3) phosphoryl compounds (fosinopril and ceronapril). In addition, there are more than 80 compounds in various earlier stages of development.

Mechanism and site of action

ACE inhibitors act competitively on the enzyme by virtue of their structural resemblance to the dipeptides cleaved by ACE. The inhibition was demonstrated in experimental animals and humans by blocking the conversion of intravenously administered angiotensin I and preventing the resulting pressor effect. This action is specific because the pressor response to exogenously administered angiotensin II or norepinephrine is not influenced by ACE inhibitors.

ACE is also responsible for the breakdown of kinins (e.g., bradykinin). Therefore enzyme inhibition causes accumulation of compounds that are known to produce vasodilatation and lowering of blood pressure. Some of the side effects (flushing, itching, coughing, etc.) can be attributed in part to accumulation of kinins.

Angiotensin II stimulates the synthesis and release of aldosterone to increase sodium–potassium exchange in the distal convoluted tubules. The reduced formation of angiotensin II during ACE inhibitor therapy may lead to a significant reduction of aldosterone plasma levels and subsequent increase in serum potassium and depletion of sodium. The reduction of ADH release will increase water elimination and contribute to volume depletion by simultaneously administered diuretics.

Proteinuria due to excessive glomerular filtration pressure, often observed in chronic hypertension, is reduced or eliminated after blood pressure reduction.

Plasma renin activity increases during ACE inhibitor administration because the angiotensin II-regulated feedback mechanism is impaired.

Therapeutic effects

In hypertensive patients, ACE inhibitors reduce blood pressure by reducing total peripheral arterial resistance and increasing compliance of large arteries, while causing no change or slight increase in cardiac output. The renal blood flow is increased, but the glomerular filtration rate remains the same because of compensatory dilatation of both afferent and efferent arterioles. The blood-pressure-reducing effects of ACE inhibitors are additive to those of thiazide diuretics. ACE inhibitors can also be combined with α-blockers, β-blockers, or calcium-channel blockers. The natriuretic effect is the result of reduced aldosterone secretion and improved renal hemodynamics. In congestive heart failure, the effects of venodilatation and reductions in pulmonary artery pressure, pulmonary capillary wedge pressure, and left atrial and left ventricular filling pressure lead to increases in stroke volume, cardiac output, and exercise tolerance. After several months of ACE inhibitor administration, in addition to the improvement in overall hemodynamics, the hypertension-induced left ventricular hypertrophy is considerably reduced. In contrast, it is not clear at the present time whether there is any long-term benefit in using ACE inhibitors following myocardial infarction.

Additional and adverse effects

In the presence of renal artery stenosis, ACE inhibitors, by lowering the blood pressure, may cause additional reduction of renal perfusion, thus increasing BUN and serum creatinine. A significant increase in serum potassium may occur in patients with renal impairment or in those receiving the ACE inhibitor together with potassium-sparing diuretics. The angiotensin II-stimulated renal prostaglandin synthesis may be reduced, causing changes in intrarenal blood distribution. Self-limiting cough and throat irritation due to kinin accumulation is very common, even in patients with low plasma renin activity. Serious hypotension following first-dose administration can be avoided by starting therapy with one-quarter or less of the usual dose and then gradually increasing the dose to the therapeutically effective level.

The most frequently observed adverse reactions are dizziness, upper abdominal pain, headache, mental confusion, urticaria, uremia, acute renal failure (in patients with renal artery stenosis), and impotence.

Toxicity

ACE inhibitors are contraindicated in pregnancy because their use has been associated with reduced amniotic fluid volume (oligohydramnios), fetal growth retardation, patent ductus arteriosus, pulmonary hypoplasia, and stillbirths. Although adverse effects resulting from first-trimester exposure have not been documented, ACE inhibitor administration should be discontinued if pregnancy is planned or suspected. Repeated ultrasound examinations should be carried out if drug administration is unavoidable during pregnancy.

Toxicity associated with ACE inhibitor administration includes transient angioedema of the face, lips, and tongue, with possible fatal outcome if the larynx is involved. In rare cases neutropenia and agranulocytosis have been reported. Therefore, patients who unexpectedly develop systemic or oral-cavity infections during therapy should be closely followed. WBC and differential blood counts should be performed, especially during the early stages of therapy. Transient or long-lasting dermatological reactions such as rash or pruritus with fever, arthralgia, and eosinophilia may occur any time during ACE inhibitor administration; this requires termination of therapy.

Proteinuria and increased BUN and creatinine occur primarily in patients with preexisting renal disease or in those who receive high doses of ACE inhibitors. Anaphylactoid reactions have been reported in dialysis patients and during desensitization treatment with Hymenoptera venom. Patients with liver disease may develop hepatitis and elevated liver enzymes. Temporary dysgeusia (perverted taste sensation) occurs often, accompanied by moderate weight loss.

Therapeutic application

ACE inhibitors alone, or in combination with thiazide diuretics or other antihypertensive agents, are used for the treatment of hypertension. They are also useful for the treatment of heart failure in patients who do not respond adequately to digitalis and diuretics. Consideration should always be given to the risk of neutropenia, agranulocytosis, or laryngeal edema. In general, patients with chronic renal failure (creatinine clearance <40 mL/min) may require only 25–50% of the normal dose, except for fosinopril, which usually requires no dose adjustment.

Drugs

Alacepril (Cetapril) is a prodrug that is rapidly converted first to desacetyl alacepril, which is not detected in plasma, and then to the active metabolite captopril. Oral bioavailability is 70% and maximum plasma concentration of captopril occurs after 1–2 hours. Maximum drop in systolic blood pressure occurs after 3–3.5 hours, and a significant blood-pressure-lowering effect is noticeable for up to 24 hours. About 50–70% of the dose is excreted in urine as captopril.

Benazepril (Lotensin) is a prodrug that is converted to the active metabolite benazeprilat by liver and plasma esterases. After oral administration, 37% is absorbed; the presence of food in the stomach does not affect bioavailability. The peak plasma concentration of benazepril is reached in 0.5–1 hour and that of benazeprilat occurs in 1–2 hours. At therapeutic concentrations, the serum protein binding of benazepril is 97% and that of benazeprilat is 95%. The conjugated drug and its free and conjugated metabolites are excreted in urine. The effective half-life is 11 hours. The usual daily dose is 10–20 mg, and the maximum is not more than 40 mg.

Captopril (Capoten, Fig. 32-2) was the first clinically useful, orally administered ACE inhibitor. It is absorbed rapidly after oral administration, reaching peak blood levels in about 1 hour. The drug should be administered 1 hour before meals because the presence of food in the stomach reduces its bioavailability. Less than 30% of the circulating drug is bound to plasma proteins. It is unevenly distributed in total body water. A minor amount crosses the blood–brain barrier in experimental animals, but it freely crosses the human placenta. The estimated serum half-life is about 2 hours. The antihypertensive effect is much longer than the demonstrable inhibition of the circulating ACE, perhaps because the ACE present in vascular endothelium is inhibited by extremely low serum concentrations. About half the absorbed dose is excreted in the urine unchanged; the rest leaves as the disulfide dimer of captopril and captopril-cysteine disulfide. Captopril may cause a false-positive urine test for acetone. Doses range from 25 to 300 mg/day.

Cilazapril (Inhibace) is a prodrug that is rapidly deesterified in liver and blood after oral administration to form the active metabolite cilazaprilat. Peak plasma concentration is reached in less than 1 hour for the parent drug and in 1.7 hours for the metabolite. The bioavailability is 29%, and it is not much influenced by food. The plasma half-life of the parent compound is 1.3 hours but that of the active metabolite is considerably longer (30–50 hours). Peak effects occur in 2–3 hours, but significant lowering of blood pressure persists for 30–50 hours. Cilazaprilat is eliminated primarily by the kidneys. Doses range from 2.5 to 10 mg/day.

Enalapril maleate (Vasotec) is the maleic acid salt of enalapril (see Fig. 32-2), which is the ethyl ester of enalaprilic acid. About 60% of the orally administered enalapril is absorbed into the systemic circulation, reaching maximum serum concentration in 60 minutes. Food does not affect the bioavailability. It is hydrolyzed to enalaprilat, which is much more potent than the parent drug. Peak serum concentrations of enalaprilat occur 4–5 hours after administration of enalapril. The drug is not biotransformed further, and 94% of the dose is excreted in urine and feces as enalapril and enalaprilat. There is a prolonged terminal phase in the serum concentration profile of enalaprilat that represents the slow elimination of the ACE-bound drug. The effective serum half-life of enalaprilat is about 11 hours. Neither the drug nor its active metabolite crosses the blood–brain barrier in experimental animals, but it freely crosses the placenta. Doses range from 2.5 to 40 mg/day.

Fosinopril (Monopril, Fig. 32-2) is a prodrug that is hydrolyzed to the active metabolite fosinoprilat by gut-wall and hepatic esterases. Peak plasma concentration of fosinoprilat occurs in 3 hours. The maximum absorption of fosinopril following oral administration is 36% of the dose. It is present in plasma as fosinoprilat (75%), its glucuronide conjugate, and a p-hydroxy metabolite. About 95% of fosinoprilat is bound to plasma proteins. The plasma half-life is 3–4 hours but the average half-life of the effect is 11.5 hours. The active metabolite and its conjugate are excreted in urine and bile. In oliguria, dose reduction is not essential because extensive biliary excretion compensates for reduced renal elimination. Usual daily doses range from 10 to 80 mg.

Lisinopril (Zestril, Prinivil) is an analog of enalaprilat, with lysine replacing alanine. Bioavailability following oral administration is 25%, and peak serum concentration occurs after 6–8 hours. Bioavailability is not affected by food, age, or coadministration of hydrochlorothiazide, propranolol, digoxin, or glyburide. Lisinopril is not a prodrug like enalapril, it is not bound to serum proteins, and it is excreted unchanged in the urine. Steady-state plasma concentration is achieved after 3 days of administration, and accumulation occurs in patients with severe renal impairment. The effective serum half-life is about 13 hours, but significant blood pressure reduction continues for more than 24 hours. The pharmacological properties are similar to those of captopril and enalapril. Usual doses range from 5 to 40 mg/day.

Perindopril (Coversyl, Electan, Procaptan) is a long-acting prodrug, 17–28% of which is hydrolyzed to the active metabolite, perindoprilat. Peak plasma concentration occurs in 1 hour for the prodrug and in 3–4 hours for the active metabolite. The plasma half-life of perindopril is 1.5–3 hours, and for perindoprilat it is 25–30 hours. The drug is rapidly absorbed following oral administration, with 65–95% bioavailability. Perindopril, some of its inactive metabolites, and perindoprilat are excreted in urine. Usual daily doses range from 4 to 8 mg.

Quinapril (Accupril), a prodrug, is well absorbed after oral administration and rapidly hydrolyzed to the active metabolite quinaprilat. Peak plasma concentration of quinaprilat occurs in 2 hours. The parent compound has a plasma half-life of 0.8 hour and the active metabolite 2 hours. The antihypertensive effect may last for 24 hours. Quinaprilat is 97% plasma protein-bound. Quinaprilat (50–60%), a small amount of quinapril, and two diketopiperazine metabolites are excreted in urine. The magnesium content of quinapril tablets may reduce the bioavailability of concurrently administered tetracycline. Daily doses range from 5 to 80 mg.

Ramipril (Cardace) is a prodrug that is rapidly hydrolyzed by liver esterases to the long-acting active metabolite ramiprilat. Maximum effect occurs in 6 hours. The plasma half-life of ramiprilat is 24–50 hours. Plasma protein binding is 73% for ramipril and 56% for ramiprilat. Oral doses range from 5 to 20 mg/day. The drug is in its final stages of clinical trials in Europe.

Zofenopril (Zoprace) is a prodrug that is hydrolyzed to the active metabolite during and after absorption. Bioavailability is 96% after oral administration. The drug and its metabolites are excreted mainly in the bile and partly in urine. Daily doses range from 30 to 60 mg.

KININS

Kinins are a separate class of peptides that are formed from kininogen precursors (which, like an-

giotensinogen, are α_2-globulins) by the proteolytic enzymes, kallikreins, and some nonspecific enzymes such as trypsin. In plasma the nonapeptide bradykinin (named for its action in producing slow contraction of the gut) is formed. In tissues, the initial product is kallidin, a decapeptide that can be converted to bradykinin by an aminopeptidase that removes a lysine residue. Bradykinin has a very short half-life (15 seconds) and is inactivated by kininases. Kininase II is identical with peptidyl dipeptidase (the enzyme that converts angiotensin I to angiotensin II, see above) and can thus be blocked by ACE inhibitors (Fig. 32-3).

Kinins act on specific receptors (B_1, B_2, and B_3) to activate phospholipase C or A_2, causing powerful vasodilatation in most vascular beds.

In addition to vasodilatation, kinins also cause increased vascular permeability and edema. Bronchoconstriction induced by kinins is selectively antagonized by acetylsalicylic acid and similar analgesics. In asthmatics, kinins may cause respiratory distress. In addition, kinins are potent pain-inducing agents. The hyperalgesia, edema formation, and vasodilatation associated with the kinins are due at least partially to increased synthesis and release of certain prostaglandins.

At present the kinins have no therapeutic use. However, the inhibition of kinin breakdown by ACE inhibitors may contribute to the antihypertensive effects of these agents (see above). At the present time, several bradykinin analogs are being tested for their kinin-receptor-blocking properties.

Aprotinin (Trasylol) is an inhibitor of the enzyme kallikrein, probably identical with the pancreatic trypsin inhibitor of Kunitz, and is used in treating acute pancreatitis, the carcinoid syndrome, and states of hyperfibrinolysis because of its action as an inhibitor of trypsin, kallikrein, and plasmin.

NONOPIOID PEPTIDES OF BRAIN AND GASTROINTESTINAL TRACT

Substance P

Substance P is an undecapeptide that was first extracted from intestine. It is also found in brain, in primary afferent neurons, and in small arterioles of the human heart. It is proposed to be a sensory neurotransmitter associated with pain transmission. Substance P binds to G protein-coupled substance P receptors and causes release of endothelium-derived hyperpolarizing factor (EDHF), resulting in vasodi-

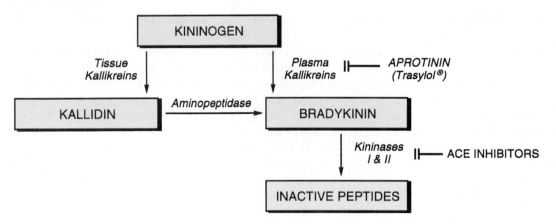

Figure 32-3. Pathways of formation and inactivation of bradykinin (‖ indicates blockade at the points shown).

latation. It contracts smooth muscles of the gut. The functions of substance P in the brain are not yet fully identified, although a cotransmitter role in some serotonin neurons has been postulated (see Chapter 20). Participation of substance P neurons in extrapyramidal motor control has also been proposed. Antagonists of substance P are not known at present.

Endothelins

Endothelins are peptides released from mammalian vascular endothelial cells. Endothelin-1 (ET-1) acts on ET_A receptors to produce intense and long-lasting vasoconstriction, but also acts on ET_{B1} receptors to cause vasodilatation by release of NO. Selective antagonists of the ET_A receptors are being explored for possible use in the treatment of vasospasm.

Cholecystokinin (CCK)

This is a peptide composed of 33 amino acids; however, a shorter (eight amino-acid) fragment of CCK also has full biological activity. CCK is localized in the brain and gastrointestinal tract. When injected into the brain, CCK causes anorectic reactions and may be a factor that triggers peripheral satiety mechanisms (see also Chapter 20).

Neurotensin

This tridecapeptide was found originally in the brain and subsequently in the intestinal mucosa. Systemic administration of neurotensin causes vasodilatation, hypotension, and increased vascular permeability. These actions may be due at least in part to histamine release.

Vasoactive Intestinal Polypeptide (VIP)

VIP consists of 28 amino acids. It is present in intestinal neurons and is also found in the brain (including coexistence in some dopamine neurons). The neurons containing VIP in the intestine may be involved in reflexes facilitating intestinal transport. VIP also causes relaxation of tracheal smooth muscles.

The central roles of the above peptides are largely unknown at present. They coexist in neurons together with classical central transmitters. They seem to act through specific individual receptors and play either a neuroregulator or a neurotransmitter role.

In the intestine, these neuropeptides likely are important in regulating intestinal motility, blood flow, and mucosal transport. If specific antagonists for the individual peptides are discovered, they may greatly assist in clarifying the roles of these peptides.

Somatostatin

The function of somatostatin is primarily to control the activity of growth-hormone-releasing hormone (GHRH), but it is also found outside of the CNS in D cells of the pancreatic islets and in gastric and duodenal mucosa. It inhibits the secretion of growth hormone, insulin, glucagon, gastrin, vasoactive intestinal peptide (VIP), and possibly others.

Octreotide (Sandostatin) is a synthetic octapeptide analog of naturally occurring somatostatin. It inhibits the secretion of peptides of the gastroenteropancreatic endocrine system (insulin, glucagon, gastrin), growth hormone, and thyrotropin-releasing-hormone-stimulated release of thyroid-stimulating hormone.

Octreotide is indicated for symptomatic treatment of carcinoid and vasoactive peptide-secreting tumors, and it is most beneficial for the control of diarrhea and flushing episodes associated with these conditions. It is administered intravenously in daily doses of between 100 mg and 600 mg. Adverse effects are local irritation, gastrointestinal disturbances, impaired glucose tolerance, and hepatic dysfunctions.

5-HYDROXYTRYPTAMINE (SEROTONIN)

The synthesis and degradation of serotonin are described in Chapter 20. (See also Fig. 32-4.) About 90% of body serotonin is found in enterochromaffin cells of the gastrointestinal tract. The remainder is localized in platelets and in specific neurons in the central nervous system.

Physiology and Pharmacology

In the central nervous system 5-HT acts as a neurotransmitter localized in neurons originating in the raphe nuclei and distributed throughout the brain. Stimulation of 5-HT_{1A}-receptors may increase or decrease adenylyl cyclase activity, resulting in increased or decreased (inhibited) K^+ conductance.

Stimulation of 5-HT_2-receptors causes excitation by activation of phospholipase C and increased synthesis of inositol trisphosphate and diacylglycerol. The central functions of 5-HT relate to regulation of mood, food intake, and sleep. It may also participate in the regulation of adenohypophysial secretions, stimulating the release of ACTH, growth hormone, and prolactin and inhibiting the release of luteinizing hormone (LH), follicle-stimulating hormone (FSH), and thyroid-stimulating hormone (TSH). In the pineal gland 5-HT serves as the precursor of the hormone melatonin.

In the periphery, 5-HT_3-receptors found in autonomic ganglia may cause increased norepinephrine or acetylcholine release, and those on sensory nerves may produce itch or pain.

The cardiovascular system may be affected directly by stimulation of 5-HT receptors or indirectly by influencing norepinephrine release. 5-HT receptors designated as 5-HT_{1A}, 5-HT_{1B}, 5-HT_{1C}, and 5-HT_{1D} are located on various blood vessels in the body and may cause vasodilatation in skeletal muscles and coronary arteries by inhibition of adenylyl cyclase, release of nitric oxide (NO, also called endothelium-derived relaxing factor, EDRF), or prostaglandins. 5-HT_2-receptor stimulation activates phospholipase C, increases intracellular calcium ion concentration, and produces vasoconstriction in the splanchnic area, lungs, and kidneys.

Stimulation of 5-HT_1-receptors in the heart increases the heart rate and force of contraction, but stimulation of 5-HT_3-receptors in the coronary arteries and baroreceptors causes significant reflex slowing of the heart rate, hypotension, and vasovagal syncope.

5-HT synthesized in enterochromaffin cells is released into the blood and is actively taken up by platelets. 5-HT and thromboxane A_2 are released from platelets during aggregation or (in vitro) after exposure to air. Hemostasis is promoted by further platelet aggregation (5-HT_2-receptors) and constriction of cutaneous blood vessels.

5-HT-receptors located in the gastrointestinal tract, uterus, and bronchial smooth muscle may have some physiological function but are also stimulated by 5-HT released from enterochromaffin cell tumors (carcinoid tumors), and are responsible for most of the cardiovascular, intestinal, bronchial, and other symptoms associated with these tumors.

5-HT is also involved in the prodromal vasoconstriction stage (aura) of classical migraine that is followed by pain due to intense vasodilatation caused by liberation of other vasoactive substances such as prostaglandins, kinins, and nitric oxide (NO).

When administered systemically, 5-HT affects the

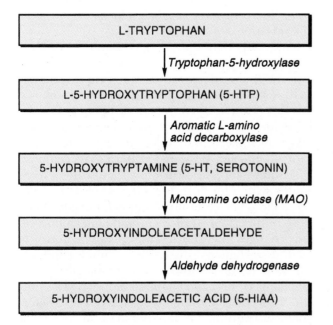

Figure 32-4. Biosynthetic pathway and metabolism of serotonin.

cardiovascular, respiratory, gastrointestinal, and other organ systems in the periphery, but it does not cross the blood–brain barrier. However, its precursors tryptophan and 5-hydroxytryptophan enter the brain fairly readily by facilitated transport.

5-HT-Receptor Agonists

Drugs with selective 5-HT-receptor-stimulating properties are of great interest for the investigation and treatment of conditions in which the function of tryptaminergic neurotransmission or receptors is implicated. Drugs with beneficial effects on mood, mentality, or certain behaviors such as excessive alcohol consumption, and without serious toxic effects, would have an enormous impact on society.

Sumatriptan succinate (Imitrex) is the first synthetic 5-HT analog that stimulates primarily 5-HT$_1$-receptors. In general, activation of 5-HT$_1$-receptor subtypes A–D may cause either vasodilatation or vasoconstriction by stimulation or inhibition of adenylyl cyclase, or, indirectly, by increased or decreased release of norepinephrine or acetylcholine. This drug is recommended for migraine therapy. It effectively relieves migraine headache by selective vasoconstriction within the carotid arterial circulation supplying the brain and meninges, mainly of dural blood vessels during the extensive vasodilatory (pain) phase of migraine.

Sumatriptan is rapidly absorbed after subcutaneous and oral administration. Mean oral bioavailability is only 14% because of extensive first-pass metabolism in the liver. Therapeutic plasma concentration is reached within 30–45 minutes after oral administration, but further absorption takes place for 4–6 hours. Mean plasma half-life is 2 hours. The plasma protein binding is low, in the 14–21% range.

Sumatriptan is not recommended for prophylactic use, and until further data are available it is contraindicated for hemiplegic or basilar migraine, for patients with ischemic heart disease, in uncontrolled hypertension, and in patients receiving treatment with MAO inhibitors, selective 5-HT reuptake inhibitors, and lithium.

Ergotamine and dihydroergotamine have been used for many decades for the treatment of migraine headache. Some of their properties, such as stimulation of 5-HT-receptors, are similar to those of sumatriptan, but they may have significant additional effects by blocking adrenergic receptors and causing vasoconstriction by a direct action on blood vessels.

Selective Serotonin Reuptake Inhibitors (SSRIs)

The use of SSRIs, including **fluoxetine, fluvoxamine, sertraline, paroxetine** and **trazodone,** in the treatment of major depressions is described in Chapter 29.

Drugs Influencing Endogenous Serotonin

Since tryptophan hydroxylase, the rate-limiting enzyme in 5-HT formation, is not saturated with its substrate, the administration of tryptophan can increase the levels of serotonin. In this manner, tryptophan may be of value in phenylketonuria.

The compounds that lower brain serotonin levels, such as parachlorophenylalanine (an inhibitor of tryptophan hydroxylase) and 5,7-dihydroxytryptamine (which destroys serotoninergic neurons), have no clinical use at present. Reserpine, a drug that depletes serotonin storage sites (but also those of other monoamines), has been used in the treatment of hypertension and psychosis. These effects are presumably exerted not via the serotoninergic system, but rather via the analogous effects of reserpine on noradrenergic and/or dopaminergic neurons.

Lysergic acid (LSD) and other hallucinogens selectively antagonize many peripheral actions of 5-HT. A similar antagonism of 5-HT actions in the brain has been suggested as the basis of the hallucinogenic effects of LSD, but this is not proven (see Chapter 30). Morphine partially blocks 5-HT action on the intestine.

Compounds that were designed and synthesized specifically to block the peripheral actions of 5-HT include methysergide, pizotifen, and cyproheptadine, as well as several newer agents described below.

Methysergide, a congener of LSD, is recommended for the prophylactic treatment of migraine. It takes 1–2 days to develop its full effect, and therapy should not be initiated during an acute attack. Continuous administration should not exceed 6 months without a drug-free interval of 3–4 weeks. Patients should be carefully monitored for side effects such as retroperitoneal or pleuropulmonary fibrosis, fibrotic changes in aortic and mitral valves, gastrointestinal disturbances, insomnia or mild euphoria, weight gain, dermatological and hematological manifestations, peripheral edema, and alopecia. The dose should be decreased gradually over 2–3 weeks before complete discontinuation in order to avoid "headache rebound."

Pizotifen was introduced for the prophylactic treatment of migraine headache. It is effective in reducing the frequency or severity of attacks. Since it is a potent serotonin and histamine antagonist and also has anticholinergic and sedative effects, the drug should be administered with caution, and drug-free intervals of 3–4 weeks should follow every 6 months of continuous therapy. The initial dose is 0.5 mg at bedtime; this is usually increased to 0.5 mg or more three times a day, but the total dose should not exceed 6 mg/24 hr. Unpleasant side effects are drowsiness, potentiation of CNS depressants (alcohol, antihistamines, etc.), headache, edema, dry mouth, and impotence. Hepatotoxic effects might occur after prolonged use.

Cyproheptadine is a potent 5-HT and histamine antagonist with mild anticholinergic and CNS-depressant properties. It is used primarily as an antipruritic agent when itching is caused by the release of 5-HT or histamine. It may cause weight gain and increased rate of growth in children. The CNS-depressant effects of other drugs may be potentiated if these are taken concomitantly with cyproheptadine. The usual adult dose is 4 mg, three to four times a day.

Ketanserin, a 5-HT$_2$-receptor blocker, relaxes vascular and tracheal smooth muscle and has been studied as a possible antihypertensive agent. It also blocks α_1-adrenoreceptors, H$_1$ histamine receptors, and dopamine receptors. It has not yet had wide clinical use.

Risperidone (Risperdal), similar to ketanserin, blocks 5-HT$_2$-receptors in low doses, and D$_2$ dopamine and α_1-adrenergic receptors in high doses. It is used primarily for the treatment of acute and chronic schizophrenic psychoses (see Chapter 28). Adverse effects include insomnia, agitation, extrapyramidal side effects, and headache. The recommended daily dose is 6 mg.

Ondansetron (Zofran) is a 5-HT$_3$-receptor antagonist used for the prevention and control of nausea and vomiting accompanying radiotherapy or antineoplastic chemotherapy. It has no extrapyramidal side effects. The most common adverse effects are headache, constipation, or transient diarrhea. The drug is available in tablets and injectable formulation. Doses range from 4 to 8 mg as required.

SUGGESTED READING

Antonaccio MJ. Angiotensin converting enzyme (ACE) inhibitors. Annu Rev Pharmacol Toxicol 1982; 22:57–87.

Case DB. Angiotensin-converting enzyme inhibitors: are they all alike? J Clin Hypertens 1987; 3(3):243–256.

Gregory RA, ed. Regulatory peptides of gut and brain. Br Med Bull 1982; 38(3):219–313.

Harrington MA, Zhong P, Garow SJ, Ciaranello RD. Molecular biology of serotonin receptors. J Clin Psychiatry 1992; 53 (Suppl 10):8–27.

MacKenzie ET, Scatton B. Cerebral circulatory and metabolic effects of perivascular neurotransmitters. CRC Crit Rev Clin Neurobiol 1987; 2(4):357–419.

Nathan C, Rolland Y. Pharmacological treatments that affect CNS activity: serotonin. Ann NY Acad Sci 1987; 499:277–296.

Opie LH. Angiotensin converting enzyme inhibitors. New York: Wiley-Liss, 1992.

Salvetti A. Newer ACE inhibitors. A look at the future. Drugs 1990; 40(6):800–828.

Serotonin in cardiovascular regulation. Satellite symposium to the 11th meeting of the International Society of Hypertension (several papers). J Cardiovasc Pharmacol 1987; 10 (Suppl 3).

Timmermans PB, Wong PC, Chiu AT, et al. Angiotensin II receptors and angiotensin II receptor antagonists. Pharmacol Rev 1993; 45:206–251.

Von Euler US, Pernow B, eds. Substance P. New York: Raven Press, 1977.

Weber C, Schmitt R, Birnboeck H, et al. Pharmacokinetics and pharmacodynamics of the endothelin-receptor antagonist bosentan in healthy human subjects. Clin Pharmacol Therap 1996; 60:124–137.

Zusman RM. Effects of converting-enzyme inhibitors on the renin-angiotensin-aldosterone, bradykinin and arachidonic acid-prostaglandin systems: correlation of chemical structure and biologic activity. Am J Kidney Dis 1987; 10 (Suppl 1):13–23.

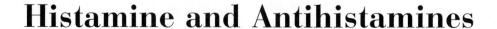

CHAPTER 33

Histamine and Antihistamines

D. KADAR

CASE HISTORY

A 48-year-old female in early menopause, but in good health on hormone replacement therapy, had suffered from seasonal hay fever in late summer and early autumn for several years. Self-medication with diphenhydramine or related antihistamines gave sufficient relief of symptoms for many years but was accompanied by a moderate degree of tolerable sedation. Recent newspaper and TV advertising convinced her that newer antihistamines would cause significantly less or no daytime sedation, whereupon she changed to terfenadine 60 mg three times a day. Because this drug is sold over-the-counter, she did not bother to inform her physician. She was happy with her choice because she experienced no sedation or any other side effects with this drug. Toward the end of the hay fever season she came down with an acute bacterial upper respiratory tract infection, for which her physician prescribed clarithromycin 250 mg twice daily. After 3 days of taking both terfenadine and clarithromycin, she complained of fatigue, headache, palpitation, and unusual weakness. ECG showed a significantly prolonged QT interval with ventricular dysrhythmia (torsade de pointes). On questioning, she told her physician about the terfenadine and it was replaced by diphenhydramine for the duration of the antibiotic therapy. She was warned not to mix the so-called low-sedating antihistamines with any other medication without prior consultation with her physician.

HISTAMINE AND ALLERGIC PHENOMENA

Histamine is widely distributed in nature. It occurs in practically all mammalian tissues and body fluids in varying concentrations.

Histamine is an amine formed by decarboxylation of the amino acid histidine (Fig. 33-1). Decarboxylation occurs in the same tissues in which histamine is stored, chiefly the lungs, skin, and gastrointestinal mucosa. In these tissues, histamine is present in the mast cells as small, dense granules of an inactive histamine–anionic polymer (heparin) complex along with other pharmacologically active chemicals and enzymes. It is also present in blood platelets and basophilic leukocytes (as chondroitin sulfate complex), as well as in the CNS and fetal liver. Histamine in tissues not containing mast cells is of lesser importance than in the mast cells and has a rapid turnover because of lack of a storage mechanism.

Histamine is released from tissues in free, active form by:

1. Destruction of cells, e.g., from bee sting venom, bacterial toxins, cold, injury
2. Dissolution of cytoplasmic granules, e.g., by surfactants, radiation
3. Histamine liberators, e.g., drugs (d-tubocurarine, morphine), foreign proteins, dextran, X-ray contrast media

Despite its wide distribution and potent pharmacological actions, the physiological role of histamine is not yet clear. Its effects are mediated through special histamine receptors that are designated as H_1, H_2, and H_3 types. A number of structural analogs of

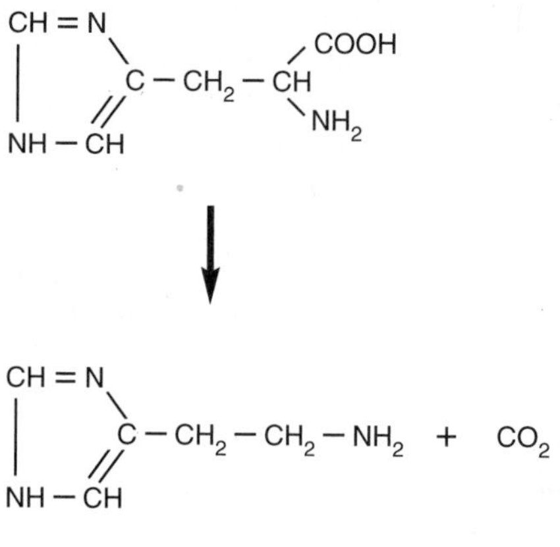

$$CH = N$$
$$| \qquad C - CH_2 - CH \begin{array}{c} COOH \\ \\ NH_2 \end{array}$$
$$NH - CH$$

↓

$$CH = N$$
$$| \qquad C - CH_2 - CH_2 - NH_2 \ + \ CO_2$$
$$NH - CH$$

Figure 33-1. Formation of histamine from histidine.

histamine have been synthesized, and more or less specific agonists have been identified for the H_1 (2-methylhistamine)-, H_2 (4-methylhistamine)-, and H_3 (N-α-methylhistamine)-receptors.

Mechanism of Action

Histamine H_1-, H_2-, and H_3-receptors are located on the cell surface, and the stimulus-response coupling is mediated through altered Ca^{2+} flow into the cell or increased utilization of intracellular calcium.

1. In general, H_1-receptor stimulation that results in contraction of the organ increases cyclic GMP concentrations and activates phospholipase C, thus causing increased formation of inositol-1,4,5-trisphosphate and 1,2-diacylglycerol, which in turn leads to increased cytosolic Ca^{2+} concentration and activation of protein kinases.
2. However, when H_1-receptor stimulation leads to smooth muscle relaxation, the mechanism of this action may involve activation of phospholipase A_2, release of arachidonic acid, and increased prostaglandin production. In addition, NO (now believed to be the endothelium-derived relaxing factor, EDRF) may activate guanylate cyclase to increase cyclic GMP levels to activate protein kinases and reduce calcium ion concentration.
3. H_2-receptor stimulation, leading to gastric acid secretion, smooth muscle relaxation, or inhibition of basophil degranulation, acts through cyclic AMP accumulation in the responding cell. In addition, H_2-receptors appear to have an autoregulatory role since their stimulation by histamine prevents further histamine release in some experimental preparations. Histamine may stimu-

late T-cell H_2 receptors, resulting in elevated cyclic AMP concentration and reduced T-cell-mediated cytotoxicity. Lymphocyte proliferation may also be reduced or suppressed. The suppressor-cell function is inhibited by H_1-receptor stimulation.

4. Histamine H_3-receptors are located in the CNS and in the periphery and act both as inhibitory autoreceptors on histamine-containing terminals and as inhibitors of release of various other neurotransmitters. The mechanisms of signal transduction underlying these actions are not yet fully known but appear to involve a G protein (G_i/G_o) and reduction of Ca^{2+} influx through an N-type calcium channel.

Pharmacological Effects

Combination of histamine with both H_1- and H_2-receptors leads to capillary dilatation and greatly increased permeability, with leakage of plasma proteins and fluid and their accumulation in extracellular spaces. In the skin this gives rise to the classical "triple response" to local injury: local reddening, wheal formation, and flare ("halo"). Urticaria is the cutaneous reaction to systemic histamine release or to allergens. On the other hand, histamine action on H_2-receptors blocks the degranulation of basophils by IgE.

The heart responds to medium-high systemic doses of histamine with positive chronotropism (H_2-receptors) and positive inotropism (H_1- and H_2-receptors).

Histamine stimulates exocrine secretions through action on both H_1-receptors (e.g., nasal and bronchial mucus) and H_2-receptors (stimulation of gastric HCl secretion; see Chapter 44).

Histamine stimulation of H_1-receptors on chromaffin cells causes the release of epinephrine from the adrenal medulla.

Stimulation of sensory nerve endings by histamine produces itch and pain (mainly H_1-receptors).

Histamine appears to play an important role in the production of certain types of migraine (vascular) headaches.

Histamine seems to have some as yet poorly understood neurotransmitter and neuroendocrine function in the CNS; H_1-, H_2-, and H_3-receptors appear to be involved (see Chapter 20).

Biotransformation

The inactivation of histamine occurs in many tissues by N-methylation or oxidative deamination (Fig. 33-2). The respective products, methylhistamine and imidazole acetic acid, are converted further to a number of other derivatives.

Allergy and Anaphylaxis

There is a marked similarity between the symptoms elicited by intravenous injection of histamine and those of anaphylactic shock and allergic reactions. In both conditions contraction of smooth muscle, dilatation and increased permeability of capillaries, stimulation of secretions, and action on sensory nerve endings occur. It is generally felt, although without complete agreement, that allergic and anaphylactic reactions are due to the release from storage sites of mediators of anaphylaxis such as histamine, 5-hydroxytryptamine, leukotrienes (SRS-A), eosinophil chemotactic factor of anaphylaxis (ECFA), prostaglandins, thromboxane A_2, neutrophil chemotactic factor, platelet activating factor (PAF), kinins, and protease enzymes.

The differences between localized allergic reactions (e.g., cutaneous, respiratory) and generalized anaphylactic reactions presumably depend upon the sites and rates of mediator release. If localized release of histamine is slow enough to permit inactivation of any that gets into the bloodstream, only a local allergic reaction is presumed to occur. However, if the release is too rapid and explosive for inactivation to keep pace, the reaction will be of the anaphylactic type.

Drug-induced histamine release can be triggered by antigen–antibody reactions, but most often the presence of circulating (IgG) or cell-bound (IgE) antibodies cannot be detected. X-ray contrast media in the absence of antibodies may liberate massive amounts of histamine, causing anaphylactoid reactions, often with fatal outcome.

Measures for the control of allergy and anaphylaxis may be either prophylactic or therapeutic and may be either specific or symptomatic depending on their locus of action.

Prophylactic treatment of asthma and certain allergic conditions with nedocromil sodium or cromolyn sodium (sodium cromoglycate) hinders the release of histamine and other autacoids from mast cells and other cell types (see Chapter 40).

Ketotifen fumarate (Zaditen), a prophylactic-antiallergic agent against pediatric asthma, blocks H_1-receptors but in addition has an apparently separate anti-inflammatory effect in the lungs. It inhibits release of leukotrienes, prevents bronchoconstriction induced by leukotrienes and by PAF, and decreases PAF-induced platelet and eosinophil accumulation in the airways.

Specific therapy would be the avoidance or elimination of offending antigens or the desensitization of the sensitive individual.

Symptomatic therapy with H_1-receptor blockers ("antihistamines") will relieve the effects of histamine release, as in hay fever. If H_1-receptor blockade is not effective or not practical, physiological antagonists such as epinephrine, specific β_2-adrenoceptor stimulants, or theophylline can be used. In serious cases beclomethasone by inhalation or nasal spray for localized effects can be as effective as systemic glucocorticoid therapy.

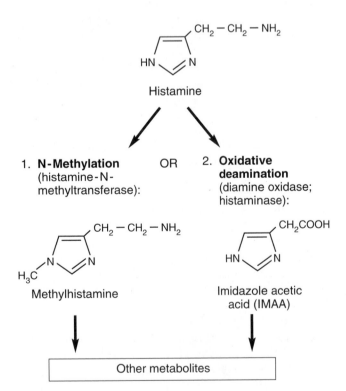

Figure 33-2. Biotransformation of histamine.

Clinical Uses

Histamine is used occasionally to assess the ability of the stomach to secrete acid and to test bronchial reactivity. Pentagastrin, a synthetic analog of gastrin, is now preferred for stimulation of gastric HCl secretion; it has fewer unwanted effects than either histamine or other histamine analogs.

Histamine can be used to test the integrity of sensory nerves and as a provocative agent for the diagnosis of pheochromocytoma.

HISTAMINE H$_1$-RECEPTOR BLOCKERS

In 1937 Bovet and Staub detected histamine-blocking activity in one of a series of amines with a phenolic ether function. This substance (2-isopropyl-5-methylphenoxyethyldiethylamine) protected guinea pigs against lethal doses of histamine, antagonized histamine-induced spasms of smooth muscle, and lessened the symptoms of anaphylactic shock (these are now known to be H$_1$-receptor-mediated reactions). It was too weak and too toxic for therapeutic use, but the synthesis of related substances resulted, in 1942, in the first clinically employed antihistamine, phenbenzamine (Antergan). Other highly effective histamine antagonists followed rapidly.

Classification

All antihistamines have the same basic structure, consisting of two aryl rings attached to one end of a three-atom (C, O, S, or N) chain or its steric equivalent, with a dimethylamine group at the other end, as shown in Fig. 33-3. In addition, the terminal dimethylamine group may be incorporated into a ring structure, as in chlorcyclizine (Figs. 33-3 and 33-4).

From all these possible constituents, a tremendous number of combinations can be made. There have been more than 4000 such compounds synthesized and tested, and several dozen are in clinical use. However, none of these will inhibit the histamine-induced stimulation of gastric acid secretion, an H$_2$-receptor-mediated reaction. Table 33-1 lists the most-often-used histamine H$_1$-receptor blockers, of which some examples are shown in Figure 33-4.

Mechanism and Site of Action

The mechanism and site of action are virtually identical for all H$_1$-receptor blockers. The basic structure of conventional antihistamines contains a portion that is similar to the essential structure of histamine

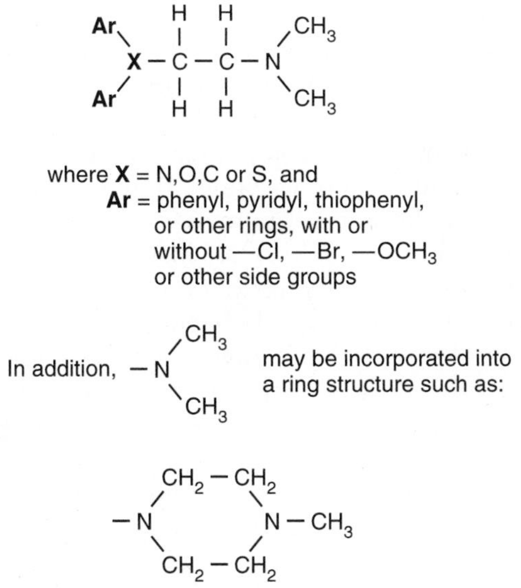

Diphenhydramine

Chlorpheniramine

Chlorcyclizine

Promethazine

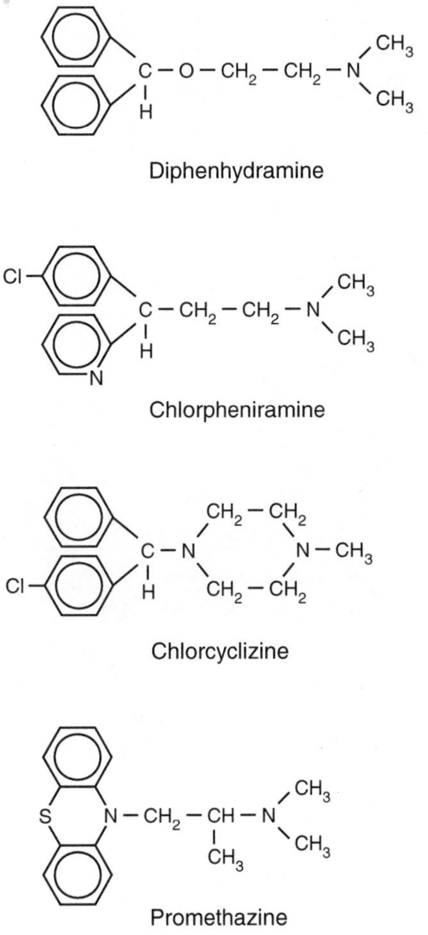

Figure 33-4. Examples of antihistamines (H$_1$-receptor blockers).

where **X** = N,O,C or S, and
Ar = phenyl, pyridyl, thiophenyl, or other rings, with or without —Cl, —Br, —OCH$_3$ or other side groups

In addition, a dimethylamine group may be incorporated into a ring structure such as:

Figure 33-3. Basic structure of antihistamines (H$_1$-receptor blockers).

Table 33-1 Most Often Used Antihistamines (H$_1$-Receptor-Blocking Agents) by Class, Nonproprietary Name, Brand Name, Routes of Administration

Ethanolamines
Diphenhydramine (Benadryl)
   oral, parenteral
*Dimenhydrinate (Dramamine, Gravol)
   * oral, rectal, parenteral

Ethylenediamines
Tripelennamine (Pyribenzamine)
   oral, topical
Antazoline (Antistine)
   oral
Naphazoline (Privine)
   nasal

Alkylamines
Chlorpheniramine (Chlor-Tripolon)
   oral, parenteral
Brompheniramine (Dimetane)
   oral

Piperazines
*Cyclizine (Marzine)
   oral, rectal, parenteral
*Meclizine (Antivert, Bonamine)
   oral
Cetirizine (Reactine)
   oral

Phenothiazine
Promethazine (Phenergan)
   oral, rectal, parenteral

Piperidines
Astemizole (Hismanal)
   oral
Loratadine (Claritin)
   oral
Terfenadine (Seldane)
   oral

*Used primarily for prevention of nausea, vomiting, and motion sickness.

itself. This similarity is sufficient to permit the antihistamines to compete for the histamine receptor sites on target cells, while the differences are such as to render them inactive as histamine substitutes; i.e., they are competitive blockers of histamine. This can be demonstrated with isolated tissues in vitro.

In vivo, conventional antihistamines, i.e., H$_1$-receptor blockers, antagonize all the actions of histamine, except the stimulation of HCl secretion in the stomach and that part of the vasodilatation that is mediated by H$_2$-receptors.

Pharmacokinetics

All H$_1$-receptor blockers are well absorbed following oral administration, and maximum serum levels are achieved within 1–2 hours. The bioavailability is high, except that of rectally administered preparations, which depend on too many variables to be predictably absorbed. The older antihistamines, such as diphenhydramine and chlorpheniramine, are distributed in all tissues including the CNS, but the newer agents (e.g., loratidine, astemizole) do not appear to enter the CNS as readily. Plasma protein binding is variable. The major site of biotransformation of all antihistaminic drugs is the liver, and minute amounts of the unchanged drugs and most of the metabolites are excreted in the urine. Some of the metabolites are active and contribute to the total duration of action of the parent compound. Cetirizine is itself a metabolite of the anxiolytic agent hydroxyzine, which also has H$_1$-receptor-blocking activity (see Chapter 27). The plasma half-life varies widely: For many of the older compounds it is in the range of 4–6 hours, but for the piperazine and piperidine groups it tends to be closer to 24 hours or even longer.

Pharmacological Effects

Antihistamines offer almost complete protection against the effects of injected histamine, but their effectiveness is less complete against endogenously liberated histamine. The histamine-induced contraction of gastrointestinal or respiratory smooth muscle is diminished or abolished both in vivo and in vitro. The H$_1$-receptor-mediated component of increased capillary permeability and vasodilatation is inhibited, especially if the antihistamine is administered before liberation of, or exposure to, histamine. This latter consideration is particularly important for astemizole, because its full clinical effects develop only after 2–3 days of medication. Salivary, lacrimal, and bronchial secretions are reduced or arrested if the activity of the glands was due to excessive histamine stimulation.

The H$_1$-receptor blockers have limited effectiveness in severe allergic or anaphylactic reactions. In serious cases, or in the presence of laryngeal edema, epinephrine remains the drug of choice.

The effects of H$_1$-receptor blockers on the CNS

are unpredictable. Most often they cause CNS depression, but in some patients agitation or restlessness may occur. The pharmacological effect involved in the prevention of motion sickness is not fully understood, and not all H_1-blockers are equally effective against motion sickness.

Additional and Adverse Effects

All antihistamines have some **CNS-depressant** effects, but these are much less marked with astemizole, loratadine, and terfenadine, presumably because of their reduced entry into the CNS. Some antihistamines are good sedatives or hypnotics (e.g., promethazine, which has a phenothiazine nucleus). Others have antitussive properties (e.g., diphenhydramine). The relative prominence of these effects varies from one antihistamine to another.

All antihistamines have **local anesthetic** activity, and some are quite potent in this respect. The dimethylaminoethanol group, either in ester or ether linkage, is common to the local anesthetics and to many antihistamines (see Chapter 11).

Like the local anesthetics, the antihistamines in high doses cause central stimulation and may cause convulsions, as may sometimes be observed in attempted suicide with antihistamines.

Also like the local anesthetics, and like procainamide and quinidine (which also share the dialkylaminoethyl group), the antihistamines are cardiac depressants when given in high dosage.

Some of the antihistamines, and especially those in Figure 33-3 in which $X = O$, are potent **anticholinergics**. If the acetyl group in acetylcholine is replaced by progressively larger groups, the acetylcholine-like action becomes less and less, and it is finally converted into an anticholinergic effect. Benzilic acid esters of choline (e.g., oxyphenonium) are good examples. Oxygen-containing antihistamines have a chemical resemblance to these choline esters, which suggests a basis for this anticholinergic activity.

Some antihistamines, especially the phenothiazine derivatives, are adrenergic blockers, while others have a weak ganglioplegic effect.

Thus, all antihistaminic drugs have adverse effects to some degree. It is obvious that the side effects differ for different drugs, because they derive from chemical features other than those responsible for antihistaminic action. The incidence and severity of side effects also vary greatly between individual subjects. Therefore, in prescribing a given antihista-

mine, it is essential to know the particular constellation of side effects for that drug and to expect that about one person in four will experience some bothersome reaction during antihistamine therapy.

The most frequently observed side effect common to most histamine antagonists is **sedation.** Other untoward reactions, including dizziness, tinnitus, lassitude, incoordination, fatigue, blurred vision, and tremors, are referable to central actions of the antihistamines. Some side effects involve the digestive tract (loss of appetite, nausea), and these drugs may cause dryness of the mouth (atropine-like effect). All of these troublesome symptoms may or may not disappear with continued therapy.

The most recently introduced antihistaminic drugs, cetirizine, astemizole, loratadine, and terfenadine, are claimed to be generally free of CNS-related side effects and to have a lower incidence of other side effects. In addition, they do not appear to intensify the CNS-depressant effects of other drugs or alcohol. Side effects recorded in some clinical trials have been not much greater in frequency than those of placebo. Nevertheless, patients with heart disease should be watched for any changes in cardiac performance.

The simultaneous administration of metronidazole, systemic antifungals (e.g., ketoconazole, fluconazole), macrolide antibiotics (e.g., erythromycin), or any other drug that inhibits the cytochrome P450 isozyme responsible for the biotransformation of terfenadine or the other nonsedating antihistamines is contraindicated. Severe interference with cardiac rhythm was reported in susceptible individuals taking these medications concurrently.

The antihistamines can themselves evoke allergic reactions, presumably by acting as haptens that combine with some tissue protein to form antigen complexes. The usual drug allergies, including agranulocytosis and chronic dermatoses, are thus occasionally produced by these drugs, especially if used topically or intermittently, as against the common cold, in which they have relatively little beneficial effect.

Interactions of antihistamines with other drugs can have serious consequences. The older antihistaminics potentiate the central effects of all other CNS-depressant drugs including alcohol. Patients taking antihistamines, even if only one dose, should be warned not to drink alcohol, or to drive, or to operate dangerous machinery while under the influence of the drug. In many countries, including the United States and Canada, the use of antihistamines, as in cough and cold preparations, is generally not a mitigating factor in impaired-driving charges. Almost all cough and cold preparations contain substances that are banned by Olympic and other sports organizations.

Acute Poisoning

Although the margin of safety of antihistamines is relatively high, and chronic toxicity is rare, acute poisoning with these drugs is not uncommon, especially in young children.

In acute poisoning, central effects predominate and are the greatest danger. The syndrome includes hallucinations, excitement, ataxia, and convulsions. The latter are difficult to control. In the child, the picture includes fixed dilated pupils, flushed face and fever, and is remarkably similar to that of atropine poisoning. If untreated, deepening coma and cardio-respiratory collapse may lead to death within a few hours. In the adult, fever and flushing are less severe, and drowsiness and coma often precede the excitatory (convulsive) phase. Since there is no specific therapy for antihistamine poisoning, treatment is generally symptomatic and supportive.

Therapeutic Applications

Suppression of allergic phenomena

Antihistamines give good results in nasal allergies (hay fever), acute skin reactions (urticaria, drug rashes), and systemic allergic reactions (serum sickness, transfusion reaction, etc.), but they are almost without effect against asthma and chronic skin allergies. Perhaps it is a matter of differential ability of these drugs to penetrate to the sites of endogenous release of histamine and other "autacoids" (5-HT, prostaglandins, etc.). It is also conceivable that different and as yet unrecognized receptor variants are involved.

Antiparkinsonian use

Atropine and various synthetic atropine-like drugs have an antiparkinsonian effect that generally parallels their anticholinergic activity (see Chapter 21). The oxygen-containing antihistamines, which have anticholinergic side effects as already noted, also have useful antiparkinsonian properties. Orphenadrine is used almost exclusively for this purpose. It

is possibly more useful in the short-term treatment of parkinsonian symptoms that may occur as a side effect of phenothiazine neuroleptic therapy than in the long-term treatment of postencephalitic parkinsonism, because the drug tends to lose its effectiveness after a few months.

Anti–motion-sickness use

Nausea and vomiting can result from several different types of stimuli. The phenothiazine neuroleptics are effective suppressants of the chemoreceptor trigger zone, but they do not block the effects of vestibular stimuli. Some, but not all, antihistamines do prevent or diminish nausea and vomiting mediated by both the vestibular and the chemoreceptor pathways. Among the most effective ones are promethazine, cyclizine, meclizine, and dimenhydrinate. These are different chemical types, with different side effects, so the antiemetic action appears to be independent of the antihistaminic and other actions mentioned before.

Recent approaches to the control of hyperemesis of multifactorial origin also employ other agents. Nabilone (Cesamet) and dronabinol (Marinol) are cannabinoid antiemetics used in cancer chemotherapy to control nausea and vomiting (see Chapter 30). However, they also have sedative and psychotropic properties which limit their usefulness in many patients. Transderm-V, a thin multilayer circular film containing 1.5 mg scopolamine, is applied to the skin behind the ear approximately 12 hours before an antiemetic effect is required. There is a sustained absorption of scopolamine for about 3 days while the tape is in contact with the skin. Scopolamine produces all the side effects of atropine (see Chapter 15).

HISTAMINE H_2-RECEPTOR BLOCKERS

The H_2-receptor-blocking agents constitute a clinically important group having very little if any affinity for H_1-receptors. Unfortunately, the first two agents (burimamide and metiamide) that were found to be clinically effective in blocking the stimulatory effects of histamine and of pentagastrin on gastric HCl secretion may cause agranulocytosis; therefore their use has been discontinued. However, safer new H_2-receptor-blocking drugs are now in use. Their molecular structure contains a portion that resembles the histamine molecule, but the five-membered ring varies: cimetidine retains the imidazole ring of histamine, but in newer drugs of this class it is replaced by furan or thiazol rings.

Cimetidine

Mechanism of action

This drug acts on H_2-receptors located in stomach, blood vessels, and other sites in the body. It is a competitive antagonist of histamine, and its effect is fully reversible. It has no affinity for H_1- or other known receptors.

Cimetidine (Tagamet, Peptol) (Fig. 33-5) completely inhibits gastric acid secretion induced by histamine, gastrin, or pentagastrin; that induced by acetylcholine or bethanechol is only partly inhibited. In therapeutic concentrations it inhibits gastric HCl secretion in all phases following solid, liquid, or sham food feeding, or after insulin and caffeine administration. Extremely high doses paradoxically facilitate histamine release by blocking the H_2-receptor-mediated negative-feedback mechanism.

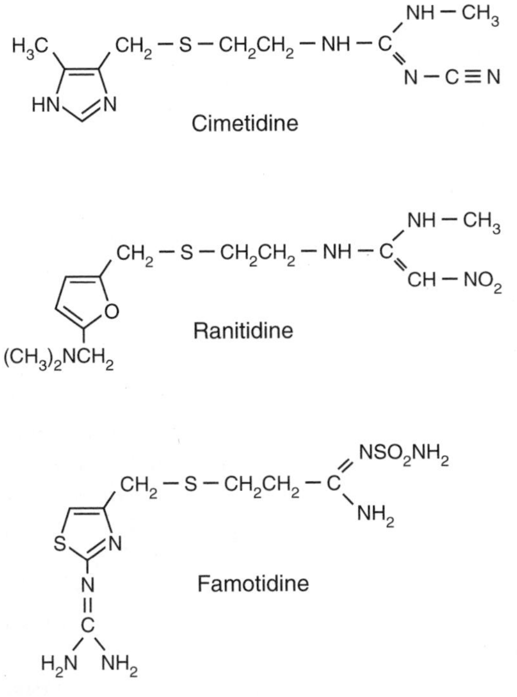

Figure 33-5. Structural formulae of cimetidine, ranitidine, and famotidine (H_2-receptor blockers).

Pharmacokinetics

Close to 80% of an orally administered dose is absorbed, and maximum blood concentrations appear in 1–1.5 hours. The therapeutic plasma concentration is about 2 μmoles/L. It is unevenly distributed in the various organs of the body; it crosses the placental barrier, but it does not cross the blood–brain barrier easily because of its high water solubility. It can be found in the CSF in concentrations about 30% of those in plasma. Less than 25% is bound to plasma proteins. Cimetidine has two major metabolites, which are excreted in urine together with about 50% of unchanged drug. The serum half-life is short, about 1–1.5 hours, but longer in renal failure.

Adverse effects

The adverse effects of cimetidine are usually minor and are mainly associated with the reduced gastric juice production. Headache, confusion, hallucinations, dizziness, or other CNS-related side effects may occur primarily in the elderly or following prolonged administration, as for treatment of the Zollinger-Ellison syndrome, a chronic gastric hypersecretory state. A few cases of mild gynecomastia have been reported, but no endocrine basis for it has been found. Cimetidine can bind to androgen receptors, and at very high doses it can reduce the sperm count. It is practically nontoxic, even following accidental overdose of 10 g or so. The heart rate may be increased, probably as a reflex response to mild reduction in blood pressure. Cimetidine reduces the rate of hepatic cytochrome P450-dependent biotransformation of a number of drugs. It also may competitively inhibit the renal tubular secretion of other organic bases (e.g., procainamide). The circulating gastrin concentration is elevated during cimetidine administration.

Ranitidine

Mechanism of action; pharmacokinetics

Ranitidine (Zantac) is a very potent H_2-receptor blocker. Its mechanism and site of action, as well as its pharmacological effects, are similar to those of cimetidine, but ranitidine is five to 10 times more potent. Only 50% of an orally administered dose is absorbed and maximum plasma concentration occurs 1–2 hours later. The plasma half-life is 3 hours. The distribution and plasma protein binding are similar to those of cimetidine. Ranitidine has two minor metabolites, which are excreted in urine, but most of the drug is eliminated unchanged.

Adverse effects

Adverse effects of ranitidine include mild and infrequent gastrointestinal complaints, and rare CNS side effects. Drug interactions at the renal or hepatic level are less frequent than with cimetidine, because ranitidine does not inhibit cytochrome P450. Endocrine-related symptoms have not been reported, and ranitidine does not block androgen receptors. Ranitidine is considered to be practically nontoxic, although elevation of serum transaminase levels and possible hepatocellular injury have been reported in a few cases.

Famotidine

Famotidine (Pepcid), another member of the group of very potent H_2-receptor blockers, has a thiazole ring in place of the imidazole (see Fig. 33-5).

Mechanism of action; pharmacokinetics

The mechanism of action, pharmacological effects, site of action, indications, and clinical use are the same as for the other H_2-receptor antagonists. Famotidine is three to 20 times as potent as ranitidine. Less than 45% of an oral dose is absorbed; maximum plasma concentration occurs 1–3 hours later. The plasma half-life is 2.5–3.5 hours in patients with normal kidney function; but with creatinine clearance of less than 10 mL/min the elimination half-life can be 12 hours or longer, and 20 hours or more in anuric patients. About 30% of an oral dose and 65–70% of an intravenous dose are eliminated in the urine unchanged, and the rest is eliminated as sulfoxide metabolite. The recommended single daily dose of 20–40 mg at bedtime inhibits up to 94% of nocturnal gastric acid secretion, and 25–30% for another 8–10 hours later. The nocturnal intragastric pH is between 5.0 and 6.4.

Adverse effects

Adverse effects of famotidine observed during controlled clinical trials were few and of minor importance. They are similar to those of ranitidine. The frequency of these reactions was comparable to those recorded in the placebo group, and a causal relation-

ship could not be established. Most often observed were headache, dizziness, constipation, and diarrhea. Treatment of accidental or intentional overdosage should be symptomatic and supportive. Daily doses of up to 640 mg, administered to patients with pathological hypersecretory conditions, had no serious adverse effects. With chronic treatment, gastric emptying and exocrine pancreatic functions are not affected, but an increase in gastric bacterial flora may occur. Because adverse effects can emerge after years of extensive clinical use of new drugs, careful observation of patients treated with famotidine is advised. In healthy volunteers famotidine in clinical doses caused significant increases in cardiac preejection period and decreases in stroke volume and cardiac output without significant change in heart rate or blood pressure.

Nizatidine

Nizatidine (Axid) is the most recently approved H_2-receptor blocker for the treatment of acute duodenal and benign gastric ulcers. It is absorbed rapidly after oral administration, reaching peak serum concentrations in 0.5–3 hours. Food has no significant effect on bioavailability. About 35% is protein-bound, mainly to α_1-glycoprotein. The volume of distribution is between 0.8 and 1.5 L/kg, plasma half-life is 1–2 hours, and 60% of the dose is excreted in the urine as unchanged drug. The average plasma clearance is about 50 L/hr, which can be reduced to 7–14 L/hr in patients with creatinine clearance of 10 mL/min or less, giving rise to a plasma half-life of 4–11 hours. An oral dose of 300 mg at bedtime can suppress gastric acid secretion for 10–12 hours.

In short-term trials nizatidine was found to be free of hormonal interference and had no effect on the drug-metabolizing P450 enzymes. In clinical trials the frequency of observed side effects such as headache, somnolence, and pruritus was somewhat higher than in the placebo group, but a relationship to nizatidine administration could not be established. Serum cholesterol, serum uric acid, serum creatinine, and platelet and WBC counts showed statistically significant differences from the placebo group, and serum transaminases have been elevated in a few cases, but the clinical importance of these changes is not clear. In healthy volunteers nizatidine was shown to have a negative chronotropic influence with increased cardiac preejection period and decreased heart rate and cardiac output, without change in stroke volume.

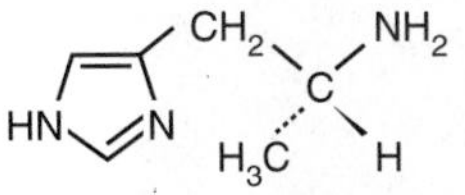

(R)α - Methylhistamine

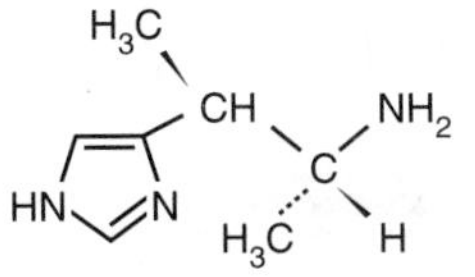

(αR, βS)α, β - Dimethylhistamine

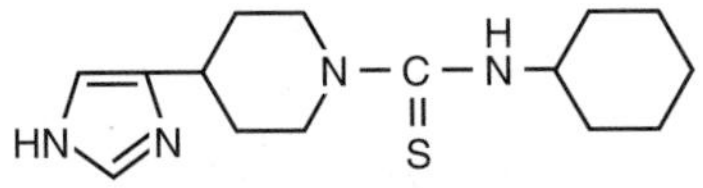

Thioperamide

Figure 33-6. Structural formulae of H_3-receptor agonists and the H_3-receptor-blocker thioperamide.

Clinical Uses of H_2-Receptor Blockers

Therapeutic applications of these agents are identical. H_2-receptor blockers are useful in the treatment of conditions that require a reduction of gastric acid secretion, such as treatment of duodenal ulcer, non-malignant gastric ulcer, gastroesophageal reflux disease, pathological hypersecretion states associated with Zollinger-Ellison syndrome, systemic mastocytosis, and multiple endocrine adenomas. They are also described in this specific context in Chapter 44.

Histamine H_3-Receptor Agonists and Blockers

Histamine H_3-receptors found in the CNS are located on presynaptic histaminergic neurons and modulate

the synthesis of histamine and its release into the synaptic cleft. H_3-Agonists ([R]α-methylhistamine and [$αR$, $βS$]α,β-dimethylhistamine) (Fig. 33-6) are used to study the distribution of H_3-receptors in the brain and peripheral tissues and to determine their physiological and pathological role.

Thioperamide (N-cyclohexy-4-[imidazol-4-yl]-1-piperidine carbothioamide) (Fig. 33-6) is the most often used histamine H_3-receptor blocker. It appears that most but not all histamine-induced actions in vitro, and in animal models, are blocked by H_1-, H_2-, and H_3-receptor blockers. In the periphery, additional distinct histamine receptors are expected to be discovered shortly.

SUGGESTED READING

Estelle F, Simmons R, Simmons KJ. Pharmacokinetic optimisation of histamine H_1-receptor antagonist therapy. Clin Pharmacokinet 1991; 21:372–393.

Feldman M, Barton ME. Histamine H_2 antagonists. N Engl J Med 1990; 323:1672–1680.

Hill SJ. Distribution, properties, and functional characteristics of three classes of histamine receptor. Pharmacol Rev 1990; 42:45–83.

O'Connor BJ, Lecomte JM, Barnes PJ. Effect of an inhaled histamine H_3-receptor agonist on airway responses to sodium metabisulphite in asthma. Br J Clin Pharmacol 1993; 35:55–57.

Pounder R, ed. Histamine H_2-receptor antagonists. London: Science Press, 1990.

Raud J, Thorlacius J, Xie X, Lindbom L, Hedqvist P. Interactions between histamine and leukotrienes in the microcirculation. Aspects of relevance to acute allergic inflammation. Ann NY Acad Sci 1994; 744:191–198.

Rimmer SJ, Church MK. The pharmacology and mechanisms of action of histamine H_1-antagonists. Clin Exp Allergy 1990; 20 (Suppl 2):3–17.

Timmerman H, van der Goot H, eds. New perspectives in histamine research. Basel: Birkhauser Verlag, 1990.

CHAPTER 34

Anti-Inflammatory Analgesics

D. KADAR

CASE HISTORY

A 64-year-old man who had been treated for several years with hydrochlorothiazide 25 mg every other day for moderate hypertension began to experience mild pain and discomfort in the hip area. He started self-medication with ibuprofen 600 mg at bedtime. During a routine checkup 2 months later his blood pressure was found to be moderately elevated, and the dose of diuretic needed to be increased to 50 mg for adequate control. Ibuprofen was replaced with enteric-coated acetylsalicylic acid (ASA) 650 mg to control the discomfort of the patient's arthritis. A few weeks later the patient complained of epigastric pain and painful swelling of one of his big toes. He was found to have hyperuricemia, and ASA was replaced with acetaminophen 500 mg. The diuretic was changed to furosemide 40 mg every other day, and allopurinol 100 mg daily with food was added to control the hyperuricemia. After 2 months the antihypertensive medication was changed to the more specific agent fosinopril 10 mg daily, and allopurinol was discontinued because the blood uric acid concentration had normalized and the pain and swelling of the toe had subsided. The pain and discomfort in the hip area were well controlled by the administration of a combined preparation of diclofenac sodium 50 mg and misoprostol 200 μg twice daily, supplemented by occasional acetaminophen if needed. Blood uric acid tests and general follow-up examinations were ordered at 3-month intervals.

(Note: Other designations for this group of drugs are: antipyretic-analgesics, anti-inflammatory agents, nonsteroidal anti-inflammatory drugs [NSAIDs], and nonnarcotic analgesics.)

The beneficial effect of willow bark extract in fever and pain was known to ancient civilizations, but the first reliable description of its antipyretic effect is attributed to Edmund Stone, who was searching for an inexpensive substitute for cinchona bark in the 18th century. The active ingredient, salicin, a bitter glycoside, was isolated in 1827, and various derivatives were later found in other plants. Acetylsalicylic acid (ASA) was synthesized by Gerhardt in 1853 and introduced into medicine by Dreser in 1899 under the Bayer Pharmaceutical Co. trade name of Aspirin. (In Canada, "Aspirin" is still a patented trade name, but in the United States and many other countries "aspirin" is a nonproprietary name.)

The sharp increase in the number of anti-inflammatory drugs released for medicinal use during the last 20 years can be attributed to the ease and reliability of modern in vitro and in vivo testing for the desired pharmacological action. All of these drugs inhibit prostaglandin synthesis and prevent the development of carrageenan-induced rat paw edema (Table 34-1). With these two rather simple experimental models, hundreds of chemicals can be screened in relatively short time. Since prostaglandin synthesis is tissue- and species-specific, however, the final evaluation of the beneficial and toxic properties of such drugs requires extensive long-term experience in human subjects.

Pain is essential for survival. It can serve as a

Table 34-1 Comparison of Prostaglandin Synthase Inhibitory Activity and Anti-inflammatory Potency of Selected Nonopioid Analgesics

Drug	Inhibition of Prostaglandin Synthase (IC_{50}, μg/mL)	Reduction of Carrageenan-Induced Rat Paw Edema (ED_{50}, mg/kg)
Piroxicam	0.06	4.0
Indomethacin	0.06	6.5
Mefenamic acid	0.17	55.0
Phenylbutazone	2.23	100.0
ASA	6.62	150.0
Acetaminophen	100	Inactive

warning of impending or actual tissue or organ injury. Humans usually do not "adapt" to pain. The sensation originates from stimulation of naked nerve endings found in all parts of the body. The pain receptors (nociceptors) can be stimulated by mechanical or chemical means. Pain-producing substances such as histamine or kinins stimulate the naked nerve endings directly, while prostaglandins lower the pain threshold by increasing the sensitivity of the receptors to the stimulus. PGE_2 and $PGF_{2\alpha}$ are known to cause local pain at sites of injection, vascular pain, and headache.

The sensation of pain is transmitted from the periphery through the spinal cord to higher integrative centers in the CNS by "fast" myelinated Aδ fibers at 10–30 m/sec, and by nonmyelinated "slow" C fibers at 0.5–2 m/sec. When first-order sensory neurons from a diseased organ and from another area of the body synapse on the same second-order neurons in the spinal cord, pain actually originating in the diseased organ may be perceived as coming from the other area; this is known as "referred pain." The intensity of pain sensation can be influenced by distraction (e.g., "white noise"), hypnosis, placebo or suggestion, acupuncture, local anesthetics, nerve section, or analgesic drugs. Anxiolytics and neuroleptics may diminish the emotional response to pain through action on the limbic system and hypothalamus. Morphine and other opioid analgesics act on opiate receptors in the gray matter around the cerebral aqueduct and adjacent to the third and fourth ventricles (see Chapter 23).

Fever is the body's response to exogenous or endogenous substances called pyrogens. Bacteria, molds, yeasts, and viruses elaborate high-molecular-weight lipopolysaccharides capable of stimulating the release of "pyrogens" such as cytokines (interleukin-1 [IL-1]) from polymorphonuclear leukocytes and monocytes, and tumor necrosis factor from other cells. These pyrogens act on the thermoreceptive region in the preoptic anterior hypothalamus to release arachidonic acid, stimulate prostaglandin synthesis (see Chapter 31), and raise the set point of the temperature-regulating center, which in turn will lead to vasoconstriction in the skin, decreased heat loss, and increased body temperature. Administration of type E prostaglandin to the cerebral ventricles of experimental animals causes fever. Fever arising from extensive tissue damage, autoimmune disease, neoplasia, or following thromboembolism is thought to be due to the release of a leukocyte-type pyrogen from the involved tissue. Salicylates and other antipyretic drugs appear to act by inhibiting the synthesis or release of prostaglandins in the thermoregulatory center.

The **inflammatory process** can be initiated by invading microorganisms, immunological reactions, tissue decay, and many other less-known phenomena. Mediators of inflammation are thought to cause increased release of fatty acid precursors of prostaglandins and to increase the rate of prostaglandin synthesis. Prostaglandins may cause inflammation on their own, or they may aggravate a preexisting inflammatory condition. Endogenous mediators of inflammation may originate from the plasma (such as bradykinin, C_3 and C_5 fragments, $C_{\overline{567}}$ complex, fibrinopeptides, fibrin degradation products) and from tissues (such as histamine, serotonin, leukotrienes [SRS-A], prostaglandins, lysosomal proteases, migration inhibitory factor, chemotactic factors, lymphotoxin, skin reactive factors, mitogenic factors, lymph node permeability factor, interleukin-1, platelet activating factor [PAF]). Endogenous pyrogens and leukocytosis factors may be liberated, causing local redness, swelling, heat, pain, and disturbed function of the involved organ. Most prostaglandins are known to cause peripheral vasodilatation with local redness and edema formation and to synergistically increase the effect of bradykinin. Practically every part of the body may suffer damage as the result of an inflammatory process. Drugs do not reverse the damage, but they may arrest the process or slow its progress. In addition, the intensity of the pain may be significantly reduced or eliminated.

Anti-inflammatory drugs reduce pain and tissue damage by inhibiting prostaglandin synthesis (Table 34-1). In addition, one or more of the following may contribute to the anti-inflammatory effect: (1) inhibition of leukocyte migration and phagocytosis, during which histamine, serotonin, and other substances (autacoids) may often be released; (2) stabilization of lysosomal membranes, thus preventing the escape of lysosomal enzymes into the cytoplasm, and damage to cell structures; and (3) inhibition of plasmin, a plasma proteolytic enzyme that may activate kinin formation. The composition, biosynthesis, or metabolism of connective tissue mucopolysaccharides can also be affected.

The suppression of antigen–antibody reactions by anti-inflammatory drugs may be due to depressed antibody production, interference with antigen–antibody reactions, reduced histamine release, or cell membrane stabilization.

SALICYLATES

Acetylsalicylic acid (ASA) is the most frequently used member of this class of drugs. The others are salicylic acid, sodium salicylate, choline salicylate, choline magnesium salicylate, salicylamide, methylsalicylate, salsalate, 5-aminosalicylate, and diflunisal. The chemical structures of salicylic acid, ASA, and diflunisal are shown in Figure 34-1.

Mechanism and Site of Action

The analgesic, antipyretic, and anti-inflammatory actions of salicylates are attributed primarily to their ability to inhibit cyclooxygenase, the enzyme responsible for the conversion of arachidonic acid to prostaglandin peroxides. This action of the drugs is exerted both in the periphery and at the hypothalamic ther-

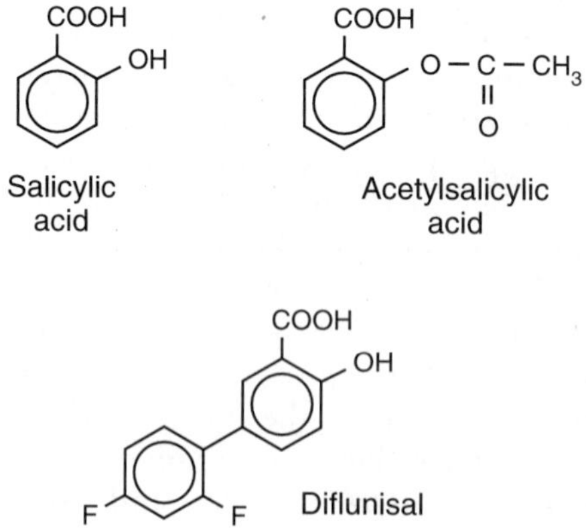

Figure 34-1. Structural formulae of three salicylates.

moregulatory center (see Chapter 31). ASA acetylates the serine moiety at or near the active center of the enzyme; the inhibition is irreversible, and restoration of prostaglandin production requires biosynthesis of new enzyme. In addition, salicylates may inhibit formation of plasmin, and thereby of bradykinin. They also block the production of pain by kinins acting on chemoreceptors.

Pharmacokinetics

Orally administered ASA is absorbed by passive diffusion, partly in the stomach but to a large extent also in the small intestine. The absorption of all acidic drugs including the salicylates is influenced by the pH of the aqueous layer next to the mucous membrane. In the stomach, the low pH enhances absorption because the uncharged molecules of weakly acidic drugs are able to penetrate lipid membranes with relative ease. In the intestines, at almost neutral pH, the effect of reduced absorption due to ionization is offset by the greater solubility in water, which aids in the dispersal of these drugs over the large absorbing surface, thereby enhancing absorption. Antacids may reduce the rate of ASA absorption from the stomach by increasing the pH of the gastric juice, but the increased rate of gastric emptying may make more drug available for intestinal dissolution and absorption. The end result on ASA absorption may be negligible. Rectal absorption is slow and unreliable. Salicylates, especially methylsalicylate, are absorbed through the intact skin.

After oral administration of usual therapeutic doses of ASA, absorption is more than 90%. Enteric-coated preparations are designed to release the drug at the pH of the small intestine. Occasionally the acid-resistant coating fails to dissolve and the intact tablet is found in the feces. The amount of drug available for absorption from delayed-release preparations is greatly influenced by gastrointestinal motility.

Salicylates are unevenly distributed in the body. High levels of ASA are found in organs of the central compartment, such as blood, renal cortex, and liver, and considerably less (one-sixth to one-tenth that of the plasma concentration) in other sites, such as brain, spinal fluid, muscle, intestine, aqueous humor, lens, and semen. The ASA concentration in synovial fluid taken from an inflamed joint is about five times as high as the plasma concentration of free ASA, and the half-life of the drug is considerably longer in synovial fluid. Salicylates cross the placenta and also appear in the milk. Salicylate competes with other drugs and bilirubin for serum albumin binding sites.

The liver is the principal site of salicylate biotransformation by the microsomal and mitochondrial enzymes. ASA is first hydrolyzed to salicylic acid and then converted to salicyluric acid, the acyl and phenolic glucuronides of salicylic acid, and gentisic acid.

The metabolites, along with a fraction of the unchanged salicylic acid, are excreted in the urine. Excretion of the unchanged drug is enhanced by sodium bicarbonate administration, because in alkaline urine the drug is ionized and cannot back-diffuse from the renal tubules. This procedure is especially useful to hasten excretion after an overdose.

The plasma half-life of ASA is about 15 minutes. That of salicylic acid is longer and dose-dependent—about 2–3 hours after a 600-mg dose and 6–12 hours after larger doses. At therapeutic doses the elimination follows first-order kinetics, but after toxic doses it follows a mixed order because of enzyme saturation, and the plasma half-life may increase to 15–30 hours.

Diflunisal, the most recently introduced substituted salicylic acid derivative, has powerful analgesic and anti-inflammatory activity but mild and unreliable antipyretic properties. It is completely absorbed after oral administration, is distributed similarly to ASA, and has a plasma half-life of 8–12 hours. The pharmacokinetics of diflunisal are dose dependent, and doubling the dose more than doubles the plasma concentration. Steady state is achieved only after several days of administration. More than 99% is bound to plasma proteins. The drug may appear in human milk at a concentration of up to 7% of the total plasma concentration.

The major pharmacokinetic features of salicylates are summarized in Table 34-2.

Pharmacological Effects

Analgesia

Low-intensity pain, such as headache, myalgia, arthralgia, and other pain arising from integumental structures rather than from viscera, is alleviated by salicylates. Part of the analgesia arises from actions on subcortical sites of the CNS, probably the hypothalamus, because at therapeutic concentrations mental function or alertness is not affected. In contrast to the opioid analgesics (see Chapter 23), these drugs do not produce tolerance or physical dependence during chronic administration. Paradoxically, salicylates cause headache in toxic overdose. ASA is frequently combined with codeine or other opioid analgesics and sedatives; such combinations are claimed to give more pain relief with less toxicity than any of the ingredients given alone in effective doses, although this claim has not been clearly proven. The analgesic dose range is between 300 and 1000 mg three or four times a day.

Antipyresis

Salicylates lower the body temperature in febrile patients by direct action on the hypothalamic thermoreceptive region and the temperature-regulating center concerned with heat production and heat loss. Normal body temperature is not affected by therapeutic doses. The increased heat loss produced by salicylates in febrile patients is due to secondary peripheral vasodilatation, especially in cutaneous areas, and to increased sweating. Sweating is important but not essential in this process, because atropine (which prevents sweating; see Chapter 15) does not prevent salicylates from lowering the elevated temperature. Heat production is not inhibited, and toxic doses of salicylates actually produce fever. The antipyretic dose range is similar to the analgesic range.

Effects on rheumatic, inflammatory, and immunological processes

Salicylates in large doses (5–8 g daily) are used for the treatment of rheumatoid diseases and other inflammatory conditions. The increased capillary permeability during inflammation is reduced by salicylates, which thereby prevent edema formation, cellular exudation, and pain. Their ability to block cellular immune responses appears to contribute to the therapeutic effect.

Uricosuric effect

Salicylates in doses of 500 mg inhibit both the renal tubular secretion of uric acid and the uricosuric effect of probenecid and sulfinpyrazone by competition for the same proximal tubular transport systems. In large doses of 5–10 g daily, however, the tubular reabsorption of uric acid is also inhibited by competition with uric acid for more distal active transport sites in the tubule. The net effect of the larger doses is that most of the uric acid filtered by the glomeruli is excreted and the uric acid concentration in the blood is low-

Table 34-2 Recommended Dosages and Known Pharmacokinetic Data for the Anti-inflammatory Analgesics Described in this Chapter*

Generic Name	Trade Name	Recommended Daily Dose (mg)	Bioavail-ability (%)	Time to Maximum Serum Concen-tration (hours)	Serum Half-Life (hours)	Protein Binding (%)
Salicylates						
Acetylsalicylic acid (ASA)	Aspirin,† others	325–1000	70	1–2	0.2‡	80
Sodium salicylate		350–1000	—	1–2	2–30	80
Choline salicylate	Arthropan, Teejel	1000–7000	—	1–2	2–30	80
Choline magnesium salicylate	Trilisate	1000–3000	—	1–2	9–18	80
Diflunisal	Dolobid	500–1000	95	2–3	8–12	99
Para-aminophenol						
Acetaminophen	Tylenol, others	325–3900	60–90	0.5–1	1–5	10
Pyrazolones						
Phenylbutazone	Butazolidin	300–800	95	2	36–168	98
Oxyphenbutazone	Tandearil (withdrawn in most countries)	50–200	90	2	55–90	98
Sulfinpyrazone	Anturan	200–800	95	1–2	3–8	98
Indoles						
Indomethacin	Indocid, Indocin	50–200	95	3	4–12	90
Sulindac *(Indene)*	Clinoril	150–400	90	1 (met2)	7‡ (met18)	93‡
Etodolac	Ultradol	400–600	80	1–2	7	99
Phenylpropionic Acids						
Fenoprofen	Nalfon	900–2400	90	1.5	2.5	99
Flurbiprofen	Ansaid	150–200	95	1.5	4	99
Ibuprofen	Advil, Motrin, Ruefen, others	600–2400	98	1–2	2	99
Ketoprofen	Orudis	100–200	98	1–2	1–35	91
Oxaprozin	Daypro	600–1200	95	1–2	26–92	99
Tiaprofenic Acid	Surgam	600–1800	—	0.5–1.5	1.7	99
Naphthylpropionic Acids						
Naproxen	Naprosyn	500–1000 }	99	2–4	12–15	99
Naproxen sodium	Anaprox	825–1375				
Naphthylalkanones						
Nabumetone	Relafen	600–1200	—	3–6	26–92	99
Anthranilic Acids						
Meclofenamate	Meclomen	300–600	99	0.5–2	2	99
Mefenamic acid	Ponstan	1000	99	2–4	2–4	99
Floctafenine	Idarac	600–1200	—	1–2	8	99
Pyrrole-acetic Acid						
Tolmetin	Tolectin	600–1800	99	0.5–1	1–6	99
Ketorolac tromethamine	Toradol	30–40 p.o. 90–120 i.m.	80	0.5–1	5	99
Phenylacetic Acid						
Diclofenac sodium	Voltaren	75–150	95	2.5	1–2	99
Oxicam						
Piroxicam	Feldene	20	99	2–4	35–90	99
Tenoxicam	Mobiflex	20	99	0.5–6	72	99

*Abbreviations: Bil = biliary; Con = conjugation; Dem = demethylation; Hyd = hydrolysis; Hyx = hydroxylation; Oxi = oxidation; Red = reduction; Ren = renal; AN = analgesic; AP = antipyretic; AS = ankylosing spondylitis; D = dysmenorrhea; JA = juvenile arthritis; OA = osteoarthritis; RA = rheumatoid arthritis; met = active metabolite.
†In Canada only.
‡See text for variations.

V_d (L/kg)	Biotrans-formation	Excretion	Therapeutic Use	Side Effects
0.1–0.35	Hyd Con Oxi	Ren	AN, AP, RA, OA, AS, JA	GI, tinnitus, hypersensitivity, hyperuricemia, Reye's syndrome, salicylism
0.1–0.35	Con Oxi	Ren	AN	GI, salicylism
0.1–0.35	Con Oxi	Ren	AN, AP, RA, OA	GI, salicylism
0.1–0.35	Con Oxi	Ren	AN	GI, salicylism
0.09	Con	Ren	AN, RA, OA, JA, AS	GI, headache, rash, jaundice, drowsiness, confusion, hypersensitivity
1.0	Con Oxi	Ren	AN, AP	Skin rash, hepatic necrosis, renal tubular necrosis
0.08	Oxi Con	Ren Bil	RA, AS, gout	GI, blood dyscrasias, hepatic and renal necrosis, edema, agranulocytosis
0.08	Con	Ren Bil	OA, RA, AS, gout	GI, blood dyscrasias, edema, agranulocytosis
0.16	Oxi Con	Ren	Thrombosis, gout	GI, ↓ renal function, blood dyscrasias
1.0	Oxi Con Dem	Ren Bil	Gout, AS, RA, OA	GI, headache, dizziness, tinnitus, somnolence, agranulocytosis
2.0	Oxi Red	Ren Bil	Gout, AS, OA, RA	Same as indomethacin but milder
0.41	Hyd Con	Ren Bil	AN, OA	GI, chills, fever, nervousness, depression, blurred vision
0.08	Oxi Con Dem	Ren	AP, AN, RA, OA, D	GI, dizziness, nervousness, palpitations, somnolence
0.1	Oxi Con	Ren	RA, OA	GI, headache, edema
0.12	Oxi Con	Ren Bil	AN, AP, OA, D	GI, dizziness, rash, edema, blurred vision, agranulocytosis
0.1	Oxi Con	Ren	AP, AN, RA, OA, D	GI, renal, headache
0.25	Con	Ren	OA, RA	GI, rash, depression, tinnitus
0.1	Unchanged	Ren	OA, RA	GI, dizziness, drowsiness, headache, rash, edema
0.1–0.35	Dem	Ren	OA, RA, AS, AN, D, gout	GI, edema, headache, drowsiness, tinnitus
0.25	Con	Ren	OA, RA	GI, dizziness, headache, rash, edema, tinnitus
Not available	Oxi Con	Ren Bil	AN, D, RA, OA	GI, edema, rash, headache, dizziness, tinnitus
Not available	Oxi Hyx	Ren Bil	AN, D	GI, dizziness, agranulocytosis
Not available	Oxi Con	Ren Bil	AN	GI, dysuria, polyuria, drowsiness, dizziness, headache
0.1	Con Hyx	Ren	RA, OA, AS	GI, hypersensitivity, edema, headache, dizziness, ↑ BP
0.25	Con Hyd	Ren	AN	GI, headache, dizziness, rash, edema
0.13	Con	Ren Bil	RA, OA	GI, dizziness, headache, palpitations, rash, edema
0.12	Hyx Con Hyd	Ren	RA, OA, AS, D	GI, headache, rash, edema, ↓ hemoglobin, ↑ liver enzymes
Not available	Oxi Con	Ren	RA, OA, AS	GI, rash, headache, dizziness, edema

ered. When this happens, the urate crystals already deposited in joints (in cases of gout) are slowly eliminated.

Additional and Adverse Effects

Respiration

Salicylates in medium or large therapeutic doses directly stimulate the respiratory center, leading to respiratory alkalosis that is normally compensated by increased urinary elimination of bicarbonate. In toxic doses salicylates cause central respiratory depression, as well as increased CO_2 production by mitochondria in muscle. These effects result in a combination of uncompensated respiratory and metabolic acidosis. Reduction of plasma bicarbonate level by the salicylates, which are acidic, may also contribute to the acidosis.

Gastrointestinal

Epigastric distress, nausea, and vomiting are quite common complications of salicylate therapy, and microscopic bleeding is almost universal. Exacerbation of peptic ulcer symptoms, gastrointestinal hemorrhage, and blood loss occur in sensitive patients on prolonged salicylate therapy. Pain of gastritis from other causes (e.g., alcoholic gastritis) should not be treated with salicylates because of the increased danger of bleeding.

All anti-inflammatory drugs have the potential to cause damage to the gastrointestinal tract. Weakly acidic drugs such as salicylate may be trapped intracellularly in high concentrations because at intracellular pH the ionized form predominates and cannot readily diffuse out of the cell. High intracellular salicylate levels may contribute to the production of gastric mucosal erosion. This is similar to gastritis following excessive consumption of vinegar or vinegar-containing salad dressing.

Prostaglandins, especially PGE_2, act cytoprotectively on the gastrointestinal mucosa by increasing blood flow and the formation of mucus and sodium bicarbonate while reducing the release of HCl and digestive enzymes. Inhibition of prostaglandin synthesis by salicylates therefore may also contribute to damage of gastrointestinal epithelium.

Corticosteroids, which are powerful anti-inflammatory drugs that are not acidic, also cause gastric ulceration on long-term use because they inhibit the phospholipase A_2-induced release of ara-

chidonic acid, thus secondarily reducing prostaglandin synthesis.

Blood

Large doses of salicylates administered over a prolonged period of time shorten erythrocyte survival and interfere with iron metabolism. In addition, the plasma prothrombin level is reduced, and anticoagulants may have to be given in reduced dosage. Since ASA acetylates the active site of cyclooxygenase responsible for prostaglandin endoperoxide synthesis and subsequent thromboxane synthesis in platelets, platelet aggregation is inhibited and the bleeding time is prolonged. Platelets do not synthesize new enzyme; therefore this action is irreversible, and the effect lasts until new platelets are formed.

Metabolic processes

Oxidative phosphorylation is inhibited by large doses of salicylates, and the energy normally used for ATP production is dissipated as heat. This explains the pyretic effect of toxic overdose. The occasionally observed hyperglycemia may be caused by increased epinephrine release through activation of central sympathetic centers, and resulting increase of glucose-6-phosphatase activity. Salicylates are also known to cause hypoglycemia, probably by increased utilization of glucose and inhibition of gluconeogenesis.

Endocrine functions

In addition to stimulating epinephrine release, ASA increases plasma adrenocorticosteroid levels by increasing the release of ACTH from the hypothalamus. It also competes with thyroid hormones for binding sites on plasma proteins. This effect leads to higher tissue uptake of thyroxine and triiodothyronine, which may contribute to the higher metabolic rate seen with overdoses of salicylates.

Pregnancy

Some data show correlation between consumption of large doses of ASA during the first 16 weeks of pregnancy and the incidence of fetal malformations. If taken regularly during the last trimester it may contribute to prolonged gestation, prolonged labor, and increased maternal blood loss during delivery. There is no evidence, however, that occasional use of small doses of ASA during pregnancy is harmful.

Hypersensitivity

The incidence of hypersensitivity reactions to ASA is about 5%, but true allergy is estimated at less than 1%. It is usually manifested as bronchoconstriction, urticaria, or angioneurotic edema; fatal anaphylactic shock is rare. Many patients sensitive to salicylates also may be sensitive to the other anti-inflammatory drugs and to tartrazine, a yellow dye used in numerous pharmaceutical and food preparations. Some foods and beverages containing salicylate, such as curry powder, paprika, licorice, Benedictine liqueur, prunes, raisins, gherkins, and tea, may contribute to allergic reactions.

Drug interactions

The combination of salicylates with oral anticoagulants or heparin can lead to hemorrhage for reasons already mentioned.

Absorbed ASA is hydrolyzed to salicylic acid, and about 80% is bound to serum albumin. Other drugs that are also bound to albumin, such as sulfonamides, can be displaced by salicylates, raising the concentration of free drug in the plasma and therefore increasing the toxicity. For the same reason, infants with incompletely developed bilirubin-conjugating enzyme systems may develop kernicterus after salicylate administration (see Chapter 4).

The risk of toxicity of methotrexate, a cancer chemotherapeutic agent, is increased by salicylates because they inhibit the active renal tubular secretion of methotrexate and displace the antineoplastic compound from plasma protein binding sites. This type of interaction may also be a limiting factor when low doses of methotrexate are used in combination with nonsteroidal anti-inflammatory drugs in the treatment of rheumatoid arthritis.

Interaction with the uricosuric effects of probenecid and sulfinpyrazone may effectively cancel urate excretion, as explained above, but this risk is very small with the occasional use of ASA for headache or other minor pain.

Increased gastrointestinal blood loss following simultaneous ingestion of alcohol and ASA is probably due to additive but independent effects of the two agents on the gastric mucosa.

Ammonium chloride, acid sodium phosphate, and ascorbic acid may acidify the urine and thus increase the reabsorption of salicylic acid. The resultant cumulation can be hazardous with large ASA doses.

The interaction of oral hypoglycemic agents and ASA is complex; the plasma concentration of both drugs may increase through competition for plasma protein binding sites and reciprocal interference with urinary elimination.

ASA increases the plasma half-life of penicillin because it competes with penicillin for the active transport (secretory) mechanism in the renal tubules.

Toxicity

Salicylism, a mild form of intoxication, is characterized by headache, dizziness, mental confusion, tinnitus, nausea, and vomiting. Marked hyperventilation is also present, resulting from the direct stimulatory effect of salicylates on the respiratory center. Prolonged hyperventilation leads to respiratory alkalosis, but compensatory increases in sodium and potassium bicarbonate excretion may produce a slight improvement in the condition of the patient. The improvement is only temporary if a large dose has been ingested. Serum salicylate concentration and pH should be measured to indicate the type of procedure required for further treatment.

If the dose is large enough, and the condition remains untreated, the preceding symptoms are followed by respiratory and metabolic acidosis, restlessness, delirium, hallucinations, convulsions, coma, and death from respiratory failure.

Symptomatic treatment is sufficient in mild cases of poisoning. Alkalinization of the urine will enhance salicylate elimination. In serious cases intravenous administration of fluids, frequent measurement and correction of acid–base and electrolyte imbalance, and hemodialysis or peritoneal dialysis are mandatory. Methyl salicylate, the methyl ester of salicylic acid, is nonionizable and therefore rapidly crosses cell membranes, including those in the CNS. Therefore it is the most toxic salicylate: one teaspoonful (4 g) may cause death in children.

The occurrence of nephropathy following long-term analgesic therapy is not rare and may lead to a requirement for long-term hemodialysis. The mechanism of development of this toxicity is not clear. The formation of a reactive metabolite that depletes glutathione and binds to cellular macromolecules in the renal tubules may only partly explain the observed cell damage. ASA may cause transient shedding of renal tubular cells, alteration in excretion, and reduced glomerular filtration with consequent retention of water, sodium, and potassium. Patients with active systemic lupus erythematosus, advanced liver cirrhosis, and chronic renal insufficiency appear to be most at risk.

Prostaglandins have an important role in the maintenance of cellular integrity and renal blood circulation. Inhibition of prostaglandin synthesis may cause renal vascular constriction and alteration in vasomotion. In addition, chloride reabsorption in the renal tubules is more complete, and antidiuretic hormone activity (via production of cyclic AMP) is unaffected, resulting in increased water reabsorption. This may cause significant water retention, especially in patients with congestive heart failure, and diminished effectiveness of diuretics. Most patients with analgesic nephropathy are middle-aged women with histories of peptic ulcer, anemia, psychiatric disorders, headaches, and arthralgias. If the renal abnormalities are diagnosed early, the condition may stabilize or improve after drug withdrawal.

The recently observed increase in the number of infants and young children suffering from Reye's syndrome (an often fatal fulminating hepatitis with cerebral edema following a prodromal viral infection) has been attributed to the indiscriminate use of antipyretic medication. Although other factors also have been implicated, this highlights some of the risks of prescribing antipyretics such as ASA, especially for children.

Finally, it is important to know that salicylate intoxication is a leading cause of accidental poisoning in all age groups, particularly in children.

Therapeutic Applications

Sodium salicylate, choline salicylate (available in liquid formulation), choline magnesium salicylate, and ASA are used as antipyretics and analgesics and for the treatment of gout, acute rheumatic fever, and rheumatoid arthritis. Salsalate (salicylsalicylic acid) is a weak inhibitor of prostaglandin synthesis that is used only for the treatment of arthritis. ASA also inhibits platelet aggregation irreversibly. Salicylic acid is used topically as a keratolytic agent (corns and calluses) and for the treatment of epidermophytosis and hyperhidrosis. Salicylamide is included in a number of over-the-counter analgesic and sedative preparations, but its effect is not reliable. Methyl salicylate is a colorless or yellowish liquid used in liniments for cutaneous counterirritation.

Extensive clinical trials involving several thousand patients were carried out to determine the beneficial effect of ASA, administered alone or in combination with dipyridamole, for the prevention or treatment (secondary prevention) of cerebral and coronary thrombosis. In most studies of coronary thrombosis the mortality rates of the treated and placebo groups were not significantly different, but the rate of reinfarction was significantly reduced by drug treatment. The inability to define precisely the etiology of the disorders is partly responsible for the equivocal results and interpretation. However, ASA administration is beneficial in the prevention of strokes in patients who have experienced transient ischemic attacks and visual disturbances (see also Chapter 42). Several other inhibitors of thromboxane synthesis are in advanced clinical trials as candidates for the treatment of conditions in which vasoconstriction, platelet aggregation, and bronchoconstriction may endanger the life of the patient.

Diflunisal is recommended for the relief of mild to moderate pain accompanied by inflammation in conditions such as musculoskeletal trauma, pain after dental extraction, postepisiotomy pain, and osteoarthritis. It has a slow onset (2–4 hours for maximum analgesia) and long duration of action (8–12 hours). Only large doses inhibit platelet function, and the inhibition is reversible. Diflunisal in daily doses of 500 mg or more increases uric acid elimination, but on prolonged use it may cause serious fluid retention. Drug interactions may occur with oral anticoagulants, tolbutamide, diuretics, and other anti-inflammatory drugs. The most-often-reported side effects are gastrointestinal complaints, headache, drowsiness, cholestatic jaundice, skin eruptions, and confusion. The drug is not recommended during pregnancy or breast feeding, it should not be administered to patients with ASA hypersensitivity or allergy, and upward dose adjustments should not be made without proper instructions to the patient.

Recently, adhesive patches containing 15% salicylic acid were made available for transdermal systemic administration.

Misoprostol (a synthetic prostaglandin E_1 analog, see Chapter 31) increases the secretion of mucus and bicarbonate by secretory cells of the stomach, and it increases capillary blood flow. These properties are utilized for the prophylaxis and treatment of gastric and duodenal ulcers and to prevent the gastrointestinal complications induced by long-term use of anti-inflammatory analgesics. The usual dosage and frequency of administration of misoprostol is 0.2 mg given simultaneously with the prescribed anti-inflammatory agent for the prevention of gastrointestinal complications, but more frequently for the treatment of established NSAID-associated gastric ulceration.

5-Aminosalicylic acid (5-ASA) and its analogs are widely used as approved medications for the treatment and prevention of relapses of inflammatory bowel disease. The dosage forms are designed to release the medication in the terminal ileum and colon (see Chapter 45).

PARA-AMINOPHENOLS

The antipyretic analgesic action of **acetanilid** was discovered by accidental mixup in compounding a prescription. The drug was introduced into medicine in 1886 but abandoned several decades later because of its toxicity. **Acetaminophen** and **phenacetin** are congeners of acetanilid, with analgesic and antipyretic effects similar to those of ASA, but they have no therapeutically significant anti-inflammatory or antirheumatic properties. Acetanilid and phenacetin are no longer used in North America because of their toxic side effects.

Acetaminophen

Mechanism and site of action

Acetaminophen (Fig. 34-2) is similar to ASA except that it is a very weak cyclooxygenase inhibitor in vitro. However, it is quite possible that the sensitivity of the enzyme is different in various parts of the body and that sufficient inhibition does occur with acetaminophen to produce analgesia and to reduce fever in environments that have low peroxide concentration.

Pharmacokinetics

Acetaminophen is rapidly absorbed from the gastrointestinal tract, and peak plasma levels are reached in 30–60 minutes. The bioavailability is influenced by the rate of absorption because significant first-pass biotransformation takes place in the luminal cells of the intestine and in the hepatocytes. From ordinary doses of less than 1 g, only 60% of the drug will reach the central compartment in active form. From doses greater than 1 g, up to 90% or more is available for distribution after absorption. The drug diffuses quickly into most tissues and concentrates mainly in the liver. The apparent volume of distribution is 1 L/kg, and less than 10% is bound to plasma proteins (see Table 34-2).

Acetaminophen is conjugated in the liver to form inactive metabolites. Following ordinary clinical doses, 54% is conjugated with glucuronic acid, 33% with sulfuric acid, 4% with cysteine, and 5% as a mercapturic acid (see Chapter 4). A minor amount of acetaminophen is converted in the hepatocytes (and probably in other organs with significant cytochrome P450 activity) to a chemically reactive intermediary metabolite. Under normal circumstances the active metabolite reacts with glutathione to form a harmless end-product. Following the consumption of large doses, glutathione is depleted and the active metabolite will attach covalently to macromolecules that have an essential role in the normal biochemical processes of the cell. In some individuals this leads to liver-cell death, which constitutes a very serious and life-threatening toxicity (see also Chapters 46 and 74).

The plasma half-life of acetaminophen depends on the dose, rate of absorption, and biotransformation. The average normal half-life is 1–2 hours, which may increase to 4–5 hours following large doses or in severe hepatic insufficiency. Mild or moderately severe liver disease does not affect the biotransformation. About 2–5% of the dose is eliminated unchanged in the urine; the rest is conjugated mainly to the glucuronide or sulfate.

Pharmacological effects

The antipyretic and analgesic properties of acetaminophen are very similar to those of ASA, but the duration of action is slightly shorter. It is an ideal analgesic for patients who suffer from gastric complaints or who cannot tolerate ASA. The analgesic effect appears to be mediated entirely by an action on the central nervous system.

Adverse effects and toxicity

At ordinary dosage, acetaminophen is virtually free of significant adverse effects. Its only significant drug interaction is increased risk of hepatotoxicity (see below) in alcoholics or users of other hepatotoxic drugs.

Skin rash or other minor allergic reactions occur infrequently, and minor alterations in the leukocyte count are transient. Renal tubular necrosis and hypo-

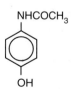

Figure 34-2. Structural formula of acetaminophen.

glycemic coma are rare complications of prolonged large-dose therapy. Renal damage is independent of hepatic toxicity. Potentially fatal hepatic necrosis may occur from overdose of 10 g or more for an adult. The reactive metabolite formed in the liver can easily deplete the normal glutathione supply and cause irreversible cell damage. In this case the administration of N-acetylcysteine can be life-saving if administered within 12–20 hours (see also Chapters 46 and 74). Currently available N-acetylcysteine preparations are administered orally, but they are equally effective when administered intravenously.

Phenacetin is still marketed in a number of countries as a substitute for acetaminophen. Its pharmacological and toxicological properties are similar to those of acetaminophen, but in addition it may cause hemolytic anemia, methemoglobinemia, and in toxic overdose cyanosis, respiratory depression, and cardiac arrest.

NONSTEROIDAL ANTI-INFLAMMATORY DRUGS (NSAIDs)

The drugs in this section are commonly known as NSAIDs. Although they share many properties and applications with the salicylates (notably ASA), they are by convention regarded as a separate group. Personal preference by the physician or the patient, and individual tolerance, are the main criteria for selecting one or other of these similar drugs.

The NSAIDs are chemically diverse (i.e., pyrazolones, indoles, phenylpropionic acids, naphthylpropionic acids, naphthylalkalones, anthranilic acids, pyrrole-acetic acids, phenylacetic acids, oxicams; see Table 34-2), but they share to a large extent the mechanisms of action and adverse effects. These are therefore discussed collectively for the group. Pharmacokinetic data are summarized in Table 34-2.

Mechanisms of Action of NSAIDs

All NSAIDs inhibit the cyclooxygenase required for conversion of arachidonic acid to endoperoxide intermediates (PGG_2 and PGH_2). In contrast to ASA, the inhibition is either readily or slowly reversible, depending on the compound and the tissue source of the microsomal enzyme tested. The antipyretic, analgesic, and platelet-inhibitory effects in most cases are primarily a function of cyclooxygenase inhibition. The actions on rheumatic, inflammatory, and

immunological processes, as well as acute gout, depend to various degrees on inhibition of cyclooxygenase and on many other poorly understood processes, such as inhibition of leukocyte migration and phagocytosis, stabilization of lysosomal membranes, inhibition of plasmin, increased cell-wall integrity, uncoupling of oxidative phosphorylation, inhibition of phosphodiesterase, depression of mucopolysaccharide biosynthesis, and increased release of epinephrine and adrenocorticosteroids.

Adverse Effects and Toxicity Attributed to Inhibition of Cyclooxygenase

These are more or less the same as those produced by ASA, but they are probably less frequently encountered and are of reduced intensity. However, NSAIDs may occasionally cause agranulocytosis, which is not observed with salicylates.

Gastrointestinal

Like ASA, the NSAIDs are weak organic acids and can cause gastric mucosal damage, both by inhibiting prostaglandin synthesis and by accumulating intracellularly because of the low pH in the gastric lumen. The following adverse effects have been reported: occult gastrointestinal bleeding with anemia, gastritis, epigastric pain, hematemesis, dyspepsia, ulcerative esophagitis, acute and reactivated gastric and duodenal ulcer with perforation and hemorrhage, and ulceration and perforation of the large bowel and rectum. These effects are delayed if the drugs are administered rectally, parenterally, or in enteric-coated formulations, and the coadministration of H_2-receptor blockers or of prostaglandin analogs (e.g., misoprostol) will increase gastric tolerance during chronic administration of NSAIDs.

Platelet function

The synthesis of thromboxane A_2 (TXA_2), derived from cyclic endoperoxides (PGG_2 and PGH_2) that are synthesized from arachidonic acid by cyclooxygenase, is reversibly inhibited by most NSAIDs. Platelets may fail to aggregate. Prostacyclin (PGI_2) formation, which opposes platelet aggregation, is also inhibited by NSAIDs, but because of abundance of cyclooxygenase in endothelial cells and the cells' ability to synthesize new enzyme, the reduction of PGI_2 production during long-term NSAID administration is of minor significance. The interaction of NSAIDs with warfarin, however, may have serious consequences.

Renal

The participation of prostaglandins in renal function is complex. PGI_2 and PGE_2 cause direct renal vasodilatation and increased cortical and medullary blood flow, which results in increased glomerular filtration rate, decreased renal vascular resistance, increased natriuresis, and reduced medullary hypertonicity with decreased water reabsorption in the loop of Henle. Also, prostaglandins may indirectly moderate or prevent the action of antidiuretic hormone (ADH) on tubular epithelium by negative feedback, resulting in increased water elimination. Thus, prostaglandins favor the formation of dilute urine and enhanced water excretion.

NSAIDs, by inhibiting prostaglandin synthesis, remove the negative feedback on ADH (allowing excessive water retention and edema formation), and they permit humoral or neurogenic renal vasoconstriction and sodium and water reabsorption. The administration of NSAIDs to patients with normal renal hemodynamic function may cause temporary water retention and "weight" gain. Patients suffering from marginal or significantly reduced renal function, congestive heart failure, hypertension, or conditions that require the administration of a diuretic, however, are at great risk of serious adverse effects. These adverse effects usually consist of edema, fluid and electrolyte disturbances, sodium and chloride retention, and plasma dilution. NSAID-induced renal failure is usually temporary, and normal renal function returns shortly after drug administration is terminated. Of the presently used NSAIDs, sulindac appears to be the least-nephrotoxic drug.

Respiratory

The administration of NSAIDs to persons suffering from asthma or other respiratory ailments may provoke acute rhinitis, angioneurotic edema, urticaria, bronchial asthma, bronchoconstriction, hypotension, and shock. These reactions do not appear to have an antigenic component, but they may be due to inhibition of cyclooxygenase and a consequent overabundance of leukotriene production.

Pregnancy and labor

NSAID administration during the last trimester of pregnancy may prolong gestation, delay labor, and cause excessive postpartum bleeding and hemorrhage by inhibition of PGE_2, $PGF_{2\alpha}$, and TXA_2 synthesis.

Side Effects That Appear to be Unrelated to the Inhibition of Cyclooxygenase

The rate of occurrence of these side effects is different for each drug. Without regard for rank order or frequency and severity, they can be summarized as follows.

Allergic: Hypersensitivity reactions, bronchospasm, anaphylactic/anaphylactoid reactions, serum sickness, arthralgia, fever.

Cardiovascular: Vasodilatation, pallor, elevation of blood pressure, palpitation, angina, arrhythmias, pericarditis, perivascular granulomata.

CNS: Headache, dizziness, dry mouth, sweating, nervousness, excessive thirst, inability to concentrate, insomnia, stimulation, vertigo, confusion, light-headedness, convulsions, syncope, paresthesia, peripheral neuropathy, psychic disturbances, tiredness, disorientation, nightmares, hallucinations, migraine, speech disorder, tremor, muscle twitch.

Dermatological: Urticaria, rash, erythema, pruritus, angioedema, angiitis, loss of hair, photosensitivity, erythroderma, Stevens-Johnson syndrome, toxic epidermal necrolysis.

Ear: Tinnitus, vertigo, impaired hearing, hearing loss.

Endocrine: Hyperglycemia, hypoglycemia, thyroid hyperplasia, toxic goiter, gynecomastia.

Eye: Macular and corneal deposits, corneal opacity, blurred vision, orbital and preorbital pain, diplopia, optic neuritis, retinal hemorrhage, retinal detachment, toxic amblyopia.

Gastrointestinal: Flatulence, gastritis, diarrhea, constipation, gastrointestinal fullness, epigastric distress, stomatitis, glossitis, coated tongue, abnormal taste, salivary gland enlargement, ulcerative stomatitis, colitis.

Hematological: Purpura, leukopenia, thrombocytopenia, agranulocytosis, pancytopenia, hemolytic anemia, bone marrow depression, aplastic anemia.

Liver: Liver function abnormalities, elevated liver enzymes, reversible hepatitis and jaundice, fulminant hepatitis.

Musculoskeletal and whole body: Myalgia, asthenia.

Renal: Interstitial nephritis, glomerulonephritis, acute tubular necrosis, papillary necrosis, proteinuria, oliguria, anuria, nephrotic syndrome, bilateral renal cortical necrosis, renal calculi, renal failure with azotemia.

Respiratory: Dyspnea, asthma, respiratory distress, respiratory alkalosis, pharyngitis, rhinitis, sinusitis, voice alteration.

Urogenital: Increased urinary frequency, oliguria, hematuria, glycosuria, vaginal bleeding.

Others: Impotence, pancreatitis, metabolic acidosis.

NSAIDs BY CATEGORY

Pyrazolones

Antipyrine and **aminopyrine** have been used extensively in the past for the treatment of rheumatic fever. In hypersensitive patients aminopyrine causes agranulocytosis; therefore its use is restricted. However, a number of chemically related compounds are widely used as anti-inflammatory agents.

Phenylbutazone and oxyphenbutazone

Phenylbutazone (Fig. 34-3) is an antipyrine congener. Oxyphenbutazone is one of the active metabolites of phenylbutazone with all the same properties as the parent compound. They are discussed together.

Mechanism and Site of Action; Pharmacokinetics. Phenylbutazone, beside inhibiting prostaglandin synthesis, stabilizes lysosomal membranes, thereby reducing the release of ribonuclease and acid phosphatase. The uricosuric effect produced by large

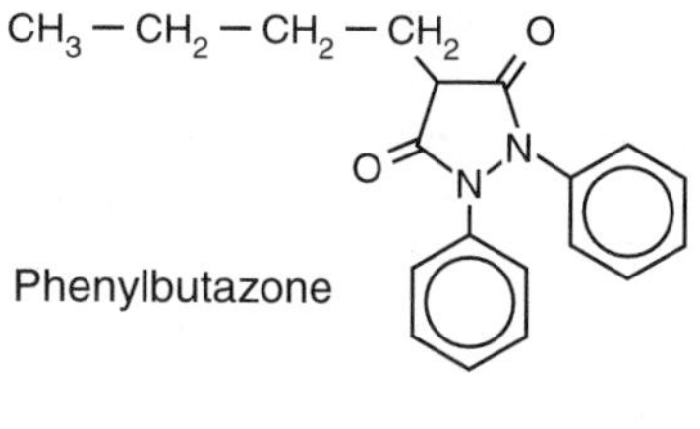

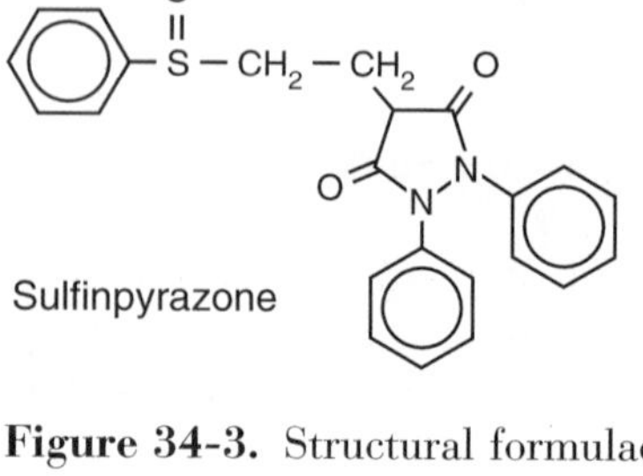

Figure 34-3. Structural formulae of pyrazolones.

doses is due primarily to the inhibition of uric acid reabsorption in the proximal convoluted tubules by hydroxyphenylbutazone, a metabolite of phenylbutazone.

Phenylbutazone is converted slowly to hydroxyphenylbutazone and oxyphenbutazone, both of which are active. The metabolites are further conjugated with glucuronic acid.

Pharmacological effects; adverse effects. Phenylbutazone has powerful anti-inflammatory effects, which are comparable in magnitude to those of the adrenocorticosteroids. The analgesic and antipyretic effects are relatively weak, and the drug should not be used for these purposes because of its potential side effects, which are mainly gastrointestinal.

Drug interactions may be significant with any drug that can be displaced from binding to plasma proteins, such as other anti-inflammatory agents, oral anticoagulants, oral hypoglycemics, phenytoin, and sulfonamides. Phenylbutazone may cause induction of hepatic microsomal drug-metabolizing enzymes.

The most serious but infrequent toxic effects are fatal aplastic anemia and agranulocytosis. These may occur at any time during treatment, or when treatment is resumed after a drug-free period. Patients taking phenylbutazone should be supervised closely and should have frequent blood examinations.

Sulfinpyrazone

Sulfinpyrazone (Fig. 34-3) is a phenylbutazone derivative without antirheumatic, antipyretic, analgesic, or sodium-retaining activity. It is a powerful uricosuric agent used for the treatment of chronic gout. The drug is also used to inhibit platelet aggregation in the treatment of transient ischemic attacks, of thromboembolism associated with vascular or cardiac prostheses, of recurrent venous thrombosis, and of arteriovenous shunt thrombosis (see also Chapter 42). The side effects and toxicity of sulfinpyrazone are similar to those of phenylbutazone, the most frequent being gastrointestinal complaints. Concurrent salicylate therapy is not recommended because salicylates and citrates antagonize the uricosuric effect of sulfinpyrazone, and ASA may prolong bleeding time.

Apazone

Apazone is one of the recently developed pyrazolone derivatives with analgesic, antipyretic, and powerful anti-inflammatory properties similar to those of phenylbutazone. It is a strong uricosuric agent with various side effects. It is used primarily for acute gout, rheumatoid arthritis, and osteoarthritis. The drug is not available in North America.

Indoles

From the many compounds containing an indole group that have been tested for antipyretic, analgesic, and anti-inflammatory actions, indomethacin and etodolac were found to be clinically useful. Sulindac is an indene, chemically related to indomethacin but lacking the indole nitrogen (Fig. 34-4).

Indomethacin

The analgesic, antipyretic, and anti-inflammatory actions of indomethacin are similar to those of the

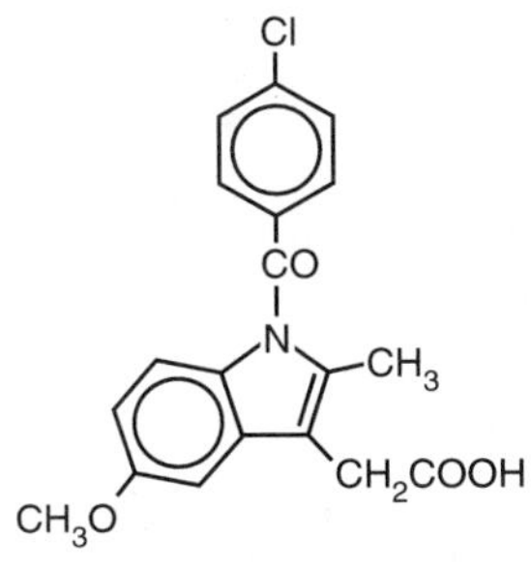

Indomethacin

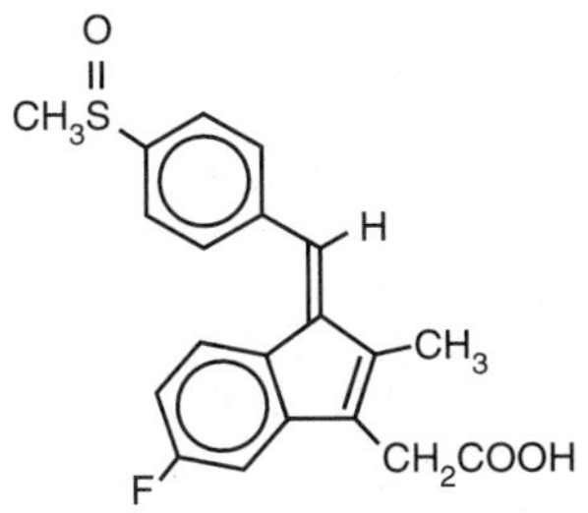

Sulindac

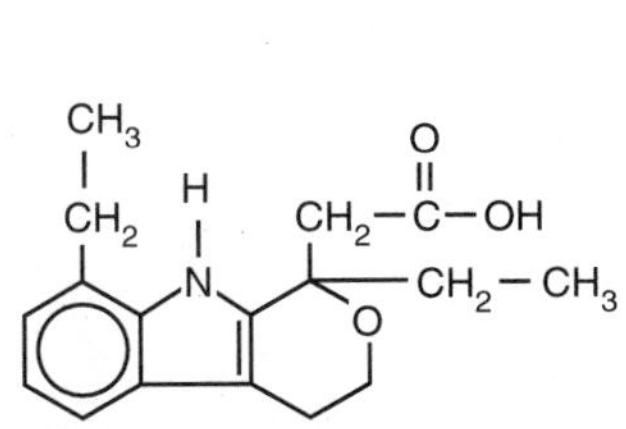

Etodolac

Figure 34-4. Structural formulae of indole compounds.

salicylates. It is a very potent inhibitor of cyclooxygenase. It also uncouples oxidative phosphorylation, depresses the biosynthesis of mucopolysaccharides, inhibits phosphodiesterase, and inhibits the motility of polymorphonuclear leukocytes. The drug is *O*-demethylated and conjugated with glucuronic acid by hepatic microsomal enzymes.

Indomethacin is a very potent anti-inflammatory agent. Although it has antipyretic and analgesic properties, it also tends to cause serious gastrointestinal and other complications. Therefore it should be used only for the treatment of rheumatoid arthritis, ankylosing spondylitis, osteoarthritis, and acute gout and for the control of pain in uveitis and postoperative ophthalmic pain.

Sulindac

Sunlindac (Fig. 34-4), which is closely related to indomethacin, requires in vivo transformation to become active. Hepatic microsomal enzymes oxidize the molecule to a sulfone and reduce it to a sulfide, which is the active form of sulindac. It inhibits prostaglandin synthesis and is about half as potent as indomethacin. The absorption, distribution, and plasma protein binding are also similar to those of indomethacin (see Table 34-2). The plasma half-life of sulindac is about 7 hours, but for the sulfide metabolite it is about 18 hours. Sulindac spares the kidney because it does not affect renal PGI_2 synthesis.

Etodolac

This drug is similar to indomethacin but requires higher doses for equivalent effects. It is a potent inhibitor of cyclooxygenase isoforms of prostaglandin synthesis that are involved in inflammatory conditions. Gastric prostaglandin synthesis appears to be less affected.

The drug is well absorbed orally, it is unevenly distributed, and it is eliminated after conjugation as unchanged drug (20%) and as hydroxylated metabolites (45%) in urine (73%) and feces (14%).

Etodolac is a potent anti-inflammatory, analgesic, and antipyretic drug recommended for the management of rheumatoid arthritis, osteoarthritis, and pain. The dose should not exceed 1200 mg in 24 hours, and it should be reduced if renal function is significantly impaired.

Gastrointestinal disturbances are the most frequent adverse effects, but they are usually less serious than those associated with most other NSAIDs. Drug interactions with other highly protein-bound drugs may occur, but preliminary observations with glyburide, phenytoin, and warfarin were negative. The phenolic metabolites of etodolac may produce a false-positive urinary bilirubin test.

Phenylpropionic Acid Derivatives and Analogs

The drugs in this group (Fig. 34-5) share many pharmacological and toxicological properties. They are all substituted phenyl-, naphthyl-, or thienyl-propionic acids, which are chemically and pharmacologically analogous. The drugs inhibit prostaglandin biosynthesis in vitro and in vivo but differ in their potency, which is reflected in the respective doses

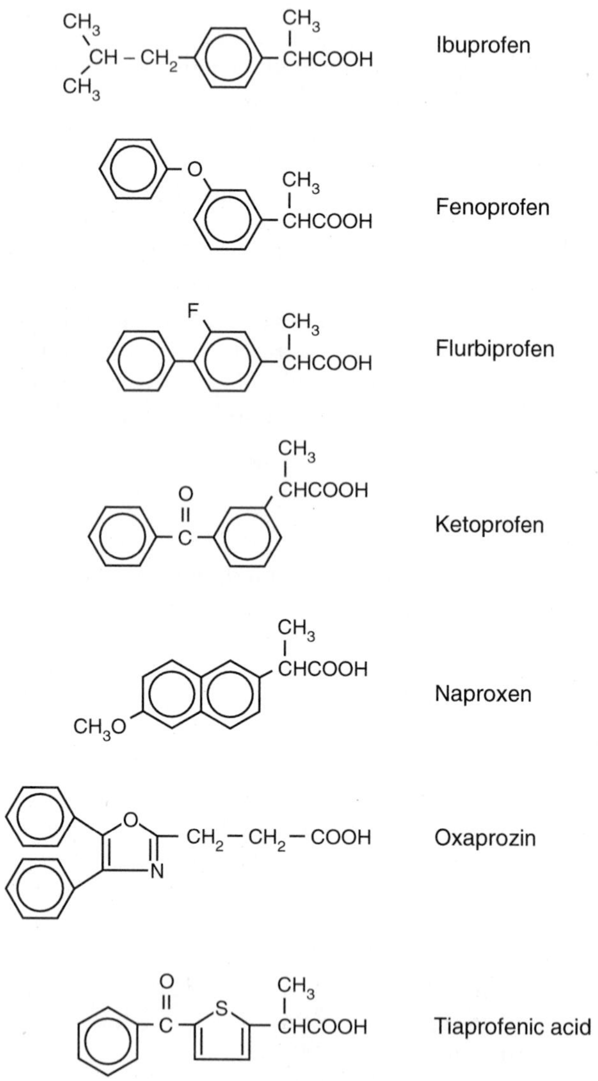

required to produce analgesia, reduce fever, and inhibit inflammatory processes. Table 34-2 summarizes the pharmacokinetics, the uses, and the most significant side effects.

Ibuprofen is probably the best tolerated on long-term use, even by patients who cannot tolerate ASA because of gastric complaints. Oral absorption is complete, but rectal absorption is slow and erratic.

Fenoprofen is less popular than the other members of this group, probably because of less intensive commercial promotion. Oral absorption is fast, but it is not complete in the presence of food.

Ketoprofen is absorbed rapidly and completely after oral administration, but it is distributed unevenly in body water. The plasma half-life may vary between 1 and 35 hours; the causes of this variability are unknown.

Flurbiprofen cannot be tolerated by a small number of patients because of side effects occuring after a few days of administration.

Naproxen is well tolerated and completely absorbed after oral or rectal administration. Antacids containing magnesium oxide or aluminum hydroxide reduce the rate of absorption.

Oxaprozin is a long-acting NSAID recommended primarily for the symptomatic treatment of rheumatoid arthritis and osteoarthritis. It has analgesic, anti-inflammatory, and antipyretic properties. Care must be taken to avoid overdosage because of the drug's long plasma half-life of 26–92 hours. The adverse effects are similar to those of other NSAIDs. Drug interaction with other highly protein-bound drugs is a distinct possibility.

Tiaprofenic acid is one of the most recently introduced members of this group. It is rapidly absorbed from the stomach and duodenojejunal area, and the drug can be detected in synovial fluid for up to 11 hours. Over 90% of the dose is excreted unchanged in the urine. Therefore the dose should be reduced for patients with impaired renal function.

Naphthylalkanones

Nabumetone (Fig. 34-6) is a prodrug that requires biotransformation by liver enzymes to form the active metabolite, 6-methoxy-2-naphthylacetic acid (6-MNA), which is a potent inhibitor of cyclooxygenase

Figure 34-5. Structural formulae of propionic acid derivatives.

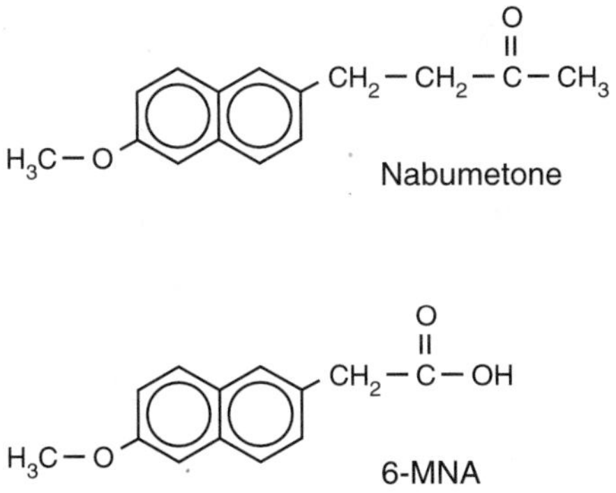

Figure 34-6. Structural formula of nabumetone and its active metabolite 6-methoxynaphthylacetic acid (6-MNA).

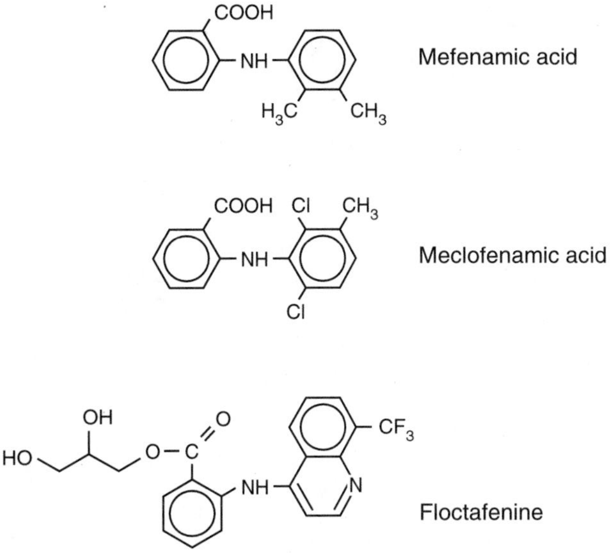

Figure 34-7. Structural formulae of anthranilic acids.

and has anti-inflammatory, analgesic, and antipyretic effects.

Orally administered nabumetone is absorbed mainly in the duodenum. Maximum concentration of 6-MNA is achieved in serum in 3–6 hours and in synovial fluid in 4–12 hours. Free and conjugated 6-MNA as well as other active free and conjugated metabolites are excreted in urine (80%) and feces (10%).

Nabumetone is used for its anti-inflammatory and analgesic effect in the symptomatic treatment of rheumatoid arthritis and osteoarthritis. Clinical evaluation for other conditions, such as ankylosing spondylitis and self-limited soft-tissue and musculo-skeletal conditions, is in progress.

Adverse effects are similar to those of other NSAIDs. Hepatic or renal impairment and cross-sensitivity with other NSAIDs should be evaluated before commencement of treatment. Drug interactions with other highly protein-bound drugs (e.g., warfarin, tolbutamide, chlorpropamide) or with digoxin, lithium, and methotrexate are possible.

Anthranilic Acids

Mefenamic acid (Fig. 34-7 and Table 34-2), in addition to inhibiting prostaglandin synthesis, appears to inhibit the action of $PGF_{2\alpha}$ on isolated bronchial smooth muscle. It is unevenly distributed in body water, and it has several metabolites that are eliminated in urine along with the unchanged drug. Mefenamic acid has analgesic, antipyretic, and anti-inflammatory properties, but because of gastrointestinal side effects, including occasionally severe diarrhea, the drug is used primarily for short-term analgesia and dysmenorrhea.

Meclofenamate sodium (meclofenamic acid, Fig. 34-7 and Table 34-2) acts similarly to mefenamic acid. It produces significant analgesia in about 30 minutes.

Floctafenine (Fig. 34-7 and Table 34-2) is a recently introduced anti-inflammatory analgesic. It is completely absorbed after oral administration, attains peak plasma levels in 1–2 hours, and has an initial plasma half-life (α phase) of 1 hour and a β phase of 8 hours. The drug is recommended primarily for the short-term treatment of mild to moderately severe pain.

Pyrrole-acetic Acid and Phenylacetic Acid Derivatives

Tolmetin (a substituted pyrrole-acetic acid derivative; Fig. 34-8 and Table 34-2) has analgesic, antipyretic, and anti-inflammatory properties similar to those of ASA. Tolmetin is recommended as an anti-inflammatory drug, but many patients cannot tolerate the side effects (gastric erosion, ulceration, bleeding; nervousness, drowsiness, insomnia).

Ketorolac tromethamine (a substituted pyrrolizine-carboxylic acid; Fig. 34-8 and Table 34-2) is a potent analgesic with minimal anti-inflammatory or antipyretic activity. It is recommended as an analgesic for mild to moderately severe pain, to be used for up to 3–4 weeks. Side effects are mainly gastrointestinal and somnolence.

Diclofenac sodium (a substituted phenylacetic

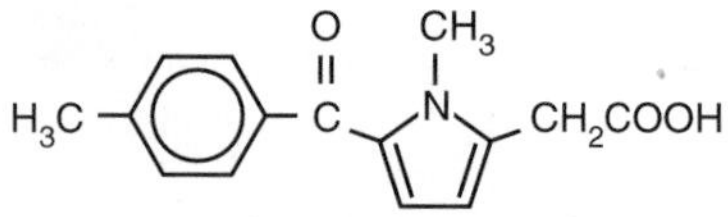

Tolmetin

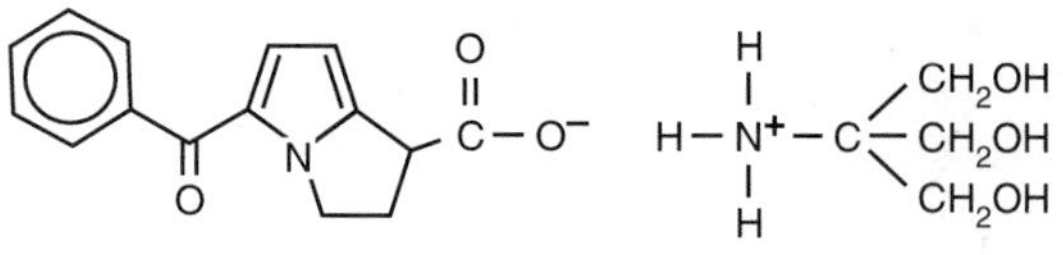

Ketorolac tromethamine

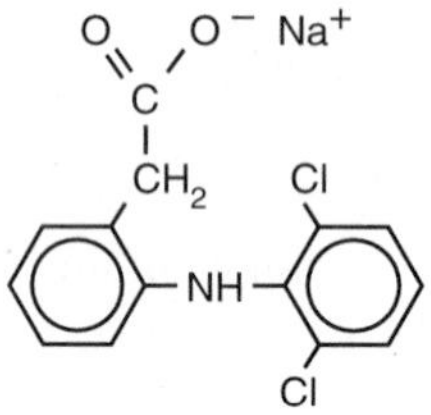

Diclofenac sodium

Figure 34-8. Structural formulae of pyrrole- and phenylacetic acid derivatives.

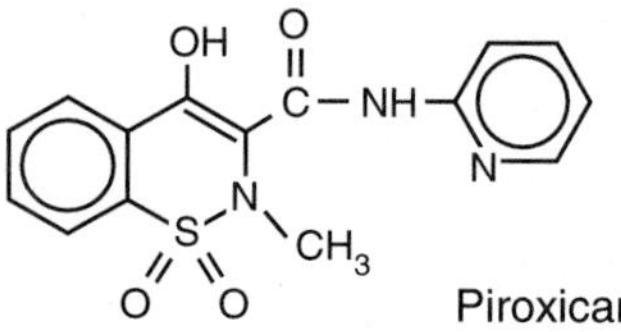

Piroxicam

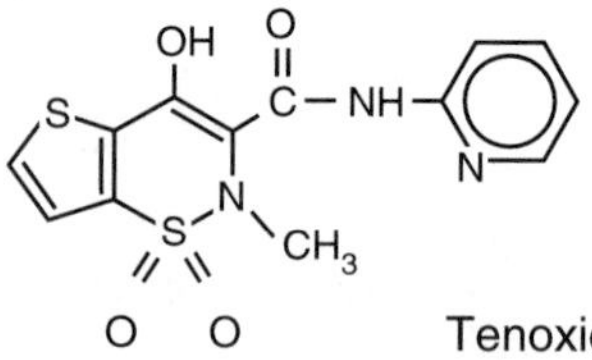

Tenoxicam

Figure 34-9. Structural formulae of oxicams.

acid derivative; Fig. 34-8 and Table 34-2) has analgesic, antipyretic, and anti-inflammatory properties similar to those of ASA. It is recommended for the treatment of rheumatoid arthritis and severe osteoarthritis, including degenerative joint disease of the hip. It has many side effects commonly encountered with this group of drugs, the most serious being gastrointestinal bleeding, cardiac arrhythmias, water retention, and reversible depression of the hematopoietic system. Enteric-coated tablets or a combination product with misoprostol is recommended for oral administration to reduce gastric irritation.

Bromfenac (an aminobenzoylphenylacetic acid), an orally active analgesic with anti-inflammatory and antipyretic properties, is in an advanced stage of clinical testing.

Oxicams

Piroxicam (Fig. 34-9 and Table 34-2) is an amphoteric compound and may behave either as a weak acid or a weak base. It is absorbed slowly after oral administration. Because of its long half-life (in excess of 40 hours), with daily doses of 20 mg the plasma levels rise for about 5–7 days to reach a steady state. Food in the stomach does not influence bioavailability. Because of its potential for cumulation, caution is required when the drug is administered to patients with impaired hepatic or renal function.

Tenoxicam (Fig. 34-9 and Table 34-2) is an anti-inflammatory agent with analgesic and antipyretic properties. It inhibits prostaglandin synthesis in vitro and in vivo, and it may act as a scavenger of active oxygen at the site of inflammation. The plasma half-life may vary from 32 to more than 100 hours. Steady-state plasma concentration is reached within 10–15 days with daily doses of 20 mg. The main hydroxy metabolite is excreted in urine, but appreciable amounts of the glucuronide conjugates are excreted in bile.

GOLD COMPOUNDS

Gold compounds, such as **auranofin** (Ridaura), **aurothioglucose** (Solganal), and **sodium aurothiomalate** (Myochrysine), are strictly reserved for the treatment of patients with rapidly progressive rheumatoid arthritis who respond poorly to conventional drug treatment. Reliable results are obtained after intramuscular administration of a solution or oily suspension of the gold compound at weekly or longer time intervals. The bioavailability of orally administered preparations is low but sufficient for maintenance therapy. Clinically significant improvements may take months to develop and may last for a year after discontinuation. The distribution of gold in the body is unpredictable; it tends to accumulate in inflamed tissues and joints. After termination of treatment the concentration in blood will gradually diminish over 2–3 months, but significant amounts are excreted in the urine for a year or longer. The mechanism of action is uncertain, the most acceptable theory being that gold compounds suppress immune responsiveness by inhibition of mononuclear phagocyte function. There are numerous side effects including dermatitis, proximal tubular damage, blood dyscrasias, and encephalitis. Gold is contraindicated for patients with heavy-metal hypersensitivity, diabetes mellitus, renal disease, and many other conditions including pregnancy and breast feeding.

DRUGS USED IN THE TREATMENT OF GOUT

A variety of analgesics, uricosuric agents (probenecid and sulfinpyrazone), and corticosteroids are used in the symptomatic or specific treatment of gout. Acute attacks of gout respond well to colchicine, and the chronic form may be controlled by reducing plasma uric acid with allopurinol.

Probenecid (see Chapter 7) inhibits the proximal renal tubular secretion *and reabsorption* of uric acid. Therefore the whole filtered load of uric acid is eliminated in the urine. The active tubular secretion of penicillin, indomethacin, cephalosporins, thiazides, and other weakly acidic drugs is also blocked by probenecid. The uricosuric effect of probenecid and of sulfinpyrazone is antagonized by ASA.

Colchicine is an alkaloid obtained from the autumn crocus. It is used as an anti-inflammatory drug in the prevention and treatment of acute gouty arthritis. It causes the disappearance of the fibrillar microtubules in granulocytes and leukocytes, thereby preventing their mobilization to the site of inflammation. It inhibits the release of histamine and the secretion of insulin, and it arrests cell division in metaphase. It may cause nausea, vomiting, hemorrhagic gastroenteritis, and, following chronic administration, alopecia, agranulocytosis, and aplastic anemia. The usual oral adult dose is about 1 mg initially, but not more than 3 mg in 24 hours. For prophylaxis a daily dose of 0.5 mg, 2–4 days per week, is usually adequate to prevent flareups. It is also administered together with allopurinol or uricosuric drugs.

Allopurinol and its primary metabolite alloxanthine reduce plasma uric acid concentration by inhibiting xanthine oxidase, the enzyme catalyzing the final steps of uric acid synthesis. Thus, hyperuricemia of almost any cause, including that induced by other drugs, is normalized. This facilitates the dissolution of tophi and prevents the development or progression of chronic gouty arthritis. Allopurinol and its metabolites are excreted in dose-dependent fashion by glomerular filtration, but there is significant tubular reabsorption, which is sensitive to probenecid inhibition. The drug is well tolerated, but hypersensitivity reactions may occur even after months or years of continuous medication. The usual daily dose is 100 mg, which may be increased to 300 mg/day.

SUGGESTED READING

Aspirin and acetaminophen. Arch Intern Med 1981; 141(3) (special issue with 26 articles).

Brooks PM, Day RO. Nonsteroidal anti-inflammatory drugs—differences and similarities. N Engl J Med 1991; 322:1716–1725.

Buckley MM-T, Brogden RN. Ketorolac. A review of its pharmacodynamic and pharmacokinetic properties, and therapeutic potential. Drugs 1990; 39:86–109.

Chaffman M, Brodgen RN, Heel RC, et al. Auranofin. A preliminary review of its pharmacological properties and therapeutic use in rheumatoid arthritis. Drugs 1984; 27:378–424.

Flower JR, Vane JR. Inhibition of prostaglandin biosynthesis. Biochem Pharmacol 1974; 23:1439–1450.

Fowler PD. Aspirin, paracetamol and nonsteroidal anti-inflammatory drugs. A comparative review of side effects. Med Toxicol Adverse Drug Exp 1987; 2:338–366.

Gonzales JP, Todd PA. Tenoxicam. A preliminary review of its pharmacodynamic and pharmacokinetic properties, and therapeutic efficacy. Drugs 1987; 34:289–310.

Lanza FL. Gastrointestinal toxicity of the newer NSAIDs. Am J Gastroenterol 1993; 88:1318–1323.

Petro R, Gray R, Collins R, et al. Randomized trial of prophylactic daily aspirin in British male doctors. Br Med J 1988; 296:313–316.

Rainsford KD. Mechanisms of gastrointestinal damage by NSAIDs. Agents Actions Suppl 1993; 44:59–64.

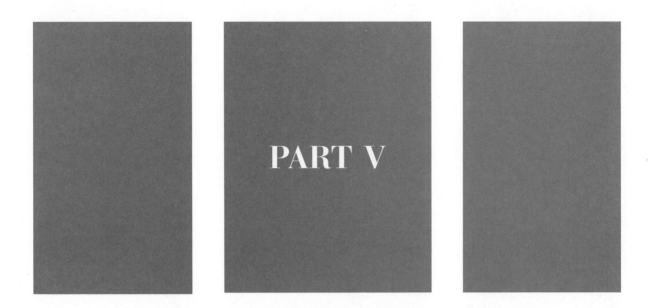

PART V

CARDIOVASCULAR SYSTEM

CHAPTER 35

Cardiovascular System Overview and Organization

U. ACKERMANN

At present, pharmacological treatment of cardiovascular dysfunction is directed at five classes of functional disturbance affecting (1) rhythm, (2) cardiac contractile performance, (3) blood vessel function, (4) blood pressure regulation, and (5) blood clotting. To appreciate present and potential future strategies for therapeutics, one must know something about the interrelationships among these five functional components of cardiovascular performance. This chapter relates to the first four of these functions. The principles of hemostasis are discussed in Chapter 42.

OVERVIEW

The cardiovascular system consists of a four-chambered pump, the heart, and a flow-distributing network of blood vessels. Its two primary functions are to provide to all tissues at all times the supply of nutrients required to sustain the metabolic activity of the tissue, and to remove from all tissues the products of their metabolic activity.

Cardiac function is initiated by electrical events in the heart. The processes of excitation-activation-contraction coupling convert electrical activity into mechanical actions that propel blood from the right ventricle into the pulmonary artery and from the left ventricle into the aorta. Viscoelastic properties of the arterial network convert the pulsatile output of the heart into a smooth, uninterrupted capillary flow. The viscoelastic properties of the venous network

function mainly to modulate, on a time scale of seconds to minutes, the flow that returns to the heart from the capillary beds. The venous system and the pattern of cardiac relaxation after each contraction are the two major influences on the filling of the ventricles with blood in preparation for the next ejection. Relaxation, like contraction, is initiated by electrophysiological and biochemical events in cardiac cells.

CARDIAC ELECTROPHYSIOLOGY

The electrical activity of the cardiac cell can be measured as periodic changes in the electrical potential difference between the inside and outside of the cell. The polarity, amplitude, and pattern of change of this potential difference are determined by the transport, both passive and active, of ions across the cell membrane. Passive transport through ion-selective channels determines cell behavior on a time scale of milliseconds, while active transport mechanisms are the dominant influence on long-term electrical behavior of the cells.

Ion Channels

Voltage-gated ion channels, located in the sarcolemma, undergo periodic changes in conductance that lead to crucial alterations in the intracellular ionic and metabolic milieu. Voltage-dependent activation (channel opening) is followed within milliseconds by a process of inactivation (channel closure). In addition, channel conductance is influenced over longer time periods by the action of neurotransmitters or hormones.

Voltage-gated, ion-selective channels are members of a closely related family of intrinsic cell membrane proteins. They typically consist of a principal subunit which, in the case of both Na^+ and Ca^{2+} channels, is made up of several homologous domains (Fig. 35-1), each consisting of several transmembrane segments. The segments and domains are serially linked in the extracellular space and in the cytosol by polypeptide chains (Fig. 35-1). The domains of the Na^+ and Ca^{2+} channels are thought to be arranged around a central "pore" through which the ion travels after each of the surrounding domains has undergone a voltage-driven conformational change to activate the channel. The most significant ion currents involved in the cardiac action potential are Na^+, Ca^{2+}, and K^+. The interactions of these ion currents determine the various features of the action potential (described below).

Sodium channels

Channel activation. The main functional component of the Na^+ channel is a large (269 kDa) transmembrane protein known as the α subunit (shown in Fig. 35-1). It contains the binding site for tetrodotoxin and saxitoxin, both of which will inhibit channel conductance. In different excitable tissues the α subunit can occur in association with a variable number of smaller subunits, termed β_1 and β_2, that may modulate channel structure or function but are not essential for ion transport. It is believed that the S4 segment in each transmembrane domain functions as the voltage-sensing element in the channel.

Upon depolarization of the membrane, the S4 segments of the four domains undergo rotational movements that permit the conformational change that opens the channel for the passage of ionic current.

Channel inactivation probably involves a further conformational change in the Na^+ channel, but the details of the process are not yet known.

Long-term modulation. Modulation on a time scale that is longer than a few milliseconds occurs via phosphorylation of the channel protein by protein kinase C and by cAMP-dependent protein kinase A. The greatest effect is on channel inactivation.

Calcium channels

Most excitable cells have many types of Ca^{2+} channels, but the L type is prominent in cardiac muscle. Sinoatrial cells and Purkinje cells also show T-type channels. The L channel mediates long-lasting Ca^{2+} currents. Membrane depolarization causes the L channel to admit an influx of Ca^{2+} that is capable of triggering intracellular responses. It is inhibited by external multivalent cations (Mn^{2+}, Mg^{2+}, Ni^{2+}, etc.), by H^+, and by at least three structurally different classes of antagonists. These antagonists are the dihydropyridines (for example, nifedipine and nisoldipine), the phenylalkylamines (such as verapamil), and the benzothiazepines (for example, diltiazem). T channels differ from L channels in that they have (1) a more negative activation threshold voltage; (2) more rapid, voltage-dependent inactivation; (3) an insensitivity to the common L-channel blockers but a high sensitivity to blockade by nickel ions; and (4) a high resistance to β-adrenergic stimulation.

The purified Ca^{2+} channel consists of up to five subunits, one of which is a tissue-specific 175-kDa subunit, termed α_1 (shown in Fig. 35-1). The positively charged S4 segment of this protein probably forms the voltage-sensing element in a manner analogous to that described for the Na^+ channel. Both L- and T-type channels have a distinct threshold voltage: At membrane potentials more positive than threshold, channels are activated quickly, permitting Ca^{2+} current to flow. Activation reaches a peak and then diminishes slowly during an inactivation phase that lasts up to 300 msec in myocardial cells. Inactivated channels undergo a process of reactivation, returning to the closed state to be available for activation in a subsequent depolarization.

Channel activation occurs at a threshold level that is influenced by the extracellular concentration (C_o) of divalent cations such as Ca^{2+}; higher concentrations move the threshold voltage toward positive values because these ions shield the external surface charge. The L-type channel threshold is near -40 mV (at 2 mM $[Ca^{2+}]_o$) and the T-type threshold is -50 to -65 mV. Observations on families of channels show that not all available channels are activated by a given depolarizing voltage.

Channel inactivation increases the fraction of channels in a population that remain closed. In myocyte L channels the process of inactivation is slow, lasting a few hundred milliseconds, and is influenced by both membrane voltage and Ca^{2+} entry into the cell. In T channels the inactivation process is much

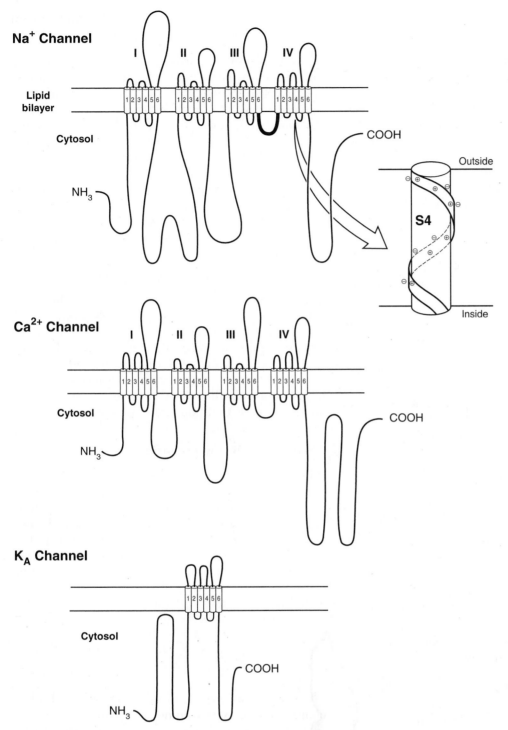

Figure 35-1. Typical structure of the principal subunits in ion-selective membrane channels. The α subunit of the Na$^+$ channel, the α_1 subunit of the Ca^{2+} channel, and the A-current K$^+$ channel are shown. Each domain is identified by a Roman numeral (I–IV), and each domain consists of six segments (S1 to S6). The inset shows a model of the S4 segment within domain IV. It is thought to be the voltage-sensitive component in each of the four domains. It has positively charged amino acids (which are generally arginine, but may occasionally be lysine) arranged within an α-helix across the membrane. The spiral of positive charges is held in place by negatively charged amino acids on neighboring S1, S2, and S3 segments. The cytosolic chain linking S6 (III) to S1 (IV) has been emphasized in the diagram of the Na$^+$ channel. Integrity of this chain is essential for channel inactivation to occur after an action potential. (Modified from Catterall WA. "Molecular Properties of Voltage-Gated Ion Channels in the Heart." In Fozzard HA, et al. (eds.) Raven Press, 1991, Chapter 37.)

more rapid, lasting a little less than 50 msec, and it appears to be primarily voltage-dependent.

Channel reactivation. Channels that have gone through an activation-inactivation cycle following membrane depolarization can be made available again by membrane repolarization. The time required for this restoration of availability is on the order of 100 msec at −80 to −100 mV, but it increases with lower intracellular Ca^{2+} concentration.

Modulation of channel behavior. Apart from the complete blockade described above, Ca^{2+} channel behavior can be altered by a variety of neurohumoral influences.

- **β-Adrenoceptor** stimulation enhances L-type Ca^{2+} current ($I_{Ca,L}$) via a protein kinase A-dependent mechanism.
- Modulation by **muscarinic receptor** stimulation is a controversial matter because muscarinic activation stimulates a transient outward K^+ current that overlaps $I_{Ca,L}$. Basal $I_{Ca,L}$ appears to be unaffected by acetylcholine, but catecholamine-stimulated $I_{Ca,L}$ is inhibited by it.
- Modulation by G_s **proteins** may stimulate $I_{Ca,L}$ by a cytoplasmic pathway identical to the one that follows β-adrenoceptor stimulation.
- Elevation of $[Ca^{2+}]_i$ inhibits L-type calcium channels.

Potassium channels

The arrangement of the transmembrane segments of the K^+ channel (shown in Fig. 35-1) is similar to that found in each of the domains of the Na^+ channel. *Channel activation* also involves conformational changes of the S4 segment. *Channel inactivation*, however, depends critically on a sequence of amino acids at the NH_3 terminal of the protein. Although the structure of the K^+ channel is simpler than that of the Na^+ or Ca^{2+} channels, less is known about the details of its function. Several **functional subtypes** have been identified:

- Channels that are opened by extracellular acetylcholine and by adenosine.
- Acetylcholine-insensitive channels that appear to be the major carrier of basal potassium current in human heart cells. Their "open" times are longer than those of the acetylcholine-sensitive channels.
- Channels carrying the delayed rectifier current, I_K, that provides outward current for repolarization of

the membrane towards its diastolic potential. Its threshold is near −50 mV and it continues to activate up to potentials as high as +50 mV. It is not affected by acetylcholine, but β-adrenoceptor agonists (1) move its threshold 5–10 mV more negative, (2) increase the magnitude of the fully activated current, and (3) slow the kinetics of channel deactivation.

- Channels that are inactivated by ATP. These channels contribute negligibly to the basal potassium current, but may become important during ischemia when cellular ATP levels are low.

Membrane Potentials

Cardiac cells are excitable cells and are, therefore, capable of generating action potentials. Most muscle cells in the atria and ventricles tend to have stable resting membrane potentials in the intervals between action potentials. Some cardiac cells, called **pacemaker cells,** never rest; they have unstable membrane potentials that allow them to reach threshold and generate action potentials spontaneously.

Resting membrane potentials

When they are not excited, most cardiac cells maintain a stable resting membrane potential between −80 and −95 mV. It arises from passive ion fluxes and electrogenic transport (Fig. 35-2) and is largely determined by the ratio of intracellular to extracellular K^+, because the resting membrane is far more permeable to K^+ than to the other ions in the resting state. An approximation of the steady-state resting membrane potential (E_m) can be calculated from the Goldman-Hodgkin-Katz equation:

$$E_m = \frac{RT}{F} \ln \frac{P_K\,[K^+]_o + P_{Na}\,[Na^+]_o + P_{Cl}\,[Cl^-]_i}{P_K\,[K^+]_i + P_{Na}\,[Na^+]_i + P_{Cl}\,[Cl^-]_o}$$

where R = universal gas constant, T = absolute temperature, F = Faraday's constant, P_x = membrane permeability for ion "X," $[X]_o$ = extracellular concentration of ion "X," and $[X]_i$ = intracellular concentration of ion "X."

This equation, based on a simplified model of ion transport through membranes, has guided much experimental design and interpretation and has led to the realization that the resting membrane potential is determined by the behavior of ion channels. It is, therefore, influenced by changes in the ionic milieu and by any neurohumoral factors or drugs that affect ion transport across cell membranes.

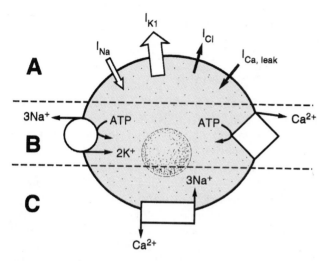

Figure 35-2. Ion currents contributing to cardiac cell resting membrane potentials. The resting membrane potential in cardiac cells results from a balance among ion fluxes that result from passive diffusion down electrochemical gradients, active transport, or coupled transport. A. *Passive diffusion mechanisms.* Four currents contribute significantly: An inwardly directed sodium current (I_{Na}); an outwardly directed potassium current (I_{K1}); a small chloride current that is directed outwardly, against the concentration gradient, because the chloride equilibrium potential is positive with respect to the resting membrane potential; a small inward calcium leakage current ($I_{Ca,leak}$). B. *Active transport mechanisms.* The Na^+-K^+ pump transports 2 K^+ into the cell while extruding three Na^+ ions for each molecule of ATP hydrolyzed. The coupling ratio of 3:2 prevails over a wide range of conditions. There also is an ATP-consuming Ca^{2+} pump that helps to maintain low resting intracellular calcium concentration. C. *Coupled transport.* The Na^+-Ca^{2+} exchanger operates through a sarcolemmal protein and is driven by the Na^+ electrochemical gradient. Reversal to a Na^+-out/Ca^{2+}-in state occurs at a membrane potential just slightly positive to the normal resting membrane potential.

Action potentials

Cardiac muscle cells respond to an appropriate stimulus with a sequence of electrophysiological changes that constitute the phases of the action potential. All of these phases occur during the cardiac systole, i.e., the period in which ventricular contraction is expelling blood into the large arteries. The period between action potentials corresponds to diastole, in which atrial contraction is refilling the ventricles with blood, in readiness for the next systole. The phases are as follows:

- *Phase 0*, the action potential upstroke. Application of an effective stimulus causes activation of enough

ion channels (mostly Na^+) to produce rapid depolarization, shown by a steep upstroke in the membrane potential recording (Fig. 35-3A) that moves rapidly toward the Na^+ equilibrium potential. The

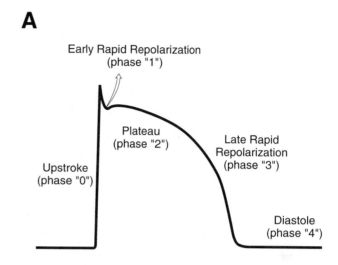

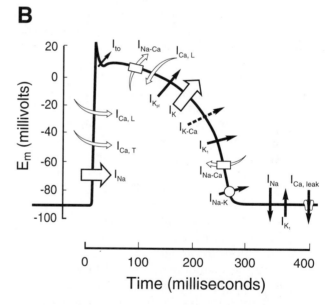

Figure 35-3. Cardiac action potential. A. Landmarks of the action potential in most cardiac muscle cells. B. The transient change in membrane potential, termed action potential, results from a coordinated sequence of ion movements. The significant currents that contribute to each phase of the action potential are identified by arrows that indicate whether the current (flow of positive charge) is being carried into the cell (arrow pointing into the area under the action potential) or out of the cell (arrows pointing out). (Modified from Ten Eick RE, Walley DW, Rasmussen HH, 1992.)

increase in Na^+ flux lasts only 1–2 msec because the channels carrying it undergo voltage-dependent inactivation. Channels carrying Ca^{2+} currents are activated when the membrane potential reaches their gating thresholds: about -70 mV for $I_{Ca,T}$ and about -40 mV for $I_{Ca,L}$. $I_{Ca,T}$ is inactivated quickly, but $I_{Ca,L}$ remains activated well into the next two phases (Fig. 35-3B). It triggers and controls the release of Ca^{2+} from intracellular sarcoplasmic stores in the process of excitation-activation-contraction coupling.

- *Phase 1*, early rapid repolarization. At the peak of the upstroke the membrane potential reaches about $+30$ to $+40$ mV and then undergoes rapid repolarization by a transient outward current that is carried mostly by K^+. The end of phase 1 is marked by a small notch, the point at which the outward current has been almost completely inactivated.

- *Phase 2*, the action potential plateau. The plateau occurs because the depolarizing and repolarizing currents are nearly in balance during this phase. The major depolarizing influence is the inward Ca^{2+} current carried through L channels that were opened during the action potential upstroke and remain open for 200–300 msec. The repolarizing influence is an outward flow of positive charge via two routes: (1) the Na^+-Ca^{2+} exchanger located in the sarcolemma, operating in the Ca^{2+}-inward mode at this membrane potential, and (2) an outward K^+ current carried by at least four types of K^+ channels. While the plateau is maintained, the cell cannot be reexcited. Because of this prolonged period of refractoriness, cardiac muscle cannot be tetanized as skeletal muscle can (see Chapter 19).

- *Phase 3*, late rapid repolarization. The plateau terminates because the L channels are inactivated by processes dependent on time, voltage, and $[Ca^{2+}]_i$. Repolarization then occurs rapidly because the influence of outward K^+ currents dominates. As the membrane potential approaches its resting value and the electrochemical gradient for K^+ decreases, the K^+ current diminishes and the Na^+-Ca^{2+} exchanger returns to its Ca^{2+}-outward mode. As the Na^+ and other channels that were inactivated by membrane depolarization return to the activatable state, membrane excitability is restored in preparation for the next action potential. The end result of the cycle is a net gain of $[Na]_i$ and a net loss of K^+ during the entire action potential. This imbalance is corrected by the sarcolemmal $(Na^+ + K^+)$-ATPase, which uses the energy from the splitting of ATP to transport Na^+ back out of the cell and K^+ back in.

Pacemaker potentials

In contrast to the muscle cells, pacemaker cells do not have a stable resting membrane potential. Instead, their membrane potential spontaneously becomes less negative throughout diastole (**phase 4 depolarization**) until it reaches the threshold for triggering an action potential (Fig. 35-4). This property is known as **automaticity.** Phase 4 spontaneous depolarization is the result of an inward positive current (I_f) carried primarily by Na^+. The phase 0 depolarization in pacemaker cells is also different from that of myocardial cells; it is largely caused by Ca^{2+} influx, resulting in a less-steep rise of potential than in myocardial cells.

The two main populations of pacemaker cells are found in the region of the sinoatrial (S-A) node and in the atrioventricular (A-V) node and Purkinje fibers. S-A node cells normally show the steeper diastolic rise in potential, because they have the lowest density of the K^+ channels that carry the major stabilizing current in the muscle cells. Hence, they are the earliest to depolarize, have the highest discharge rate, and are therefore the dominant pacemaker. When, for any reason, the A-V node takes over the pacemaker role, the heart rate is lower.

Modulation of S-A node pacemaker rate

Physiological modulation of pacemaker activity is achieved by extremely subtle changes in transmembrane ion currents. Catecholamines released from the adrenal medulla or from adrenergic nerve terminals increase the frequency of pacemaker action potentials and thus cause an increase in heart rate (**positive chronotropic effect**). The catecholamines increase the levels of cAMP, activating protein kinase A and leading to changes in several transmembrane currents:

- Increase in $I_{Ca,L}$ leads to an accelerated upstroke in the pacemaker potential.
- Increase in I_K shortens the action potential and begins the diastolic rise of membrane potential earlier.
- Steeper rise of the diastolic potential towards threshold occurs.

Parasympathetic stimulation of **muscarinic receptors** causes a reduced level of cAMP and increases

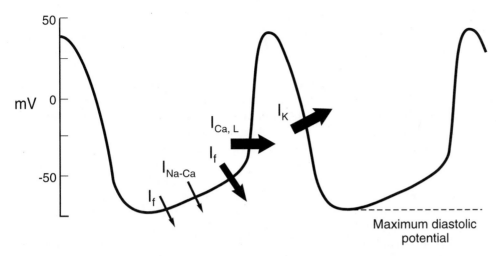

Figure 35-4. Cardiac pacemaker potential. The significant currents that contribute to each phase of the S-A node pacemaker potential are identified by arrows that indicate whether the current (flow of positive charge) is being carried into the cell (arrows pointing into the area under the trace) or out of the cell (arrow pointing out). I_f is a time-dependent inward current that is activated by hyperpolarization. I_{Na-Ca} is the current carried by the Na^+-Ca^{2+} exchanger. It is an inward current when the exchanger operates in the Ca^{2+}-out mode. $I_{Ca,L}$ is carried by L-type calcium channels. I_K is an outward time- and voltage-dependent delayed rectifier potassium current. It differs from I_{K1} in its activation kinetics.

the activity of cytosolic phospholipase C, which activates the acetylcholine-sensitive K^+ channel and initiates an outward K^+ current. The resultant hyperpolarization and slower rise of diastolic potential both contribute to a decrease in pacemaker frequency.

CARDIAC MUSCLE FUNCTION

Cardiac Metabolism, Oxygen Consumption, and Work

Although cardiac myocytes are capable of utilizing a variety of metabolic substrates, under normal conditions fatty acids supply two-thirds of myocardial ATP. They are, therefore, the key source of energy required for the performance of cardiac work. Fatty acids are actively taken up by the myocardial cell and converted to fatty acyl-CoA, transported into the mitochondria, converted to acetyl-CoA, and oxidized by the Krebs tricarboxylic acid cycle and the electron transport chain to yield CO_2, water, and ATP.

Sustained increase in cardiac work requires an increase in the rate of ATP production and utilization. Therefore anything that impairs coronary blood flow, or reduces pulmonary blood flow or oxygen-ation, will indirectly decrease myocardial performance.

The processes of **excitation-activation-contraction coupling** link electrical events of the myocyte action potential to the mechanical events of tension development and subsequent diastolic relaxation. Ionized calcium plays a crucial role in these processes, rising from a resting cytosolic concentration near 100 nM to a peak of about 1 μM during normal ventricular contraction.

Sources of Calcium

Although the large concentration gradient across the membrane causes some passive inward leak of Ca^{2+}, $I_{Ca,L}$ carries most of the calcium that enters the myocyte at the start of an action potential. It contributes no more than 10% of the total Ca^{2+} needed for a maximal contraction, but it provides the trigger for releasing calcium from intracellular stores (sarcoplasmic reticulum) during systole (see below) and supplies extracellular calcium for replenishing the intracellular stores during diastole.

Another source of intracellular Ca^{2+} is the **sodium-calcium exchanger,** which uses the Na^+ electrochemical gradient to transport one Ca^{2+} ion in exchange for three Na^+ ions moved in the opposite direction. Thus, the exchanger acts to transport net positive charge in the direction of the sodium movement. When depolarization raises the intracellular potential, the exchanger carries Na^+ out and Ca^{2+} in. Therefore, agents that increase $[Na^+]_i$ will reduce Ca^{2+} extrusion in the resting phase and enhance Ca^{2+} entry during the action potential. This movement may be too slow to play a major role in the contractile mechanism itself (see below), but it is probably important for the replenishing of intracellular calcium stores during diastole.

The **sarcoplasmic reticulum (SR)** functions as the major intracellular source and storage site for ionized calcium. A small influx of Ca^{2+} from the extracellular space operates to release Ca^{2+} from the SR. In a single contraction the SR is the major source of Ca^{2+}. However, it is the Ca^{2+} transport mechanisms across the sarcolemma that create the intracellular stores and that make repeated contraction-relaxation cycles possible.

Reuptake of Calcium

When the action potential has passed and the myocyte has repolarized, calcium is removed from the cytosol. Both the Na^+-Ca^{2+} exchanger (now working in the reverse direction) and Ca^{2+}-ATPase are significant contributors to Ca^{2+} removal from the cytosol.

A **Ca^{2+}-ATPase-dependent transporter** that is present in both the sarcolemma and the membrane of the SR transfers two Ca^{2+} per ATP. It is modulated by agents such as **phospholamban,** a protein found in juxtaposition with SR Ca^{2+}-ATPase. When it is in the unphosphorylated state, it inhibits Ca^{2+} uptake by the SR, but when it is phosphorylated it is an important promoter of Ca^{2+} transport into the SR. Phosphorylation of phospholamban is promoted by several kinases, each of which is activated by different agents, including cAMP, cGMP, and Ca^{2+}-calmodulin.

The Contraction Process

Interaction of free intracellular Ca^{2+} with protein constituents of cardiac muscle cells initiates the processes that lead to the development of tension. These protein constituents are myosin, actin, tropomyosin, and troponin. Their organized arrangement in a cardiac muscle cell is shown in Figure 35-5.

Myosin forms the thick filament. It is a long molecule that consists of two immunologically distinct heavy chains intertwined with three pairs of light chains. Each heavy chain has a globular "head," and the heads of the two heavy chains are at the same end of the myosin molecule. A single thick filament consists of about 400 myosin molecules, arranged in parallel and distributed symmetrically with half of the molecules on each side of the M-line in the sarcomere (see Fig. 35-5). The head-groups of the myosin are at the end of the molecule that is furthest from the M-line.

Actin is an almost globular molecule (G-actin) that contains specific, high-affinity binding sites for ATP and for divalent metal ions. The latter site is preferentially occupied by Mg^{2+}. The G-actin/ATP/Mg^{2+} complex aggregates to form a polymer that resembles two strands of intertwined pearls and forms the major protein of the thin filament. Thick and thin filaments alternate with each other in parallel arrays. The thin filaments have binding sites to which the globular heads of the thick filaments can attach and form cross-linkages. In the relaxed state of the muscle, however, there is no physical contact between myosin and actin because the myosin binding site on the actin molecule is shielded (Fig. 35-6).

Tropomyosin is a rod-shaped protein that lies near the actin filament and competes for the myosin binding sites during the relaxed phase of the sarcomere.

Troponin exists in muscle as a complex of three dissimilar subunits, designated Tn-C, Tn-T, and Tn-I. Tn-T binds to tropomyosin and holds the complex in place. Tn-I inhibits the actin–myosin interaction in resting conditions. Tn-C is a Ca^{2+}-binding protein.

When $[Ca^{2+}]_i$ increases after membrane depolarization, Ca^{2+} interacts with troponin C and changes the conformation of the actin-troponin-tropomyosin complex in a way that exposes the myosin binding site (see Fig. 35-6), permitting a momentary interaction between actin and myosin in the presence of ATP.

Tension development: the sliding-filament hypothesis

When the cross-bridging of myosin with actin filaments occurs, the head-groups of the myosin molecule tilt (i.e., change their angle) relative to the tail of the molecule (Fig. 35-7). This process converts chemical energy into mechanical work, pulling the thin filament toward the M-line and thus shortening the muscle fiber, or increasing its tension, or both. However, this process also activates the actomyosin-ATPase activity and disengages the cross-linkage,

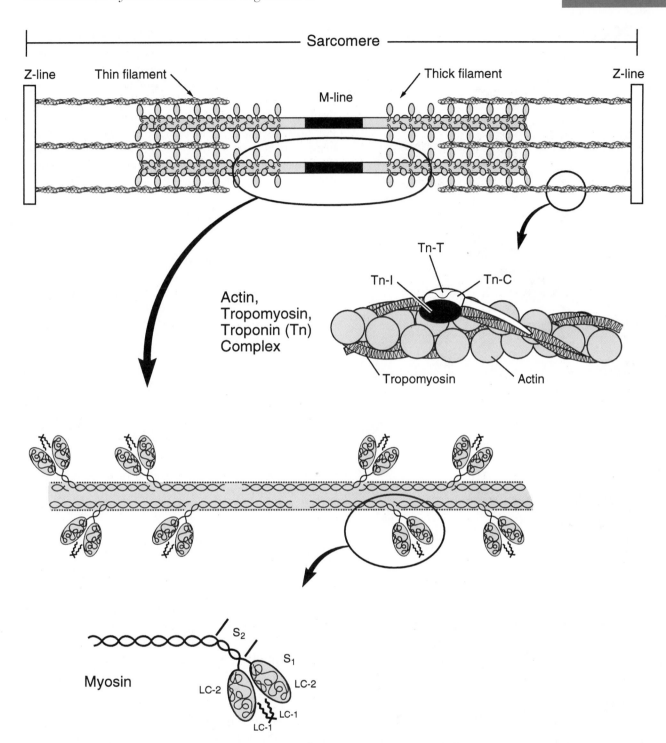

Figure 35-5. Contractile and regulatory proteins in cardiac muscle. Cardiac muscle consists of two contractile proteins, myosin and actin, as well as the regulatory proteins, tropomyosin and troponin. Myosin and actin are arranged in an interdigitating pattern of thick and thin filaments.

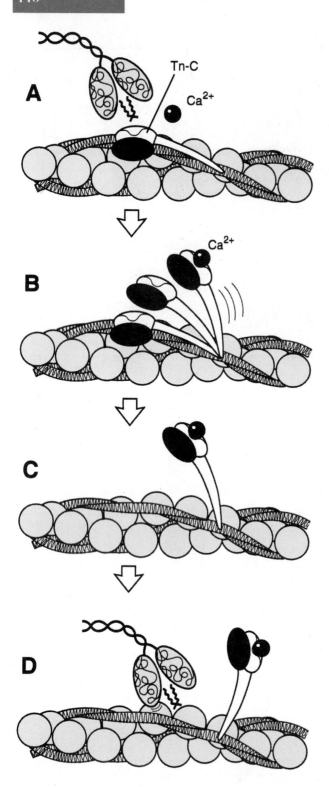

Figure 35-6. Actomyosin cross-bridge formation. When troponin-C (Tn-C) interacts with calcium, the conformation of the troponin–tropomyosin complex changes and the actin-myosin binding site is exposed. A. Tropomyosin is held in place by the troponin complex. They form a steric hindrance that shields the actomyosin binding site.

allowing the fiber to relax. The sequence shown in Figure 35-7 represents the simplest model that explains currently known features of the mechanism of muscle contraction. The sequence repeats as long as sufficient Ca^{2+} is present to expose the myosin binding site and as long as sufficient ATP is present not only to supply the energy that "cocks" the S_1 head, but also to permit disengagement of the actomyosin complex (Fig. 35-7C). Lack of ATP arrests the heart in a contracted state ("stone heart").

Cardiac Performance

All tissues receive their blood flow from a common source, the cardiac output (CO), which is the amount of blood pumped from each side of the heart each minute. CO is determined by the heart rate (HR) and the volume ejected from each ventricle with each contraction (the stroke volume, SV):

$$CO = HR \times SV$$

HR is set by the activity of the pacemaker cells. SV is determined by the effectiveness of ventricular emptying in systole. That effectiveness is termed cardiac performance and is determined by four factors:

- The degree of sarcomere stretch prior to actomyosin cross-linkage (preload).
- The efficacy of actomyosin interaction (contractility).
- The resistance to ventricular contraction (afterload).
- The interval between contraction-relaxation cycles (heart rate).

These factors apply equally to the left and right ventricles, but in the following descriptions the focus is placed on the left ventricle because it is the ultimate source of blood flow to the periphery.

Preload

Cardiac performance is normally proportional to the degree of diastolic stretch in the ventricles, as de-

Therefore, an actomyosin crossbridge cannot form. B and C. Ca^{2+} binds to Tn-C and changes the conformation of the troponin/tropomyosin complex, allowing tropomyosin to move into the actin "groove." This exposes the binding site. D. An actomyosin crossbridge forms because the S_1 head of myosin has a high affinity for actin.

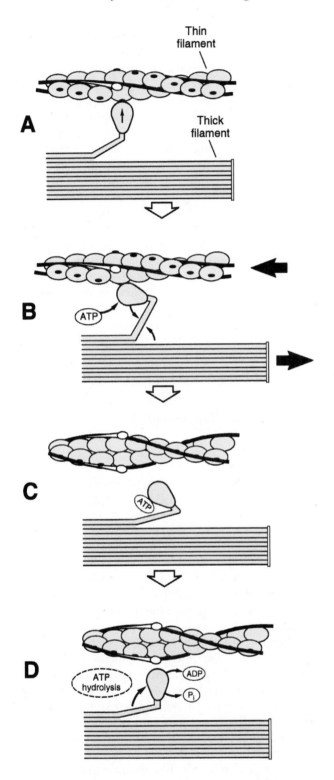

Figure 35-7. The sliding-filament hypothesis. The process of converting chemical energy to mechanical work depends on changes in protein conformation. A. Interaction of Ca^{2+} with troponin-C has caused a conformation change in the actin-tropomyosin-troponin complex that results in the exposure of myosin binding sites on the actin

scribed by the Frank-Starling law of the heart. At rest, the Starling mechanism helps to adapt cardiac performance to postural changes and to match left heart output to right heart output during respiratory changes in venous return. During exercise, responses to changes in preload contribute to the increase in cardiac output, although reflex mechanisms that operate via catecholamines can overshadow the effect of sarcomere stretch in altering cardiac performance. With advancing age, as the effectiveness of catecholaminergic modulation of cardiac performance diminishes in humans, the preload mechanism becomes increasingly important in matching cardiac output to the oxygen demands of the body.

Cellular basis of the preload mechanism. The force developed during muscle contraction is directly related to four general factors: (1) change in the number of actomyosin cross-bridges; (2) modulation of the transient increase in $[Ca^{2+}]_i$ that occurs after excitation; (3) modulation of Ca^{2+}-troponin interactions at a given $[Ca^{2+}]_i$; and (4) modulation of the degree of synchronization among individual contractile units.

It was formerly thought that the most important mechanism of the Starling effect was the increase in the number of cross-linkages between actin and myosin that is made possible by stretching the sarcomere. However, this seems unlikely, and more importance is now attributed to the increase in $[Ca^{2+}]_i$ that occurs with stretching of the fiber, and the increased calcium sensitivity of the myofilaments, resulting in a greater force generated at a given $[Ca^{2+}]_i$.

Determinants of preload. The degree of ventricular filling in diastole is a function of filling pressure, ventricular compliance, and time available for filling.

- **Filling pressure** is the difference between atrial pressure and ventricular pressure. Left ventricular

molecule. As a result, myosin binds to actin. B. The actomyosin complex undergoes a conformation change in the S_1, S_2 regions. This change accomplishes three things: (1) It moves the thick filament relative to the thin filament. (2) It allows the actomyosin complex to bind ATP. (3) It brings ATP closer to the myosin ATPase activity. C. ATP binding facilitates dissociation of myosin from actin because the ATP-myosin-actin complex is highly unstable compared to the myosin-actin complex. D. ATP is hydrolyzed by the myosin ATPase activity. This "cocks" the S_1 head in readiness for the next power stroke (see B).

filling pressure depends greatly on pulmonary vascular pressure. This, in turn, is influenced by right ventricular output as well as intrathoracic pressure.

- **Ventricular compliance** is a measure of the ease with which the ventricle expands while it accepts diastolic inflow. It can be altered by factors that alter the properties of cardiac muscle itself or by factors that alter conditions in the pericardial space. Both occur on a time scale that affects only long-term regulation.
- **Time available for ventricular filling** is inversely related to heart rate. At heart rates in excess of 150 bpm, the time available for rapid diastolic flow from the atria into the ventricles is significantly reduced.

Afterload

The term afterload was coined in isolated muscle experiments. There it refers to the load the muscle is required to lift during contraction. In the cardiovascular system, afterload is the load against which the left ventricle ejects its stroke volume, designated the aortic input impedance. This load determines left ventricular wall tension during ejection, which is the major determinant of myocardial oxygen consumption.

An increase in afterload, due to increased blood volume in the vascular bed or to decreased compliance of the arterial walls, reduces the volume of ventricular ejection at a given force of contraction.

Rate

Over most of the physiological range of heart rates, peak tension increases as the rate increases (the Bowditch effect). The shorter the interval between successive beats, the higher the residual $[Ca^{2+}]_i$, because the reuptake of Ca^{2+} after excitation-activation is a time-dependent phenomenon, driven by the rate of phosphorylation of phospholamban in the sarcoplasmic reticulum. The increased residual Ca^{2+} results in stronger contraction.

Contractility

An increase in contractility, most easily brought about by **β_1-adrenoceptor stimulation**, is associated with increased velocity of wall shortening, reduced time to peak tension, more rapid relaxation, shorter duration of systole, greater extent of fiber shortening, greater stroke volume, higher ejection fraction, and decreased end-systolic volume. If the ventricle is made to contract isovolumetrically rather than isotonically, there is, in addition to many of the above changes, an increase in peak tension.

Since all myocytes participate in a normal cardiac contraction, the measurable whole-organ changes that accompany changes in contractility cannot be due to changes in the number of active myocytes but must arise from properties associated with Ca^{2+} dynamics, the effectiveness of actin-myosin interactions, and the nature of the contractile proteins themselves. Stimulation of β_1-adrenoceptors leads to increased $[Ca^{2+}]_i$ by both direct and indirect mechanisms, as described earlier. In addition, the increase in cAMP resulting from β_1-adrenoceptor stimulation promotes the phosphorylation of troponin and hence the tension development, but it also leads to more rapid release of Ca^{2+} from the phosphorylated troponin, so diastolic relaxation and ventricular filling are facilitated.

BLOOD VESSEL FUNCTION

Vascular Smooth Muscle

Structure

Vascular smooth muscle cells are spindle-shaped or branched and make extensive electrical and metabolic contact with adjacent cells by means of gap junctions (see Chapter 2). In addition to the gap junction region, the plasma membrane shows histologically (and, presumably, functionally) different portions. One portion has surface invaginations (caveolae), another has closely apposed sarcoplasmic reticulum, and a third has attachments to intracellular dense bodies.

Caveolae greatly increase the surface area of smooth-muscle cells, but they appear to have no other function. The plasma **membrane apposed to sarcoplasmic reticulum** is probably a major site of signal transduction via voltage-gated or receptor-mediated mechanisms. Within this region there are electron-dense structures that appear to couple the plasma membrane to the sarcoplasmic reticulum (SR). Smooth-muscle SR, like cardiac-muscle SR, is the major intracellular depot for Ca^{2+}, and it plays a corresponding role with respect to Ca^{2+} movements in relation to contraction and relaxation.

The contractile machinery of smooth muscle is not as well organized as that of striated muscle, but it resembles the latter in most of the important features, including the thick and thin filaments, their involvement in a sliding-filament mechanism, the presence of both voltage-gated and ligand-gated ion channels, and the role of ion movements in the contraction-relaxation cycle.

Function

However, there are a number of important differences between the contraction of the myocardium and that of vascular smooth muscle, such as in the coronary vessels and systemic arterioles.

- Most vascular smooth-muscle cells differ from myocytes in that their action potential upstroke is caused primarily by Ca^{2+} influx rather than Na^+ influx. Three electrically distinct types of vascular smooth muscle have been identified:
  1. Some smooth muscle generates action potentials spontaneously.
  2. Some smooth muscle generates action potentials in response to an appropriate stimulus.
  3. Some smooth muscle responds to excitatory stimuli with a sustained, nonregenerating electrical response that resembles a skeletal muscle end-plate potential.

  Types 1 and 2 exhibit phasic contractions whereas type 3 shows more sustained contractions.
- Chemomechanical excitation-activation-contraction coupling accounts for drug-induced contractions of vascular smooth muscle. Its two major components are stimulation of intracellular Ca^{2+} release (predominantly by inositol trisphosphate [IP_3]) and modulation of the Ca^{2+} sensitivity of the actin–myosin interaction. Of these two, the IP_3 mechanism is by far the more important.
- The processes of cross-link formation, ATP hydrolysis, sliding filaments, and cross-link detachment are thought to be identical in smooth and striated muscle. However, in smooth muscle, there is a cascade of many more biochemical steps intervening between Ca^{2+} entry and eventual energy production by activation of myosin ATPase. These steps can be regulated to allow various degrees of tension to be developed for varying durations.

  The first step involves a small (15,000 Da) calcium-binding protein, **calmodulin.** Smooth muscle has no troponin that Ca^{2+} can bind to. Instead, when the $[Ca^{2+}]_i$ reaches approximately 10^{-6} M, Ca^{2+} binds to calmodulin and the complex activates the enzyme myosin kinase. This in turn phosphorylates the myosin light chain and permits myosin to interact with actin, leading to contraction of

the smooth muscle cell. However, in both myocardium and vascular smooth muscle it is the Ca^{2+} influx that activates the contractile process, and contraction is proportional to the Ca^{2+} influx.
- Relaxation of smooth muscle occurs when Ca^{2+} is removed from the cytosol and the myosin light chain is dephosphorylated by the action of a myosin phosphatase.
- Prolonged maintenance of contractile force with low energy consumption is a characteristic feature of smooth muscle. Various models have been proposed to explain this feature, but no consensus has been reached yet.

Vascular Endothelium

The endothelial lining of blood vessels forms autocrine and paracrine substances that serve two main functions: They prevent intravascular thrombus formation, and they modulate the tone of the underlying smooth muscle. Both relaxing and constricting factors are synthesized by the endothelium and participate in the local regulation of tissue blood flow. They can also influence the effectiveness of neurotransmitters released by autonomic nerve endings on the vascular smooth muscle and thus modulate the effect of the central nervous system on vascular tone.

Endothelium-dependent relaxation

The three important dilating factors derived from the endothelium (see Fig. 35-8) are endothelium-derived relaxing factor (EDRF), prostacyclin (PGI_2), and endothelium-derived hyperpolarizing factor (EDHF). Of these three, EDRF makes by far the greatest contribution. Its role appears to be the continuous regulation of resistance vessels and, hence, of arterial blood pressure.

Endothelium-derived relaxing factor (EDRF) is thought to be either nitric oxide or *S*-nitrosocysteine. Both are synthesized from the terminal guanidino nitrogen atom(s) of the amino acid L-arginine in vascular endothelial cells during the metabolism of arginine to citrulline. The stimulus for the formation of EDRF can be flow-induced shear stress or a variety of receptor-coupled agonists. It is likely that both operate via elevation of $[Ca^{2+}]_i$. Most agonists that release EDRF do so via activation of phospholipase C.

Prostacyclin (PGI_2) is a major intermediary product in the metabolism of arachidonic acid by cyclooxygenase in vascular smooth muscle (see Chapter 31). It is rapidly converted to prostaglandin

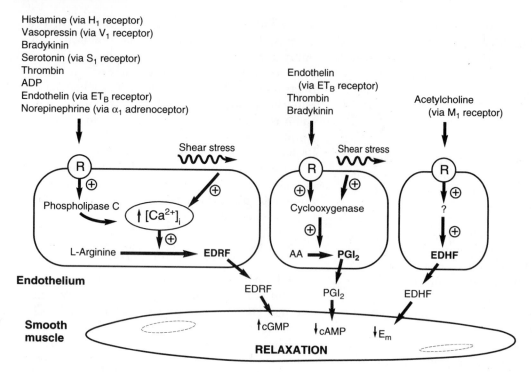

Figure 35-8. Relaxing factors derived from vascular endothelium. Three notable dilator agents are synthesized by the endothelial cells that line blood vessels. They are endothelium-derived relaxing factor (EDRF), prostacyclin (PGI$_2$), and endothelium-derived hyperpolarizing factor (EDHF). Of these, EDRF is the most significant. *Endothelium-derived relaxing factor* (EDRF) synthesis is promoted by elevated cytosolic calcium concentration. Agonists promoting its release are shear stress and a variety of receptor-mediated activators of phospholipase C. EDRF causes vascular smooth-muscle relaxation via an increase in cGMP levels. *Prostacyclin* (PGI$_2$) synthesis is enhanced by shear stress, thrombin, bradykinin, and endothelin. It operates via cAMP to relax vascular smooth muscle. *Endothelium-derived hyperpolarizing factor* (EDHF) has been identified as a short-lived product of M$_1$ muscarinic receptor activation. It desensitizes smooth muscle by hyperpolarizing its membrane potential (E_m).

ADP = adenosine diphosphate; AA = arachidonic acid.

F$_{1\alpha}$, which has no biological activity. PGI$_2$, however, causes vasodilatation. This action results from depression of cytosolic cAMP in smooth-muscle cells.

The chemical nature of **endothelium-derived hyperpolarizing factor (EDHF)** has not yet been identified. It is probably a G protein that operates by opening an acetylcholine-sensitive K$^+$ channel.

Endothelium-dependent constriction

The vascular endothelium also produces smooth-muscle-constricting factors under certain circumstances. Such production varies greatly among species and also among different vascular beds within a given species. The major contracting factors are the endothelins, locally produced angiotensin II, prostaglandin H$_2$, thromboxane, and an as-yet-unidentified contracting factor, EDCF, that is produced and released in response to hypoxia. Figure 35-9 summarizes the control of endothelial constrictor release.

Endothelin is a 21-amino-acid peptide cleaved from a 203-amino-acid precursor called pre-proendothelin. Four forms of endothelin have been identified, of which only one, endothelin-1, is produced by endothelial cells. When this agent interacts with the ET$_A$-receptor on vascular smooth muscle, it activates phospholipase C and leads to elevated [Ca^{2+}]$_i$ via the IP$_3$ pathway, causing powerful, long-lasting vasoconstriction. Endothelin-1 also potentiates the vasoconstrictor effects of hormones and neurotransmitters such as serotonin or norepinephrine.

Angiotensin-converting enzyme is located in endothelial cells, which are the major site of conversion of angiotensin I to *angiotensin II* in the circulation (see Chapters 32 and 38).

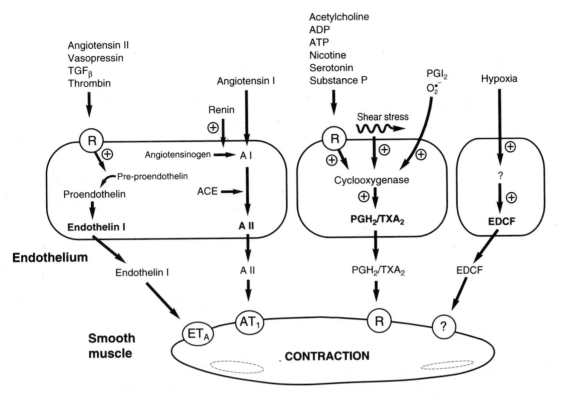

Figure 35-9. Contracting factors derived from vascular endothelium. *Endothelin I* is a 21-amino-acid peptide that is generated from the 203-amino-acid precursor pre-pro-endothelin. It is a powerful vasoconstrictor that is preferentially released toward the luminal side of endothelial cells. It is a regulator of local function as opposed to one of general systemic cardiovascular function. *Angiotensin II (AII)* is produced in endothelial cells because they are the locus for angiotensin-converting enzyme (ACE). *Prostaglandin H_2 and thromboxane (TXA)* both bind to the TXA_2-receptor. They are produced when cyclooxygenase is activated by mechanical or various chemical stimuli.

Preference for production of one or the other is determined by local concentrations of promoters and inhibitors. PGH_2 has an extremely short half-life. *Endothelium-derived contracting factor (EDCF)* is responsible for hypoxic vasoconstriction. Its chemical nature has not yet been identified.

A I = angiotensin I; A H = angiotensin II; ACE = angiotensin-converting enzyme; ADP = adenosine diphosphate; ATP = adenosine triphosphate; PGI_2 = prostaglandin I_2 (prostacyclin); TGF_β = transforming growth factor β; $O_2{}^{\cdot-}$ = superoxide anion; PGH_2 = prostaglandin H_2; TXA_2 = thromboxane A_2.

Thromboxane A_2 (TXA_2) is the major vasoconstrictor product of arachidonic acid metabolism via the cyclooxygenase pathway (see Chapter 31). Both mechanical and chemical stimuli promote its formation. In some tissues, cyclooxygenase-dependent contraction can be evoked even when thromboxane synthase is inhibited. This suggests that release of **prostaglandin H_2**, which also binds the thromboxane receptor, is involved.

Endothelium-derived contracting factor is a constrictor agent that is released from endothelial cells in response to hypoxia. Its release requires activation of voltage-gated Ca^{2+} channels. Its chemical nature has not yet been identified.

Functional Integration of Endothelium-Derived Factors

A suggested model of functional integration of control of blood flow in microvascular units, by the endothelial factors described above, is as follows:

- The smallest arterioles are controlled mainly by metabolic factors; the importance of metabolic control diminishes in larger upstream vessels.
- Midsized arterioles are influenced most strongly by pressure-dependent myogenic responses.
- Large arterioles are most responsive to blood flow, which exerts its endothelial effects via shear stress.

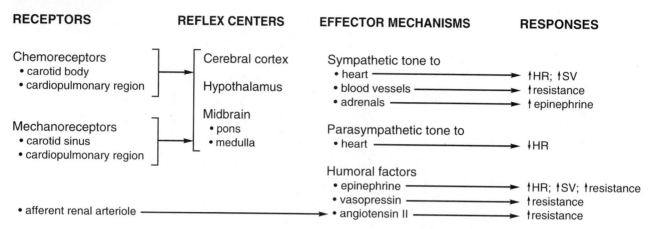

Figure 35-10. Summary of the important features of cardiovascular reflex regulation. HR = heart rate; SV = stroke volume.

Receptor-mediated release of endothelial factors has not yet been incorporated into an integrated scheme.

Cardiovascular Regulation

Regulation of **vascular** function in individual tissues results from a complex interplay among locally produced vasoactive factors and remote influences exerted by nerves and blood-borne agents (hormones and autacoids). The effect of such influences is to alter the hydraulic resistance of the tissue vasculature by altering the effective diameter of the vascular bed. The objective of such local regulation is to ensure an adequate supply of blood to support metabolic activities of that individual tissue.

Regulation of **cardiovascular** function, on the other hand, is a whole-body phenomenon, the purpose of which varies with conditions.

- When conditions are normal, the processes of cardiovascular regulation ensure that all tissues receive a flow of blood that is adequate for their metabolic needs under a variety of demands that range from sleep to intense exercise.
- When conditions are critical, cardiovascular regulation ensures survival of the organism by diverting all available flow to the two crucial vascular beds, brain and heart.

The two major aspects of cardiovascular regulation are the regulation of cardiac output (CO) and the maintenance of normal perfusion pressure (ABP). Pressure regulation can be accomplished independently of cardiac output regulation by the modulation of total peripheral resistance (TPR). The following mnemonic summarizes the essential features:

$$[HR \times SV = CO] \times TPR = ABP$$

Short-term regulation is accomplished, in part, through intrinsic mechanisms such as the cardiac responses to varying preload or afterload, and in part through the reflex regulation of autonomic nervous outflow and circulating catecholamines. Long-term adaptation to changing needs takes place via the processes of atrophy or hypertrophy. Figure 35-10 shows a schematic summary of the important features of cardiovascular reflex regulation.

SUGGESTED READING

Fozzard HA, Jennings RB, Haber E, Katz AM, Morgan HE, eds. The heart and cardiovascular system. New York: Raven Press, 1991.

Francis GS. Neuroendocrine activity in congestive heart failure. Am J Cardiol 1990; 66:33D–39D.

Katz AM. Physiology of the heart. New York: Raven Press, 1992.

Moncada S, Palmer RM, Higgs EA. Nitric oxide: physiology, pathophysiology and pharmacology. Pharmacol Rev 1991; 43:109–142.

Rowell LB. Human cardiovascular control. New York: Oxford University Press, 1993.

Ten Eick RE, Whalley DW, Rasmussen HH. Connections: heart disease, cellular electrophysiology, and ion channels. FASEB J 1992; 6:2568–2580.

CHAPTER 36

Digitalis Glycosides and Other Positive Inotropic Agents

W.A. MAHON AND C. FORSTER

CASE HISTORY

A 64-year-old male came to the physician's office because of increasing shortness of breath and the development of peripheral edema. He had a 20-year history of non–insulin-dependent diabetes mellitus and had been treated with oral hypoglycemic drugs for the past 10 years. In the past he had had two myocardial infarctions and had been treated with captopril 50 mg twice daily and occasional furosemide 40 mg as required. On this occasion he was found to have atrial fibrillation, which had not been present previously. The heart rate was 130 bpm at the apex and 100 bpm at the wrist. Physical examination revealed pitting edema of both legs up to the knees and fine rales at the bases of both lungs. The patient was given digoxin in a dose of 0.25 mg/day, and furosemide 40 mg twice daily, and he was urged to reduce his salt intake.

Ten days after the original visit, the patient returned with a complaint of "palpitations," by which he meant periods of irregular heartbeat that he felt in his chest several times a day. An electrocardiogram (ECG) showed multiple ventricular premature beats with occasional self-limited runs of ventricular tachycardia. He was sent to a cardiologist in the hospital emergency room, where his serum creatinine was found to be twice the upper limit of normal. Serum digoxin level was 3.8 nmol/L (therapeutic range is 1.0–2.6 nmol/L); the serum K^+ was normal. The cardiologist discontinued the digoxin and admitted

the patient to hospital for ECG monitoring. After 6 days the ventricular arrhythmias were no longer present and the serum digoxin level was 1.8 nmol/L. The patient was discharged on 0.125 mg of digoxin daily, which kept the heart rate at 80–90 bpm.

The drugs included under the generic term digitalis (or cardiac) glycosides are used primarily to treat cardiac failure. Many extracts from plants containing cardiac glycosides have been used at various times in different parts of the world. Digitalis, which is extracted from the foxglove plant, was used before 1785 in folk medicine, but in that year William Withering published his celebrated book *An Account of the Foxglove and Some of Its Medical Uses: With Practical Remarks on Dropsy, and Other Diseases*. Withering thought that foxglove was a diuretic but recognized that the heart was affected and that the drug produced cardiac slowing in patients with generalized edema (dropsy).

Digitalis is extracted from the dried leaf of the foxglove plant, *Digitalis purpurea*. Seeds and leaves of *Digitalis lanata*, a number of other digitalis species, and a variety of other plants also contain cardiac glycosides.

Although the beneficial clinical effects of these agents have been known empirically for over two centuries, their mechanisms of action have not been well understood until recently. It is now generally acknowledged that their most clinically significant direct action is augmentation of contraction of the

447

atrial and ventricular myocardium. A good understanding of the pharmacology of these agents is important because they are widely used and they have a narrow margin of safety; i.e., there is a very small difference between the therapeutically effective dose and the toxic or fatal dose. Several studies have indicated that approximately 20% of patients taking digitalis show some form of drug-induced toxicity. These toxic manifestations are more pronounced in elderly patients: The incidence is 24% for those over 60 years of age as compared to 14% for those under 60.

PATHOPHYSIOLOGY OF HEART FAILURE

Normal Physiology

The normal physiology of myocardial contraction, including the generation of the action potential (Fig. 36-1), the characteristics of the ion channels involved, excitation-contraction coupling, the contractile process itself, and the relaxation process, are described in detail in Chapter 35. This chapter deals with the consequences of disturbances in these pro-

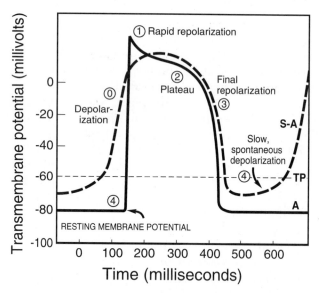

Figure 36-1. Comparison of action potentials of an atrial muscle cell (A) and a cell from the sinoatrial (S-A) node; depolarization (phase 0), repolarization (phases 1, 2, 3), resting membrane potential or diastolic depolarization (phase 4). Differences in amplitude, duration, and general configuration in the two tissue types can be seen. The slow depolarization (phase 4) of the S-A fiber diminishes its membrane potential (toward 0 mV) to reach the threshold potential (TP) and thus initiates spontaneous firing.

cesses and the pharmacology of agents used to correct them.

Heart Failure

Basically, heart failure is the inability of the heart to pump efficiently enough to meet the metabolic demands of the body. The main cause of cardiac failure is a decrease in the force of contraction of myocardial fibers, which results in a slower rate of pressure rise within the ventricle during the isovolumic phase of the contraction *(dP/dt)*, a lower peak systolic pressure, an enlarged diastolic size, and a higher filling pressure. The sequence of events resulting from the failing heart is illustrated in Figure 36-2.

Compensatory mechanisms available to the failing heart include an increase in ventricular end-diastolic pressure that enhances cardiac output (Starling's law of the heart), myocardial hypertrophy, increased sympathetic activity, and activation of the renin-angiotensin system.

In conditions where these mechanisms can produce adequate cardiac output, the heart failure is said to be compensated. Starling's curve (Fig. 36-3) shows that, at similar end-diastolic pressures, the cardiac output is lower in the failing heart than in the normal heart. Consequently, the heart enlarges to maintain cardiac output, and the heart rate increases to compensate for the poor cardiac function. In the decompensated heart, compensatory mechanisms fail to maintain cardiac output. Abnormalities occur in cardiac adrenoceptors and cyclic AMP pathways that affect both contraction and relaxation. It has been found repeatedly that the β_1-adrenoceptor is down-regulated and the β_2-adrenoceptor is uncoupled. Therefore the normal compensatory mechanism is impaired.

Administration of digitalis improves cardiac performance, shifting the cardiac function curve to the left so that it approximates the normal curve. By increasing the force of myocardial contraction, digitalis reduces the diastolic pressure, and consequently the diastolic volume. This decrease in ventricular volume increases the efficiency of contraction. Digitalis thus reduces the ratio of myocardial oxygen consumption to contractile force. The effect is largely due to decreased myocardial fiber length and diastolic wall tension. Because of the improvement in circulation, sympathetic activity is reduced, in turn reducing arterial resistance and venous tone. The reduced arterial resistance lowers the afterload on the left ventricle and permits further improvement of heart function. The decrease in heart rate is attrib-

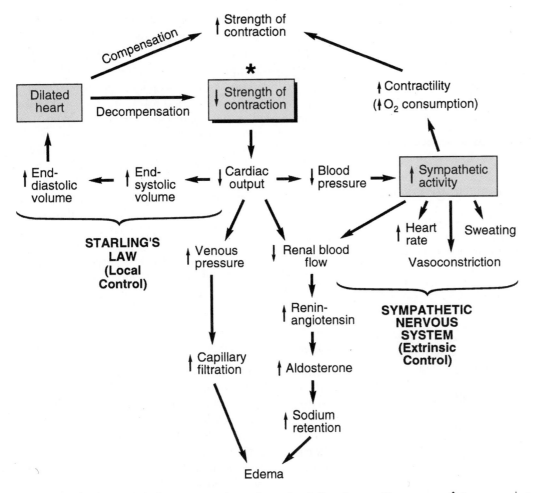

Figure 36-2. Sequence of events resulting from the failing heart. (Starts at ∗. ↑ Increase, ↓ decrease.)

uted to both direct and indirect effects on the heart. Digitalis not only reduces sympathetic tone by reflex mechanisms but also stimulates the vagus by sensitizing the baroreceptors and/or the afferent nerve activity.

In contrast to the action of digitalis in the failing heart, in the normal heart its positive inotropic effect is negated by compensatory autonomic reflexes. Digitalis also elicits peripheral vasoconstriction, therefore causing the blood pressure to rise. Again by reflex mechanisms, the myocardial activity and cardiac output are reduced in the normal individual.

DIGITALIS GLYCOSIDES

Structure

All the digitalis glycosides have three structural components (Fig. 36-4): a steroid nucleus, a series of

sugar residues in the C-3 position, and a five- or six-membered lactone ring in the C-17 position.

The steroid nucleus and the lactone ring together are called a genin or **aglycone.** This aglycone moiety elicits the cardiotonic effects, which are qualitatively similar for all the aglycones. However, absorption, onset, and duration of action vary among different glycosides in relation to the sugar portion of the molecule.

Preparations

Several compounds with digitalis-like activity are commercially available. However, only a few enjoy widespread clinical use and confidence, and it is entirely reasonable to practice medicine using only one digitalis preparation, digoxin. At least 90% of digitalis therapy in North America is carried out with digoxin, but two other digitalis preparations are official and are occasionally prescribed. Table 36-1

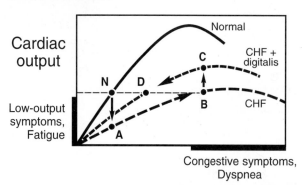

Ventricular end-diastolic pressure

Figure 36-3. Ventricular function curves in the normal heart, in congestive heart failure (CHF), and in CHF treated with digitalis, showing the operation of the Frank-Starling mechanism in the preload compensation for heart failure. Arrows linking point N to point A through D indicate, in sequence, depression of contractility with decompensated heart failure (A), Frank-Starling compensation (B), increase in contractility with digitalis (C), and reduction in use of Frank-Starling preload compensation, which digitalis allows (D). Points N, D, and B indicate the same cardiac output on the vertical axis, but each point is at a different end-diastolic pressure on the horizontal axis. The excessive end-diastolic pressure causing congestive symptoms, and the lowered levels of cardiac performance resulting in low-output symptoms, are indicated by bars on the respective axis. (From Mason 1973)

summarizes the pharmacokinetic data for three digitalis preparations, deslanoside (Cedilanid), digoxin (Lanoxin), and digitoxin (Crystodigin). It is important to recognize that the values in Table 36-1 are averages and that variations in measurements such as half-life are substantial even in normal subjects.

Mechanism of Action

Positive inotropic effects

The fundamental mechanisms by which digitalis glycosides stimulate the contractile forces within the cardiac cell have been widely debated. Present evidence suggests that this action is mediated through potentiation of the process of coupling the electrical excitation and the mechanical contraction (excitation-contraction coupling).

There is at present a consensus that the inotropic effects of cardiac glycosides result from binding of the glycoside to a subunit of the sarcolemmal $(Na^+ + K^+)$-ATPase. This causes a partial inhibition of the enzyme, impairing active transport of Na^+ and K^+ across the membrane as long as the cardiac

glycoside molecule remains associated with the site. This is the only site in cardiac tissue with the binding properties required of a "digitalis receptor." Since the glycosides have no primary effects on cyclic AMP, myocardial contractile proteins, or intermediary metabolism, the inhibition of $(Na^+ + K^+)$-ATPase must be seen as the means whereby these drugs may alter Ca^{2+} movement and hence contraction.

Cardiac glycosides, by inhibiting $(Na^+ + K^+)$-ATPase activity, increase the intracellular sodium concentration. As a result, there is more Na^+ to be exchanged for Ca^{2+} by the sodium–calcium exchanger. The small increase in intracellular Ca^{2+} concentration acts as a positive feedback signal to increase Ca^{2+} entry through Ca^{2+} channels. This sequence of events leads to a greater increase of intracellular Ca^{2+} when cardiac glycosides are present (Fig. 36-5) and underlies the inotropic response to digitalis.

Electrophysiological effects

Some of the therapeutic and most of the serious toxic effects of digitalis can be related to its action on the electrophysiological properties of the heart. The drug acts directly and indirectly on automaticity, conduction velocity, and effective refractory period of cardiac tissues. Also, digitalis indirectly increases cholinergic (vagal) tone in normal persons and decreases adrenergic nerve action on the failing heart. As mentioned above, digitalis inhibits the $(Na^+ + K^+)$-ATPase and there is a resultant decrease in intracellular K^+. This effect is dose-related. An increasing body concentration of digitalis ultimately leads to toxicity manifested by cardiac dysrhythmias. The decrease

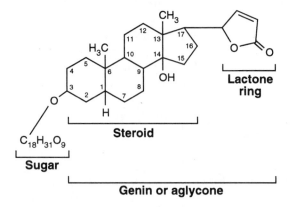

Figure 36-4. Structural formula of digitoxin. The structure of digoxin is similar except that there is an OH group on the C-12 position.

Table 36-1 Cardiac Glycoside Preparations

	Deslanoside	*Digoxin*	*Digitoxin*
Gastrointestinal absorption (%)	Unreliable	60–85	90–100
Onset of action (minutes)	10–30	15–30	25–120
Peak effect (hours)	1–2	1.5–5	4–12
Average half-life	33 hours	36 hours	4–6 days
Principal metabolic and/or excretory pathway	Renal excretion	Renal; some GI excretion	Hepatic biotransformation; renal excretion of metabolites
Protein binding at therapeutic concentration	—	25%	90%
Average digitalizing dose, oral	—	1.25–1.5 mg	0.7–1.2 mg
Average digitalizing dose, intravenous	0.8 mg	0.75–1.0 mg	1.0 mg
Usual daily oral maintenance dose	—	0.25–0.5 mg	0.1 mg

in intracellular K^+ leads to an increase in the slope of phase 4 depolarization and a decrease in maximal diastolic membrane potential (i.e., it becomes closer to zero membrane potential). This phenomenon leads to increased automaticity and development of ectopic rhythm. Not only are many of the electrophysiological and dysrhythmic effects of digitalis related to intracellular K^+ depletion, but it also appears that

K^+ and digitalis compete for binding sites on myocardial $(Na^+ + K^+)$-ATPase. K^+ is relatively loosely bound to the enzyme, but it delays subsequent digitalis binding. Once digitalis is bound, however, K^+ does not increase its rate of dissociation.

The various phases of the action potential recorded from the sinoatrial node and the atrium are shown in Figure 36-1. The frequency of firing of the

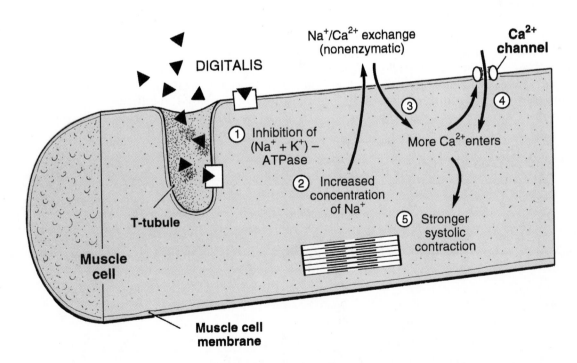

Figure 36-5. Inhibitory action of digitalis glycoside on $(Na^+ + K^+)$-ATPase. Numbers 1 to 5 indicate the sequence of events.

pacemaker cell can be altered by (1) altering the threshold potential while maintaining a constant rate of depolarization, (2) altering the rate of depolarization while maintaining the threshold potential, or (3) increasing the maximal diastolic potential of the pacemaker.

The action of digitalis on **automaticity**, i.e., the property that allows a single cell to spontaneously depolarize without outside influences, is dose-dependent. In therapeutic concentrations, digitalis has little effect. In toxic concentrations, the slope of phase 4 diastolic depolarization is increased in all cardiac tissues, and ectopic foci of impulse formation may develop. Indirectly, via vagal stimulation, digitalis causes decreased impulse formation in the S-A node.

Conduction velocity, i.e., the rate at which an impulse is conducted through cardiac tissue, is a function of the amplitude of the action potential and its rate of rise (phase 0). Both of these variables are related to the resting membrane potential present at the onset of the action potential; the more negative the membrane potential, the steeper the slope of phase 0. All concentrations of digitalis diminish conduction velocity, but different parts of the heart respond to different degrees. The A-V node is most sensitive, followed in descending order by atrial muscle, the Purkinje system, and ventricular muscle. The effect on the A-V node is partly direct and partly indirect. It is most prominent when the initial vagal tone is low and adrenergic tone is high, as in congestive heart failure. It should be noted that the direct effect of digitalis on atrial muscle (i.e., decreased conduction velocity) predominates over its indirect vagotonic effect (i.e., increased conduction).

The **refractory period,** consisting of phases 1, 2, and 3 in the transmembrane potential recording (see Fig. 36-1), includes the periods in which a cell is inexcitable (effective refractory period, ERP) and poorly excitable (relative refractory period, RRP; see also Chapter 37). The digitalis-induced increase in vagal activity causes a marked decrease in the duration of the ERP in the atria, producing greater discharge frequency of fibrillating atria (or it may convert atrial flutter to fibrillation). However, an increase in vagal activity reduces conduction velocity and prolongs the ERP. As a result, the ventricular rate is lowered. This prolongation of the ERP of the A-V node is the main beneficial effect of cardiac glycosides when used for the treatment of atrial flutter or fibrillation.

The effects of digitalis on the electrophysiology of the heart are summarized in Table 36-2. These are the basis for slowing of the compensatory tachycardia of congestive heart failure, decreasing the ventricular rate during atrial dysrhythmias, and converting supraventricular dysrhythmias to normal sinus rhythm.

The tendency of digitalis glycosides to *cause* cardiac dysrhythmia may be related to the depletion of intracellular K^+. As intracellular K^+ falls, the resting membrane potential moves toward zero. The cell now undergoes depolarization more readily as the resting membrane potential comes closer to the depolarization threshold, resulting in greater likelihood of susceptibility to dysrhythmia.

Neural effects

The three most important neural effects of digitalis glycosides are increased **vagal activity** (which can be blocked by atropine), sensitization of carotid sinus

---

Table 36-2 Electrophysiological Effects of Digitalis

	Automaticity		Conduction Velocity		Effective Refractory Period (ERP)	
	Direct	*Indirect*	*Direct*	*Indirect*	*Direct*	*Indirect*
S-A node	↑*	↓				
Atrium	↑*		↓*	↑	↑	
A-V node			↓↓	↓↓	↑↑	↑↑
Purkinje system	↑*		↓*		↓	↑
Ventricles	↑*		↑↓*		↓↓	

*At high or toxic doses; ↑ = increase; ↓ = decrease; ↑↑ or ↓↓ denotes therapeutically important effects.

baroreceptors, and increased **sympathetic outflow** from the CNS at high doses.

Extracardiac hemodynamic effects

While the direct cardiac actions of digitalis are the most apparent, there are also extracardiac effects. Cardiac glycosides constrict arterial and venous segments in isolated preparations, and arteriolar and venous constriction has been demonstrated in intact animals. It has been suggested that digoxin inhibits endothelial-dependent relaxation and that this may contribute to the vasoconstrictor action of the drug. Total systemic arteriolar resistance is also elevated in normal human subjects.

Pharmacokinetics

The pharmacokinetics of digoxin have been extensively studied. In tablet preparations, 60–80% of the digoxin content is absorbed from the gastrointestinal tract; an encapsulated gel is available that has improved bioavailability (90–100%). The major site of absorption appears to be in the small intestine. There is some enterohepatic circulation of digoxin (Fig. 36-6). Intramuscular injection of digoxin should be avoided because it produces severe pain.

The bioavailability of digoxin in tablet form varies widely between commercial preparations. In addition, even well-standardized preparations show variable absorption within and between patients. Diarrhea, malabsorption syndromes, or food in the stomach may also influence absorption significantly.

Digoxin is excreted principally in unchanged form in the urine; it is apparent, therefore, that renal insufficiency will delay excretion and thereby influence digoxin half-life. There is an almost linear relationship between the clearance of digoxin and the clearance of creatinine in human subjects. Similarly, an elevated blood urea nitrogen (BUN) is associated with diminished clearance of digoxin (Fig. 36-7), and it is possible to extrapolate from the BUN to an appropriate digoxin dosage.

About 25% of digoxin is bound to plasma albumin, compared to more than 90% for digitoxin (see Table 36-1). This difference in binding contributes to the difference in speed of onset and duration of action of the two drugs. Digitoxin is **biotransformed** in the liver and its metabolites are excreted by the kidneys.

Digoxin also appears to be metabolized by anaerobic bacteria in the gut, and the extent of this metab-

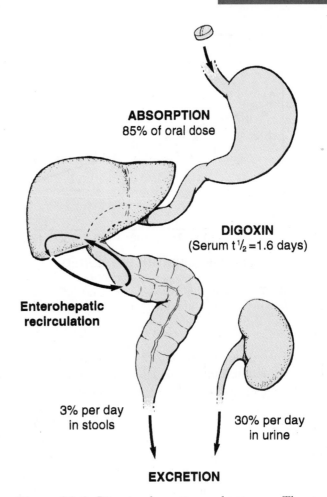

Figure 36-6. Digoxin absorption and turnover. The percentage values are calculated in terms of any given oral dose.

olism shows interethnic variation. For example, bacterial alteration of digoxin was found to be more active in Americans than in Bangladeshis, and the difference persisted even in those who migrated.

Therapeutic Applications

Cardiac glycosides are effective in the treatment of patients with congestive heart failure whose state is complicated by the presence of atrial fribrillation. In the absence of supraventricular tachycardia, however, it is not so clear that the patient with congestive heart failure and normal sinus rhythm benefits from cardiac glycosides. Patients with dilated failing hearts and impaired systolic function have subjective and objective improvement after receiving digitalis, whereas patients with elevated filling pressures due to

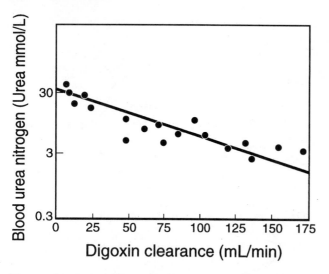

Figure 36-7. Relationship between clearance of digoxin and blood urea nitrogen in human subjects.

reduced ventricular compliance, but with preserved systolic function, may not benefit from digitalis therapy unless supraventricular tachycardia coexists.

Pregnancy

Controversy surrounds the measurement of plasma digoxin levels in pregnancy, partly because of an increase in endogenous digitalis-like substances both in pregnant women and in the neonates. These substances interfere with the usual assay for exogenous digoxin. Long-term digoxin treatment during pregnancy may shorten the duration of pregnancy and retard intrauterine growth, resulting in low birth weight and shorter labor. Nevertheless, digoxin is the drug of choice for fetal supraventricular tachycardia (SVT). It is generally considered a safe drug during pregnancy, with no risk of teratogenicity, but overdose can be detrimental to the mother and lethal to the fetus.

Pediatrics

Digoxin is often used as the initial therapy for SVT in the neonate and early infant. For infants under 2 months of age, intravenous digoxin may be used: Half of the total digitalizing dose is given i.v., followed by one-quarter of the dose 6 hours later, and the final quarter after a further 6 hours. Caution is required during concomitant therapy with quinidine or amiodarone (see Chapter 37). Care should also be exercised with the postoperative use of digoxin in the

pediatric patient. Side effects are most often seen in hypokalemic patients. Digoxin may impair myocardial function after cardiac arrest in the newborn, and therefore a full digitalizing dose is rarely given after cardiac surgery.

The Elderly

Digoxin therapy in elderly patients may be associated with states of confusion, and the potential for drug interactions and higher toxicity is increased (see below).

Drug Interactions

Digitalis action may be *enhanced* by substances that (1) slow gastrointestinal motility and thereby increase gastrointestinal absorption of slowly absorbed preparations (e.g., antispasmodics, such as atropine-like agents); (2) disturb body electrolytes by lowering plasma potassium levels, eliciting hypomagnesemia and hypercalcemia (e.g., diuretics, amphotericin B, oral or parenteral glucose); (3) change renal clearance and/or alter plasma protein binding (e.g., quinidine, verapamil, amiodarone and other antiarrhythmics); (4) stimulate β-adrenoceptors and cause cardiac dysrhythmias (e.g., epinephrine, ephedrine); and (5) elicit cardiac dysrhythmias by unknown mechanisms (e.g., succinylcholine, anticholinesterases).

Digitalis action may be *reduced* by substances that (1) reduce gastrointestinal absorption (e.g., kaolin-pectin, antihyperlipidemic agents, antacids); (2) increase gastrointestinal motility (e.g., metoclopramide); and (3) stimulate hepatic microsomal enzymes and thus enhance the biotransformation of digitoxin (e.g., spironolactone, phenytoin, ASA, phenylbutazone, barbiturates).

Side Effects and Toxicity

The toxic manifestations of digitalis may be divided into cardiac and extracardiac. The prime danger is dose-related progressively more severe **dysrhythmia** terminating in ventricular fibrillation. The common predisposing factor is a decrease in intracellular K^+. Potassium depletion may be hastened by concurrent treatment with certain diuretics or corticosteroids, or by conditions such as severe vomiting and diarrhea. Cardiac irregularities such as coupled beats (bigeminy) are usually signals calling for a reduction in digitalis dosage. Such irregularities are a sign not only that toxicity is imminent but also that the upper limit of attainable inotropic effect has been reached. Other cardiac manifestations of digitalis toxicity are premature ventricular contractions, premature atrial contractions, atrioventricular block, paroxysmal atrial tachycardia with block, paroxysmal atrial tachycardia, and ventricular tachycardia.

The principal **extracardiac** manifestations of digitalis toxicity are gastrointestinal. Vomiting is caused by stimulation of the chemoreceptor trigger zone. Diarrhea results from the activation of the dorsal motor nucleus of the vagal nerve, increasing gastrointestinal motility.

A variety of **central nervous system** side effects occur, including anorexia, weakness, lethargy and fatigue, and visual complaints. The visual disturbances include hazy vision, difficulty in reading, various types of scotoma, altered or disturbed color perception, and photophobia. Other neurological symptoms of digitalis toxicity include dizziness, headache, paresthesias and, with massive overdose, convulsions, delusions, stupor, and coma.

Treatment of Digitalis Toxicity

Digitalis must be discontinued immediately if toxic manifestations occur. Often these symptoms may persist for some time because of slow elimination of the drug. Since there is usually a loss of K^+ from the myocardium during treatment with digitalis glycosides, and since the loss of K^+ is the probable cause of dysrhythmias, immediate relief is often obtained from the intravenous administration of potassium salts. This measure raises the extracellular K^+ concentration and thus decreases the slope of phase 4 depolarization, so problems due to excessive automaticity are diminished. There are, however, hazards associated with potassium administration when there is depressed automaticity or decreased conduction, because this may lead to complete A-V block. Digitalis-induced second- or third-degree heart block is the only type of dysrhythmia in which potassium is contraindicated. In addition to potassium, digitalis-induced cardiac dysrhythmias usually respond to drugs such as lidocaine or phenytoin.

Life-threatening arrhythmias and heart block produced by digoxin or digitoxin can be safely treated with digoxin-specific Fab fragments that have been purified from antibodies raised in sheep by immunization against digoxin. The crude antiserum from sheep is fractionated to separate the IgG fraction, which is cleaved into Fab and Fc fragments by papain digestion. The Fab fragments are not antigenic and complement-binding. They are excreted fairly rapidly by the kidney as a digoxin-bound complex. In patients with life-threatening arrhythmias, treatment with digoxin-specific Fab fragments brings about rapid disappearance of the arrhythmias.

Measurement of Serum Concentration of Digoxin; Digoxin Dosage

Nanomolar concentrations of digoxin can be measured in a patient's serum, or in tissues postmortem, by means of a sensitive radioimmunoassay for digoxin. Using this technique, it has been found that the ratio of myocardial tissue concentration to serum concentration is extremely variable, but typically about 30:1. Figure 36-8 is a plot of the serum levels of digoxin in 100 consecutive patients, subdivided into a group with and a group without clinical signs of toxicity. In the majority of patients, serum levels of more than 3.8 nmol/L produced clinical toxicity. However, there is considerable overlap: Some pa-

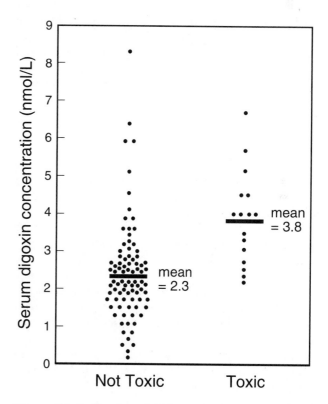

Figure 36-8. Results of 100 serum digoxin radioimmunoassay measurements. Sixteen patients were believed to show clinical toxicity; their mean serum level was 3.8 nmol/L (right). Of the patients without clinical toxicity (left), seven also had serum levels of more than 3.8 nmol/L (3ng/mL). Overlap of normal and toxic values does occur; therefore, judgment must be used when evaluating results.

tients with levels of more than 3.8 nmol/L were not adversely affected, and in some, levels as low as 2.3 nmol/L seemed to be toxic. It must be appreciated that toxicity may occur with normal serum levels in some situations such as following myocardial infarction or in association with hypoxemia, hypokalemia, or hypomagnesemia. People with hypothyroidism (myxedema) are particularly prone to develop digitalis toxicity.

The therapeutic index for digitalis is low; consequently dosage must be carefully controlled for each individual. It may be difficult to estimate the initial and maintenance doses because it would depend very much on the clinical condition of the patient—in particular, the hepatic and renal functions.

If no emergency exists, the daily maintenance dose may be given by mouth; steady-state concentration and therapeutic effect are reached in approximately five elimination half-lives. The dose may be adjusted at appropriate intervals. In an emergency requiring prompt digitalization, an initial loading dose may be given by mouth or by slow intravenous infusion. The required total body content of drug (0.7–1.2 mg) should be divided into three doses given at 6-hour intervals; then the patient is started on daily maintenance doses. Maintenance doses of digoxin for an individual with normal renal function would be approximately 0.25 mg daily.

OTHER POSITIVE INOTROPIC AGENTS

Some sympathomimetic agents, such as **dopamine** and **dobutamine,** have been used in the treatment of heart failure under certain circumstances in order to compensate for the down-regulation of the cardiac β_1-adrenoceptors. However, positive inotropes may actually worsen the congestive heart failure syndrome by increasing the energy demands of the myocardium. Phosphodiesterase inhibitors, such as **amrinone** and **milrinone,** were proposed as useful adjuncts to sympathomimetic agents, to improve myocardial function. However, these agents were found to increase mortality in heart failure. This observation supports the notion that positive inotropic therapy may hasten the progression of the heart failure syndrome as well as increase the incidence of

dysrhythmias. Low doses of **vesnarinone,** a new phosphodiesterase inhibitor, have been reported to reduce morbidity and mortality and to improve the quality of life in patients with symptomatic heart failure. However, these beneficial effects were reversed when high doses of vesnarinone were used.

CONCLUSION

Cardiac glycosides have been invaluable in the treatment of congestive heart failure. However, the highly beneficial effects of newer drugs such as the angiotensin-converting enzyme (ACE) inhibitors (see Chapter 38) have raised the question of whether the addition of a cardiac glycoside improves the total clinical benefit in patients with heart failure. The continuing role of digoxin in the treatment of heart failure is therefore uncertain and is currently under clinical investigation.

SUGGESTED READING

Bristow MR, Hershberger RE, Port JD, et al. β-Adrenergic pathways in non-failing and failing human ventricular myocardium. Circulation 1990; 82 (Suppl):I 12–25.

Kim R-SS, Labella FS. Endogenous ligands and modulators of the digitalis receptor: some candidates. Pharmacol Ther 1981; 14:391–409.

Kulick DL, Rahimtoola SH. Current role of digitalis therapy in patients with congestive heart failure. JAMA 1991; 265:2995–2997.

Langer GA. Effects of digitalis on myocardial ionic exchange. Circulation 1972; 46:180–187.

Larosa G, Armstrong PW, Seeman P, Forster C. β-Adrenoceptor recovery after heart failure in the dog. Cardiovasc Res 1993; 27:489–493.

Mason DT. Regulation of cardiac performance in clinical heart disease: interactions between contractile state mechanical abnormalities and ventricular compensatory mechanisms. Am J Cardiol 1973; 32:437–448.

Packer M, Carver JR, Rodeheffer RJ, et al. Effect of oral milrinone on mortality in severe chronic heart failure. N Engl J Med 1991; 325:1468–1475.

Schlant RC, Sonnenblick EH. Pathophysiology of heart failure. In: Hirst JW, ed. The heart, arteries and veins. New York: McGraw-Hill, 1990:387–418.

Smith TW. Digitalis: mechanisms of action and clinical use. N Engl J Med 1987; 318:358–365.

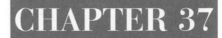

CHAPTER 37

Antiarrhythmic Drugs

P. DORIAN

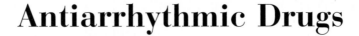

CASE HISTORY

A 55-year-old man developed a spontaneous sustained ventricular tachycardia with presyncope, for which he was admitted to hospital. He had had an anterior wall myocardial infarction 5 years previously, which was asymptomatic during treatment with acetylsalicylic acid 325 mg once a day and metoprolol 50 mg twice a day.

Investigation revealed moderate left ventricular dysfunction with an ejection fraction of 42%. There was no inducible myocardial ischemia, but Holter monitoring showed frequent short runs of nonsustained ventricular tachycardia. Soon after, he developed sustained atrial fibrillation with a resting ventricular rate of 110 bpm. Oral digoxin, 0.25 mg/day, was begun, as well as anticoagulation with warfarin to maintain an International Normalized Ratio (INR) of 2.5–3.5 (see Chapter 42). In order to prevent the risk of recurrence of sustained ventricular tachycardia and to attempt to restore and maintain sinus rhythm, amiodarone 1200 mg/day was administered orally in divided doses for 7 days in hospital with no untoward effects. The patient was then discharged with the instruction to take 400 mg/day of amiodarone for 4 weeks and to reduce the dose to 200 mg/day thereafter. Medication with digoxin and warfarin was continued. At the time of discharge, the rhythm was atrial fibrillation with a resting ventricular rate of 70 bpm. The INR was 2.9.

Three weeks later, the patient came to the Emergency Department with bleeding from the gums, very easy bruising, intermittent epistaxis, as well as extreme fatigue, nausea, and visual disturbances. Physical examination and ECG showed sinus bradycardia with 30 bpm, regular, with no evidence of heart failure. The INR was 6.5, and trough serum dixogin level was 4.5 nmol/L. Thus, the patient had clear-cut clinical evidence of excess warfarin and digitalis effects.

The doses of digoxin and warfarin were titrated downward and adjusted to the minimum required to restore a therapeutic INR of 2.5–3.5 and to correct overdigitalization in the presence of amiodarone. Once these adjustments had taken effect, the patient was discharged with exact ambulatory dosing instructions and a closely spaced recall schedule.

Comment: The patient's recovery demonstrated that amiodarone was very effective at restoring sinus rhythm in atrial fibrillation and preventing recurrence of ventricular tachycardia. However, the clearance of both digoxin and warfarin was markedly reduced during coadministration of amiodarone. In addition, some of the pharmacodynamic effects of digoxin, such as bradycardia or atrioventricular block, were likely additive with those of amiodarone. Because of these known interactions of amiodarone with drugs that are eliminated by the hepatic microsomal enzyme system, such as warfarin and digoxin, the doses of these drugs should have been reduced by one-half soon after amiodarone was started, and clinical effects and plasma concentrations should have been monitored more carefully.

The management of cardiac arrhythmias is primarily concerned with reducing symptoms from continuous arrhythmias, restoring and maintaining sinus rhythm, and preventing the occurrence or recurrence of symptomatic and/or life-threatening arrhythmias.

MECHANISMS OF ARRHYTHMOGENESIS AND THE EFFECTS OF ANTIARRHYTHMIC INTERVENTION

The normal physiology of the cardiac action potential, including the ionic currents underlying it (Table 37-1), and the differences between myocardial cells and pacemaker cells, was described in detail in Chapter 35. This chapter deals with abnormal automaticity and the drugs used to correct it.

Basic Mechanisms of Arrhythmogenesis

Once depolarization of the membrane begins, and the action potential has started, the cell becomes refractory to other stimuli. Initially, it will be totally refractory irrespective of the strength of the stimulus (**absolute refractory period**), but during the latter part of the action potential, depolarization can be induced in response to a stronger-than-normal stimulus (**relative refractory period**) (Fig. 37-1). Because excitation and recovery do not occur simultaneously in all cardiac cells, asynchrony of repolarization may occur. This results in a vulnerable period during which the heart is susceptible to the induction of arrhythmias since some cells will be able to conduct impulses whereas others will not, thus allowing for the possible occurrence of reentry phenomena, as described in the following section. The application

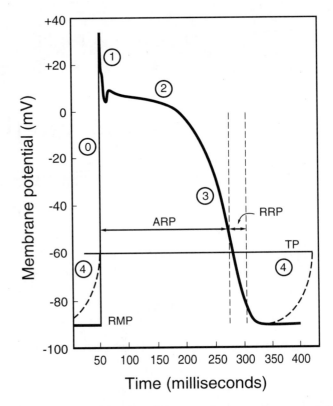

Figure 37-1. Diagram of the ventricular action potential. Phase 0 = depolarization; phase 1 = rapid repolarization; phase 2 = plateau; phase 3 = final repolarization; phase 4 = spontaneous depolarization in pacemaker cells. ARP = absolute refractory period. RRP = relative refractory period. TP = threshold potential. RMP = resting membrane potential.

of a strong single stimulus at this time may elicit an abnormal response such as ventricular fibrillation. This vulnerable period corresponds approximately to the peak of the T wave on the electrocardiogram (see Fig. 37-6A). Antiarrhythmic drugs may alter the duration of the vulnerable period or its magnitude, thus altering the likelihood of an arrhythmia developing in response to a given stimulus.

There are two putative causes of arrhythmias: alterations in impulse formation leading to **enhanced or abnormal automaticity,** and alterations in impulse conduction resulting in **reentry phenomena.** Although most common arrhythmias such as sustained ventricular tachycardia in patients with coronary disease, atrial and ventricular fibrillation, and paroxysmal supraventricular tachycardias are caused by reentry, the specific mechanism by which many clinical antiarrhythmic agents act on the factors initiating and maintaining reentry is not known.

Table 37-1 Major Ion Fluxes During the Cardiac Action Potential

Name	Ion	Current	Phase of Action Potential	
I_{Na}	Na^+	Inward	0,	(depolarization)
I_{t_o}	K^+	Outward	1,	(rapid repolarization)
I_{Ca}	Ca^{2+}	Inward	2,	(plateau)
I_K	K^+	Outward	3,	(repolarization)
I_{K_1}*	K^+	Outward	3, 4	(repolarization, diastole)
I_f	Na^+	Inward	4,	(spontaneous depolarization)

*I_{K_1} during the resting phase (diastole in cells without spontaneous depolarization) maintains the equilibrium responsible for the resting potential at or near the Nernst potential.

Effect of Antiarrhythmic Agents on Automaticity

Spontaneous phase 4 depolarization is a property of the sinus node, A-V node, His-Purkinje system, and certain specialized atrial fibers. The ability of these cells to depolarize spontaneously is called **normal automaticity**. Arrhythmias caused by alterations in automaticity are thought to arise from **enhanced normal automaticity** at any one of these sites other than the sinus node. Normal myocardial cells do not depolarize spontaneously and, therefore, arrhythmias due to enhanced normal automaticity cannot originate in these cells.

Damaged myocardial cells often remain partially depolarized, and this failure to reach maximum negative diastolic potential may induce abnormal automatic discharges. Unlike enhanced normal automaticity, arrhythmias due to **abnormal automaticity** can occur in myocardial cells as well as in specialized conduction tissue. In the presence of myocardial cell necrosis, hypoxia, or potassium imbalance, the cell fails to repolarize fully and the resting potential only reaches -30 to -40 mV.

Most antiarrhythmic agents suppress automaticity by decreasing the slope of phase 4 spontaneous depolarization and/or shifting the voltage threshold to a less negative level (see Fig. 37-1). Although this effect also decreases the frequency of discharge of normal pacemaker cells (e.g., the sinus node), it has a more pronounced action on ectopic pacemaker activity. The relatively selective suppression of ectopic pacemaker foci may abolish an arrhythmia due to abnormal automaticity at doses of a drug that have little effect on normal sinus node function. However, in states where the sinus node or conducting tissue exhibits impaired function (e.g., sick sinus syndrome), suppression of phase 4 depolarization may result in a reduction of the heart rate or possible asystole.

Another form of abnormal automaticity is called **triggered activity.** Under certain pathological conditions, a transient depolarization may occur before a cell is fully repolarized, causing early or delayed afterdepolarizations (EADs or DADs) (see Fig. 37-2). These low-amplitude oscillatory depolarizations may give rise to or "trigger" propagated action potentials. Arrhythmias caused by digitalis toxicity, and possibly catecholamine excess, or arrhythmias induced by antiarrhythmic drugs that prolong repolarization, may be examples of this mechanism. Arrhythmias caused by triggered automaticity can in general not be induced by premature extra stimuli, but they can be induced by continuous rapid stimulation. These oscillations in membrane potential can be suppressed by calcium antagonists, magnesium, and restoring physical or electrolyte balance to the cell milieu.

Effect of Antiarrhythmic Agents on Reentry

Reentry depends on the existence of two anatomically or physiologically distinct pathways, as shown in Figure 37-3. For example, the normal A-V node and an accessory atrioventricular bypass tract (Kent bundle) are anatomically distinct. In the presence of myocardial scarring (e.g., from a previous myocardial infarct), scarred tissue can exhibit slowed conduction or prolonged refractoriness. Normally, impulses from higher centers in the conducting system (e.g., the A-V node) will be conducted in the same direction down both pathways, bifurcating to cover the entire ventricular surface. However, should there be a unidirectional block (e.g., from conduction failure or functional refractoriness) in pathway 2, the impulse may only be conducted down pathway 1. If the block in pathway 2 is in the forward direction only (as would be caused by functional as opposed to "anatomical" block), it may be possible for the impulse to return in a retrograde fashion through this pathway, reaching the initial point of bifurcation, provided that the transit time through the circuit exceeds the refractory period in the circuit. Under these circumstances, reexcitation of the myocardium may occur via this "short-circuiting" of the conducting tissue, thus causing a ventricular premature contraction. If this reentry mechanism becomes repetitive, a sustained ventricular arrhythmia such as ventricular tachycardia occurs. Similar reentry mechanisms have been proposed in the atria as a common cause of atrial flutter, and near the A-V node as a cause of A-V nodal reentry tachycardia. Arrhythmias in patients with accessory atrioventricular connections (Wolff-Parkinson-White syndrome) usually arise from reentry with anterograde conduction through the A-V node and retrograde conduction through the atrioventricular bypass tract.

Antiarrhythmic agents most likely abolish reentry by depressing membrane responsiveness, slowing conduction so that propagation around the reentrant circuit cannot occur, or increasing refractoriness so that the reentrant wavefront impinges on refractory tissue, halting its further progress. Most antiarrhythmic drugs appear to act by slowing conduction and/or increasing refractoriness, converting unidirectional into bidirectional block.

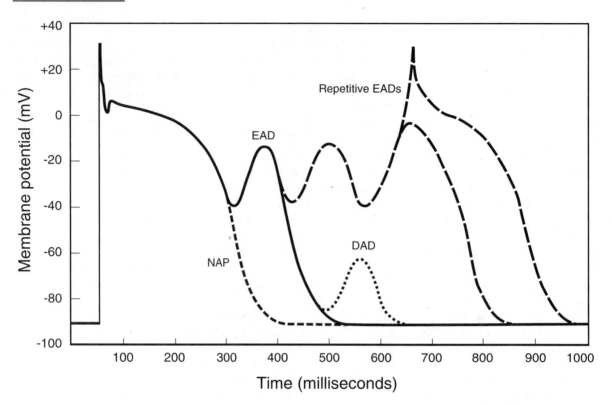

Figure 37-2. Schematic representation of an action potential with repolarization interrupted by an early afterdepolarization (EAD), and the end of the action potential followed by a delayed afterdepolarization (DAD). NAP = normal action potential.

ANTIARRHYTHMIC DRUGS

The most widely accepted classification of antiarrhythmic drug action was initially proposed by Vaughan Williams (and later modified), who separated the action of various agents according to their predominant electrophysiological effects on the action potential. It is important to understand that this classification is descriptive, and its clinical relevance has not yet been clarified. Many of the antiarrhythmic drugs shown in Figure 37-4 have actions relating to more than one class or subclass in the classification. Moreover, many antiarrhythmic drugs have active metabolites with a different class of action than that of the parent drug. The classification in Table 37-2 is used in the following paragraphs.

Drugs with Class I antiarrhythmic properties: These drugs, of which quinidine is the prototype, slow the rate of rise of phase 0 ($\dot{V}_{max}$) of the action potential by blocking membrane sodium channels and thus decreasing the rate of entry of Na^+. These drugs have little or no effect on the resting membrane potential in doses used in clinical practice. They cause a decrease in excitability and conduction velocity; some also prolong the effective refractory period (and may block K^+ channels), and may decrease the slope of phase 4 spontaneous depolarization in pacemaker cells. Quinidine, procainamide, and lidocaine also exhibit local anesthetic activity on the myocardial membrane.

Drugs with Class II mechanism of action: These drugs include the β-adrenoceptor antagonists. They depress phase 4 depolarization and exert their antiarrhythmic effects through competitive inhibition of the β-adrenoceptor site. In high concentrations, many of these agents also show local anesthetic properties, but this action is not usually seen in clinical practice.

Drugs with Class III mechanism of action prolong the duration of the action potential with a consequent increase in the absolute and effective refractory period. Some of these agents (e.g., bretylium) have no significant effect on phase 4 depolarization, whereas others (e.g., amiodarone) may depress it.

Drugs with Class IV properties decrease the inward current carried by calcium across the cell

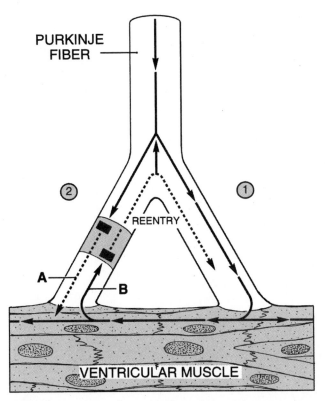

PURKINJE FIBER

② ①

REENTRY

A

B

VENTRICULAR MUSCLE

Figure 37-3. Mechanism of reentry and effect of antiarrhythmic intervention. The impulse is conducted unimpeded down pathway 1 but encounters an area of anatomical or functional block in pathway 2. The impulse can then be conducted retrogradely through pathway 2, and reentry into pathway 1 may be established. Drugs can abolish the arrhythmia by improving forward conduction (A) or by preventing retrograde conduction (B).

mic drugs are summarized in Table 37-3. Table 37-4 lists the important pharmacodynamic mechanisms, properties, and toxicities of the agents discussed in the following paragraphs. For simplicity, drugs are listed under the "class" pertaining to their predominant mechanism of action.

Given the difficulty with the commonly used modified Vaughan Williams classification of antiarrhythmic drug action, a new approach to classifying drugs with potential antiarrhythmic activity has been proposed. Termed the "Sicilian Gambit," it proposes to identify a number of potential targets for drug action, to include various ion-conducting channels (Na^+, K^+, Ca^{2+}, Cl^-), receptors (α-, β-adrenergic, muscarinic, purinergic), and pumps ($[Na^+ + K^+]$-ATPase). All antiarrhythmic drugs or substances that affect cardiac electrophysiology would then be characterized by their actions on each of these channels, receptors, or pumps. (These actions may be activation or inhibition with varying kinetics and intensity.) If the most appropriate "target" for drug action for a given arrhythmia or a given patient were known, therapy could be tailored for that specific situation. Unfortunately, the precise mechanisms of arrhyth-

membrane. In the sinus node, this results in less net inward (depolarizing) current during the latter part of spontaneous diastolic depolarization. The result is a decrease in the rate of rise (slope) of phase 4 spontaneous depolarization and a slowing of the heart rate. In addition, these drugs slow conduction in tissues dependent on calcium currents (e.g., A-V node), thus prolonging the PR interval in electrocardiograms.

Subclassification of class I mechanism of action is shown in Table 37-2. It is important to emphasize that many drugs (e.g., amiodarone) possess actions pertaining to more than one class of antiarrhythmic drug action and that drugs with a similar mechanism of action are not necessarily interchangeable with respect to clinical efficacy.

The pharmacokinetics of the main antiarrhyth-

Table 37-2 Classification of Antiarrhythmic Drug Action

Class	Predominant Action	Drugs
Ia	Slowing of rate of rise of phase 0, slowing of conduction, prolongation of refractoriness	Quinidine Procainamide Disopyramide
Ib	Slight slowing of conduction, no change in refractoriness	Lidocaine Mexiletine Tocainide Phenytoin
Ic	Marked slowing of conduction, little or modest prolongation of refractoriness	Flecainide Propafenone
II	β-Adrenoceptor antagonism	β-blockers (e.g., propranolol)
III	Prolongation of action potential duration, and of refractoriness	Bretylium Amiodarone Sotalol
IV	Blockade of calcium entry, decrease of slope of phase 4	Verapamil Diltiazem

Modified from Vaughan Williams EM. *Pharmacol Ther* 1975; 1:115–138.

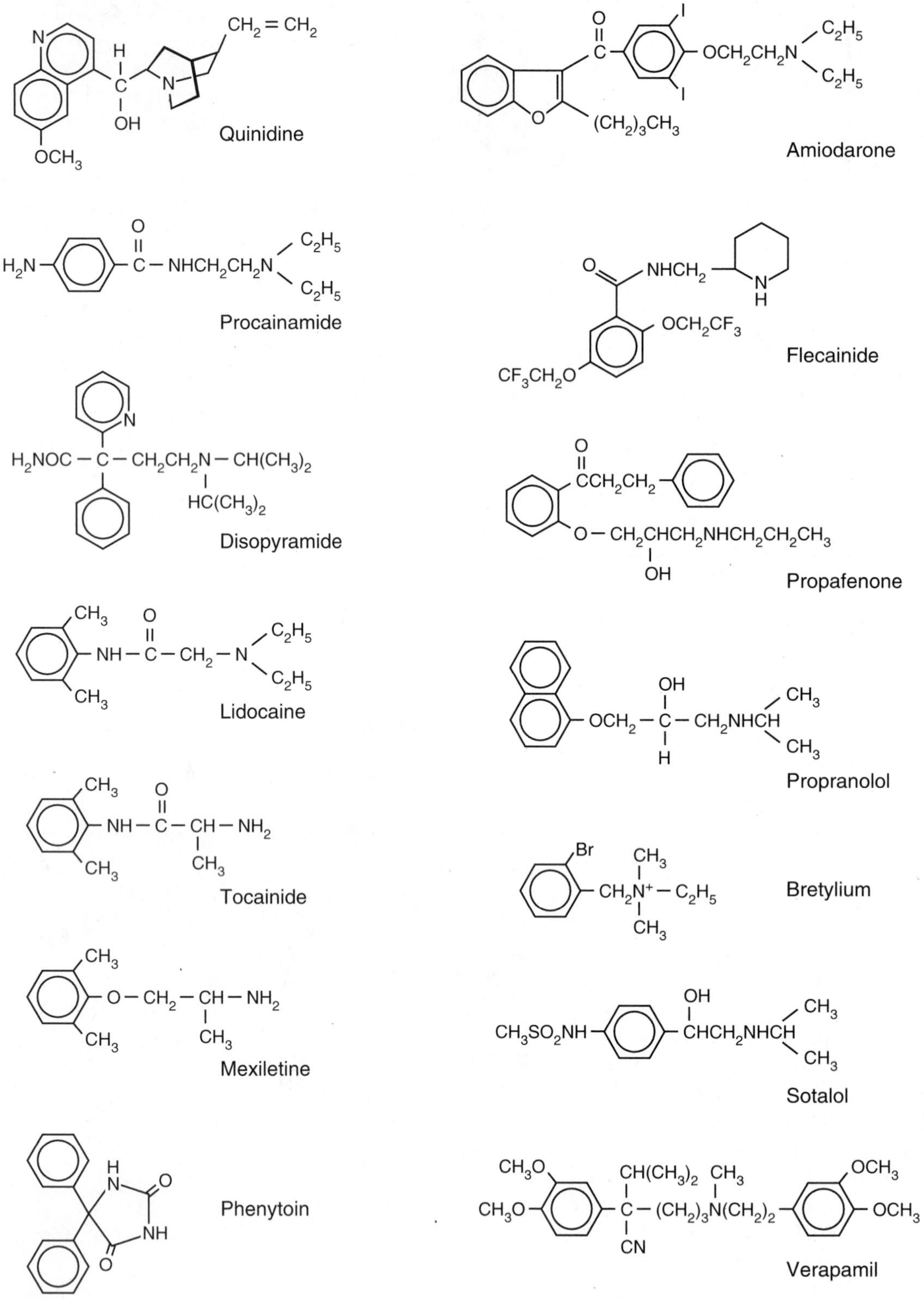

Figure 37-4. Antiarrhythmic drugs in current clinical use.

Table 37-3 Pharmacokinetics of Antiarrhythmic Drugs

Drug	Bioavail-ability (%)	V_d (L/kg)	Protein Binding (%)	Half-Life (hours)	Therapeutic Range	Biotransformation and Excretion	Metabolites
Quinidine	75	2–3	75–90	4–8	2–6 µg/mL (7.3–21.9 µmol/L)	Liver: 80% Kidney: 10–20% unchanged	Hydroxyquinidine, slight activity
Procainamide	75–95	1.5–2.5	15–25	2–4	4–10 µg/mL (17–42.5 µmol/L)	Liver: acetylation Kidney: 60% unchanged	N-acetylprocainamide (NAPA): class III activity
Disopyramide	90	0.5–1.5	35–95	6–9	2–5 µg/mL	Liver: 25–35% inactive compound Kidney: 50% unchanged	N-dealkyl disopyramide, less active than parent compound
Lidocaine	—	1–2	65–75	0.3–2	1.5–5 µg/mL (5.7–21.3 µmol/L)	Liver: 90% dealkylated	Monoethylglycylxylidine (MEGX), glycine xylidine (GX): relatively inactive
Mexiletine	90	5–9	75	9–12	0.5–2 µg/mL	Liver: 90% Kidney: 10% unchanged (↑ with acid urine)	Inactive
Tocainide	100	2–3	2–22	11–15	4–10 µg/mL	Liver: 60% Kidney: 40% unchanged	Inactive
Phenytoin	Variable	0.5–1	90	18–36	10–20 µg/mL (39.6–79.2 µmol/L)	Liver: 95% hydroxylated to inactive compound	Inactive
Flecainide	95	9	50	14–50	200–1000 ng/mL (0.42–2.11 µmol/L)	Liver: >95%	Inactive
Propafenone	5–12 dose-dependent	3	>95	3–5	500–1000 ng/mL	Liver: >99% genetic variation in biotransformation	5-OH propafenone: active
Propranolol	25–50	3–4	85–95	3–6	50–100 ng/mL (0.19–0.39 µmol/L)	Liver: High first-pass extraction	4-OH propranolol: slight activity
Bretylium	15–30	5–6	<10	6–10	0.5–1.5 µg/mL	Kidney: 80% unchanged	None
Amiodarone	20–50	Very large	Probably high	20–50 days	0.5–3 µg/mL	Liver: De-ethylation	Desethyl amiodarone (DEA): active
Sotalol	>95	1.5	Negligible	13	1–2 µg/mL (3.7–7.4 µmol/L)	Kidney: 100% unchanged	None
Verapamil	15–30	4–5	90	3–7	≈100 ng/mL	Liver: High first-pass extraction	Norverapamil: moderately active

Table 37-4 Pharmacological Mechanisms, Effects, and Toxicity of Antiarrhythmic Agents*

Drug	Antiarrhythmic Effects	ECG	Hemodynamic Properties	Toxicity

Quinidine		↑ HR
		↑ PR ↑ QRS
		↑ QT
			Minimal:
			  Negative inotropism
			  Vasodilatation
			  Decreased blood
			    pressure
				Impaired conduction/
				  asystole
				Ventricular arrhythmias
				Gastrointestinal intolerance
				Cinchonism
				Thrombocytopenia
				Drug fever

	↓ Rate of rise, phase 0
	  ($\dot{V}_{max}$)
	↓ Slope, phase 4
	Prolong ERP, but
	  modest effect on APD			

Procainamide	Decrease normal
	  automaticity
	Abolish reentry by
	  producing bidirectional
	  block
		↑ HR
		↑ PR ↑ QRS
		↑ QT
			Minimal:
			  Negative inotropism
			  Vasodilatation
				Impaired conduction and
				  ventricular arrhythmias
				Gastrointestinal intolerance
				Agranulocytosis
				Drug-induced systemic
				  lupus erythematosus

Disopyramide		↑ HR
		↑ PR ↑ QRS
		↑ QT
			Marked negative
			  inotropism
			Vasoconstriction
				Anticholinergic effects:
				  dry mouth, constipation,
				  urinary retention, blurred
				  vision
				Ventricular arrhythmias

Lidocaine		± ↓ QT	No impairment
			  of normal
			  contractility
				Drowsiness, confusion,
				  irritability
				Respiratory arrest
				Convulsions

	↓ Rate of rise, phase 0 ↓ Slope, phase 4 Shorten APD and ERP			

Mexiletine	Abolish abnormal
	  automaticity
		QT ← →	Minimal or no
			  impairment of
			  contractility
				Gastrointestinal disturbance
				Dizziness, ataxia, tremor

Tocainide	Abolish reentry by
	  producing bidirectional
	  block
		↓ QT		

Phenytoin		↓ QT	Decreased blood
			  pressure on i.v.
			  administration
				Nystagmus, ataxia
				Lethargy
				Gastrointestinal intolerance

Flecainide	Marked ↓ $\dot{V}_{max}$	↑ PR
		↑ QRS
			Moderate
			  depression of
			  contractility
				Weakness
				Dizziness
				Proarrhythmia

mias and the specific consequences of actions on particular channels or receptors are poorly understood. Nevertheless, the "Sicilian Gambit" is a very useful conceptual framework for classifying antiarrhythmic drugs and helps clinicians to understand the multiplicity of drug actions; it may ultimately allow a "dissection" of the components of drug activity and definition of the best targets for specific arrhythmias and specific situations. A summary of drugs and their effects is illustrated in Figure 37-5.

Class Ia Drugs

Quinidine

Pharmacokinetics. Quinidine sulfate (Quinidex) is rapidly and nearly completely absorbed after oral administration; the gluconate salt is absorbed more slowly and less completely. An intravenous preparation is available but can cause severe hypotension

Table 37-4 *(Continued)*

Drug	Antiarrhythmic Effects	ECG	Hemodynamic Properties	Toxicity
Propafenone	Marked ↓ $\dot{V}_{max}$ ↑ ERP	↑ PR ↑ QRS ↑→ QT	Moderate depression of contractility	Dizziness Altered taste *Proarrhythmia*
Propranolol	↓ Slope, phase 4 Competitive β-adrenoceptor blockade Abolishes catecholamine-dependent arrhythmias	↓ HR	Negative inotropism Decreased blood pressure	Impaired A-V conduction/ asystole Bronchospasm Nightmares, insomnia
Bretylium	Prolongs APD Little effect on normal automaticity	↓ HR ↑ QT	Decreased blood pressure	Gastrointestinal disturbance Parotid swelling
Amiodarone	Prolongs APD and ERP Noncompetitive β-adrenoceptor blockade Diminishes normal automaticity Abolishes reentry by producing .bidirectional blockade	↓ HR ↑ QT	No impairment of normal contractility Decreased blood pressure and increased coronary blood flow on i.v. administration	Photosensitivity Skin pigmentation changes Thyroid function abnormalities Corneal microdeposits
Sotalol	↓ Slope, phase 4 β-Adrenoceptor blockade ↑ APD, ↑ ERP	↓ HR ↑ QT	Negative inotropism Decreased blood pressure	Fatigue, lethargy Proarrhythmia (torsade de pointes)
Verapamil	↓ Slope, phase 4 ↑ Refractoriness of A-V node Diminishes normal automaticity Abolishes reentry by producing bidirectional blockade	↑ PR	Negative inotropism Vasodilatation Decreased blood pressure	Impaired conduction/ asystole Gastrointestinal intolerance Constipation

* APD = action potential duration; ERP = effective refractory period; HR = heart rate; PR, QRS, QT = respective ECG intervals; ↑/↓ = increase/decrease.

and must be administered with caution. Approximately 80% of a quinidine dose is hydroxylated in the liver, and the metabolites are cardioactive. The remainder of the drug is excreted unchanged by the kidney.

Antiarrhythmic effects. As already described, quinidine slows the rapid sodium current, thereby decreasing the rate of rise of phase 0 of the action potential ($\dot{V}_{max}$). It also decreases the slope of phase 4 spontaneous depolarization, thus tending to inhibit ectopic rhythms due to automaticity. Although quinidine suppresses ventricular arrhythmias caused by increased normal automaticity, it has little effect on abnormal automaticity. Quinidine may also abolish reentrant arrhythmias: It produces bidirectional block (Fig. 37-3, example B) by depressing membrane responsiveness and prolonging the effective refractory period.

In the presence of an intact autonomic nervous

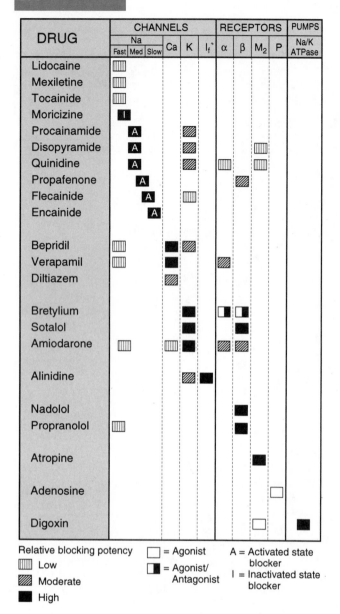

Figure 37-5. Summary of the most important actions of drugs on cardiac electrical activity. Sodium-channel block is divided into fast, medium, and slow, according to the kinetics of its development and dissipation, and results in little, modest, or marked QRS prolongation at ordinary sinus rates, respectively. Agonists are shown as open squares and antagonists as filled squares. Bretylium has initial agonist action (norepinephrine release) followed by antagonism of α- and β-receptors. Note that for simplicity α- and β-receptor subtypes are not separated out in this scheme. (Adapted from Rosen MR, Schwartz PJ 1991.)

system, quinidine may cause an increase in heart rate either by a reflex increase in sympathetic activity or by a decrease in vagal tone. In patients with sick sinus syndrome, quinidine may produce severe sinus node depression, causing an aggravation of the bradycardia.

Quinidine is useful in the treatment of a wide variety of arrhythmias including atrial, A-V junctional, and ventricular tachyarrhythmias.

Effect on the electrocardiogram. Quinidine may increase the heart rate. In therapeutic concentrations it has little effect on the PR interval, but prolongation of the QRS complex and QTc (QT interval corrected for heart rate) occurs. These effects become more pronounced with increasing plasma concentrations. (Examples of normal and abnormal ECGs are given in Figure 37-6.)

Cardiovascular and hemodynamic effects. Quinidine decreases myocardial contractility (negative inotropic effect). However, therapeutic concentrations of quinidine do not usually impair myocardial performance since the negative inotropism is minimal. If administered intravenously, quinidine may produce vasodilatation and marked hypotension.

Cautions and toxicity. With increasing plasma levels of the drug, the risk of A-V block or asystole increases. Toxic concentrations may induce abnormal automaticity and ventricular tachycardia. Another ventricular arrhythmia may be observed in patients who exhibit excessive QT prolongation; this is known as "torsade de pointes" polymorphic ventricular tachycardia (see Fig. 37-6) and may occur at therapeutic plasma concentrations of quinidine.

When administered to patients in atrial fibrillation or flutter, quinidine may occasionally cause a paradoxical increase in the ventricular rate. This is because the drug may decrease the number of atrial impulses reaching the A-V node to such an extent that 1:1 conduction through the A-V node becomes possible, and because quinidine may shorten A-V nodal refractoriness through its anticholinergic effect. In clinical practice, most patients receive digitalis preparations before quinidine is administered in order to avoid this phenomenon.

It is important to note that quinidine can interact with other drugs. In particular, it will cause a twofold increase in serum digoxin concentration in patients at steady state, as a result of decreased renal and nonrenal clearance of digoxin and the displacement of digoxin from tissue binding sites by the quinidine molecule.

Gastrointestinal intolerance (nausea and diarrhea) is common, and large doses of the drug may produce cinchonism, which is characterized by a spectrum of symptoms including blurred vision, tinnitus, headache, and gastrointestinal upset. Drug fever and rare idiosyncratic reactions, such as thrombocytopenia secondary to antiplatelet antibodies, have also been reported.

Procainamide

Pharmacokinetics. Procainamide (Procan, Pronestyl) is more than 75% bioavailable after oral administration. The intravenous preparation is relatively frequently used but can cause hypotension if rapidly administered. Procainamide has a relatively short half-life of 2–3 hours.

A variable proportion of the drug is acetylated in the liver to *N*-acetylprocainamide (NAPA). NAPA, unlike the parent drug, has little effect on $\dot{V}_{max}$ of Purkinje fibers but prolongs the duration of the action potential, thus having the properties of class III drug action. The concentration–response relationship for NAPA is different from that for procainamide; it is therefore not useful to add the concentrations of the parent drug and its metabolite when using plasma level monitoring to estimate drug effect.

The NAPA metabolite is eliminated primarily via the kidneys. Hence the patient's acetylation status (see Chapter 12) and renal function will be important in determining the plasma concentration at steady state, and dosages will need to be adjusted in renal failure.

Antiarrhthmic effects. The antiarrhythmic properties of procainamide are similar to those of quinidine; it has comparable effects on automaticity, excitability, responsiveness, and conduction. This results in **electrocardiographic features** *similar to those of quinidine*, at both therapeutic and toxic plasma concentrations.

Hemodynamic properties. Procainamide is comparable to quinidine in its minimal negative inotropic effects at usual oral clinical doses. Intravenous administration may produce vasodilatation and hypotension in addition to more marked negative inotropism.

Cautions and toxicity. Excessive concentrations of procainamide markedly impair conduction, which may result in asystole or the induction of ventricular arrhythmias. Hypersensitivity reactions include occasional drug fever and, rarely, agranulocytosis. A more common and troublesome reaction is the development of a syndrome resembling systemic lupus erythematosus (SLE), which presents with arthralgia, fever, and pleural-pericardial inflammation. The drug-induced SLE may be accompanied by LE cells in the blood smear. An antinuclear factor is often present in the blood of patients receiving procainamide and is not by itself diagnostic of the SLE syndrome. This syndrome usually disappears on withdrawal of the drug, although cases of persistent SLE have been reported following procainamide therapy. The SLE phenomenon is dose- and time-related and is more likely to occur in patients who exhibit slow hepatic acetylation resulting in higher plasma drug concentrations of the parent compound.

Rare CNS side effects include depression, hallucinations, and psychosis, but gastrointestinal intolerance is less frequent than with quinidine.

Disopyramide

Pharmacokinetics. As 50% or more of orally ingested disopyramide is excreted unchanged by the kidneys, the dosage will require adjustment downward in renal insufficiency. Approximately 30% of the drug is converted by the liver to the less active mono-*N*-dealkylated metabolite.

Antiarrhythmic effects. Disopyramide (Norpace, Rythmodan) has properties similar to those of quinidine, in that it slows the rate of rise of phase 0 ($\dot{V}_{max}$) of the action potential and causes a concentration-dependent decrease in the slope of phase 4 depolarization. Disopyramide also slows the rate of discharge of the sinus node and may cause serious bradyarrhythmias in patients with preexisting sinus node dysfunction. The **electrocardiographic features** are *similar to those of quinidine and procainamide.*

Hemodynamic effects. In comparison with quinidine and procainamide, disopyramide exerts a marked *negative inotropic effect* and may produce clinically important decreases in myocardial contractility and cardiac output in patients with preexisting impairment of left ventricular function. This property limits the usefulness of the agent in patients with a history of congestive heart failure.

Cautions and toxicity. Most of the side effects seen with disopyramide relate to its anticholinergic activity (e.g., dry mouth, urinary hesitancy or retention, blurred vision, and constipation). As with quinidine, patients who demonstrate an excessively prolonged QT interval with disopyramide are at risk of developing ventricular arrhythmias related to the therapy itself. In addition, when disopyramide is used as the sole agent in the management of atrial fibrillation it may produce an increase in the ventricular rate by a mechanism similar to that described for quinidine.

Class Ib Drugs

Lidocaine

Pharmacokinetics. Lidocaine is given intravenously because extensive first-pass transformation by the liver prevents the attainment of clinically effective plasma concentrations by the oral route. The drug is dealkylated and eliminated almost entirely by the liver, so dosage adjustments are necessary in the presence of hepatic disease or dysfunction.

Antiarrhythmic effects. Lidocaine (Xylocard) causes a reduction in $\dot{V}_{max}$ (phase 0) of the action potential. It also shortens the duration of the action potential and the effective refractory period of normal Purkinje fibers and ventricular myocardial cells. The shortening effect on the action potential is greater than that on the effective refractory period, and thus the effective refractory period is lengthened relative to the action potential duration. Lidocaine has little activity on the action potential duration in atrial tissue.

Sinus-node function is not altered in normal subjects but may occasionally be depressed in patients with preexisting sinus-node dysfunction. Unlike quinidine, lidocaine is capable of suppressing abnormal automaticity in conditions such as digitalis excess. Lidocaine abolishes ventricular reentry by a mechanism similar to that for quinidine (see Fig. 37-3, example B). The drug slows conduction most in diseased (hypoxic or ischemic) tissues and at high rates of stimulation ("use-" or frequency-dependent effect). Lidocaine is especially useful in treating ventricular arrhythmias arising during myocardial ischemia, such as during myocardial infarction. Although lidocaine is of proven benefit in preventing ventricular fibrillation early after myocardial infarction, there is no evidence that it reduces mortality in this setting. It has little effect on atrial or A-V junctional arrhythmias.

Electrocardiogram. Lidocaine has minimal effects on the ECG, although shortening of the QT interval is occasionally seen.

Hemodynamic effects. In clinical practice, lidocaine does not impair left ventricular function and

A

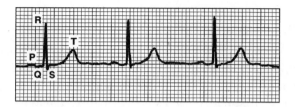

B

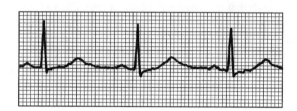

C

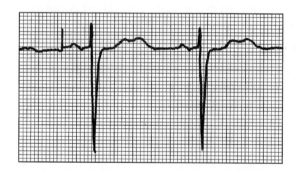

Figure 37-6. Illustrative electrocardiogram tracings.
A. Normal electrocardiogram, showing the P-QRS-T complex. (PR interval = 150 msec; QRS duration = 80 msec; QT interval = 410 msec.)
B. Prolonged QT interval of 600 msec as seen following a drug with class III antiarrhythmic action.
C. First-degree A-V block (PR interval of 210 msec), QRS prolongation (QRS duration of 135 msec), and QT prolongation (QT interval of 650 msec). These are typical ECG features of amiodarone therapy, which has class I (QRS-prolonging), class III (QT-prolonging), and class IV (calcium-channel-blocking, PR-prolonging) activity. Note

D

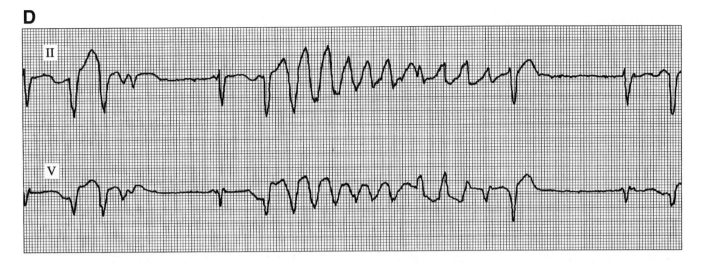

Figure 37-6, (cont'd)
also the sinus bradycardia (50 bpm) typical of a drug with antiadrenergic activity (class II).
D. Polymorphic ventricular tachycardia with QT prolongation. Note the underlying bradycardia with wide complex escape after a pause. The QT intervals after pauses are greater than 700 msec, and the coupling interval from the QRS to the first beat of ventricular tachycardia is 700 msec. This "pause-dependent" polymorphic ventricular tachycardia is termed "torsade de pointes."

has little or no negative inotropic effect. Unlike class Ia drugs, lidocaine does not alter autonomic function.

Toxicity. CNS side effects predominate; drowsiness, slurred speech, paresthesias, agitation, and confusion are most common. These symptoms may progress to convulsions and respiratory arrest (compare with cocaine, Chapter 25) if higher plasma concentrations of the drug develop.

Mexiletine

Pharmacokinetics. Mexiletine (Mexitil) is an orally effective structural analog of lidocaine. It is well absorbed and biotransformed by the liver to inactive metabolites; the half-life is relatively long (about 12 hours).

Antiarrhythmic effects. The drug has electrophysiological effects similar to those of lidocaine, shortening the action potential duration in normal tissues but slowing conduction, especially in diseased tissues. Mexiletine also suppresses abnormal automaticity in Purkinje fibers. Like lidocaine, it is effective in the treatment of ventricular arrhythmias and relatively ineffective for atrial or A-V junctional arrhythmias.

Electrocardiogram. Mexiletine has minimal effects on the ECG.

Hemodynamics. Very little negative inotropic effect is seen, and the drug can be given to patients with significant left ventricular dysfunction.

Toxicity. Gastrointestinal (nausea, anorexia) and CNS side effects (tremor, ataxia, dizziness, diplopia, insomnia, confusion) are common and respond to a decrease in dose. As with lidocaine, drug-induced arrhythmias are uncommon.

Tocainide

Tocainide (Tonocard) is another oral analog of lidocaine with a very similar profile of electrophysiological effects and clinical efficacy to that of lidocaine.

It is well absorbed and has high systemic bioavailability, with a half-life of approximately 12 hours.

Side effects are similar to those of lidocaine and mexiletine, but the drug can on rare occasions cause *agranulocytosis*. It is recommended by the manufacturer for use only when other antiarrhythmic agents are ineffective.

Phenytoin

This drug is described in greater detail as an antiepileptic agent in Chapter 22 (see also Table 37-3).

Antiarrhythmic effects and electrocardiogram. The antiarrhythmic properties of phenytoin generally resemble those of lidocaine. This drug is rarely used as an antiarrhythmic agent in adults, with the possible exception of the treatment of rhythm disturbances secondary to digitalis overdose. It is more often used in children with ventricular arrhythmias. Phenytoin shortens the QT interval in the ECG.

Hemodynamic effects. As with lidocaine, clinically useful doses of phenytoin produce little or no alteration in left ventricular function.

Class Ic Drugs

Flecainide

Pharmacokinetics. Flecainide (Tambocor) has a long half-life of 16–20 hours after oral administration; it undergoes partial biotransformation to inactive metabolites. Both the unchanged parent drug and the metabolites are eliminated renally.

Antiarrhythmic effects. The drug is a potent suppressant of $\dot{V}_{max}$ in Purkinje and myocardial fibers, causing marked slowing of conduction in all cardiac tissues with relatively small and variable effects on action potential duration and refractoriness. Automaticity is reduced by an elevation in threshold potential rather than a decrease in the slope of phase 4 depolarization. Like other class Ic agents, the drug is effective in a wide variety of atrial, A-V nodal, and ventricular arrhythmias. It is a particularly potent suppressant of premature ventricular contractions ("PVC killer") and is highly effective in slowing conduction over accessory atrioventricular bypass tracts in the Wolff-Parkinson-White syndrome. It is also effective in restoring and maintaining sinus rhythm in cases of atrial fibrillation. In atrial tissues, there is a more marked prolongation of refractoriness.

Electrocardiogram. Flecainide causes a dose-dependent increase in PR and QRS intervals; QTc intervals are little changed. QRS intervals may in-crease by up to 50%, and excessive increases appear to be associated with drug toxicity.

Hemodynamic effects. Flecainide has negative inotropic effects and can cause worsening of congestive heart failure, especially in patients with severe preexisting left ventricular dysfunction.

Toxicity. The most common side effects include dizziness, blurred vision, headache, and nausea. Like other drugs with class Ic action, *flecainide can cause a severe worsening of preexisting arrhythmias or de novo appearance of life-threatening ventricular tachycardia resistant to treatment. In patients with frequent PVCs following myocardial infarction, flecainide increases mortality compared to placebo.*

Propafenone

Pharmacokinetics. Propafenone (Rythmol) undergoes extensive first-pass transformation to a hydroxylated metabolite with reduced electrophysiological effects. The clearance is dose-dependent, and higher doses exhibit lower clearance and prolonged half-life; clearance is impaired in patients with liver disease.

Antiarrhythmic effects. Propafenone, like flecainide, markedly slows conduction in all cardiac tissues. It also prolongs action potential duration in atrial and ventricular tissues, thus also prolonging refractoriness. It decreases the slope of phase 4 in Purkinje fibers but has little effect on sinus node automaticity. Like flecainide, propafenone is a "broad-spectrum" antiarrhythmic that is effective in a wide variety of arrhythmias.

Electrocardiogram. The drug causes an increase in all ECG intervals, including PR, QRS, QT, and QTc duration.

Hemodynamic effects. Negative inotropism with worsening of congestive failure is occasionally seen.

Toxicity. Propafenone is usually well tolerated but can cause nausea, weakness, and a metallic taste. It may also have severe *proarrhythmic effects,* similar to those of the other agents with class Ic properties.

Many antiarrhythmic drugs, of which those with primarily class I action have been the best studied, are biotransformed by the hepatic microsomal enzyme system (CYP2D6). The activity of this enzyme system is genetically determined (see Chapter 12); there may be wide differences between individuals in the rate of biotransformation and therefore in the concentration of parent drug and metabolites. The electrophysiological effect of a given dose of drug may therefore be very different between individuals, due to differences in drug disposition as well as differing concentration–effect relationships at the site of drug action.

Class II Drugs

Propranolol (and other β-blockers, e.g., metoprolol, atenolol, timolol, nadolol, acebutolol).

Although propranolol is not a potent suppressant of premature ventricular contractions, it has been shown to reduce the incidence of sudden, presumably arrhythmic, death following myocardial infarction. As with metoprolol and timolol, this effect may be a direct antiarrhythmic and/or an indirect anti-ischemic effect of chronic β-adrenoceptor blockade.

This drug, and other β-adrenoceptor antagonists like it, are described in greater detail in Chapter 17 (see also Table 37-3).

Antiarrhythmic effects. Propranolol exerts its major antiarrhythmic effect through competitive inhibition of β-adrenoceptors, which also results in a relative prominence of vagal effects on the heart. Although the drug also possesses a local anesthetic action, this property does not contribute to its role as an antiarrhythmic agent in therapeutic doses. Propranolol decreases the slope of phase 4 depolarization of the sinus node. This action characteristically results in sinus bradycardia. In conditions where catecholamine excess is responsible for generating autonomous ectopic rhythm disturbances (e.g., pheochromocytoma, and exercise-induced ventricular tachycardia) propranolol is useful in abolishing the arrhythmia.

Hemodynamic and adverse effects. Other properties of propranolol, its hemodynamic effects and its toxicity, are discussed in Chapter 17. In brief, the adverse cardiac effects of propranolol are generally predictable, the most important being left ventricular failure, hypotension, bradycardia, and, rarely, A-V block.

Class III Drugs

Bretylium

Pharmacokinetics. Bretylium tosylate (Bretylate) is poorly absorbed from the gastrointestinal tract and is therefore generally administered parenterally. The drug is excreted unchanged in the urine and dosage adjustment is required in the presence of renal failure.

Antiarrhythmic effects. Bretylium differs from class I antiarrhythmic agents in that it does not slow the rise of phase 0 ($\dot{V}_{max}$) of the cardiac action potential and does not reduce the slope of phase 4 depolarization. Furthermore, therapeutic serum concentrations do not alter membrane responsiveness appreciably. The drug does, however, prolong both the duration of the action potential and the effective refractory period in Purkinje fibers.

Bretylium is generally reserved for use in life-threatening ventricular arrhythmias, especially recurrent ventricular fibrillation.

Electrocardiogram. The drug reduces the sinus rate and prolongs the QT interval.

Hemodynamic effects. Bretylium initially displaces catecholamines from sympathetic terminals but then usually causes hypotension as a result of its adrenergic neuron-blocking action (see Chapter 18). Severe postural hypotension can be seen after prolonged administration, most commonly in patients with preexisting impairment of left ventricular function, and it may cause or worsen congestive heart failure.

Toxicity. Nausea and vomiting may occur after rapid intravenous administration, and long-term oral therapy has been reported to produce painful parotid gland enlargement.

Amiodarone

Amiodarone (Cordarone) is a very complex and incompletely understood drug originally introduced as an antianginal agent.

Pharmacokinetics. Amiodarone is incompletely absorbed after oral administration. It is very extensively taken up by tissues, especially fatty tissues, and has a half-life of up to 60 days after long-term administration. The drug is extensively de-ethylated in the liver to *N*-desethyl amiodarone, which has significant electrophysiological effects. Full clinical effects may not be achieved for up to 6 weeks after initiation of treatment, with a slower onset for some effects (increases in refractoriness) than others (slowing of A-V nodal conduction).

Antiarrhythmic effects. The drug has complex effects and possesses class I, II, III, and IV actions. Its dominant effect is probably through prolongation of action potential duration and refractoriness. It also slows cardiac conduction, acts as a calcium-channel blocker and as a weak β-adrenoceptor blocker, and may have central antiadrenergic effects. The high iodine content of amiodarone exerts an antithyroid action, which may in itself have antiarrhythmic effects. Amiodarone can be used in the treatment of virtually any clinical tachyarrhythmia.

Electrocardiogram. Amiodarone causes an increase in the QT interval and smaller increases in PR and QRS intervals. Sinus bradycardia can occur. (Illustrated in Fig. 37-6C.)

Hemodynamic effects. The drug is a vasodilator and an effective antianginal agent. Although it has modest negative inotropic properties, it rarely causes clinically evident hemodynamic impairment, even in patients with severe left ventricular dysfunction.

Toxicity. Amiodarone has a very wide spectrum of toxic effects. After use of several years' duration, more than 25% of patients will suffer limiting side effects, often requiring drug discontinuation. Some of the more common effects include GI intolerance, tremor, ataxia, dizziness, hyper- or hypothyroidism, corneal microdeposits (invariable) with disturbance of night vision (occasional), liver toxicity, photosensitivity, slate-gray facial discoloration, neuropathy, muscle weakness, weight loss, symptomatic bradycardia, and proarrhythmia (rare). The most dangerous side effect is pulmonary fibrosis, which occurs in 2–5% of patients.

Sotalol

Sotalol (Sotacor) is a β-adrenoceptor blocker that also prolongs action potential duration and refractoriness in all cardiac tissues.

Pharmacokinetics. Sotalol has a half-life of about 12 hours after oral administration. It is eliminated largely by the kidneys and doses need to be lowered substantially in patients with renal dysfunction.

Electrocardiogram. Sotalol prolongs the QT interval and causes sinus bradycardia.

Antiarrhythmic effects. The drug suppresses phase 4 spontaneous depolarization and may produce severe sinus bradycardia. It also slows A-V nodal conduction. Action potential duration and refractoriness are prolonged in atrial and ventricular myocardium. The combination of β-adrenoceptor blockade and prolongation of action potential duration may be especially effective in the prevention of sustained ventricular tachycardia.

Hemodynamic effects. Significant left ventricular dysfunction can occur when sotalol is administered, especially in patients with previous left ventricular enlargement and congestive heart failure.

Toxicity. Fatigue, dizziness, and insomnia can occur. Drug-induced polymorphic ventricular tachycardia can develop in patients with excessive QT prolongation, especially if hypokalemia is present. This form of proarrhythmia is dose-dependent and is more common in women.

Class IV Drugs

Verapamil, diltiazem

These drugs are described in greater detail in Chapter 38 (see also Table 37-3).

Antiarrhythmic effects. Verapamil (Isoptin) and diltiazem (Cardizem) block the inward current carried by Ca^{2+} and exert their main antiarrhythmic action by slowing A-V node conduction and prolonging its effective refractory period; they thus slow the ventricular response to atrial fibrillation. Phase 0 of the action potential is not altered, and neither is the duration of the action potential. The slope of phase 4 depolarization is decreased, and heart rate is slightly reduced. Verapamil, when given intravenously, abolishes reentry rhythms involving the A-V node, such as A-V nodal reentrant tachycardia.

Electrocardiogram. The PR interval may increase, but QRS duration and the QT interval are not altered.

Hemodynamic effects. Verapamil, and to a lesser extent diltiazem, have negative inotropic properties and may impair left ventricular performance in patients with preexisting myocardial dysfunction. The drugs also cause peripheral vasodilatation with a resultant fall in blood pressure.

Cautions and toxicity. Both verapamil and diltiazem may cause bradycardia, and asystole has been reported, particularly if the drugs are used in combination with a β-blocker. Side effects include gastrointestinal intolerance and constipation. Diltiazem on rare occasions may cause headache, flushing, and ankle swelling.

Digoxin

Although extensively described in Chapter 36, some aspects of digoxin are worthy of consideration in the management of arrhythmias. Digoxin prolongs the effective refractory period and diminishes conduction velocity in Purkinje fibers while conversely shortening the refractory period in atrial and ventricular myocardial cells. Prolongation of the effective refractory period of the A-V node causes PR interval prolongation in the presence of sinus rhythm and permits digoxin to control the ventricular response rate in atrial fibrillation and flutter, its most important antiarrhythmic action. Digoxin also increases vagal activity and thus reduces the rate of discharge of the S-A node. If present in toxic serum concentrations, digoxin causes increased abnormal automaticity with resulting ventricular rhythm disturbance, which may be potentiated by hypokalemia. This arrhythmia has traditionally been treated with lidocaine or phenytoin.

Adenosine

Adenosine is a naturally occurring substance that attaches to receptors in the atrioventricular and sinus nodes. Intravenously administered adenosine is inactivated in the blood within seconds and thus has a very short duration of action. At therapeutic doses, A-V nodal conduction is markedly slowed or interrupted, producing transient A-V block. This makes adenosine almost universally effective for reentrant arrhythmias that use the A-V node as a portion of

the circuit. Transient bradycardia, flushing, and slight hypotension may also occur, although serious side effects are very rare. This drug can be considered first-choice therapy for A-V nodal and atrioventricular reentrant arrhythmias.

Magnesium

Although not directly antiarrhythmic in most models of arrhythmia, magnesium very effectively abolishes polymorphic ventricular arrhythmias that occur in the context of QT prolongation, i.e., torsade de pointes ventricular tachycardia such as is caused by quinidine, procainamide, sotalol, or other drugs that prolong the QT interval (e.g., disopyramide, tricyclic antidepressants, i.v. erythromycin, terfenadine, or astemizole in overdose). It interferes with calcium transfer across the cell membrane and within the cell, and at high doses reduces heart rate, slows A-V nodal conduction, and may slow intraventricular conduction.

CLINICAL MANAGEMENT OF ARRHYTHMIAS

Atrial Premature Beats

These generally do not require treatment. However, if they cause severe symptoms or are responsible for initiating paroxysmal atrial arrhythmias, they can be suppressed with quinidine or other class I agents (see Table 37-5).

Atrial Fibrillation and Flutter

In the acute state, sinus rhythm may be restored by means of electrical cardioversion. Alternatively, drugs with class I, II, and III action may terminate the arrhythmia. Drugs that slow conduction through the A-V node, such as digoxin, verapamil, propranolol, and amiodarone, will tend to control the ventricular response, and thus reduce the heart rate (see Table 37-5). Digoxin and verapamil are not useful in restoring or maintaining sinus rhythm.

Paroxysmal Supraventricular Tachycardia

This often arises via a reentry phenomenon using the A-V node. Accordingly, drugs with A-V nodal

Table 37-5 Therapeutic Choices for the Management of Common Arrhythmias*

Arrhythmia	Acute		Chronic	
	First-Line	*Alternatives*	*First-Line*	*Alternatives*
Atrial premature beats	Usually do not require treatment		Quinidine	Disopyramide Procainamide
Atrial flutter/fibrillation	DC-cardioversion Digoxin (to control ventricular response)	Diltiazem Verapamil (to control ventricular response)	Digoxin + Quinidine	Propafenone Sotalol Flecainide Amiodarone
Paroxysmal supraventricular tachycardia	Adenosine	Verapamil Propranolol	Digoxin Sotalol Verapamil	Quinidine Flecainide Amiodarone Propafenone
Ventricular premature beats	Usually do not require treatment		β-Blockers	Quinidine Procainamide Mexiletine Propafenone Flecainide
Ventricular tachycardia	DC-cardioversion	Lidocaine Procainamide Quinidine Amiodarone Bretylium	Amiodarone Quinidine Sotalol	Procainamide Propafenone Flecainide

*Note: No antiarrhythmic drug, in any patient population, has been definitively shown to prolong life for any arrhythmia. Drug therapy is therefore used to treat ongoing symptoms and prevent symptomatic recurrences of arrhythmias.

blocking properties (e.g., verapamil) will often terminate this arrhythmia. Quinidine, sotalol, propafenone, flecainide, and occasionally amiodarone have been used on a chronic basis for prophylaxis of such arrhythmias (see Table 37-5).

Ventricular Premature Beats

Ventricular premature beats do not usually cause symptoms. There is no specific indication for treating ventricular premature beats per se in any situation. Following acute myocardial infarction, intravenous lidocaine may prevent the occurrence of ventricular fibrillation. Although there is evidence that frequent ventricular premature beats late after myocardial infarction are associated with an increased risk of subsequent sudden death from ventricular tachycardia or fibrillation, there is no evidence at this time that suppressing these premature beats reduces the risk of sudden death.

Ventricular Tachycardia

If this arrhythmia occurs acutely with circulatory collapse, it is treated by direct current (DC) cardioversion. In less severe cases, reversion to sinus rhythm may be accomplished by means of intravenous lidocaine or possibly other class I agents. All of the class I and III agents listed have been used for long-term control and suppression of this arrhythmia (see Table 37-5).

The treatment of ventricular tachycardia and prevention of ventricular tachycardia or fibrillation are undergoing rapid evolution. It is advisable to refer to an up-to-date textbook of cardiology or recent periodicals for further discussion.

SUGGESTED READING

Gillis AM, Kates RE. Clinical pharmacokinetics of the newer antiarrhythmic agents. Clin Pharmacokinet 1984; 9:375–403.

Kavanagh KM, Wyse DG. Recent advances in pharmacotherapy: Ventricular arrhythmias. Can Med Assoc J 1988; 138:903–913.

Nattel S. Antiarrhythmic drug classifications: a critical appraisal of their history, present status, and clinical relevance. Drugs 1991; 41(5):672–701.

Nattel S, Talajic M, Fermini B, Roy D. Amiodarone: pharmacology, clinical actions, and relationships between them. J Cardiovasc Electrophysiol 1992; 3:266–280.

Rosen MR, Schwartz PT, eds. The Sicilian Gambit. A new approach to the classification of antiarrhythmic drugs based on their actions on arrhythmogenic mechanisms. Circulation 1991; 84:1831–1851.

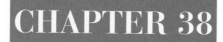

CHAPTER 38

Vasodilators

W.A. MAHON

CASE HISTORY

A 55-year-old woman who had smoked 20 or more cigarettes per day until 3 months previously began to experience chest pain. The pain was located behind the sternum and radiated to the left arm; it occurred on walking upstairs and was also noted when she walked on the level against a cold wind. Relief occurred within 2–3 minutes after she stopped. The exertion could be continued at that point and the pain did not seem to recur. These symptoms had been present for 3–4 months when she was first seen.

On physical examination, the patient was found to be overweight (30% above her ideal body weight), her blood pressure was 180/100 mmHg (taken after 4 minutes in the supine position), and the heart was clinically enlarged. An echocardiogram showed some left ventricular enlargement but no evidence of valvular heart disease and no evidence of segmental hypokinesia.

The patient was instructed in how to use nitroglycerin sublingually, to be taken at the onset of chest pain and prior to any activity that was known to induce the pain.

She remained well for several months during the summer and fall, but with the onset of winter some increase in the pain developed. It again occurred on exercise. She also reported being wakened in the morning because of chest pain. A calcium-channel-blocking drug (diltiazem) was therefore added, starting with a dose of 180 mg daily of Cardizem CD, and this produced some significant reduction in the frequency and severity of chest pain on exercise. No further early morning pain has occurred since then.

The properties of blood vessels, including the innervation and contraction of vascular smooth muscle and the role of endothelial factors in regulation of vascular function, were reviewed in detail in Chapter 35. Drugs that may be used to enhance contraction of vascular smooth muscle are described in Chapter 16. Drugs used to decrease excessive vasoconstriction by reducing sympathetic tonus are described in Chapters 17 and 18. This chapter deals with agents that produce vasodilatation mainly by direct action on the vascular smooth muscle itself.

Vasodilatation may be produced by various types of pharmacological agents. Nitroglycerin and various nitrates have been in use for the treatment of cardiac disease for more than 100 years. These agents have a profound venodilating effect, so even low doses produce an increase in vascular capacitance. Other drugs used for the same purpose include pre- or postganglionic blockers of the sympathetic nervous system, α-adrenoceptor blockers, β_2-adrenoceptor agonists, histaminergic or dopaminergic receptor agonists, blockers of calcium channels in the muscle-cell membrane, angiotensin-converting enzyme (ACE) inhibitors, and drugs that relax vascular smooth muscle directly without acting on any specific receptors. It has come to be realized that nitrate-induced venodilatation is mediated by nitric oxide ion (NO); nitrates provide an exogenous source of NO in the vascular cells, which induces vasodilatation even when endogenous production of NO is impaired, as occurs in coronary artery disease.

As the list of agents implies, the drugs differ widely in chemical structure, in specificity of action, and in primary clinical application. The three main clinical indications for the use of vasodilators are angina pectoris, hypertension, and refractory heart failure. Nitrites are used primarily for angina pectoris; hydralazine, diazoxide, sodium nitroprusside, and minoxidil are used chiefly for treatment of hypertension; calcium-channel blockers are used for both purposes; and various other agents are useful in the treatment of heart failure that is refractory to conventional treatment.

Many other drugs, including papaverine, nicotinic acid, ethanol, cyclandelate, guancycline, and theophylline and related compounds, have been used in the past as direct-acting vasodilators for the treatment of peripheral or cerebral vascular obstructive diseases. However, these are no longer considered valid indications. If blood flow in a peripheral artery is diminished because of partial or complete obstruction of a vessel, these drugs will be of no value. Indeed, they may further impair the perfusion in an ischemic area by diverting blood to areas supplied by healthy vessels which can respond to the drugs. Therefore a number of drugs have been developed to deal with the problem of vascular obstructive disease by altering the metabolism of lipids, which form the atheromatous plaques in the walls of the blood vessels (see Chapter 39).

For convenience of discussion, the drugs in current clinical use will be divided into three sections dealing respectively with vasodilators, antianginal drugs, and calcium-channel blockers.

VASODILATORS

Characteristics of Drug-Induced Vasodilatation

Relaxation of smooth muscle is a basic action of all direct-acting vasodilators, but there are considerable differences among them with respect to their relative effects in various tissues and also on different segments within the same vascular bed. The difference in their action on arteries versus veins is of particular importance in the therapeutic application of these drugs. Nitrites and nitrates have a pronounced effect on the veins, whereas sodium nitroprusside acts both on arteries (arterioles) and on veins, and hydralazine and diazoxide act mainly on arteries. The reason for

this interesting difference in vasodilatory effects on arteries and on veins is not clear.

In addition, vasodilators can differ in their action in various vascular areas; i.e., some will increase blood flow mainly in the coronary arteries while others act chiefly in the renal, mesenteric, or skin vessels. The explanation for such regional differences of action is probably complex. One factor is the relative effect of the various vasodilators on cardiac function. Blood flow in all tissues depends on the balance between vascular resistance (regulated by local factors such as adrenergic innervation, metabolites, etc.) and cardiac output. The relative contribution of cardiac and local factors to the regulation of blood flow is quite different in various tissues. Hence, it is easy to understand that a vasodilator that increases cardiac output (directly, through baroreceptor reflexes, or by enhancing venous return to the heart) may increase blood flow more in a particular vascular area in which perfusion depends mainly on the cardiac output, than another vasodilator that is without such cardiac effect.

The extent of vasodilatation also depends a great deal on the preexisting state of the vessels. Drug-induced relaxation in vitro can be best demonstrated in vessels that have been previously contracted, and it will not be demonstrable in those already relaxed. This property of the vasodilators has important consequences in clinical use.

Clinical Indications for the Use of Vasodilators

Hypertension

This is the main indication for the use of vascular smooth-muscle relaxants other than the nitrites. The last decade brought an upsurge of interest in these drugs for the treatment of arterial hypertension. Diastolic hypertension is consequent to increased peripheral resistance, and therefore the rationale for lowering arterial pressure by using drugs that relax vascular smooth muscle is obvious. Previously their use was limited because they tended to cause tachycardia and increased cardiac contractility by activating baroreceptor reflexes. These compensatory changes counterbalance the antihypertensive effect of the vasodilators. Since the discovery of β-adrenoceptor-blocking drugs, however, the reflex tachycardia and the increase in cardiac output can be counteracted. Today vasodilators are used, as a rule, together with β-blockers to treat hypertension.

The antihypertensive effect of vasodilators is enhanced by the concomitant use of diuretics. Oral diuretics are an integral part of antihypertensive therapy and can by themselves effectively control blood pressure in at least one-third of hypertensive patients. In more severe hypertension, diuretics are used in combination with β-adrenoceptor-blocking drugs, vasodilators, or some other drugs acting on the sympathetic nervous system. Diuretics decrease extracellular and plasma volume; this action and their vascular effects enhance the lowering of blood pressure caused by vasodilators. In addition, diuretics prevent retention of salt and water, which is a frequent consequence of the excessive capillary permeability to Na^+ that is caused by vasodilators (see also Chapter 41).

Refractory heart failure

Recently, vasodilators have been used with good results in patients with severe chronic heart failure refractory to digitalis and diuretics. This use of vasodilators is based on the concept that the clinical features of heart failure are related not only to severe impairment of myocardial contractile function but also to excessive peripheral vasoconstriction, which further impairs myocardial performance. Vasodilators are used to overcome the vasoconstriction and thus diminish the myocardial workload and oxygen requirement. Heart rate (unlike that in hypertensive patients) is not increased in these patients because blood pressure does not fall and therefore baroreceptor reflexes are not activated. Impressive results have been reported to follow the use of angiotensin-converting enzyme (ACE) inhibitors (see below), sodium nitroprusside, isosorbide dinitrate, and prazosin, a postsynaptic α-adrenoceptor blocker. ACE inhibitors are the drugs of choice because they lower the mortality in refractory heart failure.

Vasodilators in Clinical Use (Fig. 38-1)

Hydralazine

Hydralazine (Apresoline) has been widely used for many years to treat moderate or severe hypertension, although seldom as the sole antihypertensive agent. It lowers blood pressure by relaxing vascular smooth muscle and decreasing peripheral resistance, without exerting any central action such as had been proposed in earlier times. The mechanism of action of hydralazine is not known. It has little effect on veins; therefore orthostatic hypotension is rarely a problem with this drug. Hydralazine reduces renal vascular

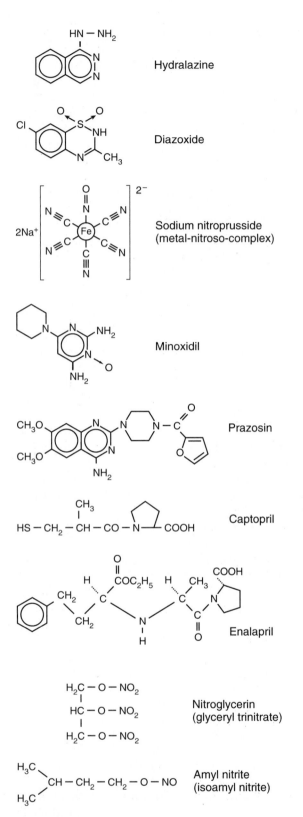

Figure 38-1. Structural formulae of drugs used to reduce peripheral vascular resistance. Calcium-channel blockers also used for this purpose are shown in Figure 38-2.

resistance and tends to maintain renal blood flow. It is well absorbed from the gastrointestinal tract and, interestingly, it yields higher blood levels when given after meals. Termination of its effect ($t_{1/2} = 2.5$ hours) is mainly by acetylation, with a higher rate of disappearance in patients who are fast acetylators (see Chapters 4 and 12).

Hydralazine is suitable for prolonged treatment of hypertension, particularly in combination with β-adrenoceptor-blocking agents and diuretics.

Adverse effects include headache, gastrointestinal complaints, palpitation, arrhythmia, precipitation of angina, and other consequences of vasodilatation. In addition, when given in large doses (at or above 200 mg/day) hydralazine can cause lupus syndrome, particularly in patients of the slow acetylator phenotype.

Diazoxide

Diazoxide (Hyperstat) is a nondiuretic congener of the thiazide diuretics. Its absorption from the gastrointestinal tract is unreliable, and today it is given only by the intravenous route. When given intravenously, diazoxide has a powerful relaxant effect on arteriolar smooth muscle, resulting in a prolonged reduction of blood pressure in the majority of hypertensive patients. A high threshold concentration is required for the action on smooth muscle, and the drug injection is therefore given rapidly to achieve this concentration during the short period before extensive redistribution of drug occurs. The same dose, injected slowly, may produce a much weaker or shorter-lasting effect. The maximal hypotensive effect develops within 10 minutes, making the drug of particular value in the *treatment of hypertensive emergencies*. It is highly bound to plasma protein, and the plasma $t_{1/2}$ is correspondingly long (28 hours), but the duration of its action is variable, generally in the range of 8–12 hours (occasionally longer).

Reflex tachycardia and increase in cardiac output can be prevented by β-adrenergic blockade. Diazoxide also has an antidiuretic action, producing salt and water retention that may interfere with its hypotensive effect but that can be controlled by the simultaneous administration of a diuretic. Hyperglycemia is rarely severe enough to cause problems during short-term therapy with diazoxide.

Sodium nitroprusside

Sodium nitroprusside (Nipride) is a very potent vasodilator that acts directly on vascular smooth muscle. Like diazoxide, it has to be given intravenously and is used mainly for *treatment of hypertensive emergencies*. Unlike diazoxide, it acts also on the veins and can reduce cardiac preload. Its effect begins almost immediately after the start of an intravenous infusion, but it ends less than 10 minutes after the infusion is stopped. The dose of sodium nitroprusside required to decrease arterial pressure is quite variable, and therefore its administration requires careful supervision and adjustment of the infusion rate.

Because of its vasodilator action, sodium nitroprusside has been given with good results to patients with low cardiac output following myocardial infarction and also to patients with chronic refractory heart failure. It was shown to reduce right atrial, pulmonary arterial, and capillary pressure, to decrease left ventricular end-diastolic pressure, and to increase cardiac output. Heart rate is not altered significantly by sodium nitroprusside in patients with cardiac failure when baroreceptor reflexes are already activated.

Most of the **adverse effects** of sodium nitroprusside are relatively minor ones, such as nasal stuffiness, nausea, vomiting, and headache. The ferrous iron in the nitroprusside molecule reacts with sulfhydryl components in red blood cells, resulting in the release of cyanide. The cyanide is reduced in the liver to thiocyanate, which is excreted by the kidneys. There is, however, a potential danger of lethal cyanide poisoning in subjects with rhodanese deficiency. Thiocyanate may accumulate in renal failure and cause seizures and coma.

Minoxidil

Minoxidil (Loniten) has a powerful blood-pressure-lowering effect with long duration of action. It produces arteriolar dilatation and hence lowers peripheral vascular resistance.

The drug is well absorbed orally, it reaches peak plasma concentrations in about 1 hour, and maximal pharmacological effects are seen in 2–3 hours. The antihypertensive effect continues for 1–3 days beyond the drug's plasma half-life of 3 hours. Minoxidil undergoes hepatic biotransformation to the glucuronic acid conjugate. Metabolites as well as small amounts of unchanged drug are excreted primarily by the kidneys.

As a "last resort," it is given orally (together with a β-blocker and a diuretic) to control severe hypertension refractory to other antihypertensive drugs.

Unfortunately, the good antihypertensive qualities of minoxidil are associated with frequent side effects. In most patients it causes hypertrichosis, fatigue, marked fluid retention, and often pericardial effusion. In animals, large doses of minoxidil cause subendocardial and subepicardial degenerative lesions with hemorrhage.

The production of hypertrichosis as a side effect of systemic minoxidil therapy was the stimulus to its use as a topical solution applied to the scalp to encourage hair growth in some types of baldness. Vasodilatation of vessels supplying the hair follicles has been suggested as one mechanism of its claimed hair-growth-promoting effect. The long-term value of this treatment is not yet clear. Enough percutaneous absorption of minoxidil can occur to cause systemic side effects in some cases.

Prazosin

This drug previously was classified as a direct-acting vasodilator. Although it does inhibit phosphodiesterase, its main action is through blockade of postsynaptic α_1-adrenoceptors (see Chapter 17). Since it does not block presynaptic α_2-receptors, norepinephrine feedback remains intact and no increase in sympathetic drive occurs (in contrast to pre- and postsynaptic α-adrenoceptor blockers such as phenoxybenzamine and phentolamine). Therefore, tachycardia and increased renin release do not occur.

The drug is well absorbed following oral administration. Serum half-life is 3–4 hours; antihypertensive effects last for up to 12 hours. There is extensive protein binding (up to 97%). Elimination is via hepatic biotransformation and excretion in the bile.

Prazosin (Minipress) is moderately effective in hypertension, to about the same degree as hydralazine. When combined with a diuretic, it has been used in patients with impaired left ventricular function.

Adverse effects may consist of orthostatic hypotension (in less than 15% of patients), especially in a hot environment or after exercise. Another possible adverse reaction is the "first-dose phenomenon"; about 30–60 minutes after the first dose, or after a significant increase in dose, postural hypotension occurs, together with transient palpitations, dizziness, and faintness (up to syncope!), especially in patients who have been depleted of salt and water. The cause is not defined, but it may be related to an abrupt change in the role of sympathetic activity in the maintenance of blood pressure. Therefore, the first dose should be given at bedtime, and treatment should be started with low doses.

Captopril and other ACE inhibitors

These drugs prevent the conversion of angiotensin I to angiotensin II by inhibiting the angiotensin-converting enzyme (ACE), a peptidyl dipeptidase (see Chapter 32). ACE inhibitors cause a reduction in peripheral arterial resistance with consequent lowering of blood pressure. Because ACE (albeit under another name) is also the enzyme that breaks down bradykinin, the vasodepressor effects of elevated bradykinin levels may contribute to the overall picture of peripheral vasodilatation produced by ACE inhibitors.

There is little change in cardiac output, and baroreceptor reflexes are not compromised. In patients with heart failure, ACE inhibitors reduce preload, afterload, and pulmonary vascular resistance, and they increase cardiac output. As noted above, they reduce mortality.

Captopril (Capoten) is given orally before meals for maximum bioavailability. It has a relatively short half-life of about 2 hours, being eliminated almost totally in the urine, about half as unchanged drug and half as metabolites. The drug may be combined cautiously with other antihypertensive agents such as diuretics and β-adrenoceptor blockers. Because of its primary excretion by the kidneys, appropriate dose reductions apply in cases of renal impairment. **Enalapril** (Vasotec) and **lisinopril** (Zestril) have longer half-lives and can be given once daily. **Cilazapril, fosinopril, quinapril,** and **remipril** are examples of newer ACE inhibitors recently introduced to clinical use. With the exception of captopril and lisinopril, all ACE inhibitors mentioned above are prodrugs with active metabolites of enhanced potency (see Chapter 32).

Adverse effects consist of exaggerated therapeutic effects (hypotension) if ACE inhibitors are combined indiscriminately with other antihypertensive agents and vasodilators. Also, all agents that affect the neuronal or humoral control of vascular tone have the potential for functional drug interactions with ACE inhibitors. Elevations in BUN and serum creatinine may occur in volume-depleted patients or those with renovascular hypertension.

Adverse Effects of Vasodilators

As with other drugs, the therapeutic value of vasodilators is limited by the frequency and severity of adverse effects. All vasodilators can cause fluid and salt retention consequent to altered capillary permeability or increased renal tubular reabsorption. Another adverse effect common to all the drugs mentioned (except prazosin and ACE inhibitors) is the reflex increase in cardiac rate and contraction. This effect, together with a sudden decrease in blood pressure caused by large doses, can precipitate angina pectoris, coronary insufficiency, and even myocardial infarction in patients with coronary heart disease in whom the coronary perfusion is already compromised. Some more specific adverse effects are shown in Table 38-1.

ANTIANGINAL DRUGS

Nature of the Problem

Angina pectoris is a characteristic chest pain occurring because of an imbalance between oxygen delivery to, and utilization by, the myocardium. The imbalance can result from spasm of the vascular smooth muscle of the coronary arteries so that they do not dilate adequately in response to increased myocardial work. Coronary blood flow may be adequate at rest even though the coronary arteries are narrowed, but inadequate when the demands of the heart are increased. Inadequate coronary blood flow

also can result from atheroma of the coronary arteries, which narrows the lumen and restricts blood flow. Both spasm and atheroma may be present in varying degrees. The strategy for relief of angina is to produce either redistribution of blood flow to or within the heart muscle, relaxation of the coronary arteries, or a decrease in the oxygen demand of the heart.

Drugs that decrease coronary vasoconstriction or spasm are of two types: the classical "antianginal drugs" covered in this section and the newer calcium-channel blockers described in the next section.

Because the presenting manifestation is a symptom, and that symptom is pain, there is significant variation in individual response and reaction, and emotional factors and expectations may play a large role in the apparent effect of treatment. One of the great difficulties in assessing drugs in angina is the high rate of response occurring with placebo. Controlled clinical trials that include placebo as well as an active drug have found that 30–50% of patients with angina pectoris respond favorably to placebo. It may be difficult to determine, therefore, whether a supposedly active drug is really more effective than a placebo.

The first pharmacological observations on or-

Table 38-1 Some Properties and Adverse Effects of Clinically Used Vasodilators[a]

Drug	Route of Administration	Main Indication	Veno-dilatation	Cardiac Output	Adverse Effects
Nitrites	Sublingual, oral, cutaneous	Angina pectoris, refractory heart failure	Yes	↑↓	Headache
Hydralazine	Oral (i.m.)	Hypertension	No	↑	Lupus syndrome
Diazoxide	Intravenous	Hypertensive emergency	No	↑	Hyperglycemia
Sodium nitroprusside	Intravenous	Hypertensive emergency	Yes	(↑)*	Cyanide poisoning (potential danger)
Minoxidil	Oral	Severe hypertension	No	↑	Hypertrichosis, fluid retention
Calcium-channel blockers	Oral (verapamil also intravenous)	Angina pectoris, hypertension, arrhythmia	No	↑↓	Headache
ACE inhibitors	Oral	Hypertension, congestive heart failure	Yes	↑↓	Headache, hyperkalemia, cough

[a]*Key to symbols:* *Only in congestive heart failure; ↑ = increase; ↑↓ = varies with drug, dose, method of administration.

ganic nitrates were made in the mid-1800s, but it was not until 1857 that an English physician, Brunton, administered amyl nitrite by inhalation and noted that anginal pain was relieved within 30–60 seconds. However, that particular nitrite was difficult to administer, and a major improvement occurred in 1880, when nitroglycerin was administered sublingually for the relief of acute angina.

In the 1960s, James Black, a British pharmacologist, synthesized propranolol and other β-adrenoceptor blockers and demonstrated that reducing cardiac work by slowing the heart rate and reducing contractility in response to exercise was also an effective method to prevent angina.

Calcium-channel-blocking drugs became known in the 1970s when Fleckenstein, in Germany, reported that verapamil was active in relaxing vascular smooth muscle; subsequently, various calcium-channel blockers have proved to be effective agents for the treatment of angina.

Nitrites and Nitrates

These drugs (see Fig. 38-1), which are marketed under a variety of brand names, have been used for many decades in the treatment of angina.

Chemistry

Nitrates and nitrites are simple nitric and nitrous acid esters of mono- or polyalcohols. They vary from extremely volatile liquids (amyl nitrite) to moderately volatile liquids (nitroglycerin, considered the prototype of the group). The formulations of nitroglycerin used in medicine are not explosive. The conventional sublingual tablet form of nitroglycerin may lose potency during storage as a result of volatilization and adsorption to plastic surfaces.

Structure–activity studies indicate that all therapeutically active agents in this group are capable of releasing nitrite ion in vascular smooth-muscle target tissues. Unfortunately, they all also appear to be capable of inducing cross-tolerance when given in large doses.

Pharmacokinetics

Organic nitrate esters are quite lipid-soluble, and therefore they are readily absorbed through the well-vascularized sublingual mucosa. They are hydrolyzed by hepatic enzymes that convert the organic nitrate esters into water-soluble partially denitrated metabolites and inorganic nitrite. These are considerably

less potent vasodilators; they continue to be found in the blood for several hours after a dose of nitroglycerin, but are eventually excreted in the urine.

The effectiveness of organic nitrates is strongly influenced by the existence of a high-capacity hepatic organic nitrate reductase that inactivates the drug. Therefore, bioavailability of all orally administered organic nitrates is very low (typically less than 10%). Consequently, the sublingual route is preferred for achieving a therapeutic blood level rapidly. Nitroglycerin and isosorbide dinitrate are both absorbed efficiently by this route and reach therapeutic blood levels within a few minutes. However, the total dose administered by this route must be limited to avoid excessive effects; therefore, the total duration of effect is brief, typically 15–30 minutes. When much longer duration of action is needed, oral preparations are available that contain an amount of drug sufficient to result in sustained systemic blood levels of drug or active metabolites despite the high first-pass effect in the liver. Other routes of nitroglycerin administration include transdermal absorption when it is applied to the skin as an ointment or patch and buccal absorption from slow-release buccal preparations.

Pharmacological Effects

In normal individuals, the exact mechanism whereby these drugs produce vascular relaxation is unknown. Low concentrations of nitroglycerin produce venodilatation, which predominates over arteriolar dilatation. As a direct consequence of venodilatation, there is a decreased venous return, with immediate fall in left and right ventricular end-diastolic pressure. This is greater on a percentage basis than the reduction of afterload that follows the fall in systemic arterial pressure. Heart rate increases, but the systemic pressure declines, and pulmonary vascular resistance is reduced. There is a decrease in cardiac output. The effects are readily visible, because there is facial flushing due to arteriolar dilatation in the face and neck, and in normal individuals headache is a very common symptom.

High intravenous or oral doses of nitrates or nitrites decrease systolic and diastolic blood pressure and cause a fall in cardiac output, with resultant hypotension and dizziness, and activation of compensatory sympathetic responses including tachycardia. Coronary blood flow increases transiently because of direct vasodilatation in the coronary vascular bed; but if a significant decline in arterial blood pressure results, there is a reduction in coronary blood flow.

The effects are particularly evident when the individual is in the upright position.

A demand for increased oxygen delivery to the heart is normally met by increasing the blood flow rather than by more complete extraction of oxygen, because the myocardial oxygen extraction is almost complete. Ischemia is the major stimulus for coronary vasodilatation, and it is believed that regional blood flow is adjusted by autoregulatory mechanisms.

In patients with organic stenosis of the coronary artery, nitrates may not increase total coronary blood flow but may alter the distribution in favor of more hypoxic regions. It is believed that nitrates cause redistribution of coronary blood flow to the ischemic subendocardial areas by selective vasodilatation of the large epicardial vessels.

Whatever the exact mechanism or combination of mechanisms of action, nitrates cause rapid reduction in myocardial oxygen demand and rapid relief of angina.

Tolerance to Nitrates

With continuous exposure to nitrates, isolated smooth muscle may develop complete tachyphylaxis (tolerance), and the intact human becomes at least partially tolerant. Continuous exposure to high levels of nitrates can occur in the chemical industry, especially where explosives are manufactured. When contamination of the workplace with volatile organic nitrate compounds is severe, workers find that, upon starting their work week (Monday), they suffer headache and transient dizziness. After a day or so, these symptoms disappear because of the development of tolerance.

Nitroglycerin is probably denitrated in the smooth-muscle cell. The resulting nitric oxide (NO) is thought to bind to a specific receptor on vascular smooth-muscle cells, stimulating guanylate cyclase to form cyclic GMP. This nucleotide causes vasodilatation either by inhibiting Ca^{2+} entry or increasing Ca^{2+} exit. Sulfhydryl (–SH) groups are required for the stimulation of guanylate cyclase. Tolerance to NO-mediated vasodilators occurs when –SH groups are oxidized by NO. Tolerance can be reversed with sulfhydryl-regenerating agents such as dithiothreitol or N-acetylcysteine, both of which act as –SH-group donors. This process suggests that an increase in cGMP is the first link in vascular smooth-muscle relaxation. Other studies implicate the production of prostaglandin E or prostacyclin (PGI_2) as an important intermediate step (see Chapter 31). There is no evidence that autonomic receptors are involved in the primary nitrate response (although autonomic reflex responses are evoked when hypotensive doses are given).

CALCIUM-CHANNEL BLOCKERS

Mechanism of Action

As described in detail in Chapter 35, the application of an effective stimulus to a muscle cell results in the influx of Ca^{2+} which in turn triggers the intracellular events leading to muscle contraction. Several different types of antagonists (Fig. 38-2) can block this sequence of Ca^{2+}-dependent steps.

Inorganic cations, such as manganese, cobalt, and lanthanum, can function as general calcium antagonists. They probably do so by substituting for calcium at a variety of binding sites and either block Ca^{2+} channels or enter the cell where they substitute for Ca^{2+} at intracellular Ca^{2+} receptors. Of much greater importance from a clinical viewpoint, however, are the organic calcium-channel blockers. These agents exert their actions at low (nanomolar) concen-

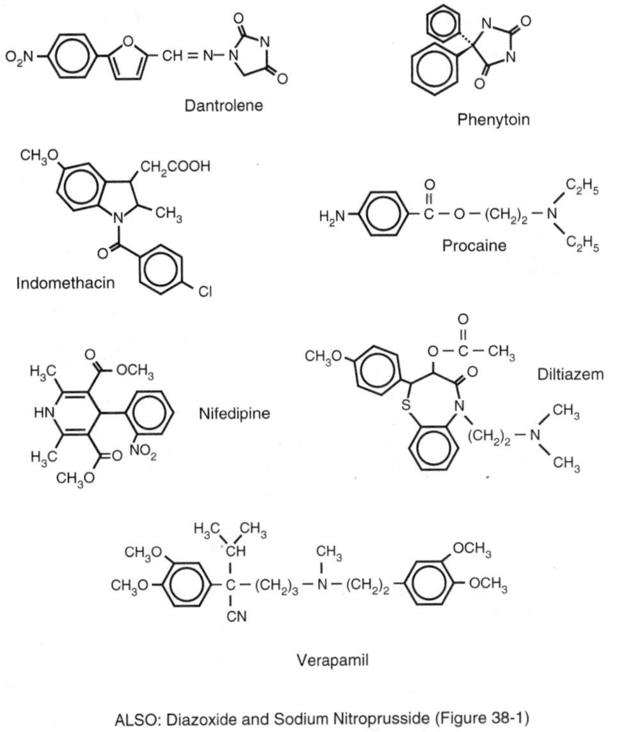

ALSO: Diazoxide and Sodium Nitroprusside (Figure 38-1)

Figure 38-2. Structural formulae of drugs having calcium-channel blocking properties. Only nifedipine, diltiazem, and verapamil are used clinically for their vasodilating action based on calcium-channel blockade.

trations and exhibit stereospecificity; it appears likely that they are recognized by specific structures in the Ca^{2+} channel. The diversity of molecular structure of the organic calcium-channel blockers is consistent with different mechanisms and sites of action. Although the therapeutic effect of nifedipine, diltiazem, and verapamil is the same, it appears likely that nifedipine acts at a different site within the Ca^{2+} channel than verapamil and diltiazem.

There is evidence at present of three different types of voltage-dependent calcium channels. These are at present designated as L-type, T-type, and N-type. They are characterized by L being large in conductance, T being transient in duration of opening, and N being neuronal in distribution. It appears that the L-type is the most frequent in cardiac and smooth muscle. It is known to contain binding sites that differ for different calcium-channel blockers and has thus been interpreted as containing several drug receptors. L-type channels are found in neurons, glandular cells, and muscle cells and are involved in excitation-contraction coupling. N-type channels appear to be limited to neuronal membranes, especially at axon terminals where they mediate the Ca^{2+} influx that triggers neurotransmitter release. This process is not sensitive to dihydropyridine-type blockers.

Effects on Smooth Muscle

Transmembrane calcium influx is responsible for normal resting tone and contractile responses in most types of smooth muscle. Such cells are relaxed by the calcium-channel blockers. Although relaxation can be demonstrated in bronchial, gastrointestinal, and uterine smooth muscle, smooth muscle in vascular tissues appears to be the most sensitive. Blood pressure is thus reduced, particularly with nifedipine. Reduction of coronary arterial tone has been demonstrated in patients who have coronary artery spasm.

Effects on Cardiac Muscle

Calcium influx is particularly important for normal cardiac function. The calcium-dependent action potentials occurring in the S-A and A-V nodes may be reduced or blocked by most of the calcium-channel blockers. Similarly, there is a reduction in excitation-contraction coupling in cardiac cells exposed to calcium-channel blockers. Cardiac contraction velocity and cardiac output may be reduced in a dose-dependent fashion by calcium-channel blockers. Thus, patients with angina may benefit by at least two mecha-

nisms: (1) the reduction in peripheral vascular resistance and (2) the reduction in cardiac output with an accompanying reduction in oxygen requirement.

The different calcium-channel blockers (Fig. 38-2) differ in the results of their interaction with Ca^{2+} and Na^+ channels. For example, Na^+ channels are blocked by verapamil, but less than are Ca^{2+} channels; sodium-channel block is much less marked with diltiazem and nifedipine. Bepridil, an investigational drug, blocks Na^+ channels as well as Ca^{2+} channels in an effective manner. Dihydropyridines such as nifedipine block vascular smooth-muscle Ca^{2+} channels at concentrations below those required for cardiac Ca^{2+}-channel blockade. Other dihydropyridines are even more effective in their smooth-muscle action than their cardiac action.

Hemodynamic Effects

Nifedipine (Adalat; Procardia) at an oral dose of 20 mg causes a reduction of systemic vascular resistance and therefore a fall in blood pressure. This leads to a reflex rise in heart rate and a consequent rise in cardiac output. The fall in blood pressure is directly related to the preexisting pressure; the higher the initial pressure, the greater the fall. Other dihydropyridines have similar, but not identical, effects.

Verapamil HCl (Isoptin), in contrast to nifedipine, in a dose of 160 mg produces a lesser fall in blood pressure, some reduction in heart rate and cardiac output, but virtually no change in systemic vascular resistance.

Diltiazem HCl (Cardizem) in a dose of 120 mg given by mouth produces a slow, progressive decline in heart rate and blood pressure and a fall in cardiac output.

Present Therapeutic Uses

Chronic stable angina

A variety of controlled studies have shown that nifedipine, diltiazem, and to a lesser extent verapamil are effective in treating this disorder. The mechanism is probably a reduction in myocardial oxygen requirement produced by reduction of the heart rate with verapamil and diltiazem, systemic vasodilatation produced by nifedipine and diltiazem, and negative inotropism particularly with verapamil. Coronary vasodilatation also occurs, and therefore coronary blood flow increases.

In double-blind studies in which a placebo was compared with verapamil, nifedipine, or diltiazem, these agents have been shown to reduce the frequency of anginal attacks, the consumption of nitroglycerin, and the frequency of deviations of the S-T segment in the electrocardiogram.

Unstable angina

This is a form of angina occurring at rest, not relieved by simple measures, and requiring hospitalization. Verapamil, diltiazem, and nifedipine all have been shown to be effective in unstable angina. This is probably due to their suppression of coronary vasospasm.

Variant angina (Prinzmetal's angina)

This is another type of angina unrelated to exercise; it occurs at rest, often during the night. It is thought to be caused by coronary artery spasm.

Nifedipine produces benefit in over 85% of patients with variant angina. The side effects are mild but relatively frequent, ranging between 15% and 20% in different studies. They consist of facial flushing, hypotension, palpitations, and peripheral edema, which is sometimes quite marked but can usually be reversed by diuretics. Nifedipine is contraindicated when severe fixed coronary artery stenosis exists. The fall in blood pressure may result in a decline in blood flow through the stenotic artery, where flow is dependent on pressure difference.

Diltiazem produces benefit in over 70% of patients with variant angina. It has a low frequency (10%) of side effects, which include facial flushing and headache as well as bradycardia and abdominal discomfort.

Verapamil produces benefit in 70% of patients with variant angina. Side effects occur in 10–20% of cases and consist of constipation, nausea, facial flushing, and headache. This drug is contraindicated in the presence of congestive heart failure and in the presence of conduction abnormalities.

Hypertension

Nifedipine and diltiazem are potent hypotensive drugs. They relax vascular smooth muscle and produce a rapid fall in blood pressure. There are many other drugs available to treat hypertension, and at present the calcium-channel blockers cannot be regarded as first-line drugs for this purpose. However, sublingual and oral nifedipine can produce a dramatic decline in blood pressure in the emergency treatment of severe hypertension. Although it is common practice to use intravenous drugs under these circumstances, the effect of sublingual nifedipine is almost as potent and rapid as that of intravenous nitroprusside, diazoxide, or hydralazine.

SUGGESTED READING

Fisher M, Grotta J. New uses for calcium channel blockers. Drugs 1993; 46:961–975.

Flaherty JT. Nitrate tolerance. A review of the evidence. Drugs 1989; 37:523–550.

Fleckenstein A. Specific pharmacology of calcium in myocardium, cardiac pacemakers, and vascular smooth muscle. Annu Rev Pharmacol Toxicol 1977:149–166.

Fleckenstein A. History of calcium antagonists. Circ Res 1983; 52 (Suppl I):3–16.

Hurwitz L. Pharmacology of calcium channels and smooth muscle. Annu Rev Pharmacol Toxicol 1986; 26:225–258.

Janis RA, Silver PJ, Triggle DJ. Drug action and cellular calcium regulation. Adv Drug Res 1987; 16:309–591.

Schwartz A, Triggle DJ. Cellular action of calcium channel blocking drugs. Annu Rev Med 1984; 35:325–339.

Triggle DJ. Calcium antagonists. Stroke 1990; 21(Suppl IV):49–58.

Triggle DJ, Janis RA. Calcium channel ligands. Annu Rev Pharmacol Toxicol 1987; 27:347–369.

Yednak KC. Use of calcium channel antagonists for cardiovascular disease. Am Pharm 1993; NS 33:49–64.

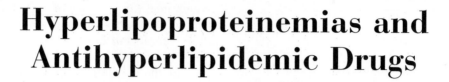

CHAPTER 39

Hyperlipoproteinemias and Antihyperlipidemic Drugs

C. FORSTER

CASE HISTORY

A 50-year-old woman recently suffered a myocardial infarction. She had a previous history of hypertension that was originally diagnosed 5 years ago. Her blood pressure had been controlled at 122/78 mmHg with hydrochlorothiazide and atenolol. She has also been receiving warfarin and low-dose ASA since the recent myocardial infarction. Postinfarction laboratory results indicated that her cholesterol levels were elevated (total cholesterol 10.1 mmol/L), and she was placed on a low-fat/low-sodium diet. She does not drink but smokes a pack of cigarettes a day. Her mother also had elevated cholesterol and coronary artery disease at age 50, and her father died of a heart attack at age 60.

Despite her diet, which complied with the American Heart Association Step-2 diet, her lipoprotein levels remained high (LDL 6.9 mmol/L and HDL 1.7 mmol/L). Lovastatin treatment was therefore initiated at a dosage of 20 mg once daily, increasing gradually to 40 mg twice daily, and her lipoprotein profile improved: LDL cholesterol was reduced by 45% to 3.8 mmol/L. However, her HDL remained low (1.5 mmol/L). Currently, her blood pressure is still controlled at 118/74 mmHg; she has no signs of xanthoma or corneal arcus and no angina or other chest pain. Although her risk for coronary artery disease has been reduced, she has failed to quit smoking and her HDL levels remain low at 1.5 mmol/L.

Clinical observation has revealed that increased concentrations of lipoproteins can accelerate the development of atherosclerosis, coronary artery disease, and myocardial infarction. To minimize these risks, both dietary and pharmacological measures need to be applied in efforts to reduce the incidence of lipoprotein disorders.

Up to the 1980s, the recommended classification of the lipoprotein disorders rested entirely on the basis of total cholesterol concentrations, or total cholesterol and triglycerides. Hypertriglyceridemia and hypercholesterolemia are now defined in terms of the specific lipoproteins that are elevated in each and the relationship each has with the other. The following sections outline the various processes leading to the development of hyperlipoproteinemias, and their classification.

LIPOPROTEIN TRANSPORT

Cholesterol and triglycerides are transported in the plasma in the form of lipoproteins, of which there are five classes differing in size, density, electrophoretic mobility, lipid and lipoprotein composition, and in the nature of the apolipoprotein moieties. These occur in a sequence of progressively smaller and denser particles beginning with the initial absorption of fats in the intestine and ending in their final disposition in the tissues (see Fig. 39-1). The lipoprotein structure consists of a nonpolar central core containing hydrophobic cholesteryl esters and triglycerides. This

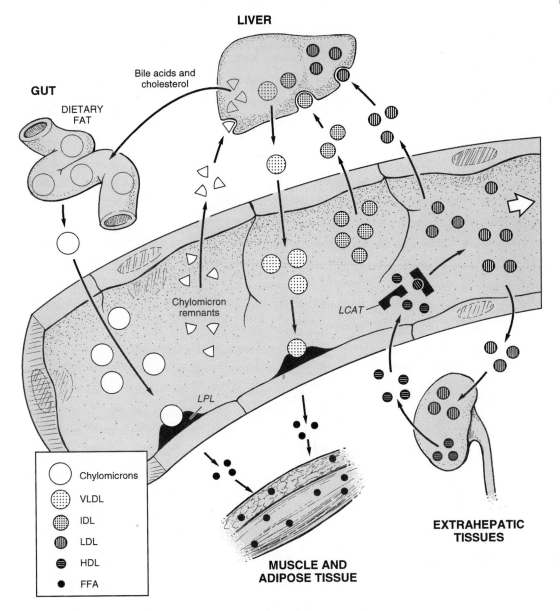

LIVER

Bile acids and cholesterol

GUT

DIETARY FAT

Chylomicron remnants

LCAT

LPL

○	Chylomicrons
⊙	VLDL
◉	IDL
▥	LDL
⊖	HDL
●	FFA

MUSCLE AND ADIPOSE TISSUE

EXTRAHEPATIC TISSUES

Figure 39-1. Schematic overview of lipoprotein transport and turnover. VLDL = very-low-density lipoproteins; IDL = intermediate-density lipoproteins; LDL = low-density lipoproteins; HDL = high-density lipoproteins; FFA = free fatty acids; LPL = lipoprotein lipase; LCAT = lecithin:cholesterol acyltransferase.

is surrounded by a hydrophilic or polar monolayer of phospholipids, free cholesterol, and proteins. This hydrophilic coating allows the transport of the insoluble cholesteryl esters and triglycerides in the aqueous phase of plasma.

The five major classes of lipoproteins in Table 39-1 have specific physiological and anatomical significance. They are often secreted in one form and rapidly transformed to others by interaction with specific enzymes such as lecithin cholesterol acyl-transferase (LCAT), lipoprotein lipase (LPL), and hepatic triglyceride lipase (HTGL).

There are separate metabolic pathways for the degradation of exogenous (dietary) lipoproteins and of endogenous lipoproteins formed by hepatic metabolism (see Fig. 39-1). Triglycerides and cholesterol in food are incorporated, in the small intestine, into large-diameter low-density lipoprotein micelles called chylomicrons. The rate of secretion of chylomicrons into plasma reflects the rate of fat absorption.

Table 39-1 Physicochemical Characteristics of the Major Lipoprotein Classes

Lipoprotein	Density (g/dL)	MW (daltons)	Diameter (nm)	Lipid (%)*		
				TG	Chol	PL
Chylomicrons	0.95	400×10^6	75–1200	80–95	2–7	3–9
VLDL	0.95–1.006	10–80×10^6	30–80	55–80	5–15	10–20
IDL	1.006–1.019	5–10×10^6	25–35	20–50	20–40	15–25
LDL	1.019–1.063	2.3×10^6	18–25	5–15	40–50	20–25
HDL	1.063–1.21	1.7–3.6×10^6	5–12	5–10	15–25	20–30

*Percentage of composition of lipids; apolipoproteins make up the rest.
TG = triglycerides; Chol = cholesterol; PL = phospholipids.
From: Ginsberg HN, Arad Y, Goldberg IJ. 1990.

The endogenous pathway involves lipoproteins that are synthesized in the liver, which serve to transport triglycerides and cholesterol to extrahepatic tissues. Both pathways provide energy to peripheral tissues by hydrolysis of triglycerides and release of free fatty acids, as well as cholesterol, to meet the metabolic and structural requirements of cells.

Apolipoproteins (Apo)

These represent the protein constituents of the lipoproteins and have important structural and functional properties. They possess both polar and nonpolar regions. The polar region is turned toward the aqueous medium and the nonpolar region binds and surrounds the insoluble triglycerides and cholesteryl esters. They function as cell ligands that allow the binding of the lipoprotein to specific cell-surface receptors; abnormalities in binding properties can lead to *dyslipidemia*. Apolipoproteins also function to activate and inhibit enzymes. For instance, LPL is activated by Apo CII and inhibited by Apo CIII. A deficiency in Apo CII causes a defect in activation of LPL and, hence, defective hydrolysis of chylomicrons and of very-low-density lipoprotein (VLDL). Apo AI is a cofactor for activation of LCAT, which must be activated before esterification of cholesterol can occur.

Chylomicrons

These are the largest particles (75–1200 nm) of low density; they are synthesized in the intestine and are used to transport triglycerides and cholesterol to the periphery.

Dietary triglyceride is hydrolyzed in the lumen of the intestine, and the resulting fatty acids and monoglycerides are taken up by gastrointestinal mucosal cells. The triglyceride is then reassembled and combined with specific apolipoproteins before being released into the lymphatics. Some important apolipoprotein exchanges occur within the chylomicrons. At first, they contain *only* Apo A and Apo B-48 and are said to be "incomplete." When they reach the circulation, they interact with circulating high-density lipoproteins (HDL). The HDL provides Apo C and Apo E in exchange for Apo AI and Apo AII. High-density lipoprotein, therefore, is an important reservoir for critical apolipoproteins that are required for normal metabolism of chylomicrons.

Hydrolysis occurs by the action of LPL, which releases free fatty acids, and the size of the chylomicron is decreased. The protein and phospholipid constituents dissociate and Apo C and Apo E are returned to new HDL particles for reuse at a later stage. This important HDL mechanism is sometimes referred to as the "HDL pathway" and has been suggested to be the third pathway in lipoprotein metabolism. When no more Apo C remains with the chylomicron, the particle is referred to as a *chylomicron remnant* that binds to a specific hepatic receptor and is removed from the circulation.

The half-life of chylomicrons is only 5–30 minutes, and therefore wide fluctuations in plasma triglyceride levels are seen. As the chylomicron remnant becomes smaller, the triglyceride content is decreased and the particle becomes relatively enriched in cholesterol and cholesteryl esters. When the remnant is removed by the liver, its cholesterol is incorporated into the hepatic cholesterol pool. Hepatic cholesterol inhibits the synthesis and expression of the LDL receptor, thus reducing the metabolic removal of LDL cholesterol and leading to hypercholesterolemia.

Very-Low-Density Lipoproteins (VLDLs)

VLDLs are synthesized in the liver and have a half-life of approximately 12 hours. They function to transport free fatty acids from the liver to peripheral tissues. VLDLs contain Apo C, Apo E, and Apo B-100. They also interact with HDL to obtain more Apo C and more Apo E, as the chylomicrons do. When this occurs, the particle is termed a *mature VLDL.* VLDLs are metabolized by LPL on the surface of capillary endothelial cells where, as the particle size decreases, they are transformed into intermediate-density lipoproteins (IDLs). These contain only Apo B-100 and Apo E, the Apo C being transferred back onto the HDL particle (see schemas in Figs. 39-2 and 39-3). As the size of the VLDL decreases, Apo B has a much more important role, and the surface expression of Apo B and Apo E changes in a way that favors binding to the LDL receptor. Fifty percent of IDL binds to and is taken up into the hepatocyte. The other 50% of IDL is converted to the cholesterol-enriched LDL particles by HTGL, which is located in the vascular endothelium of the liver. Any abnormality in HTGL will lead to an increase in IDL concentrations and a *dyslipidemia.*

An abnormality in the structure of Apo E can interfere with the binding of IDL and lead to retention of IDL and some larger particles (β-VLDL) in the plasma. The result is *type III hyperlipoproteinemia,* also known as *"broad beta disease"* or *dysbetalipoproteinemia.*

VLDL plays an important role in substrate homeostasis and is the precursor of LDL.

Low-Density Lipoprotein (LDL)

LDL has a half-life of approximately 3 days. It contains about 65% cholesterol and serves to transport cholesterol from the blood to the liver and extrahepatic tissues. The only apolipoprotein associated with LDL is Apo B-100. It contains about 1500 cholesteryl ester molecules, and the LDL particle binds to the LDL surface receptor which recognizes Apo B-100. It is then internalized and disassembled by lysosomal hydrolysis. At this stage, the LDL receptor can be recycled, but the LDL is degraded in the cell to form cholesterol and amino acids. Two-thirds of the total LDL can be removed by this pathway. The remaining one-third is bound by scavenger receptors in the liver. There are four major LDL subspecies based on the densities of the particles. LDL-1 is the largest particle. In normal individuals, there is a predominance of LDL-1 and LDL-2 subspecies. LDL-1 and LDL-2 can be positively cor-

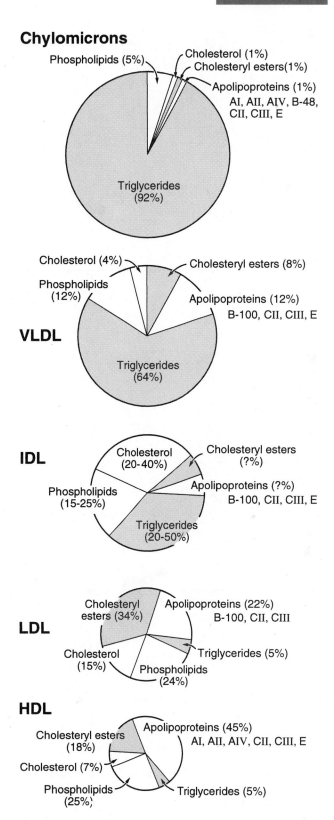

Figure 39-2. Approximate composition of lipoproteins (rounded to total 100%).

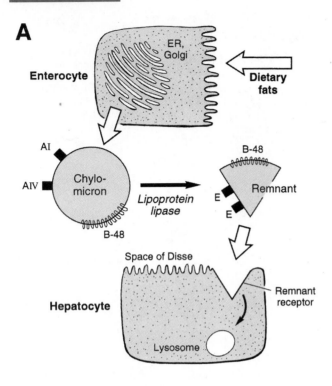

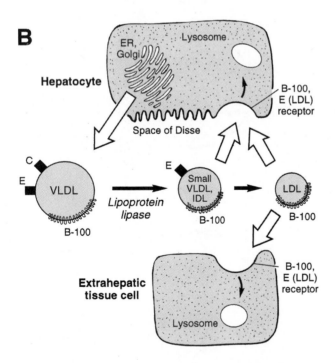

Figure 39-3. A. Metabolism of lipoproteins containing apolipoprotein (Apo) B-48. B. Metabolism of lipoproteins containing Apo-100. (From: Young SG, 1990.)

related with VLDL levels and are inversely correlated with HDL. Four mutations have been described in the LDL gene, leading to abnormalities in the receptor that give rise to a condition termed *familial hypercholesterolemia.* The LDL receptor has high affinity and low capacity. Only very low concentrations of LDL are required to meet the structural and metabolic needs of the cells. With increasing age of individuals, there is a progressive decrease in LDL receptors and, therefore, an increase in LDL cholesterol.

The intracellular level of free cholesterol in the liver determines the rate of synthesis of cellular cholesterol and LDL receptors. When the amount of free cholesterol is high, LDL receptor synthesis is inhibited, and synthesis of cholesterol by 3-hydroxy-3-methylglutaryl-CoA (Hmg-CoA) reductase is also reduced.

Some hormones can influence LDL receptors and cholesterol levels. Thyroxine and estrogen have been shown to increase LDL receptors. In menopause, when estrogen levels are low, there is an increase in LDL cholesterol. Estrogen therapy in postmenopausal women decreases LDL cholesterol by about 10–20%.

High-Density Lipoprotein (HDL)

HDL is synthesized in the liver and intestine. Ninety percent of the protein consists of Apo AI and Apo AII, but Apo C and Apo E are also present. HDL is the smallest of the lipoprotein particles. It is also known as α-lipoprotein, and it migrates rapidly during electrophoresis. HDL is also heterogeneous and consists of several subspecies. HDL_{2a}, HDL_{2b}, and HDL_3 are the most common in normal individuals. HDL_3 is cholesterol-poor and represents the newly synthesized HDL. HDL_3 can accept unesterified cholesterol, esterify it, and incorporate it into the particle. As it acquires more lipid content, the HDL_3 is converted to HDL_{2a} and then to HDL_{2b}, which delivers its lipid cargo to the uptake sites and once again becomes HDL_3.

An HDL receptor has recently been discovered in liver and in steroid-producing tissues (adrenal cortex, ovary) that strips the cholesteryl esters from the HDL particle and transports them into the cell and then releases the fat-reduced HDL particle back into circulation. Thus, HDL participates in the process of reverse cholesterol transport; i.e., it facilitates movement of cholesterol from the periphery back to the liver. Hepatic cholesterol is then excreted in the bile or converted to bile acids. This is thought to be the reason why *high blood levels of HDL are associated with lower risk of developing coronary heart disease.*

SIGNIFICANCE OF LIPOPROTEIN (a)

Lipoprotein(a) [Lp(a)] is composed of one LDL particle with more than one molecule of Apo A covalently bound to the Apo B-100 moiety. These particles have lipid composition similar to that of LDL but, because of the Apo A component, they are larger and more dense. The site of degradation of Lp(a) is uncertain; although it binds to the LDL receptor, catabolism of Lp(a) cannot be fully accounted for by LDL-receptor activity. The plasma concentration of Lp(a) is strongly controlled by genetic factors and is strongly related to the risk of developing coronary artery disease. Lp(a) crosses the endothelium by a non-receptor-mediated process and is present within the arterial intima, particularly in association with atherosclerotic plaques. The catabolism of Lp(a) is partly controlled by the LDL receptor in the liver. Interestingly, Lp(a) is structurally similar to plasminogen, and it has been suggested, therefore, that Lp(a) may impair the oxidation of plasminogen and may also compete with tissue plasminogen activator and thus prevent plasminogen from binding to fibrin. Hence Lp(a) may prevent normal clot lysis and healing of the vessel wall in atherosclerosis. As yet, there is no good evidence to show that either dietary management or exercise can affect Lp(a) levels.

LIPID LEVELS DURING GROWTH AND DEVELOPMENT

Lipid levels in children are similar in all populations. During the first year of life, as solid foods are introduced to the child, a diet-related risk factor becomes evident. A total cholesterol level of greater than 200 mg/dL (5.17 mmol/L) places boys and girls above the 95th percentile. This includes 5% of American children 5–18 years of age.

During early adolescence, up to the age of 18 years, mean cholesterol levels are decreased by a reduction in HDL with no change in LDL. VLDL levels increase in all children during puberty, but subsequently continue to rise in white boys, compared to black boys or girls. Triglyceride levels are greater in white girls than in black girls and remain relatively constant throughout the adolescent period, lower in girls than in boys.

Lipid levels in women fluctuate because of hormonal changes associated with the menstrual cycle, pregnancy, menopause, oral contraceptive use, and hormone replacement therapy.

Tables 39-2 and 39-3 list the normal mean plasma levels of triglycerides, LDL-, and HDL-cholesterol (with 95th percentile values) in white men and women for each decade of life.

HYPERLIPOPROTEINEMIA

The different classes of hyperlipoproteinemia are listed in Table 39-4, which shows some of the main features of the most common classes of hypertriglyceridemia and hypercholesterolemia encountered clinically. All of them can occur as primary disturbances with familial inheritance patterns or as secondary disturbances associated with diabetes mellitus, liver disease, and other disorders.

CARDIOVASCULAR RISK ASSESSMENT

Cardiovascular disease is a leading cause of premature death in the industrialized world. Approximately one in four individuals has some form of cardiovascular disease. Approximately one in three men and one in nine women will die of cardiovascular disease before the age of 60. Of the 1.5 million Americans who suffer a myocardial infarction in a single year, more than 0.5 million will die in a year and, of those, 0.25 million will die before they reach hospital. Seventy-five percent of these deaths are related to **atherosclerosis**, which, in the presence of hypercholesterolemia and *other risk factors*, may escalate the

Table 39-2 Plasma Triglyceride Levels in White Men and Women

Age (Years)	Males (mmol/L)		Females (mmol/L)	
	Mean	95th Percentile	Mean	95th Percentile
<10	0.56	1.02	0.73	1.47
10–19	0.79	1.52	0.79	1.41
20–29	1.13	2.09	0.96	1.86
30–39	1.47	3.22	1.02	2.09
40–49	1.69	3.50	1.18	2.31
50–59	1.64	3.33	1.41	2.88
60–69	1.52	2.88	1.52	2.99

Table 39-3 Plasma LDL- and HDL-Cholesterol Levels in White Men and Women

Age (Years)	LDL Cholesterol (mmol/L)				HDL Cholesterol (mmol/L)			
	Males		Females		Males		Females	
	Mean	95th Percentile	Mean	95th Percentile	Mean	95th Percentile	Mean	95th Percentile
<10	2.46	3.49	2.59	3.62	1.42	1.94	1.42	1.94
10–19	2.46	3.36	2.46	3.62	1.29	1.94	1.29	1.94
20–29	2.84	4.27	2.84	4.27	1.16	1.68	1.42	2.07
30–39	3.36	4.91	2.97	4.27	1.16	1.68	1.42	2.07
40–49	3.62	5.04	3.23	4.65	1.16	1.68	1.55	2.33
50–59	3.75	5.17	3.62	5.43	1.16	1.68	1.55	2.46
60–69	3.88	5.43	3.88	5.82	1.29	2.07	1.68	2.46

Table 39-4 Classes of Hyperlipoproteinemia and Their Main Features[a]

Type	Clinical Designation	Plasma Lipid Changes	Primary Defect	Other Causes	Cardiac Risk
I	Familial hyperchylo-micronemia	↑↑ chylomicrons (↑↑ TG, ↑ cholesterol)	Lipoprotein lipase deficiency, apoprotein C II deficiency	Diabetes mellitus	—
IIa	Familial hypercholesterolemia (homozygous)	↑ LDL cholesterol	LDL-receptor deficiency	Hypothyroidism, nephrotic syndrome	↑
IIb	Combined hyperlipoproteinemia	↑ VLDL, ↑ LDL* (HDL may be ↓)	LDL-receptor deficiency, ↑ production of VLDL		↑
III	Familial hyperlipidemia	↑ IDL, ↑ β-lipoproteins (LDL) (↑ cholesterol, ↑ TG)	Apoprotein E deficiency	Hypothyroidism	↑
IV	Familial hypertriglyceridemia	↑ VLDL (↑ TG, ↑ or normal cholesterol) ↓ HDL	?	Diabetes mellitus, nephrotic syndrome, obstructive jaundice	↑(?)
V	Mixed hypertriglyceridemia	↑↑ chylomicrons, ↑↑ VLDL	?	Diabetes mellitus, obstructive jaundice, pancreatitis	↑(?)
VI	Familial hyperalphalipoproteinemia	↑ HDL	?		↓
—	Dysbetalipoproteinemia	↑ VLDL (↑ cholesterol) ↑ IDL with β- rather than pre-β-electrophoretic mobility	Atypical form of apolipoprotein E, causing poor uptake of IDL by the liver		↑

[a]*Key to symbols:* *In type IIb, the relative proportions of VLDL and LDL may change gradually, the LDL increase becoming the more prominent feature. (↑=increased; ↓=decreased)

Table 39-5 Guidelines for Classification and Follow-up Based on Total Plasma Cholesterol Concentration

Total Cholesterol mg/dL (mM)	Classification	Recommended Follow-up
<200 (<5.2)	Desirable blood cholesterol	Repeat blood test within 5 years
200–239 (5.2–6.2)	Borderline high blood cholesterol	*Without* CAD* or CAD risk factors: provide dietary information and recheck annually *With* CAD or CAD risk factors: obtain lipoprotein analysis; further action based on LDL-cholesterol value
≥240 (≥6.2)	High blood cholesterol	Obtain lipoprotein analysis; further action based on LDL-cholesterol value

*CAD = coronary artery disease.
Adapted from Guidelines of the National Cholesterol Education Panel, 1988 from: Brown MS, Goldstein JL. In: Gilman AG, Rall TW, Nies AS, Taylor P, eds. Goodman and Gilman's *The Pharmacological Basis of Therapeutics*. 8th ed. Pergamon Press, 1990: 879 (with permission of the authors).

incidence of subsequent heart disease. To control atherosclerosis, treatment should be aimed at all known factors, rather than only the hypercholesterolemia per se. Coronary heart disease incidents occur not only in individuals who have extremely high cholesterol but also in those who have moderately abnormal lipid values in association with other risk factors. Guidelines for the classification of blood cholesterol levels and their importance as risk factors are shown in Table 39-5.

LIPOPROTEINS AND VASCULAR DISEASE

Figure 39-4 indicates that (1) increase in risk is linearly related to increase in LDL cholesterol; (2) in the same group a marked fall in risk occurred as HDL levels rose; and (3) predicted risk increased with increasing LDL:HDL ratios. The presence of high LDL and/or low HDL cholesterol ultimately causes damage to specific organs. This damage results from a progressive obstruction of large arteries by atherosclerosis. A high concentration of LDL cholesterol can directly damage the endothelial surface, resulting in the accumulation, within the intima, of foam cells filled with cholesteryl esters. If the insult with LDL cholesterol is continuous or repeated, marked cellular proliferation occurs, together with increasing frequency of cell death. A marked thickening of the vascular wall slowly develops, caused by increased collagen and other substances.

The correlation between LDL levels and cardiovascular disease is significant for large populations but is less reliable in individual patients since LDL and HDL are independently variable. This has led to a greater awareness of the importance of LDL:HDL ratio. Thus a person with a very high LDL and a very low HDL has a much greater predicted risk than a person with that same high LDL together with a high HDL.

During the past few years there has been a tremendous upsurge of interest in Lp(a). High plasma Lp(a) levels have been associated with an increased incidence of atherosclerosis and coronary artery disease. Lp(a) has been shown to account for a very large percentage of the remaining risk of atherosclerosis and myocardial infarction after other factors are accounted for, and may be an independent risk factor. Therefore it is currently justified to determine plasma Lp(a) levels in patients with a history of atherosclerotic cardiovascular disease. Unfortunately, the available techniques require standardization. Unlike most other risk factors, plasma Lp(a) levels are insensitive to diet and drug treatment (with the exception of niacin in high doses).

NONPHARMACOLOGICAL (DIETARY) INTERVENTION

The general outline of dietary management for dyslipidemic persons is summarized in Table 39-6. After

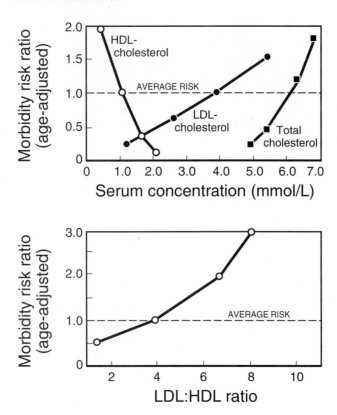

Figure 39-4. Levels of various cholesterol fractions as related to risk of coronary disease (male subjects in Framingham study).

initial assessment of the baseline diet, and the need for weight loss, a "Step 1" diet is initiated. Persons who do not achieve their therapeutic goals after several months on this diet should be put on a more stringent "Step 2" diet. Pharmacological therapy generally should be reserved for those persons who have not benefited from at least 3–6 months of dietary therapy. If the goal is achieved by diet alone, long-term monitoring is necessary.

The physician's and dietician's roles are essential in establishing dietary control in these patients. All patients should cease smoking, increase physical activity, and aim for a reduction in blood pressure.

DRUG THERAPY

Even in cases that do not show an adequate response to a careful test of dietary management, indications for drug use vary with the patient's age and clinical diagnosis. The long-term safety of these drugs in children is unclear. Some favor their use in the young in order to prevent coronary artery disease later in

Table 39-6 Recommended Diet Therapy

Nutrient	Recommended Dietary Intake	
	Step 1 Diet	*Step 2 Diet*
Total fat	Less than 30% of total calories	
Saturated fatty acids	<10% total calories	<7% total calories
Polyunsaturated fatty acids	Up to 10% of total calories	
Monounsaturated fatty acids	10–15% of total calories	
Carbohydrates	50–60% of total calories	
Protein	10–20% of total calories	
Cholesterol	<300 mg/day	<200 mg/day
Total calories	To achieve and maintain desirable weight	

From: Ginsberg HN, Arad Y, Goldberg IJ. 1990.

life, but most physicians feel that these agents should be avoided in children, except in extreme circumstances such as homozygous familial hypercholesterolemia. At the opposite extreme, the use of these drugs in an elderly person with life-threatening disease due to some other cause would obviously be inappropriate. The major indications for use of the cholesterol-lowering drugs are in young and middle-aged adults with already-diagnosed coronary artery disease. Drug therapy may also be indicated in the middle-aged person who does not yet show evidence of coronary disease, but who has an LDL-cholesterol level of 175 mg/dL (4.5 mmol/L) or more and an LDL:HDL ratio greater than 3.0.

Drugs can lower cholesterol either by decreasing production of lipoproteins or by increasing the efficiency of their removal. Seven groups of drugs are currently available that can be used as individual agents or in combinations which have synergistic effects, e.g., probucol and lovastatin given concurrently with the bile-acid-binding resins (see below). These agents are described in the following sections in relation to their different sites of action (Fig. 39-5). The drugs differ widely in structure and mechanisms of action. Historically, the common therapeutic goal of these agents was to reduce plasma triglycerides and cholesterol. However, when the protective role of elevated HDL levels became evident, the goal of drug therapy was broadened to include elevation of abnormally low HDL.

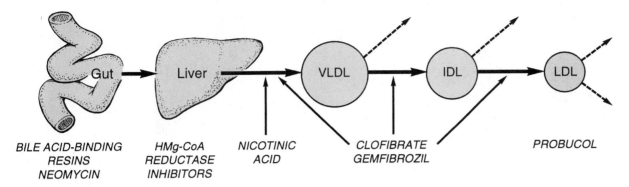

Figure 39-5. Sites of action of lipid-lowering drugs.

DRUGS THAT IMPAIR INTESTINAL ABSORPTION OF CHOLESTEROL

Bile-acid-binding Resins: Cholestyramine and Colestipol

Bile-acid-binding resins are insoluble in water, are unaffected by digestive enzymes, and are not absorbed from the intestinal tract. Their chemical structures are shown in Figure 39-6.

Mechanism of action

Cholestyramine (Questran) and colestipol (Colestid) are cationic resins that bind the bile acids and thus prevent their absorption from the intestine. The net result is increased fecal excretion of bile acids and a compensatory increase in de novo production of bile acids from cholesterol in the liver. As a consequence of reduction of cholesterol levels, there is an increase in LDL receptors and in the activity of 3-hydroxy-3-methylglutaryl-CoA (HMg-CoA) reductase, the rate-limiting enzyme in cholesterol synthesis. The increased number of LDL receptors causes increased clearance of LDL from plasma and reduction in LDL-cholesterol level. Patients (homozygotes) who suffer from a genetic defect in the production of LDL receptors cannot respond to therapy with these agents, but heterozygotes, who have one normal gene for the receptor, do respond. Body pools of cholesterol are decreased after long-term treatment and tendon xanthomas also regress.

These agents lower plasma LDL-cholesterol levels gradually, approaching 90% of the maximal effect within 2 weeks. The effect on LDL is proportional to the dose, and a 20–35% reduction in circulating LDL is seen with maximum doses of resins. Generally the level of VLDL increases by 5–20% during the first weeks of treatment and then decreases. By about 4 weeks the VLDL and triglyceride levels have returned to pretreatment levels. However, in patients whose VLDL and IDL levels are high before onset of treatment, the increase in triglycerides that occurs when the resin treatment is started may be greater and more prolonged. Therefore the resins are most effective when only LDL is elevated, as in familial hypercholesterolemia and polygenic hypercholesterolemia. Bile-acid-binding resins have no predictable effect on HDL. The efficacy of these drugs is markedly increased when they are combined with an HMg-CoA reductase inhibitor (see below).

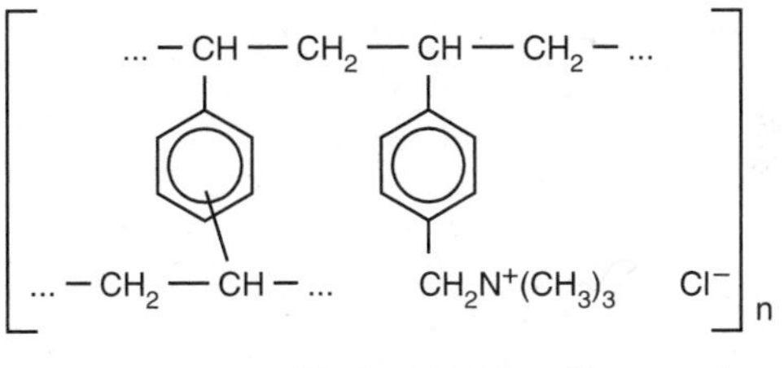

Cholestyramine (Questran)

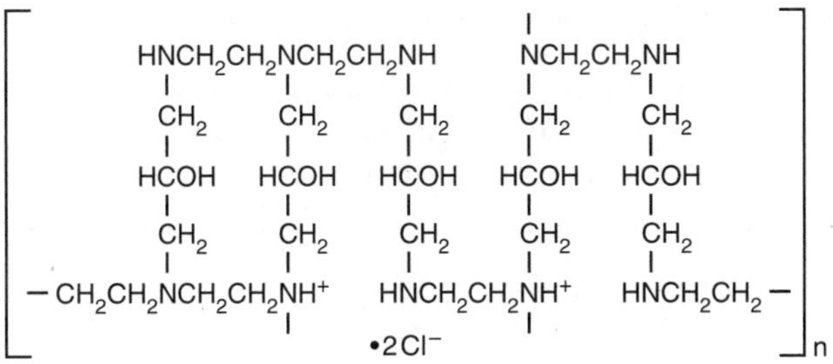

Colestipol (Colestid)

Figure 39-6. Structural formulae of bile-acid-binding resins.

Side effects

Nausea, abdominal bloating, indigestion, and constipation are common side effects. Since the resins bind the bile acids, they also impair the absorption of dietary fat; therefore, in high doses they may cause steatorrhea. Since cationic resins have high affinity for acidic compounds, they also bind to, and impair the intestinal absorption of, such drugs as warfarin and similar anticoagulants, chlorothiazide, phenylbutazone, barbiturates, thyroxine, and cardiac glycosides. Therefore, other orally administered drugs should be ingested either 1 hour before, or 4 hours after, the resins.

Neomycin

Neomycin sulfate is an aminoglycoside antibiotic (see Chapter 55) that is poorly absorbed from the intestinal tract. Like the bile-acid-binding resins, it interferes with the absorption of bile acids and cholesterol. It can reduce LDL levels without affecting HDL- or VLDL-cholesterol or triglyceride levels. Associated side effects include nausea, ototoxicity, and nephrotoxicity. Neomycin is contraindicated in patients with intestinal disease, reduced renal function, hepatic disease, or congestive heart failure, because these disorders may impair renal excretion of the small amount of neomycin that is absorbed and thus increase its toxicity. Neomycin should be considered only for patients with familial hypercholesterolemia or polygenic hypercholesterolemia who are unable or unwilling to follow other approaches.

DRUGS THAT IMPAIR SYNTHESIS OF CHOLESTEROL AND VLDL

3-Hydroxy-3-Methylglutaryl-Coenzyme A (Hmg-CoA) Reductase Inhibitors

The introduction of these compounds in North America and Western Europe has brought many promising results.

Mechanism of action

Figure 39-7 shows the chemical structures of the original HMg-CoA reductase inhibitor **mevastatin** and four agents currently used clinically—namely, **lovastatin** (Mevacor), **simvastatin** (Zocor), **pravastatin** (Pravachol), and **fluvastatin** (Lescol). These

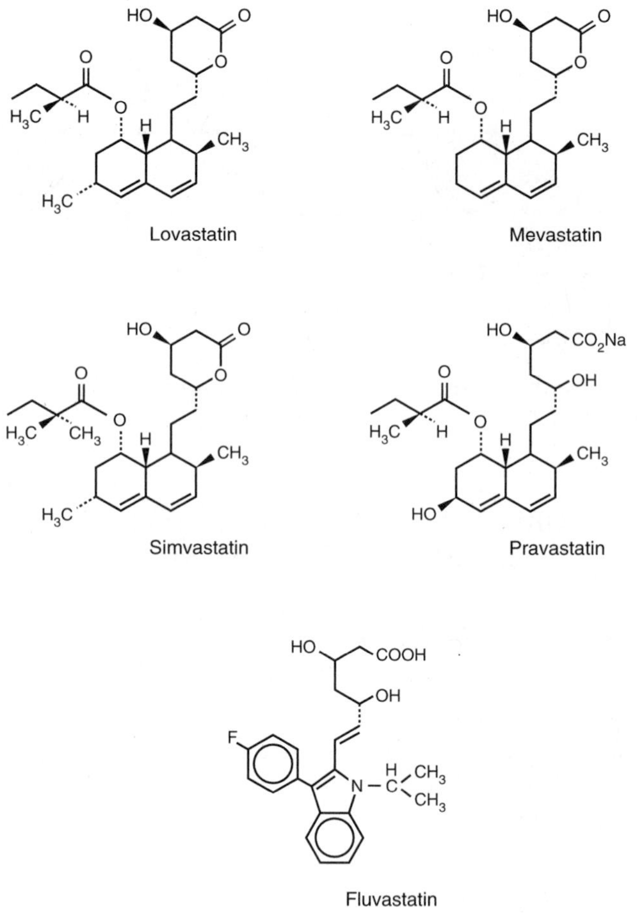

Figure 39-7. Structural formulae of HMg-CoA reductase inhibitors.

compounds act as competitive inhibitors of HMg-CoA reductase and therefore block the synthesis of cholesterol in the liver. This effect triggers a series of processes resulting in increase in LDL receptors in the liver and a corresponding reduction in plasma LDL because of receptor-mediated fractional uptake of LDL by the liver. This may be the major mechanism leading to reduced plasma LDL cholesterol in subjects with heterozygous familial hypercholesterolemia. In patients with moderate hypercholesterolemia or combined hyperlipoproteinemia, the benefits of treatment with these agents may be due to a decrease in Apo B-containing lipoproteins. Regulation of cholesterol synthesis by Apo B biosynthesis, or by assembly of Apo B into VLDL and LDL, may be implicated. Reduced VLDL formation and secretion may also be involved in the decrease of VLDL triglycerides, and removal of VLDL remnants may also play a role. It is likely that HDL levels may rise as a consequence of reduced VLDL.

Lovastatin alone, without bile-acid-binding drugs, produces dose-dependent decreases in LDL cholesterol ranging from 20% at 10 mg/day to 40% at 80 mg/day. Simvastatin and pravastatin produce similar maximum effects, but that of fluvastatin is somewhat lower. The amount of cholesterol in VLDL also declines, possibly due to a decrease in the cholesterol content of secreted VLDL. Triglyceride levels decline by up to 25% and HDL rises by up to 10%. These drugs are effective in heterozygous familial hypercholesterolemia, polygenic hypercholesterolemia, and hypercholesterolemia associated with diabetes. Since they act differently in controlling cholesterol levels, lovastatin and other HMg-CoA reductase inhibitors act synergistically with colestipol and cholestyramine, and combined therapy can reduce LDL by up to 50%.

Pharmacokinetics

Pravastatin and fluvastatin are active inhibitors of HMg-CoA reductase and are biotransformed to inactive or very weakly active metabolites. In contrast, lovastatin and simvastatin are inactive prodrugs that are biotransformed by the liver to form one or more active metabolites that are then further biotransformed to inactive products. All four drugs are well absorbed by mouth but undergo very rapid extraction by the liver and extensive first-pass metabolism. The oral bioavailability is therefore low, ranging from about 5% for lovastatin to about 25% for fluvastatin. Much of the drug extracted by the liver is excreted into the bile, so all four drugs show a mixed pattern of excretion in both the feces and the urine. All four drugs are highly protein-bound in the plasma, but the binding appears to be readily reversible, because the elimination half-life is only 1–2 hours for the active drugs fluvastatin and pravastatin, but it is longer (about 15–16 hours) for the prodrugs lovastatin and simvastatin. During combined therapy, cholestyramine has additive effects with lovastatin, pravastatin, and simvastatin. However, cholestyramine binds fluvastatin if the drugs are taken less than 4 hours apart, and it reduces its bioavailability. If the two drugs are given at least 4 hours apart, there is no interference and their therapeutic effects are additive.

Side effects

These agents are generally well tolerated, although some gastrointestinal discomfort and headache have been reported. Elevations in liver transaminases oc-

cur in 1–2% of patients. Elevations in creatinine phosphate occur in up to 10% of subjects taking lovastatin, but there is no obvious evidence of myopathies in patients without previous family history. Extremely high doses of lovastatin were shown to induce cataracts in dogs, and particular attention is being paid to the possibility of a similar effect in humans. These agents should never be given to pregnant women because of the importance of HMg-CoA reductase in the developing fetus.

Nicotinic Acid (Niacin)

Mechanism of action

The antihyperlipidemic action of nicotinic acid (niacin), discovered in 1955, is unrelated to its role as a vitamin (see Chapter 67). Although the mechanism of action is not fully understood, there is some evidence that it involves inhibition of the release of free fatty acids from adipose tissue and of their esterification to triglycerides in the liver. Nicotinic acid decreases production of VLDL in the liver, and this in turn decreases IDL and LDL levels in the plasma. Large doses can lower VLDL levels by more than 50% and reduce triglycerides correspondingly. LDL levels also fall, but much more slowly. Niacin is the only lipid-lowering drug currently available to reduce Lp(a). When niacin is given alone, LDL declines by up to 15%, but when it is given in combination with a bile-acid-binding resin, reductions of 40–60% are seen, together with some small elevation in HDL.

Side effects

Pharmacological doses of niacin can produce significant side effects that should be carefully monitored. Peripheral vasodilatation occurs in most patients and results in a cutaneous flush that can be accompanied by severe itching (pruritus). This reaction may be mediated by prostaglandins and can be relieved by ASA. Hypotension and transient vascular headaches may occur, and orthostatic hypotension caused by antihypertensive agents can be enhanced by interaction with niacin. Gastrointestinal disturbances, including peptic ulceration and bowel disease, are also common. Hepatic dysfunction, hyperglycemia, and abnormal glucose tolerance may occur even in the nondiabetic subject. Cardiac arrhythmias are also seen in patients taking this drug. Combined therapy with niacin and HMg-CoA reductase inhibitors carries an increased risk of myositis, although this appears to be less likely with fluvastatin.

DRUGS THAT IMPAIR CONVERSION OF PLASMA LIPOPROTEINS

Clofibrate and gemfibrozil are the principal drugs in this category; their structural formulae are shown in Figure 39-8.

Clofibrate

This drug (Atromid) is an ethyl ester of *p*-chlorophenoxyisobutyric acid (CPIB). After its absorption, the ester is hydrolyzed and releases free CPIB, which then is responsible for the pharmacological effects.

Mechanism of action

The primary action of clofibrate is to increase lipoprotein lipase activity. As a result, the rate of intravascular conversion of VLDL and IDL to LDL is increased and the plasma VLDL and triglyceride levels fall. This action may initially cause LDL to increase, but LDL subsequently falls, as does cholesterol. In addition, clofibrate inhibits platelet aggregation, decreases fibrinogen levels, and increases fibrinolytic activity. It inhibits the biotransformation of warfarin so that the dose of warfarin may have to be reduced. The effect on cholesterol in patients with asymptomatic hypercholesterolemia may be small,

but in familial dysbetalipoproteinemia, plasma triglyceride and cholesterol may decrease by as much as 80%. This is its main therapeutic indication. It has not been shown to have any effect on the prevention of deaths from coronary artery disease.

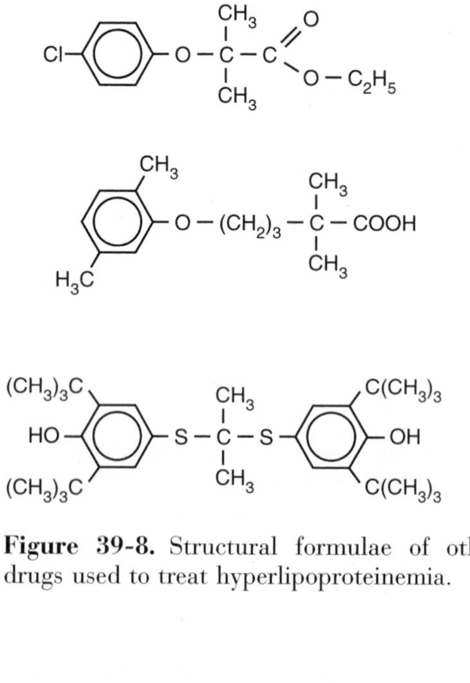

Side effects

Frequent side effects of clofibrate include epigastric and abdominal pain, nausea, and diarrhea. The incidence of gallstones (cholelithiasis) increases some two- to fourfold. Alopecia, weight gain, myositis, and leukopenia may occur with long-term use. The drug is contraindicated in patients with impaired renal or hepatic function and in pregnant and lactating women.

Gemfibrozil

This drug (Lopid) is a structural congener of clofibrate, and also lowers VLDL in hypertriglyceridemia. It can also increase HDL levels by up to 25%.

Mechanism of action

The mechanism by which gemfibrozil lowers VLDL is unknown, but it does appear to inhibit hepatic secretion of VLDL into the plasma, as well as increase the rate of its degradation by lipoprotein lipase. It has also been reported to inhibit lipolysis of triglycerides in adipose tissue and impair fatty acid uptake by the liver. These actions might contribute to a reduction in the hepatic synthesis and secretion of VLDL.

Side effects

The side effects of gemfibrozil are very similar to those of clofibrate.

DRUGS THAT INCREASE THE CLEARANCE OF LDL

Probucol

This drug (Lorelco) is chemically unrelated to any of those already described. Its structure is shown in Figure 39-8.

Figure 39-8. Structural formulae of other classes of drugs used to treat hyperlipoproteinemia.

Mechanism of action

The mechanism of action is poorly understood, and the results of its therapeutic use have been inconsistent. It is known to become incorporated into the LDL molecule and to increase LDL clearance by a nonreceptor mechanism. Probucol can decrease LDL cholesterol by 10–15%, but HDL levels are also reduced, often to a greater extent than LDL. Its maximum effect on total cholesterol levels is seen by 1–3 months after the start of therapy, but the reductions in VLDL and triglycerides are small.

Side effects

Probucol is fairly well tolerated in adults but tends to cause some gastrointestinal problems in about 10% of patients. It has also been reported to prolong the QT interval in the electrocardiograms of some patients and therefore is not recommended in patients with recent evidence of myocardial damage. Its ability to reduce plasma HDL levels makes it undesirable for use in patients with an already high LDL:HDL ratio. Its hydrophobicity may also limit its clinical usefulness.

SUGGESTED READING

Genest J, Jenner JL, McNamara JR, et al. Prevalence of lipoprotein (a) [Lp(a)] excess in coronary artery disease. Am J Cardiol 1991; 67:1039–1045.

Ginsberg HN, Arad Y, Goldberg IJ. Pathophysiology and therapy of hyperlipidemia. In: Antonaccio M, ed. Cardiovascular pharmacology. 3rd ed. New York: Raven Press, 1990:485–513.

Lipid Research Clinics Program 1984. The Lipid Research Clinics Coronary Primary Prevention Trial Results. I. Reduction in incidence of coronary heart disease. JAMA 1984; 251:351–364. II. The relationship of reduction in incidence of coronary heart disease to cholesterol lowering. JAMA 1984; 251:365–374.

Lipoprotein (a) and atherosclerosis. The Davis Conference. Ann Intern Med 1991; 115:209–218.

Paoletti R, Bernini F. Hypolipidemic agents. In: Singh B, Dzau VJ, Vanhoutte PM, Woosley RL, eds. Cardiovascular pharmacology and therapeutics. New York: Churchill Livingstone, 1994:369–384.

Report of the national cholesterol education program expert panel on detection, evaluation, and treatment of high blood cholesterol in adults. Arch Intern Med 1988; 148:23–27.

Ross R. The pathogenesis of atherosclerosis. In: Braunwald E, ed. Heart disease: a textbook of cardiovascular medicine. 4th ed. 1992:1106–1125.

Stampfer MJ, Sacks FM, Salvini S, et al. A prospective study of cholesterol, apolipoproteins and the risk of myocardial infarction. N Engl J Med 1991; 325:373–381.

Rossouw JE. An overview of lipid-lowering trials in their pharmacologic and biologic contexts. In: Singh B, Dzau VJ, Vanhoutte PM, Woosley RL, eds. Cardiovascular pharmacology and therapeutics. New York: Churchill Livingstone, 1994:1043–1089.

Steinberg D. A docking receptor for HDL cholesterol esters. Science 1996; 271:460–461.

Young SG. Recent progress in understanding apolipoprotein B. Circulation 1990; 82:1574–1594.

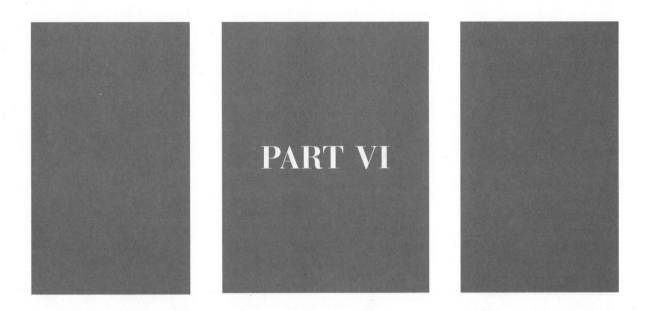

PART VI

RESPIRATORY, RENAL, AND BLOOD SYSTEMS

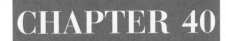

CHAPTER 40

Drugs and the Respiratory System

W.A. MAHON

CASE HISTORY

A 45-year-old woman was referred to the Emergency Department because of severe shortness of breath. Her history, provided by her husband, indicated that she has had asthma since childhood. Initially, the asthma was precipitated by exposure to pollens and domestic animals, but recently, severe asthma had occurred without any obvious precipitating stimulus. The patient had been using inhaled albuterol (salbutamol) twice daily over an extended period of time but recently had increased the dose to every 4 hours without any improvement. She was also taking oral theophylline in a dose of 200 mg twice daily in a sustained-release dosage form.

At the time she was seen, she was severely short of breath and able to speak sentences of only three to four words without stopping because of shortness of breath. She was obviously wheezing and coughing up thick, sticky mucus.

She was admitted to hospital and treated with intravenous corticosteroids, inhaled β_2-adrenoceptor agonist (albuterol) every hour, and oxygen given by mask. Intravenous theophylline (aminophylline) was given but she developed tachycardia of 160 bpm, palpitations, and nausea after 2 hours of this infusion; therefore the drug was discontinued. Thereafter, there was slow but progressive improvement over the next 36 hours. After another 72 hours had elapsed, she was able to be discharged from hospital. Intravenous corticosteroids were discontinued and replaced by inhaled steroids. At the time of her discharge, her medication consisted of inhaled corticosteroids twice daily, inhaled β_2-adrenoceptor agonists two puffs three times daily, and ipratropium two puffs twice daily. With the change in her medication, the emphasis being on inhaled corticosteroids, her asthma improved and for the next 2 years of follow-up she did not have to be hospitalized.

Drugs affect the respiratory system in a number of different ways, some by direct local action in the airways and some by remote actions in the central nervous system (CNS) with effects on the respiratory control mechanisms. The most important local drug effects on the airways are those that influence the volume and character of bronchial mucus secretion and the degree of constriction or relaxation of bronchial smooth muscle. The most important CNS effects are those that diminish the sensitivity of the cough reflex and those that alter the chemosensitivity of the respiratory control centers in the medulla and thus alter the rate and depth of respiration. These various categories of drug action are reviewed separately in the following sections.

DRUGS AFFECTING RESPIRATORY TRACT FLUID

The tracheobronchial tree is bathed in a mucus-containing fluid, a fibrous gel composed of mucoproteins, mucopolysaccharides, proteins, and fats. The fluid functions to protect the lung tissues by warming and moistening inspired air and by removing foreign airborne particles. Normal human respiratory secretion is 95% water, and adequate hydration and high relative humidity of inspired air are necessary for the production of normal mucus. The normal nasal humidification system maintains constancy of humidity and normal mucus movement as long as nasal breathing prevails. Oral breathing, in a dyspneic or unconscious patient, quickly leads to thickening of the bronchial fluid.

The rate of production of fluid averages about 100 mL/day but varies with the rate of ventilation and the quantity of airborne material inspired. Calcium ions are believed to contribute to the viscosity of sputum, and the presence of excessive calcium is the one abnormality linked to the very viscous secretions found in bronchiectasis and in cystic fibrosis. Infected or stagnant respiratory secretions contain DNA fibers from bacterial and phagocytic cells, which give purulent sputum its yellow or green color.

The respiratory-tract fluid is produced from three sources: goblet cells of the epithelium, bronchial glands in the mucosa, and serous transudate from the mucosal vasculature. In bronchitis, goblet cells are greatly increased in number and produce extremely viscous sputum. Therefore, it has been traditional practice to administer drugs to stimulate secretion of an increased volume of more watery fluid. However, any agent that increases respiratory tract secretions or decreases their viscosity may act to the detriment of the patient unless the material is propelled upward by normal ciliary activity and either expectorated by coughing or removed by mechanical suction. Otherwise, mobilized mucus will gravitate into the most dependent areas of the lungs, where it may impair respiratory function.

Antimucokinetic Agents

The reduction of respiratory-tract fluid production may be accomplished by parasympatholytic drugs such as **atropine** (see Chapter 15). This is clinically useful in some situations, such as preparation for general anesthesia (see Chapter 24).

Mucokinetic Agents (Expectorants)

Agents that increase the production of respiratory tract fluid are often used in order to prevent the drying out of secretions and the plugging of the airways with mucus, and to increase the productiveness of coughing. The most important of these agents are water and saline given as aerosols. The traditional expectorants, whether given by mouth

(e.g., **glyceryl guaiacolate**) or by vapor inhalation (e.g., **menthol, camphor,** and **lemon oils**), are of dubious value. However, **potassium iodide** solution may be effective, and **ipecacuanha** (ipecac) apparently initiates a gastric reflex that results in vagal stimulation of the bronchial glands.

Mucolytic Agents

Mucolytic inhalants are mucokinetic substances that liquefy mucus and that are usually given by aerosol to aid the elimination of excess solidified mucus in patients with respiratory disease. Excess mucus may be liquefied by proteolytic agents and disulfide bond-cleaving agents. **Acetylcysteine** is the N-acetyl derivative of the amino acid L-cysteine. It possesses a reactive sulfhydryl group that splits the disulfide bonds of the mucin molecule and thereby reduces the viscosity of mucus. This drug is an extremely effective mucokinetic agent, but it is little used because it causes many side effects such as stomatitis, nausea, vomiting, rhinorrhea, and especially bronchospasm. **Pancreatic dornase** is a hydrolytic enzyme (deoxyribonuclease) that is of value in the treatment of purulent secretions in which viscosity is due to the presence of DNA.

DRUGS AFFECTING CONTRACTION OF BRONCHIAL MUSCLE (ANTIASTHMATIC DRUGS)

Asthma

Bronchial asthma is a condition characterized by repeated attacks of paroxysmal dyspnea. It is now recognized that chronic asthma involves a characteristic inflammatory response in the airways that is present in patients with even very mild asthma. Bronchial hyperresponsiveness or an exaggerated bronchoconstrictor response to many different stimuli is characteristic of asthma. There remains considerable debate about the types of inflammatory cells and mediators involved in asthma. Presumably, mediators of inflammation also contribute to the hyperresponsiveness of the bronchi. Although mast cells may be important in the response to allergens and exercise, their exact role in chronic asthma remains less certain. Drugs that stabilize mast cells may not be useful in controlling chronic symptoms in asthma. Corticosteroids, which have no direct action on mast cells, inhibit the late response to allergens and thus may prevent or reduce bronchial hyperresponsiveness. Other inflammatory cells such as macrophages, eosinophils, neutrophils, and lymphocytes are also present in the mucosa of patients with asthma, and any of these cells may liberate inflammatory mediators. The most characteristic asthmatic cell is the eosinophil. Lymphokines may be important mediators in increasing the inflammatory response, and interleukin-5 release by lymphocytes also may be important in acting to prime the eosinophils in the mucosa. (See also Chapters 32, 34, and 61.)

Bronchodilator Drugs

The pharmacology of β-adrenoceptor agonists is described in Chapter 16. Activation of β_2-adrenoceptors on the smooth muscle of the airways causes activation of adenylyl cyclase with a subsequent increase in the intracellular concentration of cyclic AMP. In turn, this leads to activation of protein kinase A, which lowers intracellular calcium concentration and thus results in relaxation of the bronchial smooth muscle. β_2-Adrenoceptor agonists relax the bronchial smooth muscle from the trachea down to the terminal bronchioles, irrespective of the stimulus that has caused the bronchial smooth muscle to produce bronchoconstriction.

Sympathomimetic agents

Stimulation of β_2-adrenoceptors relaxes airway smooth muscle but does not produce the cardiac stimulation that results from β_1-receptor activation. Therefore β_2-selective drugs are the most important group of adrenoceptor agonists for the treatment of asthma.

Although adrenoceptor agonists (see Chapter 16) may be administered by any route, delivery by inhalation results in the greatest local effect on bronchial smooth muscle with the least systemic toxicity. Aerosol deposition depends on the particle size, the pattern of breathing (tidal volume and rate of airflow), and the geometry of the airways. Even with particles in the optimal size range of 2–5 μm, 80–90% of the total dose of aerosol is deposited in the mouth or pharynx. Particles under 1–2 μm in size remain suspended in the air within the respiratory tract and may be exhaled. Deposition can be increased by holding the breath in inspiration.

Use of sympathomimetic agents by inhalation at first raised fears about possible tachyphylaxis or tolerance to β-agonists, cardiac arrhythmias due to β_1-adrenoceptor stimulation and hypoxemia, and arrhythmias caused by fluorinated hydrocarbons in Freon propellants. However, the concept that β-agonist drugs cause worsening of clinical asthma by inducing tachyphylaxis to their own action has not been supported by sound clinical evidence.

Epinephrine (adrenaline) stimulates β_2-receptors and produces bronchodilatation in asthma. It also stimulates β_1- and α-adrenoceptors and thus produces hypertension, tachycardia, and cardiac arrhythmias. It is used for treating the acute asthmatic attack and can be given subcutaneously in a dose of 0.5–1.0 mg. The drug has also been used by inhalation, but by this route it has been replaced by more selective β_2 agents.

Albuterol (salbutamol, Ventolin) is a selective β_2-agonist. It is used as an aerosol, by intravenous infusion, and as an oral tablet. The aerosol administration minimizes side effects by delivering the drug directly to its site of action (thus permitting a lower dose) and is the method of choice for the use of this drug in the control of bronchoconstriction in chronic asthma or chronic obstructive pulmonary disease. The usual single dose delivered by an appropriate inhaler device (two puffs) is 200 μg. The onset of action of the inhaled drug is almost immediate. When the drug is given by mouth as 5-mg tablets, the action begins within 30 minutes, rises to a peak between 2 and 4 hours, and gradually declines over a period of 6 hours. The drug causes an increase in heart rate and skeletal muscle tremor when given by mouth. Other selective β_2-sympathomimetic agents with similar properties are **terbutaline (Bricanyl)**, **orciprenaline (metaproterenol, Alupent)**, **fenoterol (Berotec)**, and **isoetharine (Bronkosol)**.

These drugs are not inactivated by catechol-*O*-methyltransferase and so have a long duration of action compared to epinephrine. Table 40-1 shows the receptor activities and the durations of action of

Table 40-1 Receptor Binding Specificities and Duration of Action of Sympathomimetics

Agent	α	β_1	β_2	Duration
Epinephrine	+ + +	+ + + +	+ + +	±
Ephedrine	+	+ + +	+ +	+
Isoproterenol		+ +	+ + +	+ +
Orciprenaline		+	+ + +	+ + +
Albuterol		+	+ + +	+ + + +
Terbutaline		+	+ + +	+ + + +

the sympathomimetic drugs. Figure 40-1 shows the structural relationship between albuterol and isoproterenol. Specific β_2 stimulants are currently the drugs of first choice, and large doses in combination with methylxanthines and corticosteroids are used in the treatment of status asthmaticus.

Anticholinergic Drugs

Atropine is a competitive blocker of acetylcholine at muscarinic cholinergic receptors and thus can cause a variety of effects due to loss of parasympathetic activity, including blurring of vision, increases in heart rate, and drying of secretions in the salivary glands and respiratory tract (see Chapter 15). This limits its usefulness as a bronchodilator. Atropine is best used by inhalation, which reduces, but does not eliminate entirely, these unwanted side effects.

Ipratropium bromide (Atrovent) is a quaternary isopropyl-substituted derivative of atropine that can not cross the blood–brain barrier and therefore has practically no central effect; it also shows some degree of bronchoselectivity. The actions of ipratropium bromide are otherwise similar to those of atropine, and its therapeutic use is confined to aerosol administration. The drug is administered by inhaler and each puff contains 20 μg. The exact place of ipratropium bromide in the treatment of asthma remains somewhat uncertain, and the drug appears to have little advantage over the selective β_2-agonists.

Methylxanthines

The three important methylxanthines are theophylline, theobromine, and caffeine. Their major source of intake by humans is beverages such as tea, cocoa, and coffee, respectively. Their effects on the various organ systems are as follows.

Central nervous system. In low to moderate doses, the methylxanthines, especially caffeine, cause mild cortical arousal with increased alertness and deferral of fatigue. In unusually sensitive individuals, the caffeine contained in beverages (e.g., 100 mg in a cup of coffee) is sufficient to cause nervousness and insomnia. Nervousness and tremor are primary side effects in patients taking large doses of aminophylline for asthma.

Cardiovascular system. The methylxanthines have direct positive chronotropic and inotropic effects on the heart. At low concentrations, these effects appear to result from increased calcium influx, probably mediated by increased cyclic AMP. At higher concentrations, sequestration of calcium by the sarcoplasmic reticulum is impaired, so intracellular calcium concentration is increased and myocardial contraction is strengthened (see Chapter 35). Methylxanthines have occasionally been used in the treatment of pulmonary edema associated with heart failure. These agents also relax vascular smooth muscle except in cerebral blood vessels, where they cause contraction.

Gastrointestinal tract. The methylxanthines stimulate secretion of both gastric acid and digestive enzymes.

Kidneys. The methylxanthines, especially theophylline, are weak diuretics. This effect may involve both increased glomerular filtration and reduced tubular sodium reabsorption. The diuresis is not of sufficient magnitude to be therapeutically useful.

Smooth muscle. The *bronchodilatation* produced by the methylxanthines is the major therapeutic action. Tolerance does not develop, but side effects, especially in the central nervous system, may limit the dose. In addition to this direct effect on the airway smooth muscle, these agents inhibit antigen-induced release of histamine from lung tissue; their effect on mucociliary transport is unknown.

Skeletal muscle. The therapeutic actions of the methylxanthines may not be confined to the airways, for they also strengthen the contractions of isolated skeletal muscle in vitro (see Chapter 19) and have potent effects in improving contractility and in reversing fatigue of the diaphragm in patients with

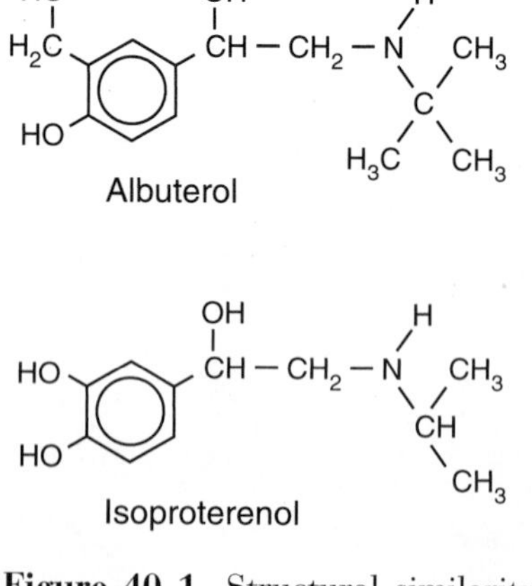

Figure 40-1. Structural similarity of albuterol (salbutamol) and isoproterenol.

chronic obstructive lung diseases. This *effect on diaphragmatic performance*, rather than an effect on the respiratory center, may account for theophylline's ability to improve the ventilatory response to hypoxia and to relieve dyspnea even in patients with irreversible airflow obstruction.

Theophylline (Pulmophylline and others)

This 1,3-dimethylxanthine (Fig. 40-2) is a plant alkaloid. It is poorly soluble and must be chemically complexed with other drugs to increase the solubility enough for clinical use (e.g., **aminophylline** = di-ethyl*amine* + the*ophylline*). It is the most selective of the methylxanthines in its effects on smooth muscle.

Mechanism of action. The major mechanism of action of theophylline as a bronchodilator is commonly believed to be its inhibition of phosphodiesterase and the consequent increase in cyclic AMP concentration in smooth muscle. However, inhibition of phosphodiesterase is not prominent at usual therapeutic doses of theophylline (10–20% inhibition occurs at blood concentrations regarded as therapeutic). It has been suggested that theophylline produces blockage of adenosine receptors, although this effect is probably not important for bronchodilatation. Alterations in smooth-muscle Ca^{2+} concentration may also be influenced by theophylline, and this may explain the relaxing effect on bronchial smooth muscles. Theophylline has also been shown to inhibit the effects of prostaglandins on smooth muscle and to inhibit the release of histamine and leukotrienes from mast cells (see Chapters 31–33). However, long-term administration does not reduce bronchial hyperresponsiveness or inhibit the release of mediators from eosinophils.

In normal subjects, intravenous administration of theophylline causes no bronchodilatation, whereas inhalation of a β_2-adrenoceptor agonist produces a definite response. In severe acute asthma, inhaled theophylline is ineffective, but intravenous theophylline has been shown to have one-third of the bronchodilator potency of inhaled isoproterenol. There is, however, no doubt about the beneficial effects of theophylline, and this improvement of airway resistance may be due to a mechanism other than bronchodilatation. For example, it has been shown that theophylline increases contractility of the diaphragm, particularly of the fatigued diaphragm (see above).

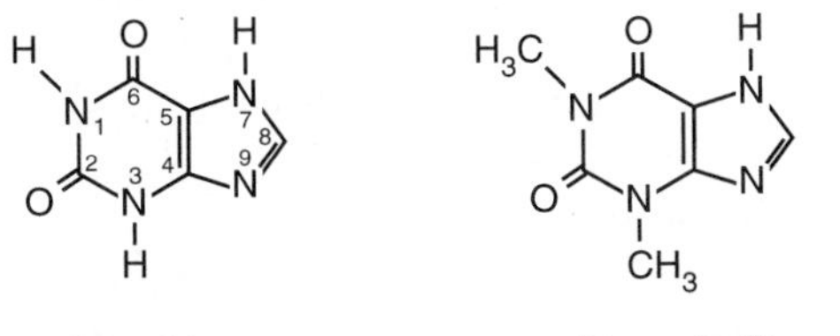

Pharmacokinetics. Theophylline is rapidly and completely absorbed when given by mouth and is distributed into all body compartments. There is marked interindividual variation in the hepatic transformation of theophylline. The clearance rate is influenced by so many different factors (Table 40-2) that it is essentially unpredictable in an individual. Therefore the dose necessary to maintain optimal serum concentrations (27–82 μmol/L, or 5–15 mg/L) varies widely and must be controlled by actual measurement of the concentrations. The clearance of theophylline in males is 20–30% higher than that in females. There may also be a circadian variation in theophylline clearance. The major routes of biotransformation are 3-demethylation by CYP1A2 and 8-hydroxylation by CYP3A3. Cigarette smoking increases theophylline elimination by inducing these hepatic enzymes (see Chapter 4), and there is decreased biotransformation of theophylline in hepatic cirrhosis, congestive heart failure, and chronic pulmonary disease.

Theophylline toxicity is largely related to dose and plasma concentration. Serious toxic effects are

Figure 40-2. Structural formulae of xanthine and theophylline.

Table 40-2 Factors Influencing Theophylline Clearance

Factor	*Theophylline Clearance Is* Decreased	Increased
Age	Prematurity >65 years	
Sex	Females	Males
Habits		Cigarette smoking
Drugs	Erythromycin	Phenobarbital
Diseases	Liver cirrhosis Congestive heart failure Chronic lung disease	

uncommon at concentrations below 110 μmol/L (20 mg/L), although a significant percentage of patients have unacceptable side effects even when the plasma concentration does not exceed the usual therapeutic range. The most serious toxicities are cardiac arrhythmias, seizures, and respiratory or cardiac arrest. Minor adverse effects occur frequently; the most common are headache, anorexia, nausea, vomiting, and anxiety.

Calcium-Channel Blockers

Calcium-channel blockers (see Chapter 38) are effective in relaxing bronchial smooth muscle and are particularly useful for the treatment of exercise-induced asthma.

Asthma Prophylaxis

Anti-inflammatory steroids

Glucocorticoid drugs such as **prednisone, prednisolone,** and **dexamethasone** (described in Chapter 51) are known empirically to relieve airway obstruction in bronchial asthma, but the mechanism of their action is complex and not fully understood. The possible actions include:

- Anti-inflammatory activity
- Reduction of tissue sensitivity to antigens
- Inhibition of contraction of bronchial smooth muscle
- Mucolytic action
- Increased responsiveness of β_2-adrenoceptors

In addition to their use for the relief of asthmatic attacks that are already in progress, glucocorticoids also find a prophylactic use for the prevention of attacks in patients who are subject to almost constant recurrence. However, the glucocorticoids can produce serious side effects such as Cushing's syndrome, peptic ulcer, osteoporosis, steroid myopathy, diabetes mellitus, sodium retention, hypertension, increased susceptibility to infection, and decreased responsiveness to stress (see Chapter 51). Therefore the chronic use of glucocorticoids must be avoided if at all possible. If it is necessary to use these drugs, minimum effective doses should be employed and therapy should be given on alternate days in order to minimize adrenal suppression. Short-term therapy is rarely harmful except in patients with concurrent disease exacerbated by glucocorticoids, e.g., diabetes mellitus.

Because many patients taking oral steroids for asthma suffer some degree of adrenal suppression, reduction or discontinuation of their oral dose must be done very slowly. For a period of up to a year after discontinuation of chronic oral steroid therapy, oral or parenteral steroids must again be administered during episodes of severe infection or trauma to prevent additional crises.

Cromolyn sodium (sodium cromoglycate, Intal and others)

Unlike the preceding drugs, this drug is used **exclusively** for the **prophylaxis,** rather than the treatment, of asthmatic attacks. It inhibits the release of mediators such as histamine and leukotrienes from the secretory granules of mast cells following the challenge of antigen interacting with specific IgE antibodies. The exact mechanism underlying the action of cromolyn sodium is not clear, but the drug is active only against type I (immediate) allergic reactions and not against delayed or immune reactions. Therefore it is used primarily for the prevention (rather than the symptomatic treatment) of allergic asthma, hay fever, and other acute allergic reactions.

However, cromolyn sodium is also effective in asthma induced by exercise and by exposure to cold dry air. Interaction of antibodies with mast cells is probably not involved in either of these types of asthma, but both are associated with rapid respiratory loss of heat, which may be a physical stimulus to mast cell degranulation. Therefore it is suggested that cromolyn sodium acts as a nonspecific stabilizer of the mast cell membrane and/or granules.

Cromolyn sodium is absorbed poorly from the gastrointestinal tract and therefore is effective only when deposited directly into the airways. Two methods of administration are currently used for asthma. In adults, the drug can be given by a "Spinhaler" apparatus that causes a capsule to be punctured so that its powdered contents are entrained into inspired air and deposited in the airways. The usual dose is 20 mg inhaled four times daily. In children, who may have difficulty in using this device, the drug may be given by aerosol. Other formulations, for topical use in the eye or nose, are intended for the prophylaxis of allergic rhinitis and conjunctivitis (hay fever).

About 10% of the inhaled dose is gradually absorbed from the lungs into the blood, from which it is cleared, unchanged, by urinary and biliary excretion, with a plasma half-life of about 1.5 hours. There are very few toxic effects of cromolyn sodium, because very little is absorbed systemically. Local side effects such as throat irritation and cough may follow inhalation of the dry powder. Rashes have been reported, as well as rare cases of anaphylactic reaction.

Use of Inhaled Bronchodilator Drugs

Selective β_2-adrenoceptor agonists such as albuterol (salbutamol), terbutaline, and fenoterol have a rapid onset of action and are effective for up to 6 hours following inhalation, if the asthma is not severe. Little difference exists between the various agents, as the duration of action and selectivity are similar. β_2-Adrenoceptor agonists such as formoterol and salmeterol (Serevent) may be effective for up to 12 hours and are therefore preferred by patients, particularly those with nocturnal symptoms.

Side effects are uncommon when the drugs are given by inhalation but are more frequent when they are taken orally. Tremor, tachycardia, and palpitations are the most common side effects; hypokalemia has been noted when higher doses are taken.

Anticholinergic agents block muscarinic receptors, thus inhibiting vagal cholinergic tone and resulting in bronchodilatation. Although several types of muscarinic receptors have been recognized in bronchial smooth muscle, the currently available anticholinergic inhalants do not discriminate between these receptors. The anticholinergic drugs inhibit only the component of bronchoconstriction that is due to cholinergic stimulation. In contrast to β_2-adrenoceptor agonists, they have no action against the direct effects of mediators on bronchial smooth muscle. Thus, anticholinergic agents are on the whole less effective than β_2-adrenoceptor agonists in the treatment of chronic asthma. They are therefore used most frequently in combination with other bronchodilators. Side effects are those caused by systemic anticholinergic activity, such as dry mouth, blurred vision, and urinary retention, but they do not occur with ipratropium bromide because it is poorly absorbed.

Recently, glucocorticoid drugs such as **beclomethasone dipropionate** and **beclomethasone valerate** have been developed for administration by inhalation. Inhalation of these compounds is as effective as oral prednisone in patients starting on steroids. Only a small amount of the steroid administered in this manner is systemically absorbed. Therefore there is little or no systemic effect or adrenal suppression and the problem of growth suppression in children may be avoided. The major problem with this form of therapy to date has been the development of fungal infections (candidiasis) in the oropharynx in about 10% of patients because of suppression of phagocytic activity by the high local concentrations of corticosteroid.

The **inhaled corticosteroids** are remarkably effective in suppressing the inflammatory process occurring with asthma. In single doses, they do not block the early response to allergens but do block the late response and the bronchial hyperresponsiveness. This effect is gradual in onset but occurs to a greater extent with inhaled steroids than with orally administered steroids. Inhaled corticosteroids produce a reduction in the number of mast cells in the airway. They also reduce the microvascular leakage caused by inflammatory mediators, although the exact molecular mechanism of their beneficial action is unclear.

Side effects are uncommon when low doses of inhaled steroids (less than 400 μg daily) are given but become more frequent at higher doses.

DRUGS AFFECTING THE COUGH REFLEX

The cough reflex is mediated by receptors located in the mucosa or deeper structures of the larynx, trachea, and major bronchi, and by mechanoreceptors that detect changes in bronchial intramural tension. Stimuli are transmitted via the vagus to the cough center in the medulla. Efferent impulses originating from the cough center are transmitted through cholinergic pathways to the abdominal and intercostal muscles and to the diaphragm, producing sudden explosive expiratory movements. The effect of coughing is to expel foreign particles that have entered the bronchial tree and to expectorate sputum from the bronchial lumen. This may be beneficial to the patient, protecting against damage by foreign bodies or bacteria and helping to clear the airways. However, repeated nonproductive coughing (i.e., coughing that fails to clear mucus from the lower respiratory tract) exhausts the patient and disturbs sleep. Long term coughing also may lead to the breakdown of elastic tissue in the lung or to damage to the tracheobronchial epithelium. It is therefore often helpful to give drugs to suppress the cough reflex.

Antitussive Drugs

Opioid antitussive agents

Opioid analgesics (see Chapter 23) are most effective in depressing the cough center. Although the precise mechanism by which they exert their effects is uncertain, they appear to react with a variety of receptors identified at numerous sites in the central and peripheral nervous systems. There is some specificity found among various opioids with respect to their antitussive potency. For example, the ED_{50} for analgesia compared to the ED_{50} for cough suppression yields a ratio of 6.62 for codeine, 4.60 for hydrocodone, and 2.87 for morphine. **Codeine** thus appears to be a more effective cough suppressant relative to its analgesic activity. The antitussive dose of codeine is relatively low, and 10 mg may produce a 62% elevation of threshold to ammonia-induced cough for 60 minutes. The usual antitussive dose is 15–20 mg as required. Codeine also has significantly less respiratory depressant effect than morphine. The development of tolerance and physical dependence is a major drawback to morphine-like drugs, and for this reason, their long-term use as antitussive agents is discouraged. They can, however, be used for short-term cough suppression. Because of the low dose of codeine required, and its relatively low addiction liability, it may be more suitable than other opioid drugs for long-term antitussive use.

Nonopioid antitussive agents

Dextromethorphan is a synthetic opioid derivative that is an effective antitussive agent, suppressing the response of the cough center but lacking analgesic or habituating properties. It is the *d*-isomer of levomethorphan, which is a potent opioid analgesic. This demonstrates that the analgesic activity, as well as the addictive properties, are exerted through receptors with stereospecificity, while the antitussive receptor sites lack the opioid stereospecificity (see Chapter 23). **Levopropoxyphene** is similarly an antitussive that lacks the analgesic activity of its isomer, dextropropoxyphene. Other nonopioid drugs that have some antitussive activity in addition to their other pharmacological actions include **phenothiazines, antihistamines,** and **benzononatate.**

SUGGESTED READING

Barnes PJ. A new approach to the treatment of asthma. N Engl J Med 1989; 321:1517–1527.

Drazen JM, Austen KF. Leukotrienes and airway responses. Am Rev Respir Dis 1987; 136:985–998.

McFadden ER, Gilbert IA. Asthma. N Engl J Med 1992; 327:1928–1937.

Piafsky KM, Ogilvie RI. Dosage of theophylline in bronchial asthma. N Engl J Med 1975; 292:1218–1222.

Robuschi M, Riva E, Fuccella LM, et al. Prevention of exercise-induced bronchoconstriction by a new leukotriene antagonist (SKF 104353). Am Rev Respir Dis 1992; 145:1285–1288.

Taburet AM, Schmit B. Pharmacokinetic optimization of asthma treatment. Clin Pharmacokinet 1994; 26:396–418.

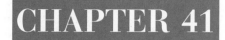

CHAPTER 41

Diuretics

C. WHITESIDE AND A. MARQUEZ-JULIO

CASE HISTORY

A 60-year-old businessman presented to his family physician with the complaint of increasing shortness of breath, weight gain of 10 kg, and swelling of the feet and legs for 4 months. He had suffered a myocardial infarction 2 years ago and anginal attacks had occurred over the past 2 months. Past history also included hypertension for 10 years, non–insulin-dependent diabetes (managed by diet) for 5 years, and hypercholesterolemia. Current medications included atenolol 100 mg/day and nitroglycerine 0.3 mg when needed for angina.

On physical examination, the moderately obese patient appeared short of breath on mild exertion and had symmetrical pitting edema (4+) to the midthighs. On auscultation both lung fields were filled with diffuse inspiratory crackles. The internal jugular vein was distended to 5–6 cm above the sternal angle (at 45° inclination). The blood pressure was 210/120 mmHg. On cardiac examination the point of maximal impulse was diffuse and displaced laterally beyond the midclavicular line. On auscultation a loud S_2 was heard along with third and fourth heart sounds. A chest X-ray revealed an increased cardiac–thoracic ratio, vascular redistribution to the upper lung fields, and diffuse interstitial infiltrate in keeping with left ventricular failure. Laboratory data included serum creatinine 300 μmol/L, urine protein 2.0 g/day (with inactive urine sediment), serum sodium 130 mmol/L, serum chloride 100 mmol/L, serum potassium 5.2 mmol/L. An abdominal ultrasound demonstrated a tortuous and mildly enlarged

aorta and bilateral small (9 cm) kidneys with thinned cortices.

The patient was admitted to hospital for evaluation and treatment. The diagnoses included congestive heart failure, severe hypertension, and chronic renal failure likely due to diabetic glomerulosclerosis and renal vascular atherosclerosis. He was treated initially for 4 days with intravenous furosemide 120 mg/day, which resulted in a weight loss of about 1–1.5 kg/day. After 4 days, furosemide treatment was changed to the same dose taken orally. A low-potassium and no-added-salt diabetic diet was instituted. The hypertension was treated with enalapril 15 mg/day and long-acting nifedipine 20 mg twice daily. Atenolol was discontinued. During this treatment the symptoms of congestive heart failure disappeared, blood pressure decreased to 160/90 mmHg, but serum creatinine increased to 390 μmol/L. Enalapril was reduced to 7.5 mg/day and furosemide to 80 mg/day. On discharge the serum electrolytes were normal and creatinine had decreased to 320 μmol/L.

Two months later, while on enalapril and furosemide maintenance therapy, he returned with a blood pressure of 190/95 mmHg and serum creatinine of 300 μmol/L. Metolazone 5 mg/day was added for improved blood pressure control. One month thereafter, his blood pressure was 150/90 mmHg, but he complained of severe weakness. His serum electrolytes revealed sodium 132 mmol/L, chloride 88 mmol/L, potassium 2.6 mmol/L, and bicarbonate 32 mmol/L. The dietary potassium restriction was withdrawn and he was placed on oral potassium supplements. Within 2 weeks serum potassium returned to normal and the weakness disappeared. He continued to work full time, played golf, and was free of angina for the next 3 years.

Diuretics are used to treat excessive water and sodium retention (edema states), hypertension, and electrolyte disorders, e.g., hypokalemia. These drugs are classified according to the renal tubular site of action. To understand the therapeutic and side effects of diuretics it is important to review renal tubular function and the maintenance of extracellular fluid and electrolyte homeostasis.

REVIEW OF RENAL PHYSIOLOGY

The kidney regulates sodium and water excretion to maintain extracellular fluid (ECF) volume within narrow limits despite an irregular and often excessive dietary intake of sodium. The filtered load of sodium first entering the nephron is equal to the product of the glomerular filtration rate (GFR) and the plasma concentration of sodium. Table 41-1 provides an estimate of sodium reabsorption in a 70-kg adult with a GFR of 180 L/day and normal antidiuretic hormone (ADH) activity. Sodium reabsorption occurs at four major sites along the nephron: the proximal tubule, the ascending limb of the loop of Henle, the distal convoluted tubule and cortical collecting duct, and the medullary collecting duct (Fig. 41-1). The first three nephron segments each reabsorb at least two-thirds of the sodium chloride that is delivered to them. The bulk of sodium reabsorption occurs in the proximal tubule and loop of Henle, whereas the final

amount of sodium excreted is dependent on the fine-regulation at the distal sites.

Sodium and water homeostasis are regulated by "sensor" and "effector" systems. The sensor limb includes intravascular stretch receptors in the low-pressure capacitance areas (intrathoracic great veins and atria) and high-pressure resistance arterial vessels, which are capable of detecting pressure as a measure of effective intravascular volume. The renal baroreceptors, including the juxtaglomerular apparatus (JGA), sense the renal perfusion pressure. Both extra- and intrarenal sensors stimulate the effector limb, which is composed of multiple neural and hormonal factors that modulate GFR and tubular transport of sodium and water. The glomerular afferent and efferent arteriolar resistance is autoregulated by vasoactive hormones and the sympathetic nervous system to maintain relatively constant renal plasma flow and GFR over a wide range of mean arterial pressure. Since the filtered load of sodium remains essentially unchanged, regulation of tubular reabsorption is the major determinant of final sodium excretion.

The renal microcirculation is composed of two capillary beds in series. The glomerular efferent arterioles feed the peritubular capillaries where the proximal tubular reabsorbate enters the circulation. In states of ECF volume contraction or decreased renal perfusion, both afferent and efferent glomerular arterioles constrict. The increase in efferent tone leads to a net change in peritubular capillary hydrostatic force, enhancing the movement of sodium and water across the epithelium of the proximal tubules into the peritubular capillaries.

The tubular epithelial cells are joined by tight

Table 41-1 Sodium and Water Reabsorption Along the Nephron

Nephron Segment	Sodium mmol/day)			H$_2$O (L/day)		
	Delivered	Reabsorbed	Exit	Delivered	Reabsorbed	Exit
Proximal tubule	27,000	18,000	9000	180	120	60
Loop of Henle	9000	8000	1000	60	40	20
Distal convoluted tubule and cortical collecting duct	1000	667	333	20	15	5
Medullary collecting duct	333	33–323	10–300	5	3–4.5	0.5–2

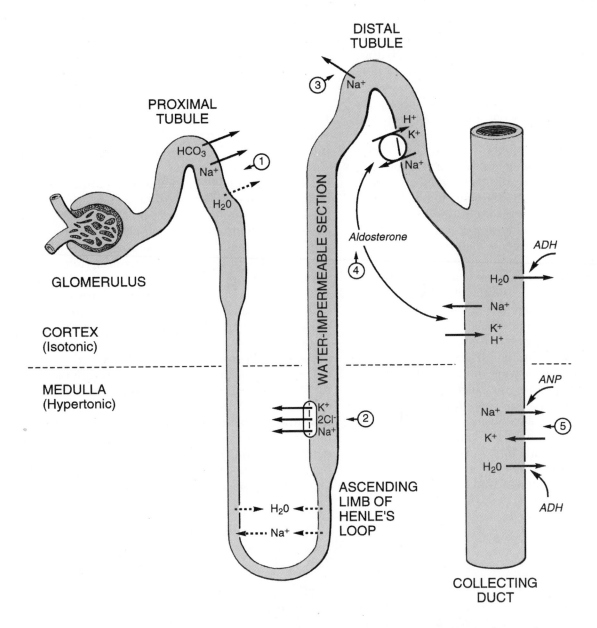

Figure 41-1. Sites of action of diuretic agents in the nephron: (1) carbonic anhydrase inhibitors, osmotic diuretics; (2) "loop" diuretics; (3) thiazide diuretics; (4) aldosterone antagonists; (5) other potassium-sparing diuretics; (⟶) specific membrane transport mechanisms; (----≫) passive transfer. ADH = antidiuretic hormone; ANP = atrial natriuretic peptide.

junctions which polarize the plasma membrane into luminal and antiluminal surfaces that differ in their transport protein composition. Along the length of the nephron $(Na^+ + K^+)$-ATPase is located on the antiluminal (basolateral) membrane, actively transporting sodium out of the cells into the extracellular space, from which it reenters the blood. There is

evidence that this ATPase activity is modulated by a prostaglandin-sensitive pathway. The resultant electrochemical gradient is the driving force for uptake of ions, including sodium, at the luminal surface by facilitated transport or through specific ion channels. At the proximal tubular luminal surface, sodium is cotransported with glucose and amino acids. The sodium-proton antiporter in the luminal membrane accounts for up to 25% of proximal tubular sodium entry (Fig. 41-2). Intracellular carbonic anhydrase enables the proximal tubular cells to generate protons and bicarbonate. Carbonic anhydrase is also located in the brush-border membrane and catalyzes the conversion of secreted protons and filtered bicarbonate to H_2O and CO_2 (Fig. 41-2).

The thick ascending limb of Henle's loop in the renal medulla is a major site of sodium reabsorption. Here, chloride, sodium, and potassium are transported out of the lumen by the same luminal carrier. The rate of reabsorption is accelerated by increased delivery of sodium chloride to the carrier sites (Fig. 41-1). Transport at this site is the principal force for the generation of the countercurrent concentrating mechanism. Since the ascending loop is water impermeable, the movement of sodium chloride out of the lumen without water creates hypertonicity of the medullary interstitial fluid. This establishes the osmotic driving force for the movement of water from the collecting duct (in the presence of ADH) to produce a concentrated urine. Inhibition of chloride and sodium transport in the thick ascending limb (e.g., by loop diuretics) prevents the nephron from producing a concentrated urine. The transport of sodium and chloride out of the lumen of the cortical segment of the ascending limb of Henle's loop results in the formation of hypotonic fluid or "solute-free water." Inhibition of sodium transport in this portion of the nephron (e.g., by thiazide diuretics) prevents the excretion of a dilute urine.

Reduced renal perfusion pressure sensed by the JGA causes renin release. The subsequent synthesis of angiotensin II results in increased renal arteriolar tone and the stimulation of aldosterone secretion from the adrenal glands. Aldosterone-sensitive sodium-channel activity occurs in the cortical collecting tubule and duct. Aldosterone also enhances potassium and proton secretion.

The final modulation of urinary sodium occurs in the medullary collecting duct, under the control of atrial natriuretic peptide action. This hormone enhances sodium excretion, in part through inactivation of electrogenic amiloride-sensitive sodium channels by a cGMP-dependent mechanism (Fig. 41-3).

In normal physiological states of sodium and water homeostasis small amounts of neurohumoral factors (e.g., angiotensin II, endothelin, prostaglandins, bradykinin, nitric oxide) regulate intrarenal blood flow and sodium reabsorption. However, in pathophysiological conditions these agents are produced in larger quantities in an attempt to maintain the systemic perfusion pressure (or effective intravascular volume). Under conditions of low perfusion pressure both vasoconstricting and vasodilating factors are synthesized at high levels to simultaneously maintain peripheral vascular resistance and GFR. For example, the use of nonsteroidal anti-inflammatory drugs (cyclooxygenase inhibitors) in the pres-

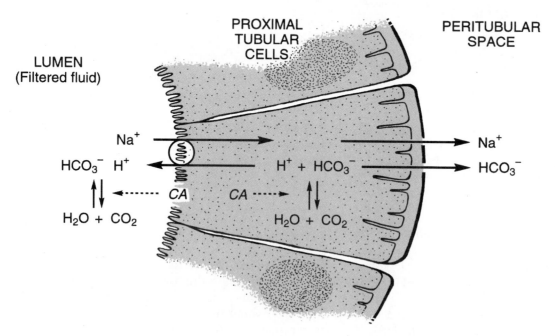

Figure 41-2. Proximal tubular reclamation of filtered HCO_3^-. Action of carbonic anhydrase (CA).

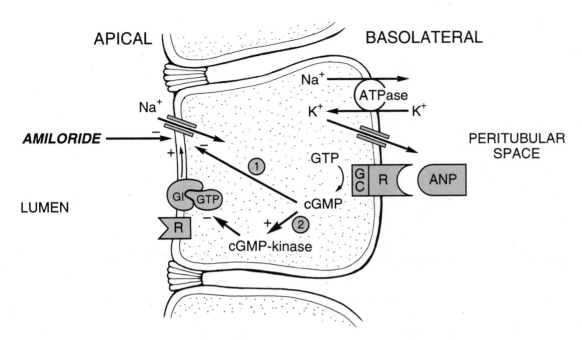

Figure 41-3. Modulation of Na$^+$ reabsorption in the medullary collecting duct by atrial natriuretic peptide (ANP). Amiloride blocks the Na$^+$ channel in the apical membrane, which is also inactivated by ANP through two cGMP mechanisms—one acting directly and another acting through a G protein linked to an unidentified receptor. (From Stanton BA. *Can J Physiol Pharmacol* 1991; 69:1546–1552.)

ence of low cardiac output, e.g., congestive heart failure, may lead to profound reduction in renal plasma flow and glomerular filtration rate. Sodium and water retention is enhanced because of reduced filtration and increased tubular reabsorption. The decreased delivery of sodium and chloride to the loop of Henle and distal tubule prevents optimal action of diuretics at these sites.

DIURETICS

Diuretic agents have been classified according to chemical structure and/or site of action (Fig. 41-1). A more clinically useful approach is to consider them also according to efficacy, as listed in Table 41-2.

Loop Diuretics

Mechanism and site of action

The loop diuretics (Fig. 41-4) directly inhibit the facilitated chloride, sodium, potassium cotransport at the luminal membrane of the medullary segment of the thick ascending limb of Henle's loop (Fig. 41-1).

Pharmacokinetics

Furosemide (Lasix, Furoside) is rapidly but incompletely absorbed from the gastrointestinal tract. In the circulation it is 98% protein-bound. Excretion is primarily via proximal renal tubular secretion, at the organic-acid secretory site. As with most diuretics, renal tubular secretion of furosemide is necessary for pharmacological effect of the drug at the luminal membrane.

Bumetanide (Bumex) is a sulfamoyl benzoic acid derivative like furosemide. It is almost completely absorbed from the gastrointestinal tract, reaching peak blood concentrations within 30 minutes after an oral dose. In plasma, it is 90% protein-bound. The drug is partially metabolized by the liver, but more than 50% is excreted unchanged in the urine within 6 hours of administration.

Ethacrynic acid (Edecrin) is well absorbed from the gastrointestinal tract, and in the circulation it is 97% protein-bound. It undergoes partial hepatic metabolism. The major portion is secreted via the

Table 41-2 Classification and Uses of Diuretic Agents

Class	Relative Natriuretic Efficacy	Chief Site(s) of Action	Major Indications	Major Complications
"Loop" diuretics	High (20–25%)*	Medullary ascending limb of Henle's loop	Pulmonary edema Resistant edema states	Vascular collapse, hypokalemia, hypochloremia, metabolic alkalosis
Thiazide diuretics	Moderate (5%)	Cortical ascending limb of Henle's loop Distal tubule	Edema states Hypertension	Hypokalemia, metabolic alkalosis, carbohydrate intolerance
Carbonic anhydrase inhibitors	Low (1–3%)	Proximal tubules	Urinary alkalinization Glaucoma	Hypokalemia, metabolic acidosis
Potassium-sparing diuretics	Low (1–3%)	Collecting tubules Collecting duct	Ascites (spironolactone) Potassium-sparing effects	Hyperkalemia
Osmotic diuretics	Dose-dependent	Proximal tubules Loop of Henle	Cerebral edema Acute renal failure	Acute volume overload Hypokalemia Hyponatremia

*Maximum % of filtered Na^+ load excreted (in parentheses).

proximal renal tubular organic-acid transport sites and can then be reabsorbed at more distal nephron sites via pH-dependent nonionic diffusion (see Chapter 7).

Torsemide (Demadex), known as **torasemide** outside of the United States, is very well absorbed from the gastrointestinal tract and reaches peak plasma concentrations within 30 minutes. It is largely metabolized by the liver, only 20% being excreted unchanged in the urine, so it is less likely than the other drugs in this group to accumulate on repeated administration in patients with impaired renal function. It also has a longer half-life than the other agents of this class, so once-daily administration is sufficient.

The onset and duration of effect of these four drugs are summarized in Table 41-3.

Pharmacological effects

Loop diuretics are highly efficacious natriuretic agents that have the capacity to inhibit reabsorption of up to 20–25% of the filtered sodium load. This efficacy is related to the relatively large magnitude of sodium chloride transport occurring in this nephron segment and to efficiency of the chloride transport blockade.

The kaliuresis observed with loop diuretics is proportional to the increased rate of urine flow caused by these agents.

Since loop diuretics impair sodium chloride reabsorption in a water-impermeable segment of the nephron, they prevent the formation of medullary hypertonicity. Maximal urinary concentration is, therefore, impaired. Furthermore, in the presence of the diuretic, sodium chloride remains within the tubular lumen and "free water" cannot be formed. Thus, these agents also impair free water clearance (i.e., the renal capacity to form dilute urine).

All loop diuretics produce major calciuresis, which accompanies the increase in sodium excretion. There is evidence to suggest that this effect is due to inhibition of calcium reabsorption in the thick ascending limb of the loop of Henle.

Adverse effects and toxicity

The most commonly encountered adverse effects of loop diuretics are intravascular volume depletion (which can lower blood pressure excessively) and

Table 41-3 "Loop" Diuretics (Also Known as "High-Ceiling" Diuretics)

Drug and Route of Administration	Onset of Effect (minutes)	Peak Effect	Duration of Action (hours)
Furosemide (Lasix, Furoside)			
p.o.	15	1–2 hours	4–6
i.v.	5	30 minutes	~2
Bumetanide (Bumex)			
p.o.	30	1–2 hours	4½–6
i.v.	10	45 minutes	~3
Ethacrynic acid (Edecrin)			
p.o.	20	2 hours	6–8
i.v.	15	45 minutes	~3
Torsemide (Torasemide; Demadex)			
p.o.	10–15	1–2 hours	12–16
i.v.	10–15	30 minutes	~6

hypokalemia (which may be associated with cardiac arrhythmias and muscle weakness). Chronic use usually leads to hypochloremic metabolic alkalosis. This is a result of large chloride loss in the urine coupled with distal sodium reabsorption in exchange for potassium and hydrogen ions (enhanced by aldosterone if intravascular volume depletion has occurred).

Hyperuricemia is frequently observed and is primarily a consequence of enhanced proximal tubular reabsorption of solute (including uric acid) when intravascular volume contraction occurs.

Carbohydrate intolerance is observed occasionally in patients with prediabetic states. Hyponatremia is infrequent: The mechanisms involved in its genesis are similar to those that cause hyponatremia with thiazide diuretics (see below).

Acute administration of loop diuretics, usually when large doses are infused rapidly by the intravenous route, has produced deafness. The exact mechanism of this adverse effect is unknown, but there may be impairment of sodium extrusion from the endolymph to the perilymph in the inner ear. Although deafness is usually transient when caused by furosemide, there are reports of permanent hearing loss following ethacrynic acid administration.

Intravenous administration of ethacrynic acid has been associated with an increased frequency of gastrointestinal hemorrhage. This has been attributed to impairment of platelet aggregation.

Rare adverse effects of the loop diuretics include agranulocytosis, thrombocytopenia, and allergic reactions including skin rash and interstitial nephritis.

Drug interactions

Three major groups of drug interactions are well recognized with loop diuretics. The most recently described, and likely the most common, is the blunting of the natriuretic effect of loop diuretics by most nonsteroidal anti-inflammatory agents. Inhibition of intrarenal prostaglandin synthesis by the latter is purported to be the mechanism of this interaction (as described in the review of renal function).

Less frequently, these diuretics potentiate the ototoxicity of aminoglycoside antibiotics and the nephrotoxicity of first-generation cephalosporins (cephaloridine, cephalothin).

Drug interactions with other organic acids have been described and are due to competition between drugs for the secretory transport system. For example, probenecid, a uricosuric agent, delays the renal tubular secretion of the loop diuretics, thereby retarding their diuretic effect. High doses of furosemide have been reported to delay the excretion of tubocurarine and prolong its action.

Thiazide Diuretics

Currently available benzothiazide diuretics (Fig. 41-5) were developed during attempts to synthesize

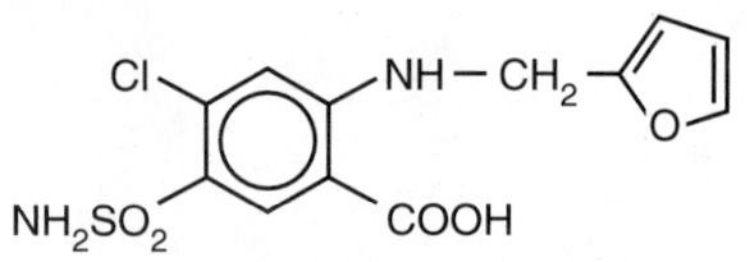

Furosemide
(Lasix, Furoside)

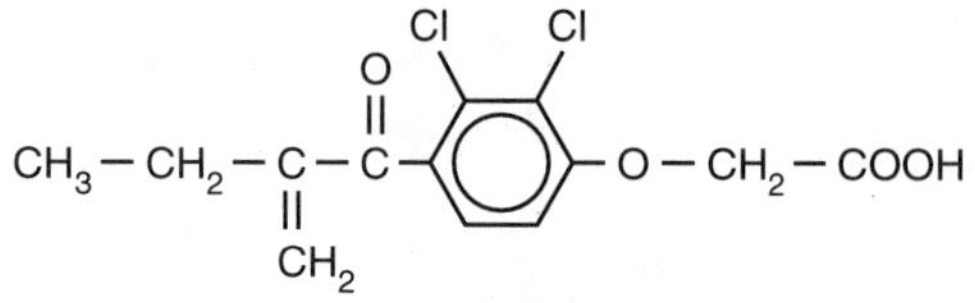

Ethacrynic acid
(Edecrin)

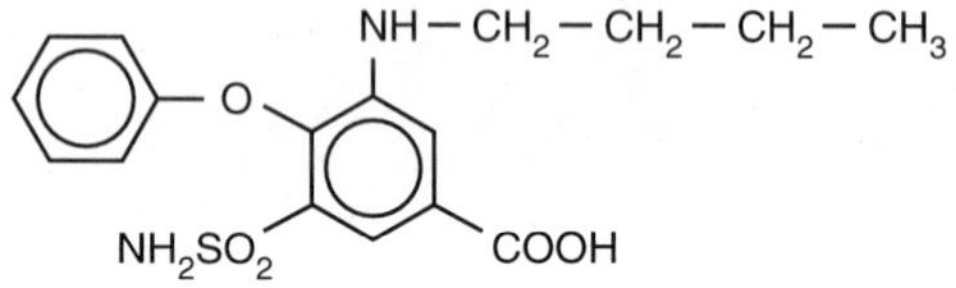

Bumetanide
(Bumex)

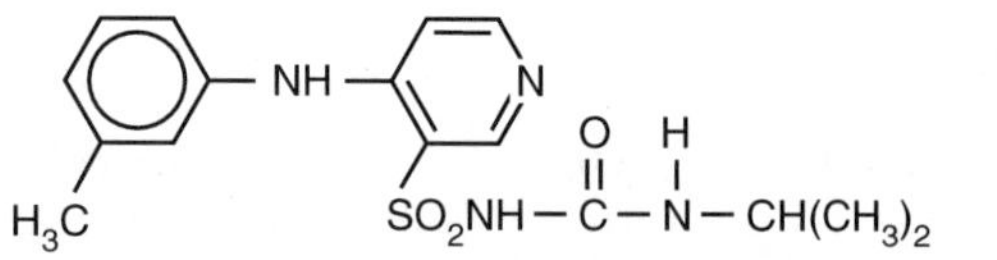

Torsemide (U.S.A.)
Torasemide (elsewhere)
(Demadex)

Figure 41-4. Structural formulae of loop diuretics.

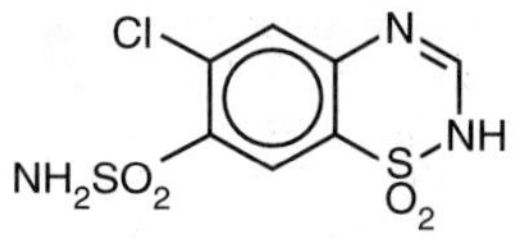

Chlorothiazide
(Diuril)

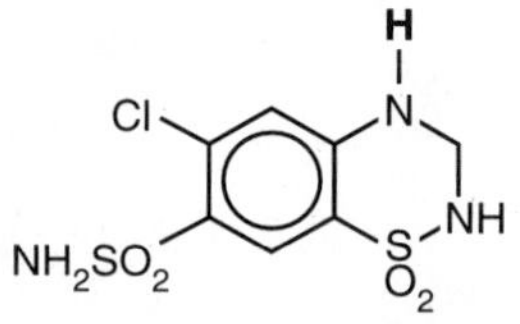

Hydrochlorothiazide
(HydroDiuril, Urozide,
Esidrix, etc.)

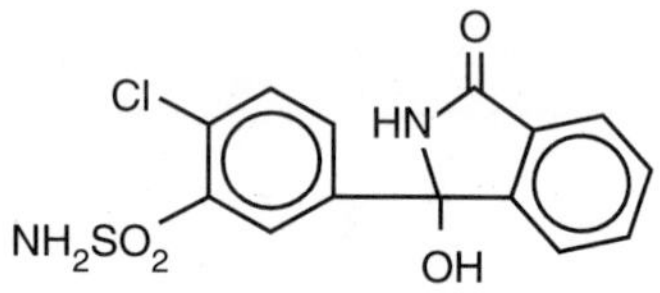

Chlorthalidone
(Hygroton, Uridon,
Novothalidone)

Figure 41-5. Structural formulae of thiazide diuretics and chlorthalidone.

limb of Henle's loop and the distal convoluted tubule (Fig. 41-1). The exact cellular mechanism of action is uncertain. Inhibition of glycolysis and diminution of energy supplies (ATP) required for transport have been implicated.

Pharmacokinetics

Thiazide diuretics are rapidly absorbed from the gastrointestinal tract. The more substituted drugs (i.e., with hydrophobic side-chain) are more highly bound to plasma proteins. As well, they are more lipid-soluble and have a greater apparent volume of distribution. Thiazides are weak acids and are secreted into the proximal renal tubular lumen by a transport system for organic acids. Protein binding decreases the rate of tubular secretion. Lipid solubility enhances reabsorption along the distal nephron. Most of these agents are excreted unchanged in the urine. The duration of action of the thiazide diuretics is noted in Table 41-4.

more effective carbonic anhydrase inhibitors (see also Fig. 11-4). The first member of this group to be studied extensively was chlorothiazide (Diuril); the basic pharmacological action of other analogs is similar to that of this agent. Somewhat different in structure, but with very similar pharmacological profiles, are agents such as chlorthalidone (Hygroton), quinethazone (Hydromox), and metolazone (Zaroxolyn). Currently available thiazide diuretics are listed in Table 41-4.

Mechanism and site of action

Thiazide diuretics inhibit reabsorption of sodium from the lumen in the cortical ascending (diluting)

Table 41-4 Thiazide and Sulfamoyl Benzamide Diuretics Available in North America

Nonproprietary Name	Trade Name	Approximate Relative Potency	Usual Oral Dose (mg/day)	Duration of Effect (hours)
Thiazides				
Hydrochlorothiazide*	HydroDiuril, Esidrix, and others	1	25–100	6–12
Bendroflumethiazide	Naturetin	10	2.5–15	6–12
Chlorothiazide	Diuril	0.1	500–2000	6–12
Methyclothiazide	Duretic	10	2.5–10	6–24
Polythiazide	Renese	10	2–15	24–48
Sulfamoyl benzamides				
Chlorthalidone*	Hygroton	0.8	25–200	48
Indapamide	Lozol, Lozide	1	2.5	14–24
Metolazone	Zaroxolyn	10	2.5–10	12–24
Quinethazone	Hydromox	1	50–100	18–24

*Agents most frequently used, least expensive.

Pharmacological effects

Thiazide diuretics are considered moderately efficacious natriuretic agents, capable of inhibiting reabsorption of up to 5% of the total filtered sodium load. The sites of action are proximal to the nephron segments responsible for potassium secretion. The increased sodium delivery to the collecting tubule results in increased sodium/potassium exchange and therefore in increased kaliuresis.

Since thiazide diuretics inhibit sodium chloride reabsorption in the water-impermeable cortical ascending limb of Henle's loop, they impair the ability of this nephron segment to generate solute-free water (i.e., they impair free-water clearance).

Acutely administered thiazide diuretics decrease urine calcium excretion. Micropuncture and microperfusion studies suggest that this phenomenon is due to direct enhancement of calcium absorption in the distal convoluted tubule. Chronic thiazide administration significantly reduces urine calcium not only because of this distal reabsorption effect, but also because of enhanced fluid and solute reabsorption in the proximal nephron secondary to extracellular volume depletion.

Adverse effects and toxicity

As with loop diuretics, thiazide diuretics frequently cause acute and chronic intravascular volume deple-

tion and dose-related hypokalemia, metabolic alkalosis, and hyperuricemia.

Hyperglycemia and glucose intolerance have been observed with chronic use of thiazide diuretics. Controversy exists as to whether this occurs only in patients with prediabetic states. Recent studies suggest that this adverse effect may be common but that it is slowly reversible in up to 60% of patients once the diuretic is discontinued. When sustained fasting hyperglycemia occurs in patients receiving thiazide diuretics, the benefits of continued diuretic use must be carefully weighed against long-term risks of diabetes mellitus. Many factors are postulated to contribute to glucose intolerance, including direct or hypokalemia-related inhibition of insulin release, as well as inhibition of insulin release and enhancement of glycogenolysis due to reflex sympathetic activity caused by intravascular volume depletion.

A recent randomized crossover trial in a hypertensive population has established that high doses of thiazide diuretics significantly increase plasma total cholesterol, VLDL cholesterol, and plasma triglycerides. The magnitude of the lipid profile change is dose-related and can be prevented by weight reduction and a low-cholesterol diet. The cause of these changes in lipid levels is unknown.

Hyponatremia may arise as a complication of thiazide diuretic therapy, even when edema is still present. A combination of factors contributes to this untoward effect. In edema states with reduced effective circulating volume, intrarenal factors such as decreased GFR and increased proximal tubular sodium and fluid reabsorption diminish the delivery of tubular fluid to the diluting segments of the nephron. Inhibition of sodium chloride transport in the water-impermeable portions of the nephron (i.e., diluting segments) impairs its capacity to generate free water (i.e., dilute urine). If the nephron is unable to generate free water, excess extracellular-fluid water cannot be excreted efficiently. Intravascular volume contraction increases ADH secretion, overriding the effect of hyposmolarity. In the presence of ADH, water reabsorption in the collecting duct continues. Water accumulates in the ECF compartment and sodium concentration decreases (hyponatremia).

In an elderly population receiving thiazide diuretics for nonedematous pathological states, profound hyponatremia has been reported. Although the same hormonal and intrarenal mechanisms are operative, it is unclear why this side effect may be more prevalent in older patients.

Sustained hypercalcemia is very occasionally seen with thiazide diuretic use. This is partly due to the increased calcium reabsorption by the kidney. Its presence should alert the physician to pathological states that cause increased serum calcium (hyperparathyroidism, neoplastic disease; see also Chapter 68).

Thiazide diuretics occasionally produce gastrointestinal intolerance (nausea and vomiting), pancreatitis, and allergic manifestations (e.g., skin rashes). Thrombocytopenia and agranulocytosis are rare toxic phenomena.

Drug interactions

The major drug interaction currently recognized is the inhibition of the natriuretic and antihypertensive effects of the thiazide diuretics when nonsteroidal anti-inflammatory agents are used concomitantly. Inhibition of intrarenal prostaglandin synthesis is felt to be part of the mechanism involved in this untoward effect.

Carbonic Anhydrase Inhibitors: Acetazolamide

Mechanism and site of action

Acetazolamide (Fig. 41-6) inhibits proximal renal tubular and luminal brush-border carbonic anhydrase. Normally carbonic anhydrase catalyzes the reaction:

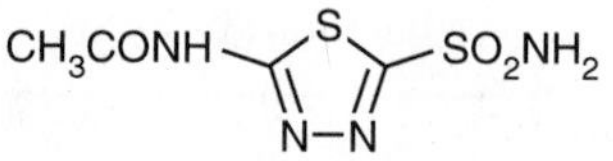

Figure 41-6. Structural formula of acetazolamide (Diamox, Acetazolam).

$$H^+ + HCO_3^- \rightleftharpoons H_2CO_3 \rightleftharpoons CO_2 + H_2O$$

as shown in Figure 41-2.

Inhibition of carbonic anhydrase results in delayed conversion of intraluminal carbonic acid (H_2CO_3) to CO_2 and H_2O. The rise in luminal H^+ concentration provides a gradient against H^+ secretion from the tubular cell. The intracellular hydration of CO_2 to H_2CO_3 and subsequent production of H^+ and HCO_3^- is retarded. Therefore, intracellular H^+ available for secretion into the tubular lumen is also decreased. Proximal tubular reclamation of filtered bicarbonate (HCO_3^-) occurs indirectly by combination of secreted H^+ with filtered HCO_3^- to ultimately form CO_2 and H_2O, which are immediately reabsorbed. Carbonic anhydrase inhibition causes HCO_3^- to remain in the tubular fluid. Furthermore, since sodium is the cation that accompanies the entry of HCO_3^- into the peritubular circulation, carbonic anhydrase inhibition results in some natriuresis. This natriuresis is mild, partly because proximal sodium reabsorption is proportionately larger with other solutes, and because of sodium uptake at more distal sites.

Pharmacokinetics

Carbonic anhydrase inhibitors, like thiazide diuretics, are well absorbed from the gastrointestinal tract and excreted via proximal renal tubular secretion within 24 hours.

Pharmacological effects

Acetazolamide is only a very mild natriuretic agent because of its proximal site of action, which does not alter sodium or water reabsorption in the more distal nephron.

Acutely, this drug increases urinary bicarbonate excretion. Once sufficient bicarbonate losses accrue, a systemic metabolic acidosis occurs. Distal tubular secretion of H^+ is then sufficient to combine with luminal HCO_3^- to ultimately form H_2O and CO_2 and thus permit little HCO_3^- to appear in the urine. When carbonic anhydrase inhibitors acutely inhibit proximal sodium reabsorption, the sodium presented to distal sites (including collecting duct) enhances kaliuresis.

In the eye, carbonic anhydrase is responsible for the transport of sodium and bicarbonate ions, together with the osmotically equivalent amount of water, into the anterior chamber. Inhibition of carbonic anhydrase therefore decreases the formation of aqueous humor and can be used to treat some forms of glaucoma.

Adverse effects

The most frequent adverse effects seen with carbonic anhydrase inhibitors are hypokalemia and systemic metabolic acidosis.

Allergic and toxic effects are similar to those of other thiazide diuretics. Acute renal failure caused by nephrolithiasis (acetazolamide may crystallize in acidic urine) has been described during chronic acetazolamide use in the treatment of glaucoma. A more recent congener, methazolamide (Neptazane), has not caused this side effect.

Drug interactions

No recognizable adverse drug interactions have been described for these agents. When carbonic anhydrase inhibitors are combined with thiazide and loop diuretics, the natriuretic and kaliuretic effects of the drugs can be augmented.

Potassium-Sparing Diuretics

Aldosterone antagonists: spironolactone

Mechanism and site of action. Normally, aldosterone acts on nephron segments beyond the distal convoluted tubule, stimulating sodium reabsorption in exchange for potassium and hydrogen ions. Spironolactone (Aldactone, Fig. 41-7) and its major metabolite, canrenone, inhibit the effect of aldosterone on the kidney. Both bind competitively to cytosolic receptor sites for aldosterone prior to translocation into the nucleus.

Pharmacokinetics. Spironolactone is well absorbed from the gastrointestinal tract and rapidly undergoes hepatic biotransformation to canrenone, the major metabolite. Canrenone is highly protein-bound and has an elimination half-life of approximately 18 hours, so it contributes to the total duration of action of spironolactone. Excretion occurs via the kidneys and the gastrointestinal tract.

Pharmacological effects. Aldosterone-stimulated sodium reabsorption in exchange for potassium and hydrogen ion, in the distal collecting tubules and ducts, accounts for only 2–3% of total sodium reabsorption. Spironolactone therefore causes only a mild natriuresis.

Adverse effects. The most potentially dangerous adverse effect of spironolactone is hyperkalemia. This occurs frequently because of inadvertent administration of spironolactone together with potassium supplementation, or because of administration to patients with moderate-to-severe renal insufficiency.

Other frequent side effects of spironolactone include an unpleasant peppermint aftertaste and nausea/vomiting. Its steroid molecular structure has been implicated in painful gynecomastia, frequently noted in men. Other side effects related to the steroid structure include loss of libido, impotence, and menstrual irregularities.

Other potassium-sparing diuretics: triamterene and amiloride

Mechanism and site of action. Triamterene (Dyrenium; Fig. 41-8) and amiloride (Midamor) inhibit sodium transport in nephron segments beyond the distal convoluted tubule. They do not interact with aldosterone receptors. The specific mechanism of action of triamterene is still unknown. Amiloride directly inhibits the luminal sodium channel. Since

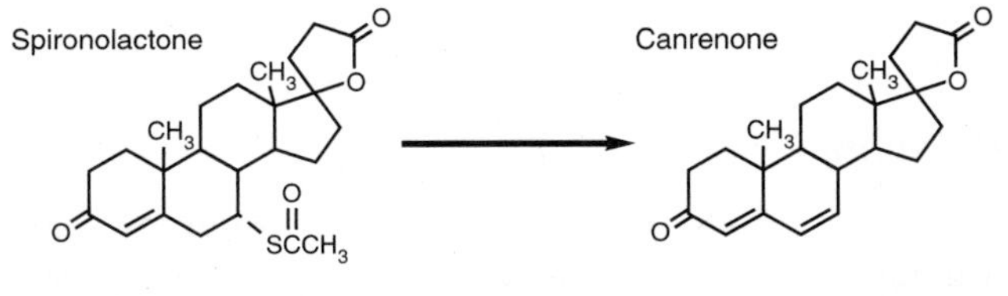

Figure 41-7. Structural formulae of spironolactone (Aldactone) and its active metabolite, canrenone.

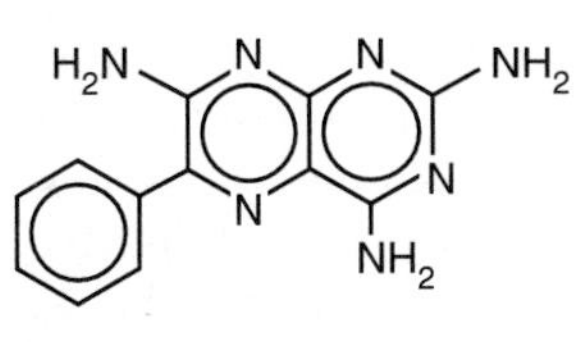

Figure 41-8. Structural formula of triamterene (Dyrenium).

sodium uptake enhances potassium secretion in the collecting duct, inhibition of sodium uptake reduces potassium loss.

Pharmacokinetics. Triamterene undergoes fast and essentially complete gastrointestinal absorption, whereas only 50% of amiloride is absorbed. Onset of diuretic effect is similar for the two drugs, occurring some 2 hours after ingestion. Duration of effect for triamterene is 7–9 hours and up to 24 hours for amiloride.

Pharmacological effects. Since sodium uptake by the collecting tubules and ducts accounts for only 2–3% of total sodium reabsorption, only a mild natriuresis will occur with these potassium-sparing diuretics. The natriuresis is coupled with decreased potassium excretion.

Adverse effects. The major adverse effect is hyperkalemia, which frequently occurs because of inadvertent concurrent potassium supplementation, coadministration of ACE inhibitors, or because of moderate to severe renal insufficiency. Another frequent adverse effect is gastrointestinal intolerance.

Drug interactions. Although not extensively studied, nonsteroidal anti-inflammatory agents oppose the natriuretic effect of triamterene. Furthermore, use of indomethacin together with triamterene has been reported to cause reversible renal insufficiency.

Osmotic Diuretics

Mannitol and **urea** have been utilized as osmotic diuretics. For this purpose these agents are administered intravenously; they are rapidly and freely filtered by the glomerulus. The hyperosmolality caused by the high intratubular concentration of these solutes prevents sodium reabsorption by effectively diluting the intraluminal sodium concentration and by markedly increasing the tubular fluid flow rate. The overall effect is increased sodium and water excretion.

The adverse effects encountered with osmotic diuretics include hypokalemia and acute intravascular volume overload. The latter effect occurs because the osmotic agent increases the transfer of fluid to the intravascular compartment from interstitial sites. The principal indications for the use of mannitol are to reduce brain edema (e.g., head trauma) and to acutely expand the intravascular volume (e.g., during cardiovascular surgery).

THERAPEUTIC APPLICATIONS

Edema

Diuretic agents are utilized primarily to enhance renal sodium excretion in abnormal clinical situations when the kidneys avidly reabsorb sodium and water despite the presence of an expanded ECF compartment (edema states).

Edema is the clinical manifestation of excess interstitial fluid. This is formed as an ultrafiltrate of plasma across capillary walls and has essentially the same sodium concentration as plasma. Increased accumulation of interstitial fluid occurs in disorders causing elevated hydrostatic pressure (e.g., congestive heart failure), reduced capillary oncotic pressure (hypoalbuminemia), or increased capillary permeability. Each of these conditions is associated with reduced mean arterial pressure due to either cardiac failure or reduced intravascular volume. This state of reduced "effective" circulating volume triggers the control systems regulating sodium balance; avid renal sodium reabsorption is the overall result of the attempt to restore a normal circulating volume.

Another mechanism of edema formation is primary sodium retention due to kidney disease (e.g., acute glomerulonephritis). Inability of the kidney to respond appropriately to the increased effective circulating volume results in positive sodium and water balance. Also, reduction in GFR and increased activity of the renin-angiotensin system may play a role in certain renal disease states. Expansion of both intravascular and interstitial compartments of the ECF rapidly becomes manifest as hypertension and edema.

The rational approach to the treatment of increased total body sodium and edema states includes dietary sodium and water restriction and the judicious use of diuretics. The underlying disorder and the physical state of the patient on examination will determine the management and, when required, the appropriate choice of diuretic.

Pulmonary edema

This is a life-threatening emergency that requires, among other therapeutic measures, a potent, rapidly acting diuretic agent. The diuretics of choice are the loop diuretics, and by convention furosemide is used most frequently. Its immediate vasodilatory action on venous capacitance vessels rapidly decreases cardiac preload while slightly decreasing total peripheral resistance and increasing renal blood flow. This transient effect, coupled with the prompt, large diuresis, has made furosemide a mainstay of therapy.

Congestive cardiac failure

Cardiac failure, from whatever cause, implies impairment of cardiac output. As a consequence of the reduced "effective" renal blood flow, retention of sodium and water occurs through both reflex and hormonal effector pathways. Gradually, as sodium and water accumulate, extracellular volume expands, ultimately leading to edema formation.

Therapy includes measures to enhance cardiac output (cardiotonic agents such as digoxin, arteriovenous dilators to decrease preload and afterload) and to minimize sodium and water retention (dietary sodium and fluid restriction, plus diuretics).

Diuretics in this setting have to be used with care and close monitoring of the patient's clinical condition (orthostatic blood pressure changes, jugular venous pressure). The danger is that excessive use will cause contraction of intravascular volume with subsequent reflex vasoconstriction (mediated by catecholamines and angiotensin II). The attendant increase in preload and afterload will be detrimental to cardiac output. Furthermore, rapid contraction of intravascular volume may lead to symptoms of cerebral, coronary, and renal insufficiency, particularly in the elderly.

Diuretic "resistance" may be encountered with both loop and thiazide diuretics. A common reason is unsuspected excessive dietary intake of sodium and water. However, the other major cause of reduced natriuretic effectiveness relates to intravascular volume contraction. Once initial diuresis has occurred, time must be permitted for interstitial fluid to shift into the intravascular compartment before further diuretic intake is prescribed. For most diuretics this implies use on alternate days.

When diuretics are used in patients with cardiac disease, hypokalemia should be prevented, particularly if the patients are also receiving digoxin. They usually require 60–80 mmol of potassium supplementation/day, through dietary manipulation and/or KCl replacement. Alternatively, potassium-sparing diuretics can be used concomitantly to maintain serum potassium above 3.5 mmol/L. Digitalis toxicity and inherent cardiac arrhythmias are more likely in the presence of hypokalemia.

Cirrhosis with ascites

Hepatic cirrhosis frequently gives rise to portal hypertension, which impairs the venous return from the splanchnic bed. Hypoproteinemia may be present because of lymphatic exudation in the peritoneal cavity and diminished hepatic production of albumin. The net balance of hydrostatic and osmotic forces then favors interstitial fluid formation in the peritoneal cavity, i.e., the formation of ascites. The exact onset and mechanism of sodium and water retention by the kidney in cirrhosis are still controversial. ECF volume redistribution into the peritoneal cavity may reduce "effective" renal plasma flow, leading to sodium and water retention. Furthermore, hepatic insufficiency decreases aldosterone degradation, and secondary hyperaldosteronism is enhanced.

The control of ascites by means of diuretics makes life more tolerable for the patient. The diuretic of choice, in the absence of renal insufficiency, is spironolactone. Doses of up to 400 mg/day may be required. Thiazide diuretics may be added if spironolactone is insufficient to control the ascites. The loop diuretics should be reserved for resistant sodium retention.

Use of diuretics in cirrhotics can be associated with complications. Fluid shift from the peritoneal compartment is limited to about 700–900 mL/day. Danger of intravascular volume depletion exists if diuresis is too brisk. The resultant intravascular volume contraction will lead to renal hypoperfusion. If this is persistent, renal failure (hepatorenal syndrome) may occur.

Renal diseases

In those renal diseases associated with the nephrotic syndrome, peripheral edema may be severe and require diuretic use. Dietary sodium restriction, and in severe cases loop diuretics, are required. As in all other edematous states, excessively brisk diuresis may only lead to acute intravascular volume contraction and, possibly, to renal hypoperfusion.

Acute glomerulonephritis, with or without the nephrotic syndrome, is associated with avid renal sodium and water retention. Diuretic resistance is frequently encountered, and loop diuretics may be required to control the acute intravascular volume expansion (manifested as hypertension, plus pulmonary edema if severe) and the peripheral edema.

In progressive chronic renal failure the remaining functional nephrons reabsorb less sodium and water and thus maintain ECF balance. Nevertheless, if the primary renal injury is associated with nephrotic syndrome and/or abnormal renal sodium and water retention, the patients may have an excess of extracellular fluid volume requiring the use of diuretics. Thiazides are effective as long as GFR is about 20–30 mL/min. Below this level, only the more potent loop diuretics are effective.

Other Uses

Hypertension

Diuretic therapy is still one of the cornerstones of current antihypertensive therapy, and it is effective monotherapy in 60% of essential hypertensive patients (see also Chapter 38). In the absence of severe renal insufficiency (i.e., if GFR >30 mL/min), thiazide diuretics are the preferred drugs: They are more effective than potassium-sparing diuretics or loop diuretics.

The antihypertensive action of diuretics is multifactorial. If the drugs are given in diuretic quantities (e.g., hydrochlorothiazide or chlorthalidone 50–100 mg), the fall in blood pressure parallels the initial decrease in intravascular fluid volume. With continued use, despite the return of the intravascular volume to normal, blood pressure remains decreased. This sustained decrease has been ascribed to autoregulatory vasodilatation.

Recent studies have demonstrated that the antihypertensive effect of thiazide diuretics occurs with much smaller doses (e.g., hydrochlorothiazide or chlorthalidone 12.5–25 mg), normally not associated with sufficient diuresis to decrease intravascular volume. The antihypertensive action in this circumstance may occur through vasodilatation resulting from direct molecular or sodium effects on the vasculature.

In otherwise-healthy hypertensive populations, thiazide diuretic-induced hypokalemia and serum lipid abnormalities may be detrimental. Serious ventricular arrhythmias have been recorded in prospectively studied hypertensive subjects who become hypokalemic. Both the serum lipid abnormalities and the hypokalemia are dose-dependent. Therefore, smaller doses of thiazide diuretics should be used, and the agents chosen should have demonstrated peak antihypertensive effects at doses well below those needed for diuretic effects (e.g., chlorthalidone: maximum antihypertensive dose 25 mg, diuretic dose 50–200 mg).

Calcium nephrolithiasis

In patients with idiopathic recurrent calcium nephrolithiasis, whether or not associated with abnormally elevated urine calcium (hypercalciuria), thiazide diuretics were demonstrated to be effective in preventing or significantly decreasing the frequency of stone formation. As reviewed earlier, this is due to both direct and reflex enhancement of urinary calcium reabsorption.

When thiazides are used for this purpose, moderate dietary sodium restriction is advised to maximize the hypocalciuric effect. States of hypercalcemia should be ruled out prior to onset of therapy, and serum calcium should be monitored.

Hyperparathyroidism

High serum calcium levels may be seen with hyperparathyroidism, either primary or secondary to malignancy (as well as with bone metastases). If serum calcium rises above 3.00 mmol/L, profound neurological disturbances and dehydration supervene, requiring emergency therapy. Together with adequate intravenous fluid replacement, loop diuretics are the treatment of choice because of their calciuric effects. Care must be taken to maintain electrolyte balance.

Diabetes insipidus

Diabetes insipidus is a rare metabolic condition in which there is partial or complete lack of ADH secretion (see also Chapter 47). Renal collecting-duct insensitivity to ADH is an equally rare condition called nephrogenic diabetes insipidus. In both states the kidneys are unable to reabsorb water from the collecting tubules and ducts. Consequently, large volumes (usually >10 L/day) of dilute urine are excreted, which require replenishment through both oral and intravenous routes.

Thiazide diuretics have been used effectively to decrease urine volume in these conditions, where natriuresis occurs along with the water diuresis. Subsequent intravascular volume contraction then enhances isotonic proximal and distal tubular sodium chloride reabsorption (i.e., accompanied by water). Less fluid reaches the collecting tubules and ducts, and urine volume decreases.

Special uses of carbonic anhydrase inhibitors

Carbonic anhydrase inhibitors are rarely used as diuretic agents because of their low efficacy.

They are used as urinary alkalinizing agents when it is desirable to maintain acidic substances in solution (e.g., uric acid, cysteine, hemoglobin, myoglobin).

These diuretics have also been used to treat diuretic-induced metabolic alkalosis, and to enhance urinary excretion in patients with chronic obstructive disease of the airways and CO_2 retention (chronic respiratory acidosis).

SUGGESTED READING

Brater DC. Clinical pharmacology of loop diuretics. Drugs 1991; 41 (Suppl 3):14–22.

De Bold AJ, Ledsome JR, Levy M, Sonnenberg H, eds. Symposium: a decade of ANF research. Can J Physiol Pharmacol 1991; 69:1478–1635.

Ellison DH. The physiologic basis of diuretic synergism: its role in treating diuretic resistance. Ann Intern Med 1991; 114(10):886–894.

Ellison DH, Biemesderfer D, Morrisey J, et al. Immunocytochemical characterization of the high-affinity thiazide diuretic receptor in rabbit renal cortex. Am J Physiol 1993; 264:F141–F148.

Martinez-Maldonado M, Cordova HR. Cellular and molecular aspects of the renal effects of diuretic agents. Kidney Int 1990; 38(4):632–641.

Murphy MB, Kohner E, Lewis PJ, et al. Glucose intolerance in hypertensive patients treated with diuretics: a fourteen-year follow-up. Lancet 1982; 2:1293–1295.

Rose BD. Diuretics—clinical conference. Kidney Int 1991; 39(2):336–352.

Suki WN, Eknoyan E. Physiology of diuretic action. In: Seldin D, Giebisch G, eds. The kidney: physiology and pathophysiology. 2nd ed. New York: Raven Press, 1992:3629–3670.

Velazquez H, Wright FS. Effects of diuretic drugs on Na, Cl, and K transport by rat renal distal tubule. Am J Physiol 1986; 250:F1013–F1023.

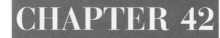

CHAPTER 42

Drugs Affecting Hemostasis

W.H.E. ROSCHLAU

CASE HISTORY

A 58-year-old white man with a number of ongoing medical problems was seen in the Emergency Room because of painful swelling of his left calf for the preceding 24 hours. Two days before this, he had made a transcontinental flight, returning to his home from a visit to his son on the West Coast. He noted and complained of progressive swelling of the left calf muscle associated with soreness. He had no shortness of breath, cough, or chest pain.

His medical problems included obesity, non–insulin-dependent diabetes mellitus for which he took oral hypoglycemic agents, and occasional angina pectoris for which he had taken a β-adrenergic blocker (metoprolol) and enteric-coated ASA.

Physical examination showed pain, redness, and swelling of the left calf, and a venogram revealed clots in the veins of the left calf and thigh. No abnormalities were detected in the arterial system, and the remaining physical examination revealed no abnormality.

Initial laboratory investigation showed a normal hemoglobin, normal prothrombin time, and a platelet count of 255,000/mm³.

As the patient gave no history of peptic ulceration, he was started on anticoagulant therapy: heparin in a bolus of 10,000 units followed by a maintenance infusion of 1400 units/hr.

Forty-eight hours after the above regimen began, his clinical symptoms had improved and the treatment was changed to oral warfarin. After 7 days of oral warfarin the INR (international normalized ratio) was between 2.5 and 3.0, which indicated that anticoagulation had achieved a satisfactory therapeutic level. His follow-up treatment included oral warfarin therapy for another 3 months.

One year later the man developed retrosternal chest pain while at an out-of-town business meeting. The pain resolved spontaneously but recurred when he was walking to his hotel. Conscious of his illness a year ago, he went to the Emergency Room, where an electrocardiogram proved to be consistent with myocardial ischemia. His chest pain again resolved spontaneously, but because of the earlier history of angina he was labeled as suffering from unstable angina in need of investigation. He was admitted to hospital and ASA was administered orally in a dose of 325 mg four times daily prior to his investigation by coronary arteriography.

Two days later, while still in hospital, the patient suffered renewed severe retrosternal chest pain. The electrocardiogram showed changes consistent with an acute anterior wall myocardial infarction. Nitroglycerin was administered sublingually with negligible relief of symptoms. He was transferred to the Coronary Care Unit and streptokinase was administered intravenously, as the onset of the latest chest pain was less than 3 hours earlier. The patient made a full recovery, but he remembers having had episodes of chills and malaise during streptokinase infusion.

The process of arresting the loss of blood from injured blood vessels (hemostasis) is of fundamental significance in health and disease. It involves vascular, platelet, and coagulation events, of which the response of blood platelets and the formation of fibrin are the most important (Fig. 42-1). Usually the first or *primary* manifestation of hemostasis is the temporary closure of a vascular lesion by a "hemostatic plug" of aggregated platelets. *Secondary* or permanent hemostasis (referred to as blood coagulation and comprising the plasma phase of hemostasis) consists of the sequential interaction and activation of normally inactive plasma clotting factors that lead to the generation of prothrombin activator (also known as thromboplastic activity), the transformation of prothrombin into thrombin, and the formation of fibrin from fibrinogen. Permanent repair of a vascular lesion is achieved by endothelialization, organization of the platelet–fibrin seal, phagocytosis, and fibrinolysis.

Disturbances of the hemostatic process may result in increased bleeding or increased clotting of blood.

Increased bleeding may be caused by clotting factor deficiencies or blood platelet abnormalities. Examples of inherited disorders are hemophilia A (classical hemophilia, factor VIII deficiency), hemophilia B (Christmas disease, factor IX deficiency), and von Willebrand's disease (factor VIII deficiency coupled with vascular and platelet defects). Acquired disorders of coagulation may be due to lack of vitamin K, or they may be associated with liver disease.

Increased clotting generally gives rise to **thrombosis**, which is the term applied to the excessive deposition of blood platelets and fibrin in the vascular system. In arteries, the process occurs most frequently on the basis of atherosclerosis. In veins, it is usually a consequence of diminished circulation, stasis, or inflammation. Blood vessel grafts, heart-valve replacements, and extracorporeal circulation are frequently complicated by thrombus formation. This is a misplaced response of the hemostatic process to hemodynamic alterations, foreign surfaces, or lesions of the vessel walls. Depending on the underlying cause and location, thrombi may be platelet-rich or platelet-poor, solitary or multiple, microscopically small or filling whole vessel segments. The term **clotting** is normally applied to blood coagulation in the test tube or during extravasation, but it is also used colloquially in reference to intravascular thrombus formation when there is a relative absence of platelets and an abundance of fibrin in the coagulum. **Embolism** occurs when blood clots or thrombi become dislodged from their site of origin and are carried to remote parts of the circulatory system. Arterial emboli will travel toward the periphery, causing vascular occlusions and ischemia of the perfused organ or tissue. Venous emboli invariably reach the lungs via the pulmonary arterial circulation, with the predictable consequence of pulmonary embolism.

AGENTS AFFECTING PLATELET FUNCTION

Many different compounds inhibit the aggregation of blood platelets both in vitro and in vivo, thereby reducing the likelihood of thrombus formation when administered to patients at risk. As shown in Table 42-1, these compounds comprise nonsteroidal anti-inflammatory agents (NSAIDs), pyrimidopyrimidine and thienopyridine compounds, and a variety of unrelated agents that were found coincidentally to have effects on blood platelets.

The mechanisms of action vary between these groups of drugs, but they all in some way inhibit the release of platelet ADP that occurs after platelets are stimulated to aggregate. This "release reaction," which has been studied extensively and is shown schematically in Figure 42-2, can be elicited in vitro (and presumably also in vivo) by collagen, adenosine diphosphate, epinephrine, thrombin, and a variety of other substances. Platelet aggregation follows a set pattern (see also Chapter 31). Upon stimulation, platelets undergo membrane changes that lead to the intracellular synthesis of prostaglandin endoperoxides and thromboxane A_2 (from platelet phospholipids by the action of platelet cyclooxygenase). Thromboxane A_2 (TXA_2) is considered to be the specific stimulus for aggregation reactions. Also involved is a system of regulation of cyclic AMP content of platelets, which is thought to influence the transport of Ca^{2+} into platelets. Cyclic AMP acts to inhibit platelet adhesion, aggregation, and release of ADP.

Inhibition of platelet cyclooxygenase by NSAIDs will prevent prostaglandin endoperoxide synthesis; inhibition of platelet phosphodiesterase by pyrimidopyrimidine compounds will maintain high intracellular cAMP; in addition to inhibition of the ADP pathway, thienopyridine compounds will interact with platelet glycoprotein and inhibit the binding of fibrinogen to the membranes of activated platelets. These mechanisms then interfere with normal platelet responses and are the basis for clinical use of platelet inhibition by "antithrombotic" drugs (Table 42-1).

NSAIDs, including acetylsalicylic acid (ASA, aspirin), are described in detail in Chapter 34.

Dipyridamole (Persantine), a pyrimidopyrimidine compound, was originally introduced as a vasodi-

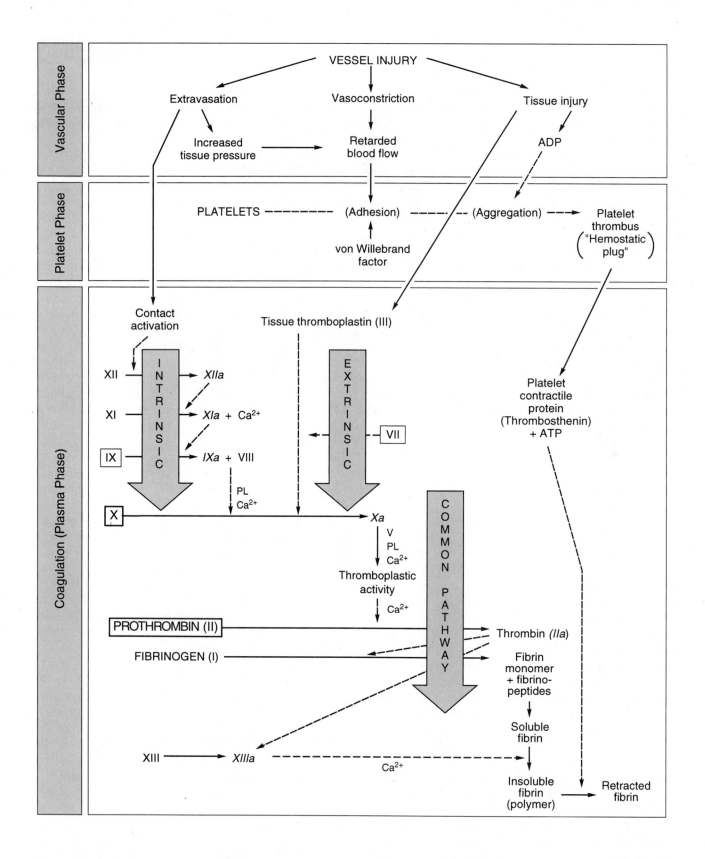

Figure 42-1. The hemostatic process. (Omitted for simplicity is the participation of prekallikrein and high-molecular-weight kininogen in the activation of factor XII.) Roman numerals designate clotting factors in the order of their discovery. Italicized (active) clotting factors are subject to inactivation by heparin. Hepatic synthesis of boxed clotting factors is inhibited by coumarins. (PL = phospholipid; a = activated factor; ----≫ acts upon; ——≫ produces or transforms into.)

Table 42-1 Inhibitors of Platelet Function (Antithrombotics)

Compounds	*Mechanisms of Action*
Nonsteroidal anti-inflammatory drugs (Acetylsalicylic acid, indomethacin, phenylbutazone, sulfinpyrazone)	Inhibit the ADP release reaction by inhibition of platelet cyclooxygenase, thus preventing synthesis of endoperoxides (PGG_2, PGH_2) and thromboxane (TXA_2); variably inhibit platelet adhesion to collagen and subendothelium
Pyrimidopyrimidine compounds (dipyridamole)	Inhibit the ADP release reaction by inhibition of platelet phosphodiesterase, resulting in increased platelet cAMP; inhibit platelet adhesion to collagen; prolong platelet survival
Thienopyridine compounds (ticlopidine HCl)	Inhibit the ADP pathway for platelet activation; interact with platelet glycoprotein, inhibiting the binding of fibrinogen to activated platelets and thus inhibiting aggregation
Prostaglandin I_2 (prostacyclin)	Opposing system to thromboxane A_2; prevents platelet adhesion to vessel wall components
Hydroxychloroquine (antimalarial) Clofibrate (antihyperlipidemic agent) Propranolol (β-adrenoceptor blocker) Cyproheptadine (antihistamine) Penicillins (antibiotic) Hydrocortisone (steroid)	Various mechanisms are proposed for these compounds, including: inhibition of thromboxane synthesis; prolongation of platelet survival; inhibition of the ADP release reaction; nonspecific platelet membrane actions

lator with predominant action on the small resistance vessels of the coronary circulation. Its vasodilator action in the treatment of anginal attacks appears to be linked to the metabolism of adenosine and adenine nucleotides, adenosine being a coronary vasodilator and signal for coronary blood flow regulation. The drug does not appear to be of significant value in the prophylaxis and treatment of angina pectoris. Its current use is for prophylaxis of thromboembolism in patients with heart-valve prostheses, to be given in combination with warfarin.

Ticlopidine HCl (Ticlid), a thienopyridine compound, was developed specifically as a platelet inhibitor. It is readily absorbed from the gastrointestinal tract and begins to inhibit platelet aggregation within 48 hours, with a maximal effect after about 1 week. The drug is rapidly and extensively biotransformed in the liver and excreted in the urine. Its half-life at steady state is 4–5 days; antiplatelet activity persists for a week or longer after treatment is discontinued.

Ticlopidine has numerous gastrointestinal side effects, and neutropenia, agranulocytosis, and thrombocytopenia have been reported. White blood cell counts need to be monitored every 2 weeks in the first 3 months of therapy, as should liver function. Other rare adverse effects are aplastic anemia, cholestatic jaundice, and elevated serum cholesterol (by 5–10%), although the HDL- and LDL-to-total-cholesterol ratios are unchanged. The absorption of ticlopidine may be decreased when antacids are taken concurrently.

Ticlopidine is approved for use to decrease the risk of thromboembolic stroke, and it has been used, primarily in Europe, for the prevention of myocardial infarction.

Since antiaggregating agents are capable of profoundly disturbing the normal hemostatic mechanisms, their use may unmask unrecognized abnormalities in hemostasis resulting from hereditary absence of, or defects in, coagulation factors coexisting with normal bleeding time. Prolonged bleeding and possible spontaneous hemorrhage may result. Because of prolongation of bleeding time (in particular by ASA and ticlopidine, but also to a lesser extent by other antiaggregating agents), the combination of these agents with anticoagulant drugs may occasionally result in serious spontaneous hemorrhage.

ANTICOAGULANTS

Many substances are capable of preventing the coagulation of blood. The clinically useful anticoagulants are those that can be administered in vivo without undue toxicity. Depending on their mechanism of action, they are classified as (1) direct anticoagulants, which act on blood constituents and prevent their normal interaction in the streaming blood (e.g., heparin), and (2) indirect anticoagulants, which interfere with the synthesis of clotting factors in the liver (e.g., vitamin K antagonists).

Heparin (Calcilean, Calciparine, Hepalean, and others)

Heparin prolongs the clotting time of blood both in vitro and in vivo. The substance was discovered and originally extracted from dog liver in Howell's laboratory in Baltimore; it was named heparin in 1918. Subsequent development of the drug occurred in Toronto (Best, Charles, Scott) and Stockholm (Jorpes). Procedures for the commercial preparation of heparin were established by Charles and Scott (Toronto, 1933), and the first recorded use for this product was in 1935–1936 by the Toronto surgeon Gordon Murray, who went on to introduce and clinically evaluate heparin as a systemic anticoagulant of phenomenal versatility.

Origin and chemistry

Heparin is a macromolecular, polymeric substance found in abundance in liver, lung, and intestinal mucosa. It is commercially extracted from bovine lung tissue and from hog and cattle intestinal mucosa. Heparin is a mucopolysaccharide and is the strongest organic acid found in the body. Its chemical structure is difficult to express, because it is a bundle of components of different chain lengths and molecular weights (average MW 15,000 Da; low-molecular-weight heparins have been prepared and are available for clinical use as anticoagulants and antithrombotics). The three principal monosaccharide building blocks are D-glucosamine, D-glucuronic acid, and L-iduronic acid, in addition to sulfuric acid. The drug is standardized in international and U.S.P. units: One unit has the activity of 0.01 mg of a sodium salt standard.

Mechanism and sites of action

Heparin interferes with clotting factor activations in both the intrinsic and extrinsic pathways of thromboplastin generation, and it has a strong antithrombin effect (see Fig. 42-1, in which *italicized* numerals indicate the factors that are subject to inactivation by heparin). The principal anticoagulant actions are due to the binding to, and acceleration of, a plasma α_2-globulin, antithrombin III, which acts as heparin cofactor and serine protease (thrombin) inhibitor. The specific sites of action in the coagulation sequence are:

1. Inactivation of factors IIa, IXa, Xa, XIa, XIIa, and XIIIa (especially factor Xa)
2. Complexing of thrombin (factor IIa)
3. Neutralization of tissue thromboplastin (factor III)

All of these anticoagulant effects of heparin take place in the blood itself, both in the circulating blood and in isolated blood samples in vitro, which distinguishes heparin from other anticoagulants that act as inhibitors of clotting factor synthesis in the liver.

Low-molecular-weight substances (MW 4,000–6,000 Da), oligosaccharide chains extracted from heparin, are available for use as anticoagulants/antithrombotics as **enoxaparin** and **tinzaparin Na.** These agents in general have an approximate ratio of anti-Xa:anti-IIa activity that is greater than 4, whereas that of heparin is equal to 1. This property was shown to permit the use of somewhat smaller doses than heparin for comparable antithrombotic effects with reduced bleeding tendency.

There is evidence that heparin is taken up against a concentration gradient and concentrated in vascular endothelium, where it reaches concentrations several hundred times greater than those in plasma; the endothelium may therefore be considered the "target organ." As described by Jaques (1982, 1985), vessel walls are athrombogenic because endothelial surfaces carry a strong electronegative charge that is produced and maintained by hydrodynamic forces as well as by metabolic processes. Loss of electronegativity is a powerful stimulus to thrombus formation, similar to that produced by injuries of the vascular endothelium and intima. Because of the strong electronegative charge of the heparin molecule, it serves to enhance or restore the negative electrostatic charge on the endothelium. This property of heparin is cited to explain its effectiveness in thrombosis prophylaxis

CIRCULATING
PLATELETS

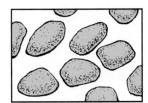

ADHESION TO
VESSEL WALL
AND TO
EACH OTHER

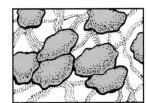

Exposure to collagen

↓

Platelet phospholipase A₂

↓

Platelet phospholipids ⟶ Arachidonic acid

Platelet cyclooxygenase ⤍ ⟶

Prostaglandin
endoperoxides
(PGG₂ & PGH₂)

Thromboxane synthase ⤍⟶

RELEASE
REACTION

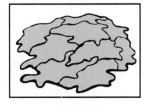

*Prostacyclin
synthase*

Thromboxane A₂
(in platelets)

ADP   Serotonin

Catecholamines

Prostacyclin
(in blood vessel walls)

AGGREGATION
(HEMOSTATIC
PLUG)

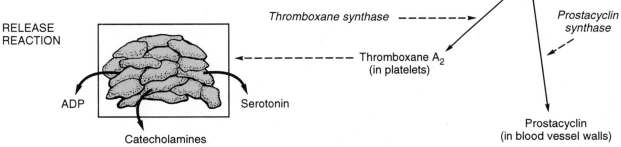

Degranulation
Shape change
Pseudopod formation

AGGREGATION **PROMOTED** by:	AGGREGATION **INHIBITED** by:
ADP	Prostacyclin (PGI₂)
Collagen	ASA
Serotonin	Indomethacin
Epinephrine	Phenylbutazone
Thrombin	Sulfinpyrazone
Fatty acids	Dipyridamole
Prostaglandin G₂	Ticlopidine
Thromboxane A₂	
Immune complexes	
Endotoxins	

Figure 42-2. Schematic representation of platelet aggregation, the principal biochemical processes, and the agents at present known to promote or inhibit aggregation (see also Chapter 31). ⤍ activates or acts upon; ⟶ is transformed into.

when used in doses too small to cause detectable systemic anticoagulation during "low-dose" heparin therapy.

In addition to its anticoagulant activity, heparin has poorly defined effects on blood platelets: Both stimulation and inhibition of aggregation have been reported. Mediated by increased electronegativity of cell membranes, heparin causes the appearance of lipoprotein lipase (which clears postprandial hyperlipemia), lecithinase, diamine oxidase, acid ribonuclease, and β-glycerophosphatase in the circulation. It protects against toxic conditions and some effects of trauma and stress; it inhibits sensitivity reactions in many systems; and a variety of effects on hormones have been reported. The effects of heparin on cellular elements of blood include mobilization of eosinophils, activation of macrophages, lymphocytosis, and increased migration of B lymphocytes. It must be stressed, though, that none of these additional actions of the drug hinder its use as an anticoagulant, nor are they of particular therapeutic value.

Pharmacokinetics

Because heparin is very strongly ionized, and because of its molecular size, it is not readily absorbed by the gastrointestinal mucosa. Also, it is destroyed in the gastrointestinal tract and must therefore be given in aqueous solution by intravenous injection or infusion, or by subcutaneous injection. Anticoagulant effects are obtained within minutes of single intravenous application. (For specific routes and dosage regimens see the end of the chapter.)

In humans, heparin has an approximate dose-dependent half-life of 1.5–2.5 hours. The elimination rate decreases with increasing dose, probably due to saturable metabolism. The drug is bound extensively to globulins and fibrinogen, but only sparingly to albumin. It is confined to the plasma volume. Due to this binding to inert carriers, but also to specific substrates, there is no correlation between the half-life determined by bioassay and the half-life of the anticoagulant effect of the drug.

A major pathway of elimination from the blood is the transfer of heparin to some extravascular compartment, such as the reticuloendothelial system. Heparin is also transformed to varying extent by hepatic sulfatase and heparinase, and a partially degraded form is excreted in the urine. The large molecular size precludes rapid renal excretion of the unchanged form in significant amounts; after very large intravenous doses, however, some unchanged heparin may appear in the urine. Heparin does not cross the placenta, and it is not secreted in milk.

Adverse effects and toxicity

Heparin is remarkably free of undesirable side effects, and even large doses over long periods of time do not normally cause difficulties other than those arising when the blood is rendered temporarily incoagulable. A rare type of hypersensitivity has been observed, particularly with impure preparations, and prolonged use may in rare instances result in reversible osteoporosis or alopecia. Heparin-induced thrombocytopenia, which is presumed to be an autoimmune type, is a potentially dangerous complication.

The practically important danger, however, lies in serious hemorrhage from **overdose.** If hemorrhage occurs, the administration of heparin must be discontinued. This will in most instances be sufficient to control hemorrhage because of the relatively short duration of action of the drug. Infusions of fresh whole blood or fresh-frozen plasma (containing most of the elements required for coagulation) may sometimes be indicated to hasten restoration of coagulability.

The specific **antidote** for heparin is **protamine sulfate.** This strongly basic substance is used to neutralize excess heparin by formation of an inactive complex; this is its only use in medicine. Note, however, that protamine must be given with caution, since it is an anticoagulant in its own right.

Vitamin K Antagonists (Coumarin Compounds)

In the 1920s Schofield described a bleeding disease in cattle that were fed spoiled sweet clover silage ("sweet clover disease"). The hemorrhagic agent responsible for this condition was identified by Campbell and Link in 1939 as bishydroxycoumarin (dicumarol). Further developments yielded many congeners, such as warfarin sodium. All coumarin compounds are similar in structure and properties, but **racemic warfarin** (Coumadin, Warfilone) has become the most widely used of the group following its initial marketing as a rodent poison.

Mechanism and site of action

The anticoagulant effect of all coumarin compounds depends on the depression of the vitamin K–dependent synthesis of clotting factors in the liver, thereby reducing their availability in the plasma. These are factors II (prothrombin), VII, IX, and X. There is a certain structural resemblance of coumarin compounds and vitamin K (Fig. 42-3).

A significant physiological role of vitamin K is to promote the synthesis of these clotting factors (see Chapter 67), most likely by acting as an essential cofactor for microsomal enzyme systems that activate precursors by conversion of peptide-bound glutamic acid to γ-carboxyglutamic acid. This newly formed amino acid enables the activated protein to bind Ca^{2+}, and this binding permits the protein to interact with phospholipid-containing membranes, an important step in the activation of these clotting factors during coagulation.

Warfarin and other coumarin-type anticoagulants interfere with the ability of the vitamin to catalyze the carboxylation and subsequent activation of clotting factor precursors. Thus, the administration of these drugs causes the accumulation of biologically inactive precursors of the clotting factors in liver and plasma.

Because the inhibition of vitamin K-dependent synthesis of clotting factors is competitive, vitamin K administration will result in displacement of coumarin compounds and resumption of normal clotting factor production. Vitamin K therefore is a specific antagonist used to reverse coumarin anticoagulant effects.

Dicumarol

Warfarin sodium

Vitamin K₁

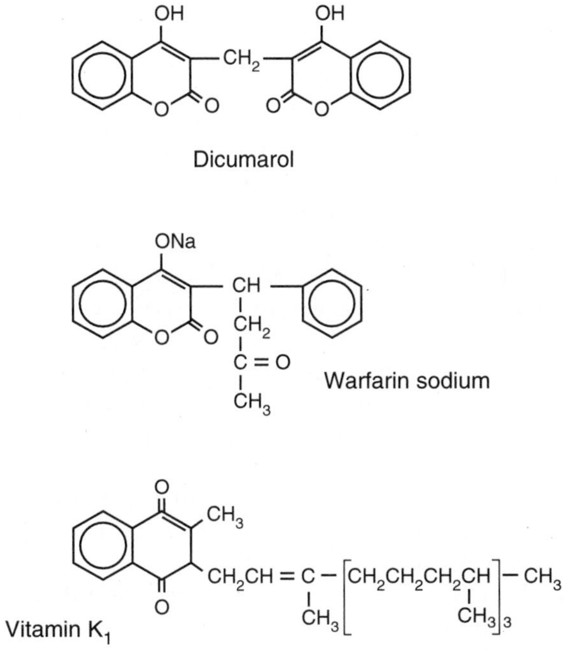

Figure 42-3. Coumarins and vitamin K₁.

Pharmacokinetics

Coumarin compounds show varying rates of absorption from the gastrointestinal tract, that of dicumarol being slow and erratic, while warfarin is rapidly and completely absorbed (Table 42-2). This absorption is a clinically important property, allowing oral administration of these drugs in routine anticoagulant therapy. The drugs are therefore also referred to as *oral* anticoagulants. Depending on the individual drugs, peak plasma levels are usually reached within 2–12 hours, the exact concentration varying from person to person. Peak anticoagulant effects (as measured with the prothrombin time), however, will not become apparent until about 24 hours after peak plasma levels have been attained. This is because the inhibition of clotting factor synthesis does not directly affect the preexisting clotting factor activity in the circulating plasma, which must decrease at its spontaneous turnover rate until a new, lower steady-state level is reached. *Clinically significant anticoagulant effects cannot be expected for about 30–60 hours,* depending on the dosage regimen (Fig. 42-4). Similarly, on cessation of treatment, it takes 2–5 days before sufficient new synthesis has occurred to restore normal clotting activity.

Within the circulation, the drugs are almost entirely bound to plasma albumin, so exceedingly small amounts of free drug are present after therapeutic doses (Table 42-2). Of racemic warfarin, the most extensively investigated member of this group of drugs, the dextrorotatory form is converted to a secondary alcohol and the levorotatory form to 7-hydroxywarfarin. These inactive metabolites undergo some enterohepatic circulation and are excreted in urine and stool.

Factors Affecting Activity; Drug Interactions

There are many factors that can affect the activity of these drugs (Fig. 42-5), and many drugs, when given concurrently, alter coumarin anticoagulant effects. This is of great clinical importance, since it involves a class of drugs with a narrow margin of safety and complex pharmacokinetic properties. Drug interactions can thus lead to serious hemorrhagic complications, or they may be the cause of therapeutic failure.

Pathophysiological conditions that increase the anticoagulant response because of induced vitamin K deficiency are inadequate diet, intestinal disease, and inadequate bile flow. Hepatic disease may predispose to defective clotting factor synthesis,

Table 42-2 Pharmacokinetics of Coumarins in Humans

Compound	Gastrointestinal Absorption	Plasma Protein Binding (%)	Plasma $t_{1/2}$ (hours)	Usual Daily Dose (mg)	Time to Peak Anticoagulant Effect* (hours)	Duration of Effect After Stopping Drug (days)
Acenocoumarol (Nicoumalone)	Rapid, complete	?	~20	2–10	36–48	1.5–2
Dicumarol	Slow, variable	99	10–30†	25–150	36–48	5–6
Phenprocoumon	Complete	99	~160	1–4	48–72	7–14
Warfarin Na	Rapid, complete	99.3	~45	2–15	36–72	4–5

*As measured with the prothrombin time.
†Plasma $t_{1/2}$ increases with plasma concentration.

and chronic alcoholics may therefore experience bleeding episodes while on anticoagulant therapy. However, they are also prone to experience an inadequate therapeutic response because of behavioral unreliability and noncompliance with medical instructions about the use of the drug. In addition, induction of smooth endoplasmic reticulum in the livers of alcoholics can increase the rate of warfarin biotransformation and thus reduce the anticoagulant effect. Although contraindicated in pregnancy because warfarin crosses the placental barrier, its administration during pregnancy would cause a *decreased anticoagulant response* in the mother because of increased clotting factor activity. The fetus, however, would remain highly susceptible to the drug and would likely require vitamin K antidotal therapy at birth (see below).

Among the **drugs that enhance the response** to oral anticoagulants are acetylsalicylic acid and other compounds with platelet-inhibitory activity, as well as clofibrate; these agents inhibit platelet adhesion and aggregation and thus add to the hemostatic defect resulting from inhibition of clotting factor synthesis. Phenylbutazone has the added effect of inhibiting warfarin biotransformation, and to some extent also displacing warfarin from its albumin binding sites, and thus may cause severe hemorrhage during anticoagulant therapy. Disulfiram and trimethoprim-sulfonamide preparations inhibit the conversion and prolong the half-life of warfarin. Other drugs that prolong the prothrombin time by a variety of mechanisms are cimetidine, sulfinpyrazone, D-thyroxine, and anabolic steroids.

Drugs that diminish the response to oral anticoagulants by induction of hepatic microsomal enzymes are barbiturates and glutethimide. Their co-administration with oral anticoagulants requires significantly higher doses of the latter for therapeutic anticoagulation. These patients are then at risk of serious hemorrhagic complications if the dosage of the interacting drug is reduced without simultaneous adjustment of the dose of anticoagulant. Rifampin reduces blood levels of oral anticoagulants, and hence anticoagulant activity, by induction of hepatic microsomal enzymes. Cholestyramine increases the elimination of anticoagulants in the stool. Any drug or substance that interferes with the absorption of anticoagulants will also delay the attainment of therapeutic plasma levels or diminish the effects. (See Chapter 64 for further examples of drug interactions.)

Adverse Effects, Contraindications, and Toxicity

Obvious contraindications for oral anticoagulant therapy are a bleeding tendency due to any cause; cerebrovascular hemorrhage; ulceration or bleeding from the gastrointestinal, genitourinary, or respiratory tract; surgery on the central nervous system; and pregnancy. Dicumarol and warfarin pass the placental barrier, leading on occasion to severe hypoprothrombinemia with cerebral injury in the newborn. These drugs are also secreted in the milk, and can thus affect the breast-fed infant. Warfarin-associated skin necrosis has been reported.

The most important complication of oral anticoagulant therapy is *hemorrhage*. Since **vitamin K** begins to reverse excessive coumarin activity within a few hours and fully corrects the coagulation defect within 24 hours, it is regarded as the **specific antidote.** Modest doses (5–10 mg vitamin K_1, also known as phytomenadione or phytonadione) are preferred

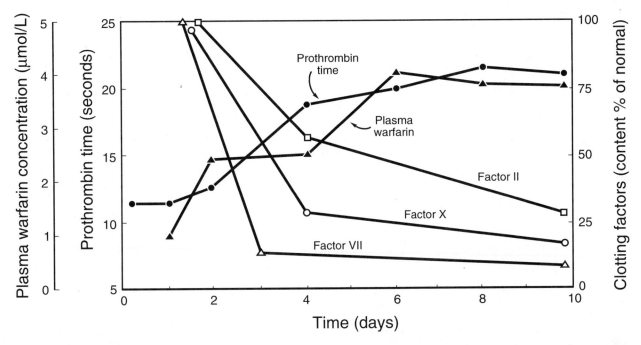

Figure 42-4. Schematic representation of the relationships between the administration of daily small doses of warfarin, fall in plasma clotting factor content, and prothrombin time response. Clotting factor $t_{1/2}$: factor II = 60 hours, factor X = 40 hours, factor VII = 6 hours. Note the disappearance of clotting factors from the plasma in relation to their half-lives. Also note the initial lag between the measured plasma warfarin levels and prothrombin times, showing that the latter is a more meaningful indicator of the degree of induced clotting factor inhibition and coagulation impairment. Note also that a steady state is eventually obtained.

because of long-lasting coumarin resistance after high doses of the vitamin. Fresh plasma transfusions facilitate the reversal of excessive anticoagulation.

In Vitro Anticoagulants

Calcium ions (factor IV) are ubiquitous participants in almost all stages of the hemostatic process. They are required for the generation of prothrombin activator (thromboplastin) and in the conversion of prothrombin to thrombin. Removal of Ca^{2+}, therefore, will prevent coagulation of blood or plasma in vitro without interference with, or destruction of, the potential activities of other coagulation factors.

Calcium-removing agents such as sodium citrate, sodium oxalate, sodium fluoride, chelating agents, and ion-exchange resins are therefore used extensively for anticoagulation of transfusion blood, in the preparation of blood plasma, and in the performance of hematological tests. Addition of molar equivalents of calcium (usually in the form of calcium chloride) to blood or plasma anticoagulated with these substances will restore the ability to clot. (Conserved anticoagulated transfusion blood will re-

acquire its coagulation characteristics when mixed with the calcium in the recipient's blood.)

FIBRINOLYTIC AND ANTIFIBRINOLYTIC AGENTS

The removal of blood clots in the organism is normally accomplished by the physiological process of fibrinolysis. This fibrinolysis is controlled in vivo by enzymatic processes involving the conversion of an enzyme precursor, **plasminogen,** into the proteolytic enzyme **plasmin,** a reaction that is mediated through activators or **kinases** (Fig. 42-6). Plasminogen activator is found in plasma as plasma activator, in urine as urokinase, in various tissues (including blood vessels) as tissue activator, and in body secretions. Therapeutic fibrinolysis (i.e., thrombolysis, the dissolution of intravascular blood clots) can be achieved by administration of activators of plasminogen or via proteolytic enzymes. Because therapeutic fibrinolysis is complex and not without danger to the patient, its use is reserved for clearly defined, limited indications.

Fungal proteases had been identified, investi-

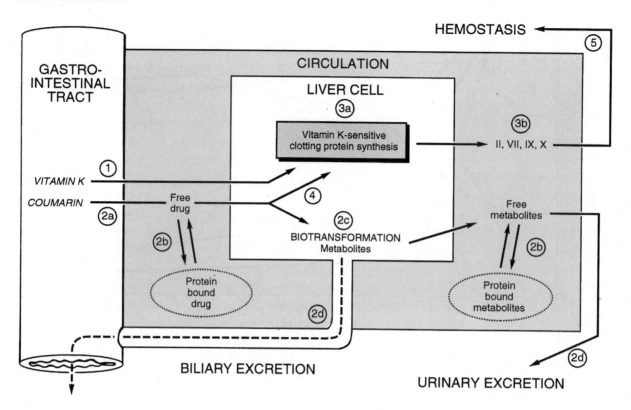

Figure 42-5. Sites at which drugs may modify the anti-coagulant action of coumarins. (1) Vitamin K bioavailability; (2a) coumarin absorption; (2b) coumarin binding to albumin; (2c) coumarin biotransformation; (2d) coumarin excretion; (3a) prothrombin complex synthesis; (3b) prothrombin complex catabolism; (4) receptor affinity for coumarins; (5) hemostasis. (Modified from Koch-Weser J, Sellers EM. *N Engl J Med* 1971; 285:487–494; 547–558.)

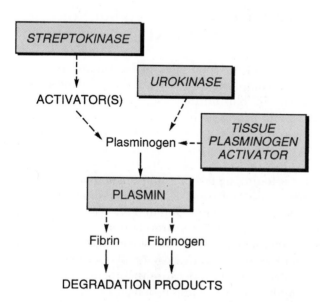

Figure 42-6. Fibrinolysis and sites of action of fibrinolytic agents. ---> activates or acts upon; ——> is transformed into.

gated, and prepared for therapeutic fibrinolysis in the 1960s and 1970s. Proteases of *Aspergillus oryzae*, *Aspergillus ochraceus*, *Armillaria mellea*, and *Trichothecium roseum* attained clinical investigational status for limited use in thrombotic conditions usually associated with extracorporeal circulation and hemodialysis. However, these enzyme preparations were eventually determined to be too difficult to use because of broad and nonspecific proteolytic spectra, complex inhibitor systems in mammalian plasma, and the need for specialized hematological support of patients. Newer products (see below) do not have these disadvantages.

Streptokinase (Kabikinase, Streptase)

This is a plasminogen activator derived from hemolytic streptococci. It has the longest history of clinical use, and the important concepts of thrombolytic therapy, indications, contraindications, and technique have been established with this agent in international collaborative trials. Streptokinase is antigenic because of its bacterial origin, and fever and allergic reactions are among the known risks and complications during its use in therapy. Naturally occurring antistreptococcal antibodies cross-react with streptokinase and reduce its activity. Following its systemic administration, patients experience periods of increased hemorrhagic risk from generalized lysis of fibrin and fibrinogen.

Streptokinase interacts with plasminogen, forming an active complex with protease activity that catalyzes the conversion of plasminogen to plasmin. The drug is usually administered intravenously as a loading dose of 250,000 I.U. over 30 minutes, followed by continuous infusion of 100,000 I.U./hr for 24–48 hours. Therapy is monitored by the thrombin time, which should be two to five times the control value. There are, however, variations to this usual treatment regimen depending on the location, severity, and duration of the vascular occlusion.

Intravenously administered streptokinase is rapidly distributed in the blood. Its plasma clearance exhibits a biphasic course. The drug is inactivated by binding to streptokinase antibodies in the blood and by accumulation in the liver. Rapid antibody binding eliminates small amounts from the blood with a half-life of about 20 minutes. Thereafter, the main portion of the drug interacts with plasminogen. This process eliminates streptokinase with a half-life of about 80 minutes. Most of an administered dose is excreted by the kidneys as amino acids and peptides. The drug does not readily cross the placental barrier.

Urokinase (Abbokinase)

This enzyme is derived from human urine, where it occurs in relative abundance, or from cultures of human kidney cells, or most recently by employing recombinant DNA technology in bacteria. It is used similarly to streptokinase to activate the patient's own plasminogen. The activator is nonantigenic, highly specific, but apparently quite costly to manufacture.

Urokinase is administered intravenously, usually in a loading dose of 4000 I.U./kg over 10 minutes, followed by infusion of 4000 I.U./hr for 12 hours. Because fibrinolytic therapy with urokinase is expensive, it should be reserved for patients who are allergic to streptokinase.

Tissue-Type Plasminogen Activator (Activase)

This agent of human origin is manufactured by means of recombinant DNA technology. It has undergone extensive multicenter trials and is promoted as specific therapy for fresh thrombotic coronary artery occlusions. Tissue plasminogen activator is claimed to act preferentially on fibrin-bound plasminogen and to have less systemic activity than streptokinase and urokinase on circulating fibrinogen. The drug is very expensive, and this fact, together with its currently narrow indication, restricts its use.

Plasmin

Plasmin is the naturally occurring species-specific fibrinolytic enzyme of mammals; it is prepared by in vitro activation of human plasminogen with streptokinase. It is inactivated by naturally occurring antiplasmins in plasma and serum, and it is unstable in solution. Its use in therapy, therefore, is limited.

Aminocaproic Acid (Amicar)

ε-Aminocaproic acid, a lysine analog, is a synthetic inhibitor of fibrinolysis that is used as a specific antidote for overdose of fibrinolytic agents. It inhibits the formation of plasmin from plasminogen, and large doses also inhibit the action of plasmin. Other uses are in the treatment of pathological hyperfibrinolytic states that result in life-threatening hemorrhage or hematuria (e.g., prostatic, cardiac, hepatic surgery; urinary tract neoplasia; hemophilia).

THERAPEUTIC APPLICATIONS OF ANTITHROMBOTICS AND ANTICOAGULANTS

Abnormal tendencies of premature clotting and thrombus formation may be influenced therapeutically at various stages of the hemostatic process (Table 42-3).

Antiaggregating Agents

Typically, arterial thrombi consist predominantly of platelet aggregates, and platelets tend to be primarily responsible for thromboembolic disorders in cerebral vessels, vessel grafts, and heart-valve prostheses. It is therefore quite rational that antiaggregating agents are used with increasing frequency in the prevention and treatment of such disorders. This therapeutic approach has gained wide acceptance since numerous randomized trials have shown the usefulness of pharmacological suppression of platelet activity in preventing strokes, transient ischemic attacks, and

Table 42-3 Characteristics of the Main Classes of Antithrombotic Drugs

Characteristic	Heparin	Coumarins	Platelet Inhibitors
Source	Natural	Synthetic	Synthetic
Principal use	Short-term, intensive, controlled anticoagulation	Long-term, sustained, controlled anticoagulation (thrombosis prophylaxis)	Long-term inhibition of platelet function (thrombosis prophylaxis)
Site of action	Circulating blood (in vivo and in vitro)	Liver (in vivo only)	Circulating blood (in vivo and in vitro)
Mechanism of action	Activates plasma antithrombin III. Inactivates factors IIa, IXa, Xa, XIa, XIIa, XIIIa. Complexes thrombin. Neutralizes tissue thromboplastin. Enhances negative charge on endothelium	Inhibit hepatic synthesis of factor II, factor VII, factor IX, factor X (all vitamin K-dependent)	Inhibit platelet cyclooxygenase and synthesis of TXA_2, causing failure to aggregate. Inhibit platelet phosphodiesterase, elevating platelet cAMP and causing failure to aggregate
Tests for evaluating the degree of clinical effect	In vitro: Activated partial thromboplastin time; whole-blood clotting time	In vitro: Prothrombin time	In vitro: Platelet aggregation. In vivo: Bleeding time
Route of administration	Parenteral	Oral	Oral
Onset of action	Immediate (10–20 minutes)	Delayed (after 12–24 hours)	Rapid (1–4 hours)
Duration of action	2–4 hours i.v. 8–12 hours s.c.	2–5 days	5–7 days
Antidotes	Protamine sulfate (rapidly acting)	Vitamin K_1 (slow acting)	No specific antidotes (fresh plasma)

recurrent myocardial infarction. The drugs most extensively investigated are **acetylsalicylic acid** (ASA, in doses ranging from 30 mg/day to 300 mg four times daily, depending on conditions of use and still-controversial recommendations for "high" versus "low" dose from various clinical trials), **sulfinpyrazone** (800 mg/day), **dipyridamole** (200–400 mg/day), and **ticlopidine** (250 mg twice daily). Therapeutic inhibition of platelet aggregation can be estimated by measuring drug-induced prolongations of the **bleeding time** or by automated instrumented measurements of aggregation with reagents such as ADP, epinephrine, and collagen.

Heparin

The almost instantaneous and predictable anticoagulant effects of heparin through its direct interference with circulating procoagulants, as well as its relatively short duration of action and consequent safety, have made it the most attractive and useful agent in the prevention and treatment of the majority of thromboembolic disorders. The drug is particularly useful in short-term prophylaxis of thrombosis and in the acute treatment of a variety of life-threatening conditions of thromboembolic origin. The drug does not dissolve existing thrombi, but it prevents the extension of thrombotic vascular obstructions and aids in the maintenance of blood circulation.

In order to obtain therapeutic anticoagulation, the drug is preferably introduced directly into the bloodstream, and the dose is titrated by repeated measurements of anticoagulant effects. The methods of measurement are the **activated partial thromboplastin time** or, now rarely, the **whole-blood clotting time.** The therapeutic objective is a prolongation of clotting times to approximately two or three times normal (pretreatment) values, depending on clinical circumstances.

Depending on clinical circumstances, various treatment schemes are used; for example:

- Intravenous injection—10,000-unit bolus, followed by 5000–10,000 units every 6 hours
- Intravenous infusion—5000–10,000-unit loading dose, then continuous infusion at a rate of 1000 units/hr (20,000 units/day)
- Subcutaneous injection ("low-dose heparin")— 5000 units every 12 hours

Intramuscular injections are painful, are frequently associated with hematoma formation, and should not be used.

Low-molecular-weight heparin (**enoxaparin**) is used for the prophylaxis of thromboembolic disorders following hip or knee replacement surgery and in the management of postoperative venous thromboembolism following general surgery. The preparations are standardized in anti-factor Xa international units, and administration is by subcutaneous injection according to manufacturers' recommendations. The dosage schedules vary according to specific indications.

Oral Anticoagulants

These agents are used primarily in the long-term (sometimes life-long) prophylaxis of thrombosis in individuals at risk and to prevent the recurrence of thrombophlebitis, venous thrombosis, or pulmonary embolism in patients with a previous history of such thromboembolic disease. Because of the chronic nature of therapy, absolute compliance must be assured, and patients are usually thoroughly instructed in the type and use of their medication for reasons of safety and efficacy of anticoagulation.

The objective of oral anticoagulation is to obtain *maximal interference with coagulation with minimal risk of hemorrhage for long periods of time.* Dosages vary among individual drugs (Table 42-2). Therapy with warfarin, which is the drug of choice over all other coumarin-type agents, is usually initiated by administration of small doses and not a large loading dose. In this way the gradual development of hypoprothrombinemia may be observed, maintenance doses may be titrated, and the accidental occurrence of hemorrhage can be prevented (Figure 42-4). This method may also prevent the occurrence of skin necrosis.

The commonly used method of control of therapy at present is based on the one-stage **prothrombin time** (PT) ("Quick time" or variations thereof). It is essential that measurements be performed daily until a steady-state anticoagulation has been achieved and the patient has stabilized. Periodic measurements must then be performed for the duration of anticoagulant therapy. Results of measurements are reported in terms of international normalized ratio (INR) values according to the following formula: $INR = (PT_{patient}/PT_{mean})^{ISI}$. The INR thus is the prothrombin time ratio of a given patient measurement to the mean prothrombin time of a representative "normal" population of the respective institution's laboratory, corrected by the international sensitivity index (ISI) of the commercial thromboplastin reagent used in the test. Depending on clinical circumstances and patient characteristics, therapeutic anticoagulant INR values are in the range of 2.0 to 4.0.

SUGGESTED READING

Antiplatelet Trialists' Collaboration. Collaborative overview of randomised trials of antiplatelet therapy—I: prevention of death, myocardial infarction, and stroke by prolonged antiplatelet therapy in various categories of patients. Br Med J 1994; 308:81–106.

Antiplatelet Trialists' Collaboration. Collaborative overview of randomised trials of antiplatelet therapy—II: maintenance of vascular graft or arterial patency by antiplatelet therapy. Br Med J 1994; 308:159–168.

Antiplatelet Trialists' Collaboration. Collaborative overview of randomised trials of antiplatelet therapy—III: reduction in venous thrombosis and pulmonary embolism by antiplatelet prophylaxis among surgical and medical patients. Br Med J 1994; 308:235–246.

deProst D. Heparin fractions and analogues: a new therapeutic possibility for thrombosis. TIPS 1986; 4(12):496–500.

Fuster V. Coronary thrombolysis—a perspective for the practicing physician (Editorial). N Engl J Med 1993; 329:723–724.

Green D, Hirsh J, Heit J, Prins M, Davidson B, Lensing AWA. Low molecular weight heparin: a critical analysis of clinical trials (Review). Pharmacol Rev 1994; 46:89–109.

GUSTO Investigators. An international randomized trial comparing four thrombolytic strategies for acute myocardial infarction. N Engl J Med 1993; 329:673–682.

Hirsh J, Fuster V. Guide to anticoagulation therapy. Part 1: heparin (Review). Circulation 1994; 89:1449–1468.

Hirsh J, Fuster V. Guide to anticoagulation therapy. Part 2: oral anticoagulants (Review). Circulation 1994; 89:1469–1480.

Jaques LB. Heparin: a unique misunderstood drug. TIPS 1982; 3(7):289–291.

Jaques LB. The new understanding of the drug heparin. Chest 1985; 88:751–754.

Markwardt F, ed. Fibrinolytics and antifibrinolytics. Handbook of experimental pharmacology, vol 46. Berlin: Springer-Verlag, 1978.

Ogston D. The physiology of hemostatis. Cambridge: Harvard University Press, 1983.

Roschlau WHE. Fungal proteases. In: Markwardt F, ed. Fibrinolytics and antifibrinolytics. Handbook of Experimental Pharmacology, vol 46. Berlin: Springer-Verlag, 1978; 337–450.

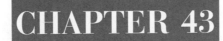

CHAPTER 43

Drugs Affecting Erythropoiesis

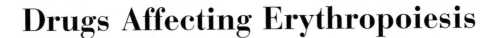

W.H.E. ROSCHLAU

CASE HISTORIES

Case 1

A 35-year-old woman consulted her physician because of complaints of weakness, dizziness, and epigastric discomfort. She gave a history of peptic ulcer, first diagnosed 5 years earlier, for which she was taking antacids. She also had a longstanding (more than 20 years) history of headaches, for which she took two 325-mg tablets of ASA, sometimes two or three times daily. In addition, she had significant acne, for which she took tetracycline 250 mg twice daily.

On physical examination, she was pale and lethargic but no abnormality was detected in any organ system.

Lab studies revealed a hemoglobin of 8 g/dL. The blood smear showed hypochromic red cells and the stools were positive for occult blood. At 800,000/mm^3 the platelet count was higher than the normal range, and the reticulocyte count was 0.2%. A diagnosis was therefore made of iron deficiency anemia due to GI blood loss. This was thought to be secondary to chronic use of salicylate for the treatment of headache and/or to recurrent peptic ulcer. The treatment therefore involved oral iron in the form of ferrous sulfate, 500 mg three times daily for 3 weeks, then reduced to 100 mg twice daily for 2 months, to restore optimal hemoglobin production. The patient was counseled on the use of ASA and tetracycline, and a medical investigation searching for the possible upper-GI site of blood loss was begun.

Case 2

A 42-year-old man presented with a longstanding history of excessive alcohol intake and a 5-year history of seizures that have been treated with phenytoin 400 mg/day and phenobarbital 90 mg/day. It was estimated that the patient habitually consumes alcohol in amounts equivalent to a pint of whiskey per day.

Laboratory investigation showed that his hemoglobin was 7 g/dL, and the white blood cell count was 3500/mm^3. The reticulocyte count was 1% and the smear showed hypersegmented granulocytes. Serum folate was 2 ng/mL. A diagnosis of folic acid deficiency was made, contributed to by alcoholism and the accompanying nutritional folate deficiency. The ingestion of phenytoin for the seizure disorders may also have contributed to the reduced serum folate.

The patient was treated with oral folic acid, 5 mg twice daily, and recalled for laboratory tests every 2 weeks to monitor the effects of this therapy on hemoglobin, white and red blood cells, and serum folate. Counseling was begun in order to address the patient's chronic drinking problem, which was recognized as the main cause of his folate deficiency anemia.

Erythrocytes are formed in the sinusoids of red bone marrow from differentiating precursor cells; undifferentiated (i.e., multipotential) stem cells proliferate and develop into proerythroblasts, and these mature and develop through three successive stages of erythroblasts (normoblasts) into reticulocytes. During maturation the original stem cell nuclei and cytoplasmic organelles degenerate and disappear, and increasing amounts of hemoglobin are laid down in the cytoplasm. Reticulocytes, the immediate precursors of mature erythrocytes, are somewhat larger than erythrocytes, contain a network of endoplasmic reticulum, are metabolically active, and can synthesize proteins. Their proportion in the blood is about 2% of red blood cells. Once fully developed, mature erythrocytes have lost the reticulum and most of the characteristics of living cells.

Erythropoiesis is stimulated by *erythropoietin*, a glycoprotein that is synthesized mainly in renal cortical cells and is responsive to varying demands of erythropoiesis during life (see later in this chapter). During optimal erythropoiesis in the adult, *vitamin B_{12}* and *folic acid* are required for purine and pyrimidine synthesis in the synthesis of DNA (see Chapter 67). A deficiency in these vitamins will result in faulty cell division and maturation with the appearance in the bone marrow of megaloblasts (in place of erythroblasts), and of macrocytic erythrocytes in the blood.

Hemoglobin, composed of heme and globin, is a tetrameric structure that contains two α and two β polypeptide chains, to which are attached four heme molecules. Heme is protoporphyrin that is bonded with one atom of iron in ferrous form. One molecule of hemoglobin, therefore, contains four atoms of iron. Of these, each atom of iron takes up one molecule of oxygen when reduced hemoglobin is converted to oxyhemoglobin. This uptake of oxygen is oxygenation (rather than oxidation), which allows for the reversibility of the uptake of oxygen by *ferrous iron* (Fe^{2+}). A deficiency in ferrous iron interferes with normal hemoglobin synthesis: Red blood cells are paler (hypochromic) and smaller (microcytic) than normal, and the ability of erythrocytes to carry oxygen is greatly reduced.

"Anemia" is the collective term applied to conditions that manifest themselves in deficient numbers of circulating red blood cells or in abnormally low total hemoglobin content per unit of blood volume. Table 43-1 provides a partial classification of anemias; it indicates that the variety in etiology may require combinations of symptomatic and specific therapy for rational treatment and that lasting thera-

Table 43-1 Etiological Classification of Anemias*

Excessive loss of blood
  Acute or chronic posthemorrhagic anemia
Deficient red blood cell production
  Deficient hemoglobin or DNA synthesis
    Iron deficiency
    Vitamin B_{12} deficiency ⎫ So-called
    Folic acid deficiency   ⎬ nutritional anemias
    Other nutritional deficiencies ⎭
    Thalassemia
  Bone marrow abnormalities
    Hypoplastic and aplastic anemias
    Endocrine disorders
    Chronic renal failure
    Sideroblastic anemia
Excessive red blood cell destruction
  Due to intrinsic erythrocyte defects
    Hereditary enzyme deficiencies and/or membrane
      defects
    Hemoglobinopathies (e.g., sickle-cell anemia)
  Due to extraerythrocytic factors
    Reactions to incompatible blood, to chemicals and
      drugs, to infectious agents, to physical agents,
      antibody-mediated, hypersplenism, etc.

* Only the so-called nutritional anemias are discussed in this chapter.

peutic benefits can usually not be expected unless the causative factors are identified and corrected.

The blood and the blood-forming organs are affected by a large number of drugs, either directly or indirectly, and many drugs exert known toxic effects on blood cells, hemoglobin, and hematopoietic organs. These are mentioned in the respective chapters in which these drugs are described. It is axiomatic that a drug with known hematotoxicity should not be administered unless the risks are recognized and weighed against the benefits and unless proper hematological surveillance is carried out.

NUTRITIONAL ANEMIAS

Many dietary factors are important for normal hematopoiesis, and a chronic lack or deficiency of one or more of these might eventually be reflected in deficient erythropoiesis and anemia. These "nutritional anemias" (see Table 43-1) are a large group of disorders of the erythropoietic system and are most responsive to specific drug therapy.

Any nutrient deficiency arises from one or more of five basic causes: inadequate ingestion, absorption or utilization, or increased excretion or requirement. Nutritional anemias are all treatable by providing the deficient nutrient in appropriate form and dosage as a "drug." In addition, the therapeutic goal is to determine and, if possible, eliminate the cause of the deficiency.

Iron Deficiency Anemia

In states of constant blood volume and red blood cell values the amount of iron required daily is determined by the average lifespan of erythrocytes and the total quantity of circulating hemoglobin. Iron is preserved in the body by recycling from broken-down red blood cells into the bone marrow and then reutilized for hemoglobin production.

About 0.8% of circulating red blood cells are broken down daily. The quantity of hemoglobin thus removed and replaced daily is approximately 7.65 g, corresponding to 26 mg of iron. Total iron loss per day (intestine, urine, sweat) is probably not more than 1 mg, which is easily replaced from dietary sources (variously estimated at about 1.5–2 mg/day).

However, iron requirements are greatly increased during growth, menstruation, pregnancy, blood donations, and pathological bleeding, i.e., during periods of increased hematopoietic demands. Active growth and menstruation may require iron supplementation in addition to iron from dietary sources. During pregnancy up to 6 mg of iron may be required daily, which cannot be met by diet alone (Table 43-2).

Thus, iron deficiency anemia is a symptom of diminished essential body iron rather than a primary disease. It begins with the gradual depletion of iron stores and leads, when untreated, to the development of **hypochromic microcytic anemia** accompanied by low plasma iron level and elevated plasma iron-binding capacity (Table 43-3). The only effective therapy is supplementation of iron intake to correct the deficiency.

Iron physiology

Absorption of elemental iron and inorganic iron salts, whether dietary or medicinal, occurs from the gastro-intestinal tract beyond the stomach. It must be ionized and divalent (ferrous, Fe^{2+}) for easiest absorption. Conversion of trivalent (i.e., ferric) to divalent iron occurs readily in the gastrointestinal tract through gastric acid, ascorbic acid in food, and –SH or other reducing groups. Iron may pass directly into and through the mucosal cells of the duodenum and upper small intestine into the bloodstream, where it is attached to transferrin (a β_1-globulin that binds two atoms of iron per molecule) for transport from sites of absorption or storage to sites of utilization. Alternatively, iron may be bound to apoferritin to form a complex called ferritin, which is stored in the intestinal mucosal cells for elimination by exfoliation. During situations of high iron demand, when iron stores become depleted, the absorption of iron is increased. Conversely, during iron overload the absorption of iron can be blocked by increased ferritin storage in mucosal cells. Iron absorption is controlled by a combination of factors, such as serum iron levels, the amount of ferritin in duodenal mucosal

Table 43-2 Estimated Iron Requirements to Balance Iron Losses

	Estimated Losses (mg/day)				Amount That Must be Absorbed to Maintain Optimal Hemoglobin Synthesis (mg/day)
	Normal Excretion	*Menses*	*Pregnancy*	*Growth*	
Men and postmenopausal women	1.0				1.0
Menstruating women	1.0	1.0			2.0
Pregnant women	1.0		3.0–5.0*		4.0–6.0
Children (average)	0.5			0.5	1.0
Girls (adolescent)	0.5	0.5		0.5	1.5

*Demand increases throughout pregnancy and fetal development.

Table 43-3 Main Features of Nutritional Deficiency Anemias

Iron Deficiency Anemia (Hypochromic/Microcytic Anemia)

Iron requirements
  Greatest during growth, menstruation, pregnancy, blood donation, pathological bleeding (likely conditions for iron supplementation).

Development of anemia
  Decreased, and then depleted, tissue iron stores
  Decreased hematocrit values (= fewer red blood cells; some paler, some smaller than normal)
  Decreased hemoglobin values (= hypochromic, microcytic red blood cells)

Therapy
  Correction of iron deficiency:
    To restore hemoglobin synthesis and red blood cell production
    To replenish depleted tissue iron stores
  Oral: 200–300 mg elemental iron/day for weeks or months
  Parenteral: 150 mg iron for each gram of hemoglobin deficit, plus 600 mg to replenish tissue stores, given over 1–3 weeks

Megaloblastic/Macrocytic Anemias:	*Vitamin B_{12}*	*Folic Acid*
Required for	Hematopoiesis; production of epithelial cells; maintenance of myelin	Purine and pyrimidine synthesis; amino acid interconversions
Symptoms common to both types of deficiency	*Megaloblastosis:* Affects all proliferating tissues, specifically the hematopoietic system	
	Macrocytosis: Large stem cells in bone marrow; large cells with short lifespan in peripheral blood: "anemia"	
Additional symptoms	Defective maintenance of myelin sheath with peripheral and other neurological deficits	
Development of anemia	Mainly due to impaired absorption of vitamin B_{12} (pernicious anemia)	Mainly due to inadequate nutritional intake or utilization of folic acid
Therapy	Cyanocobalamin (i.m.)	Folic acid (p.o./i.m.)

cells, the degree of transferrin saturation, the state of iron stores, and the rate of erythropoiesis.

In the normal adult with about 4–5 g total body iron, iron turnover is approximately 35 mg/day. Of this, most enters the bone marrow for use in erythropoiesis, and about 1 mg goes into storage, extracellular fluid, and excretion. Iron entering the plasma under conditions of normal turnover is that salvaged from aged red blood cells, returned from storage and extracellular fluid, and absorbed from the intestinal tract. Iron storage sites are the marrow, spleen, liver, and other reticuloendothelial structures, where iron is present as ferritin and hemosiderin (ferritin aggregates holding additional iron). Excretion is by desquamation of iron-containing cells from bowel, skin,

and genitourinary tract and in bile, urine, and sweat. The normal loss is probably not more than 1 mg/ day, but it is at least double that amount during menstruation. Iron provided from maternal stores to the fetus and placenta during pregnancy, together with losses during delivery and lactation, result in a net deficit of 200–500 mg for each pregnancy.

Pharmacological effects of iron

Medicinal iron enters the total body pool and, in patients with iron deficiency anemia, oral administration of iron preparations increases the rate of red cell production and rapidly improves the subjective symptoms. The correction of hemoglobin iron deficiency is accomplished with ease and efficiency by administering the greatest amount of iron that can be utilized. This amount is usually determined by the ability of the patient to tolerate the medication and by the absorptive capacity of the small intestine. The commonly accepted ceiling for iron absorption in a moderately severe anemia is about 150 mg of elemental iron per day. This requires the oral administration of at least twice that amount because of incomplete absorption. If this amount enters the erythroid marrow, the rate of red cell production will increase to two to three times normal. To replenish completely the depleted iron stores requires several more months of continued iron therapy after the anemia is corrected.

Adverse effects of oral iron preparations; drug interactions

These are localized mainly in the gastrointestinal system and are a result of physical intolerance. A dose–effect relationship has been shown for the incidence of nausea and upper abdominal pain, while the frequency of constipation and diarrhea is apparently unrelated to the size of dosage.

A potential drug interaction is the chelation of iron in the gastrointestinal tract. Tetracyclines, for example, are strong chelators of both iron and calcium (see Chapter 55). The absorption of tetracycline as well as of iron may be significantly impaired, and discontinuation of iron therapy may therefore be required during periods of oral medication with tetracycline antibiotics.

Toxicity

Acute effects from ingestion of toxic doses of iron (which may be any dose in excess of 1 g, usually about 5–10 g in fatal cases) appear in 30–60 minutes and consist of abdominal pain, nausea, vomiting, acidosis, and cardiovascular collapse, followed by coma and death if untreated. There is usually severe tissue damage to the gastrointestinal tract, the liver, and the kidneys, such as ulceration of the bowel, hepatic parenchymal cell necrosis, renal vascular congestion, and tubular degeneration. Treatment of this acute toxicity consists of rapid removal of the excess iron by gastric lavage and intravenous administration of iron-binding chelating agents (e.g., deferoxamine, see Chapter 74), symptomatic therapy of peripheral vascular collapse, and fluid and electrolyte replacement.

Chronic administration of iron to persons without

iron deficiency may eventually lead to hemochromatosis, a condition characterized by excessive iron accumulation in all iron storage sites and in liver and pancreas. Iron has a corrosive action and causes cell necrosis. The resulting damage to these organs takes the form of cirrhosis, fibrosis, and diabetes; skin pigmentation may also occur.

Iron compounds and therapeutic applications

Iron is usually administered orally as one of the iron salts. The oldest and most commonly prescribed form is **ferrous sulfate**, which also serves as the standard with which new iron preparations are compared. Other iron salts for oral administration, marketed under many trade names, are **ferrous ascorbate**, **ferrous fumarate**, **ferrous gluconate**, and **ferrous succinate**. Parenteral iron preparations are **iron dextran** (for deep intramuscular or intravenous administration) and **iron sorbitol** (to be used only intramuscularly).

Iron dosage must be calculated in terms of elemental iron rather than of the iron salt. Approximate elemental iron equivalents per 100 mg of the orally administered salts are:

ferrous fumarate	32 mg
ferrous gluconate	12 mg
ferrous succinate	35 mg
ferrous sulfate	20 mg

Average oral elemental iron requirements in deficient adults are, with great individual variations, about 100–150 mg/day (about 200–300 mg/day if allowance is made for incomplete absorption), which determines the size and frequency of dosage with the respective iron salts.

The dosage of parenterally administered iron must be calculated more precisely. For example, each gram of hemoglobin deficiency requires 150 mg of iron, and to this must be added 600 mg to replenish tissue stores. This total calculated dose is then divided into convenient daily doses and is given by injection over a period of 1–3 weeks.

Vitamin B$_{12}$ Deficiency Anemia

Defective gastrointestinal absorption of vitamin B$_{12}$ for very long periods of time (usually measured in years) will cause megaloblastosis (see Chapter 67). Megaloblastosis is the result of blocked DNA synthesis but continued RNA and protein synthesis in replicating cells and occurs throughout the gastrointestinal tract, the cervix and vagina, and the hematopoietic tissues. The bone marrow of vitamin B_{12}-deficient patients shows a proliferation of erythrocyte precursors, and in the peripheral blood a combination of macroovalocytes, hypersegmented polymorphonuclear leukocytes, and giant platelets is found. These macrocytes have an abnormally short lifespan, and the condition is appropriately named **megaloblastic** or **macrocytic anemia.** In addition, vitamin B_{12} deficiency may cause neurological problems from the inhibition of methylmalonyl-CoA mutase (for which vitamin B_{12} is a cofactor) and the consequent accumulation of abnormal fatty acids in myelin, which results in defective maintenance of the myelin sheath and consequent functional deficits in peripheral nerves and posterior or lateral columns of the spinal cord (Table 43-3). The basal metabolic rate is usually increased and hyperpigmentation of the skin may occur.

A familial, apparently immunologically based, abnormality of vitamin B_{12} absorption, historically named **pernicious anemia** or Addisonian anemia, may develop from lack of the gastric intrinsic factor first described by Castle. This is a glycoprotein which binds ingested vitamin B_{12} and protects it against destruction in the upper gastrointestinal tract, thus permitting its absorption from the ileum. However, even in the presence of intrinsic factor a number of intestinal diseases or defects can interfere with the absorption of the intrinsic factor–B_{12} complex. Gastric atrophy and gastric surgery are common causes.

Vitamin B_{12}, described in Chapter 67, is a cobalt-containing compound of rather complex structure; the term cyanocobalamin is accepted interchangeably with vitamin B_{12} as the name of the active compound in humans. All requirements are usually met by a normal diet, and about 1–2 μg/day will maintain balance if gastric secretions are normal. Cyanocobalamin is stored in the liver (up to 90% of total). These stores become depleted very slowly, and it takes years for the development of megaloblastosis (see also Chapter 67).

Cyanocobalamin (vitamin B_{12}) is available for both oral and parenteral administration. The only established therapeutic use is in the treatment of vitamin B_{12} deficiency. In pernicious anemia the preferred route of administration of cyanocobalamin is by subcutaneous or intramuscular injection in monthly doses of 60–100 μg, since oral preparations cannot be depended upon because of the patient's inability to absorb the vitamin. Preparations of cyanocobalamin are nontoxic.

Folic Acid Deficiency Anemia

Folic acid (folate; described in Chapter 67) is required as a cofactor for purine synthesis, pyrimidine nucleotide synthesis, and amino acid interconversions. It is an essential vitamin for humans, but in bacteria it must be synthesized from para-aminobenzoic acid (see Chapter 56). The biologically active form is the tetrahydro derivative, folinic acid, produced by the action of dihydrofolate reductase on folic acid following its absorption. (It is this step which makes folic acid vulnerable to the action of antibacterial and antineoplastic agents. See also Chapters 56 and 60.)

Folate deficiency results in **megaloblastic hematopoiesis** that is hematologically indistinguishable from that caused by vitamin B_{12}-deficiency. A striking clinical difference, however, is the absence of myelin damage, and its neurological consequences, in folic acid deficiency (see Table 43-3).

All physiological requirements for folic acid (about 200 μg/day in adults) are usually met by a normal diet (see also Chapter 67). However, in situations of inadequate diet for long periods of time, chronic alcoholism (i.e., interference with the intermediate metabolism of folic acid), vitamin C deficiency (i.e., inability to reduce folic acid to its metabolically active form, tetrahydrofolic acid), chronic liver disease, and intestinal malabsorption, a **macrocytic anemia** from folic acid deficiency may develop.

Total body stores of folic acid are about 5–10 mg, of which about half is found in the liver. The main therapeutic use of folic acid is in the treatment of folate deficiency. Other established and proposed uses are discussed in Chapters 60 and 67.

SOME OTHER DEFICIENCIES MANIFESTING AS ANEMIAS

Copper and Cobalt

Deficiencies in these metals are rare but can be produced experimentally. Copper deficiency has been described following extensive intestinal bypass surgery, in patients receiving parenteral nutrition, and in severely malnourished infants. A therapeutic trial with daily doses of 0.1 mg/kg of copper is indicated in identified copper deficiency.

Although primary cobalt deficiency has not been reported in humans, the metal may improve hematocrit, hemoglobin, and erythrocyte values in various types of refractory anemia not responding to conventional therapy.

Ascorbic Acid

Although quite rare, severe vitamin C deficiency may be associated with hypochromic anemia, which can be microcytic in conditions of chronic blood loss, or macrocytic when associated with folic acid deficiency.

Pyridoxine

Pyridoxine, one of the three forms of vitamin B_6, produces a beneficial hemoglobin response in individuals suffering from a form of sideroblastic anemia that is characterized by abnormally large amounts of nonhemoglobin iron in erythrocyte precursors, hypochromic microcytic anemia, and other signs of severely disturbed blood regeneration. This pyridoxine-responsive anemia occurs sporadically in adult males as a possible familial condition; it is not due to nutritional pyridoxine deficiency. Pyridoxine therapy is thought to compensate for other unknown deficiencies in enzymes involved in normal hemoglobin synthesis (see also Chapter 67).

ERYTHROPOIETIN

Hematopoietic processes for all blood cell lines depend on the presence of various growth factors that stimulate proliferation, differentiation, and maturation of precursor stem cells. An important factor that is responsible for the regulation and modulation of erythropoiesis during the early stages of erythrocyte development is a substance known as erythropoietin, which attaches to erythropoietin receptors (EPO-R) on the stem cell's outer membrane. Almost all (90%) of this glycoprotein is synthesized in renal cortical cells. The remainder is synthesized in the liver. Riboflavin (vitamin B_2) is necessary for its synthesis and function.

Erythropoietin synthesis is responsive to the varying demands of erythropoiesis. Renal synthesis is stimulated, and normally low plasma levels during periods of stable hematopoiesis are greatly elevated in the presence of hemorrhage, anemia, hemolysis, pregnancy—i.e., in conditions that result in hypoxia. Erythropoietin production is also promoted by conditions of increased tissue oxygen demand (e.g., ischemia, hyperthyroidism). The resultant actions of erythropoietin on colony-forming units of erythroid cell lines are demonstrated by increased release from the bone marrow of reticulocytes and erythrocytes.

Conversely, the maturation of multipotential stem cells into red blood cells is slowed or stopped by the binding of a recently identified down-regulating enzyme (SH-PTP1) to a specific site adjacent to stem cell EPO-R, which terminates signal transduction. This process of inhibition of erythropoietin action is recognized as a precise control mechanism that regulates the number of circulating red blood cells.

Erythropoietin deficiency, i.e., greatly reduced or absent renal synthesis resulting in diminished red blood cell production and extremely low hematocrit values, is a life-threatening complication of end-stage kidney disease.

The amino acid sequence of biologically active erythropoietin has been determined (166 amino acids, MW 35,000 Da), and the agent is produced commercially by recombinant DNA methods (Eprex) for intravenous or subcutaneous use. Its therapeutic value lies in the maintenance of near-normal erythropoiesis in patients requiring long-term hemodialysis, and as an adjunct in the treatment of anemias of complex origin, such as during cancer chemotherapy or the treatment of acquired immunodeficiency (AIDS).

Commercial human erythropoietin is nonallergenic. Adverse effects are related primarily to changes in blood viscosity and hemodynamics in response to rapidly rising red cell volumes.

SUGGESTED READING

Babior BM. The megaloblastic anemias. In: Williams WJ, Beutler E, Erslev AJ, Lichtman MA, eds. Hematology. 4th ed. New York: McGraw-Hill, 1990:453–481.

Bridges KR, Seligman PA. Disorders of iron metabolism. In: Handin RI, Lux SE, Stossel TP, eds. Blood: Principles and practice of hematology. Philadelphia: Lippincott, 1995:1433–1472.

Cooper BA, Rosenblatt DS. Disorders of cobalamin and folic acid metabolism. In: idem, 1399–1432.

Eckardt K-U, Bauer C. Erythropoietin in health and disease. Eur J Clin Invest 1989; 19:117–127.

Eschbach JW, Kelly MR, Haley NR, et al. Treatment of the anemia of progressive renal failure with recombinant human erythropoietin. N Engl J Med 1989; 321:158–162.

Fairbanks VF, Beutler E. Iron deficiency. In: Williams WJ, Beutler E, Erslev AJ, Lichtman MA, eds. Hematology. 4th ed. New York: McGraw-Hill, 1990:482–505.

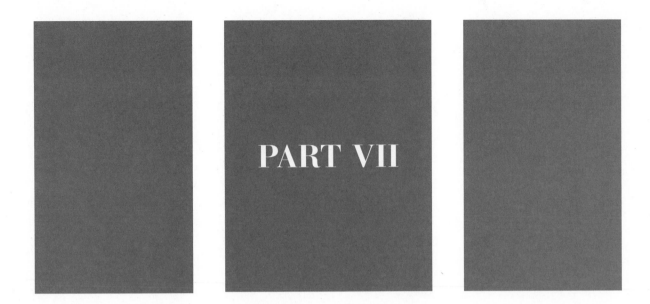

PART VII

GASTROINTESTINAL SYSTEM

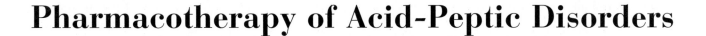

CHAPTER 44

Pharmacotherapy of Acid-Peptic Disorders

E.A. ROBERTS

CASE HISTORY

A 30-year-old man complained of dull epigastric pain that sometimes awakened him at night. In general, it did not extend through to his back or around either side. He said he could eat fatty foods without getting the pain, although he had avoided very spicy, hot foods for some time. Indeed, the pain was more likely to occur when he had not eaten recently, and eating sometimes made him feel better. He occasionally took a liquid antacid if it was handy, but he could not say that this actually helped. He denied having heartburn, water brash, dark tarry stools, or having vomited blood.

Physical examination revealed a muscular, well-nourished male. The abdomen was not distended, but there was epigastric tenderness on palpation. Laboratory tests were performed. The hemoglobin was somewhat low at 122 g/L and the platelet count was slightly elevated. Endoscopy of the stomach and duodenum showed a nodular gastritis and a 1-cm ulcer in the duodenal cap. Biopsies of the antrum were obtained for histology and culture.

The patient was started on ranitidine 300 mg at bedtime. He felt somewhat better. Several days later further laboratory data were available: the gastric biopsies were positive for *Helicobacter pylori*. Accordingly, the treatment was changed: The ranitidine was stopped, and triple therapy including an acid suppressor and antibiotics was substituted. Since the patient was allergic to penicillin, clarithromycin was substituted for amoxicillin. On the combination of omeprazole, clarithromycin, and metronidazole, the patient felt generally unwell and complained of persistent nausea. When he tried to drink some wine with dinner, he vomited. After 2 weeks, the treatment was stopped and he felt well.

Six months later, his dyspeptic symptoms returned. Endoscopy of the upper gastrointestinal tract was repeated, but the stomach and duodenum looked near normal. In particular, no ulcers were found. Gastric biopsies were taken and these proved positive again for *H. pylori*. Treatment was reinstituted with bismuth subsalicylate, clarithromycin and tetracycline. This was discontinued after 2 weeks, and his symptoms did not recur.

DISTURBANCES OF GASTROINTESTINAL FUNCTION

The gastrointestinal tract consists of four hollow viscera (esophagus, stomach, small intestine, and colon) and two solid organs (pancreas and liver). All of the hollow viscus organs contribute to digestion but have somewhat different functions. The pancreas produces enzymes and hormones. The liver has multiple functions that are not all related to digestion. For example, synthesis of albumin and other proteins occurs in the liver, as well as activation and detoxification of various chemicals, hormones, and drugs (see Chapter 46). Not only does the gastrointestinal tract consist of multiple disparate organs with diverse functions, but diseases of the gastrointestinal tract are also numerous and diverse. Apart from neoplasia and infections, the spectrum of disease includes ulcer formation in the upper gastrointestinal tract, inflammatory bowel disease, pancreatitis, abnormal intestinal motility, viral hepatitis, autoimmune liver disease, and inherited metabolic diseases, to name just a few.

Many different drugs are used to treat diseases of these organs. Corticosteroids, immunosuppressive drugs such as azathioprine, methotrexate, cyclosporine, antibiotics, and antivirals are discussed in other chapters, but it is important to recognize that these drugs are also used to treat gastrointestinal and hepatic diseases. The scope of this chapter is limited to drugs used mainly or exclusively in the treatment of gastrointestinal acid-peptic disorders. Nutritional treatments, including pancreatic enzyme supplements and vitamins, will not be discussed in this chapter.

DEVELOPMENT OF ACID-PEPTIC DISEASE

Acid-peptic disease can affect various organs in the GI tract including the esophagus, stomach, and duodenum. Although a bacterium, *H. pylori*, has recently been shown to cause duodenal ulcers and other types of acid-peptic disease, gastric acid plays a major role in the development of these problems, and suppression of acid production is an important element in their therapy. Gastric acid production reflects three stages of stimulation to the gastric parietal cell. (1) In the cephalic stage, the thought of eating initiates secretion by stimulation via the vagus nerve, acetylcholinergic neurons in the local nerve plexus, and M_1 muscarinic receptors in the parietal cell-membrane. (For a discussion of the various subtypes of muscarinic receptors see Chapters 13, 14, and 20.) (2) In the gastric phase, acid production is stimulated by gastrin, a polypeptide hormone released from specific cells in the antral mucosa in response to both mechanical and chemical stimuli generated by the presence of food in the stomach. The gastrin acts as a local hormone and is carried in the blood to the acid-secreting cells in the mucosa of the body of the stomach. (3) In the intestinal phase of gastric acid secretion, a small amount of gastrin is also secreted by the duodenal mucosa and carried in the blood to gastrin receptors on the parietal cell. The final common pathway for acid production is the proton pump on the parietal cell membrane, which is a unique $(H^+ + K^+)$-ATPase (Fig. 44-1). This is activated through the combined effects of acetylcholine acting on muscarinic receptors, histamine acting on H_2-receptors, and gastrin acting on the gastrin receptors, all located on the parietal cell surface. The receptor

activation leads to increases in concentration of various intracellular messengers including cAMP and calcium, which stimulate the ATPase activity. In the acidic gastric fluid, pepsinogen, which is secreted by gastric chief cells, is converted to pepsin at acid pH (0.8–3.5). Thus a secondary effect of decreased gastric acid production is decreased pepsin production. It is important to note that the stomach can employ multiple protective measures to guard against acid-induced injury—notably, the barrier created by gastric mucus and the mainly alkaline microenvironment along the gastric epithelium.

DRUGS FOR ACID-PEPTIC DISEASE

The general pharmacological approaches to treating acid-peptic disorders are directed at the various steps in the physiology of acid production. The main strategies include (1) use of antacids to neutralize acid already secreted in the stomach; (2) interference with the production of acid by blocking the histamine H_2-receptor (H_2-receptor blockers), the muscarinic receptor (pirenzepine), or the proton pump itself (omeprazole); (3) increase of mucosal defenses (prostaglandin analogs, sucralfate); and (4) eradication of *H. pylori* (bismuth plus antibiotics). Prostaglandin analogs also work in part by inhibiting acid formation (Fig. 44-1), and sucralfate may work by increasing local concentrations of prostaglandins. Colloidal bismuth subcitrate may also work by enhancing the trophic effects of epidermal growth factor on gastric mucosa.

Antacids

Antacids, the original drug treatment for acid-peptic disease, are still widely used. Bicarbonate of soda (sodium bicarbonate) is rarely used medically as an antacid, and sodium citrate has limited application, because they both can cause systemic alkalosis. The three categories of antacids in general use are those containing primarily calcium, magnesium, or aluminum salts. Calcium-containing antacids usually contain calcium carbonate. Magnesium hydroxide and magnesium trisilicate are the major magnesium salts used, and aluminum hydroxide and aluminum phosphate are the usual aluminum salts. The neutralizing chemical reaction with hydrochloric acid results in formation of calcium, magnesium, or aluminum chloride and water. Antacids vary in their buffering capacity and side effects.

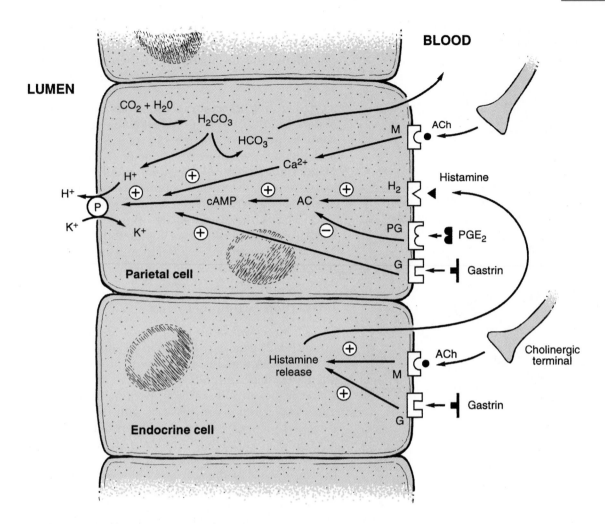

Figure 44-1. Schematic representation of control of acid secretion by the gastric parietal cell. Acetylcholine (ACh) and gastrin, acting on M_1 muscarinic (M) and gastrin (G) receptors, stimulate release of histamine by the endocrine cell. The parietal cell is then stimulated by the combined action of (1) ACh on M receptors to increase Ca^{2+}, (2) histamine on H_2-receptors to increase cAMP production by adenylyl cyclase (AC), and (3) gastrin acting on G receptors. All three increase activity of the $(H^+ + K^+)$-ATPase proton pump (P). PGE_2 decreases acid secretion by inhibiting AC.

Efficacy

The relative antacid strength of a number of liquid antacids was first quantified in terms of the acid-neutralizing capacity (ANC), defined as the amount of 0.1 N HCl (100 mEq H^+/L) that can be added to 1 ml of liquid antacid over a 2-hour period without lowering the pH below 3.0. This in vitro technique showed that antacids containing calcium carbonate are extremely effective, and those containing primarily aluminum hydroxide are very ineffective for neutralizing acid. The effectiveness of magnesium-containing antacids depends upon the particular combination and chemical formulation of the magnesium and other salts used (Table 44-1). The in vitro acid-neutralizing capacity may guide the choice and dosage of a particular antacid, but the effectiveness of an antacid in vivo also depends on other factors, including the presence of food or other buffers in the stomach and the rate of gastric emptying. The sodium content of antacids is important for patients with clinical conditions prone to sodium retention, because large quantities may be administered in a high-volume antacid regimen. The antacids that are

Table 44-1 In Vivo Neutralizing Capacity for Some Aluminum- and Magnesium-Containing Liquid Antacids

Antacid (Proprietary Name)	Capacity (mEq/L)	Volume for 80 mEq (mL)	Na⁺ in 80 mEq (mg)
Ducon	7.0	11.4	40.8
Mylanta II	4.1	19.3	30.9
Camalox	3.6	22.3	11.5
Aludrox	2.8	28.5	28.5
Maalox	2.6	31.0	34.7
Creamalin	2.6	31.1	18.7
Mylanta	2.4	33.6	26.2
Win Gel	2.2	35.6	8.8
Gelusil M	2.2	35.9	40.9
Riopan	2.2	36.2	5.1
Amphojel	1.9	41.4	49.7
A-M-T	1.8	44.7	53.6
Trisogel	1.6	43.5	155.2
Gelusil	1.3	60.1	85.6
Robalate	1.1	70.8	43.2
Phosphaljel	0.4	190.5	495.3

most commonly used currently are mixtures of mainly magnesium and some aluminum hydroxides, formulated to maximize potency and palatability.

Side-effects

Complications differ with each category of antacid. Antacids containing mainly calcium salts may cause *rebound acidity* through a mechanism involving release of gastrin, mediated by the increased intragastric calcium concentration released from the antacid. The clinical importance of this phenomenon (so-called "acid rebound"), however, is disputed. Chronic use of carbonate antacids together with large amounts of milk may also be associated with the *milk-alkali syndrome* (i.e., increased systemic absorption of calcium, possibly facilitated by a component of milk, leads to hypercalcemia, mild alkalosis, and calcific renal stone formation, which may cause chronic renal failure). The major problem with antacids containing mostly magnesium salts is *diarrhea*. In addition, up to 5% of magnesium may be absorbed and will accumulate when there is renal failure, since excretion of magnesium is mainly renal. Therefore, these antacids cannot be used in patients with renal insufficiency. Antacids containing exclusively alumi-

num hydroxide bind phosphates in the intestinal tract. In some patients this is useful for removing phosphate, but in other patients hypophosphatemia may develop. Absorption of aluminum may also be toxic.

Other side effects of these drugs are related to *disturbed intestinal motility.* Alkalinizing the gastric content increases both the rate of gastric emptying and the lower esophageal sphincter (LES) pressure. Magnesium enhances intestinal motility and may cause severe diarrhea. Aluminum-containing antacids relax gastric and intestinal smooth muscle by interfering with calcium fluxes, so motility is slowed. Gastric emptying may be so impaired that an antacid bezoar, a concretion of antacid and nonabsorbable food contents, forms in the stomach.

Interactions with other drugs

Drug interactions between antacids and other drugs (Table 44-2) generally lead to interference with drug absorption. Antacids are not inert. In most, but not all, cases these interactions lead to lower plasma concentrations of the drug in question. Antacids can affect absorption by interacting with the medication itself or by altering its rate of absorption as a result of change in gastric or intestinal pH. Antacids containing magnesium and/or aluminum salts reduce the absorption of digoxin and chlorpromazine from the gastrointestinal tract, in part by adsorption of the drug. In contrast, magnesium hydroxide can enhance absorption of dicumarol. Antacids interfere with tetracycline bioavailability by forming chelates with

Table 44-2 Important Drug Interactions With Antacids

Effect	Antacid Component	
	Al(OH)₃	Mg(OH)₂
Decreased drug level or action	Aspirin Chlordiazepoxide Chlorpromazine Isoniazid Propranolol Tetracycline Vitamin A	Aspirin Chlordiazepoxide Cimetidine Digoxin Tetracycline
Increased drug level or action	Levodopa Quinidine	Levodopa Quinidine Dicumarol Sulfonamides

tetracycline, but an increased gastric pH may also interfere with the dissolution of tetracycline tablets. Antacid-induced reduction in gastric emptying may influence the rate of absorption of isoniazid and cimetidine. Antacids may decrease glucocorticoid bioavailability. If enough antacid is taken, it may affect drug excretion by alkalinizing the urine. This will decrease the excretion of the basic drug quinidine, leading to toxic serum concentrations, but accelerate the excretion of acetylsalicylic acid.

Administration and dosage

Antacids should be taken 1 hour after a meal, again 2 hours after that if another meal is not forthcoming, and again at bedtime. This regimen takes advantage of the natural neutralizing effect of food. The usual dose of most liquid preparations (suspensions) is 30 ml, but for the newer high-potency antacids it is 10–15 ml, and with an average of six to seven doses daily this adds up to a large volume of antacid each day. Given the potential for developing diarrhea, especially with antacids containing high proportions of magnesium salts, and the inconvenience of taking a liquid medication, compliance can be imperfect. Antacid tablets may be as effective, and their convenience may increase compliance. The sodium content per dose of the major aluminum-plus-magnesium antacids is 4–7 mg/dose, in low-sodium antacids less than 1 mg/dose, and in aluminum hydroxide antacids as high as 20 or more mg/dose.

H₂-Blockers

H$_2$-blockers were developed specifically to be competitive inhibitors of the histamine H$_2$-receptor (see also Chapter 33). They are examples of "designer drugs" and chemically they resemble histamine. The major drugs of this class currently in use are cimetidine, ranitidine, famotidine, and nizatidine (Table 44-3, Fig. 44-2). Typically all these drugs inhibit basal and nocturnal gastric acid secretion, as well as gastric acid secretion provoked by administration of histamine, acetylcholine, or (penta)gastrin. They also decrease pepsin production. Cimetidine also affects the character of gastric mucus.

Cimetidine (Tagamet)

Structurally, cimetidine is very similar to histamine, with a substituted imidazole ring (Fig. 44-2). Cimetidine is almost 100% absorbed after oral administration, but a comparatively large hepatic first-pass effect results in systemic bioavailability of only 60–70%. After intravenous administration, the elimination half-life is about 2 hours in adults. Urinary excretion is fairly rapid, and 60–70% of the absorbed cimetidine is excreted unchanged. Given this extensive renal excretion, dosage must be modified when there is renal impairment. Dose adjustment is not needed in patients with liver disease except when liver failure occurs. Cimetidine is a potent inhibitor of cytochrome P450; this property underlies many of its drug interactions (see below).

Ranitidine (Zantac)

Ranitidine has a furan ring where cimetidine has the imidazole group (Fig. 44-2). Originally, the imidazole group was thought to be essential for the H$_2$-blocking function, but in fact ranitidine is a stronger blocker of histamine H$_2$-receptors than is cimetidine. At equal doses, ranitidine has between four and nine times more effect than cimetidine in suppressing gastric acid secretion, and on a molar basis it appears to be five to 12 times more potent, depending on the

Table 44-3 Pharmacokinetic and Other Features of Major H₂-Receptor Blockers

	Cimetidine	*Ranitidine*	*Famotidine*	*Nizatidine*
Ring	Imidazole	Furan	Thiazole	Thiazole
Bioavailability	60–70%	50%	40–50%	90%
Elimination $t^{1/2}$	2–2.5 hours	2.5–3 hours	3–3.5 hours	1–1.5 hours
Excretion	Renal	Renal	Renal	Renal
Adverse effects	Many	Few	Few	Few
Drug interactions	Many	Few	None	None
Dose (once daily)	800 mg	300mg	40mg	300 mg

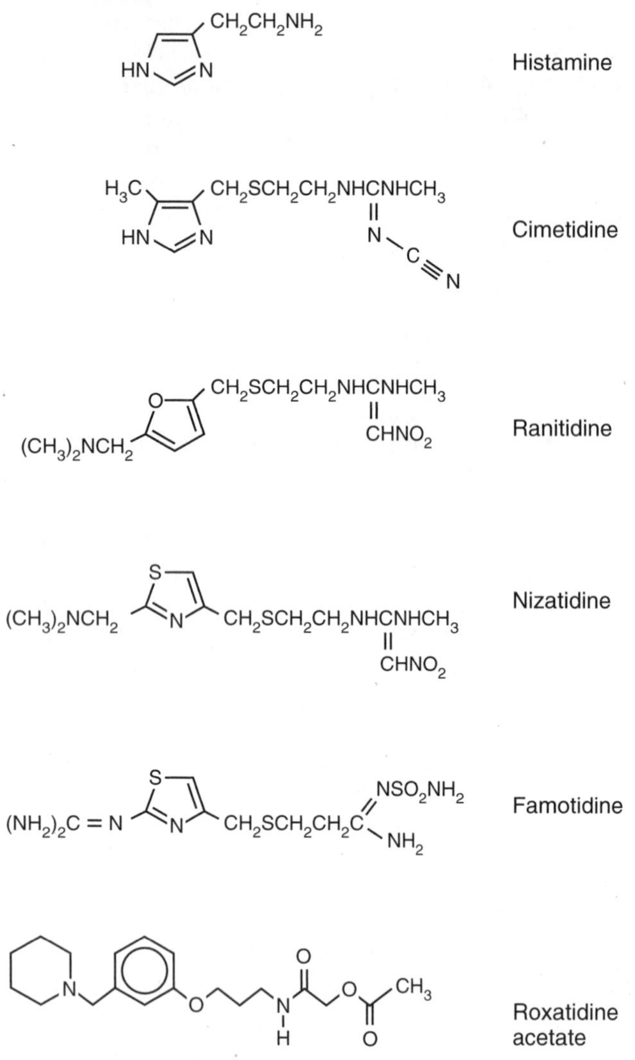

Figure 44-2. Structural formulae of histamine and a number of H$_2$-receptor blockers (see also Chapter 33.)

test secretagogue. However, the duration of action of ranitidine seems to be comparable to that of cimetidine.

The pharmacokinetic characteristics of ranitidine are similar to those of cimetidine. In adults there is a considerable first-pass effect after oral administration, and systemic bioavailability is approximately 50%. The elimination half-life of ranitidine after parenteral administration is 2–2.5 hours. Most of the drug (50–70%) is excreted in the urine unchanged.

Famotidine (Pepcid)

Famotidine (Fig. 44-2) is noteworthy because it is very potent and has prolonged action due to its guanidinothiazole ring, which gives it much greater affinity for the H$_2$-receptor. Its bioavailability is approximately 40–50% (less than that of the other drugs in this group), and its plasma excretion half-life is longer (3–3.5 hours).

Nizatidine (Axid)

Nizatidine has a thiazole ring in place of the furan ring of ranitidine (Fig. 44-2). In many respects nizatidine is similar to ranitidine, but nizatidine has a much higher bioavailability in adults (>90%). However, its elimination half-life is shorter than that of cimetidine, ranitidine, or famotidine. It does not inhibit cytochromes P450.

Roxatidine (Roxit)

Roxatidine (Fig. 44-2) is administered as the prodrug roxatidine acetate, which must be deacetylated by small intestinal or hepatic esterases to the active drug. It has a high bioavailability. Its elimination half-life is 1–3 hours, depending on how it is formulated. Roxatidine does not interact with hepatic cytochromes P450. It has been tested mainly in Europe.

Side effects

A problem with long-term cimetidine treatment is the high incidence of side effects. Common side effects include elevated serum creatinine or aminotransferases during treatment. Central nervous system syndromes occur: Confusion is the principal problem, especially in the elderly, but it may also occur in children. Cimetidine has an antiandrogen effect due to displacement of dihydrotestosterone from androgen binding sites. This competitive inhibition is reflected by increased basal level of serum testosterone. Impotence and gynecomastia have developed in some adult male patients. Cimetidine may cause increased serum prolactin, although only after a large bolus dose.

By contrast, ranitidine and famotidine have fewer side effects. Common side effects of ranitidine are relatively trivial, including skin rash, headache, and dizziness. Ranitidine hardly penetrates into the central nervous system, and therefore side effects such as confusion are infrequent. Ranitidine does not appear to exert antiandrogenic effects; reported frequencies of gynecomastia or impotence are low. Famotidine is relatively free of side effects despite its high potency.

Drug interactions

Adverse drug interactions with drugs biotransformed via cytochromes P450 are common with cimetidine. This is due to a direct binding of cimetidine to cytochromes P450, probably because of its imidazole group. These drug interactions may be clinically important when the drug involved itself has a narrow therapeutic index, such as theophylline. Clinical studies have shown that cimetidine inhibits the biotransformation of warfarin, phenytoin, diazepam, and theophylline (Table 44-4). Although ranitidine appears to interact with some species of cytochromes P450, it causes little interference with hepatic microsomal drug metabolism. No disturbance of metabolism of the probe drugs such as theophylline, warfarin, or antipyrine has been found, but recently some clinically significant interactions with theophylline have been reported. Famotidine does not interfere with cytochromes P450.

Therapeutic uses

H_2-receptor blockers are very effective treatment for reflux esophagitis and for duodenal and gastric ulcers. The recurrence rate in these latter conditions, however, is high when the drug is stopped. Smaller maintenance doses are customarily used. They can be used for prophylaxis against stress ulceration in acutely ill patients with head trauma or compromised respiration. In high doses they are suitable for treatment of Zollinger-Ellison syndrome (gastrinoma). H_2-receptor blockers are also prescribed to prevent gastrointestinal complications induced by long-term use of anti-inflammatory analgesics (see Chapter 34).

Table 44-4 Drug Interactions with H_2-Receptor Blockers

Drug	Cimetidine	Ranitidine	Famotidine
Theophylline	Yes	No	No
Warfarin	Yes	?	No
Phenytoin	Yes	?	No
Propranolol	?	No	No
Diazepam	Yes	No	No
Lidocaine	Yes	No	No

? = uncertain.

Pirenzepine

Classic anticholinergics such as atropine and propantheline are not used for gastric acid suppression because of their adverse side effects. Pirenzepine (Fig. 44-3) is a complex tricyclic compound, chemically related to tricyclic antidepressants, which selectively inhibits postganglionic M_1 muscarinic receptors. It thus reduces both acid and pepsin secretion and can act synergistically with H_2-blockers. Additionally, it may have mucosal protective properties.

After oral administration, bioavailability is comparatively poor—only 25% of the drug is absorbed. Peak plasma concentrations are found approximately 4 hours after administration; little (12%) is protein-bound. The elimination half-life is 11 hours. Most of the drug is excreted unchanged in the urine, as there is little hepatic metabolism.

Pirenzepine appears free of major side effects. Many patients develop some degree of dry mouth. Intestinal motility, apart from gastric emptying, is not affected. Pirenzepine is quite hydrophilic and does not cross the blood–brain barrier.

Pirenzepine can be used as effective treatment for peptic ulcer disease and may have a role in prophylaxis against stress ulceration; however, actual clinical use of this drug has been limited.

Omeprazole

Mechanism of action

This substituted benzimidazole (Fig. 44-4) is important because of its novel mode of action: It blocks the proton pump, the $(H^+ + K^+)$-ATPase, on the parietal cell membrane. It is extremely potent, because in the highly acidic milieu around the proton pump this drug becomes protonated and undergoes molecular rearrangement to highly reactive deriva-

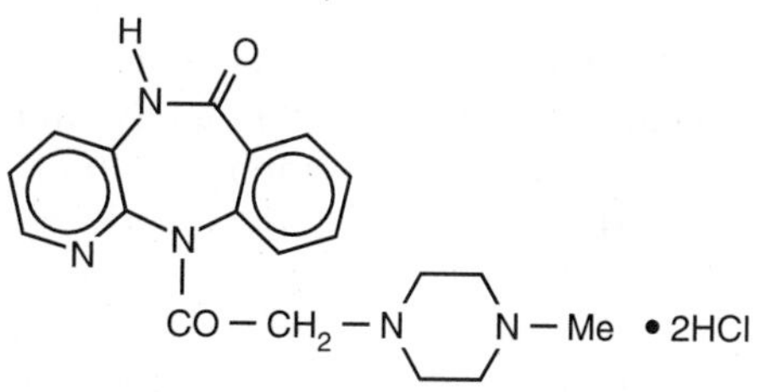

Figure 44-3. Structural formula of pirenzepine dihydrochloride (Gastrozepin), an anticholinergic agent related to the tricyclic antidepressants.

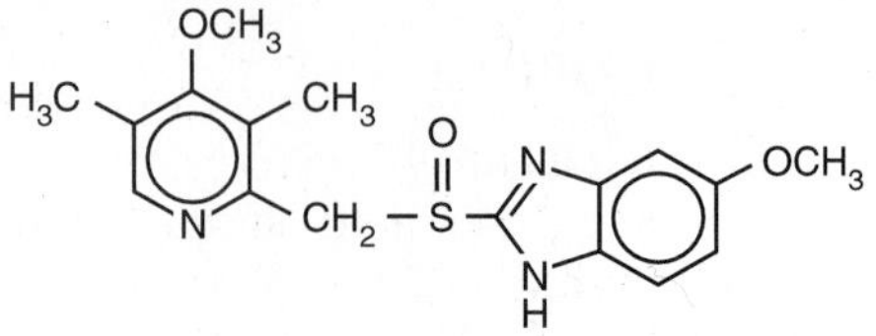

Figure 44-4. Structural formula of omeprazole (Losec).

tives that bind irreversibly to the ATPase. Thus omeprazole effectively blocks both basal and stimulated gastric acid secretion.

Pharmacokinetics

Omeprazole is well absorbed but has to be protected from degradation by gastric acid. Bioavailability improves after a few days of treatment, presumably because gastric acid production declines. It is highly (95%) protein-bound. It undergoes extensive biotransformation in the liver, and virtually no unchanged drug is found in the urine. Its serum half-life in adults is approximately 1 hour (range 0.27–2.52 hours), but its duration of action is considerably longer (approximately 24 hours). This is due to irreversible binding to its target. Its pharmacokinetics are not affected by renal failure or hemodialysis.

Therapeutic uses

Omeprazole is even more effective than the H_2-blockers for treating acid-peptic disease. It may be curative in cases of peptic ulcer disease that do not respond to H_2-blockers. In severe reflux esophagitis omeprazole has a success rate for healing of approximately 80%, compared to approximately 60% for H_2-blockers. Relapse after stopping treatment occurs at about the same rate as with H_2-blockers.

Adverse effects

Omeprazole has potentially serious adverse side effects. It abolishes acid production so completely that serum gastrin levels rise. In rodents enterochromaffin-like cell tumors and carcinoid tumors have developed. It is not known whether this drug is carcinogenic in humans by a similar mechanism. Moreover, bacterial overgrowth may develop in the stomach in the absence of acid. Bacterial metabolism of dietary nitrites may then lead to production of N-nitroso compounds that are carcinogenic. This risk is not limited to chronic omeprazole treatment; it can theoretically occur with any effective long-term antacid regimen. Moreover, omeprazole appears to affect the cytochromes P450. Although initial studies suggested an inhibitory effect, more recent studies indicate that omeprazole may induce the cytochrome P450 1A subfamily that is associated with activation of certain chemical procarcinogens, such as polycyclic aromatic hydrocarbons.

In clinical practice, however, omeprazole is well tolerated and has a low frequency of minor side effects, of which the most common are gastrointestinal upset, tiredness, dizziness, headache, and skin rashes. Nevertheless, the safety of prolonged chronic use remains uncertain.

Mucosal Protectors

Drugs that increase mucosal defenses, independently of any effect on acid secretion, represent an important complement to treating acid-peptic disease by removing or neutralizing gastric acid. The major drugs that act as mucosal protectors are prostaglandin E analogs and sucralfate.

Prostaglandin E analogs (misoprostol, enprostil, arbaprostil; see also Chapter 31) are used as mucosal protectors although it is evident that they have multiple actions. Several modes of action that result in "mucosal protection" are increased bicarbonate secretion, increased mucus secretion, increased mucosal blood flow, and enhanced epithelial regeneration. With respect to inhibition of gastric acid production, prostaglandin analogs bind to a specific receptor on the parietal cell (not the histamine H_2-receptor) and prevent activation of adenylyl cyclase by histamine (Fig. 44-1). They also inhibit release of gastrin by gastrin-producing cells.

Of the various prostaglandin analogs available, misoprostol is the only one in common use. It is absorbed rapidly after oral administration, is highly (85%) protein-bound, undergoes some hepatic biotransformation, and is mostly excreted via the kidneys. Its elimination half-life is 1.5 hours. Major side effects are diarrhea and intestinal cramps. It increases uterine contractility and may cause uterine bleeding or loss of pregnancy; this limits its use in women of child-bearing potential. Although as effective as cimetidine for ulcer healing, misoprostol is less effective than ranitidine and may provide little immediate symptomatic relief. The main indication for misoprostol is as prophylaxis against gastritis due to nonsteroidal anti-inflammatory drugs.

Sucralfate is a complex basic salt of sucrose sulfate and aluminum hydroxide (Fig. 44-5). It polymerizes to form a paste (a viscous polyanionic gel with a strong negative charge) that adheres selectively to ulcerated areas in the mucosa. Its mucosal protective effect may be due in part to enhanced local prostaglandin action as a result of increased mucosal cyclooxygenase activity and increased release of prostaglandins directly from the mucosa by mechanisms involving aluminum and/or epidermal growth factor. However, its other possible modes of action include (1) inactivating pepsin, (2) providing a physical barrier over the ulcerated area, (3) changing the composition of gastric mucus, and (4) increasing bicarbonate output from the gastric mucosa (by both prostaglandin-dependent and prostaglandin-independent mechanisms). Trophic effects involving epidermal growth factor and/or fibroblast growth factor (which it binds to gastric tissue) and increased mucosal blood flow may also be critically important. Sucralfate does not affect gastric acidity and it has no antibacterial action.

Sucralfate is effective in various sorts of acid-peptic disease and has few side effects. Constipation may occur. It blocks the absorption of some drugs including warfarin, digoxin, and phenytoin, and these drugs should not be taken at the same time as sucralfate. It should not be used simultaneously with fluoroquinolone antimicrobial agents, because it greatly reduces their effectiveness. Although there is little convincing evidence of short-term absorption of aluminum, aluminum accumulation associated with prolonged chronic use of sucralfate may turn out to have clinically important adverse side effects. In summary, sucralfate is an effective medication but its unique place among antacid treatments is still being determined.

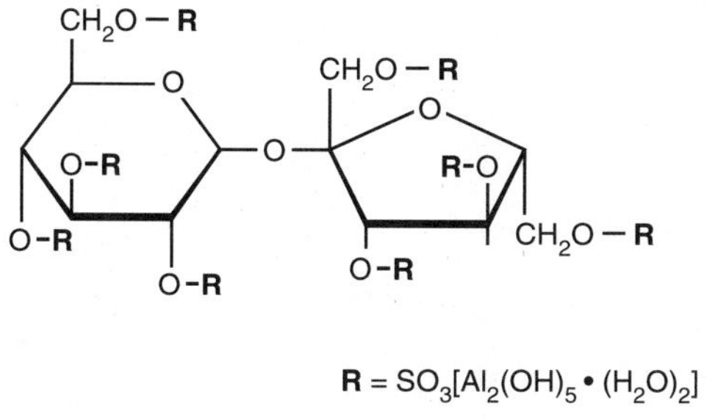

$$R = SO_3[Al_2(OH)_5 \bullet (H_2O)_2]$$

Figure 44-5. Chemical structure of the basic unit of sucralfate (Sulcrate).

Agents Targeting H. pylori

The role of *H. pylori* bacterial infection in causing acid-peptic disease has been appreciated only recently. As a result antibacterial agents are now used in the treatment of this condition. Agents containing bismuth, colloidal bismuth subcitrate (CBS, De-Nol), and colloidal bismuth subsalicylate (BSS, Pepto-bismol) appear to be intrinsically bactericidal to *H. pylori*.

Colloidal bismuth subcitrate is a complex of bismuth and citric acid that precipitates preferentially in eroded mucosa to form a glycoprotein–bismuth complex. This has mucosal protective properties and fosters healing much in the same way as sucralfate. Pepsin production is decreased. In addition to being bactericidal to *H. pylori*, CBS counteracts the adverse effects of *H. pylori* on gastric mucus by inhibiting bacterial proteolytic enzyme activity.

CBS appears to remain largely in the intestinal tract, exerting only local effects. Little of the bismuth in CBS is soluble, and only minimal amounts are absorbed in normal individuals, even with chronic administration. Any bismuth that is absorbed is excreted in the urine, and thus patients with renal insufficiency may be at risk of bismuth accumulation. Most of the bismuth in CBS is excreted in feces as bismuth sulfide.

Colloidal bismuth subsalicylate (BSS) contains nearly equal amounts of bismuth and salicylate per milliliter of liquid preparation. In the stomach at pH < 3.5, BSS reacts with hydrochloric acid to form bismuth oxychloride and salicylic acid. Very little (<1%) of the bismuth is absorbed, but most of the salicylic acid is absorbed. In the small intestine, BSS, bismuth oxychloride, and other bismuth salts react with hydrogen sulfide to form bismuth sulfide, which turns the stool a dark, nearly black color.

Little is known about adverse effects due to bismuth compounds. A single case of toxic encephalopathy after prolonged chronic use has been reported with CBS. Reye's syndrome, a theoretical risk with BSS, has not been reported. Less-severe side effects, such as bad taste, blackening of the tongue, mild tinnitus, and constipation, are common. CBS may impair absorption of tetracycline, iron, and calcium.

These drugs are effective in acid-peptic disease associated with *H. pylori* infection. Resolution of disease will not occur without eradication of the bacterial infection. Current regimens include a bismuth compound and one or more antibiotics, of which the most frequently used are a tetracycline, metronidazole, amoxicillin, and clarithromycin (see Chapters 53, 55, 57).

SUGGESTED READING

Ching CK, Lam SK. Antacids: indications and limitations. Drugs 1994; 47:305–317.

Grant SM, Langtry HD, Brogden RN. Ranitidine. An updated review of its pharmacodynamic and pharmacokinetic properties and therapeutic use in peptic ulcer disease and other allied diseases. Drugs 1989; 37:801–870.

Hawkey CJ, Rampton DS. Prostaglandins and the gastrointestinal mucosa: are they important in its function, disease, or treatment? Gastroenterology 1985; 89:1162–1188.

Howard JM, Chemros AN, Collen MJ et al. Famotidine, a new potent, long-lasting histamine H_2-receptor antagonist: comparison with cimetidine and ranitidine in the treatment of Zollinger-Ellison syndrome. Gastroenterology 1985; 88:1026–1033.

Jensen SL, Funch Jensen P. Role of sucralfate in peptic disease. Dig Dis 1992; 10:153–161.

Mahachai V, Walker K, Thomson ABR. Comparison of cimetidine and ranitidine on 24-hour intragastric acidity and serum gastrin profile in patients with esophagitis. Dig Dis Sci 1985; 30:321–328.

Maton PN. Omeprazole. N Engl J Med 1991; 324:965–975.

Rost KL, Brosicke H, Heinemeyer G, Roots I. Specific and dose-dependent enzyme induction by omeprazole in human beings. Hepatology 1994; 20:1204–1212.

Somogyi A, Gugler R. Drug interactions with cimetidine. Clin Pharmacokinet 1982; 7:23–41.

Walsh JH, Peterson WL. The treatment of Helicobacter pylori infection in the management of peptic ulcer disease. N Engl J Med 1995; 333:984–991.

Walt RP. Misoprostol for the treatment of peptic ulcer and antiinflammatory-drug-induced gastroduodenal ulceration. N Engl J Med 1992; 327:1575–1580.

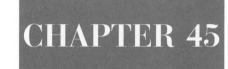
Drugs Used in the Treatment of Intestinal Motility Disorders and Inflammatory Disease

E.A. ROBERTS

CASE HISTORY

A 10-year-old boy presented with a 6-week history of bloody diarrhea, crampy lower abdominal pain, and a 5-kg weight loss. Previously he had been entirely well and had enjoyed a trip to Mexico a few months earlier. He described having to get up at night because of the diarrhea, and in the course of a single day, he would have 10–15 small bowel movements, which were mainly blood. He looked pale and chronically ill. On examination the abdomen was scaphoid and diffusely tender, but there were no masses and there was no rebound tenderness.

The child was hospitalized and treated with total parenteral nutrition. Examination of the stool revealed abundant leukocytes in it. Cultures for enteric pathogens including *Clostridium difficile* were negative; *Entamoeba histolytica* was not found on examination of the stool for ova and parasites. Colonoscopy revealed friable mucosa and confluent ulceration throughout the colon; colonic mucosal biopsies were consistent with ulcerative colitis. The patient was started on oral prednisone. The diarrhea resolved over the next 2–3 weeks, and the prednisone was then tapered off slowly. Sulfasalazine was begun incrementally; nevertheless, the patient developed headaches transiently. Eventually the prednisone was stopped altogether, and he was maintained asymptomatically on only sulfasalazine.

Some months later the boy developed fever, chills and cough. Chest X-ray showed a right lower lobe infiltrate. He was treated for community-acquired pneumonia with amoxicillin. After 4 days of treatment he developed bloody diarrhea again despite taking his sulfasalazine regularly.

He was switched to olsalazine but did not improve. Finally he was given 5-aminosalicylic acid in enteric release form, and his diarrhea resolved. When treatment with amoxicillin was completed, he continued taking the pure 5-aminosalicylic acid. Later he tried taking sulfasalazine and found that it was once again effective in controlling his symptoms.

DRUGS AFFECTING GASTROINTESTINAL MOTILITY

The physiology of GI-tract motility is currently an area of intensive research. The GI tract has smooth muscle with intrinsic and variable contractions. There are sphincter-like structures at the gastro-esophageal junction, the pylorus, and the ileocolonic junction. The various contractile functions should normally be smoothly coordinated throughout the gastrointestinal tract so that the contents are moved along as on a well-regulated conveyor belt. Muscular

561

Table 45-1 Prokinetic Agents

	Metoclopramide	Domperidone	Cisapride
Structure	Benzamide class	Benzimidazole class	Benzamide class
Mechanism	Antidopaminergic (central and peripheral) Augments ACh release	Antidopaminergic (peripheral) No cholinergic activity	Augments ACh release in myenteric plexus
Lower esophageal sphincter tone	Increase	Increase	Increase
Gastric motility	Increase	Increase	Increase
Intestinal motility	? Increase small bowel	No effect	Increase throughout
Side effects	Many	Few	Occasional

propulsive activity should also change with swallowing or with ingestion of food. Nervous system control of the enteric smooth muscle accounts for some of this adjustment. Hormonal factors also affect GI-tract motility. Motilin, a gastrointestinal hormone acting on specific motilin receptors in the enteric nerve plexuses, helps to initiate the "major migrating complexes" in the proximal bowel. Other external factors sometimes play a role, e.g., osmotic retention of excessive fluid in the lumen, due to nonabsorbable salts such as magnesium.

This section of the chapter deals with several types of drug used to correct or relieve the consequences of disturbed contractile function. Drugs affecting GI-tract motility include the so-called prokinetic agents, laxatives and antidiarrheals.

PROKINETIC AGENTS

Metoclopramide, domperidone, and cisapride (Table 45-1) are the major prokinetic agents that work by affecting neural control of enteric smooth-muscle activity. A simplified version of this mechanism is shown in Figure 45-1. Enteric nerve plexuses operate by release of acetylcholine. Dopamine antagonizes their action. Thus a prokinetic drug may work by enhancing the cholinergic effect directly (i.e., as a cholinergic agonist) or indirectly (either by enhancing acetylcholine release or by sensitizing the muscarinic receptors of the enteric smooth muscle so that the threshold for acetylcholine action is lower), or by interfering with the action of dopamine (i.e., as a dopamine antagonist). The overall outcome on

smooth-muscle activity varies from species to species and may vary somewhat from one part to another of the human GI tract.

Metoclopramide (Reglan)

This is a derivative of procainamide and is a central dopaminergic (D_2-receptor) and serotonergic (5-HT_3-receptor) antagonist. The structure of metoclopramide is shown in Figure 14-6. Its **mechanism of action** is complicated. It appears to enhance coordinated transmission in cholinergic nerve plexuses that finally release acetylcholine at muscarinic M_2-receptors on the muscle cells, since its effect is abolished by atropine. It may also sensitize muscarinic receptors on the smooth muscle of the upper gastrointestinal tract so that there is a lower threshold for acetylcholine and histamine action. Since it is a dopaminergic neuron antagonist in the central nervous system, it may possibly also have a direct influence on dopaminergic or other innervation of gastrointestinal smooth muscle.

In the upper gastrointestinal tract, metoclopramide causes a dose-related rise in the lower esophageal sphincter (LES) pressure (tone). It increases the amplitude of peristaltic contractions in the esophagus, slightly increases their duration and speed of propagation, but does not disturb synchrony of contractions. It does not interfere with LES relaxation in the course of swallowing. It also does not influence gastric acid secretion. Metoclopramide increases gastric emptying in most people. It also has a good antiemetic effect arising from its central D_2- and 5-HT_3-blocking actions.

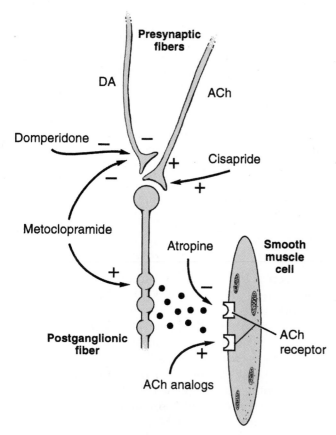

Figure 45-1. Mechanisms of action of prokinetic agents. Acetylcholine (ACh, top) stimulates postganglionic fiber to release more ACh, which acts on an ACh receptor on a smooth-muscle cell. *Atropine blocks* the ACh receptor on a muscle cell; *ACh analogs stimulate* the receptor on muscle cell. Dopamine (DA, top) *inhibits* release of ACh by presynaptic ACh fiber; *cisapride stimulates* release of ACh. Domperidone and metoclopramide block the effect of DA on preganglionic ACh release. (Adapted from Reynolds JC, 1989).

Pharmacokinetics

Metoclopramide is rapidly absorbed after oral administration. Its excretion is predominantly renal, partly as the unchanged drug and partly as the sulfate or glucuronide. Its elimination half-life is 4–6 hours. It is not highly bound to plasma proteins, and it crosses the blood–brain barrier easily.

Adverse effects

Metoclopramide has adverse side effects such as fatigue, dizziness, faintness, and various extrapyramidal syndromes caused by its central antidopaminergic activity (Table 45-2). Increased irritability may be an important side effect in infants because the drug may aggravate gastroesophageal reflux. In children, the major extrapyramidal syndrome is an oculogyric crisis with torticollis and neck pain. Children who develop phenothiazine-induced oculogyric crisis may be more prone to this with metoclopramide. Phenothiazines, monoamine oxidase inhibitors, tricyclic antidepressants, and sympathomimetic drugs should not be given along with metoclopramide. With chronic use, metoclopramide may also cause increased serum prolactin levels in adults, which may result in gynecomastia. Because it accelerates gastric emptying, it may increase the rate of absorption of some drugs.

Domperidone (Motilium)

This benzimidazole derivative is a peripheral dopamine antagonist. The structure of domperidone is shown in Figure 28-8. It has no procholinergic effects. It is also effective in reducing gastroesophageal reflux, and it increases gastric emptying. Unlike metoclopramide, domperidone has few side effects. It is thought to be well tolerated mainly because the quaternary N does not permit it to cross the blood–brain barrier as readily as metoclopramide. Dystonic

Table 45-2 Estimated Frequency of Side Effects With Metoclopramide

Side Effects	Patients (%)
Central nervous system	
Drowsiness, lethargy	4–10%
Dizziness, faintness	1–6%
Dystonic reactions	1%
↑ Prolactin secretion, galactorrhea	Occasional
Anxiety, agitation	Rare
GI tract	
Diarrhea, constipation, abdominal cramps	1%
Others	
Rashes	<1%
Oropharyngeal edema	Rare
Hypertensive crisis with pheochromocytoma	3 cases
Cardiac arrhythmia	Occasional

symptoms are rare; however, it may be associated with elevated serum prolactin, occasionally resulting in galactorrhea and menstrual irregularities.

Cisapride (Propulsid; in Canada, Prepulsid)

This drug is not an antidopaminergic. It releases acetylcholine in the myenteric plexus by an indirect effect, apparently via an action on enteric serotonin 5-HT_4-receptors. It increases LES pressure and increases motility in the stomach, small intestine, and colon. These effects, like those of metoclopramide, can be blocked by atropine. It may also affect the motility of the biliary tree.

Pharmacokinetics

Cisapride is absorbed rapidly after oral administration but undergoes extensive first-pass biotransformation so only 40–50% of the dose is available. Absorption is impaired by coadministration of antacids or H_2-blockers. It is extensively biotransformed in the liver, via N-dealkylation and aromatic hydroxylation; dose modifications may be required in patients with severe liver disease. It is largely bound to plasma proteins and has an elimination half-life of approximately 10 hours in healthy adults. It is excreted in both the urine and the feces and is secreted into breast milk.

Adverse effects

Cisapride appears to be well tolerated by most patients. The major side effect is diarrhea, but dizziness, headache, vomiting, and rhinitis have also been reported. Since it is not antidopaminergic, it does not cause abnormal movement disorders. It is susceptible to drug interactions associated with changes in the absorption of certain drugs, including enhanced absorption of diazepam.

Cisapride is effective in treating esophageal reflux and certain severe intestinal motility disorders presenting as intestinal pseudo-obstruction in children and adults. Cisapride improves intestinal function in children with cystic fibrosis and distal intestinal obstruction syndrome. In adults it has been shown to promote gastric emptying in patients with dyspepsia, or with gastric motility disorders such as those associated with diabetes or scleroderma.

Bethanechol

This direct muscarinic cholinergic agonist can be used to treat esophageal and intestinal motility disorders. However, its efficacy is questionable, at least in children. It has important contraindications, including esophageal stricture and asthma; these make it a poor candidate for treatment of adults. Its adverse effects are due to the nonselectivity of its action in increasing parasympathetic tone. Among the frequent side effects are abdominal cramps, diarrhea, increased salivation, flushing, bradycardia, and blurred vision.

Macrolides

Erythromycin, a macrolide antibiotic, is representative of a new group of prokinetic agents that appear to work mainly through a unique mechanism. It increases gastrointestinal contractility mainly by acting as an agonist at the motilin receptor, for which it is a competitive ligand. It may also act at the neuromuscular junction. Current research is aimed at developing macrolides with predominantly prokinetic activity and little antibiotic effect.

Erythromycin increases LES pressure and enhances esophageal contractility. It speeds gastric emptying and improves the coordination of antral and duodenal contractions. It appears to increase contractility of the gallbladder. In the colon, it induces major migrating complexes as motilin does. Its main clinical use is in enhancing gastric emptying. It also can be used to treat constipation due to abnormal colonic motility, but it works best if there is some vestige of major migrating complexes prior to treatment. It is clinically ineffective for treating disorders of esophageal motility.

Adverse reactions to erythromycin include rare but well-documented cases of hepatotoxicity. There is, at least theoretically, a risk of selecting resistant bacterial strains with prolonged use. Tachyphylaxis develops for this and other prokinetic drugs. Since erythromycin is metabolized via CYP3A4, interactions with other drug substrates for CYP3A4 are possible.

LAXATIVES

Laxatives can be considered prokinetic agents for the colon. Indeed, certain prokinetic agents enhance colonic motility. However, laxative action of this class of drugs is somewhat more complicated than simply affecting motility because these drugs lead to increased water content in the stool. Laxatives may promote colonic secretion of water by indirect or irritative effects or by modifying cellular processes for sodium and water secretion (Table 45-3). They may increase the excretion of water in the stool by either osmotic or bulk action. Certain laxatives retain water and block its colonic absorption. Colonic distension by hydrated luminal contents may then enhance colonic motility.

The average diet should contain sufficient nonabsorbable fiber to ensure regular bowel action. The average healthy person should not need or use chemical laxatives to obtain a daily bowel movement. Laxatives should not be given to anyone with abdominal pain because they may aggravate an undiagnosed bowel obstruction. Chronic routine use of chemical laxatives can lead to hypokalemia and to structural changes in the colon that result in hypomotility. In contrast, patients with pseudo-obstruction syndromes may require multiple prokinetics to maximize colonic motility.

Laxatives That Increase Secretion

Anthraquinones

Anthraquinones are found in the leaves, roots, or seed pods of various plants, such as aloe, cascara, and rhubarb, and they are present as glycosides as well as in the free forms. The glycoside conjugates are absorbed only after hydrolysis, yielding the free anthraquinone and glucose. Hydrolysis occurs only in the large intestine by the action of the indigenous bacterial flora of the colon; this accounts, in part, for the delay in onset of action of these agents. The free anthraquinone is then reduced by the intestinal flora to the active anthral form. **Danthron** (1,8-dihydroxyanthraquinone) is a synthetic derivative that may be absorbed by the small intestine and/or alter the function of this portion of the bowel. **Cascara sagrada,** in usual doses, is the mildest of the anthraquinone laxatives. It is effective in about 8 hours and seldom causes colic. **Senna** is more active, is effective in about 6 hours, and usually causes some colic. **Aloe** is the most irritant and can stimulate other visceral smooth muscles including the uterus. It acts in about 8–12 hours and usually causes considerable colic. **Rhubarb** is a relatively mild laxative that causes little discomfort.

Table 45-3 Classification of Laxatives According to Their Effects on Intraluminal Fluid Accumulation

Laxatives that increase secretion
  Anthraquinones
  Castor oil (ricinoleic acid)
  Diphenylmethane laxatives
  Dioctyl sodium sulfosuccinate
  Bile acids
  Plant resins
  Magnesium salts
  Fiber

Laxatives that decrease absorption
  Liquid petrolatum
  Fiber
  Hydrophilic colloids

Laxatives that increase osmolarity
  Magnesium salts
  Lactulose
  Fiber

These agents appear to work by inhibiting colonic mucosal $(Na^+ + K^+)$-ATPase, leading to accumulation of salt and water in the lumen. At higher doses they may stimulate colonic myenteric nerve fibers.

Castor oil

The active constituent of castor oil, extracted from the **castor bean** (*Ricinus communis*), is ricinoleic acid, an 18-C aliphatic, monohydroxyl fatty acid. It is present as a triglyceride that is hydrolyzed by pancreatic lipase to yield free ricinoleic acid. The laxative action takes place especially in the small bowel, the contents of which may be emptied into the colon within only 2 hours. A dose of castor oil is effective within 2–6 hours. Because the remaining unhydrolyzed oil is also eliminated, the effects tend to be self-limiting.

Ricinoleic acid acts rapidly on the small intestine and colon to increase the intraluminal fluid content. It inhibits mucosal $(Na^+ + K^+)$-ATPase, thus decreasing the absorption of Na^+ and of the actively cotransported solutes (sugars, amino acids, etc.). It increases intracellular cyclic AMP, either as a response to an increased synthesis of prostaglandin E_2 that stimulates adenylyl cyclase activity or by a competitive inhibition of soluble cAMP-phosphodiesterase activity, or both. It damages enterocytes directly. On electron microscopy, disintegration of microvilli and damaged villus tips have been observed.

Diphenylmethane Laxatives

Phenolphthalein

Before this agent causes laxation, it must be absorbed, conjugated with glucuronide by the endoplasmic reticulum of the liver, and excreted in the bile. Enterohepatic circulation also prolongs its duration of action. It loses the laxative effect in obstructive jaundice or after ligation of the bile duct.

Bisacodyl

This agent (Dulcolax) is chemically similar to phenolphthalein. It is an effective laxative, acting 6–8 hours after oral administration. It is active only after deacetylation, absorption from the small intestine, and excretion in the bile. When given in a rectal suppository, it is effective in 20–60 minutes. Like phenolphthalein, it has no laxative effect after bile duct ligation.

The mechanism of action of these drugs is essentially similar to that of ricinoleic acid. (1) Both drugs inhibit $(Na^+ + K^+)$-ATPase. (2) Bisacodyl increases adenylyl cyclase activity and intracellular cyclic AMP. This direct effect is controversial in the case of phenolphthalein. (3) Both compounds increase the synthesis and release of PGE_2, resulting in an indirect increase in cyclic AMP. The role of PGE_2 in the laxative effects of phenolphthalein and bisacodyl explains the reduction of their laxative effect after pretreatment with indomethacin. (4) They may damage intestinal mucosa and increase permeability. (5) Bisacodyl has also been shown to cause a two- to threefold rise in K^+ efflux across the colonic mucosa. It has been proposed that this effect depends on raised levels of intracellular Ca^{2+}, and it probably reflects an increase in mucosal K^+ permeability. There is evidence that both cyclic AMP and Ca^{2+} may have a role in modulation of mucosal border K^+ permeability.

Dioctyl Sodium Sulfosuccinate (DSS)

This compound (Colace) was developed for use as a synthetic wetting agent—as a stool softener; this action is attributed to its ability to decrease surface tension and thus increase exposure of the stool surface to luminal water, resulting in fecal hydration. More recent studies have shown that DSS also acts through an increase in intraluminal water by mechanisms similar to those described for ricinoleic acid (inhibition of $(Na^+ + K^+)$-ATPase, increase in cyclic AMP, and cellular damage).

Laxatives That Decrease Water Absorption (Emollient Cathartics): Liquid Petrolatum

Some oils literally "lubricate" the fecal mass, prevent excessive dehydration of the material, and may inhibit water reabsorption by coating the gut wall. The only oil preparation now in use is **liquid petrolatum (mineral oil)**, a mixture of liquid hydrocarbons. It is indigestible but, nevertheless, in some people it is slightly absorbed. It interferes with the absorption of fat-soluble vitamins. It should always be taken at night on an empty stomach.

Mineral oil may leak past the anal sphincters. It has also been reported to interfere with healing of wounds in the anorectal area. It should not be used in very debilitated patients, the elderly, or patients with swallowing abnormalities because of the risk of aspiration and lipoid pneumonia.

Hydrophilic Colloids, Bulk-Forming Laxatives

This group includes both natural and semisynthetic polysaccharides and cellulose derivatives that dissolve or swell in water, forming a viscous solution or emollient gel. These gelatinous masses, of greatly increased bulk when moistened with water, exert a mildly laxative action. In addition, bulk-forming agents may actually promote colonic fluid accumulation by delivering bile acids and fatty acids to the colon where they may interfere with water and electrolyte transport. Cases of esophageal obstruction, fecal impaction, and even intestinal perforation have occurred when these drugs are taken in the dry form. Fluids should always be administered concurrently. These agents have occasionally been used to provide relief in acute diarrhea because they form an emollient intestinal mass and absorb water. Because of their bulk, they have also been suggested as appetite suppressants in the management of obesity. **Agar, psyllium (plantago), methylcellulose,** and **sodium carboxymethylcellulose** are examples of hydrophilic cellulose derivatives.

Laxatives That Increase Osmolarity

Magnesium salts

Laxatives such as **magnesium sulfate** (Epsom salts) and **magnesium hydroxide** (Milk of Magnesia) contain ions that are only slowly absorbed from the intestine, such as Mg^{2+} and SO_4^{2-}. These ions retain fluid in the bowel lumen by virtue of their osmotic action and therefore increase the rate of transit in the small intestine and cause a larger volume of fluid to enter the colon. This distends the colon, thereby stimulating it so that catharsis occurs quickly. Magnesium laxatives may increase release of cholecystokinin (CCK), which in turn stimulates pancreatic and duodenal secretion and decreases water, sodium, and chloride reabsorption. CCK causes an increase in cyclic GMP without affecting cyclic AMP. As the kidneys normally handle whatever ions are absorbed, these laxatives can also act as diuretics. When absorbed in sufficient quantity, Mg^{2+} can depress the central nervous system; however, this rarely happens unless there is impaired renal function or prolonged retention of the saline solution in the intestine.

Lactulose (4-β-galactoside-(1,4)-D-fructose)

This disaccharide is resistant to hydrolysis by the small-intestinal disaccharidases. It has an osmotic effect in the small bowel, drawing water into the intestinal lumen. Thus, a large volume of fluid enters the colon. Once in the large intestine, lactulose is acted upon by the endogenous flora of the colon with the production of lactic acid and of short-chain, volatile fatty acids. As these acids have a low lipid solubility, their colonic absorption is very limited; therefore, they also have an osmotic effect. Like lactic acid, they increase colonic mucosal secretion.

This mechanism applies also to other nondigestible disaccharides and to lactose in people with lactose intolerance (low intestinal lactase activity). The latter condition is common in all populations, although more so in African and East Indian populations than among Caucasians. Its prevalence tends to increase with age, and the symptoms of diarrhea and flatulence may be troublesome after use of milk or milk-containing foods. In such cases, either these foods must be eliminated from the diet or lactase can be used—in the form of tablets taken with the meals or as drops that are added to milk 1 or 2 days before it is used.

Side Effects of Laxatives

Cathartic colon syndrome

This is a frequent cause of diarrhea, abdominal pain, and cramps. In radiographs the colon appears dilated, hypomotile, with few or absent haustral margins; sometimes areas of pseudostricture are observed. Morphologically, there is mucosal inflammation, hypertrophy of the muscularis mucosae, thinning or atrophy of outer muscle layers, and damage to submucosal and myenteric plexuses.

Hypokalemia

The loss of Na^+ and water in stools results in a reduction of plasma volume, stimulation of the renin-angiotensin system, and increased serum levels of aldosterone. In the colon and kidney, aldosterone increases the reabsorption of Na^+ in exchange for K^+ that is then lost in stools and urine, respectively. Abnormal release of insulin and carbohydrate intolerance may occur as a consequence of hypokalemia.

Malabsorption

Chronic and continuous use of laxatives can lead to malabsorption of xylose and other carbohydrates, fat, fat-soluble vitamins, and calcium and thus to the production of osteomalacia.

Liver abnormalities

Chronic hepatitis has been reported after use of the combination of dioctyl calcium sulfosuccinate (Surfak) and the anthraquinone laxative danthron. DSS may have contributed to the liver damage caused by the laxative oxyphenisatin, which was withdrawn from the market because of hepatotoxicity. Phenolphthalein may also be directly hepatotoxic.

Increased loss of proteins through the intestine

With the sole exception of fiber and lactulose, all laxatives have been reported to cause an excessive loss of proteins through the intestine.

Indications for Laxatives

Most cases of constipation can be treated without the use of pharmacological agents simply by substituting whole wheat flour for white flour; by reducing the intake of food that contains no fiber; by eating plenty of fruits and vegetables; and by taking extra fiber in the form of unprocessed bran.

Laxatives should never be used on a regular basis simply to produce a daily bowel movement. Taking the above into consideration, nearly the only indications for the use of these potentially risky pharmacological agents are (1) to empty the bowel before elective colonic or rectal surgery or radiological or endoscopic examinations; (2) to minimize straining at stool in patients with cardiovascular disease or with hernia; and (3) to prevent hard, abrasive bowel movements that elicit pain (the last of which may best be achieved with emollient laxatives).

All laxatives must be avoided in persons with nausea, vomiting, cramps, colic, or other unexplained abdominal discomfort.

ANTIDIARRHEALS

Antidiarrheals are a heterogenous group of drugs used for the symptomatic relief of diarrhea. These agents have limited utility. The etiology of the diarrhea usually dictates specific, not symptomatic, treatment. In general, mild diarrhea due to enteric viral infections should be allowed to run its course. Bacterial enteric infections, if treated at all, should be treated etiologically. Patients with diarrhea due to colonic spillage of bile acids usually respond to administration of a resin that binds bile acids. Giving opioids to a patient with diarrhea caused by ulcerative colitis may precipitate toxic megacolon. In general, antidiarrheals are reserved for patients who cannot cope anatomically with their colonic contents because of a short gut, altered rectal or anal tone, or other structural motility problems as in Crohn's disease.

Opioid Analogs

Diphenoxylate (Lomotil) and loperamide (Imodium) (Fig. 45-2) are the opioid analogs used most specifically as antidiarrheals. Both are synthetic opioids of the piperidine group, and diphenoxylate is closely related to meperidine (see Chapter 23).

These drugs resemble morphine in their effect on the small intestine and colon. They are thought to decrease fluid secretion by the small intestine and decrease intestinal motor activity generally.

Diphenoxylate acts as an agonist at opioid receptors at two locations in the GI tract. (1) Those on

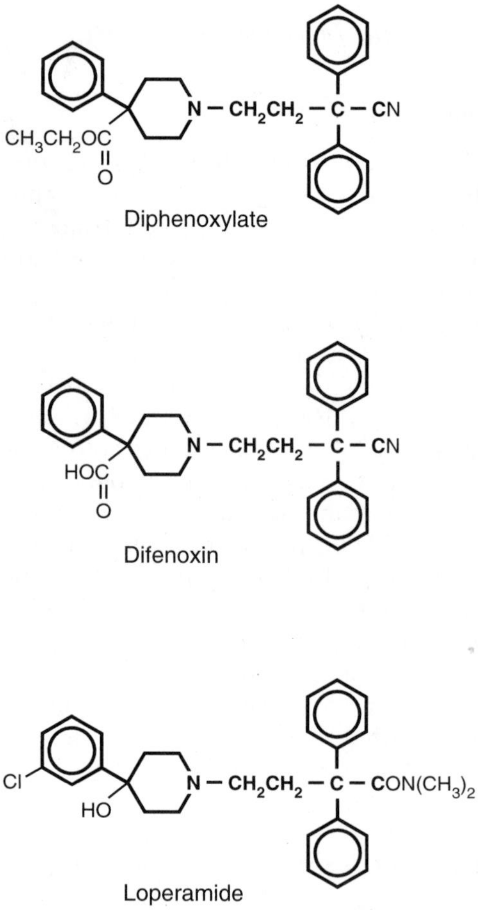

Figure 45-2. Structural formulae of diphenoxylate, difenoxin, and loperamide. (Common elements are emphasized.)

cholinergic terminals inhibit the release of acetylcholine and thus decrease propulsive contractions of the longitudinal muscle. (2) Those on presynaptic terminals of inhibitory neurons inhibit the release of vasoactive intestinal peptide, thus *dis*inhibiting the sphincter-like segmental contractions of circular muscle. Both effects contribute to decreased propulsive motility of the GI tract.

Diphenoxylate is well absorbed after oral administration but does not cross the blood–brain barrier as easily as most opioids do and therefore is relatively selective for peripheral opioid receptors. However, at high doses or when used for more than a few days, it can produce drowsiness, depression, and potentiation of the effects of ethanol, barbiturates, benzodiazepines, and other CNS depressants. Overdose can cause respiratory depression that is reversible by naloxone. It can also produce an opioid-like euphoria, and a small amount of atropine is therefore added to the diphenoxylate preparation (Lomotil) to prevent abuse by causing disagreeable symptoms if too much is taken.

The elimination half-life of diphenoxylate is about 12 hours, but the drug is biotransformed in the liver to the active metabolite **difenoxin,** which is more potent than diphenoxylate. Therefore overdose effects can occur after many hours have passed and the concentration of difenoxin has risen.

Loperamide has largely replaced diphenoxylate as the drug of choice. It is effective, nonhabituating, and safe. It is similar chemically to both diphenoxylate and haloperidol. Loperamide has high affinity for both peripheral and central opioid receptors but enters the brain even less readily than diphenoxylate. It acts in the intestinal tract, principally in the jejunum, via opioid receptors of the μ class, and its effects can be blocked by naloxone. It is demethylated in the intestinal wall, and little is absorbed systemically. Its elimination half-life is about 10–15 hours. About 7% of the drug is excreted in the urine; significant hepatic biotransformation and biliary excretion occur, and substantial amounts of the unchanged drug and metabolites are found in the feces.

Loperamide is two to three times more potent than diphenoxylate, and its action is more rapid in onset and more prolonged. It has no analgesic effects. It has not been reported to have central nervous system or cardiovascular effects. Side effects are uncommon but include dizziness, dry mouth, and fatigue.

DRUG TREATMENT OF INFLAMMATORY BOWEL DISEASE

Sulfasalazine (Salazopyrin)

Sulfasalazine (Fig. 45-3) is the name commonly used for salicylazosulfapyridine, i.e., salicylate linked to a sulfonamide via an azo linkage. The salicylate is 5-aminosalicylic acid (5-ASA), an anti-inflammatory agent, which was invented in the 1940s as a possible treatment for rheumatoid arthritis, for which it proved to have rather limited utility. It is valuable as chronic treatment for ulcerative colitis and for initial treatment of Crohn's disease with a prominent colonic involvement.

Sulfasalazine is a good example of a **prodrug.** The 5-ASA, which is in fact the active ingredient, is linked to the sulfonamide so that it can be delivered to the colon. Sulfasalazine is not absorbed in the

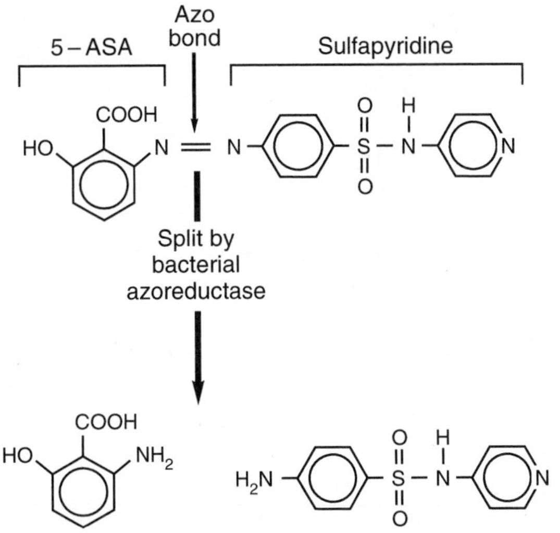

Figure 45-3. Structural formula of sulfasalazine. The azo bond between 5-ASA and sulfapyridine is split by intestinal bacterial action, liberating the active anti-inflammatory component 5-ASA.

stomach; what is absorbed in the small intestine is subject to enterohepatic circulation and ends up in the colon eventually. In the colon the bacterial flora cleaves the azo bond, which separates the 5-ASA from the sulfapyridine. The sulfapyridine is absorbed, biotransformed in the liver, and excreted. The 5-ASA is mostly retained locally in the colon, where it exerts its anti-inflammatory effect.

The mechanism of this anti-inflammatory effect has been the subject of much recent research. The inflammatory response in ulcerative colitis and Crohn's disease includes such diverse features as cellular infiltration, increased vascular permeability, and variable local tissue damage. Increased concentrations of soluble mediators of inflammation can be detected. Principal among these are the products of arachidonic acid metabolism: prostaglandins, thromboxanes (via the cyclooxygenase pathway), and leukotrienes (via the 5-lipoxygenase pathway) (see Chapter 31). Prostaglandins have numerous effects: They are vasodilators and enhance the effects of other inflammatory mediators, such as histamine, but they also decrease phagocyte activation and cytokine production. Thromboxane A_2 is a vascular constrictor. Leukotriene B_4 has potent chemotactic effects, and other leukotrienes increase smooth-muscle contraction and vascular permeability. With respect to these agents, the main action of 5-ASA is to inhibit leukotriene production. Effects on prostaglandins appear to be unimportant. 5-ASA also interferes with production of platelet-activating factor, and it decreases production of cytokines such as interleukin-1 (see Chapter 61). 5-ASA also appears to neutralize, or scavenge, activated oxygen species produced in the inflammatory response; it may inactivate nitric oxide that contributes to vasodilatation and local tissue damage. 5-ASA interferes with secretion of antibodies and with bacterial action. Which of these actions is most important for its anti-inflammatory effect remains to be established.

The problem with sulfasalazine is that the sulfapyridine component causes significant toxicity; as a result sulfasalazine may be poorly tolerated. Nausea, abdominal upset, and headache are mostly avoided by using enteric-coated tablets and an incremental dosage to build up gradually to the maintenance dose. Hemolytic and other anemias, rashes, Stevens-Johnson syndrome, pancreatitis, fibrosing pulmonary disease, hepatitis, and even acute liver failure have been reported. These tend to be worse in slow acetylators (see Chapter 12). Sulfasalazine has been shown to impair male fertility; fortunately, sperm morphology and motility revert to normal when the drug is stopped. Known hypersensitivity to sulfonamides, or glucose-6-phosphate dehydrogenase deficiency, precludes the use of sulfasalazine.

5-Aminosalicylic Acid (5-ASA)

Since 5-ASA (or a metabolite) is the active component, and the sulfonamide portion of sulfasalazine causes most of the side effects, it seemed reasonable to link two molecules of 5-ASA together via an azo bond and exclude sulfapyridine altogether. This resulting drug is called olsalazine (Dipentum). Olsalazine and sulfasalazine both have some predictable problems because they are dependent on bacterial degradation (Table 45-4). Whenever intestinal transit is too fast, there is less bacterial degradation. If a patient is treated with broad-spectrum antibiotics, reducing the bacterial flora, olsalazine and sulfasalazine are ineffective.

A second strategy to avoid the need for sulfapyridine is to develop special formulations of 5-ASA to favor delivery to the distal ileum or colon. These are called collectively mesalamine in the United States and mesalazine in Canada. These drugs are unusual in that the pharmaceutical preparation itself is important in determining the pharmacological characteristics, and thus it is often necessary to refer to these drugs by trade name, rather than by official or nonproprietary name. Likewise, each requires separate clinical testing, which is currently underway. The preliminary impressions are that they are effective (like sulfasalazine) and well tolerated. Optimal doses have not been completely determined.

Current formulations of mesalamine are detailed in Table 45-4. Some preparations consist of 5-ASA coated with an acrylic resin that disintegrates at a fixed pH. When the acrylic coating is Eudragit S, the resin breaks down at pH >7, releasing 5-ASA in the distal ileum or right colon. When the acrylic coating Eudragit L is used, the resin breaks down at pH >6, and the 5-ASA is released in the proximal ileum and onward. When 5-ASA is packaged in microgranules coated with an ethylcellulose membrane, it acts as a timed-release preparation and is gradually released throughout the entire small intestine and colon. The-

Table 45-4 Preparations of 5-Aminosalicylate Used in the Treatment of Inflammatory Bowel Disease

Nonproprietary Name	Trade Name	Formulation	Release Mechanism	Site of Release	Systemic Absorption
Olsalazine	Dipentum	Two 5-ASA moieties joined via azo bond	Bacterial action on azo bond	Colon	20–40%
Mesalamine (USA)	Asacol	Acrylic resin coating (Eudragit S)	pH-dependent from resin	pH >7, distal ileum onward	34–44%
Mesalazine (Canada)	Salofalk Claversal	Acrylic coating (Eudragit L)	pH-dependent from resin	pH >6, proximal ileum onward	44%
	Pentasa	Microgranules with ethyl cellulose membrane	Timed release	Entire small intestine, colon	60%

oretically these drugs have the same efficacy as sala-zopyrine but none of the toxicity associated with sulfapyridine.

Pure 5-ASA preparations are not, however, entirely free of adverse side effects, although the incidence of these is much lower than with salazopyrine. Watery diarrhea is an adverse effect of olsalazine; it occurs at higher doses and with severe or more extensive disease. The probable mechanism is promotion of ileal fluid secretion, which is not reabsorbed by the inflamed right colon. Olsalazine may cause renal toxicity, manifested either as nephrotic syndrome or as increased serum creatinine. The important side effects of 5-ASA remain undetermined; nephrotoxicity, myocarditis, and pancreatitis have also been reported. Occasional patients have identical adverse reactions to sulfasalazine and 5-ASA. Therefore 5-ASA should be used cautiously in patients who do not tolerate sulfasalazine, although the general experience is that most will tolerate 5-ASA.

Pure 5-ASA is also formulated as suppositories and enemas. These are effective treatment for ulcerative proctitis and distal ulcerative colitis.

SUGGESTED READING

Demol P, Ruoff HJ, Weihrauch TR. Rational pharmacotherapy of gastrointestinal motility disorders. Eur J Pediatr 1989; 148:489–495.

Greiff JM, Rowbotham D. Pharmacokinetic drug interactions with gastrointestinal motility modifying agents. Clin Pharmacokinet 1994; 27:447–461.

Hanauer SB. Inflammatory bowel disease. N Engl J Med 1996; 334:841–848.

McCallum RW, Prakash C, Campoli-Richards DM, Goa KL. Cisapride: a preliminary review of its pharmacodynamic and pharmacokinetic properties, and therapeutic use as a prokinetic agent in gastrointestinal motility disorders. Drugs 1988; 36:652–681.

Peppercorn MA. Advances in drug therapy for inflammatory bowel disease. Ann Intern Med 1990; 112:50–60.

Reynolds JC. Prokinetic agents: a key in the future of gastroenterology. Gastroenterol Clin North Am 1989; 18:437–457.

Riley SA, Turnberg LA. Sulphasalazine and the aminosalicylates in the treatment of inflammatory bowel disease. Quart J Med 1990; 75:551–562.

Thompson WG. Laxatives: clinical pharmacology and rational use. Drugs 1980; 19:49–58.

CHAPTER 46

Drugs, Alcohol, and the Liver

H. KALANT AND E.A. ROBERTS

CASE HISTORY

A 14-year-old girl was found to have a moderately enlarged liver and a palpable spleen on routine examination. She was well and had never been jaundiced. She denied fatigue, pruritus, or easy bruisability. On slit-lamp examination of the eyes, definite Kayser-Fleischer rings were found. Neurological examination was normal.

Laboratory studies showed that the hemoglobin was 110 g/L, with a mildly elevated reticulocyte count. The direct Coombs' test was negative; serum haptoglobin was low at 0.22 g/L. Abnormal liver function tests included elevated AST (92 U/L) and ALT (56 U/L), low albumin (29 g/L), and prothrombin time prolonged to 5 seconds beyond normal control. Serum copper was 8.2 μmol/L and ceruloplasmin was 68 mg/L (both subnormal). Basal 24-hour urinary copper excretion was extremely elevated at 18.4 μmol/day. Serological tests for viruses commonly causing hepatitis were negative. The patient was diagnosed as having Wilson's disease, and treatment was begun with penicillamine 500 mg twice daily. To minimize side effects the drug was started gradually, and the full dose was reached within 10 days. The patient's only complaint was that some foods now tasted peculiar.

Surveillance of the complete blood count showed no abnormalities over the first several weeks of treatment. However, after approximately 2 months of treatment, the child developed a vasculitic rash on her arms. White blood cell and platelet counts were normal, but urinalysis revealed proteinuria. Quantified 24-hour urine collection showed the urine protein to be twice normal for her age. There was no urinary tract infection. Serum creatinine was normal. The most likely explanation therefore was penicillamine nephrotoxicity.

The occurrence of vasculitis and nephrotoxicity required stopping the penicillamine. However, continuous treatment with a chelating agent is mandatory in Wilson's disease. Therefore the patient was treated with trien, which she tolerated well. The rash disappeared spontaneously, and the proteinuria resolved over the next few weeks.

Interactions between drugs and the liver are of pharmacological interest in relation to three different questions: (1) How do variations in liver function affect the fate of drugs? (2) How do drugs (including ethanol) affect liver function? (3) How are drugs used in the treatment of liver disease? The first question is dealt with in several other chapters of this book and will therefore be mentioned only briefly in the present context. The second question will be covered in greater detail, in particular as it relates to drug-induced liver disease. The third question is partly covered in several other chapters, and only certain drugs that are used specifically in some types of liver disease are dealt with here.

EFFECTS OF LIVER FUNCTION ON PHARMACOKINETICS

Basic Liver Functions Relevant to Drug Metabolism

Circulation

In keeping with its major metabolic role, the human liver normally receives a large blood supply, amounting to about 25–30% of the cardiac output. However, this comes from two different sources: Normally the portal vein supplies about 70–75% of the liver blood flow and the hepatic artery about 25–30%. Since the portal venous blood has already passed through the intestinal circulation, it is a low-pressure flow with a low P_{O_2} of about 55 mmHg, compared to 95 mmHg in the hepatic arterial blood. The normal oxygen tension at the confluence of the hepatic arterial and portal venous flows, at the proximal end of the sinusoid (zone I of the liver acinus), is therefore about 65–70 mmHg. As the blood moves along the sinusoid and oxygen is removed by the surrounding liver cells, the P_{O_2} falls steadily to about 30–35 mmHg at the venous end (zone III of the liver acinus). This is normally still high enough to meet the basic needs of the last liver cells along the sinusoid. However, zone III is normally in a state of relative hypoxia. If the arterial P_{O_2} falls because of conditions such as anemia, congestive heart failure, or anesthesia, or if the oxygen requirement of the liver is increased by conditions such as fever or hyperthyroidism, there may be insufficient oxygen left at the venous end. Unless the increased oxygen demand is met by a corresponding increase in oxygen delivery, the still-further-reduced P_{O_2} in zone III could result in **focal damage or necrosis** of liver cells.

The liver also has low-resistance shunts that connect the junction of the portal venous and hepatic arterial flows directly to the terminal hepatic venule (central vein), bypassing the sinusoid. These shunts probably serve to permit portal venous blood to reach the systemic circulation when the perfusion pressure is too low to ensure flow through the sinusoids. The cost of this safeguard is that blood passing through the shunts is not exposed to the hepatocytes. Variations in blood flow and in intrahepatic shunting, therefore, markedly affect the delivery of drug to the liver. The importance of this factor in drug clearance is explained in Chapter 7.

Cellular uptake mechanisms

Free drug can enter the hepatocyte by passive diffusion or active transport; protein-bound drug can be taken up by pinocytosis. More than one mechanism may be involved in the uptake of the same drug. For example, free *d*-tubocurarine, which is actively transported across the cell membrane into the cytoplasm, is secreted into the bile, but protein-bound tubocurarine, which is taken up by pinocytosis, finds its way into lysosomes, where it is stored and from which it can be displaced by quinacrine and other competing drugs. Mathematical analysis of hepatic uptake of drugs is considered in Chapter 7.

Storage

Storage can occur in lysosomes, as mentioned above, or by binding to intracellular proteins, as in the case of the antimalarial drugs. It seems likely that highly lipid-soluble drugs can also be stored within intracellular fat droplets.

Biotransformation

This is dealt with in detail in Chapter 4. As noted there, biotransformation can inactivate many drugs, but it can activate others and convert them into toxic compounds. The latter process will be of special interest in this chapter.

Biliary secretion

Two separate phases contribute to the formation of the bile that is finally put out by the liver. The canalicular phase involves active secretion of Na^+, bile pigments, and drugs and their metabolites by the hepatocytes; this phase is induced by chronic treatment with phenobarbital. The bile-duct phase involves movement of electrolytes and water across the bile-duct epithelium; it is under endocrine control and regulates the concentration and volume of the bile, and therefore its rate of movement down the biliary duct system. Biliary secretion may be an important factor in the fate of some drugs and of negligible significance to others.

Effects of Disturbed Liver Function on Pharmacokinetics

Circulation

Shock causes a fall in visceral blood flow and portal pressure, and within the liver the blood is diverted from the sinusoids to the low-pressure shunts. This reduces the delivery of drug to the liver cells and also decreases the supply of oxygen needed for most drug biotransformations. Both effects tend to prolong the half-life of the drug in the body. The same results can be produced by an extrahepatic portocaval shunt or by intrahepatic obstruction of blood flow due to swelling of the liver cells (e.g., inflammation, fat accumulation, hypertrophy of endoplasmic reticulum, osmotic swelling) or fibrosis (e.g., portal cirrhosis). Similar effects can be produced temporarily by vasoconstrictor drugs such as catecholamines and vasopressin, which can therefore alter the hepatic uptake of other drugs.

While the major effect of such circulatory disturbances is to reduce the rate of drug delivery to the liver, they can also decrease the rate of absorption of drug from the intestinal lumen. Increased intrahepatic pressure, with corresponding decrease in hepatic blood flow, also decreases the rate of flow through submucosal capillaries in the GI tract, and thus decreases the concentration gradient that maintains diffusion of drug from the lumen to the blood. For example, in one study of patients with portal hypertension, the time to reach peak plasma concentration after an oral dose of the anti-inflammatory agent sulindac (see Chapter 34) was increased to 2.5 hours from a normal time of 1.2 hours.

The effect of such changes in drug delivery depends on the relative importance of hepatic biotransformation versus other routes of elimination for the individual drug in question. For example, the fate of digoxin will be unchanged because it is eliminated by renal excretion, while the half-life of digitoxin will be prolonged because it depends primarily on hepatic biotransformation. Similarly, the fate of ether will not be affected appreciably because it is primarily cleared by the lung, whereas halothane and methoxyflurane will have a longer sojourn in the body because they undergo a substantial degree of biotransformation in the liver. For most drugs, the effect of decreased hepatic circulation will be a decreased rate of elimination from the body, and therefore an increased risk of toxicity. However, this same effect can be protective if the drug is transformed into a toxic material in the liver.

Hepatocellular uptake

A reduction in functional liver cell mass can have two competing effects on the hepatic uptake of drugs:

1. Decreased plasma protein concentration, which often results from liver disease, can cause a significant increase in the free fraction of a drug that is normally extensively protein-bound, and this in turn can result in increased hepatic uptake. Many different types of drug are affected in this way. Some well-studied examples are amobarbital, cefoperazone, diazepam, morphine, phenytoin, propranolol, tolbutamide, and various nonsteroidal anti-inflammatory drugs. The increase in hepatic uptake of the drug is sometimes greater than the reduction in plasma albumin concentration; this suggests that a qualitative change in the albumin may result in lower drug-binding affinity.

2. The decreased liver cell mass can mean a decreased uptake capacity. The actual result in any given case depends on the balance between the effects of reduced liver cell mass and decreased plasma protein binding. Usually, in severe liver disease the effect of reduced cell mass predominates, and drug uptake is diminished. Several studies of patients with severe liver disease have shown a significant decrease in the clearance of antipyrine that is closely correlated with the decreased clearance of indocyanine green (a marker of liver cell function) and with decreased liver size as estimated by ultrasonic scan. Severe cirrhosis also greatly prolongs the serum half-life for phenobarbital, amobarbital, and hexobarbital.

Severe liver disease may also be accompanied by an increase in the apparent volume of distribution (see Chapter 5) for some drugs. This can be due to reduced plasma protein binding or to the accumulation of ascitic fluid, into which the drug can equilibrate.

Biotransformation

The effect of liver disease on the biotransformation of drugs after their uptake depends on the stage and severity of the disease. In mild disease, during the stage of recovery, there may be proliferation of liver cells to replace those previously damaged. In this regeneration phase, all constituents of the cytochrome P450 pathway (see Chapter 4) may be increased, and the rate of biotransformation of barbiturates and many other drugs may actually be greater than normal.

However, in severe liver disease, punch biopsies have shown a 40–50% reduction in the cytochrome P450 content and in the activities of *N*- and *O*-demethylases, pseudocholinesterase, and glucose-6-phosphate dehydrogenase. Such changes are found in alcoholic hepatitis and active cirrhosis, but not in uncomplicated fatty liver or mild viral hepatitis. These factors may require a decrease in dosage for some drugs. For example, patients with active liver disease may require from 15% to 65% reduction in dosage of various opioid analgesics, nonsteroidal anti-inflammatory agents, long-acting benzodiazepines, digitoxin, β-blockers, and verapamil.

Similar decreases in drug biotransformation by the liver may result from endocrine or other factors affecting the liver secondarily. For example, progesterone and synthetic progestogens used in oral contraceptive pills prolong the sleeping time after a test dose of hexobarbital in the rat. Experimental kidney disease, in the stage of uremia, causes a fall in hepatic content of cytochrome P450 and a decrease in drug-metabolizing activity. The mechanism of this effect is not clear; it may be due to endocrine disturbances or possibly result from the accumulation of some hepatotoxic material that is normally excreted in the urine.

Bile flow

The importance of reduction in rate of bile flow varies greatly from drug to drug. Some drugs (e.g., *d*-tubocurarine) or drug metabolites, (e.g., hydroxybarbiturates) are secreted in high concentration in the bile and are significantly affected by changes in bile flow rate. For example, an infusion of saline or of sodium taurocholate, which increased the canalicular bile formation, resulted in a 40% increase in biliary excretion of pentobarbital and its metabolites. The ratio of pentobarbital to pentobarbital metabolites was not altered, so the effect must have been exclusively on the flushing out of the biliary tree rather than on the biotransformation reactions in the liver cell. Ligation of the bile duct caused the opposite change: The duration of action of thiopental, hexobarbital, or zoxazolamine was doubled 24 hours after bile-duct obstruction. In contrast, other drugs (e.g., digitoxin) are biotransformed in the liver, but the metabolites are passed back into the circulation and excreted by the kidney. Neither biliary obstruction nor bile flow stimulation affects their duration of action.

Very closely related drugs may differ markedly with respect to their biliary excretion pattern. For example, after a test dose of the anticancer drug doxorubicin (see Chapter 60), only 20% of the drug appeared in the bile in 24 hours, mainly as unaltered drug; with the analog trifluoroacetyldoxorubicin, over 80% appeared in the bile, mainly as metabolites.

A general problem in such studies is that biliary excretion of a drug is normally investigated in animals or surgical patients with bile-duct drainage via a catheter to the exterior. Therefore the results do not indicate what would happen in the intact subject when the bile reaches the intestine. If there is a significant degree of enterohepatic recirculation (see Chapter 1), the half-life for whole-body clearance might not be appreciably altered by a change in biliary secretion rate.

MECHANISMS OF DRUG-INDUCED LIVER DISEASE

Drugs can cause pathological changes in liver histology and liver function by at least three different mechanisms. The type of damage differs according to the mechanism involved; the speed of onset and the dose–effect relations also differ.

Indirect Extrahepatic Mechanisms

Drugs that produce major effects on circulation or respiration can cause liver damage by sharply decreasing the blood or oxygen supply to the liver, even temporarily. For example, a massive release of norepinephrine or epinephrine causes a temporary **constriction of the splanchnic arterial bed**, including the hepatic artery. Production of shock by overdose of drugs that **impair myocardial contractility** (e.g., quinidine) can produce an equivalent effect by decreasing the perfusion pressure. **Respiratory depression**, by large doses of barbiturates or other hypnosedative drugs, causes poor oxygenation of the blood, so oxygen supply to the liver is decreased even if the blood flow is not markedly affected.

All of these disturbances can lead to hypoxia of the liver. If severe enough, this may result in degenerative changes or necrosis of liver cells. Because of the special features of hepatic circulation described above, the damage tends to be periacinar, i.e., in the region of the terminal hepatic venule.

Drugs can also reduce hepatic blood flow by producing lesions of the intrahepatic blood vessels themselves. Oral contraceptives (see Chapter 49) and various anticancer chemotherapeutic agents (see Chapter 60) have been incriminated in the production of **thrombosis** of the large hepatic veins (Budd-Chiari syndrome) and of **veno-occlusive disease** of the small intrahepatic veins. The latter is a gradual constriction of the small veins by deposition of connective tissue around them. The same drugs, as well as a number of metallic poisons and vinyl chloride, have also been linked to perisinusoidal fibrosis and to gradual fibrous occlusion of the branches of the portal vein (hepatoportal sclerosis). Intravenous use of methamphetamine has been reported to cause **necrotizing angiitis,** a condition characterized by the formation of inflammatory nodules and microaneurysms in the walls of arterioles in the liver, brain, kidney, and other organs. These drug-induced vascular lesions are relatively rare but can be fatal when they do occur.

Indirect Intrahepatic Mechanisms

Many drugs can cause liver injury by **interfering with an important metabolic pathway** and depriving the liver cell of an essential product. For example, tetracyclines and chloramphenicol (see Chapter 55) are antibiotics that can interfere with the synthesis of cell proteins, including the very-low-density lipoproteins that normally transport triglycerides out of the hepatocyte. Anticancer drugs (e.g., methotrexate, urethane, 6-mercaptopurine) can inhibit the synthesis of nucleic acids in normal cells as well as in malignant ones.

These metabolic disturbances typically lead to the production of fatty liver and other degenerative changes, and only occasionally (in severe cases) to liver cell necrosis. The effects are generally dose-dependent, but with a high degree of variability that possibly reflects differences in the degree of metabolic activity in the liver at the time the drug was given. The latency between the administration of the drug and the appearance of the damage ranges from several hours to several days. The percentage of exposed individuals who actually suffer liver damage is relatively low.

Indirect cell damage can also be caused by **cholestasis** (obstruction of bile flow by precipitation of bile pigment within the bile canaliculi). Several ste-

roids that are alkylated at C-17, such as the anabolic steroids and the synthetic estrogens and progestins used in oral contraceptives (Fig 46-1), can inhibit the uptake of bile pigment from the plasma into the liver cell and its secretion into the bile. In addition, they inhibit the $(Na^+ + K^+)$-ATPase of the liver cell and thus decrease active secretion of Na^+ into the bile. They also increase the permeability of the canalicular membrane to back-diffusion of water and some solutes from the bile canaliculi into the liver cell. Other compounds, such as halogenated hydrocarbons, or chlorpromazine and a number of its derivatives, increase the permeability of the ductal epithelium, thus reducing the volume and the rate of bile flow along the canaliculi, permitting the conjugated bile pigments to precipitate and form solid plugs. These plugs block the canaliculi and lead to obstructive jaundice and mild degenerative changes in the liver cells. These effects are reversible when the drug is stopped.

Jaundice can also be caused by drugs that **interfere with the uptake of unconjugated bile pigments** from the circulating blood into the hepatic parenchymal cells. Examples include the antibiotics novobiocin and rifampin, and various radiopaque dyes used for X-ray visualization of the gallbladder. Since the bile pigments are prevented from being taken up into the liver and conjugated, they remain poorly water-soluble, are not readily excreted by the kidney, and remain largely bound to serum proteins, where they can compete against the binding of other drugs.

Direct Hepatic Toxicity

A number of agents including chloroform, carbon tetrachloride, furosemide, phenacetin, and acetaminophen are directly toxic to the liver cell. Unlike the indirect hepatotoxins, these direct-acting compounds show a **strict dose dependence** with very **high reproducibility** experimentally and with a very **high incidence of damage** in exposed individuals. There is a **very short latency** between drug administration and onset of damage, on the order of a few hours.

Some drugs appear to cause direct damage to the cell membrane and mitochondrial membranes. For example, an Asian hornet venom was found to cause leakage of mitochondrial enzymes, accompanied by electron-microscopic evidence of mitochondrial and plasma membrane damage, in humans who had been stung repeatedly. Acetaminophen-induced hepatotoxicity in the rat was reported to cause a selective

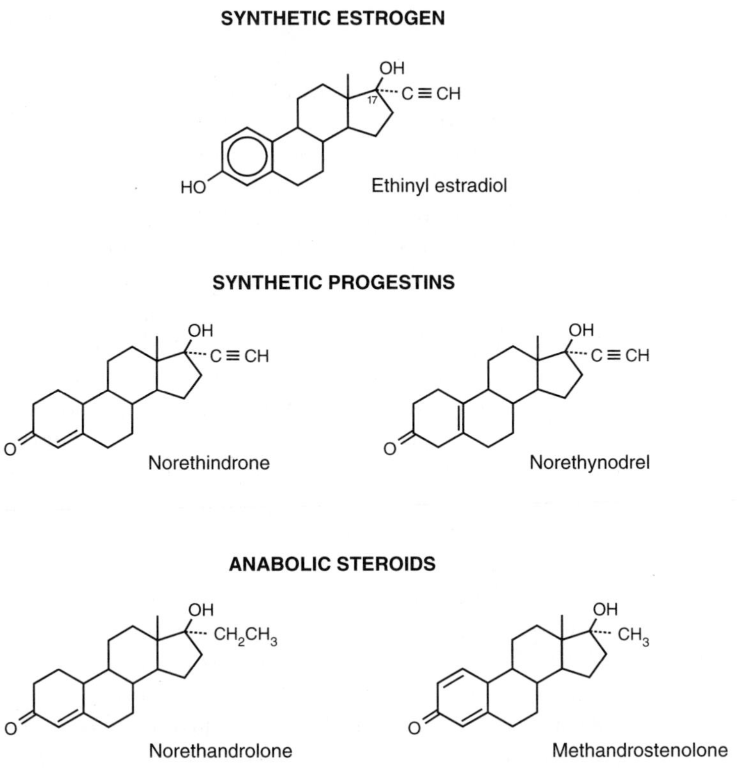

SYNTHETIC ESTROGEN

Ethinyl estradiol

SYNTHETIC PROGESTINS

Norethindrone

Norethynodrel

ANABOLIC STEROIDS

Norethandrolone

Methandrostenolone

Figure 46-1. Examples of C-17 alkylated steroids capable of causing cholestatic jaundice.

52% drop in hepatocyte membrane $(Na^+ + K^+)$-ATPase 3 hours after the drug administration, whereas leakage of alanine aminotransferase and microscopic signs of necrosis were not found until 24 hours later. However, the typical lesion is **necrosis** (rather than fatty change, as caused by the indirect mechanisms). It tends to be widespread throughout the liver and indiscriminately located, although with a few of these drugs it may be zonal (periportal with some drugs, and surrounding the terminal hepatic venule with others).

With a number of the direct hepatotoxins there is a **threshold dose** necessary to cause damage. For example, acetaminophen does not cause liver cell necrosis until the dose exceeds 300 mg/kg; beyond that, the damage is proportional to the dose. The reason for this appears to be that the damage is caused by a minor but highly reactive metabolite (Fig 46-2) that can be inactivated by glutathione conjugation (see Chapter 4) to yield a mercapturic acid derivative that is excreted harmlessly in the urine. No damage occurs until the available glutathione is all used up and the toxic material is then free to react with essential constituents of the cell. Therefore, the damage is increased by metabolic factors that reduce the cellular content of reduced glutathione and thus prolong the half-life of the toxic metabolite.

Numerous other drugs can produce direct hepatocellular damage by mechanisms involving the production of reactive intermediates by cytochrome P450 reactions. For example, **α-methyldopa** is converted to an epoxide intermediary metabolite, which acts as an arylating agent. **Halothane** is generally a safe anesthetic, but a certain number of patients, especially those who undergo repeated exposure to it, develop fever, muscle and joint pains, nausea, anorexia, abdominal discomfort, and jaundice, which progresses to a zone III hepatocellular necrosis. The explanation again appears to be the formation of a reactive metabolite. Under normoxic conditions the cytochrome P450 system oxidizes the halothane to trifluoroacetate, but under hypoxic conditions it acts as a reducing system (see Chapter 4) and produces a toxic free radical (Fig. 46-3).

The mechanism of damage in all these cases appears to involve covalent bonding of the toxic metabolite to a vital cell constituent, possibly a membrane protein or a nucleic acid. Extent and severity of damage are proportional to the amount of covalent

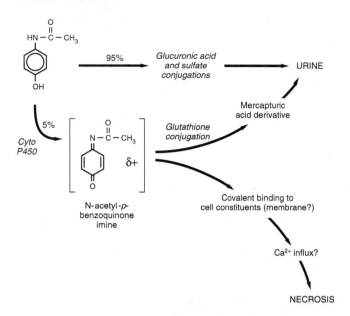

Figure 46-2. Probable mechanism of hepatotoxicity of acetaminophen. Covalent binding appears to occur only when the capacity of glutathione conjugation has been exceeded.

binding, which can be shown to occur about 1–2 hours before the appearance of cytological damage. Glutathione can protect against such damage in at least three different ways: (1) detoxification of H_2O_2 and organoperoxides by a glutathione peroxidase reaction, (2) noncatalyzed nucleophilic reaction of glutathione and drug to form stable adducts, and (3) the glutathione transferase reaction (see Chapter 4). Cell destruction can be prevented if reducing substances, such as cysteine or dimercaprol, are given early enough after the hepatotoxic drug. These substances can react with the toxic metabolite and prevent it from bonding to the target constituents in the cell. In the case of CCl_4 poisoning, the toxic metabolite is the free radical, $CCl_3\cdot$, which can be "mopped up" by N-acetyl-cysteine or cystamine given up to 12 hours after the CCl_4. In contrast, drugs such as pyrazole or aminotriazole, which prevent the free radical formation, are protective only if given before or together with the CCl_4, but can do nothing against the $CCl_3\cdot$ if given after it has formed.

After covalent binding has occurred, two different mechanisms may be responsible for immediate versus delayed cell damage. **Immediate** damage, as in the case of halothane, appears to be due to altered ion permeability. Covalent binding of reactive intermediates to membrane proteins renders the membrane permeable to Ca^{2+}, which floods in along a concen-

tration gradient and is the agent that finally kills the cell. In tissue culture, cell death can be prevented, even after covalent binding has occurred, by using a very-low-calcium medium. Chlorpromazine, which hinders Ca^{2+} entry, also has a protective effect.

Delayed cell death, however, appears to be the result of an autoimmune reaction. The proteins that have been altered by covalent binding of the reactive drug metabolites can serve as antigens, giving rise to antibodies that may be able to attack the native proteins in previously undamaged cells. There is evidence that this may explain the increased risk of hepatotoxicity with repeated exposure to halothane, as well as the relatively long latent period. Similarly, tienilic acid (ticrynafen, a diuretic and uricosuric agent now removed from the market because of hepatotoxicity) gives rise to a reactive intermediate that can alkylate a specific cytochrome P450, converting it into an antigen. This gives rise to an antibody that reacts specifically with that cytochrome P450 and decreases its ability to carry out hydroxylation of tienilic acid itself and of various other drugs. This antibody was found in the plasma of patients with ticrynafen hepatitis but not in the plasma of patients who also received the drug but did not develop hepatitis. It is believed that the hepatitis was caused by the antibody attacking the native cytochrome P450 in previously undamaged cells.

Since the damage in these cases is done by a **reactive metabolite** of the original drug, it can be prevented by blockers of the cytochrome P450 system or be increased by inducers of this system. **Zonal distribution** of damage is seen with those drugs for which the biotransformation is localized to a specific zone (Fig. 46-4). The damage tends to occur at the point where the toxic metabolite is produced. For example, allyl alcohol is converted to acrolein in the periportal zone (zone I) and produces necrosis there. In contrast, with acetaminophen the biotransformation and the damage are essentially in zone III. **Genetic variations** in drug biotransformation may also affect susceptibility to liver damage by the metabolites.

MECHANISMS OF ETHANOL-INDUCED LIVER PATHOLOGY

Alcoholic liver disease is the fourth most common cause of death in white males in the United States. World-wide, the annual mortality from alcoholic liver disease is over 300,000. The death rate due to this

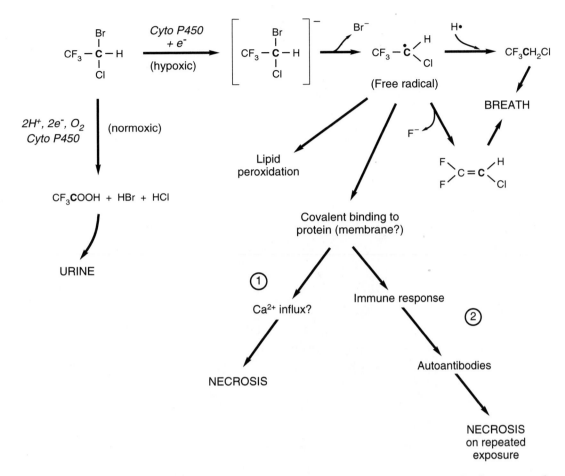

Figure 46-3. Postulated mechanism of hepatotoxicity by halothane. Pathway 1 would be the mechanism of necrosis produced by a single exposure to halothane; pathway 2 is the suggested explanation of the increased risk on subse- quent exposures. Both occur only under conditions of hypoxia in the liver, when the cytochrome P450 functions as a reductase.

disease correlates quite well with the mean per capita alcohol consumption in a population (see Chapter 72).

Traditionally, alcoholic liver disease has been classified according to morphological criteria into three categories: (1) fatty liver, (2) alcoholic hepatitis (liver cell necrosis and inflammation), and (3) cirrhosis, in which the normal lobular architecture of the liver is replaced by irregular nodules surrounded by thick, fibrous septa. In the context of this chapter, alcoholic liver disease serves to illustrate how all three types of mechanism of drug-induced liver damage described above can be activated by the same drug.

Fatty Liver

This abnormality results mainly from the change of NAD to NADH during the metabolism of ethanol and acetaldehyde (see Chapter 26). The increase in hepatic NADH inhibits the oxidation of both glycerophosphate and free fatty acids, raising their levels in the cytoplasm and stimulating formation and accumulation of neutral triglycerides in the liver. This is an *indirect intrahepatic* mechanism of liver damage. For other examples of ethanol-induced disturbances of intermediary metabolism in the liver see Chapter 26. Fatty liver, of itself, probably does not lead directly to hepatic fibrosis or cirrhosis.

Alcoholic Hepatitis

Alcoholic hepatitis is characterized by clusters or foci of necrotic liver cells, surrounded or infiltrated by inflammatory cells. Enzymes and other molecules that are normally confined within the liver cells are released into the circulation as the damaged cells

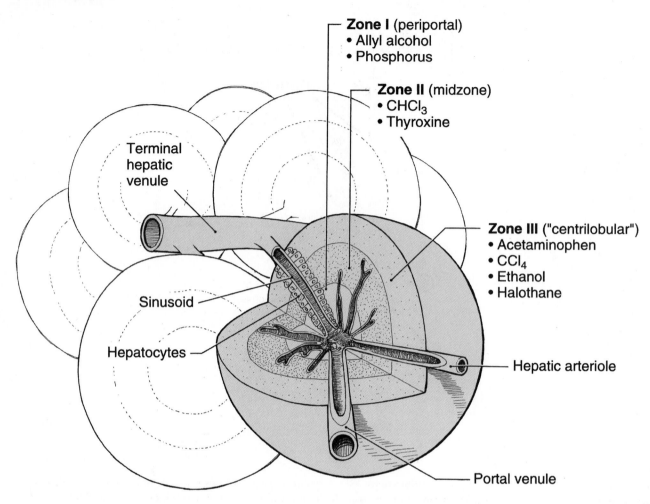

Figure 46-4. Zonal distribution of necrosis in the liver acinus, produced by various hepatotoxic agents.

break down, and they serve as diagnostic markers of the disease process. Several different effects of ethanol or its metabolism have been implicated in the production of necrosis and inflammation.

Hypoxia

As described above, the special features of hepatic blood flow make it very susceptible to hypoxic damage in zone III of the liver acinus. Both acute and chronic ingestion of ethanol lead to increased oxidative activity of the liver mitochondria and thus increase the hepatic oxygen consumption. This does not usually result in liver cell damage, because of a compensatory increase in portal blood flow induced by ethanol. However, if this increase is prevented by other factors, the degree of hypoxia in zone III becomes sufficient to cause cell death. Among such factors encountered in chronic heavy drinkers are anemia, pulmonary insufficiency, and reduced oxy-

gen-carrying capacity of hemoglobin due to heavy smoking (carbon monoxide).

In addition, hepatomegaly is a nearly constant finding in the early stages of alcoholic liver disease in humans, and is due to an increase in hepatocyte size rather than in the number of hepatocytes. The cell swelling is largely due to an increase in intracellular water caused by the osmotic effect of raised levels of intracellular K^+ and protein, secondary to disturbances of transport functions. The enlarged hepatocytes compress the sinusoids, resulting in increased resistance to blood flow and, after a threshold in cell size is exceeded, in increased intrahepatic and portal venous pressure. In humans with alcoholic liver disease, biopsies also reveal a marked reduction in the caliber of the sinusoids and in total sinusoidal cross-sectional area. The compression of the sinusoids decreases blood flow through the sinusoids and reduces delivery of oxygen to the hepatocytes.

The hypoxia resulting from all these causes thus

represents a combination of *indirect extrahepatic* and *indirect intrahepatic* mechanisms of liver cell damage.

The increase in oxygen consumption induced by both acute and chronic administration of ethanol requires thyroid hormone function as a permissive factor. Both thyroidectomy and the administration of the antithyroid drug propylthiouracil (PTU, see Chapter 48) markedly suppress or abolish both the acute and chronically induced hypermetabolic state. PTU administration markedly protected rats against liver necrosis induced by ethanol in the presence of low atmospheric oxygen tensions. Prolonged administration of PTU to patients with alcoholic liver disease resulted in an important decrease in mortality during a 2-year period of observation.

Acetaldehyde

Acetaldehyde, the initial product of alcohol oxidation, is a highly reactive metabolite that can bind to a number of molecules of biological importance, including proteins (such as hemoglobin, tubulin, and albumin), DNA, phospholipids, and serotonin. Also, it can interact with dopamine and norepinephrine, yielding pharmacologically active and potentially cytotoxic compounds.

Acetaldehyde per se can become a hapten when bound covalently to amino acid residues in macromolecules. The antibodies generated are directed against acetaldehyde-modified proteins independently of the nature of the carrier protein. If this happens on the surface of cells, it might be followed by cell lysis. Increased antibody titers against acetaldehyde-containing epitopes have been found predominantly in those alcoholics with alcoholic hepatitis characterized by cell necrosis and polymorphonuclear inflammation. Acetaldehyde might also contribute to the predominantly zone III localization of cell necrosis, since it is formed in the metabolism of ethanol along the sinusoid and is present in a higher concentration in blood leaving zone III than in zone I. All of these effects might be regarded as either *indirect intrahepatic* or *direct* mechanisms of hepatotoxicity.

Oxidative stress

As described in Chapter 26, ethanol is oxidized not only by alcohol dehydrogenase but also by CYP2E1, especially at high alcohol concentrations and in regular heavy drinkers. This pathway generates a variety of highly reactive oxidizing species, including superoxide free radicals, hydroxyl radical, and H_2O_2. In addition, the increase in NADPH:NADP and NADH:NAD ratios mobilizes free Fe^{3+}, which acts as a catalyst for peroxidation of lipids. Normally these oxidizing factors are scavenged by glutathione and other intracellular reducing agents, but ethanol tends to decrease the protection afforded by these agents. Acutely, ethanol decreases the synthesis of glutathione and increases its efflux from liver cells. Chronically, it decreases the mitochondrial content of both vitamin E and glutathione, thus decreasing the protection against superoxide radicals formed during the electron transport process.

The consequence of this loss of protection is referred to as *oxidative stress*, which includes increased risk of cell membrane lysis by lipoperoxides formed by peroxidation of fatty acids. In addition, lipoperoxides have two other actions relevant to the production of alcoholic hepatitis: (1) They act as chemotactic factors for polymorphonuclear leukocytes, thus accounting at least in part for the leukocytic infiltration, and (2) they activate Ito cells in the sinusoids, causing them to synthesize collagen and thus to contribute to the formation of increased fibrous tissue that is seen in later stages of the disease. Thus alcohol, by giving rise to toxic metabolites, can also act as a *direct* hepatotoxin.

Cirrhosis

This is the end stage of alcoholic liver disease and develops in about 10% of persons taking alcoholic beverages in excess. The condition is characterized by a loss of the normal architecture of the liver, formation of fibrous septa bridging the portal veins, and formation of regenerative nodules. As a consequence of these abnormalities, hepatic vasculature is grossly distorted: Sinusoids are transformed into capillary-like structures and blood is shunted from the portal venules to the hepatic vein. Much of the portal blood thus bypasses the hepatic parenchymal cells, and there is a progressive loss of the liver's important role as a filter for substances entering the circulation from the gastrointestinal tract.

The mechanism by which prolonged heavy intake of alcohol leads to cirrhosis probably includes all of the processes described above, in addition to others that may be described as self-aggravating "vicious cycles." For example, constriction of the sinusoids and swelling of hepatocytes cause increased portal venous pressure, which in turn results in upper gastrointestinal bleeding, increase in collateral circulation bypassing the liver, increased collagen deposition in the space of Disse, reduced functional blood perfusion of the liver, hypersplenism, and secondary anemia. All of these reduce oxygen availability to the liver and therefore, in the presence of continued alcohol intake, they increase the risk of further hypoxic necrosis of the liver.

The risk of development of cirrhosis is related to the degree and duration of excessive alcohol use. Most cirrhotics have consumed more than 250 mL of distilled spirits (equivalent to more than 80 g of absolute ethanol) daily for more than 10 years. Absolute alcohol intake seems to be the important factor, regardless of the type of beverage consumed.

DRUGS USED TO TREAT LIVER DISEASE

In recent years the drug treatment of hepatic disease has expanded rapidly. Antivirals, corticosteroids, and immunosuppressive drugs figure prominently in the treatment of various hepatic diseases. There are also specific drug treatments for Wilson's disease, cholestasis, and cholelithiasis. These include **penicillamine, trien, zinc,** and a bile acid, **ursodeoxycholic acid.**

Wilson's Disease

Wilson's disease is an autosomal recessive inherited disorder of hepatic copper metabolism. In Wilson's disease, hepatic incorporation of copper into its carrier protein, ceruloplasmin, and excretion of copper into bile, are abnormal. The defective biochemical mechanisms are not well understood, but the gene for Wilson's disease has recently been identified. Patients with this disorder accumulate copper in the liver; this leads initially to liver damage and later to systemic, principally CNS, damage when the copper begins to spill out of the liver and accumulates in other organs such as the brain, and Kayser-Fleischer rings in the eyes. Wilson's disease is treatable with chelating agents. If it is diagnosed before there is major organ damage, the patient may remain asymptomatic after treatment is begun. Untreated Wilson's disease is always fatal, with progressive hepatic and/or neurological damage.

Penicillamine

This drug chelates copper and can be taken orally. It is a sulfur-containing amino acid in which the thiol group and the amino group play roles similar to those of the two thiol groups in the classic chelator dimercaprol (Fig. 46-5). Penicillamine is quite toxic. However, the D-isomer is less toxic than the L-isomer, and D-penicillamine is the routine treatment modality. Penicillamine can bind lead, mercury, iron, arsenic, and copper. It can bind cystine and is used to treat cystinuria. It inhibits collagen-crosslinking, and it exerts an anti-inflammatory effect; therefore it is also used for the treatment of rheumatoid arthritis. It is an antivitamin for pyridoxine, lowering the plasma and tissue levels of pyridoxine. Therefore this vitamin is given along with penicillamine.

Penicillamine is fairly rapidly absorbed from the gastrointestinal tract. Approximately 50% of the oral dose is absorbed, and a peak blood concentration is reached in 2 hours. The mechanism of absorption is unusual: Penicillamine binds to a protein in the enterocyte membrane and then is absorbed through the enterocyte, perhaps by pinocytosis. The overall bioavailability is 40–70%. A meal taken with penicillamine decreases absorption of the drug by about one-half. Once absorbed, penicillamine circulates 80% bound to plasma proteins; of the 20% unbound, 6% is free penicillamine, and the rest consists of inactive disulfides. Excretion of penicillamine is largely renal; fecal excretion accounts for approximately 16%. S-methylation of penicillamine occurs in the liver, but this metabolite (S-methyl-D-penicillamine) is more common in patients with rheumatoid arthritis than in those with Wilson's disease. The elimination half-life of penicillamine varies widely between 1.7 and 7 hours. Some metabolites of penicillamine remain detectable in urine months after the drug is stopped.

Adverse side effects of penicillamine are said to be more common in patients without Wilson's disease, but the incidence in Wilson's disease is as high as 30%. Skin changes may develop, due to changes in collagen formation. Adverse cutaneous reactions include various types of rashes, pemphigus, and elastosis perforans serpiginosa. Nausea may occur and the sense of taste may change (dysgeusia); these are relatively trivial problems. Adverse hematological reactions are common but are usually reversible if caught early. Leukopenia or thrombocytopenia may occur. Rarely, severe global bone marrow failure develops. Perhaps the worst problems are autoimmune-like syndromes: nephrotic syndrome, systemic vasculitis resembling lupus erythematosus, Goodpasture's syndrome affecting the lungs, or a syndrome resembling myasthenia gravis. Severe hematological or systemic side effects require cessation of treatment. If penicillamine treatment in Wilson's disease needs to be stopped because of untoward side effects, a different chelator must be substituted.

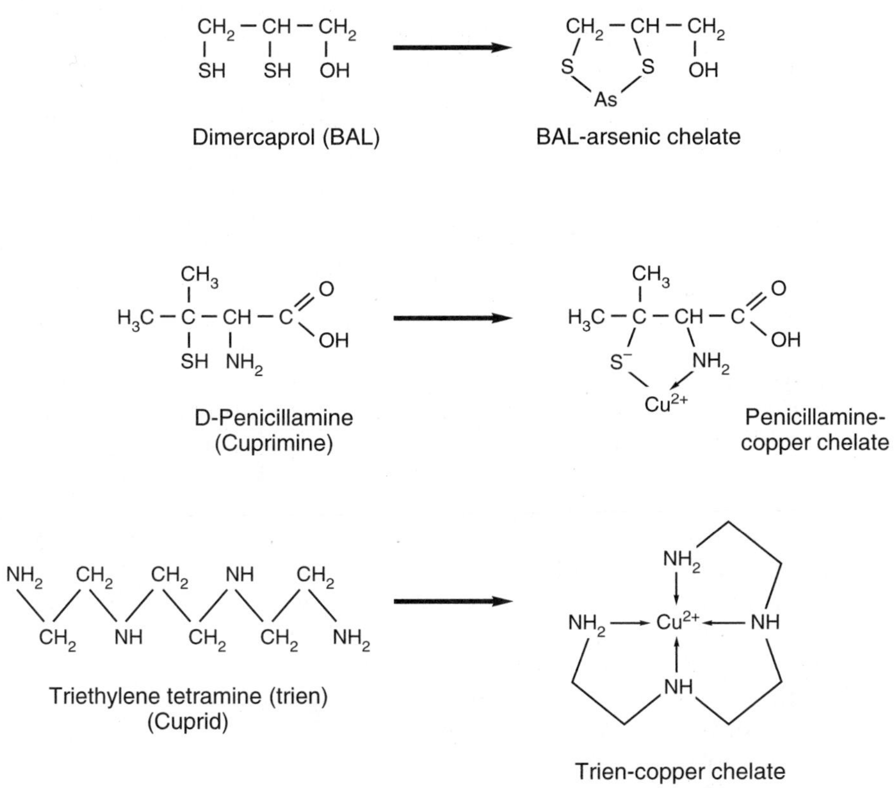

Figure 46-5. Structural formulae of dimercaprol (BAL), D-penicillamine, and triethylene tetramine (trien), and the formation of metal chelates.

Some patients develop an early hypersensitivity reaction to penicillamine in the first 7–10 days of taking it. They develop rash, fever, anorexia, lymphadenopathy, leukopenia, and thrombocytopenia. Proteinuria may also occur. If penicillamine is stopped and then reintroduced gradually, these patients may develop tolerance for the drug. Occasionally, steroids must be given briefly. Alternatively, a second-line chelator may be substituted.

Trien

The usual alternative treatment for patients with Wilson's disease who develop severe toxicity from penicillamine is triethylene tetramine dihydrochloride (2,2,2-tetramine), known by its official short name **trien** or as **trientine** (Fig. 46-5). Trien does not contain sulfhydryl groups. It chelates copper by forming a stable complex with its four constituent nitrogens in a planar ring. Trien increases urinary copper excretion and may interfere with its intestinal absorption.

Little is known about the pharmacokinetics of trien. It is poorly absorbed from the gastrointestinal tract; what is absorbed is biotransformed and inacti-vated. Chronic treatment may lead to iron deficiency. Trien may rarely cause hemorrhagic gastritis, loss of taste, and rashes. However, adverse effects due to penicillamine resolve and do not recur during treatment with trien. Although trien may be intrinsically somewhat weaker as a chelator than penicillamine, the dose can be adjusted for clinical effectiveness.

Zinc

Although zinc was used to treat Wilson's disease in the early 1960s, it has only recently received wider attention as an alternative treatment modality for this disease. Some treatment regimens are unwieldy. For adults the most practical and effective regimen is 200 mg of zinc sulfate (equivalent to 45 mg elemental zinc) orally 30 minutes before meals, three times daily. Half of this dose is used for children. The dosage regimen must then be individualized by titrating against its effect on free serum copper.

This drug therapy is important because the mechanism of action of zinc in Wilson's disease is entirely different from that of chelators. Zinc treatment interferes with uptake of copper from the gastrointestinal tract. It is postulated that excess zinc induces the formation of metallothionein in enterocytes. However, the metallothionein has greater affinity for copper than for zinc, and it preferentially binds copper present in the gastrointestinal tract. Once bound, the copper is not absorbed but rather is lost into the fecal contents as enterocytes are shed in the course of normal cellular turnover. Since copper enters the gastrointestinal tract from saliva and gastric secretions, it is possible for zinc treatment to remove stored copper. An unresolved problem with zinc therapy is the effect on hepatic copper. Patients treated chronically with zinc have been found to have higher concentrations of hepatic copper late in the treatment, despite being clinically well. Possibly this copper is complexed to hepatic metallothionein and is thus detoxified.

The major adverse effect of zinc treatment has been abdominal pain, probably reflecting gastritis. Acetate or gluconate salts of zinc may be less irritative than the sulfate. The pain is probably less likely to occur if the zinc is taken with food, but food interferes greatly with zinc absorption and thus with the effectiveness of treatment. Other long-term effects in humans are uncertain. Studies in laboratory animals suggest that high doses of zinc may be immunosuppressive, may depress polymorphonuclear leukocyte chemotaxis, and may interfere with bone formation.

Cholestasis and Cholelithiasis: Ursodeoxycholic Acid

Ursodeoxycholic acid (ursodiol, UDCA) is a hydrophilic epimer of one of the primary bile acids, chenodeoxycholic acid (CDCA). As shown in Figure 46-6, the difference is in the position of one hydroxyl group. In oral pharmacological doses, UDCA displaces more toxic bile acids from the bile acid pool, partly by decreasing intestinal absorption of the primary bile acids, cholic acid and chenodeoxycholic acid. UDCA appears to have three main pharmaco-logical effects: (1) increasing cholesterol saturation in bile; (2) causing increased bile secretion (choleresis); and (3) providing hepatic cytoprotection. The choleresis appears to be due to increased biliary bicarbonate excretion and increased contractility of the smallest bile duct radicles. UDCA was originally used for treatment of cholesterol gallstone disease, but more recently it has been used for other types of chronic liver disease including chronic cholestasis and liver disease associated with cystic fibrosis.

UDCA, administered orally as unconjugated bile acid, is absorbed rapidly from the small intestine. It is conjugated with glycine or taurine in the liver and enters the enterohepatic circulation. With repeated dosing, UDCA becomes a major constituent of the bile acid pool. Excretion is ultimately via the feces. The elimination half-life for exogenously administered UDCA is estimated to be 3–6 days.

UDCA is well tolerated when taken orally. It may cause some transient itching. Unlike CDCA, it does not cause diarrhea to any great extent because it does not stimulate colonic water secretion. It is not hepatotoxic; however, it should not be given to patients with complete blockage of bile drainage because in this situation liver damage may ensue.

With respect to **gallstone dissolution,** its original use, UDCA is effective in dissolving pure cholesterol gallstones that are not calcified. It is more likely to work when the stone is small (<1 cm diameter) and floating on the gallbladder contents. It is not effective if the gallbladder is so diseased that it does not concentrate the bile, or if the cystic duct is blocked. The mechanism of dissolution is that UDCA increases the effectiveness of micelle formation, supports cholesterol liquid crystal formation within these micelles, and increases the amount of cholesterol that can be solubilized.

As a therapy, gallstone dissolution by UDCA will likely not replace cholecystectomy, but it has a role in patients who cannot undergo an operation, or as an adjunct to lithotripsy, and for hepatolithiasis.

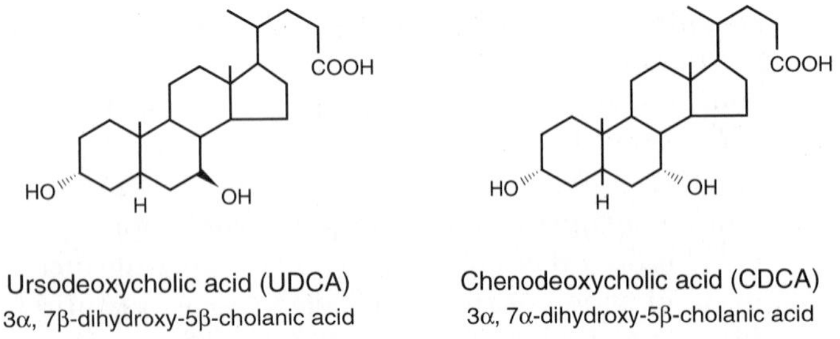

Ursodeoxycholic acid (UDCA)
3α, 7β-dihydroxy-5β-cholanic acid

Chenodeoxycholic acid (CDCA)
3α, 7α-dihydroxy-5β-cholanic acid

Figure 46-6. Structural formulae of ursodeoxycholic acid (UDCA) and chenodeoxycholic acid (CDCA).

Chronic administration of UDCA can dissolve cholesterol gallstones without producing the diarrhea and hepatotoxicity that are major side effects of chenodeoxycholic acid, which is also used for gallstone dissolution. Compared to CDCA, UDCA is safer and more effective, but surface calcification of the gallstone is more likely to develop. UDCA enhances micelle formation in the bile to a greater extent than CDCA, thus increasing the cholesterol-carrying capacity, but it does not suppress hepatic bile acid synthesis as much as CDCA does.

In the course of studying the use of UDCA for gallstone dissolution, its beneficial effects in **chronic cholestasis** were discovered. UDCA has been tried in nearly every chronic cholestatic disease and may be beneficial in some of them. In primary biliary cirrhosis, biochemical abnormalities improve at least temporarily during UDCA treatment, although the downward course of the disease is not necessarily changed. UDCA appears to improve liver function in children with liver disease associated with cystic fibrosis, and it decreases cholestasis in children with Alagille's syndrome, improving the pruritus and lowering serum cholesterol levels. UDCA appears to improve liver function in babies with certain rare inborn errors of bile acid metabolism.

Several mechanisms of action have been proposed to explain the beneficial effect of UDCA in chronic cholestatic liver disease. Its action as a choleretic may be important. Also, it prevents damage to liver cell membranes by more hydrophobic bile acids. This cytoprotective effect has been demonstrated in vitro. It also affects some immune functions, including decreased expression of class I HLA antigens on hepatocytes. It has been shown to inhibit proliferation of peripheral blood mononuclear cells in vitro.

SUGGESTED READING

Arias IM, Jakoby WB, Popper H, Schachter D, Shafritz DA, eds. The liver: biology and pathobiology. New York: Raven Press, 1988.

Cameron RG, Feuer G, de la Iglesia FA, eds. Drug-induced hepatotoxicity. Berlin: Springer-Verlag, 1996.

Farrell GC. Drug-induced liver disease. Edinburgh: Churchill Livingstone, 1994.

Gleeson D, Ruppin DC, Saunders A, et al. Final outcome of ursodeoxycholic acid treatment in 126 patients with radiolucent stones. Quart J Med 1990; 76:711–729.

Israel Y, Kalant H, Orrego H, et al. Experimental alcohol-induced hepatic necrosis: suppression by propylthiouracil. Proc Natl Acad Sci USA 1975; 72:1137–1141.

Israel Y, Orrego H. Hypermetabolic state, hepatocyte expansion and liver blood flow: an interaction triad in alcoholic liver injury. Ann NY Acad Sci 1987; 492:303–323.

Meeting Report. Current progress in studies on alcohol-induced organ injury. Alcohol 1993; 10:437–484.

Mitchell JB, Russo A. The role of glutathione in radiation and drug induced cytotoxicity. Br J Cancer (Suppl) 1987; 8:96–104.

Poupon RE, Poupon R, Balkau B, UDCA-PBC Study Group. Ursodiol for the long-term treatment of primary biliary cirrhosis. N Engl J Med 1994; 330:1342–1347.

Walshe JM. Treatment of Wilson's disease with trientine (triethylene tetramine) dihydrochloride. Lancet 1982; I:643–647.

Yarze JC, Martin P, Munoz SJ, Friedman LS. Wilson's disease: current status. Am J Med 1992; 92:643–654.

Zafrani ES, Pinaudeau Y, Dhumeaux D. Drug-induced vascular lesions of the liver. Arch Intern Med 1983; 143:495–502.

Zimmerman HJ, Maddrey WC. Toxic and drug-induced hepatitis. In: Schiff L, Schiff ER, eds. Disease of the liver. 5th ed. Philadelphia: JB Lippincott, 1987:591–667.

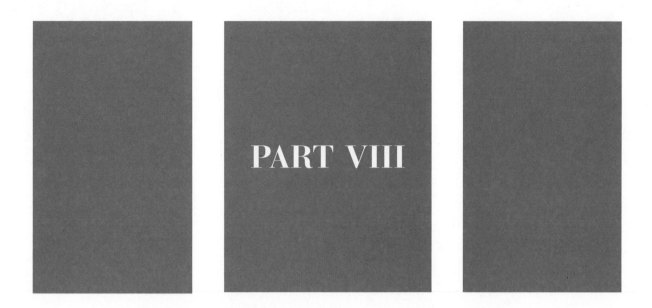

PART VIII

ENDOCRINE SYSTEMS

CHAPTER 47

Vasopressin, Oxytocin, and Uterotonic Drugs

S.R. GEORGE AND B.P. SCHIMMER

CASE HISTORY

A 32-year-old male race car driver crashed during a race and sustained a skull fracture with severe contusions of the head and loss of consciousness. In hospital, his urinary output was noted to be excessive, at a rate of 500 mL/hr. The urine was pale and dilute, with a specific gravity of 1.005. The serum sodium was elevated, with a value of 149 mmol/L (normal range 132–145), and there was hyperosmolality. A diagnosis was made of diabetes insipidus secondary to trauma. He was given desmopressin 1 μg subcutaneously, and the signs of diabetes insipidus diminished within a few hours. The treatment was repeated every 12 hours. After 3 days his general condition, including consciousness, reflexes, and movement, improved markedly and he was switched from parenteral desmopressin to the nasal spray of desmopressin, 10 μg twice daily.

After 5 weeks on this treatment, during which his injuries had continued to improve steadily, he began to complain of headache and some flushing of the face. Two days later he became rather confused and suffered a generalized tonic-clonic seizure. His plasma sodium was found to be 115 mmol/L. The desmopressin was stopped and fluid intake was restricted. Over the next 3 days he recovered fully and was able to maintain normal water and electrolyte balance without reinstatement of desmopressin therapy.

Vasopressin and oxytocin are related nonapeptides that differ from each other by only two amino acids. Both hormones may have evolved from a single ancestral peptide, vasotocin, through molecular processes involving mutation and gene duplication. Vasotocin is the natural form found in primitive species such as elasmobranchs and bony fish and has biological activities intermediate between those of vasopressin and oxytocin when tested in mammalian systems. Du Vigneaud is credited with determining the structure of these peptide hormones and with their chemical synthesis. He was awarded the Nobel Prize in 1955.

Because of their structural similarities, the two peptides have similar pharmacological activities, but these are expressed to different degrees. For example, vasopressin has greater antidiuretic and pressor activities and less uterotonic and milk-ejecting activities than oxytocin has.

Following the pioneering work of du Vigneaud, a large number of synthetic hormone analogs have been prepared and tested for separation of these various activities. Some of the analogs have markedly selective actions and have become clinically important drugs.

BIOSYNTHETIC AND ANATOMICAL RELATIONSHIPS

The hypothalamus and the posterior lobe of the pituitary gland function together as a neurosecretory unit. The anatomical relationships of this unit are shown in Figure 47-1.

Site of Synthesis

Vasopressin and oxytocin are synthesized in specialized neurons of the hypothalamus and transported to the posterior lobe (pars nervosa) of the pituitary gland. **Vasopressin** is synthesized in neural cell bodies that are localized predominantly in the **supraoptic nucleus,** while **oxytocin** is synthesized in neural cell bodies that are predominantly in the **paraventricular nucleus.**

Synthesis and Processing

Both peptides have molecular weights of approximately 1100 Da but are synthesized as larger precursor peptides (prohormones). The precursor peptides also give rise to two distinct neurophysins (approximate MW 10,000 Da), which serve as carrier proteins for vasopressin and oxytocin. The precursors are synthesized on membrane-bound ribosomes, packaged into secretory granules, and then enzymatically cleaved so that the hormones remain associated with the neurophysins through electrostatic forces. The hormone-containing granules are transported to nerve terminals via unmyelinated axons. Most axons pass through the pituitary stalk and end in the posterior pituitary. Some axons only extend to the median eminence.

Secretion

Inputs from peripheral signals and from the CNS converge on the hypothalamic nuclei. These signals trigger electrical impulses that travel down the axons of the neurosecretory fibers to the nerve terminals and stimulate hormone secretion. The secretory response is thought to involve: (1) influx of calcium to the cytosol, (2) fusion of secretory granules with the membranes of the nerve terminals, (3) emptying of the granule contents into surrounding capillaries, and (4) recapture of empty granules (as small vesicles) from the cell surface. Although vasopressin and oxytocin are synthesized in separate neurons, most stimuli for secretion may cause the release of both peptides. The type of stimulus, however, does determine the relative proportions of the secreted mixture. For example, thirst or hemorrhage causes preferential

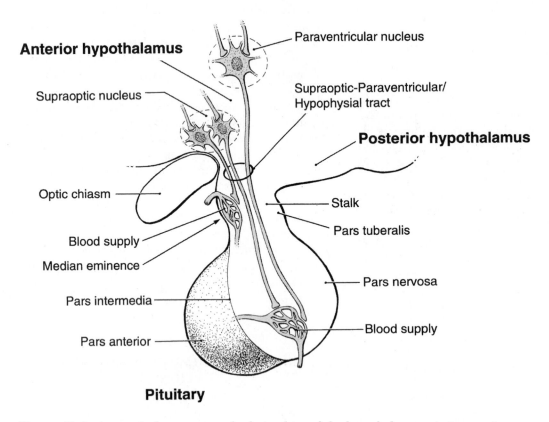

Figure 47-1. Anatomical structure and relationships of the hypothalamus-pituitary unit.

release of vasopressin; suckling stimulates the preferential release of oxytocin.

Role of the Posterior Pituitary Gland

The posterior pituitary serves as a storage site for vasopressin and oxytocin. It is a physical, as well as functional, extension of the nervous system, organized into a specialized secretory apparatus. The posterior pituitary is composed of swollen, granule-filled, nerve terminals in juxtaposition to blood capillaries (see Fig. 47-1) and supported by pituicytes (glial cells). Lesions in the hypothalamic nuclei or in the hypothalamic-neurohypophysial tract destroy the capacity for vasopressin and oxytocin synthesis. Removal of the posterior pituitary, however, generally causes only a transient deficiency, because the nerve fibers terminating in the median eminence remain functional and release amounts of these hormones sufficient for normal physiological requirements.

CHEMISTRY

Structures

The structures of vasopressin and oxytocin are shown in Figure 47-2. In both hormones, six of the amino acids form ring structures by closure of the S–S bond between cysteines at positions 1 and 6; attached to the ring of each peptide is a tail of three amino acids with an amide at the carboxyl terminus. Opening the S–S bond results in a linear nonapeptide devoid of hormonal activity. For vasopressin activity, the tail must contain a basic amino acid (arginine in most mammals, lysine in the pig) at position 8 (Fig. 47-2).

VASOPRESSIN (ADH)

Physiology and Pharmacology

Receptors

Vasopressin acts through different types of receptors, designated V_1 and V_2. The V_1 type acts through the cell membrane inositol trisphosphate cycle and results in a large increase in intracellular Ca^{2+} (see Chapter 10). The V_2 type is a G protein-coupled membrane receptor that activates adenylyl cyclase. Both types are found in the periphery, as well as in

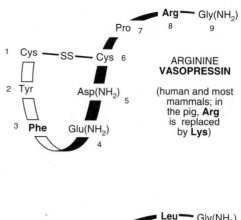

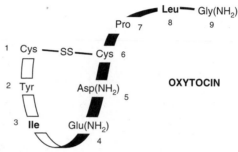

Figure 47-2. Amino acid sequences for vasopressin and oxytocin. The differences are at positions 3 and 8.

the brain. Synthetic peptides have been produced that act as specific agonists or specific antagonists for V_1- or V_2-receptors and permit a more detailed analysis of the mechanisms responsible for different effects of vasopressin.

Antidiuretic action

The major physiological action of vasopressin in the human is on the reabsorption of water by the collecting ducts of the kidney. Therefore vasopressin is also known as the antidiuretic hormone (ADH). ADH increases the permeability of the tubular epithelium to the passage of water. Water, together with sodium and urea, moves from the tubular lumen into the interstitial fluid in response to an osmotic gradient, leaving solutes behind in more concentrated urine. The antidiuretic effect is extremely potent. Less than 0.1 μg/hr, administered by slow intravenous infusion, suppresses human urine flow completely.

The mechanism of action of ADH on the collecting duct is shown in Figure 47-3. ADH, in sequential fashion, (1) interacts with a receptor of the V_2 subtype, (2) activates a stimulatory guanine nucleotide-binding protein, (3) activates adenylyl cyclase and causes cyclic AMP to accumulate, and (4) activates

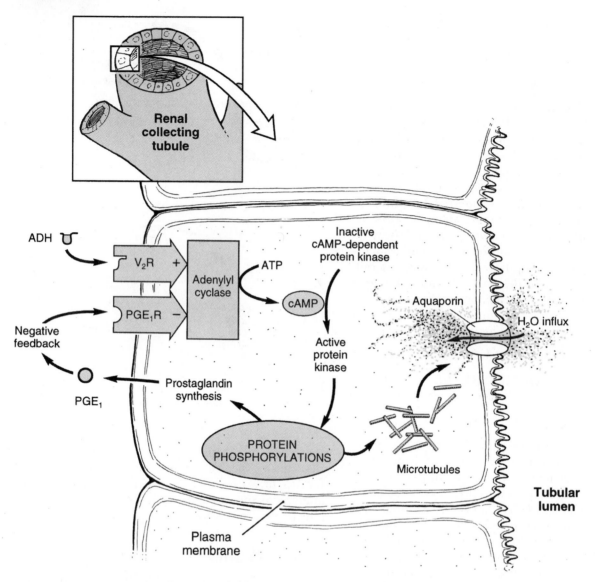

Figure 47-3. Mechanism of action of ADH on water reabsorption.

cyclic AMP-dependent protein kinase, increasing the phosphorylation of specific proteins. There is some evidence that one of the consequences of ADH-stimulated protein phosphorylation is the appearance of cell-surface water channels (aquaporins), thus increasing the permeability of the luminal membrane to water. Since this process is sensitive to microtubule poisons (colchicine, vinca alkaloids), microtubules are probably involved. As part of its action, ADH also stimulates the synthesis of prostaglandin E_1 (PGE_1), which serves in a negative-feedback loop to inhibit ADH action locally. The adenylyl cyclase system appears to be the target of the inhibitory influence of PGE_1. Atrial natriuretic peptide antago-

nizes ADH effect on water permeability in the collecting ducts and promotes diuresis through a cyclic GMP mechanism (see Chapter 41).

Secretion of ADH can be stimulated or inhibited by osmotic, volemic, or neural stimuli reaching cells in the supraoptic nucleus (Fig. 47-4).

ADH secretion is stimulated by:

- Hyperosmolality of plasma—e.g., secretion is responsive to as little as 1–2% change in osmolality. This action is exerted through **osmoreceptors** located in the hypothalamus and other brain regions.

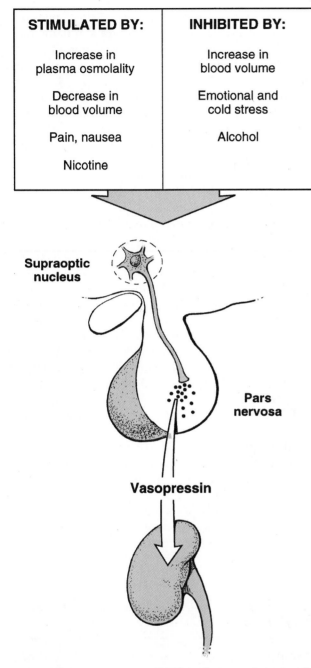

STIMULATED BY:	INHIBITED BY:
Increase in plasma osmolality	Increase in blood volume
Decrease in blood volume	Emotional and cold stress
Pain, nausea	Alcohol
Nicotine	

Figure 47-4. Factors involved in the stimulation and inhibition of vasopressin secretion.

- Volume depletion—e.g., hemorrhage or pooling of blood in the extremities on standing. As little as 6–10% change in blood volume affects ADH release by an action through stretch receptors and baroreceptors in the left atrium, carotid bodies, aorta, and pulmonary vessels.
- Drugs—e.g., cholinergic agonists (nicotine), clofi-

brate, tricyclic antidepressants, cyclophosphamide.
- Noxious stimuli—e.g., pain, nausea.

ADH secretion is inhibited by:

- Hydration—drinking large volumes of water; hypo-osmolality and increased blood volume are the operative factors.
- Alcohol—by blocking nervous impulses from the midbrain; this action can be overcome by nicotine.
- Some nervous stimuli—e.g., cold exposure.

In addition to stimulating and inhibiting ADH secretion, drugs can affect the antidiuretic action of ADH in a variety of ways, as shown in Table 47-1.

Smooth-muscle contraction

At high dose, vasopressin causes the contraction of smooth-muscle fibers in a number of tissues through

Table 47-1 Other Drugs Affecting Antidiuretic Action of ADH

Drugs	Mechanism of Action
Potentiators of ADH action	
Acetylsalicylic acid (aspirin)	Inhibit renal prostaglandin synthesis; chlorpropamide also stimulates ADH secretion
Chlorpropamide	
Indomethacin	
Inhibitors of ADH action	
Lithium carbonate	Inhibit adenylyl cyclase
Prostaglandin E_1	
Colchicine	Microtubular poisons
Vinca alkaloids	
Demeclocycline	Results in nephrogenic diabetes insipidus. Used clinically to treat SIADH*
Thiazide diuretics	
Useful in treatment of nephrogenic or partial hypothalamic diabetes insipidus	Unknown and paradoxical; effects may result from systemic depletion of electrolytes, which in turn causes enhanced resorption of salt and water from the proximal tubule (see also Chapter 41)

*Syndrome of inappropriate antidiuretic hormone.

an action on vasopressin V_1-receptors located on vascular and other smooth-muscle cells.

- It causes pronounced vasoconstriction; the effect is general and includes coronary blood vessels.
- The motility of intestinal smooth muscle, especially in the lower bowel, is increased.
- Vasopressin stimulates uterine and cervical contractions, particularly circular smooth muscle. It causes short, frequent contractions without distinction between pregnant and nonpregnant uterus.

Blood coagulation

Vasopressin increases the levels of clotting factor VIII and Von Willebrand factor. This effect may have implications in the management of some blood clotting diseases and in prophylactic control of bleeding during surgery in patients with factor VIII deficiency.

ACTH secretion

Vasopressin stimulates ACTH release from the anterior pituitary. It is synergistic with corticotropin-releasing factor (CRF), which is the principal releasing factor for ACTH.

CNS function

Vasopressin is found in other parts of the brain in association with both V_1- and V_2-receptors; this fact suggests that vasopressin has neurotransmitter or neuromodulator activity and may have various physiological roles in the CNS (see Chapter 20). When administered through normal routes, vasopressin improves the ability to learn new information and enhances long-term memory. These effects are being explored in the treatment of amnesia and in the improvement of attention and memory in the elderly. Vasopressin also has effects on autonomic function mediated via the CNS, including actions that decrease body temperature, slow the heart rate, and increase the respiratory rate.

Synthetic Analogs

Both vasopressin and oxytocin have short half-lives in the circulation (approximately 10 minutes), principally due to proteolytic degradation. An important site for proteolytic inactivation in both hormones is between the first two amino acids (Cys-Tyr). Cleavage of peptide bonds in the tail also contributes to

loss of activity. The rapid turnover of these peptides limits their duration of action. Hence synthetic analogs of vasopressin with increased duration of action have been developed and are more important clinically.

Another important rationale for the development of synthetic analogs is to achieve greater separation of the antidiuretic and pressor actions of vasopressin. As shown in Table 47-2, four modifications are important for enhanced antidiuretic activity. Combinations of these four modifications produce synergistic results. For example, 1-desamino-8-D-arginine vasopressin (DDAVP, desmopressin) has an antidiuretic activity that is 2000 times greater than its pressor effect. The analog, 1-desamino-4-valine-8-D-arginine vasopressin (DVDAVP), is even more selectively potent but has been used only experimentally so far. Deamination at position 1 also renders the peptide more resistant to proteolysis, as does the substitution of D-arginine at position 8.

Other modifications can selectively increase the pressor effect of vasopressin, yielding derivatives with clinical potential as local hemostatic agents during surgery. One such analog is 2-phenylalanine-3-isoleucine-8-ornithine vasopressin. It has a pressor:ADH ratio of 255:1; it is used for experimental purposes only.

Some of the smaller peptides produced by partial proteolytic cleavage of vasopressin have physiological activities that differ from those of vasopressin. For example, removal of the terminal glycine (NH_2) from the side-chain yields desglycinamide arginine vasopressin (DGAVP), which retains the central actions of vasopressin but has greatly reduced peripheral activity.

Table 47-2 Modifications Affecting the Ratio of Antidiuretic to Pressor Activity of Vasopressin

Modification	ADH/Pressor Ratio*
Deamination at position 1	4
Substitution of Phe for Tyr	3
Substitution of Val or Thr for Glu (NH_2)	23
Substitution of D-Arg for L-Arg	28
1-Desamino plus 8-D-Arg	2000
1-Desamino-8-D-Arg plus 4-Val	>150,000

*Results are compared with arginine vasopressin, which is assigned a normalized value of 1.0.

Preparations

Desmopressin (DDAVP), the 1-desamino-8-D-arginine synthetic analog of vasopressin, has a longer half-life than vasopressin. Since it is selective for V_2 vasopressin receptors, it has greater ADH potency and less pressor activity than vasopressin. It has to be administered in high doses when given by mouth because it is broken down by intestinal peptidases. Preparations are supplied in isotonic saline as the acetate salt (0.1 mg/mL) and are administered intranasally. DDAVP for injection (4 μg/mL) also is available. Its duration of action is 8–12 hours. An oral formulation has recently become available.

Vasopressin (Pitressin) is an aqueous solution for intravenous or intramuscular injection; the standard dosage form provides 10 I.U./0.5-mL ampoule. (The International Unit of vasopressin is defined by the pressor activity, in rats, of 0.5 mg of a U.S.P. standard posterior pituitary powder. One unit of activity corresponds to approximately 3 μg of purified arginine vasopressin.) The active principle may be purified from animal posterior pituitary (in which case it may have some contaminating oxytocic activity); more often, it is chemically synthesized. It acts for 3–4 hours.

Lysine vasopressin (Lypressin, Diapid) is a synthetic preparation of lysine vasopressin, more stable than arginine vasopressin, and available as a nasal spray or in injectable form.

Therapeutic Uses

Diabetes insipidus

This disease, caused by insufficient endogenous ADH, is characterized by excretion of large volumes of dilute urine (specific gravity about 1.002), extreme thirst, and copious intake of water. It can be congenital or can result from lesions affecting the hypothalamus, such as tumor or trauma. The treatment of choice is desmopressin (DDAVP) administered intranasally. The dose depends on the severity of the case and ranges between 2.5 and 20 μg intranasally two or three times a day. Patients intolerant to this route of administration may receive 1–2 μg twice daily by subcutaneous or intramuscular injection. The main adverse effect of nasal administration is local irritation (rhinitis).

The existence of polyuria and polydipsia is not synonymous with diabetes insipidus of hypothalamic origin. For example, similar symptoms are seen in diabetes insipidus of nephrogenic origin (failure of the kidney to respond to ADH). Small doses of vasopressin are very effective in decreasing polyuria, polydipsia, and water intake in hypothalamic diabetes insipidus; there is a corresponding increase in urine osmolality, which is diagnostic of this condition.

Local hemostasis

This is achieved by intravenous infusion of vasopressin in the treatment of bleeding esophageal varices; vasopressin causes strong splanchnic vasoconstriction, thus lowering pressure in the portal vein. Vasopressin can also be administered by local arterial infusion to control active gastrointestinal bleeding during abdominal surgery.

Coagulation disorders

Desmopressin is used to treat Von Willebrand's disease and hemophilia associated with factor VIII deficiency, particularly before elective surgery.

Enuresis (bed-wetting)

Desmopressin has also been used to treat children with primary enuresis by administering a single bedtime dose to increase nocturnal renal concentrating ability. However, the high probability of spontaneous disappearance of the problem, and the possibility of side effects of the treatment, limit the value of this therapy.

Toxicity

Symptoms of toxicity (which may occur from overdose) result from a mixture of effects at V_1 and V_2 vasopressin receptors and include hypertension, headache, cerebral or coronary arterial spasm, water intoxication, hyponatremia, pallor, nausea, abdominal cramps from increased intestinal activity, uterine cramps, and vasospasm that may result in gangrene.

Syndrome of Inappropriate Antidiuretic Hormone (SIADH)

SIADH results from the pathological overproduction of ADH as a result of CNS disorders or ectopic production by tumors. This condition is treated by demeclocycline (a tetracycline), which inhibits ADH action in the collecting ducts of the kidney.

OXYTOCIN

Physiology and Pharmacology

Milk ejection

Milk ejection appears to be the major physiological function of oxytocin. Oxytocin stimulates the contraction of myoepithelial cells of the breast during the postpartum period. These cells surround the channels of the glandular system and serve to squeeze milk out of the alveoli and ducts into larger sinuses. This is called "milk letdown" and is different from milk secretion. Suckling at the nipple of the breast is an important stimulus for the release of oxytocin.

Uterine contraction

Sensitivity of the uterus to oxytocin increases rapidly during the *last trimester of pregnancy* because of a dramatic increase in uterine oxytocin receptors. Thus, when labor is imminent, sensitivity to oxytocin is much greater than to vasopressin. Oxytocin stimulates slow, long-lasting peristaltic contractions of the upper uterine segment and relaxes the cervix. This is a useful type of contraction for the expulsion of uterine contents. Estrogen increases the sensitivity of the uterus to oxytocin; progesterone renders uterine tissue more resistant. The effect of oxytocin on the *nonpregnant uterus* is slight.

The physiological importance of oxytocin in the initiation of labor or in delivery is debatable. Arguments against the involvement of oxytocin include the observations that blood levels of oxytocin do not increase until labor is well advanced and that parturition still proceeds in the absence of oxytocin (although prolonged labor has been reported).

Effects on the corpus luteum

Recent evidence suggests that oxytocin may also regulate the lifespan of the corpus luteum and thus play a role in the regulation of fertility. Included in this evidence are the observations that oxytocin administered to experimental animals shortens the lifespan of the corpus luteum and hastens the onset of estrus, while active immunization of animals against oxytocin has the opposite effect. These observations raise the possibility that oxytocin analogs may one day provide new pharmacological approaches to contraception.

Vascular effects

Oxytocin tends to relax circular fibers of smooth muscles and in large doses will lower blood pressure. Deep anesthesia or concurrent use of ganglionic blocking drugs increases the likelihood of this potentially dangerous effect.

Mechanism of action

The hormone exerts its action through specific G protein-coupled receptors at the cell surface. Activation of the receptor is associated with increased phospholipase C activity, with consequent mobilization of intracellular calcium. Activation of voltage-sensitive calcium channels has also been demonstrated.

Preparations

Oxytocin injection (Pitocin, Syntocinon) contains synthetic, pure oxytocin and is provided as an aqueous solution for intramuscular or intravenous injection, containing 10 IU/mL. (One unit is equivalent to about 2 μg of pure oxytocin. Oxytocic activity is bioassayed by measuring the drop in blood pressure in chickens; uterotonic activity parallels the decrease in blood pressure.) **Oxytocin nasal solution** is a nasal spray containing 40 IU/mL of synthetic oxytocin.

Therapeutic Uses

Stimulation of labor at term

Oxytocin is used primarily to **induce labor.** The aim is to determine the dose that just initiates labor without producing overly strong contractions, thereby avoiding damage to the fetus or uterus in the early stages. Preferably oxytocin is administered by slow intravenous infusion. Initial doses are small (2 mU/min) and are gradually increased to a maximum of 20 mU/min if necessary. Throughout this treatment the resting uterine tone; the force, duration, and frequency of uterine contractions; and the fetal heart rate should be carefully monitored. The short half-life (minutes) of oxytocin permits effective control through changes of the infusion rate. Oxytocin may be used in selected cases to **resume labor** if the uterus shows inertia during the first stage.

Contraindications for the use of oxytocin include situations that preclude normal vaginal delivery, predisposition to uterine rupture, or signs of fetal distress.

Control of postpartum bleeding

Bleeding may occur if the uterus relaxes too much during the interval of placental expulsion. Administration of oxytocin (approximately 5 IU) after the head is delivered will prevent excessive relaxation of the uterus during this stage. If oxytocin is administered again *after* the placenta is expelled, it will cause strong tetanic contraction of the uterus and prevent postpartum bleeding.

Stimulation of milk ejection

Oxytocin is sometimes useful in relieving breast engorgement or in facilitating breast feeding when letdown is a problem. For these purposes, oxytocin is administered as a nasal spray a few minutes before feeding. Oxytocin is of no value if there is inadequate milk production.

Adverse Effects

The toxicity of oxytocin is an extension of its physiological effects and may include **tetanic uterine contractions,** which may result in fetal hypoxia. β_2-Adrenergic agonists may be used to reverse the sustained (tetanic) uterine contractions. **Hypotension** occurs as a result of relaxation of vascular smooth muscles. **Symptoms of water intoxication** may be elicited because of the structural similarity between oxytocin and vasopressin.

ERGOT ALKALOIDS AND OTHER OXYTOCIC DRUGS

A number of other agents, though chemically unrelated to oxytocin, are used clinically because of their ability to stimulate contraction of uterine muscle. Some of these agents are described briefly in this section.

Ergot Alkaloids

These compounds are derived from a fungus commonly known as ergot that grows on grain. For centuries, crude extracts of ergot were used by midwives as an obstetrical aid to hasten the onset and progress of labor. Their effects on uterine contraction, however, were vigorous and sustained. As a consequence, fetal anoxia and uterine rupture occurred with unacceptable frequency. In high concentrations, the extracts caused ergot poisoning characterized by marked vasoconstriction, giving rise to burning sensations in the extremities ("St. Anthony's Fire") and sometimes to gangrene and CNS irritation (leading to convulsions).

With the isolation and purification of the various alkaloids of ergot, **ergonovine** and **methylergonovine** were identified and were found to have a highly selective action on the uterus while causing minimal vasoconstriction. Structurally, they are simple amide derivatives of lysergic acid (Fig. 47-5).

Currently, the ergot alkaloids are never used in the early stages of labor; however, because they are so effective in "clamping down" the uterus, they are used to control postpartum hemorrhage. The actions of the two ergot alkaloids are rapid and are exerted directly on the uterus. Effects are observed 8–10 minutes after an oral dose and almost immediately after intravenous or intramuscular injection. In very high doses, the toxic symptoms of ergot poisoning become evident.

Ergonovine differs from both vasopressin and

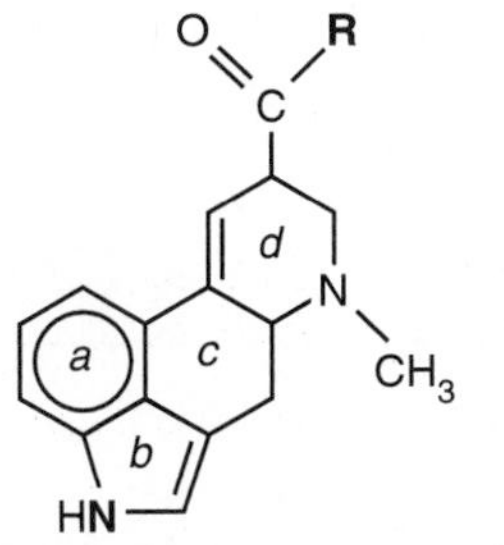

Lysergic acid	R= — OH
LSD	R= — N(CH$_2$CH$_3$)$_2$

Ergonovine (= Ergometrine)	R= — N — CHCH$_2$OH
	   |
	   CH$_3$

Methylergonovine	R= — N — CHCH$_2$OH
	   |
	   CH$_2$ — CH$_3$

Methysergide	H**N** group in *b* ring replaced by CH$_3$**N**

Figure 47-5. Ergot alkaloids.

oxytocin in its effects on the uterus (Table 47-3). In the nonpregnant uterus it stimulates short, rapid contractions of the body of the uterus and contraction of the cervix. It has a preferential action on the **pregnant uterus,** stimulating sustained contractions, and has a longer duration of action than oxytocin.

Ergonovine maleate ("ergometrine maleate"; Ergotrate maleate) and methylergonovine maleate (Methergine) are available for injection (in a usual dose of about 0.2 mg i.m.) and as tablets (0.2 mg orally every 2–4 hours).

Ergotamine tartrate (Ergomar, Medihaler-ergotamine) is an amino-acid-substituted alkaloid with prominent vasoconstrictor activity. It is a partial agonist at α-adrenergic and 5-HT-receptors. It is particularly effective in relieving migraine headaches, which are believed to be caused by dilatation of meningeal branches of the internal carotid artery. The drug is ineffective against other headaches because it is not an analgesic. It is used only in the early onset phase of the migraine, not for routine maintenance therapy. Its absorption after oral administration is erratic (30–60%), and bioavailability is only about 10% because of extensive first-pass hepatic biotransformation. Elimination is mainly by biliary excretion. Among its major acute adverse effects are nausea, vomiting, tachycardia, and anginal pain.

Bromocriptine mesylate (Parlodel) is a semi-synthetic ergot alkaloid that functions as a specific dopamine receptor agonist. It suppresses the production of prolactin and reverses effects of hyperprolactinemia including amenorrhea, galactorrhea, and infertility in women as well as impotence and infertility in men. In patients with prolactin-secreting pituitary tumors, bromocriptine causes tumor regression. Therapeutic doses range from 2.5 to 7.5 mg. It is available as 2.5-mg tablets and 5-mg capsules.

Bromocriptine is also used in the treatment of acromegaly, suppressing growth hormone production in doses ranging from 7.5 to 40 mg/day. It is also employed as an adjunct in the treatment of Parkinson's disease in doses that may range up to 100 mg/day (see Chapter 21).

The use of bromocriptine is associated with a high incidence (68%) of mild side effects including nausea, headache, postural hypotension, and dizziness. At the higher doses cited above, additional side effects are seen, including abnormal involuntary movements, hallucinations, and mental confusion.

Pergolide mesylate (Permax) is another semi-synthetic ergot alkaloid that is a dopamine receptor agonist. It is primarily used in the treatment of Parkinson's disease. It is supplied as tablets of 0.05, 0.25, and 1 mg. The adverse effects of pergolide are similar to those of bromocriptine.

Prostaglandin E_2 (see Chapter 31)

Dinoprostone (Prostin E_2, tablets of 0.5 mg, vaginal suppositories of 20 mg, or a gel of 1–2 mg) is used as an alternative to oxytocin, to induce labor when vaginal delivery is intended, or to induce abortion.

Table 47-3 Comparison of Oxytocic Agents*

| | | Smooth Muscle | | | | | |
| | | | | Uterus | | | |
	ADH Activity	Blood Vessels	Gut	Nonpregnant	Pregnant	Onset	Duration
Oxytocin (injection)	+	−	0	± (cervix −)	+ + +	Quick	Short
Ergonovine (injection, oral)	0	+	0	+ +	+ + +	Quick	Long
Ergotamine (for migraine)	0	+ +	0	+	+ +	Quick	Variable
Prostaglandin E_2, $F_{2\alpha}$							
(injection)	0	+ +	+ +	+ +	+ + +	Slow	Medium
(local)	0	0	0	+ +	+ + + (cervix −)		
Vasopressin (injection)	+ + + +	+ +	+ +	+ +	+ +	Quick	Short

*Effects: + = positive; − = negative; 0 = none.

The objective is to aim for the minimum effective concentration of prostaglandin by gradual administration of drug. Prostaglandin E_2 is equally effective on the pregnant and nonpregnant uterus; it generally has a slow onset of action and a short half-life once absorbed. Other actions include stimulation of gastrointestinal smooth muscle, leading to nausea, vomiting, and diarrhea (Table 47-3).

SUGGESTED READING

Brindley BA, Sokol RJ. Induction and augmentation of labour: basis and methods for current practice. Obstet Gynecol Surv 1988; 43:730–743.

Howl J, Wheatley M. Molecular pharmacology of V_{1a} vasopressin receptors. Gen Pharmacol 1995; 26:1142–1153.

Kovacs GL, de Wied D. Peptidergic modulation of learning and memory processes. Pharmacol Rev 1994; 46:269–291.

Manning M, Bankowski K, Sawyer WH. Selective agonists and antagonists of vasopressin. In: Gash DM, Boer GJ, eds. Vasopressin: principles and properties. New York: Plenum Press, 1987:335–368.

Margolis B, Angel J, Kremer S, Skorecki K. Vasopressin action in the kidney—overview and glomerular actions. In: Cowley AW, Liard JF, Ausiello DA, eds. Vasopressin: cellular and integrative functions. New York: Raven Press, 1988:97–106.

North WG. Biosynthesis of vasopressin and neurophysins. In: Gash DM, Boer GJ, eds. Vasopressin: principles and properties. New York: Plenum Press, 1987:175–209.

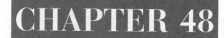

CHAPTER 48

Thyroid Hormones and Antihyperthyroid Drugs

B.P. SCHIMMER AND S.R. GEORGE

CASE HISTORY

A 47-year-old woman consulted her physician because of heart palpitations, tremulousness, weight loss of 7 lb, and heat intolerance, all of which had started 6 weeks previously. Physical examination revealed a resting heart rate of 110 bpm, BP of 150/70, and a diffusely enlarged thyroid gland. She had a fine tremor of her outstretched hands, a wide-eyed stare, and "lid lag." She was started on treatment with propranolol, 40 mg three times daily, and was sent for laboratory tests. The results showed a free thyroxine (T_4) level of 40 pmol/L and a free triiodothyronine (T_3) level of 10.6 pmol/L. Thyroid-stimulating hormone (TSH) was undetectable, but thyroid-stimulating globulins were markedly elevated, confirming the diagnosis of Graves' disease.

The patient was started on propylthiouracil 200 mg twice daily, and the propranolol was continued. She became euthyroid in 6 weeks, and the propranolol dose was gradually reduced and finally discontinued. She continued receiving a maintenance dose of propylthiouracil (50 mg twice daily) for 1 year, after which the drug was discontinued. She remained well for 3 years, but the symptoms of hyperthyroidism then recurred. Treatment with propranolol and propylthiouracil was reinitiated in the same dosages as before to normalize the thyroid hormone levels and provide symptomatic relief. However, after 7 weeks she developed an itchy, red, maculopapular rash over her whole body. The propylthiouracil and propranolol were therefore discontinued and she was given $Na^{131}I$ in a dose of 370 mBq (10 mCi) by mouth for definitive control of her hyperthyroidism.

Three months later the patient returned, complaining of lethargy, tiredness, a feeling of coldness at normal room temperature, puffiness around the eyes, and constipation. Laboratory tests showed a free T_4 level of 8 pmol/L, free T_3 level of 3.0 pmol/L, and a TSH level of 25 mU/mL, confirming a diagnosis of hypothyroidism. She was started on levothyroxine 0.1 mg daily. Six weeks later, a blood test showed a TSH level of 3.2 mU/mL, and the patient's complaints had disappeared. She has remained well on this therapy for the past 2 years.

The thyroid gland synthesizes and secretes thyroid hormones which are required for the integration of normal body function. Abnormalities of thyroid hormone can lead to impairment of growth, development, metabolic regulation, CNS function, and adaptive responses including acclimatization to heat and cold. This chapter deals with drugs used in the management of thyroid hormone deficiency and thyroid hormone excess.

SYNTHESIS AND METABOLISM OF THYROID HORMONES

Figure 48-1 shows the principal features of the biosynthesis and metabolism of thyroid hormones, which are discussed in detail below.

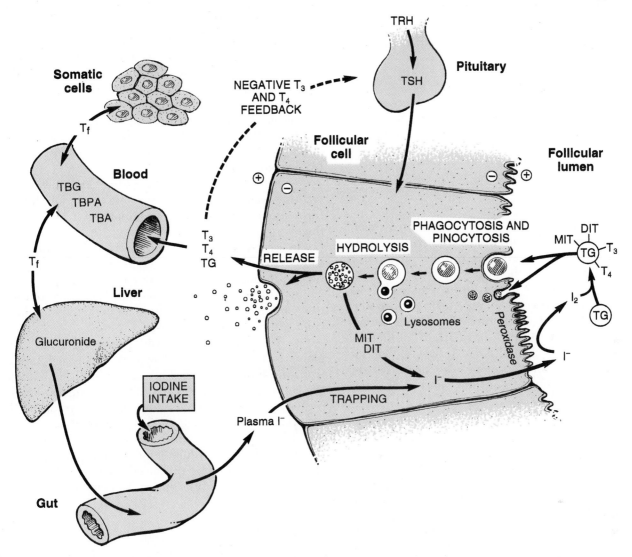

Figure 48-1. Principal features of the biosynthesis and metabolism of thyroid hormone(s) (see text for abbreviations).

Hypothalamic-Pituitary-Thyroid Unit

Thyrotropin-releasing hormone (TRH) is a hypothalamic peptide that functions via a specific G protein-coupled receptor, the TRH receptor, to stimulate the release of thyrotropin (thyroid-stimulating hormone, TSH) from the anterior pituitary (Fig. 48-1). TRH is a tripeptide with the structure L-pyroglutamyl-L-histidyl-L-prolinamide (Fig. 48-2).

TRH also stimulates the release of prolactin and growth hormone, although the physiological significance of these latter effects is uncertain. TRH has other effects within the CNS itself; for example, it increases the sense of well-being and motivation, and it counteracts the depressant effects of ethanol,

barbiturates, and other hypnotic drugs. However, these effects are not well understood and have not yet found clinical applications. Factors that increase TRH levels include circadian rhythms (highest during sleep), low ambient temperature, and norepinephrine. Nonspecific stress (trauma, anesthesia) reduces the level of TRH.

TSH is a pituitary glycoprotein (molecular weight about 28,000 Da) made up of two chains designated α and β. The α chain is identical to the α chains of FSH and LH (see Chapter 49). TSH stimulates the production of thyroid hormones through interactions with a specific G protein-coupled TSH receptor at the thyroid cell surface that activates adenylyl cyclase and phospholipase C. Cyclic AMP, Ca^{2+}, and diacyl-

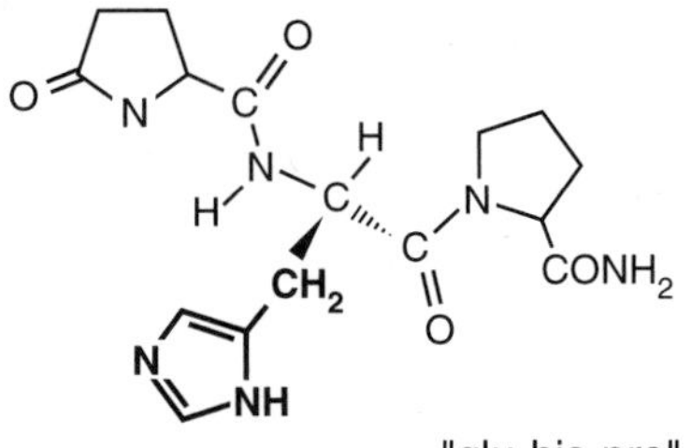

"glu-his-pro"

Figure 48-2. Thyrotropin-releasing hormone (TRH; L-pyroglutamyl-L-histidyl-L-prolinamide).

glycerol serve as the intracellular second messengers for the hormone. TSH stimulates the synthesis and secretion of thyroid hormones through actions on virtually every step of the pathway (see Fig. 48-1). TSH also stimulates the growth of thyroid cells (excess TSH causes thyroid enlargement, i.e., goiter) and maintains cellular structure. Circulating thyroid hormone exerts a negative-feedback inhibition of TSH production by inhibiting transcription of the TSH β gene. Thyroid hormone also decreases the levels of TRH receptors in pituitary and TRH secretion from the hypothalamus (see Fig. 48-1).

Structure of Thyroid Hormones

The two active hormones produced by the thyroid gland are **thyroxine** (tetraiodothyronine, T_4) and **triiodothyronine** (T_3). Their structures are shown in Figure 48-3.

The triiodinated hormone T_3 has four to 10 times the activity of the tetraiodinated compound T_4. The basic structural requirements for thyroid hormone activity include two aromatic rings with an aliphatic side-chain (an alanine side-chain gives optimum activity). The iodine atoms and the oxygen bridge maintain the two aromatic rings in the proper spatial alignment necessary for optimal interaction with the thyroid hormone receptor. A similar spatial alignment, with resultant hormonal activity, can be achieved by using other bulky groups (methyl, isopropyl) in place of iodine. For example, dimethyl isopropyl thyronine (DIMIT; see Fig. 48-3) has about 20% of the activity of T_4 and is of potential interest for transplacental hormone delivery to the fetus because it is resistant to metabolic inactivation by deiodination.

Biosynthesis of Thyroid Hormones

The points to be noted are illustrated in Figure 48-1:

1. Iodine (150 μg/day) is ingested in food and water and is absorbed into the blood as iodide.

2. Iodide is "trapped" by the thyroid gland by an active transport process leading to concentrations within the gland that are 20 to several hundred times higher than in plasma. Iodide not taken up by the thyroid is readily excreted by the kidney.

3. In the follicular lumen near the apical cell membrane, iodide is oxidized to a more reactive form by thyroidal peroxidase.

4. In successive stages the iodine combines with tyrosine residues in the glycoprotein thyroglobulin to form monoiodinated and diiodinated tyrosine residues.

In a subsequent oxidation reaction, involving the same peroxidase, the iodotyrosine residues are condensed to form the precursors for T_3 and T_4.

5. The iodinated thyroglobulin (TG) is stored in the acini of the gland and gives a characteristic pink color after staining with eosin.

6. The release of thyroid hormones from the gland is initiated by endocytosis of thyroglobulin from the lumen into the cells of the follicle. Within the cell, thyroglobulin is hydrolyzed to amino acids by lysosomal enzymes; T_4 and some T_3 are released into the circulation. The iodine associated with monoiodotyrosine (MIT) and diiodotyrosine (DIT) is reutilized. With a normal dietary intake of iodine, T_4 is the major hormone produced. When the dietary intake is low, the proportion of T_3 is increased.

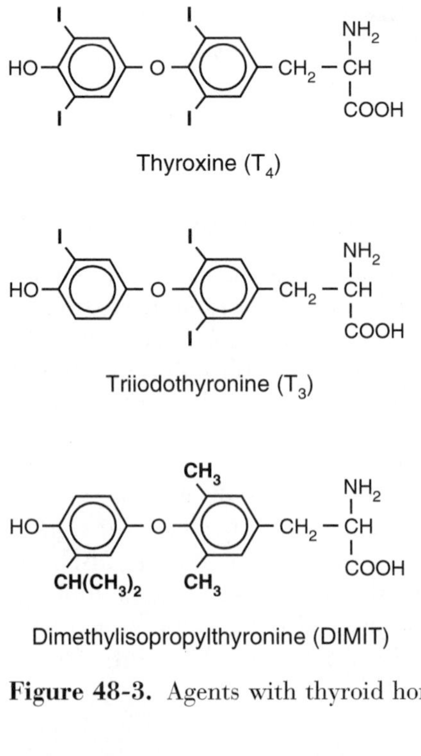

Thyroxine (T_4)

Triiodothyronine (T_3)

Dimethylisopropylthyronine (DIMIT)

Figure 48-3. Agents with thyroid hormonal activity.

Transport and Metabolism

1. Most of the thyroid hormone in the circulation (about 90%) is in the form of T_4; 5% circulates as T_3. Both hormones are tightly bound to certain plasma proteins, with only a small fraction circulating as "free" hormone. The free hormone is considered to represent the physiologically active fraction. Unbound or "free" thyroxine (T_f) accounts for approximately 0.05% of the total T_4. T_3 is bound more loosely than T_4 (0.5% is free). Since the free hormone also is metabolized more rapidly than the bound, it follows that the half-life of T_3 in the circulation (about 2 days) is shorter than that of T_4 (about 7 days).

2. Thyroxine-binding globulin (TBG) acts as a carrier for approximately 75% of the thyroid hormones. The remainder is bound to thyroxine-binding prealbumin (TBPA or transthyretin) and to albumin.

3. Measurements of free thyroid hormones and TSH levels provide a more sensitive indicator of thyroid function. Normal values for free hormone levels are FT_4 11–24 pmol/L and FT_3 3.3–8.2 pmol/L.

4. Thyroid hormones circulate to all tissues and are taken up in varying amounts. Thyroxine is metabolized by deiodination, about 35% to the more potent T_3 and about 45% to "reverse T_3" (rT_3; monodeiodinated at the inner or α-benzene ring rather than the outer ring; metabolically inactive). Further metabolism results in the appearance of acetic and propionic acid derivatives of T_3 (metabolically active), various deiodinated derivatives, and iodotyrosines. The second major pathway for disposal of thyroid hormones is via glucuronic acid conjugation in the liver and excretion in the feces (20–40% of the total amount).

5. Although the thyroid gland secretes some T_3, most of the active hormone (at least 70%) arises from deiodination of T_4 in peripheral tissues. Since T_3 is considerably more potent than T_4, it has been suggested that T_4 functions as a circulating "prohormone" for T_3.

ACTIONS

Thyroid hormones are essential for normal function of all body tissues. They have profound influences on integrated processes such as differentiation and development, growth, and adaptation to environmental stress. The importance of these actions is apparent from the signs and symptoms of hyper- and hypothyroidism.

With thyroid hormone deficiency (**hypothyroidism**) there is impairment of:

- Growth of skeletal tissues
- Growth, development, and function of the central nervous system
- Protein synthesis
- Carbohydrate absorption
- Lipid metabolism
- Adrenocortical and gonadal functions
- Cardiac and renal functions
- Overall tissue metabolism

With excessive function (**hyperthyroidism**; thyrotoxicosis) the principal effect is an increase in metabolism of most (if not all) tissues, causing an increased basal consumption of oxygen (BMR) and an increase in the amount of energy expended as heat. Most other effects of hyperthyroidism follow from these; increased appetite, loss of weight, high pulse rate, high systolic pressure, increased water turnover by sweating, dyspnea, and fine tremor of skeletal muscles. Many of these changes resemble those of excessive activity of the sympathetic nervous system.

The mechanisms underlying the diverse actions of thyroid hormone are not known precisely. In the current view, thyroid hormone binds to a specific receptor in the cell nuclei of many tissues. The thyroid hormone receptor is a member of the superfamily of nuclear hormone receptor transcription factors. Thyroid-hormone–receptor complexes recognize specific DNA sequences (thyroid hormone response elements, TRE) in the promoter regions to alter transcription of specific genes. This results in increased synthesis of several important proteins. Among these are nerve growth factors (CNS development) and β-adrenoceptors (potentiation of cardiovascular and metabolic effects of catecholamines).

Autoimmunity and Thyroid Function

Graves' disease (Basedow's disease; diffuse toxic goiter; exophthalmic goiter) is the major cause of thyroid hyperactivity (hyperthyroidism) in humans; the incidence of Graves' disease is at least three times greater in women than in men. In Graves' disease, the circulating T_4 is high and TSH is suppressed. Autoimmune disease is the underlying cause of this disorder in which circulating antibodies to the TSH receptor (TSI, thyroid stimulating immunoglobulins) are present. These antibodies bind to and activate the TSH receptor, resulting in thyroid enlargement and hormone overproduction. As might be expected, the elevated thyroid hormones do not suppress the action of TSI.

Circulating antibodies to thyroglobulin and to microsomal antigens are also increased in this disease. A significant number of cases of Graves' disease undergo spontaneous remission but often relapse.

A distinctive disorder often associated with Graves' disease is exophthalmos (Graves' ophthalmopathy), a protrusion of the eyeballs and widening of the palpebral fissures. It is produced by an enlargement of external ocular muscles and associated connective tissue; however, there is no agreement as to its cause. Exophthalmos cannot be produced experimentally by administering thyroid hormone, nor does it occur in all hyperthyroid patients. Immune mechanisms, both cell-mediated and humoral, are currently regarded as likely pathogenic factors.

Hashimoto's disease (chronic thyroiditis) belongs to the spectrum of autoimmune thyroid disorders and is usually characterized by hypothyroidism due to autoimmune destruction of the thyroid gland.

Thyroid Hormone in Pregnancy

Pregnancy, or estrogen treatment, increases the concentration of TBG, resulting in increased amounts of thyroid hormone in the bound form. Feedback regulatory mechanisms compensate, however, and thyroid hormone synthesis increases enough to maintain a normal level of free hormone.

T_4 and T_3 are rapidly degraded by a highly active deiodinase in the placenta, so only small amounts of maternal thyroid hormone reach the fetus. The amount of thyroid hormone necessary for normal development of the fetus is open to debate. Body growth is not affected in the athyreotic fetus, but proper brain development is at risk. There is agreement that, after birth, prompt and vigorous replacement treatment is essential in the management of **neonatal hypothyroidism.** Failure to treat this condition will result in severe mental retardation and other manifestations of cretinism. Even prompt treatment after birth may not reverse all the effects of hypothyroidism on brain development. Some research has been directed toward treating fetal hypothyroidism in utero. Drugs such as DIMIT, which can cross the placenta intact, are of interest in this regard.

Hyperthyroidism also is of concern in pregnancy. While TSH and thyroid hormone cannot cross the placenta, thyroid-stimulating immunoglobulins will traverse the placenta and stimulate the fetal thyroid gland. In addition, labor and delivery may precipitate "thyroid storm," an extreme and life-threatening state of hyperthyroidism, in the mother. Treatment is designed to maintain the well-being of the mother.

CLINICAL USE OF THYROID HORMONE

The administration of thyroid hormone is indicated as replacement therapy for treatment of hypothyroidism. Thyroid hormone deficiency may present with symptoms ranging from severe hypothyroidism (cretinism, myxedema), to mild hypothyroidism in which only one, or at most a few, of the symptoms are present. Laboratory tests (TSH, free T_3, free T_4) help establish the diagnosis and treatment.

Preparations

Levothyroxine (sodium); sodium L-thyroxine, U.S.P., B.P. (Eltroxin, Levothroid, Levoxine, Synthroid).

This is a synthetic crystalline compound, prepared in oral tablets, in strengths ranging from 0.025 mg to 0.3 mg; it is also available in sterile lyophilized form for injection after reconstitution. Because of its chemical purity and uniform bioavailability, levothyroxine has replaced thyroid powders and extract (e.g., desiccated thyroid).

Levothyroxine is well absorbed by mouth but is influenced by intestinal contents; bioavailability ranges from 40 to 75%. In the plasma, more than 99% is protein-bound. The normal half-life is 6–7 days, but it is increased in myxedema and pregnancy, and during treatment with estrogens (that increase the level of thyroid-binding globulin). Conversely, the half-life is shortened if protein binding is decreased by disease (hepatic cirrhosis, nephrotic syndrome) or by drugs (salicylate, dicumarol, phenytoin, carbamazepine).

Liothyronine (sodium); L-triiodothyronine (Cytomel, Triostat)

This is a synthetic crystalline compound available in oral tablets of 5 and 25 μg. A dose of 25 μg is equivalent to 0.1 mg of levothyroxine.

Liotrix (Thyrolar, Euthyroid, available in the United States, not currently available in Canada)

This is a combination of synthetic T_4 and T_3 in a ratio of 4:1; this ratio is thought to resemble closely the physiological secretion ratio. The value of this combination is not clear, since T_3 is readily derived from circulating T_4. The mixture is supplied as tablets in several strengths.

Dextrothyroxine (Choloxin)

This D-isomer of levothyroxine is used as a hypocholesterolemic agent (see Chapter 39). The rationale for this use was based on the observation that the D-isomer is approximately as potent as L-thyroxine in lowering cholesterol in blood, but it has only one-quarter the ability to increase the general rate of metabolism. However, because of its potential for unwanted metabolic and cardiovascular actions, other approaches to lowering plasma lipid are preferred.

Therapy of Hypothyroidism

The drug of choice in the treatment of hypothyroidism is levothyroxine. It is usual to begin with a low dose (e.g., 0.05 mg daily), to avoid cardiovascular complications such as tachycardia or angina pectoris.

The full effect takes several weeks to develop; therefore, because of the long half-life of levothyroxine, the dose should not be adjusted upward for 4–6 weeks. In the presence of cardiac disease, increments should be small and the intervals between them extended. By successive increments (0.025–0.05 mg L-thyroxine) the dose is eventually brought up to a maintenance level based on normalization of the TSH level. If there is concomitant adrenal steroid deficiency, glucocorticoid replacement therapy should be started before thyroid hormone replacement.

In infants and children the dosage is related to age and body weight and is adjusted to normalize TSH. Adequate dosage is extremely important for normal growth and mental development.

Triiodothyronine is much more rapid in action and more potent than L-thyroxine. Effects start to occur in 4–8 hours, reach a maximum in 24–48 hours, and wear off in a few days if medication is stopped. In contrast, thyroxine has a prolonged action that takes up to 3 months to wear off completely. Therefore, the "evenness" of effect of triiodothyronine depends more closely on regularity of dosage, which makes it a difficult agent for routine use. It is also more expensive than thyroxine. The value of triiodothyronine lies in its relatively short duration of action; in certain cases, repeated thyroid function

tests may be desirable and these can be done a few weeks after stopping triiodothyronine medication.

THERAPY OF HYPERTHYROIDISM

When the thyroid gland is overactive, secreting excessive (thyrotoxic) amounts of thyroid hormones, the therapeutic objective is to interrupt synthesis and/or release. Several methods are available.

Inhibition of Thyroid Hormone Synthesis by Thionamides

The thionamides are ringed structures derived from thiourea (Fig 48-4). They inhibit thyroid peroxidase and in this way block the iodination of tyrosyl groups and the coupling of iodotyrosines in thyroglobulin. The resultant effect is to block thyroid hormone synthesis.

They do not interfere with the processing of stored iodinated thyroglobulin or the release of thyroid hormone; therefore the onset of clinical effect is slow and depends on depletion of the stored hormone precursor. Several weeks are usually required to pro-

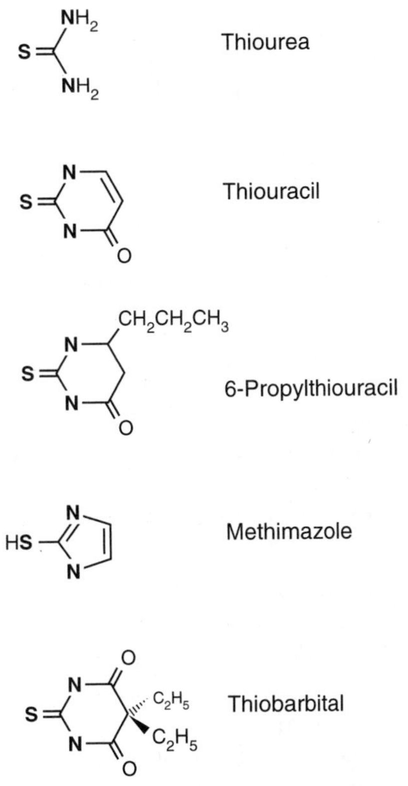

Figure 48-4. Thiourea and derivatives.

duce a maximal effect. These drugs may also have immunosuppressive effects in patients with autoimmune thyroid disease. Propylthiouracil, but not methimazole or carbimazole, inhibits deiodination of T_4 to T_3 in tissues. Some clinicians feel this is an added benefit; however, it also inhibits the deiodination (inactivation) of T_3.

Propylthiouracil (PTU; Propyl-Thyracil)

PTU is well absorbed orally (bioavailability 60–90%), reaches peak plasma concentration within 1 hour and is rapidly distributed. It is partly biotransformed and inactivated in the liver, and both the original drug and the metabolites are excreted by the kidney. The normal half-life is 1–2 hours. Initial dosage is 200–600 mg/day in divided doses; maintenance doses range from 50 to 200 mg. It is provided as 50- and 100-mg tablets.

Methimazole (thiamazole; Tapazole)

The duration of action is approximately 6 hours. Methimazole has a longer half-life than PTU and is approximately 10 times as potent. It is well absorbed orally and excreted by the kidney. Initial dosage is 15–60 mg/day depending on severity; maintenance doses are 5–15 mg. It is provided as 5-mg tablets.

Carbimazole (not available in United States or Canada) is metabolized to methimazole in vivo and behaves similarly.

Toxic Effects of Thionamides

All drugs of this group are capable of causing toxic effects (in about 3% of patients with propylthiouracil and 7% with methimazole). These include:

- Agranulocytosis (most serious, reported in 0.5% of cases)
- Drug rash, arthralgia, edema (in over 2% of cases), drug fever (very rare), alopecia, hair depigmentation
- Rare cases of hepatitis, lymph node swelling, loss of taste

Physiologically, the level of free thyroid hormone determines the secretion of TSH by feedback regulatory mechanisms. With thionamides, inhibition of thyroid hormone synthesis may cause a gradual increase in output of TSH, making the gland larger.

Thionamides cross the placenta and small amounts (<1% of the dose) are also secreted in breast milk. Infants born of mothers who are being treated with these drugs may show hyperplasia of the thyroid (goiter). If breast-fed, they may develop cretinism. Therefore, in the treatment of maternal hyperthyroidism during the perinatal period one uses the lowest possible dose and initiates bottle-feeding. If the dosage is low, the effect on the fetus is not serious because it is reversible.

Inhibition of Thyroxine Release

Iodide is thought to inhibit the lysosomal protease that releases thyroxine from thyroglobulin; treatment with iodide therefore causes large amounts of colloid to accumulate in the gland. It also inhibits other steps in the regulation of thyroid hormone synthesis, including iodide transport and iodination of thyroglobulin (Wolff-Chaikoff effect). Symptoms of hyperthyroidism are relieved rapidly, making iodide useful in the treatment of thyroid storm.

Iodide is not suitable for long-term therapy because the gland escapes from the inhibitory effect of I^-, and the release of thyroxine is resumed. Therefore it is used only for a few weeks. The available form is potassium iodide (Lugol's solution; saturated KI solution). Enough is used to provide 60 mg of I^- per day.

Lithium carbonate is also effective in preventing release of thyroid hormones from the thyroid gland. It most likely acts by inhibiting the thyroid adenylyl cyclase. Its place in the treatment of hyperthyroidism is unclear.

Inhibition of Iodide Uptake

Perchlorate ion (ClO_4^-) and thiocyanate ion (SCN^-) resemble halide ions in size and distribution of charge. Therefore they act as competitive blockers of iodide transport. SCN^- has marked hypotensive effects and is too toxic for long-term therapy. $KClO_4$ is effective, but reports of fatal aplastic anemia during continued treatment with high doses have limited its use.

Radioactive Iodine

Radioactive iodine is used to achieve nonsurgical ablation of thyroid tissue. $Na^{131}I$ is taken up and concentrated by the gland in the same way as ordinary I^-. The uptake is especially great in the hyperactive gland, as in thyrotoxicosis. Where the normal gland takes up less than 30% of an administered dose, the hyperactive one may take up 80% or more. This concentration of ^{131}I causes intense local β

irradiation that destroys glandular epithelium; the low concentration in the rest of the body causes no damage to other tissues. In some cases, more than one treatment may be required to achieve control. ^{131}I is also used to treat thyroid carcinoma, including metastases, provided the cells still retain their I$^-$-trapping mechanism (i.e., they are not too undifferentiated).

Danger: If the thyroid gland has a large store of colloid, surgical manipulation or destruction of thyroid tissue by ^{131}I may release a flood of thyroxine into the circulation and cause "thyroid storm." Therefore one usually tries to block synthesis of hormone first with a thionamide, allowing the gland to become depleted before using radioablation. ^{131}I is not used in pregnant women because it crosses the placenta and can have potentially harmful effects on fetal tissues, especially thyroid. It also is not generally used in children.

Symptomatic Relief

β-Blockers such as propranolol (see Chapter 17) can be administered to block the sympathetic effects of excess thyroid hormone. Propranolol acts quickly and is well tolerated. The usual contraindications for use of propranolol should be kept in mind, e.g., bronchial asthma, chronic obstructive lung disease, and congestive heart failure.

Glucocorticoids may be used for the rapid treatment of severe hyperthyroidism or thyroid storm; they inhibit the conversion of T_4 to T_3 in peripheral tissues.

SUGGESTED READING

Chopra IJ. New insights into metabolism of thyroid hormones: physiological and clinical implications. Prog Clin Biol Res 1981; 74:67–80.

Cooper DS. Antithyroid drugs. N Engl J Med 1984; 311:1353–1362.

Schimke NR. Hyperthyroidism. The clinical spectrum. Postgraduate Medicine 1992; 91:229–236.

Strakosch CR, Wenzel BE, Row VV, Volpe R. Immunology of autoimmune thyroid disease. N Engl J Med 1982; 307:1499–1507.

Surks MI, Sievert R. Drugs and thyroid function. N Engl J Med 1995; 333:1688–1694.

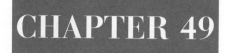

CHAPTER 49

Gonadotropic and Gonadal Hormones

S.R. GEORGE AND B.P. SCHIMMER

CASE HISTORY

A 55-year-old woman, who had been experiencing gradual lengthening of her menstrual cycles, consulted her physician after 4 months of amenorrhea. She complained of frequent hot flashes, sleep disturbance, and vaginal dryness. She was given a prescription for conjugated estrogen 0.625 mg daily, plus medroxyprogesterone 5 mg on days 16–25 of each month. This treatment produced a return of regular withdrawal (menstrual) bleeding at the end of each cycle. She initially felt slightly nauseated, and gained 3 lb in weight, but the discomfort disappeared after three cycles of treatment.

Four years later, the patient noticed a small mass, 2 cm in diameter, in her left breast. Radiological investigation and a needle aspiration biopsy revealed carcinoma of the breast. The estrogen and progestin were discontinued, and the patient underwent a lumpectomy and received a course of postoperative radiation treatments. The carcinoma proved to be strongly positive for estrogen receptors, and she was therefore started on tamoxifen 40 mg daily. She remained well on this treatment, and showed no signs of recurrence or metastasis during the next 5 years. The tamoxifen was therefore discontinued, and she has continued to feel well.

Gonadal hormones are important for conception, embryonic development, development at puberty (primary and secondary sex characteristics), and for the desire and ability to procreate. While not essential for life, they are essential for the individual's well-being. Their use in fertility control has had significant impact both socially and economically.

The production and release of the gonadal steroid hormones (estradiol, progesterone, testosterone) are controlled by the gonadotropins (luteinizing hormone, LH; follicle-stimulating hormone, FSH) of the anterior pituitary, and these are in turn under the influence of gonadotropin-releasing hormone (GnRH) from the hypothalamus.

The principal features of these relationships are shown in Figures 49-1 and 49-2.

GONADOTROPIN-RELEASING HORMONE

Gonadotropin-releasing hormone (GnRH) is a decapeptide with the structure

PyroGlu-His-Trp-Ser-Tyr-Gly-Leu-Arg-Pro-GlyNH$_2$

In the human, this peptide acts through a specific G protein-coupled receptor to stimulate the release of both LH and FSH from the anterior pituitary. The quantal release of FSH is less than that of LH. The quantitative discrepancy between release of LH and of FSH is related to differential responses of gonadotrophs to stimulation by GnRH and to feedback modulation by gonadal steroids, and by two types of polypeptide hormone (activin and inhibin) produced in the gonad.

There is evidence that endogenous opioids exert a central inhibitory regulation of GnRH secretion that may be relieved by adrenergic influences. Higher

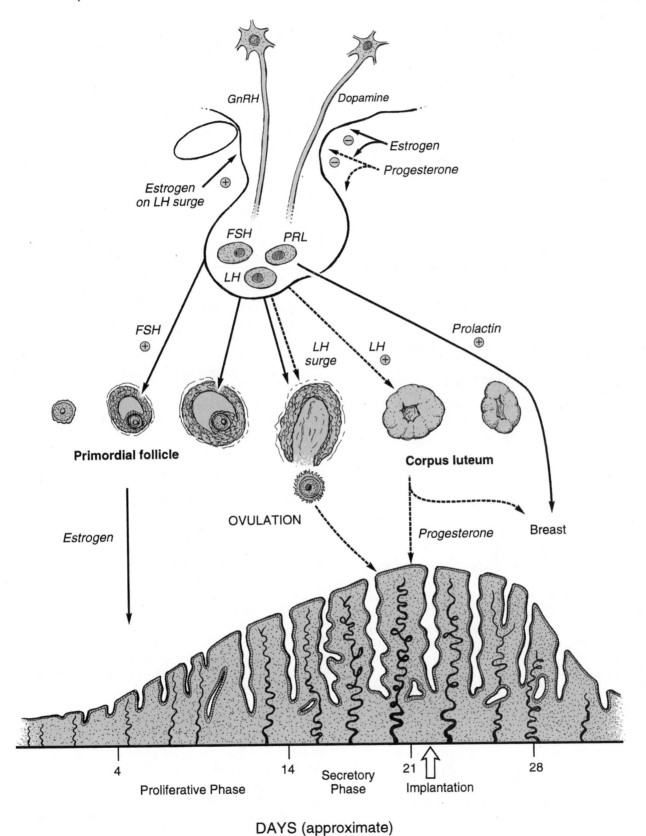

Figure 49-1. Physiological relationships of gonadotropins and gonadal hormones and their influences on the ovary, uterus, and breast.

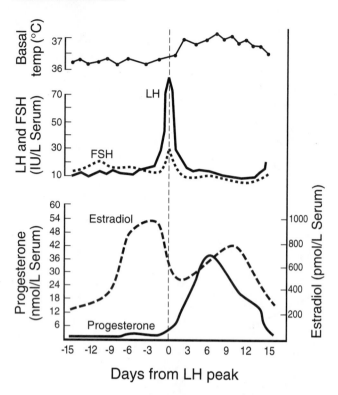

Figure 49-2. Approximate plasma concentrations of ovarian hormones and gonadotropins during a normal menstrual cycle. The change in body temperature through the cycle is shown on the top.

dopaminergic pathways may also be involved, but their role is less well defined.

The secretion of GnRH is pulsatile, the frequency and amplitude of the pulse being of major importance in the effects it produces on secretion of LH and FSH. Continuous administration initially stimulates but then inhibits the release of LH and FSH, due to desensitization of the GnRH receptors on the gonadotrophs. Pulsatile administration of GnRH maintains receptor sensitivity and has been used successfully to increase fertility in males and females.

The biological half-life of GnRH is short, but agonist analogs have been synthesized that are more stable metabolically and function as potent agonists or as inhibitors (via desensitization). GnRH analogs (Fig. 49-3) have proven useful as GnRH inhibitors in the treatment of hormone-dependent tumors (prostate, breast, uterine fibroids) and other conditions such as precocious puberty and endometriosis. They are provided as injectable (i.v., s.c.), nasal spray, and depot (i.m.) forms.

GONADOTROPINS

In the human there are two pituitary gonadotropins that act on the ovary and testis. Chemically they are complex glycoprotein hormones that consist of a common α and distinct β subunits (LH-β, FSH-β) that confer specificity. The hormones are synthesized within the same cells, the gonadotrophs of the anterior pituitary, although there is heterogeneity in the relative amounts of LH and FSH produced in each gonadotroph. FSH induces development of ovarian follicles in the female and initiates and maintains spermatogenesis in the male. LH induces estrogen and progesterone synthesis and continued follicular development, followed by ovulation and corpus luteum formation. In the male, it stimulates androgen formation by the Leydig cells of the gonad. Each of these hormones interacts with specific G protein-coupled receptors to generate cyclic AMP and other second messengers.

An LH-like gonadotropin (human chorionic gonadotropin, or hCG) is found in the chorion of the placenta. It is detectable in plasma as early as 7 days after conception and forms the basis for the test to confirm pregnancy.

Preparations

- **Human chorionic gonadotropin** (hCG; Profasi, A.P.L., Follutein, Pregnyl) has predominantly LH activity and is derived from the urine of pregnant women. It can be used in infertile women to promote ovulation by duplicating the LH "surge," in infertile men to promote spermatogenesis, in male children to stimulate Leydig cells in the treatment of undescended testicles, and as an adjunct in in vitro fertilization treatment programs.
- **Menotropin** (hMG; Pergonal) is a gonadotropin prepared from urine of postmenopausal women that has both FSH and LH activity. It is used to simulate the LH surge and produce ovulation.

Related hormones

Prolactin is closely related chemically to growth hormone. It is produced in the lactotrophs of the anterior pituitary. Its release is under inhibitory dopaminergic control from the hypothalamus. Overproduction of prolactin can occur from pituitary adenomas or from loss of dopaminergic control (e.g., pituitary stalk section, or drugs such as morphine, metoclopramide, haloperidol).

PREPARATION	STRUCTURE
Gonadorelin hydrochloride (Factrel)	PyroGlu – His – Trp – Ser – Tyr – Gly – Leu – Arg – Pro – GlyNH$_2$
Goserelin acetate (Zoladex)	PyroGlu – His – Trp – Ser – Tyr – **D-Ser** – Leu – Arg – Pro – **azaGly NH$_2$** | **(O-terbutyl)**
Buserelin acetate (Suprefact)	**5-oxo-Pro** – His – Trp – Ser – Tyr – **D-Ser** – Leu – Arg – Pro – **ethyl NH$_2$** | **(O-terbutyl)**
Leuprolide acetate (Lupron)	**5-oxo-Pro** – His – Trp – Ser – Tyr – **D-Leu** – Leu – Arg – Pro – **ethyl NH$_2$**
Nafarelin acetate (Synarel)	**5-oxo-Pro** – His – Trp – Ser – Tyr – **D-Ala** – Leu – Arg – Pro – **Gly NH$_2$** | **[3-(2-naphthyl)]**

Figure 49-3. Gonadotropin-releasing hormone (GnRH) analogs.

Prolactin, with other hormones (e.g., ovarian and adrenal steroids, placental lactogen, thyroid hormone), plays a major part in the growth and development of the breasts during pregnancy and lactation. Prolactin also inhibits the secretion of GnRH and this action contributes to the infertility seen with hyperprolactinemia.

ESTROGENS

Metabolism and Pharmacokinetics

The principal naturally occurring estrogen is 17-β-estradiol. It is formed from androstenedione or testosterone and is produced predominantly in the ovaries and placenta, but small amounts may be secreted from testes, adrenals, and adipose tissue. Estradiol circulates in plasma bound strongly to an α_2-globulin called sex-hormone-binding globulin (SHBG), and less avidly to albumin. The free estradiol (unbound hormone) is the fraction available for hormone action in target cells. The levels of urinary estrogen metabolites may be used as an index of endogenous estrogen production.

Estrogens are readily absorbed from the skin, mucous membranes, and gastrointestinal tract. After oral administration, a high proportion is biotransformed and partly inactivated during passage through the liver (first-pass metabolism). Estradiol exists in equilibrium with its oxidation product, estrone. Estradiol and estrone are irreversibly hydroxylated by a hepatic microsomal 16α-hydroxylase, leading to the formation of estriol (Fig. 49-4). Estrone and estriol retain some estrogenic activity but are much less potent than estradiol. A fraction of the estriol is conjugated with sulfuric and glucuronic acids. Estriol and its metabolites are excreted by the kidney. The conjugated estrogens are also excreted into the bile and may be recycled by bacterial hydrolysis and reabsorption from the gut (enterohepatic recirculation).

Estradiol is only very slightly soluble in water and is therefore injected (usually intramuscularly) as an aqueous suspension or as a solution in oil. However, it has enough polarity to be quickly absorbed from the injection site and metabolized. Esters of estradiol (e.g., valerate, cypionate) become less polar as the size of the ester substituent is increased, and the rate of absorption from oily solutions is decreased accordingly, leading to a less-intense but longer-lasting action.

The synthetic analogs 17-α-ethinyl estradiol and mestranol (Fig. 49-5) are well absorbed after oral administration, but unlike estradiol they are inactivated very slowly in the liver and peripheral tissues. This slow inactivation is responsible for their high potency and prolonged action.

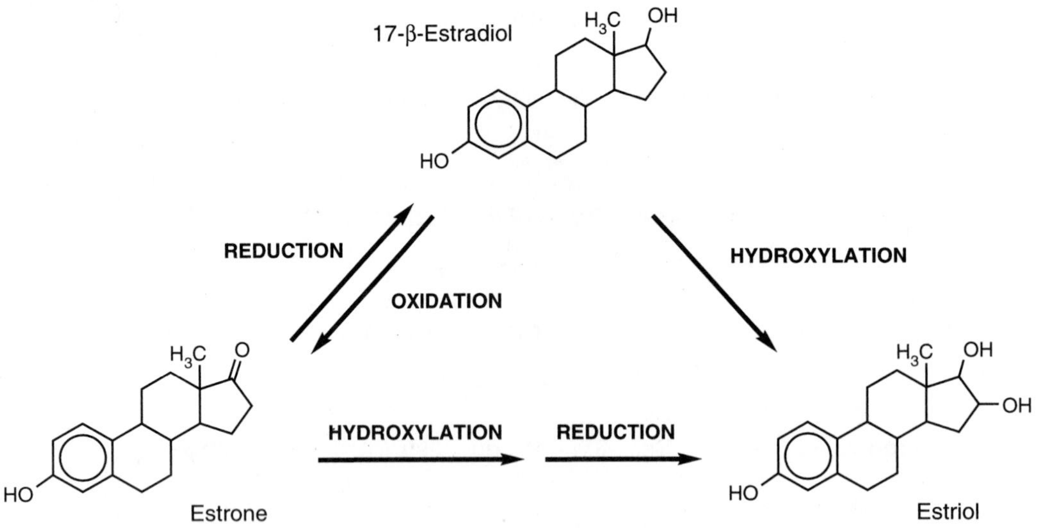

Figure 49-4. Natural estrogens and their metabolic interconversions.

Preparations

- **17-β-Estradiol** is available as dermal patches for absorption through the intact skin (Estraderm) or as micronized tablets (Estrace) and vaginal cream.
- **Conjugated estrogens** are extracted from pregnant mare's urine (Premarin, CES, Congest). This preparation contains estrogen conjugates, principally sodium estrone sulfate (60%) and sodium equilin sulfate (30%). They are effective orally or by injection.
- **Estropipate** (Ogen, piperazine estrone sulfate) is an orally active water-soluble preparation of estrone sulfate, stabilized with piperazine.
- **Esters of 17-β-estradiol** (Delestrogen, Depo-Estradiol) are given by intramuscular injection for slow absorption from the site, resulting in prolonged action.
- **Ethinyl estradiol** (Estinyl, Feminone) is a synthetic estrogen with an ethyne group at C-17 that makes this compound orally active.
- **Mestranol** (3-methoxy-17-α-ethinyl estradiol) is inactive until it is converted to ethinyl estradiol in the liver.

Equivalent replacement doses for selected estrogens are as follows:

17-β-estradiol transdermal 25–50 μg; 17-β-estradiol oral micronized 0.5–2 mg; conjugated estrogens 0.625–1.25 mg; ethinyl estradiol 5–20 μg.

Note: Estrogens are usually administered in cycles of about 21 days on estrogen and 7 days off; these doses are the daily doses during the 21-day drug portion of the cycle.

Nonsteroidal Estrogens

Certain nonsteroidal substances are highly estrogenic. These compounds resemble natural estrogens in structure or spatial arrangement sufficiently to stimulate estrogen receptors in target tissues. The first example was the stilbene derivative **diethylstilbestrol** (DES) (Fig. 49-6). Once a widely used estrogen substitute, DES is currently used only for palliative treatment of inoperable prostatic carcinoma.

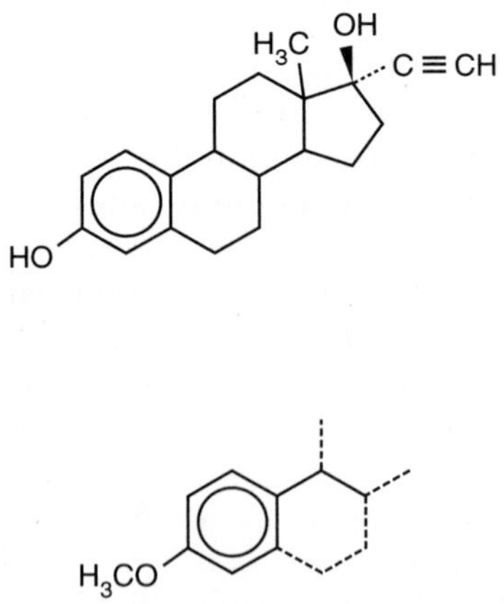

Figure 49-5. Structural formulae of (upper) ethinyl estradiol and (lower) mestranol, the C-3 methoxy derivative of ethinyl estradiol.

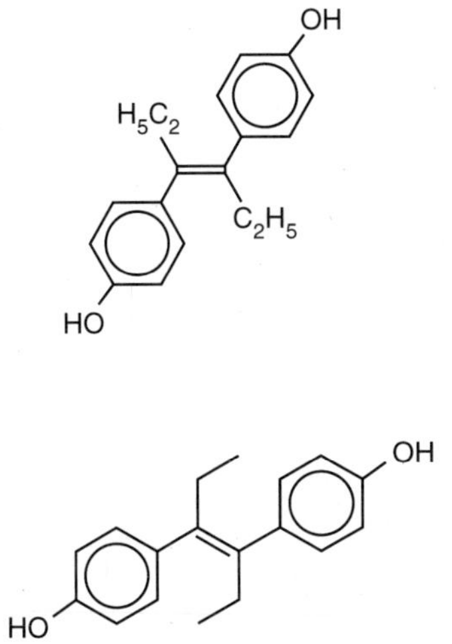

Figure 49-6. Formulae of diethylstilbestrol: (upper) structural formula; (lower) theoretical spatial arrangement (steroid-like form).

Actions

Estradiol binds to specific receptors in the nuclei of cells of estrogen-sensitive target tissues (e.g., uterine muscle, brain, breast, pituitary), which are nuclear transcription factors. In these tissues the specific estrogen receptor binds the steroid hormone and undergoes an activation process that permits interaction with specific estrogen-responsive DNA elements to alter the transcription of certain genes. Recent evidence indicates that the same estrogen–receptor complex can bind to different DNA elements that mediate different effects of the estrogens. As a consequence, the production and expression of messenger RNAs is either stimulated or inhibited, leading to changes in the production of various proteins.

The **physiological functions** of estrogens may be summarized as follows:

- Growth and development of reproductive organs in females
- Development of female secondary sex characteristics
- Linear bone growth, prevention of bone resorption and hastening of epiphyseal closure
- Behavior (sexual, maternal)
- Sensitization of tissues to progesterone by induction of progesterone receptors
- Feedback regulation of gonadotrophs, including stimulation of the preovulatory LH surge
- Other metabolic effects (increases in HDL levels, hepatic protein synthesis, secretion of binding glob-

ulins CBG, TBG, SHBG, renin substrate, and clotting factors)

Clinical Uses

Hypogonadism. An estrogen is used in replacement therapy for estrogen-deficient patients. Cyclical administration, in combination with a progestin, is recommended if the uterus is intact, to prevent endometrial carcinomas (see below).

Menopause. Following natural menopause or surgical castration, many patients show varying degrees of vasomotor instability, headache, emotional lability, sleep disturbances, and atrophy of estrogen-dependent tissues. The more severe consequences of menopause are osteoporosis and increased risk of cardiovascular disease. Estrogens are effective in alleviating these problems. For the treatment of postmenopausal osteoporosis, estrogens are often used in conjunction with calcium, vitamin D, cyclical bisphosphonates and, rarely, with androgens.

Senile atrophic vaginitis. Local therapy, in the form of vaginal creams, may be used to avoid systemic effects.

Dysmenorrhea. In severe cases, continuous estrogen therapy, alone or in combination with a progestin, suppresses ovulation. Suspension of estrogen is followed by atypical but painless menstruation.

Carcinoma of the prostate. Estrogens (e.g., DES) have been used, either alone or in combination with surgical castration, for metastatic carcinoma of the prostate. In prostatic cancer, estrogen decreases androgen synthesis by shutting off the release of LH. The use of estrogen in this condition has largely been replaced by GnRH analogs, which have fewer side effects.

Contraception. Estrogens, given together with a progestin, inhibit the production of gonadotropins and GnRH and thus prevent ovulation (see section on Fertility Control).

"Morning after" contraceptive pill. For this use, ethinyl estradiol is given within 72 hours, in two doses (100 μg each) 12 hours apart, usually in an oral contraceptive formulation. Postulated effects include acceleration of passage of the fertilized ovum along the fallopian tube as well as induction of withdrawal bleeding.

Hirsutism. Hirsutism resulting from excess androgens of ovarian origin may respond to estrogen therapy. The estrogen-induced increase in SHBG also serves effectively to decrease circulating concentrations of "free" androgens (i.e., the fraction that is not protein-bound).

Adverse and Toxic Effects

- **Gastrointestinal upset** (nausea and vomiting) is the most common disturbance.
- **Breast engorgement, endometrial hyperplasia,** and **vaginal bleeding.** The risk of endometrial carcinoma consequent to endometrial hyperplasia is increased if the estrogen is not combined with progestin.
- **Retention of Na$^+$ and water.** An increase in plasma renin substrate also occurs. Hypertension, weight gain, edema, or heart failure may occur. Caution is advisable in older patients.
- The use of estrogen predisposes in a dose-related fashion to **thromboembolic events** such as thrombophlebitis, pulmonary embolism, myocardial infarction, stroke, and mesenteric and retinal thromboses. The risk is increased in smokers, in those over age 35, and in the obese.
- Stilbestrol has been implicated as the likely cause of the rare clear-cell **vaginal or cervical adenocarcinoma** and more frequent benign abnormalities of the genital tract that have been reported in a number of young women whose mothers received stilbestrol during early pregnancy. In the male offspring, an increased incidence of genital abnormalities has been reported. The use of any exogenous estrogen in pregnancy is not recommended.
- **Cholestatic jaundice** and an increased incidence of gallstones (**cholelithiasis**) have been reported in patients taking estrogens (see Chapter 46). The formation of hepatic adenomas in long-term users is recognized.
- **Carbohydrate tolerance** may be impaired during estrogen therapy. Diabetics or patients with positive family histories of diabetes should be followed closely.
- Onset of **migraine headaches** or exacerbation of migraine is experienced by some patients. Other nonspecific headaches may also occur.
- Many other **nonspecific effects** have been documented, including appetite stimulation, depression, chloasma or hyperpigmentation, loss of scalp hair, rashes, pancreatitis, vaginal candidiasis, and post-pill amenorrhea.

Antiestrogens

Historically, substances that modify or oppose the action of estrogens have been referred to as "antiestrogenic," and in this sense both progestins and androgens were included. Currently, the term antiestrogens refers to estrogen-receptor antagonists, such

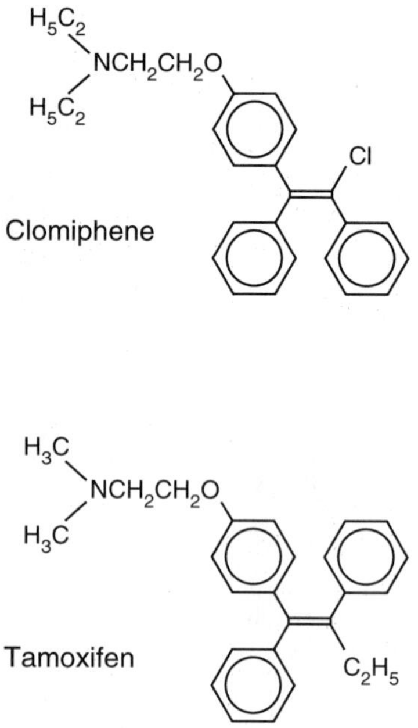

Figure 49-7. Structural formulae of clomiphene and tamoxifen.

as clomiphene and tamoxifen (Fig. 49-7). These compounds have a weak estrogenic effect and inhibit the action of potent estrogens by competing for their access to receptor sites.

Clomiphene citrate (Clomid, Serophene) interferes with the "negative feedback" of estrogens on the hypothalamus and pituitary, resulting in an increase in the secretion of GnRH and gonadotropins. This stimulates ovarian function and leads to maturation of multiple follicles, ovulation, and luteinization. It has been used successfully to treat infertility by inducing ovulation. However, the use of this drug has been associated with an increased incidence of ovarian cancer. In addition, the possibility of multiple births or ovarian hyperstimulation must be kept in mind when clomiphene is employed.

Tamoxifen citrate (Nolvadex, Tamofen,) has a greater blocking effect on peripheral target tissues than clomiphene does. For this reason it is used in the palliative treatment of carcinoma of the breast provided that estrogen receptors are present in the tumor tissue. Trials to evaluate the use of tamoxifen in the prophylaxis of breast cancer were discontinued because of an associated increase in the incidence of endometrial carcinoma, probably due to its weak estrogenic activity.

PROGESTINS

The chemical structure of **progesterone**, the natural hormone of the corpus luteum, is shown in Figure 49-8. It is also produced by the placenta, testis, and adrenal cortex.

For therapeutic use progesterone is available in a micronized oral form (Prometrium) or as an injectable in an oil-based solution. Synthetic progesterone esters (e.g., medroxyprogesterone acetate, Fig. 49-9) and 19-nor derivatives of testosterone (Fig. 49-9) also are available for use as progestational agents. The latter compounds are the progestational component of combination oral contraceptive pills.

Metabolism and Excretion

Progesterone in the circulation is bound to albumin and CBG and is almost entirely metabolized in its first passage through the liver. The 19-nor compounds (ethinyl-substituted) are more stable.

Progesterone is biotransformed to pregnanolones and pregnanediol. The latter is conjugated with glucuronic acid in the liver and excreted via the kidney.

Actions and Uses

Progesterone interacts with a specific nuclear steroid hormone receptor to influence gene transcription and protein synthesis.

In the uterus, progesterone converts the proliferative endometrium (estrogen effect) to a secretory state in preparation for implantation of a fertilized ovum. In the hypothalamus and pituitary, progesterone suppresses the production of gonadotropins and thus prevents further ovulation and follicular maturation. The abrupt fall in progesterone levels (associated with the end of the menstrual cycle, or cessation of administration of exogenous progestin) produces vascular changes in the endometrium that result in

Norethindrone

d-Norgestrel
(30-100 times the progestational activity of norethindrone)

Norethynodrel
(in Enovid)

Medroxy-progesterone acetate
(Provera)

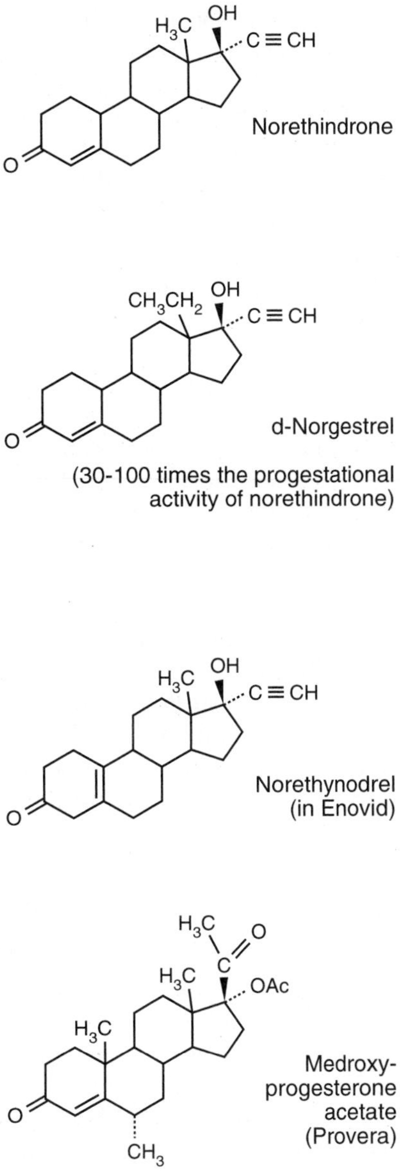

Figure 49-9. Synthetic progestogens used in oral contraceptive preparations.

shedding, with menstrual flow. If a fertilized ovum is implanted before this series of events takes place, hCG from the placenta supports the corpus luteum of pregnancy. The secretion of progesterone thus continues and the uterine endometrium is maintained, permitting the pregnancy to continue.

Progesterone, with estrogen, prolactin, and other hormones, is important in breast development and lactation. It is also responsible for the rise in body temperature that occurs close to the midpoint of the menstrual cycle, corresponding with the time of ovulation.

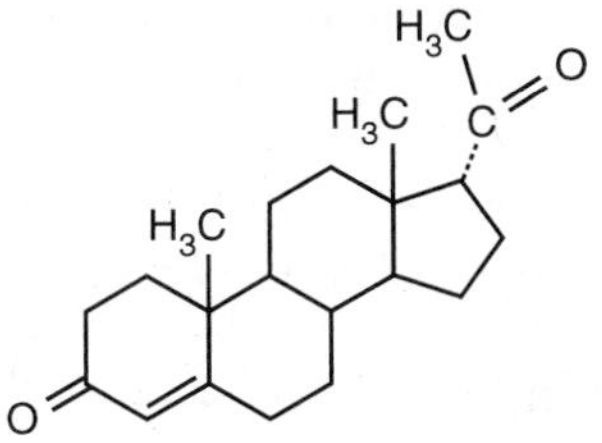

Figure 49-8. Structural formula of progesterone.

By far the greatest clinical use of progestins is as a component of **oral contraceptive pills** in combination with estrogen (discussed below in connection with fertility control). The availability of inexpensive oral progestins has also greatly extended the range of therapeutic uses, some of which are listed below:

Dysfunctional uterine bleeding. A short period of daily administration of a progestin, followed by sudden withdrawal, causes rapid shedding of endometrium and helps to control anovulatory bleeding.

Endometriosis. When progestins are given for prolonged periods, the ectopic endometrial tissue undergoes some involution and develops areas of necrosis, thus presenting a decidua-like reaction.

Progestins are used as adjunctive or palliative treatment of certain **metastatic cancers** originating from endometrial, breast, renal, and other primary cancers.

Amenorrhea. Progesterone can be used diagnostically to test for endogenous estrogen production and endometrial proliferation. If sufficient estrogen had been produced to cause endometrial proliferation, a short period of daily administration of progesterone followed by sudden withdrawal causes menstrual flow.

Adverse Effects

- Atherogenic effects. Progestins reduce HDL and elevate LDL. Thromboembolic events have been reported.
- Edema and weight gain may result from fluid retention.
- Miscellaneous effects, such as breakthrough bleeding, skin rashes, breast tenderness, and headache, have been associated with progestins.

Many side effects are attributable to the androgenic action of 19-nor testosterone derivatives, e.g., acne, hirsutism.

Antiprogestins

Mifepristone (RU-486) is a 19-nor testosterone derivative that functions as a progesterone antagonist, although it has weak partial agonist activity. Administration of this agent prevents ovulation by a central action that suppresses the preovulatory LH surge, and it can terminate early pregnancy by causing endometrial shedding. RU-486 also binds to glucocorticoid receptors to block cortisol action, but it does not bind to estrogen or mineralocorticoid receptors.

RU-486 is approved for clinical use in some countries, but not in North America. When administered together with a prostaglandin, it is effective as an abortive agent if given within 10 days of a missed menstrual cycle.

FERTILITY CONTROL

A decrease in fertility can be achieved in many ways:

- Interfering with fertilization by nonpharmacological means, e.g., behavioral control, mechanical barriers
- Interfering with maturation of gametes, e.g., by gossypol, a phenolic compound from cottonseed, which has been used in China as a male fertility inhibitor
- Impairing gametogenesis, e.g., by mitotic damage caused by alkylating agents, radiation, chemotherapy, or elevation of testicular temperature
- Preventing ovulation: suppression of gonadotropins by the use of 19-norprogestins, alone or combined with estrogens; prevention of gametogenesis by continuous dosage of long-acting analogs of GnRH
- Interference, before or at implantation, by mechanical means (e.g., intrauterine device), or alteration of the endometrium by hormones (e.g., very low dosage of a progestin)
- Interference with gestation (abortion)

All these methods have been examined, but at present preventing ovulation is the most widely used.

Drugs

The available commercial preparations (commonly known collectively as "the pill") include a small amount of a synthetic estrogen (ethinyl estradiol or mestranol), together with a progestin.

Currently used oral contraceptive preparations (see Table 49-1) consist of a combination of estrogen and progestin in a fixed daily dose or in a phasic formulation. In the fixed-dose preparation, the estrogen dose is usually 30–50 μg, and the progestational agent varies, depending on its potency. In the phasic preparation the concentration of the estrogen and/or progestin is varied through phases in the cycle to maintain optimal gonadotropin suppression and prevent breakthrough bleeding. When the oral contraceptive is discontinued, the endometrium is "shed," and menstrual flow usually results.

Combinations containing low doses of estrogen

Table 49-1 Representative Oral Contraceptive Preparations

Estrogen	Progestin	Product
Monophasic		
Ethinyl estradiol	Norethindrone	
20 μg	1 mg	Minestrin 1/20, Loestrin 1/20
30 μg	1.5 mg	Loestrin 1.5/30
35 μg	0.5 mg	Brevicon 21, Ortho 0.5/35, Modicon 21
35 μg	1.0 mg	Ortho 1/35
50 μg	1 mg, 2.5 mg	Norlestrin 1/50, 2.5/50
Ethinyl estradiol	Norgestrel	
30 μg	0.15 mg (*l*-isomer)	Minovral
50 μg	0.5 mg (racemate)	Ovral
Ethinyl estradiol	Norgestimate	
35 μg	0.25 mg	Cyclen
Ethinyl estradiol	Ethynodiol	
35 μg	1 mg	Demulen 1/35
50 μg	1 mg	Demulen 1/50, Demulen 50
Ethinyl estradiol	Desogestrel	
30 μg	0.15 mg	Marvelon, Ortho-Cept
Mestranol	Norethindrone	
50 μg	1 mg	Norinyl 1/50, Ortho-Novum 1/50
80 μg	1 mg	Ortho-Novum 1/80
100 μg	0.5 mg, 2 mg	Ortho-Novum 0.5 mg, 2 mg
Biphasic		
Ethinyl estradiol	Norethindrone	
35 μg	0.5 mg then 1 mg	Ortho 10/11
Triphasic		
Ethinyl estradiol	Norethindrone	
35 μg	0.5 mg then 0.75 mg then 1.0 mg	Ortho 7-7-7
35 μg	0.5 mg then 1 mg then 0.5 mg	Synphasic
Ethinyl estradiol	Norgestrel	
30 μg then 40 μg then 30 μg	0.05 mg then 0.075 mg then 0.125 mg	Triphasil, Triquilar
Ethinyl estradiol	Norgestimate	
35 μg	0.18 mg then 0.215 mg then 0.25 mg	Ortho Tri-Cyclen
Progestins		
None	Norethindrone	
	0.35 mg	Micronor

(less than 50 μg) are preferable, as they offer a low but effective dose with a usually acceptable level of side effects. With low-dose estrogen, "breakthrough" bleeding may occur, but other possible explanations of bleeding in patients using the pill are worth considering. For instance, the concurrent administration of substances such as tetracycline, rifampin, and ampicillin may induce hepatic cytochrome P450 and related enzymes and so accelerate the biotransformation of estrogens, thus reducing their effectiveness.

The effectiveness of the combination oral contraceptives is due to suppression of ovulation (primary action), creating an endometrium that is unfavorable for implantation of the ovum and causing a thickening of cervical mucus secretion that impairs sperm penetration. This technique is almost 100% effective. Generally, the incidence of side effects is low, and their nature depends to a large extent on the quantities of the two components in the combination pill.

The "minipill" (Micronor) consisting of norethindrone 0.35 mg is taken continuously, but does not appear to be as effective as the combination.

Implants of a progestin (medroxyprogesterone) are effective for 3 months or more.

Side Effects and Contraindications

Both components of these preparations (i.e., the estrogen as well as the progestin) contribute to the production of side effects. The most serious of the common side effects is an increase in the incidence of **thromboembolic disease** (thrombophlebitis, pulmonary emboli, cerebrovascular disease). Common but less severe side effects include weight gain, mild edema, nausea, fullness of the breasts, headache, dizziness, depressed mood.

Among young women, these hazards and the mortality associated with them are much less than the risks associated with pregnancy or abortion. These risks, however, increase with age and smoking tobacco. In women over 40 years of age, mortality risks are still less than those associated with pregnancy; but in those over 40 who smoke, the risks are nearly three times those associated with childbirth.

Thromboembolic side effects may be related to the increases in clotting factors, decrease in antithrombin III, and acceleration of platelet aggregation, and they are largely estrogen dose-dependent. Other factors, such as the progestational agent and genetic factors (e.g., blood groups A, B, and AB), may have a role.

Other side effects include changes in carbohydrate metabolism, with a decrease in glucose tolerance; occasional alteration in liver function tests; increased incidence of gallbladder disease and hepatic adenoma; acceleration of closure of epiphyses in the adolescent.

There have been several studies suggesting a link between estrogen use and an increased risk of breast carcinoma. These few reports remain controversial, and the link is unproven.

These side effects are offset by some very desirable features of oral contraceptives, including lack of fear of pregnancy, and reduced frequency of ovarian cysts, benign breast lesions, heavy and irregular periods, and dysmenorrhea. A decreased incidence of ovarian and endometrial carcinoma has been reported in users and previous users of the pill who are over the age of 40.

In terms of effectiveness and aesthetic accep-

tance, no method of contraception compares with the use of the combination pill. It seems clear that its benefits must be balanced against the costs involved. The costs are likely to be too high in the presence of the following conditions, which are considered to be **absolute contraindications:**

- Thromboembolic disease
- Cerebrovascular disease
- Impaired liver function
- Carcinoma of the breast, or other estrogen-dependent neoplasia
- Undiagnosed vaginal bleeding
- Pregnancy or suspected pregnancy
- Classical migraine

ANDROGENS

Physiology

Testosterone (Fig. 49-10) is the principal natural androgen produced in the Leydig cells of the testis. Androstenedione and dehydroepiandrosterone are weaker androgens that serve as precursors for testosterone. In some tissues testosterone acts directly, while in others it is first converted to the more potent derivative dihydrotestosterone. As discussed above, testosterone may also be converted to 17-β-estradiol. After binding to the specific androgen receptor, testosterone and dihydrotestosterone localize in the nuclei of target tissues (a similar mechanism to that of estrogens) to alter gene transcription. Testosterone plays an essential role in spermatogenesis (initiated by FSH) and has a variety of other physiological effects on male genital development (prostate, external genitalia), secondary sex characteristics (hair distribution, voice), and somatic development in general (skeletal muscle and organic matrix of bone).

Most modifications of the testosterone molecule affect all these activities in equal proportions; for example, stanolone (androstane-17-ol-3-one), which resembles testosterone except that the 4–5 double bond is saturated, is a much weaker androgen and

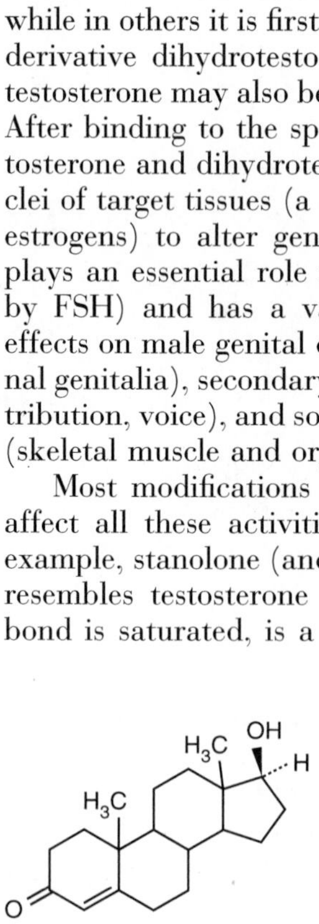

Figure 49-10. Structural formula of testosterone.

also a weaker anabolic hormone. All the modifications have a $-CH_3$ at C-19 and are often referred to as C-19 steroids.

Like estrogens, testosterone in blood is largely bound to the carrier protein, sex-hormone-binding globulin. Examples of the actions of testosterone and its metabolites on various tissues are shown in Table 49-2.

Metabolism

In various tissues, but chiefly in the liver, testosterone is biotransformed to the compounds shown in Figure 49-11. The most important metabolic changes are:

1. Oxidation of the 17-OH group to a keto group
2. Reduction of the 3-keto group to –OH
3. Saturation of the 4–5 double bond to yield 5α- and 5β-stereoisomers

These metabolites are much less potent androgens than testosterone. They are the main urinary excretion products of testicular origin; however, they represent only about 30% of total urinary 17-ketosteroids.

In the normal male, 70% of ketosteroids are derived from the adrenal cortex, the most important being dehydroepiandrosterone. In the female almost all (98%) are from the adrenal cortex.

Modified Testosterones

Testosterone is readily absorbed from the GI tract but is inactivated by first-pass metabolism in the

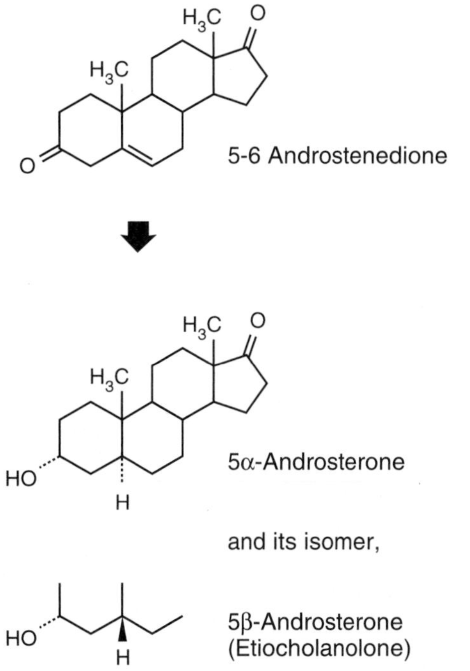

Figure 49-11. Metabolic products of testosterone.

liver. Since these natural modifications all result in loss of activity, synthetic changes for pharmacological purposes are of two different types: those that modify solubility and susceptibility to enzymatic breakdown, and hence affect route and duration of action; and those intended to give some separation between androgenic and anabolic effects. The half-life of testosterone is generally 10–20 minutes. In order to delay absorption and prolong its duration of action, testosterone has been converted to esters that are much less polar. Esterification with propionic acid (Testex) at the 17-OH position yields a product that has a steady effect when injected at 2–3-day intervals. The cypionate (cyclopentylpropionate; Depo-Testosterone cypionate) and enanthate (Delatestryl) esters are effective for periods of up to 3 weeks. Testosterone undecanoate (Andriol) is a testosterone ester that bypasses the liver via absorption through the lymphatic system and is thus orally active. Crystals in aqueous suspension may also be injected intramuscularly. A transdermal patch preparation (Androderm) is also available.

A different set of modifications consists of the addition of a methyl group at C-17 ("1" in Fig. 49-12) to yield methyltestosterone (Metandren) or the insertion of an –F at the 2 position and an –OH group at the 3 position in methyltestosterone to produce fluorohydroxymethyltestosterone (fluoxymesterone,

Table 49-2 Examples of the Actions of Testosterone and Its Derivatives

Intracellular Product	Examples of Actions
Testosterone	Development of structures derived from Wolffian duct Erythropoietin synthesis Pectoral muscle development Kidney hypertrophy
5α-DHT	Growth of genital tubercle, hair
Estradiol	Brain: behavioral effects Gonadotropin secretion Anabolic effects on some muscle
5β-DHT	Red cell production in bone marrow

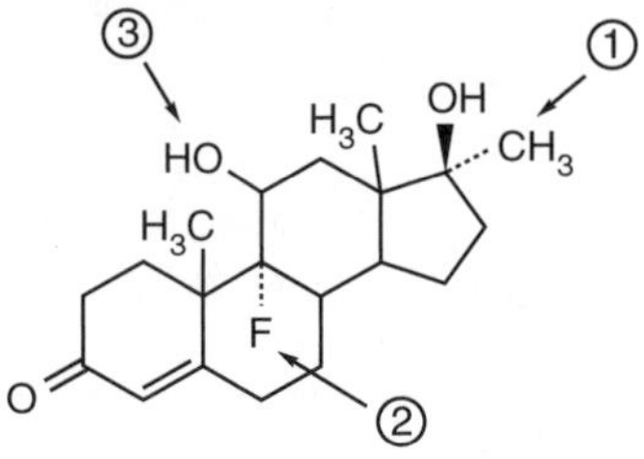

Figure 49-12. Structural formula of fluoxymesterone. See text for explanation of numbers.

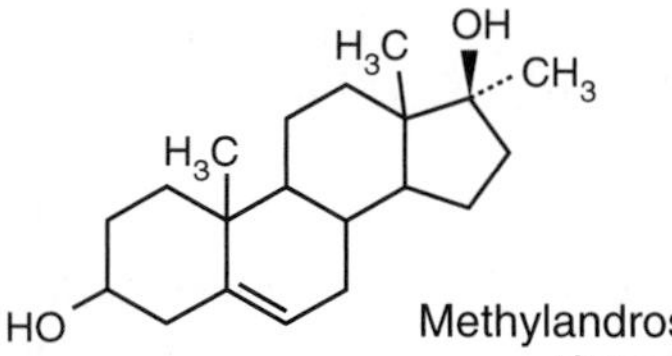

Methylandrostenediol, stenediol

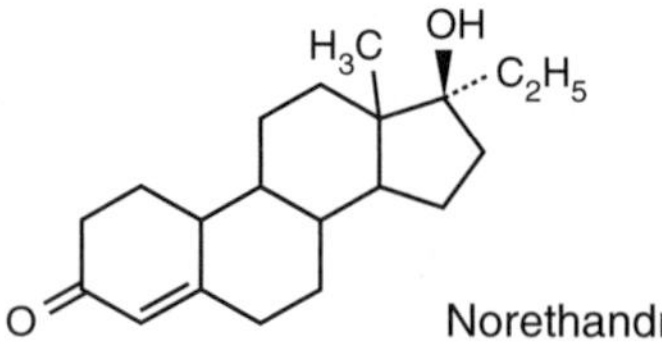

Norethandrolone (17-ethyl-19-nortestosterone)

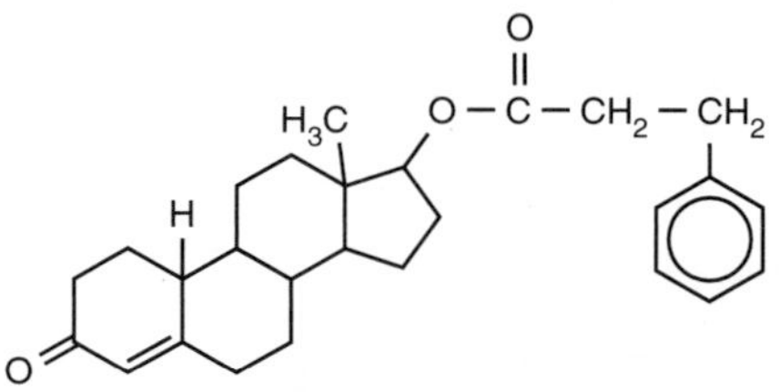

Nandrolone phenpropionate (19-nortestosterone propionate), Durabolin

Figure 49-13. Some modified androgenic preparations.

Halotestin; see Fig. 49-12). These changes facilitate absorption of the product through the oral mucosa, so that it can be administered as tablets placed under the tongue; this mode of administration bypasses the liver so that the same distribution through the body is achieved as by injection. In addition, these modifications result in slower metabolic inactivation of the compound, so the effects are prolonged.

Uses

Androgen replacement therapy. In cases of testicular hypofunction, whether primary, or secondary to pituitary failure, androgens maintain the secondary sexual characteristics and muscular development, and prevent the development of anemia.

Anabolic effects. Androgens produce an increase in the mass of skeletal muscle, an increase in the organic matrix of bone, and retention of nitrogen. These anabolic actions are used in various situations: to offset catabolic effects of adrenal cortical hormones; in burn treatment; to speed recovery from chronic debilitating diseases or operations; to promote bone matrix formation and calcification in senile osteoporosis; to increase muscle mass in athletes. Only long-term use of anabolic steroids can be expected to improve competitive athletic performance, and there are significant risks of side effects attendant on such use. National and international athletic federations disapprove strongly of the use of anabolic steroids. For these purposes, androgenic effects per se are undesirable but unavoidable side effects. If anabolic effects could be separated from virilizing effects, the androgens would be much more useful for this purpose. A selective anabolic activity is claimed for synthetic testosterone analogs such as nandrolone (Durabolin, Deca-Durabolin, Fig. 49-13), but significant androgenic effects persist.

Carcinoma of the breast. Androgens are sometimes used in premenopausal women to suppress the growth of carcinoma of the breast. Most often, these are cases with extensive metastases, especially to the skeleton.

Treatment of anemias. The mild anemia associated with hypogonadism is corrected by administration of androgens. Large doses have been observed to cause polycythemia. Androgens are used in the treatment of aplastic anemia, and sometimes for other anemias refractory to other treatments. Androgens stimulate erythropoietin production from the kidney and have stimulatory effects on other cells of the bone marrow.

Side Effects

Virilization is the most common side effect. All androgens can cause salt and water retention due to mineralocorticoid-like activity and should be used cautiously if heart failure is a threat. Androgens adversely alter the lipid profile by raising LDL cholesterol and lowering HDL cholesterol (see Chapter

39). Gynecomastia may occur, secondary to the aromatization of testosterone to estrogen in peripheral tissues.

Androgens with a methyl or ethyl group on C-17 cause hepatic dysfunction and cholestatic jaundice. This appears to be a direct effect on the liver, related to dose, and not a sensitivity reaction (see Chapter 46). A high dose or prolonged use may cause dilatation of biliary ducts, cholestasis, obstructive jaundice, and hepatic adenoma. Anabolic androgenic steroids also reduce output of testosterone and gonadotropins, thus causing a reduction in spermatogenesis.

ANTIANDROGENS

Potential antiandrogens are compounds that block the synthesis or action of androgens. Continuous administration (see above) of GnRH or its analogs effectively inhibits the whole axis and shuts off testicular production of androgens.

Cyproterone acetate (Androcur) is a progestin that potently antagonizes androgen action by competitive inhibition of androgen binding to its receptor.

Flutamide (Euflex) is a nonsteroidal antiandrogen that prevents androgen uptake and inhibits androgen binding to its receptor. However, by blocking the feedback of testosterone on LH secretion, flutamide markedly elevates LH and testosterone levels. Thus, to be effective it has to be coadministered with a GnRH analog to completely block androgen action.

These classes of compounds that function as antiandrogens have proven clinical utility in the treatment of carcinoma of the prostate (see Chapter 60). In addition, some of these drugs have potential value for the treatment of prostatic hypertrophy, male pattern baldness, acne, hirsutism, and male precocious puberty, and to decrease libido in male sex offenders.

Finasteride (Proscar) is a 5-α reductase inhibitor that blocks the conversion of testosterone to dihydrotestosterone and is used in the treatment of benign prostatic hypertrophy.

SUGGESTED READING

Bagatell CJ, Bremner WJ. Androgen and progestagen effects on plasma lipids. Prog Cardiovasc Dis 1995; 38:255–271.

Beato M. Gene regulation by steroid hormones. Cell 1989; 56:335–344.

Birkhauser M. Hormone replacement therapy and estrogen-dependent cancers. Int J Fertil Menopausal Stud 1994; 39 Suppl 2:99–114.

Breslau NA. Calcium, estrogen, and progestin in the treatment of osteoporosis. Rheum Dis Clin North Am 1994; 20:691–716.

Creasy GW, Kafrissen ME, Upmalis D. Review of the endometrial effects of estrogens and progestins. Obstet Gynecol Surv 1992; 47:654–678.

Ernster VL, Huggins GR, Hulka BS, et al. Benefits and risks of menopausal estrogen and/or progestin hormone use. Prev Med 1988; 17:201–223.

Evans RM. The steroid and thyroid hormone receptor superfamily. Science 1988; 240:889–895.

Katzenellenbogen BS, Bhardwaj B, Fang H, et al. Hormone binding and transcription activation by estrogen receptors: analyses using mammalian and yeast systems. J Steroid Biochem Mol Biol 1993; 47:39–48.

Knopp RH, Zhu Z, Bonet B. Effects of estrogens on lipoprotein metabolism and cardiovascular disease in women. Atherosclerosis 1994; 110 Suppl:S83–S91.

Kolb VM. Luteinizing hormone regulators: luteinizing hormone releasing hormone analogs, estrogens, opiates, and estrogen-opiate hybrids. Prog Drug Res 1994; 42:39–52.

Lobo RA. The role of progestins in hormone replacement therapy. Am J Obstet Gynecol 1992; 166:1997–2004.

Martucci CP, Fishman J. P450 enzymes of estrogen metabolism. Pharmacol Ther 1993; 57:237–257.

Namer M. Clinical applications of antiandrogens. J Steroid Biochem 1988; 31:719–729.

Schwartz J, Freeman R, Frishman W. Clinical pharmacology of estrogen: cardiovascular actions and cardioprotective benefits of replacement therapy in postmenopausal women. J Clin Pharmacol 1995; 35:314–329.

Shenfield GM. Oral contraceptives. Are drug interactions of clinical significance? Drug Saf 1993; 9:21–37.

Song JY, Fraser IS. Effects of progestagens on human endometrium. Obstet Gynecol Surv 1995; 50:385–394.

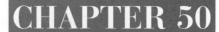

CHAPTER 50

Insulin and Oral Hypoglycemic Drugs

B.P. SCHIMMER AND S.R. GEORGE

CASE HISTORY

A 45-year-old man first consulted his physician because of nocturia, mild thirst, and some fatigue. At the time, he was somewhat overweight and sedentary in his habits. Laboratory tests showed an elevated fasting blood glucose level of 15 mmol/L (normal 4–6.5), glucose but no ketones in the urine, normal plasma electrolytes, and normal anion gap. Diabetes mellitus was diagnosed, and he was placed on a diabetic diet low in free sugar and fat. After 2 months on this diet he had a fasting blood glucose level of 9.5 mmol/L and a 2-hour postlunch glucose value of 12.8 mmol/L (normal < 8.5); glycosylated hemoglobin (Hb A_{1C}) level was 10.5% (normal < 6%). He was therefore started on glyburide at a dosage of 5 mg before breakfast and 5 mg before dinner, but the blood glucose remained elevated. The dosage was therefore raised to 10 mg twice daily, and this achieved a good result.

After 3 years on this regimen, he developed unstable angina pectoris, and the blood glucose and Hb A_{1C} levels were again found to be elevated. Addition of metformin to his treatment produced some improvement in his carbohydrate metabolism, but his cardiac symptoms gradually worsened over the next 3 years. He showed intermittent glycosuria during this time, and proteinuria appeared. His weight had fallen to a level that yielded a normal body mass index. His physician therefore decided to transfer him to insulin therapy, and he was admitted to hospital at the age of 53.

He was started on a regimen of 22 units of Lente insulin and 12 units of regular insulin every morning before breakfast. His 8:00 A.M. blood glucose was found to be 10 mmol/L and there was extensive glycosuria. In an attempt to normalize blood sugar levels, the dose of Lente insulin was raised gradually to 35 units. As a result, his 4:00 A.M. blood glucose level fell to 3 mmol/L, rising to 13 mmol/L at 8:00 A.M., before breakfast. After further adjustment of the insulin into a split A.M. and P.M. dosage, the patient's blood sugars ranged from 4.5 to 8 mmol/L before meals and from 6.5 to 13 mmol/L after meals. During the next year he had three mild hypoglycemic reactions. He was found to have stable background retinopathy, mild diabetic nephropathy, and mild numbness and tingling in both feet, but blood pressure remained normal.

In the following year, during three routine visits to his family physician, his blood pressure readings were 140/90, 145/95 and 150/100 mmHg. His physician started antihypertensive therapy with enalapril and propranolol. Three weeks later the patient was found at home in a semiconscious state resulting from severe hypoglycemia, having taken an unusually long walk earlier in the day. After being revived, he denied feeling any of his usual symptoms of hypoglycemia.

Diabetes mellitus has been recognized for centuries as a debilitating and life-threatening disease. It is a metabolic disturbance that is characterized by hyperglycemia, resulting in excretion of large volumes of urine containing sugar, and excessive thirst. Other features include altered metabolism of lipids and carbohydrates, and wasting of tissue (loss of nitrogen). In severe cases, ketoacidosis develops, leading to coma and, if uncorrected, to death. The long-term complications include vascular disease, retinopathy and other microvascular disease, atherosclerosis, nephropathy, and neuropathy.

An extract of pancreas, prepared by F.G. Banting and C.H. Best at the University of Toronto in 1921, contained an active principle (insulin) capable of controlling the hyperglycemia of diabetes. The very first diabetic patient treated with Banting and Best's pancreatic extract was a 14-year-old boy named Leonard Thompson, at the Toronto General Hospital. Thompson continued the use of insulin until death at age 76. This discovery dramatically improved the lifespan of diabetic patients. However, the long-term complications secondary to diabetes continue to cause significant morbidity. In North America, diabetes mellitus is prevalent in 2–3% of the population and has a hereditary component.

The disease is categorized into two major classes: type I, insulin-dependent diabetes mellitus (IDDM), and type II, non–insulin-dependent diabetes mellitus (NIDDM). IDDM often occurs in juveniles and is characterized by destruction of β cells of the pancreas, possibly triggered by viral and autoimmune mechanisms. This results in severe insulin deficiency leading to ketoacidosis. NIDDM typically exhibits a slow onset and occurs predominantly in older age groups. The hyperglycemia is thought to result from a failure of pancreatic β cells to produce sufficient insulin in response to glucose and from a resistance of peripheral tissues to insulin that may result from defects at different points in the signal transduction pathway that mediates insulin action. Therefore NIDDM represents a heterogeneous group of genetic disorders with similar clinical manifestations.

The objectives of treatment are the same for both types—to maintain blood glucose within normal limits so as to prevent the development of complications of diabetes mellitus.

INSULIN

Insulin is a protein with a molecular mass of about 6000 Da and is made up of two polypeptide chains (an A-chain consisting of 21 amino acids and a B-chain of 30 amino acids) linked by two disulfide bonds (Fig. 50-1). It is produced in the β cells of the islets of Langerhans, initially as a single precursor molecule, proinsulin (formed from a larger precursor, pre-proinsulin), that is cleaved by proteolytic enzymes to form insulin. Porcine insulin differs from human insulin in only one amino acid, whereas bovine insulin differs from human insulin by three amino acids. The greater similarity between pork insulin and human insulin may explain the lesser antigenicity of pork insulin in therapeutic use.

Most of the insulin in the β cells of the human pancreas (approximately 200 units) is contained in secretory granules. Under appropriate stimulation the contents of the granules are released into the extracellular space by exocytosis. Connecting peptide (C-peptide) and some proinsulin are released into the circulation along with insulin but do not contribute significantly to bioactivity.

The molecule contains a high proportion of dicarboxylic acids, which enables it to combine readily with basic proteins without affecting its fundamental structure. This property is utilized in the preparation of long-acting insulin for clinical use. In an acid medium it tends to polymerize into insoluble fibrils.

Physiology

The main physiological stimulus for insulin secretion is a rise in blood glucose level. Glucose produces a rapid release of insulin, as well as a secondary, slower release that raises blood levels of insulin for about an hour. The rapidly released insulin is from the pool stored in secretory granules present in β cells, whereas the slow release is attributed to release of newly synthesized insulin. Glucose taken orally has a greater effect on insulin secretion than glucose by injection, the likely explanation being that glucose taken orally concurrently stimulates the secretion of glucagon, ileum-derived glucagon-like peptide 1, and digestive hormones. These in turn stimulate the release of insulin additively from the islet cells. Other factors that may enhance the release of insulin include secretin, pancreozymin, gastric inhibitory polypeptide (GIP), gastrin, glucagon, some amino acids (arginine, leucine), and free fatty acids (FFA).

Autonomic mediators also influence secretion of insulin. Epinephrine and norepinephrine (acting through α_2-adrenergic receptors) inhibit the secretion induced by a rise in blood glucose. Cholinergic drugs enhance the release of insulin. Growth hormone stimulates the synthesis of insulin but probably does not have a direct effect on its release. Drugs of the sulfonylurea group (glyburide, chlorpropamide, tolbutamide) also stimulate release of insulin (Fig. 50-2).

Somatostatin, produced by the δ cells of the pancreatic islet, inhibits the secretion of both insulin and glucagon by direct actions on islet β and α

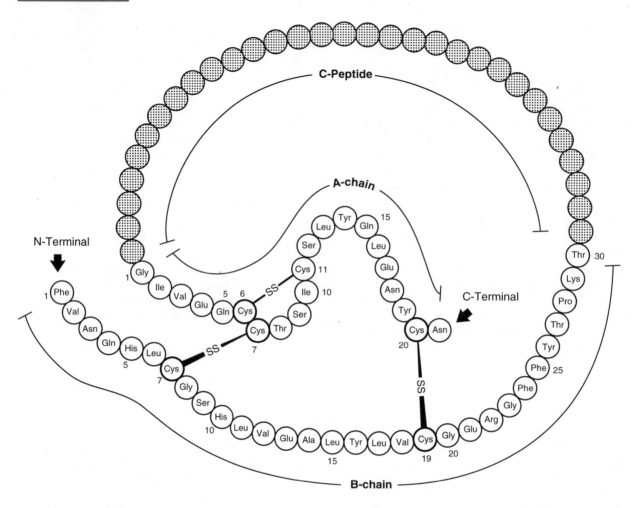

Figure 50-1. Structure of human insulin (A-chain = 21 amino acids, B-chain = 30 amino acids, connected by two of three disulfide bridges, those at positions A7–B7 and A20–B19). The proinsulin molecule contains a "C-peptide" of 31 amino acids, which is removed by proteolysis to form insulin.

cells. The physiological importance of this action of somatostatin is not clear. Somatostatin is also produced in the GI tract, where it inhibits the secretion of gastrin, secretin, cholecystokinin, pepsin, and HCl. Therefore its physiological role in glucose homeostasis may be very complex.

Insulin exerts its actions by binding to specific receptors on the surface of target cells. The insulin receptor is made up of α and β subunits and exists as an α_2-β_2 dimer. The α subunits are extracellular and provide the binding site for insulin. The β subunits are transmembrane proteins that anchor the α subunits and have intracellular tyrosine kinase activity. The binding of insulin to the α chains leads to activation of β subunit tyrosine kinase and consequent phosphorylation of other substrate proteins intracellularly. These events initiate a cascade of enzymatic reactions that are not fully understood.

Insulin-receptor activation results in the mobilization of specific glucose transporters in muscle and adipose tissue that promote the uptake of glucose. Glucose uptake in certain tissues (neurons, erythrocytes, intestinal mucosa, kidney) is mediated by different glucose transporters that are not dependent on insulin. In liver and muscle, glycogen synthase activity is increased and glycogen phosphorylase activity is inhibited, leading to increased deposition of glycogen. In the liver, insulin also inhibits the synthesis of glucose (gluconeogenesis), and increases glucose uptake, in part by stimulating glucokinase activity. In muscle, insulin promotes protein synthesis by facilitating amino acid uptake. Therefore insulin is an anabolic and anticatabolic hormone. In adipose tissue insulin promotes triglyceride synthesis and inhibits lipolysis.

Insulin increases glucose uptake and oxidative

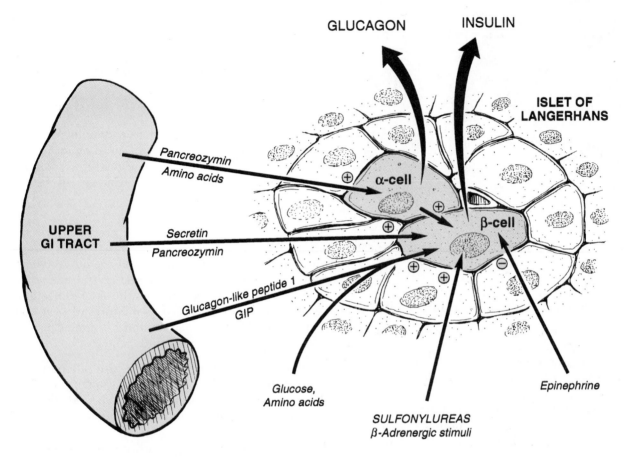

Figure 50-2. Factors involved in the stimulation (+) and inhibition (−) of insulin production and release.

metabolism by muscle and other tissues. This prevents breakdown of tissue protein and conversion of residual amino acids into glucose by the liver. Insulin thus prevents gluconeogenesis and glycogenolysis and consequently reduces glucose release from the liver. It also prevents mobilization of fatty acids from fat depots and the consequent breakdown of these fatty acids by the liver. Insulin thus prevents the formation of ketone bodies. Indeed, fat synthesis from glucose is promoted by insulin. In the diabetic subject, these actions result in a lowering of blood sugar, disappearance of glycosuria and polyuria, and disappearance of ketone bodies from the blood and urine.

Preparations and Properties

For many decades following its discovery, the world's supply of insulin for therapeutic use was derived from extracts of bovine and porcine pancreases. The procedures for purification of insulin from these sources have undergone almost continuous refine-

ment in an effort to remove contaminants such as insulin precursors and proteolytic fragments, glucagon, and other pancreatic hormones.

As a result of recent technological advances, human insulin has become available and is used widely. At present, human insulin is produced by means of recombinant DNA technology in which human proinsulin is expressed in bacteria or yeast and then hydrolyzed to yield insulin. In some formulations human insulin is produced by chemical conversion from pork insulin by substituting threonine for alanine at position 30 of the B chain (Table 50-1 and Fig. 50-1). Human insulin is more polar than insulin from animal sources, and therefore it is absorbed more quickly from its site of injection. Therefore, the duration of action is somewhat shorter and doses must be adjusted to compensate. Recombinant insulin has provided an assured supply of hormone, which is fortunate, because the world-wide incidence of diabetes is increasing.

A large variety of insulin formulations are available; they can be divided into groups on the basis of

Table 50-1 Species-Specific Structural Differences Between Human, Porcine, and Bovine Insulin (cf. Fig. 50-1)

Species	Amino Acids at			C-Peptide Amino Acids
	A-8	A-10	B-30	
Human	Thr	Ile	Thr	31
Pig	Thr	Ile	Ala	33
Ox	Ala	Val	Ala	30

different onset times, times to maximal activity (peak time), and durations of action (Table 50-2).

Crystalline zinc insulin (CZI, regular insulin)

Purified insulin is crystallized as a zinc salt and then redissolved to give a clear solution. One milligram of crystalline human insulin = 27.5 units. It is usually given subcutaneously, but the intravenous route is used in emergencies and other circumstances such as during surgery. When administered subcutaneously, it lowers plasma glucose within minutes and its effects last for 8–12 hours; however, the exact duration and magnitude of effect depend on the dose and on the individual patient. The plasma half-life of intravenous insulin is only a few minutes. Regular insulin is available as human insulin (recombinant or semisynthetic), as a mixture of beef and pork insulin, and as pork insulin.

NPH insulin (neutral protamine Hagedorn)

NPH insulin is formed by treating regular insulin with protamine and zinc at neutral pH (7.2), causing a fine precipitate of protamine zinc insulin. This fine suspension can only be given subcutaneously and is absorbed slowly and evenly. Its onset of action is 1–2 hours, its peak action occurs at 6–12 hours, and the effect wears off 18–24 hours after administration. NPH insulin is available as preparations made from human insulin (semisynthetic or recombinant), a mixture of beef and pork insulin, and pork insulin.

PZI insulin (protamine zinc insulin)

Like NPH, this is a suspension of crystalline insulin, zinc, and protamine at neutral pH. However, it contains more protamine than NPH and its duration of action is prolonged. It has no short-term action, but slowly reaches a maximum effect by about 24 hours, and then gradually wears off over the next 24 hours. This formulation is made only with animal insulin.

Insulin mixtures

These are premixed formulations containing crystalline zinc insulin and NPH insulin in different ratios, e.g., 30% CZI:70% NPH. These mixtures combine the benefits of rapid onset and prolonged duration of action.

Lente insulins

These are suspensions of insulin in acetate buffer at neutral pH. The physical state and crystal size influence the rate of absorption from the site of injection. Lente insulins are provided as mixtures of beef and pork insulin, as pork insulin, and as human insulin (recombinant or semisynthetic).

1. **Insulin (Semilente); insulin zinc suspension prompt (U.S.P.):** a suspension of amorphous insulin with rapid onset of action, a peak time of 5–10 hours, and a duration of action of 14–16 hours.
2. **Insulin (Ultralente); insulin zinc suspension extended (U.S.P.):** large crystals, slow absorption, similar to protamine zinc insulin in duration of action.
3. **Insulin (Lente); insulin zinc suspension (U.S.P.):** made up of 70% ultralente and 30% semilente insulin. Its effect is similar to that of NPH but may have a slower onset.

Sulfated insulin (beef)

Sulfated insulin is insulin treated with sulfuric acid to sulfate the tyrosine residues. Sulfated insulin is used in patients with insulin resistance who require very high insulin doses because of the presence of circulating insulin antibodies. Insulin antibodies do not appear to bind to this modified form of the hormone.

Insulin Pharmacokinetics

Insulin, like many proteins, can be hydrolyzed and inactivated in the gastrointestinal tract. Therefore, insulin is administered by injection, most commonly by the subcutaneous route. When crystalline zinc insulin is injected subcutaneously, it is absorbed and

Table 50-2 Summary of Available Insulin Preparations

Insulin Preparation	U.S.P. Official Name	Common Synonyms and Proprietary Names	Action (hours)		
			Onset	Peak	Duration
Rapid action					
Insulin (crystalline zinc)* beef, pork, beef and pork†	Insulin injection U.S.P.	Regular*; CZI* Toronto-Neutral* Insulin-Toronto Iletin Regular	0.5	3–5	8–12
Insulin (crystalline zinc)* human biosynthetic (rDNA origin)*		Humulin-R Novolin Toronto	0.5	3–5	6–8
Insulin (Semilente) beef and pork	Insulin zinc suspension prompt U.S.P.	Insulin semilente	0.5	5–10	14–16
Intermediate action					
Insulin (Isophane) beef, pork, beef and pork†	Isophane insulin suspension U.S.P.	NPH; NPH-50 Iletin NPH NPH Insulin	2.5	4–12	12–24
Insulin (Isophane) human biosynthetic (rDNA origin)		Humulin (various preparations) Novolin (various preparations)	1.5	4–12	12–24
Insulin (Lente) beef, beef and pork†	Insulin zinc suspension U.S.P.	Lente; Insulin zinc suspension intermediate Insulin lente	2.5	7–15	12–24
Prolonged action					
Insulin (protamine zinc) beef, pork, beef and pork†	Protamine zinc insulin suspension U.S.P.	PZI	4	10–30	36
Insulin (Ultralente) beef and pork	Insulin zinc suspension extended U.S.P.	Ultralente; Insulin zinc suspension prolonged Insulin ultralente	4	10–30	36
Insulin (Ultralente) human biosynthetic (rDNA origin)		Humulin-U Novolin Ultralente	4	8–24	28

*Only regular (crystalline zinc) insulin can be given intravenously.
†Available as single-species (beef *or* pork) and mixed-species (beef *and* pork) preparations.

distributed rapidly, and within minutes it can be detected in the cells of liver, kidney, and muscle. These tissues (particularly liver and kidney) contain an enzyme, insulinase, that is of primary importance in degrading the hormone. After intravenous injection the plasma half-life of insulin is less than 9 minutes. Its volume of distribution approximates that of extracellular fluid. Attempts to modify the time of onset and duration of action of injected insulin are all based on influencing the rate at which it reaches the bloodstream from the site of injection.

The fate of injected insulin is different from that of secreted insulin. About 50% of insulin secreted into the portal vein is destroyed in the liver and never reaches the general circulation. This creates a marked differential concentration gradient between the liver and the periphery, resulting in a greater effect of secreted insulin on hepatic function. Attempts to control hepatic gluconeogenesis with injected insulin therefore do not mimic the effects of secreted insulin because there is no concentration gradient. Adequate levels of insulin for hepatic effect may result in peripheral hyperinsulinemia.

The different time relations of various insulin preparations are idealized in Figure 50-3. These profiles assume a constant level of glycemia. In normal subjects, a regular eating pattern consists of taking three or four meals about 4–5 hours apart, followed by a long overnight period with little or no food intake. Therefore, there usually are three main peaks of hyperglycemia: in midmorning, midafternoon, and early evening. Plasma glucose is lower overnight and lowest in the early morning. These increases in plasma glucose stimulate peaks of insulin secretion. During the overnight (fasting) period insulin secretion is at a low basal level.

In insulin-dependent diabetic patients, combinations of regular insulin together with an intermediate or long-acting form can be administered in various proportions to approximate the normal endogenous patterns of insulin secretion. The regular insulin provides rapid, short-term effect; the longer-acting preparations provide sustained effects with peak action at later times.

Since 1975, all preparations in North America have been standardized at 100 units/mL. The standard mode of insulin administration is via a needle and calibrated 1-ml syringe. For convenience, portable injector pens with retractable needle are available that contain cartridges of insulin sufficient for multiple injections.

Clinical Uses

Diabetes mellitus

The principal use of insulin is for replacement therapy in insulin-dependent diabetes mellitus, in which the patient's own insulin supply is deficient. In the patient with diabetes mellitus, the therapeutic objective is to maintain plasma glucose concentrations in the normal range. This involves administering sufficient insulin to control the hyperglycemia associated with food intake as well as maintaining a basal level of insulin to prevent excessive mobilization of fuels between meals.

Several different insulin treatment regimens are used to achieve these objectives, usually by means of a combination of intermediate or long-acting insulin with regular insulin. In a typical regimen of insulin

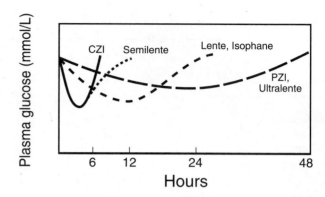

Figure 50-3. Usual patterns of blood sugar responses with different insulin preparations.

administration, an intermediate-acting insulin (Lente or NPH) in combination with regular insulin is given twice daily, usually before breakfast and before the evening meal. Additional fine adjustments to glucose homeostasis can be achieved by altering meal times to correspond better with peak insulin concentrations or by delaying the evening injection of intermediate-acting insulin until bedtime.

In NIDDM, dietary control together with regular exercise is often sufficient. Insulin may be used in these patients if they remain hyperglycemic in spite of diet and exercise.

Infections, uremia, surgical trauma, other serious illnesses, and even anxiety tend to increase insulin requirements because of increased secretion of glucagon. With appropriate treatment of the underlying condition, the insulin requirements will decrease.

As indicated earlier, insulin has dramatically increased life expectancy, but the complications of diabetes mellitus—cardiovascular, renal, neural, and ocular—remain unpleasant prospects for the diabetic. It had been assumed that good control of blood sugar would prevent such complications or slow their progression, and results from the 1993 Diabetes Control and Complications Trial (DCCT) now strongly support this assumption for the insulin-dependent diabetic. Achieving rigid control of blood sugar, however, is not without attendant difficulties, including poor patient compliance, cost, and increased frequency of hypoglycemic reactions from intensive therapy. The DCCT trial did not address the value of intensive therapy in NIDDM, and extrapolation to this form of diabetes is not currently justified.

Diabetic coma

This is an emergency situation, associated with severe dehydration and acidosis, which may be fatal. Intravenous fluid and regular insulin are the mainstay of treatment. The soluble short-acting type of insulin is needed to achieve rapid and flexible therapy, since the condition of the patient can change rapidly with massive administration of intravenous fluid and electrolytes. The usual recommended dose of insulin in this case is 0.1 unit/kg body weight/hr by infusion, preceded by an initial bolus that is equivalent to the dose in the first hour. This dosage approximates the normal rate of endogenous insulin delivery to the periphery and produces a level of venous plasma insulin (about 100 μU/mL) close to that seen after a carbohydrate meal. However, the dosage has to be titrated to individual patient requirements. As blood glucose levels fall toward normal, the rate of insulin infusion can be slowed and intravenous glucose can be started to prevent insulin-induced hypoglycemia.

Diagnostic test

Insulin-induced hypoglycemia stimulates the output of releasing factors from the hypothalamus that in turn release growth hormone and ACTH from the anterior pituitary. Injection of insulin is therefore used as a diagnostic test of the integrity of these hypothalamic and pituitary responses.

Undesired Side Effects

Hypoglycemic reactions

Mild hypoglycemic reactions are common and are seen when a meal is missed, when an overdose of insulin has been taken, or when strenuous muscular work has been done. The typical symptoms include sweating, tachycardia, tremor, weakness, hunger, "being ill at ease" (adrenergic symptoms resulting from a compensatory increase in the secretion of epinephrine), blurred vision, and mental confusion; severe cases may go on to convulsions or coma. If the latter occurs, it is important to differentiate it from diabetic coma (Table 50-3).

Laboratory tests or capillary glucose monitoring provide conclusive differentiation. If these are not available and diagnosis is uncertain, intravenous glucose will cure hypoglycemic coma in minutes and will not do much harm to diabetic coma. On the other hand, insulin administration in hypoglycemic coma may kill the patient. Glucagon injection is used for the emergency treatment of severe hypoglycemia when use of intravenous glucose is not possible.

Local lipodystrophy

Irregular atrophy and lumpiness of subcutaneous fat may occur if insulin injections are given repeatedly in the same place. To prevent this occurrence, the sites of injection should be varied.

Insulin presbyopia

This visual disturbance is due to osmotic changes in ocular fluids; it occurs early in therapy but is usually transient.

Edema

Edema lasting for a few weeks may occur on initiation of insulin therapy. This effect results in part from an insulin-dependent sodium retention by the kidney.

Insulin allergy

The most common manifestation of insulin allergy is a cutaneous reaction at the site of injection, e.g., rash or hives due to IgE-mediated histamine release from mast cells. Severe allergy, with urticaria, angioneurotic edema, and anaphylaxis, occurs in only a small percentage of patients. The allergic reaction is often due to traces of other proteins present but may also result from reactions to denatured or aggregated insulin. When mixtures of beef and pork insulin are used, most cases of allergy appear to be due to the beef component and can be eliminated if human or pure pork insulin is used. Treatment of insulin allergy may also require the use of antihistamines and glucocorticoids and a desensitization regimen.

Insulin resistance

A totally insulin-deficient diabetic usually requires from 30 to 50 units of insulin per day for control. A requirement of 200 units or more per day indicates that the patient is "resistant" to insulin. Occasionally 1000 or more units fails to control hyperglycemia and the frequent attendant ketoacidosis. Several factors may cause insulin resistance.

Immune insulin resistance is due to insulin-binding IgG antibodies. As noted earlier, the antibodies may be species-specific.

Genetic mutations in components of the insulin-signaling pathway (insulin receptor, IRS-1, glucokinase, GLUT 4 glucose transporter, etc.) occur rarely

Table 50-3 Differentiation Between "Hypoglycemic Shock" and Diabetic Coma

	Acute *"Hypoglycemic Shock"*	*Diabetic Coma*
Onset	Rapid	Gradual—over days
Acidosis, dehydration	No	Severe
Preceding infection	No	Common, often with vomiting or diarrhea
Skin	Pale, sweating	Hot, dry
Respiration	Normal or shallow	Deep—"air hunger"
CNS	Tremor, mental confusion (even coma); occasionally convulsions; may have positive Babinski sign	General depression

but have been implicated as a cause of variability in response to insulin, including insulin resistance.

Metabolic. Fewer insulin receptors are present in the cells of obese type II diabetics than of nondiabetics, and relatively high blood insulin levels are frequently observed in such individuals. This resistance is often reversible by weight loss and exercise.

Problems and Prospects

It is very important that insulin-dependent diabetics monitor plasma glucose so that periods of hyperglycemia and hypoglycemia do not go undetected. Since reliable methods for monitoring blood glucose at home, using a drop of fingertip capillary blood, are now available, such monitoring has vastly improved diabetic control.

Measurements of glycosylated hemoglobin A_{1C} provide another index of glycemic control. Fractions of hemoglobin are slowly and irreversibly glycosylated in erythrocytes by a nonenzymatic glycation reaction.

Therefore the levels of glycosylated hemoglobin reflect the glucose concentrations encountered over the lifespan of the erythrocyte (about 120 days) and provide a time-averaged measurement of plasma glucose levels. The normal Hb A_{1C} level is less than 6% of total hemoglobin. In poorly controlled diabetics, values may range from 15 to 20%.

Along with these means of assessing the degree of control, attempts have been made to develop systems for the continuous delivery of insulin from portable or implanted pumps in amounts determined by metabolic need. Two principal methods have been explored: the "closed loop," in which delivery is controlled by frequent automated measurements of

blood glucose, and the "open loop" used in ambulatory patients, in which delivery is controlled by a preset schedule based on times of food intake and physical activity.

Efforts also have been made to find more acceptable routes of insulin administration and achieve more physiological profiles of blood glucose. The nasal route of administration may offer an alternative to the parenteral route, but further work is required to identify agents that will safely increase the bioavailability of insulin from the nasal passages.

ORAL ANTIDIABETIC DRUGS

Sulfonylureas

Soon after the discovery of insulin, the search began for antidiabetic drugs that could be taken by mouth. In 1942, French workers (Janbon, Loubatières, and colleagues) found that some antibacterial sulfonamides lowered blood sugar. This discovery led to subsequent modifications of the sulfonamide molecule that enhanced hypoglycemic activity and removed the antibacterial effect (Fig. 50-4; see also Fig 11-4).

These modified drugs, termed sulfonylureas, appear to act by inhibiting potassium efflux via ATP-dependent potassium channels in pancreatic β cells. This action leads to cellular depolarization, calcium influx, and calcium-stimulated release of insulin from the pancreas. Second-generation derivatives (e.g., glyburide) also seem to potentiate the peripheral and hepatic actions of insulin and are more potent than first-generation drugs (e.g., tolbutamide, chlorpropamide). Because these drugs act as hypoglycemic

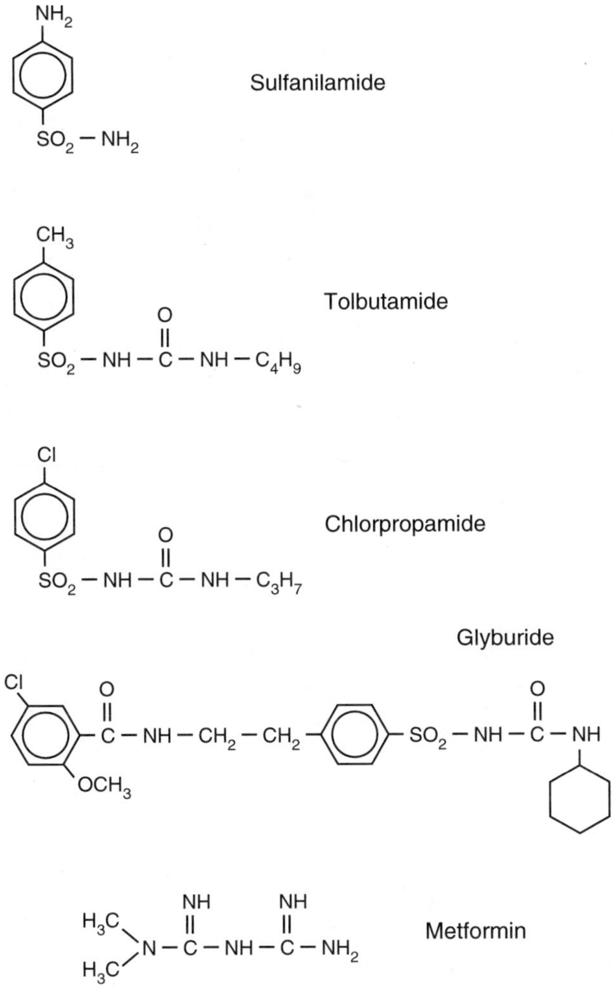

Figure 50-4. Sulfanilamide and selected oral hypoglycemics.

agents only in patients whose pancreases can produce insulin, they cannot be used as insulin substitutes in patients with IDDM. The main use of the oral hypoglycemic drugs is in moderately severe cases of NIDDM that do not respond adequately to a regimen of diet and exercise.

Preparations: first-generation drugs

Tolbutamide (Orinase, Mobenol) available in 0.5- and 1.0-g tablets; dose 1–6 tablets daily.

Chlorpropamide (Diabinese) available in 0.1- and 0.25-g tablets; usual dose 1–2 tablets daily.

Acetohexamide (Dimelor) available in 0.5-g tablets; dose 1–3 tablets daily.

Preparations: second-generation drugs

Glyburide (glibenclamide, Diaβeta, Euglucon, Micronase) available in 2.5- and 5.0-mg tablets; usual dose 5–10 mg daily.

Gliclazide (Diamicron) available in 80-mg tablets; usual dose 40–320 mg daily.

Glipizide (Glucotrol) available in 5-mg tablets; usual dose 5–40 mg daily. Not available in Canada.

Pharmacokinetics

All of the sulfonylureas are well absorbed from the small intestine, but glyburide is the most slowly absorbed unless it is subjected to a micropulverization process to reduce the particle size. These agents are mainly converted to hydroxylated derivatives that are inactive, except for the hydroxyacetohexamide metabolite, which is active and has a $t_{1/2}$ considerably longer than that of the parent drug. Chlorpropamide is the only one that is excreted unchanged in the urine to a significant degree (about 20%); about 10% of administered acetohexamide and 5% of glipizide are also excreted unchanged, as are negligible amounts of the other sulfonylureas. Some of the major pharmacokinetic data are shown in Table 50-4.

There are few significant drug interactions involving these agents. Barbiturates and rifampin have been reported to decrease the effect of some sulfonylureas by inducing their biotransformation in the liver. Tolbutamide and chlorpropamide can increase the anticoagulant effect of oral vitamin K antagonists. β-Blockers may increase the risk of hypoglycemia by preventing the adrenergic response to a fall in blood sugar.

Untoward effects and toxicity

Since these drugs cause release of endogenous insulin, they can cause **hypoglycemic reactions**; these reactions may be insidious in onset and therefore hard to recognize.

Adverse reactions most commonly encountered are nausea and vomiting, which may be severe enough to prevent use; occasional hematological and dermatological effects have been reported. An intolerance to alcohol (disulfiram-like) is common, especially with chlorpropamide, although less likely to occur with glyburide. In patients on chlorpropamide, obstructive jaundice due to plugging of fine intrahepatic biliary ducts has been reported.

Patients receiving chlorpropamide may occasionally develop hyponatremia and water retention, re-

Table 50-4 Some Pharmacokinetic Features of Sulfonylureas and Metformin

Agent	Oral Bioavailability (%)	t_{max} (hours)	$t_{1/2}$ (hours)	Excretion in Urine
1st generation				
Acetohexamide	95	1–2	1.5 (original) 4.5 (hydroxy metabolite)	10% unchanged
Chlorpropamide	90	2–6	36–40	20–25% unchanged
Tolbutamide	93	3–4	6–7	Negligible
2nd generation				
Glyburide	60–100	2–3	6–10 (terminal $t_{1/2}$ 15–20)	Negligible
Gliclazide		4–8	10	Negligible
Glipizide	95	1–2	4–7	<5% unchanged
Biguanide				
Metformin	50–60	2	1.5–4	100% unchanged

sembling the syndrome of inappropriate ADH secretion (SIADH). This is probably due to an effect on renal tubular cells, increasing their sensitivity to endogenous ADH. An increased formation and release of ADH has also been reported.

In **secondary failure,** about 75% of cases, chosen as described above, show good initial response to these drugs, but about 5–10% later stop getting any effect from them. Some will show a response if switched to another drug, but most do not. Therefore, if secondary failure occurs, the patient should be switched to insulin therapy.

Safety of sulfonylureas

In 1970, the University Group Diabetic Program (UGDP) conducted a study comparing insulin and oral hypoglycemics in the treatment of NIDDM. They found that the mortality (mainly from cardiovascular causes) among patients receiving tolbutamide was significantly higher than in those treated with insulin or with diet alone. The results of this study, however, are highly controversial, and interpretations remain unclear. Questions have been raised about the selection of subjects, and the absence of a difference in nonfatal cardiovascular complications remains a

puzzle. Because the UGDP study is considered not to be definitive, sulfonylureas continue to be used widely in cases in which diet and exercise are insufficient. The oral hypoglycemic agents (sulfonylureas or metformin) are minimally effective in preventing the long-term complications of diabetes.

Biguanides

Biguanides act directly on muscle to increase glucose uptake and utilization. They also reduce hepatic glucose production and divert intestinal glucose into lactic acid production. Since these effects of biguanides require the presence of insulin, biguanides are effective only in non–insulin-dependent diabetics. Biguanides do not cause hypoglycemia, and they tend to lower the levels of plasma lipids, especially VLDL.

Metformin (Glucophage; Fig. 50-4) is a biguanide closely related to phenformin. Phenformin was taken off the market in 1978 because it caused serious lactic acidosis in some patients. Metformin is still in use and has a much lower incidence of lactic acidosis. However, the risk of lactic acidosis is increased when renal or hepatic disease coexists. Metformin accumulates in the gastrointestinal tract and salivary glands, and its most common side effects are nausea, vomiting, epigastric distress, and diarrhea. It is reported to decrease the risk of vascular complications of diabetes by reducing platelet aggregation and increasing fibrinolytic activity.

Glucosidase Inhibitor

Acarbose (Precose) is an oligosaccharide that competitively inhibits the activity of intestinal α-glucosidases such as α-glucoamylase, maltase, and sucrase. This action results in inhibition of carbohydrate digestion and delays glucose uptake. By slowing the formation and absorption of glucose following a meal, acarbose reduces the peaks of hyperglycemia following food intake.

The major side effects are gastrointestinal, since the drug is not systemically absorbed. Doses are 150–300 mg/day.

COMBINED THERAPY

Sulfonylurea and Biguanide

This is an effective combination for patients with NIDDM, because the two drugs have very different mechanisms of action. One increases insulin release and the other promotes glucose utilization.

Sulfonylurea and Insulin

Insulin is sometimes used at bedtime to augment the effect of sulfonylureas when maximal doses of the latter are inadequate to control hyperglycemia.

SUGGESTED READING

Bailey CJ, Turner RC. Metformin. N Engl J Med 1996; 334:574–579.

Baker DE, Campbell RK. The second generation sulfonylureas: glipizide and glyburide. Diabetes Educator 1985; 11:29–36.

Bergman RN, Steil GM, Bradley DC, Watanabe RM. Modeling of insulin action in vivo. Annu Rev Physiol 1992; 54:861–883.

Boyd AE III, Aguilar-Bryan L, Nelson DA. Molecular mechanisms of action of glyburide on the beta cell. Am J Med 1990; 89(Suppl 2A):3s–10s.

Bunn HF, Gabbay KH, Gallop PM. The glycosylation of hemoglobin: relevance to diabetes mellitus. Science 1978; 200:21–27.

Clauser E, Leconte I, Auzan C. Molecular basis of insulin resistance. Horm Res 1992; 38:5–12.

Diabetes Control and Complications Trial. The effects of intensive treatment of diabetes on the development and progression of long-term complications in insulin-dependent diabetes mellitus. N Engl J Med 1993; 329:977–986.

Muller-Wieland D, Streicher R, Siemeister G, Krone W. Molecular biology of insulin resistance. Exp Clin Endocrinol 1993; 101:17–29.

University Group Diabetes Program. A study of the effects of hypoglycemic agents on vascular complications with adult-onset diabetes. Diabetes 1970; 19(2):747–830.

University Group Diabetes Program. Supplementary report on nonfatal events in patients treated with tolbutamide. Diabetes 1976; 25(6):1129–1153.

White MF, Kahn CR. The insulin-signalling system. J Biol Chem 1994; 269:1–4.

CHAPTER 51

Adrenocortical Steroid Hormones

B.P. SCHIMMER AND S.R. GEORGE

CASE HISTORY

A 35-year-old woman with a 6-year history of Hashimoto's thyroiditis (autoimmune thyroiditis) with hypothyroidism, who had been well and stable on treatment with levothyroxine 0.125 mg daily, came to see her physician with complaints of fatigue, lethargy, and loss of appetite over the preceding 3–4 months. She had lost 15 lb in that time. She also complained of intermittent nausea and dizziness on standing up from a recumbent position. Physical examination revealed a lean and rather frail person with a BP of 115/70 in the supine position and 90/60 when she stood up. She said that she had not been in the sun for at least a year, yet her skin was tanned and there was increased pigmentation in the creases of her palms and on the gum margins. The thyroid gland was at the upper range of normal size, and she was clinically euthyroid on her usual dose of levothyroxine.

Laboratory investigations revealed a mild normochromic normocytic anemia, normal T_4 and T_3 levels, but elevated serum K^+. A random plasma sample showed a cortisol level of 100 nmol/L (normal range 170–660) and an ACTH level of 330 pmol/L (normal <22). A presumptive diagnosis of Addison's disease was made. The patient was quickly stabilized with intravenous hydrocortisone hemisuccinate and rehydration with intravenous saline. Subsequently, a 3-day infusion of ACTH was given to test adrenal cortical function, but no adrenal response to ACTH was found.

She was therefore started on long-term replacement therapy with prednisone 5 mg each morning and 2.5 mg each evening, together with fludrocortisone acetate 0.1 mg twice daily. She has felt well and completely symptom-free on this therapy.

THE HYPOTHALAMIC-PITUITARY-ADRENAL AXIS

Certain nuclei in the hypothalamus, the corticotropin-producing cells of the anterior lobe of the pituitary gland, and the adrenal cortex constitute a closely integrated functional system that is often referred to as the hypothalamic-pituitary-adrenal axis. It acts as a regulatory mechanism for maintaining normal levels of adrenal cortical hormone activity, but also permits sudden increases in output of these hormones in response to physiological stresses of various types. The normal physiological relationships of the hypothalamic-pituitary-adrenal axis are summarized in Figure 51-1.

The adrenal cortex is divided into histologically and functionally distinct zones. The outermost zone, the zona glomerulosa, is the site of mineralocorticoid (aldosterone) synthesis. The inner zones, the zonae fasciculata and reticularis, produce glucocorticoids (cortisol) and weak androgens (dehydroepiandrosterone).

Glucocorticoid production is stimulated by adrenocorticotropic hormone (ACTH) secreted from the anterior pituitary gland. Secretion of ACTH is stimulated by the hypothalamic peptide corticotropin-releasing factor (CRF) and inhibited by feedback effects of the glucocorticoids, which act at the level of

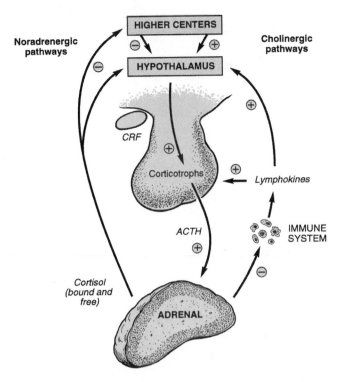

Figure 51-1. Functional relationships in the hypothalamic-pituitary-adrenal axis. (+) indicates stimulation of release; (−) indicates inhibition.

the hippocampus, hypothalamus, and pituitary. The immune system also plays important roles in the positive and negative regulation of glucocorticoid production.

Mineralocorticoid secretion is governed primarily by the renin-angiotensin system and potassium concentrations. ACTH has only a minor role.

CORTICOTROPIN-RELEASING FACTOR

Corticotropin-releasing factor (CRF) is a 41-amino-acid peptide present in high concentrations in neurosecretory cells in the paraventricular and periventricular nuclei of the hypothalamus. Cholinergic and serotonergic pathways stimulate CRF release, whereas specific noradrenergic pathways are inhibitory. The release of CRF varies in a circadian pattern under basal conditions, resulting in the occurrence of diurnal rhythms of ACTH and cortisol levels in blood (high in the morning, low in the evening). Neural stimuli brought about by stress, trauma, infection, hypoglycemia, and anxiety override the basal controls and increase the release of CRF.

Vasopressin also stimulates CRF release from the hypothalamus and potentiates the action of CRF on ACTH release from the pituitary.

ADRENOCORTICOTROPIC HORMONE

ACTH is a protein composed of 39 amino acids that is synthesized in the corticotrophs of the anterior pituitary. The first 24 amino acids of ACTH are responsible for the hormonal activity of the peptide. The basic amino acids at positions 15–18 provide a high-affinity recognition site for the ACTH receptor and amino acids 6–10 participate in receptor activation. Species variation occurs in the region from the 25th to the 33rd residue.

ACTH is derived from a larger precursor protein, proopiomelanocortin (POMC), by proteolytic cleavage. Cleavage of POMC also liberates other important regulatory peptides as shown in Figure 51-2. These include α-, β-, and γ-MSH (melanocyte-stimulating hormones), a lipid-mobilizing factor (β-lipotropin), and the opioid peptide β-endorphin (see Chapter 23).

Neural control of ACTH is demonstrated by the wide variety of stimuli that increase ACTH secretion and therefore plasma cortisol levels. Those factors that regulate the secretion of ACTH similarly regulate the production of the other peptides associated with POMC. These stimuli include both physical and psychological stresses, which can override the usual feedback control. Recent studies indicate that the immune system also is an important regulator of the hypothalamic-pituitary-adrenal axis during stress. Interleukins produced by macrophages, monocytes, and lymphocytes stimulate ACTH secretion; cortisol suppresses lymphokine production (see Fig. 51-1).

The most important physiological effect of ACTH is to stimulate the biosynthesis and output of adrenal steroid hormones. Its basic action is to stimulate the first step in the adrenal steroid hormone biosynthetic pathway, i.e., the oxidative cleavage of cholesterol to pregnenolone in adrenal mitochondria. The further metabolism of pregnenolone and the secretion of steroid products occur rapidly and are not under acute hormonal influence. The translocation of cholesterol from the cytoplasm to the inner mitochondrial membrane (where the oxidative cleavage occurs) is rate-limiting for steroidogenesis. ACTH exerts its effects through the ACTH receptor which activates adenylyl cyclase, thereby increasing cyclic AMP formation and stimulating cAMP-dependent protein kinases. The subsequent steps intervening between the cAMP-dependent protein kinase and

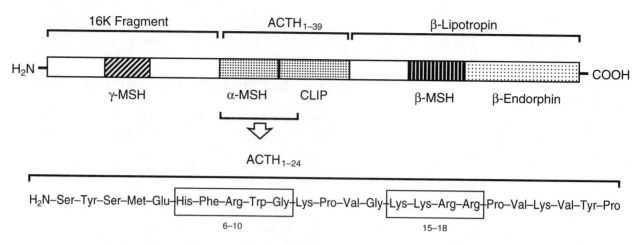

Figure 51-2. Biologically important peptides derived from proopiomelanocortin. MSH = melanocyte stimulating hormone; CLIP = corticotropin-like intermediate lobe peptide.

cholesterol metabolism are not fully elucidated but include the involvement of a "labile" protein known as StAR (*St*eroid *A*cute *R*egulator).

ACTH also maintains the levels of the adrenal steroidogenic enzymes through transcriptional control and structural integrity of the zonae fasciculata/reticularis of the adrenal cortex. When ACTH levels are suppressed for prolonged periods (e.g., following hypophysectomy or feedback inhibition by exogenous glucocorticoids), these inner zones of the cortex atrophy and secrete less steroid.

Regulation of aldosterone production involves a different mechanism. Angiotensin II and potassium are the major regulators of aldosterone production by the zona glomerulosa. Aldosterone secretion from the glomerulosa is stimulated by high levels of ACTH (equivalent to the levels encountered in response to stress), but secretion is not maintained. ACTH acts primarily to maintain the capability of the zona glomerulosa to respond to angiotensin II.

MINERALOCORTICOID ACTIONS

Mineralocorticoids are corticosteroids with relatively greater action on water and electrolyte ("minerals") metabolism than on carbohydrate and protein metabolism. They cause the renal tubule to retain Na^+, HCO_3^-, and water, and excrete more K^+; these actions ordinarily help to maintain normal concentrations of serum Na^+ and K^+. Mineralocorticoid deficiency results in the loss of Na^+ and water by the kidney, leading to dehydration and vascular collapse.

Mineralocorticoid excess results in elevated serum Na^+, decreased serum K^+, and retention of water, leading to elevated blood volume and blood pressure.

GLUCOCORTICOID ACTIONS

Glucocorticoids are corticosteroids with relatively greater effect on carbohydrate metabolism than on water and electrolyte metabolism. Despite the name "glucocorticoid", however, they have a very broad range of effects on many metabolic activities.

Metabolic Effects

Glucocorticoid receptors are found in virtually every cell in the body. As a consequence, glucocorticoids exert a wide range of physiological actions affecting virtually every organ system. Glucocorticoids are so named because of their actions on intermediary metabolism of glucose and other substances.

Under the influence of glucocorticoids, proteins in muscle, bone, and other tissues are broken down to amino acids (catabolic actions). The amino acids are carried to the liver, deaminated, and converted to glucose (gluconeogenesis). The net effect is to *increase* liver glycogen concentration, fasting blood sugar levels, and urinary nitrogen output. The proportions of carbohydrate and fat utilized by muscle are altered (increased mobilization and oxidation of depot fat; decreased utilization of glucose).

Effects on Blood and Lymphoid Systems

Erythrocyte and hemoglobin levels are increased. Circulating lymphocytes and eosinophils are decreased, due mainly to redistribution of these elements away from blood into other body compartments such as bone marrow, spleen, and lymph nodes and, to a lesser extent, to lymphocytolysis. The intensity of inflammatory responses is dampened by multiple actions. These include decreased production of vasoactive substances (e.g., prostaglandins and leukotrienes) and chemoattractants (e.g., cytokines), decreased secretion of lipolytic and proteolytic enzymes (e.g., phospholipases, collagenase, elastase), and inhibition of fibroblast growth.

Renal and Cardiovascular Effects

The ability of the kidney to excrete water is maintained by permissive effects on renal tubular free water clearance and maintenance of the glomerular filtration rate. Generally, a shift of water into cells is prevented, and extracellular volume is maintained. Cardiac contractility and vascular tone are enhanced, in part as a result of increasing sensitivity to vasoactive substances such as catecholamines and angiotensin II.

Other Physiological Effects

CNS effects include regulation of mood and an increased sense of well-being as a result of direct actions in brain and via supportive metabolic effects.

The ability of muscles to do prolonged work is maintained and includes effects on the circulatory system (independent of effects on carbohydrate and fat metabolism).

The production of gastric acid is increased. Glucocorticoids decrease total body calcium by inhibiting uptake from the intestine (competitive inhibition of the action of vitamin D_3) and stimulating renal calcium excretion.

MECHANISM OF ACTION

Many of the physiological effects of the adrenal steroid hormones have been known for years; classically they were deduced from the adrenal insufficiency states associated with Addison's disease and their reversal by steroid hormone replacement therapy. It now seems clear that most of the effects are produced by the activation of specific intracellular receptors.

In the absence of corticosteroids, the receptors are complexed with other regulatory proteins (e.g., heat-shock proteins) that restrict the receptors to the cytoplasm in an inactive state. In the presence of corticosteroids, the receptors dissociate from the inhibitory proteins, migrate to the nucleus, and act as transcription factors for specific genes to either stimulate or inhibit their expression.

Glucocorticoid and mineralocorticoid receptors are structurally related and have extensive similarities of amino acid composition. Whereas the glucocorticoid receptor is highly selective for glucocorticoids, the mineralocorticoid receptor seems to interact equally well with both glucocorticoids and mineralocorticoids. Since the circulating levels of glucocorticoids are much higher than the circulating levels of mineralocorticoids, mineralocorticoid-responsive tissues must contain additional mechanisms that provide for the specific effects of the mineralocorticoid hormones. One such mechanism seems to be the formation of an enzymatic barrier that selectively inactivates glucocorticoids before they reach the mineralocorticoid receptor. A key enzyme forming this barrier is an 11β-hydroxysteroid dehydrogenase. This enzyme inactivates cortisol by oxidizing the 11β-hydroxyl group (see Fig. 51-3) to an 11-keto group. The 11β-hydroxyl group on the mineralocorticoid may be protected from oxidation through the formation of a cyclic hemiacetal structure (see Fig.

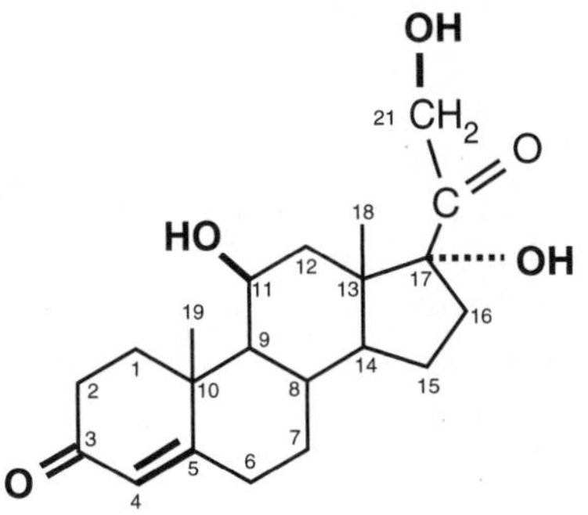

Figure 51-3. Structural formula of cortisol. The four rings that constitute the steroid nucleus are virtually coplanar. Chemical substitutions to the steroid molecule that reside above the plane of the rings are designated β and are conventionally represented by solid lines; substitutions made below the plane of the rings are designated α and are conventionally represented by broken lines, as shown above and in subsequent figures. Features that are important for glucocorticoid activity are shown in bold type.

51-6). Individuals with an inherited deficiency of the 11β-hydroxysteroid dehydrogenase exhibit symptoms of apparent mineralocorticoid excess due to the glucocorticoids acting inappropriately as mineralocorticoids. Interestingly, glycyrrhetinic acid, the active pharmacological ingredient of licorice, which inhibits the activity of the 11β-hydroxysteroid dehydrogenase, also produces similar symptoms.

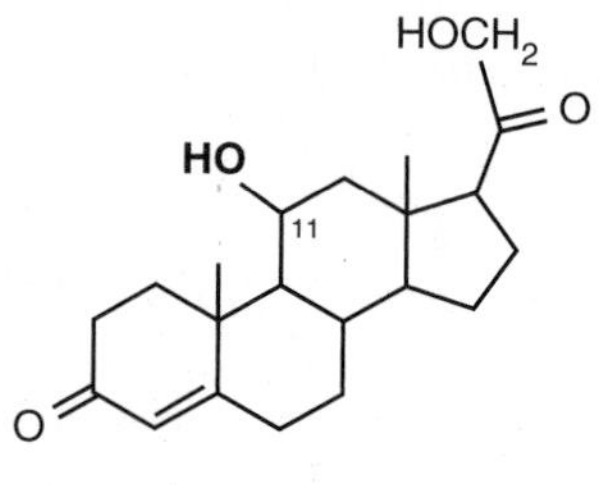

CHEMISTRY, KINETICS, AND SYNTHETIC ANALOGS

Structural Requirements

The structure of cortisol is shown in Fig 51-3. Important features that determine glucocorticoid activity are the keto group at C-3, the double bond at C-4 = C-5, and the three hydroxyl substitutions at C-21, C-17α, and C-11β. The 11β-OH is essential for glucocorticoid activity. In its absence the adrenal corticoids exhibit only mineralocorticoid activity (e.g., 11-deoxycorticosterone, Fig 51-4). A keto group at C-11 (e.g., cortisone or prednisone) also supports glucocorticoid activity because it is metabolized to an 11β-OH. The 17α-OH is not as critical, although it does have a quantitative influence; in its absence, corticosteroids exhibit weaker glucocorticoid activity and increased mineralocorticoid action, (e.g., corticosterone; Fig 51-5). The 21-OH is required for both glucocorticoid and mineralocorticoid activity. However, in some synthetic glucocorticoids, other functional groups such as Cl may be substituted for OH at C-21.

Aldosterone also has an OH at C-11, which might predict glucocorticoid activity; however, this group in aldosterone is adjacent to an aldehyde at C-18 which sequesters the 11β-OH in a cyclic hemiacetal structure (Fig 51-6). Under physiological conditions, the hemiacetal form predominates, so aldosterone exhibits negligible glucocorticoid activity.

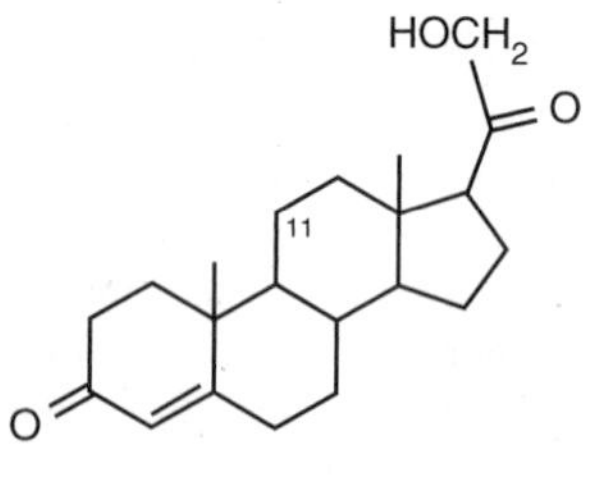

Figure 51-4. Structural formula of deoxycorticosterone (progesterone ring structure).

Figure 51-5. Structural formula of corticosterone.

Transport and Metabolism

The daily rates of secretion of adrenal steroids and their normal levels in plasma are given in Tables 51-1 and 51-2. The cortisol secretion rate is about 10 mg/day and cortisol concentrations in plasma are in the range of 10 μg/100 mL (280 nmol/L); 90–95% is bound to proteins. Most is bound with high affinity to a specific globulin called cortisol-binding globulin (CBG); the remainder is bound nonspecifically and with low affinity to albumin. Free cortisol, the active fraction, is in equilibrium with the bound forms. Aldosterone is present in plasma at much lower levels (see Table 51-2) and circulates primarily in the free form.

Cortisol has a plasma half-life of about 90 minutes, and to a large extent it is inactivated in the liver by reduction of the 3-keto, 4,5-double bond and subsequent conjugation with sulfate or glucuronate. Aldosterone is metabolized somewhat more rapidly, chiefly to glucuronides.

Synthetic Analogs

Selective modifications of the corticosteroid structure decrease the rate of metabolic inactivation of corticosteroids in the body. Analogs with a double bond between C-1 and C-2 or with a fluorine atom introduced into the molecule are biotransformed much more slowly, and the half-life is correspondingly increased. More importantly, these modifications enhance affinity for the glucocorticoid receptor, increase selective action as glucocorticoids, and reduce mineralocorticoid activity. The relative effectiveness of several synthetic analogs is given in Table 51-3, and their structures are shown in Figure 51-7. Specific modifications include:

1. Insertion of a double bond between C-1 and C-2. This changes cortisol (hydrocortisone) to prednisolone, and cortisone to prednisone, which are four times more potent than the respective precursors.

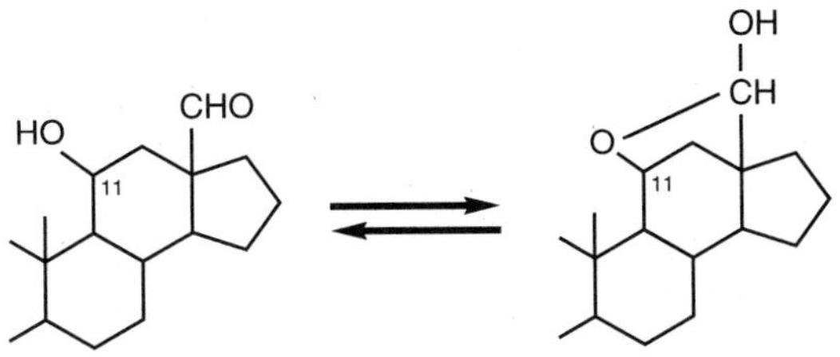

Figure 51-6. Aldehyde (left) and hemiacetal (right) forms of aldosterone.

Neither has appreciable mineralocorticoid activity. Prednisone has a half-life of 3–4 hours, is converted to prednisolone in the liver, and is ultimately degraded via the same pathways as cortisol.

2. Addition of a 6-methyl group to prednisolone gives methylprednisolone, which has slightly greater glucocorticoid potency than prednisolone.

3. Addition of fluorine to C-9 of cortisol gives fludrocortisone. This addition markedly increases both glucocorticoid and mineralocorticoid potencies, but the increase in mineralocorticoid activity is far greater, so fludrocortisone is used therapeutically as a mineralocorticoid. It is 70–80% bound to proteins in the plasma and has a half-life of 6–8 hours, although its biological effects are longer-lasting. It is biotransformed by reactions similar to those of other corticosteroids.

4. 9α-Fluoroprednisolone, analogous to the above, is not used medicinally but is a starting point for other modifications. Additions at C-16 of –OH (triamcinolone), α-CH$_3$ (dexamethasone), and β-CH$_3$ (betamethasone) all yield very potent glucocorticoids with minimal mineralocorticoid effect.

5. Addition of –F at C-6 of triamcinolone yields fluocinolone and increases glucocorticoid activity still further. Fluocinolone is used topically.

6. Beclomethasone (the 9α-chloro analog of betamethasone) is used topically and as an aerosol for the treatment of asthma. Its effectiveness by the latter route makes it possible to reduce (or even eliminate) systemic therapy in severe chronic asthma.

CLINICAL USES

Replacement and Substitution Therapy

Primary or secondary adrenocortical insufficiency, as well as congenital adrenal hyperplasia, are effectively treated with substitution of adrenocorticosteroids. Although secondary adrenal insufficiency due to pituitary or hypothalamic defects could be treated with ACTH, responses are not always predictable and are difficult to titrate. Therefore ACTH is not used, and the treatment of choice is the administration of adrenal steroids.

Congenital adrenal hyperplasia is caused in 95% of cases by 21-hydroxylase insufficiency. As a consequence of this defect, cortisol synthesis is impaired and precursor steroids, including the adrenal androgens, rise. Depending on the nature and severity of the enzyme defect, the clinical manifestations will vary and may include virilization, salt wasting, and hypertension. Treatment with synthetic glucocorticoids suppresses ACTH production by feedback regulation of the pituitary, shutting off abnormal steroid production and substituting a normal level of glucocorticoids.

Mineralocorticoid defects are the more acute threat to life because of salt-wasting, hypotension, and vascular collapse. Therefore replacement therapy

Table 51-2 Usual Steroid Plasma Levels

Steroid	Plasma Level/100 mL	
	Total	Free
Cortisol (hydrocortisone)	5–20 μg	1000 ng
Corticosterone	1 μg	100 ng
Aldosterone	3–15 ng	3 ng
Dehydroepiandrosterone	65 μg	65 μg

Table 51-1 Steroid Secretion by the Human Adrenal Gland

Steroid	Daily Secretion Rate*
Cortisol (hydrocortisone)	10–20 mg
Corticosterone	2–4 mg
Aldosterone	50–200 μg (100 μg)
Dehydroepiandrosterone	15–30 mg (20 mg)
Progesterone	0.4–0.8 mg
Androstenedione	1–10 mg
Testosterone	Trace
Estradiol	Trace

*Average values for the most significant steroids are given in parentheses. Values selected are somewhat arbitrary, and vary in different reports.

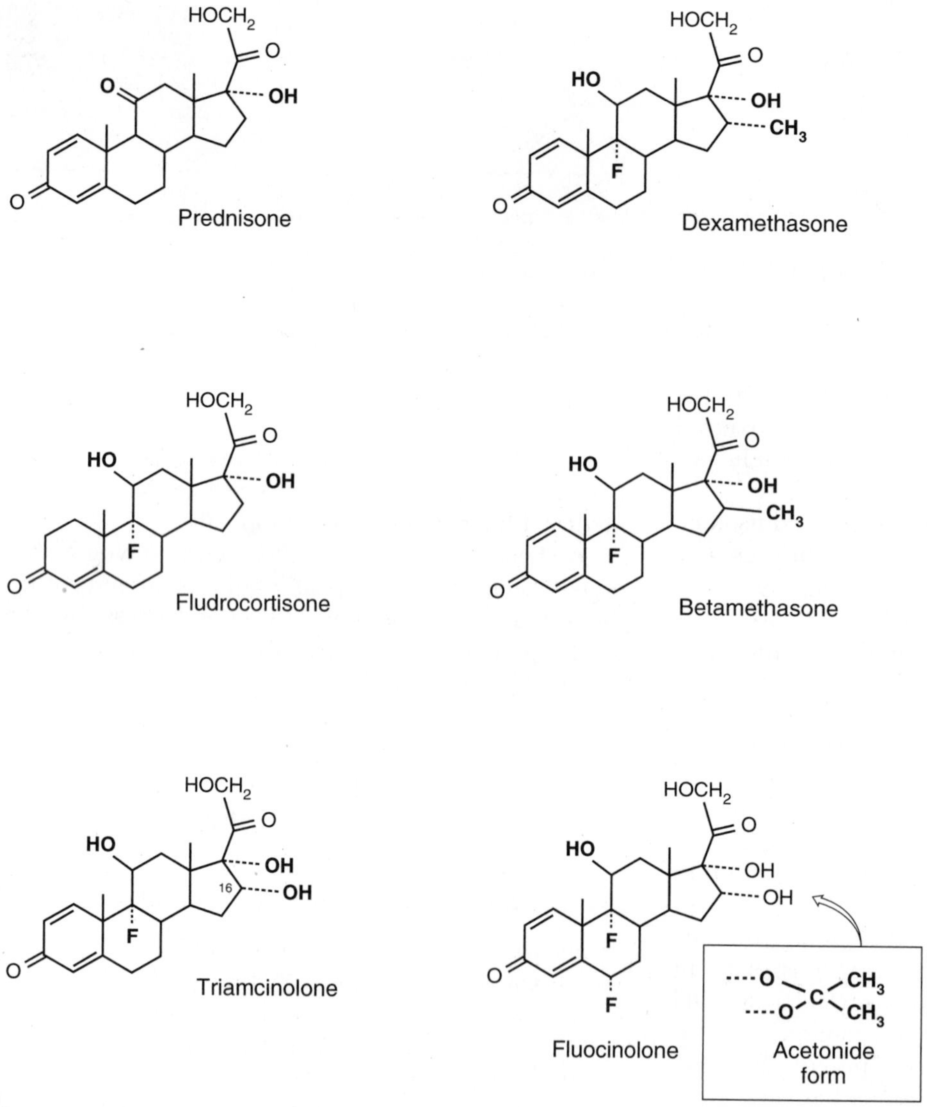

Figure 51-7 Structural formulae of synthetic corticoid analogs.

with adrenal steroid hormones must take into account both glucocorticoid and mineralocorticoid status. These must be treated separately since no single corticosteroid analog provides sufficient activity for both.

Antiallergic and Anti-inflammatory Therapy

It came as a surprise when Hench and Kendall reported, in 1949, that one of the adrenal steroids, now known as cortisone (compound "E"), relieved pain, inflammation, and disability in rheumatoid arthritis. This finding led to one of the most important clinical uses of the glucocorticoids, i.e., as anti-in-

flammatory, antiallergic, and immunosuppressive agents.

By far the most frequent use of corticosteroids today is in the treatment of inflammatory and allergic conditions in doses that range from the physiological to the pharmacological. Antibody titers seem not to be affected; instead, suppression of each stage of the inflammatory response seems to underlie both the anti-inflammatory and antiallergic actions of the glucocorticoids. Among the known components of the anti-inflammatory and antiallergic actions are decreases in capillary and leukocytic responses to local injury, inhibition of secretion of proteolytic and lipolytic enzymes, stabilization of lysosomes, inhibition

Table 51-3 Relative Potencies of Various Synthetic Analogs as Glucocorticoids (GC) and Mineralocorticoids (MC)

	Equivalent Dose	Relative GC Activity	Relative MC Activity
Cortisol (hydrocortisone) *Cortate, Cortef, others*	20 mg	1	1
Cortisone *Cortone*	25 mg	0.8	0.8
Prednisone *Deltasone, Winpred*	5 mg	4	0.3
Prednisolone *Delta-Cortef, others*	5 mg	4	0.8
Methylprednisolone *Medrol*	4 mg	5	0.5
Triamcinolone *Aristocort*	4 mg	5	0
Dexamethasone *Decadron, Dexasone*	0.75 mg	25	0
Betamethasone *Beben, Betnovate, Celestone, Diprosone, others*	0.5 mg	40	0
Fludrocortisone *Florinef*	Not applicable	10	250

of fibroblast growth, and inhibition of scar formation. For these reasons, corticosteroids are used in the treatment of many conditions, including:

- Allergic diseases such as serum sickness, urticaria, bee stings, and drug reactions
- Rheumatic diseases such as rheumatoid arthritis, rheumatic fever, and the collagen-vascular disorders, e.g., systemic lupus erythematosus, polyarteritis nodosa, and giant cell arteritis
- Respiratory diseases such as asthma and infant respiratory distress syndrome
- Dermatological disorders such as contact dermatitis, pemphigus, psoriasis, and eczema
- Ophthalmological diseases such as allergic conjunctivitis and acute uveitis
- Conditions as varied as nephrotic syndrome secondary to minimal change glomerulonephritis, inflammatory bowel diseases, cerebral edema, and organ transplantation

Malignancies

Lymphosarcoma, lymphatic leukemia, multiple myeloma, and Hodgkin's disease may respond to corticosteroid therapy, with remissions lasting from weeks to many months. These effects are in part due to lytic actions of glucocorticoids on lymphatic and related tissues.

Glucocorticoids also have been used to treat hypercalcemia associated with tumor **metastases to bone.** These metastases put out a prostaglandin-like substance that stimulates osteoclastic resorption of bone and releases calcium into the blood. Glucocorticoids lower blood calcium by decreasing calcium uptake from the intestine (anti–vitamin D_3 effect).

General Considerations About Therapeutic Uses

It must be stressed that the actions of corticosteroids against allergic and inflammatory disorders are not curative but merely palliative and aimed at relieving symptoms.

In the case of an acute allergic or inflammatory reaction, initial therapy may require administration of glucocorticoids at high doses (five to 10 times the replacement dose). If therapy is stopped abruptly, the disease may recur in full force; hence the glucocorticoid dose is tapered gradually. In the case of diseases requiring chronic glucocorticoid therapy, the objective is to provide the lowest dose of glucocorticoid necessary to keep the symptoms under control. Prolonged use of glucocorticoids (longer than a few weeks) can suppress ACTH production. Therefore withdrawal of exogenous glucocorticoid must be gradual to avoid precipitation of adrenal insufficiency. (Complete withdrawal may require 1 year or longer.)

Extreme caution must be exercised in the use of glucocorticoids because latent infections may be reactivated (see section on Toxic Effects). Systemic glucocorticoids should be used not for minor conditions, but for (1) relief of acute allergic reactions, (2) relief of severe or potentially fatal symptoms, and (3) prevention of tissue and organ damage.

In patients with adrenal insufficiency or glucocorticoid-induced ACTH suppression, stressful conditions such as trauma, surgery, or infections necessitate an increase in their glucocorticoid dosage to approximate the increased glucocorticoid output of the normal stressed adrenal.

Diagnostic Uses

CRF is used diagnostically to release ACTH and thereby test the adequacy of pituitary corticotroph function. Synthetic CRF is available only for investigational purposes at present.

ACTH is used to differentiate between primary and secondary/tertiary adrenal insufficiency. ACTH administration will stimulate cortisol production if the disorder is of hypothalamic or pituitary origin and the adrenal glands are intact. ACTH is not the preferred treatment for adrenal hormone replacement because of difficulty with dose titration, inconvenience of administration, and stimulation not only of glucocorticoid but also of mineralocorticoid and adrenal androgen secretion.

Dexamethasone is used to test the suppressibility of the hypothalamic-pituitary-adrenal axis in patients with elevated levels of cortisol. Because dexamethasone is a potent glucocorticoid, low doses (1 mg) will inhibit the release of ACTH from the anterior pituitary in normal individuals. In some depressed or psychotic patients, ACTH and cortisol production is not suppressed on the 1-mg dexamethasone dose and a higher dose may be required. In patients with elevated cortisol due to Cushing's syndrome, low doses of dexamethasone (1 or 2 mg) do not suppress ACTH or cortisol levels effectively. Higher doses of dexamethasone (8–16 mg) are used to distinguish pituitary-dependent Cushing's disease

(suppressible) from adrenal tumors and ectopic ACTH-producing tumors (not suppressible).

PREPARATIONS

ACTH is available as a purified powder, or aqueous solution for subcutaneous, intramuscular, or intravenous injection.

There are also depot forms, i.e., ACTH to which gelatin is added, to slow the absorption and so give prolonged action over 24–72 hours after a single injection. This form is used intramuscularly only.

Synthetic ACTH (cosyntropin, a peptide containing 24 amino acids, marketed as Cortrosyn or Synacthen) is available and is less likely to produce allergic reactions.

All glucocorticoids named in Table 51-3 are in clinical use. They are available in many forms, including oral tablets, ointments, lotions, ophthalmic drops, aqueous suspensions for intramuscular use, and solutions for intravenous and inhalational use. The choice of one glucocorticoid over another is not clear-cut. Perhaps the most important consideration is the degree of separation of desired glucocorticoid effects from undesired mineralocorticoid effects.

In replacement therapy the morning dose is generally twice as large as the evening dose, to mimic the diurnal rhythm. Equivalent daily replacement doses are hydrocortisone 30 mg, prednisone 7.5 mg, cortisone acetate 37.5 mg.

Fludrocortisone (Florinef) is a potent orally active mineralocorticoid. The daily replacement doses are in the range of 0.05–2.0 mg.

TOXIC EFFECTS

The adrenal cortical steroids show toxic effects that are exaggerations of their physiological actions and relate to the potency, dose, and duration of treatment. Side effects may include:

- Salt and water retention, leading to edema, hypertension, and congestive heart failure. Excessive K^+ loss in urine at the same time may cause hypokalemia, resulting in muscular weakness and cardiac arrhythmias. Excessive HCO_3^- retention may cause hypochloremic alkalosis. This is most likely to occur with mineralocorticoids, cortisone, or hydrocortisone (cortisol).
- Metabolic effects including negative nitrogen balance and impaired glucose utilization may cause

myopathy and induce a diabetic state in predisposed subjects. Redistribution of fat from the periphery to central locations results in truncal obesity, moon facies, buffalo hump, and supraclavicular fat pad enlargement.

- Osteoporosis and impaired wound healing, including impaired synthesis of collagen, result from a catabolic effect on protein metabolism. The inhibition of growth in children receiving corticosteroids over long periods probably falls into this same category.

These first three groups of toxic effects make up most of the clinical picture of "iatrogenic Cushing's syndrome" caused by exogenous adrenal steroids. The following are also important adverse effects:

- Masking of infections by inhibition of inflammatory and immune responses. Susceptibility to infection may be increased. In the presence of infection, the use of glucocorticoids may precipitate a fulminating course. Latent infections may become activated (e.g., tuberculosis). In herpetic keratitis, for instance, glucocorticoids may allow the infection to spread and cause blindness unless effective antiviral chemotherapy is used concurrently (see Chapter 58). Therefore, in the presence of infection, glucocorticoids should be used together with appropriate and effective antibiotic/antiviral therapy.
- Peptic ulceration, GI bleeding, and perforation. The association of glucocorticoids with these effects is debatable, but increased secretion of HCl and pepsin by the stomach, together with impaired healing, may contribute.
- Precipitation of mood disorders, ranging from euphoria to depression, and also psychoses in certain individuals.
- Adrenal insufficiency due to inhibition of ACTH secretion. As a consequence the adrenal cortex loses steroidogenic capacity and undergoes atrophy. Therefore therapy cannot be stopped abruptly, and dosage should be reduced gradually. There is some evidence that administration of glucocorticoids on alternate days in the treatment of chronic diseases may result in less suppression by negative feedback.
- Avascular necrosis of bone, most notably of the femoral head, has been reported. This is more likely to occur with long-term use or higher doses of glucocorticoids.
- Posterior subcapsular cataracts and increased intraocular pressure may occur.

INHIBITORS OF ADRENOCORTICOSTEROID BIOSYNTHESIS

This group of drugs is used clinically in the treatment of glucocorticoid overproduction caused by diseases such as Cushing's disease, ectopic ACTH production, and adrenal carcinoma. These agents interfere with the cytochrome P450 hydroxylases required for steroid hormone biosynthesis. They not only affect adrenal steroid hormone production but also may inhibit the biosynthesis of gonadal steroid hormones.

Aminoglutethimide

Aminoglutethimide (Cytadren) is a reversible inhibitor of the oxidative cleavage of cholesterol to pregnenolone, the first step in the biosynthesis of glucocorticoids, mineralocorticoids, and gonadal steroids. In addition, aminoglutethimide inhibits the adrenal 11β-hydroxylase as well as the aromatase that converts androgens to estrogens. Aminoglutethimide has been used to reduce glucocorticoid overproduction and also to reduce estrogen production, e.g., in the treatment of breast carcinoma.

Ketoconazole

The principal use of ketoconazole (Nizoral) is as an antifungal agent that inhibits the synthesis of sterols required for fungal cell-membrane integrity (see Chapter 54). At very high doses, ketoconazole inhibits the conversion of cholesterol to pregnenolone and therefore suppresses the synthesis of adrenal and gonadal hormones.

Metyrapone

Metyrapone (Metopirone) inhibits 11β-hydroxylase, the enzyme responsible for the final step in the synthesis of cortisol and aldosterone. Consequently the precursor of these hormones (11-desoxycortisol, compound S), which is biologically inactive and does not inhibit ACTH secretion, is excreted in the urine. Because *less* cortisol is formed, the blood level falls, and in the normal person, this causes an increased release of ACTH. The increased levels of ACTH stimulate further steroid synthesis so that with metyrapone an increased amount of 11-desoxycortisol is synthesized (and excreted).

Metyrapone has been used as a test of pituitary function, since a fall in the blood level of cortisol is expected to induce ACTH secretion. This drug is currently available both in Canada and the United States for therapeutic use only on a compassionate basis.

Mitotane

Mitotane (o,p′-DDD; Lysodren) is an organic insecticide derivative that is cytotoxic for the adrenal cortex. It is used for the treatment of inoperable metastatic adrenocortical carcinoma.

SUGGESTED READING

Boumpass DT, Chrousos GP, Wilder RL, Cupps TR, Balow JE. Glucocorticoid therapy for immune-mediated disease: basic and clinical correlates. Ann Int Med 1993; 119:1198–1208.

Corticosteroids and hypothalamic-pituitary-adrenocortical function (Editorial). Br Med J 1980; 280:813–814.

Cronstein BN, Weissman G. Targets for anti-inflammatory drugs. Annu Rev Pharmacol Toxicol 1995; 35:449–462.

Dooms-Goossens A. Sensitisation to corticosteroids. Consequences for anti-inflammatory therapy. Drug Saf 1995; 13:123–129.

Eastell R. Management of corticosteroid-induced osteoporosis. UK Consensus Group meeting. J Int Med 1995; 237:439–447.

Ellershaw JE, Kelly MJ. Corticosteroids and peptic ulceration. Palliative Med 1994; 8:313–319.

Funder JW, Pearce PT, Smith R, Smith AI. Mineralocorticoid action: target tissue specificity is enzyme, not receptor, mediated. Science 1988; 242:583–585.

Hanania NA, Chapman KR, Kesten S. Adverse effects of inhaled corticosteroids. Am J Med 1995; 98:196–208.

Imura H. Control of biosynthesis and secretion of ACTH: a review. Horm Metab Res (Suppl) 1987; 16:1–6.

Jusko WJ. Receptor-mediated pharmacodynamics of corticosteroids. Prog Clin Biol Res 1994; 387:261–270.

Munck A, Guyre PM, Holbrook NJ. Physiological functions of glucocorticoids in stress and their relation to pharmacological actions. Endocr Rev 1984; 5:25–44.

Reichlin S. Neuroendocrine-immune interactions. N Engl J Med 1993; 329:1246–1253.

Taylor AL, Fishman LM. Medical progress: corticotropin-releasing hormone. N Engl J Med 1988; 319:213–222.

Wiseman MH, Wineblatt ME. Treatment of the rheumatic diseases. Companion to the textbook of Rheumatology. Philadelphia: WB Saunders, 1995.

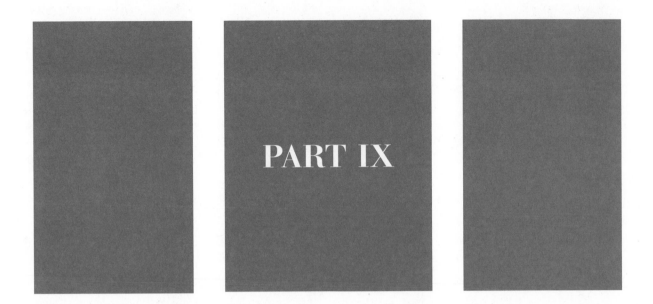

PART IX

ANTI-INFECTIVE CHEMOTHERAPY

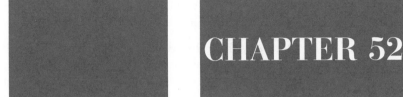

CHAPTER 52

Principles of Antimicrobial Therapy

J. UETRECHT AND S.L. WALMSLEY

One of the greatest achievements of medical science has been the control and management of infectious diseases. The role of microbes in causing severe infections was not appreciated until Louis Pasteur (1822–1895) formulated the germ theory in the years 1853 to 1867. Between 1880 and 1910, dozens of pathogenic bacteria were discovered. It was, however, not until the 20th century that therapy directed specifically against these microbes was developed.

THE ERA OF PRE-ANTIBIOTIC SYNTHETIC COMPOUNDS

Paul Ehrlich (1854–1915) was responsible for establishing a basic principle of chemotherapy. The importance of drug distribution as a determinant of drug action had been realized in the latter part of the 19th century. Struck by the observation that certain chemicals show a remarkable affinity for various materials (e.g., the affinity of dyes for the proteins of wool), Ehrlich reasoned that if chemicals with antimicrobial activity could be targeted to be taken up in certain human tissues, they would exert there a chemical action against infecting microbes. Unfortunately Ehrlich's search for such "magic bullets" was initially rather nonspecific. He utilized chemicals that fix to specific biological macromolecules, and therefore these chemicals interfered not only with the infecting microbes but also with host tissues. Ehrlich realized that a useful antimicrobial drug would have to be selectively toxic to the microbes, and he therefore began to investigate chemical modifications that would cause the toxic materials to be selectively taken up by the pathogens. This led to the introduction in 1909 of an arsenic derivative arsphenamine (**Salvarsan**) for the treatment of syphilis. Although this drug had considerable toxicity, it and its successor **Neosalvarsan** were the standard treatments for the disease throughout the world for over 40 years, until superseded by penicillin. Ehrlich not only developed an important chemotherapeutic agent but also began the systematic exploration of the molecular basis of antibacterial chemotherapy.

Within about three decades of Ehrlich's original work, Domagk and others found that a red tissue dye had antibacterial action. This substance, **Prontosil**, was the forerunner of the sulfonamides, which are still among the most important of the synthetic antibacterial compounds.

THE ERA OF ANTIBIOTICS

The term antibiosis was coined in 1889 by Vuillemin and originally meant the antagonism between living creatures. This terminology was refined by Waksman who, in 1942, defined antibiotics as substances produced by microorganisms that are, even in high dilution, antagonistic to the growth or life of other microorganisms. The first clinically useful antibiotic was penicillin, a product of a *penicillium* mold. This was discovered by Fleming in 1928 and it initiated the antibiotic era, which extends to the present. Innumerable microbial products have been investigated since the discovery of penicillin, and a great variety of them have proven to be useful antibiotic substances. Pharmaceutical companies have been extremely active in the search for these products and have made fundamental contributions to the development of antibiotic drugs.

Much work has been done in modifying the natural products (by removing some chemical groups and adding others) in attempts to enhance the beneficial effects while minimizing the toxic effects. The resultant modified end-product is termed a semisynthetic antibiotic. Most antibiotics currently used in clinical practice are semisynthetic. Some of the desirable pharmacological characteristics cultivated in these semisynthetic agents are stability, solubility, diffusibility, activity in the complex environment of the body, and slow excretion. In addition, these agents are designed to possess as large a therapeutic index as possible (i.e., the amount of drug causing toxicity exceeds by as much as possible the amount of drug necessary for a therapeutic response).

The relationships between patient, infecting pathogen, and antimicrobial agent are illustrated in Figure 52-1. The therapeutic usefulness of a given chemotherapeutic agent is usually determined by its selective toxicity toward the pathogen.

MECHANISMS OF ACTION

The mechanisms of action of antimicrobial agents are based upon an attack on targets present in bacteria and other organisms but either absent or less vulnerable in human cells (selective toxicity, a term formally introduced by Adrien Albert in 1951). These microbial targets include the cell wall, the cytoplasmic membrane, cellular proteins, cellular nucleic acids, and intermediary metabolism. It is traditional to classify antimicrobial agents by their mechanism of action, a system that is used throughout these chapters. In the following chapters the drugs to be described in relation to the sites of action mentioned above include:

- Cell wall—penicillins, cephalosporins, carbapenems, monobactams, vancomycin, bacitracin, cycloserine, isoniazid, ethambutol.
- Cell membrane—polymyxins, nystatin, amphotericin B, imidazoles, triazoles, allylamines.
- Cell proteins—aminoglycosides, spectinomycin, tetracyclines, chloramphenicol, clindamycin, macrolides.
- Cellular nucleic acids—griseofulvin, 5-fluorocytosine, rifampin, pyrazinamide, para-aminosalicylic acid, quinolones, sulfonamides, trimethoprim, pyrimethamine, sulfones.

The individual mechanisms of action are described in detail in the respective chapters.

BACTERIOSTATIC VERSUS BACTERICIDAL ANTIMICROBIALS

Bacteriostatic antimicrobial agents such as chloramphenicol, the tetracyclines, and erythromycin inhibit

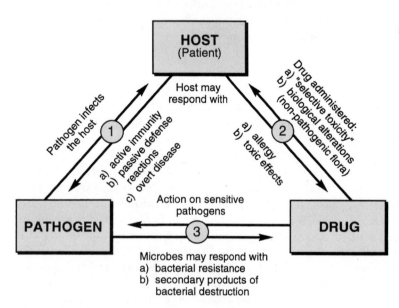

Figure 52-1. Host-pathogen-drug relationships in antimicrobial chemotherapy. (1) Pathogenesis of infectious disease process. (2) Pharmacokinetics and -dynamics (i.e., pharmacology) in the patient. (3) Microbiological processes of drug-pathogen interaction.

bacterial cell replication but do not kill the organisms; that is, they stop bacterial growth and allow the host's immune system to ultimately clear the infection. Therefore, if host immunity is suppressed, or if the infection is in an area of poor immunological surveillance (e.g., cerebrospinal fluid or vegetations of subacute bacterial endocarditis), bacteriostatic drugs may not suffice as sole therapeutic agents.

Bactericidal antimicrobial agents such as the penicillins and cephalosporins cause microbial death by lysis. They therefore rely less on host immunity for clearing of bacterial infections.

Some antimicrobial agents, such as the sulfonamides and tetracyclines, are indeterminate in the extent of their action. They are bacteriostatic or bactericidal depending on the concentration of drug, the nature of the environment, and the specific microorganisms against which they are employed.

ANTIBIOTIC RESISTANCE

Most, if not all, microorganisms are capable of developing resistance to the action of antimicrobial agents. For example, when penicillin was first introduced almost all *Staphylococcus aureus* organisms were sensitive; however, resistant strains that produce penicillinase (an enzyme that inactivates penicillin) increased over time to the point that *S. aureus* is now generally resistant to penicillin. Newer penicillins were synthesized that are resistant to penicillinase; however, some strains of *S. aureus* have developed resistance to these newer agents through a different mechanism. Some strains of *Neisseria gonorrhoeae* and *Streptococcus pneumoniae* which were previously very sensitive to penicillin have also developed resistance. Thus, there is a constant evolution of bacteria with changing patterns of antibacterial sensitivity. The parallel development of new antibiotics requires constant reevaluation to determine the optimal drug for the treatment of a given bacterial infection.

Despite the recognition that bacteria can develop resistance, the steady stream of new antibiotics made it appear as if we were gaining the upper hand against bacterial infections, and work on the development of new antibiotics almost came to a stop. But the ability of bacteria to develop resistance was underestimated, and we have actually lost ground over the last decade. Among contemporary pathogens, especially those that are hospital-acquired, resistance to a specific drug is often part of a larger package of resistance factors located on bacterial plasmids or transposons. This can result in simultaneous resistance to more than one antibiotic. Also, the use of one antibiotic may select for the emergence of bacterial strains that are resistant to another antibiotic. Changing the pattern of antibiotic use would not end the selective pressure unless all relevant drugs were withdrawn. There are now several bacteria, such as vancomycin-resistant enterococci, methicillin-resistant *S. aureus*, and multidrug-resistant mycobacteria, that are almost impossible to treat. This has led to renewed efforts by pharmaceutical companies to develop new agents. There are several promising new agents, such as oxazolidinones, which inhibit protein synthesis, and LY 333328, which inhibits cell wall synthesis; however, it will be some time before these agents are generally available and have been demonstrated to be safe and effective in clinical use.

Mutation

This is a rare, spontaneous, "normal" event that is not usually induced (although it may be selected for) by antimicrobials. However, the actions of antimicrobials may be affected by a variety of mutations, including:

- Alterations of cell walls, or cell membrane components, that prevent the entry of drugs into cells or actively exclude them

- Alteration of the target or binding site for an antimicrobial agent inside the cell

- Other indirect mechanisms (such as chromosomal mutations affecting the regulation of antibiotic resistance genes, including those encoding for β-lactamase) by which previously susceptible cells may become nonresponsive to the action of drugs

Mutationally altered cells are often metabolically inferior to wild-type cells; they tend to be suppressed and diluted out in competitive growth of a bacterial population. Thus, they rarely give rise to a resistant strain. However, mutants may become a threat when selective antibiotic pressure on the wild-type organisms is maintained by suboptimal antibiotic exposure, extensive topical use of the drug, or other factors that allow resistant mutants to gain the competitive advantage.

Inheritance

This is the most common way for microbes to acquire resistance to antimicrobials. It is selected for by exposure to antimicrobial agents, and it is transferable within a microbial population.

The genetic agents that confer antimicrobial resistance are the resistance plasmids (**R plasmids**), which may encode for resistance to as many as six or seven antimicrobial agents. Plasmids are extrachromosomal genetic elements in bacteria, ranging in size from a few daltons to more than a million daltons. Their main role is to allow bacterial evolution under greatly varying environmental conditions. They code for genetic properties that confer selective advantages for bacterial survival under particular conditions, such as the presence of antibiotics. Thus, plasmid-determined functions include bacterial replication, fertility, metabolism, virulence, and resistance to toxic metals, in addition to resistance to antimicrobials.

Resistance plasmids are believed to arise from collections of foreign genes that are not normally part of a bacterium's chromosomes. These genes may have come from a variety of unrelated bacterial or fungal sources (such as antibiotic-producing microorganisms), and the fact that they have been assembled into resistance plasmids that have survived implies that they must have experienced strong selective pressures (such as may have been created by exposure to metals, halogens, and similar antibacterial agents of the preantibiotic era). Since their description by Watanabe in 1963, R-plasmid activity and dissemination have been recognized as the major threat to continued antibiotic effectiveness.

Examples of the products of R plasmid–coded activity are:

- Products produced in cell walls or cell membranes that interfere with transport systems or block pores, so that antibiotics cannot enter the cell
- Enzymes produced by microbes that modify the site of drug action in such a way that even though the antibiotic enters the cell, the drug-binding site is lacking
- Enzymes produced by microbes that destroy the antibiotic (i.e., no active antibiotic remains)
- Substitute enzymes produced by microbes that are resistant to antibiotic action and replace antibiotic-sensitive essential enzymes. The substitute enzyme permits cell growth in the presence of antibiotic.
- Active transport systems that remove an antibiotic from the bacteria.

Dissemination of Resistance

Most R plasmids are transferable and conjugative; i.e., they possess the sex-factor activity necessary to initiate conjugation between resistance-positive (R$^+$) and resistance-negative (R$^-$) bacteria. This conjugation leads to a direct transfer of complete R plasmids from one bacterial cell to another.

R plasmids can also spread among microorganisms via a bacteriophage vector. This process, called transduction, is limited to R plasmids that can be accommodated in a bacteriophage chromosome, i.e., plasmids of smaller size.

R plasmids may be carried between microorganisms by direct DNA transfer, a process called transformation. This is the basis of recombinant DNA technology and "genetic engineering" with *Escherichia coli*. Although unproven in nature, it conceivably occurs through contact of plasmid DNA from lysed bacteria with recipient cells.

Resistance determinants can be transferred independently of the R plasmids by a process called transposition (i.e., hopping from one plasmid to another, or to a chromosome, or to a bacteriophage). This is thought to be the "natural" means of construction of R plasmids from various genetic sources; the new resistance is then permanently transferred with its new vector. This process allows previously nontransferable forms to be joined to transferable R plasmids, which may be the most common basis of resistance in hospital environments.

Some known mechanisms of antibiotic resistance, relative to the mode of action of respective drugs, are shown in Table 52-1.

LABORATORY MONITORING

As a general rule it is best to use a single agent that is specific for the organism involved, rather than "shotgun" therapy with a combination of agents, or a specific agent with a very broad spectrum of activity. Specific therapy usually decreases toxicity and reduces the emergence of resistant strains of bacteria. Nevertheless, there are exceptions to this rule. Although the use of multiple antibiotics leads to the overall risk that bacteria will develop resistance in the treatment of a specific infection, it may decrease the probability that some of the organisms in that infection will be resistant to the multiple antibiotics. This can be an important concept in the treatment of serious infections in which there is a high incidence of resistant organisms, such as tuberculosis. The tubercle bacillus is very polymorphic, and there is a high probability that a given infection will contain organisms that are resistant to any one antitubercular drug. These resistant organisms can proliferate and become the dominant organism of infection. The use

Table 52-1 Known Mechanisms of Antibiotic Resistance

Agent	Mode of Antibacterial Action	Microbial Resistance Mechanism
Sulfonamides	Block synthesis of tetrahydrofolic acid and cell-linked metabolic pathways	R plasmid-coded, sulfonamide-resistant dihydrofolic acid synthetase
Trimethoprim	Competitive inhibition of dihydrofolic acid reductase; blocks synthesis of tetrahydrofolic acid	R plasmid-coded, trimethoprim-resistant dihydrofolic acid reductase
Penicillins and cephalosporins	Interfere with cell-wall biosynthesis by interacting with penicillin-binding proteins	Hydrolysis of the antibiotic's β-lactam ring by β-lactamase enzyme
Tetracyclines	Inhibit protein synthesis by interaction with 30S and 50S ribosome subunits	Interference with transport of drug into cell; cell unable to maintain drug
Aminoglycosides	Bind to 30S (and 50S) ribosome subunit, cause translational misreading, inhibit peptide elongation	Enzymatic modification of drug by R plasmid-coded enzyme; drug has reduced affinity for ribosome; reduced transport into cell
Erythromycin and lincomycin	Bind to 50S ribosome subunit; inhibit protein synthesis at chain elongation step	Enzymatic modification of ribosomal DNA of sensitive cells renders ribosome drug-resistant
Chloramphenicol	Inhibits protein synthesis by interacting with 50S ribosome subunit	Drug inactivated by acetylation of –OH groups by chloramphenicol transacetylase; interference with drug transport into cell
Rifampin	Binds to bacterial RNA polymerase and blocks RNA synthesis (transcription)	Resistance arises by spontaneous mutation (no plasmid-coded mechanism known)

of two or more antitubercular drugs decreases the risk of such an occurrence.

Another exception is the use of synergistic combinations such as penicillin and an aminoglycoside in the treatment of enterococcal endocarditis, which is a life-threatening infection that is difficult to treat with a single agent. The combination of sulfamethoxazole and trimethoprim is also said to be synergistic, but the evidence is not compelling, and since sulfamethoxazole is associated with a relatively high incidence of serious adverse reactions, the routine use of this combination is now being questioned. A final example is an infection in an immunosuppressed patient, in which it is often difficult to culture the responsible organism; one is forced to employ broad-spectrum therapy.

The rational use of antimicrobial agents requires careful laboratory monitoring. One important aspect of this monitoring is determination of the degree of activity of the selected antimicrobial agent against the infecting bacterial strain. This is termed sensitivity testing. Though most bacteria have a predictable sensitivity pattern (to be discussed in subsequent chapters for specific antimicrobial agents), there is sufficient variation that the degree of activity of a specific antibiotic against an organism causing a serious infection should always be assessed. Knowledge of local patterns of resistance is very important because they can vary considerably between geographical regions and from one hospital to another.

The principle at work in sensitivity testing is that the activity of the antibiotic against one or several specific bacteria can be determined in vitro under conditions that simulate the environment of the bacteria in the host. The two methods of performing sensitivity testing are the disk-diffusion method and the dilution method.

Disk-Diffusion Method

This was the earliest available method and is currently the most extensively used world-wide. Commercially available paper disks impregnated with specific amounts of antimicrobial agents are placed onto agar plates containing a standardized number (inoculum) of the bacteria to be tested. The antibiotic diffuses out of the disk into the agar, establishing a linear concentration gradient from the center of the disk to some peripheral point in the agar. Bacteria growing on the agar are therefore presented with a continuous concentration gradient of antibiotic that inhibits or kills the bacteria for a variable distance around the disk. This resulting zone of antibacterial effect, the diameter of which is determined after an overnight incubation, is called the zone of inhibition.

The exact size of the zone (expressed in millimeters) reflects the degree of susceptibility or resistance, but the interpretation of the results is based upon prior studies using dilution tests (see below), which have correlated zone sizes with the minimum amount of antibiotic required to inhibit the growth of the bacterium. Results are expressed in only three susceptibility categories: sensitive, intermediate, and resistant. These categories are based upon observations of clinical outcomes in a large number of cases in which (1) the infection being treated was in the bloodstream or in tissues having approximately the same antibiotic concentrations as those in the bloodstream, (2) the patient was receiving a "standard dose" of the antibiotic in question, and (3) that dosage produced the usual concentration of that antibiotic in the bloodstream. Therefore the categories are meaningful only in cases in which the same criteria apply. If the infection is in the urinary tract, for example, it is necessary to use a different set of disks that release different concentrations of antibiotic reflecting those found in the urine in order to generate corresponding sensitivity categories.

Although it is recognized that the disk-diffusion method of sensitivity testing is rather imprecise, in general it provides sufficient information to permit choice of the appropriate antibiotic.

Dilution Method

This method of sensitivity testing can be carried out in agar or broth. A standardized inoculum of bacteria is exposed to varying concentrations (usually successive twofold dilutions) of an antimicrobial agent. The minimum concentration of antibiotic required to inhibit the growth of the bacteria can then be determined. This **minimum inhibitory concentration (MIC)** can then be compared with the measured or predicted concentration of antibiotic at the site of infection, be that the blood, urine, cerebrospinal fluid, or other site.

In addition to the MIC, the **minimum bactericidal concentration (MBC)** can also be determined, especially if the original dilutions were done in broth. To measure the MBC, aliquots of broth from tubes showing no visible growth after overnight incubation are subcultured onto antibiotic-free agar. The MBC is represented by the lowest concentration of antibiotic that completely prevents the growth of bacteria on the subculture. In general, the MIC and MBC of a bactericidal agent will be equal, whereas a bacteriostatic drug will have a large difference between the MIC and MBC. The clinical significance of the difference between MIC and MBC is unclear, and most reporting is in terms of the MIC. (MBCs are performed in hospital laboratories only under special circumstances.)

Many laboratory variables may affect the results of a sensitivity test, such as size of the inoculum of bacteria used, the temperature of incubation, and the pH and cation content of the culture medium. These and other important variables are usually controlled in consistent fashion by the laboratory providing this critically important information to clinicians; but clinicians must realize that, as with any test, extraneous factors (such as the immune status of the host, site of infection, extent of plasma protein binding, etc.) may influence the observed results. Newer methods have been developed in hospital microbiology laboratories for the automation and semi-automation of antibiotic sensitivity testing. In some cases the results are expressed as sensitive or resistant, while in other circumstances, actual MIC values are reported. These automated methods may decrease the time required for the performance of sensitivity testing and allow for large numbers of organisms to be tested.

Another important aspect of sensitivity testing relates to assessing the in vitro effects of a combination of antibiotics. Two antimicrobial drugs acting together in vitro may be indifferent, antagonistic, additive, or synergistic. When their combined action is no greater than that of the more active drug alone, they are said to be indifferent. When the activity of one is reduced by the presence of the other, they are said to be antagonistic. When their combined effect is significantly greater than that of either alone, they are said to be synergistic. Description of the precise mathematical definitions of these combined actions and of the methodologies available to test for these effects is beyond the scope of this chapter.

As early as 1952 it was suggested that the type of interaction of two drugs could be predicted on the basis of whether the component drugs were bactericidal or bacteriostatic. Two bacteriostatic drugs together would be additive, two bactericidal drugs together would be synergistic, and the combination of one of each type would be antagonistic. It has become clear, however, that those generalizations do not apply to all combinations of antimicrobial agents. When a clinician deals with serious infections, especially those caused by relatively resistant microbes, the type of interaction can only be ascertained by direct synergy testing.

Determinations of Antimicrobial Concentrations

Another aspect of laboratory monitoring in the rational use of antimicrobial agents involves the determination of the concentrations of these agents. Although the approximate concentrations that will be attained in various body sites after standard therapeutic doses can be predicted from the literature, there is considerable interpatient variability. The only way of knowing what concentrations are attained after a given dose is to measure the plasma or serum levels. This is not so important for relatively nontoxic agents, which, at usual doses, generally attain concentrations several-hundredfold greater than the MIC of the bacteria being treated (e.g., penicillin in *S. pneumoniae* bacteremia). Here the permissible margin for error is wide; however, for other agents that may attain concentrations only three- to fourfold higher than the MIC of the bacteria being treated (e.g., aminoglycosides in enteric aerobic infections), determining the attained concentrations is more important. In addition, the aminoglycosides have a low therapeutic index (i.e., narrow margin of safety), so the determination of concentrations is also important for limiting concentration-related toxic reactions.

Serum Bactericidal Titers

The ultimate control of infection not only depends on the action of the antimicrobial agents but also reflects the resultant effect of many host factors, primarily immunological. Therefore, a meaningful test of therapeutic activity should take into account all of these factors. Such a test is the measurement of serum bactericidal titer (SBT). Serum samples are obtained to coincide with anticipated maximum (peak) and minimum (trough) antimicrobial drug levels. The test is performed by adding a known inoculum of the bacterium isolated from the patient to serial twofold dilutions of the serum. The minimum concentration (highest dilution) of the serum capable of inhibiting and ultimately killing the inoculated bacteria is determined. This test, which has been most widely used for the determination of therapeutic effectiveness in bacterial endocarditis and other serious infections, permits monitoring of therapeutic response and allows modification of the choice and dosage of various antimicrobial agents. Although there is controversy about this point, for the highest probability of clinical improvement the peak SBT should represent a dilution of at least 1:8. Trough SBTs and other tests, such as the area under the concentration–time curve above the MIC, are being evaluated as methods of predicting outcome.

DETERMINANTS OF RESPONSE TO ANTIMICROBIAL THERAPY

Several factors must be considered when an antimicrobial agent is prescribed, if therapy is to be successful. Antimicrobial agents are of no value in treating viral infections or in treating noninfectious ailments. Presuming that an established bacterial infection is being treated, the antibiotic must be active against the infecting bacteria. This implies a knowledge of the most likely pathogens and a knowledge of the spectrum of activity of the selected antimicrobial agent. If a bacterium has actually been isolated, then in vitro sensitivity testing is appropriate. The appropriate dose, route of administration, and duration of therapy must be selected for the specific patient, keeping in mind the specific site of infection. This is intended to maximize the chance of attaining adequate concentrations of the antimicrobial agent at the site of the infection. For certain antibiotics, especially those with a low therapeutic index, the actual measurement of the drug concentrations attained is indicated. Finally, successful therapy requires an assurance of compliance with the prescribed agents and dosage regimens, a factor that must be remembered in outpatient therapeutics.

Successful outcome may also require the employment of ancillary modes of therapy to assist antibiotic action. This might include surgical drainage of abscesses, removal of obstructions to urinary flow, or removal of foreign bodies such as intravascular catheters.

PHARMACOKINETIC FACTORS ESSENTIAL FOR OPTIMAL ANTIMICROBIAL THERAPY

The rational use of antibiotics requires some knowledge of their pharmacokinetics. Although it may not be necessary to know all kinetic details for each agent, the following are essential:

1. The *anticipated concentration of the antibiotic that the selected dose will yield at the site of infection.* This implies knowledge of the serum concentration attained and the diffusion characteristics (distribution) of the antibiotic into the infected tissue. This concentration can then be related to the sensitivity of the infecting bacterium. It is generally desirable to attain antibiotic concentrations at the site of infection at least two- to fourfold in excess of the MIC for the infecting organism.

2. The *elimination half-life of the antibiotic.* This allows an approximation of the dosing interval that will result in maintenance of the desired concentration range.

3. The *sources of pharmacokinetic variation.* This implies some knowledge of biotransformation and elimination. If an agent is excreted primarily by the kidneys and the patient is in renal failure, it is necessary to recognize the need for dose adjustment. Similarly, if the agent is biotransformed in the liver and the patient is in hepatic failure, or if, on the contrary, the biotransforming enzymes have undergone induction by another agent, the dose may have to be adjusted. Some of the host variables influencing the kinetics of antibiotics, with examples from clinical practice, are outlined in Table 52-2.

In the chapters that follow, these variables will not be specifically considered for each antibiotic; rather, the discussion will refer to normal adult patients. It is important, however, to always consider sources of pharmacokinetic variation, for no patient will behave precisely in textbook fashion.

SUGGESTED READING

Albert A. Selective toxicity: the physicochemical basis of therapy. 7th ed. London: Chapman and Hall, 1985.

Burns JL. Mechanisms of bacterial resistance. Pediatr Clin North Am 1995; 42:497–508.

Goldfarb J. New antimicrobial agents. Pediatr Clin North Am 1995; 42:717–733.

Table 52-2 Some Variables Influencing the Kinetics of Antimicrobial Agents

Variable	Mechanism of Effect	Example
Age	Decreased renal function early in life and late in life	Need to decrease dose of aminoglycosides in neonates and elderly
Renal function	Important for drugs dependent on renal excretion	Need to decrease dose of aminoglycosides in patients with compromised renal function
Liver function	Important for drugs biotransformed in the liver	Need to decrease dose of chloramphenicol in patients with compromised liver function e.g., premature newborns
Fever/burns	Increased excretion or increased V_D* of some drugs	Need to increase dose of aminoglycosides
Acetylation status	Important for drugs being acetylated	Need to increase dose of isoniazid in rapid acetylators on regimen of once- or twice-weekly dosage
Diabetes mellitus	Reduced absorption of certain drugs after intramuscular dosing	Need to increase dose of intramuscular penicillins in diabetics
Cystic fibrosis	Increased clearance and V_D* of some drugs	Need to increase dose of aminoglycosides in these patients
	Altered absorption of some drugs	Chloramphenicol palmitate malabsorbed because of lipase deficiency
GI surgery	Altered absorption of drugs in patients with short bowel, e.g., ileal bypass	Ampicillin bioavailability is 15% of normal after small-bowel bypass

*V_D = volume of distribution

Jacoby GA, Arches GL. New mechanism of bacterial resistance to antimicrobial agents. N Engl J Med 1991; 324:601–612.

Koren G, Prober CG, Gold R, eds. Antimicrobial therapy in infants and children. New York: Marcel Dekker, 1988.

Rosenblatt JE. Laboratory tests used to guide antimicrobial therapy. Mayo Clin Proc 1991; 66:942–948.

Sanders CC. Beta-lactamases of Gram-negative bacteria: New challenges for new drugs. Clin Infect Dis 1992; 14:1089–1099.

Service RF. Antibiotics that resist resistance. Science 1995; 270:724–727.

Stager CE, Davis JR. Automated systems for identification of microorganisms. Clin Microbiol Rev 1992; 5:302–327.

Timmins KN, Gonzales-Carero MI, Sekizaki T, Rojo F. Biological activities specified by antibiotic resistance plasmids. J Antimicrob Chemother 1986; 18(Suppl C):1–10.

Wilkowske CJ, Hermans PE. General principles of antimicrobial therapy. Mayo Clin Proc 1991; 66:931–941.

CHAPTER 53

Antimicrobial Agents That Act on Bacterial Cell Wall Formation

J. UETRECHT AND S.L. WALMSLEY

CASE HISTORY

A 65-year-old man with a history of chronic obstructive lung disease and non–insulin-dependent diabetes mellitus saw his physician for the complaint of increasingly hesitant urination, nocturia, and postvoid dribbling. On physical examination, his prostate gland was palpably enlarged. He was referred to a urologist and was booked for an elective transurethral prostatectomy.

Three weeks before the date of surgery, he developed dysuria and hematuria. A urine culture confirmed *E. coli* cystitis, sensitive to ampicillin and the quinolones and resistant to trimethoprim–sulfamethoxazole. This infection was treated with oral ampicillin, 250 mg four times daily for 7 days, and full recovery occurred. Three weeks later, the patient was admitted for prostatectomy, which was performed under intravenous perioperative antibiotic prophylaxis with 1 g ampicillin and 80 mg gentamicin given once before and again 6 hours after surgery. He recovered well from this procedure.

One week after discharge, he was seen by his urologist in follow-up. A VDRL (Venereal Diseases Research Laboratory) test and confirmatory test, which had been performed as part of a routine hospital admission screen, had been reported positive. The patient could not recall a history of syphilis, but he had had intercourse with prostitutes as a young soldier in World War II. There was no clinical evidence of tertiary cardiovascular or central nervous system (CNS) syphilis. Although a false-positive VDRL test could not be ruled out, he was treated with benzathine penicillin G, 2.4 million units weekly for 3 weeks, because of the possibility of untreated late latent syphilis.

Three years later, he came to the local Emergency Room with a 3-hour history of crushing retrosternal chest pain. A diagnosis of unstable angina pectoris was made. Following an urgent coronary catheterization that confirmed triple-vessel disease, a coronary artery bypass procedure was performed, during which he received intravenous antibiotic prophylaxis with cefazolin, 1 g before and 1 g every 6 hours after surgery for 48 hours. Surgery was uneventful, but 48 hours later he developed fever and elevation of his white blood cell count as well as infiltration on his chest X-ray. A diagnosis of nosocomial pneumonia was made, and he was treated with intravenous cefotaxime, 1 g every 8 hours. This decision was based on the assumption that Gram-negative organisms are the usual pathogens in nosocomial pneumonia. A third-generation cephalosporin was chosen in this case, because the patient had experienced an elevation of serum creatinine to 300 μmol/L postoperatively and his physician wished to avoid the nephrotoxicity of the aminoglycosides. Forty-eight hours later, sputum cultures were reported positive for *Klebsiella pneumoniae* resistant to ampicillin and sensitive to cefotaxime, and a strain of *Pseudomonas aeruginosa* sensitive to tobramycin and imipenem and resistant to cefotaxime and ceftazidime. Cefotaxime was therefore changed to imipenem, 500 mg every 6 hours for 48 hours.

Despite continued antibacterial treatment, the incision at the site of the vein removal became red and warm. A swab was taken from the purulent exudate and methicillin-resistant *Staphylococcus aureus* was cultured. Intravenous vancomycin, 1 g every 12 hours, was added to the antibiotic regimen and the patient was placed in contact isolation. The wound healed, the pneumonia resolved, and the patient was discharged from hospital after 2 more weeks of therapy.

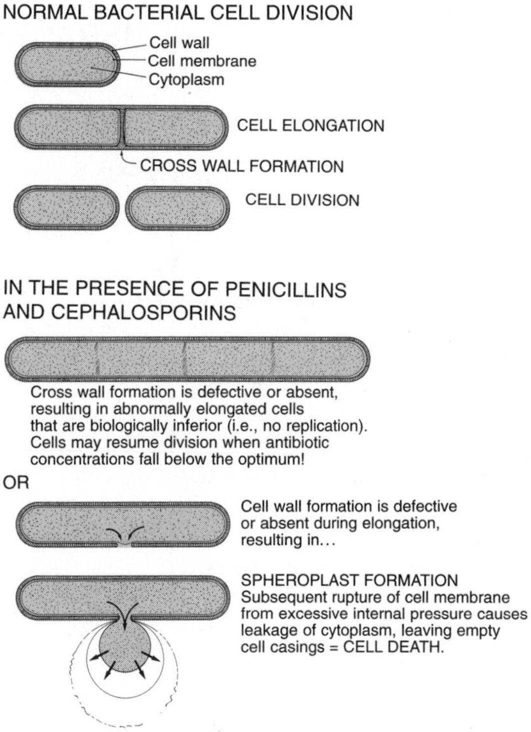

All living cells, including bacteria as well as mammalian tissue cells, have *cell membranes* (plasma membranes) that are necessary for the functional integrity of the cells. These membranes have complex lipid structures that can be disrupted by surfactants (detergents). Surfactants can therefore have antibacterial action but will also damage mammalian cells.

However, bacteria have much higher internal osmotic pressure than mammalian cells, and they require a *rigid outer cell wall*, external to the cell membrane, to prevent osmotic rupture in the isotonic medium of mammalian blood and tissues. These cell walls also maintain the shape of the bacteria. Mammalian cells do not have such cell walls.

During bacterial cell growth and division, the original cell wall must also enlarge and form a new septum (cross wall) between the two daughter cells so that, when they separate, each has a complete outer wall. This requires the synthesis of new wall material. Inhibitors of bacterial cell wall biosynthesis will therefore render growing bacteria vulnerable to osmotic rupture, without affecting mammalian cells (Fig. 53-1). Since cell wall biosynthesis is complex, inhibitors can act at different points in the sequence.

MECHANISMS OF ACTION

The process of cell wall formation begins in the bacterial cytoplasm with conversion of L-alanine into D-alanine. Two D-alanine molecules are then linked together. **Cycloserine** competitively inhibits the conversion of L-alanine into its D-form and the linking of the two D-molecules. Since the D-ala–D-ala unit is needed for the synthesis of all bacterial cell walls, cycloserine is effective against Gram-positive and Gram-negative bacteria alike, as well as the tubercle bacillus. However, other antibiotics are superior in treating infections caused by most organisms; the use of cycloserine is limited to the treatment of infections

NORMAL BACTERIAL CELL DIVISION

Cell wall
Cell membrane
Cytoplasm

CELL ELONGATION

CROSS WALL FORMATION

CELL DIVISION

IN THE PRESENCE OF PENICILLINS AND CEPHALOSPORINS

Cross wall formation is defective or absent, resulting in abnormally elongated cells that are biologically inferior (i.e., no replication). Cells may resume division when antibiotic concentrations fall below the optimum!

OR

Cell wall formation is defective or absent during elongation, resulting in…

SPHEROPLAST FORMATION
Subsequent rupture of cell membrane from excessive internal pressure causes leakage of cytoplasm, leaving empty cell casings = CELL DEATH.

Figure 53-1. Principal structural effects of penicillins and cephalosporins on bacterial (*E. coli*) replication.

caused by the tubercle bacillus resistant to first-line agents, and even that use is uncommon.

The next step in cell wall synthesis is the linkage of the D-ala dipeptide to three other amino acids and an amino sugar, *N*-acetylmuramic acid, to form a sugar-pentapeptide. This in turn is coupled to a molecule of another amino sugar, *N*-acetylglucosamine (Fig. 53-2). The whole sugar-peptide structure, linked to a lipid carrier molecule, isoprenyl phosphate, is then transported from the cytoplasm to the exterior of the cell membrane, where the sugar-peptide unit is added on to the lengthening polymer chains (peptidoglycan strands) from which the new cell wall is being built. **Bacitracin** interferes with this process by binding to the isoprenyl phosphate to form an unusable complex inside the bacterial cell. **Vancomycin** prevents the transfer of the sugar-pentapeptide from the carrier molecule to the growing polymer chain on the outside of the cell membrane.

The terminal event in cell wall synthesis is a cross-linking of the peptidoglycan strands by connecting a D-ala of a sugar-peptide in one strand to a diaminopimelic acid unit in a sugar-peptide of an adjacent strand (Fig. 53-3). This is a transpeptidation reaction, which is catalyzed by various enzymes

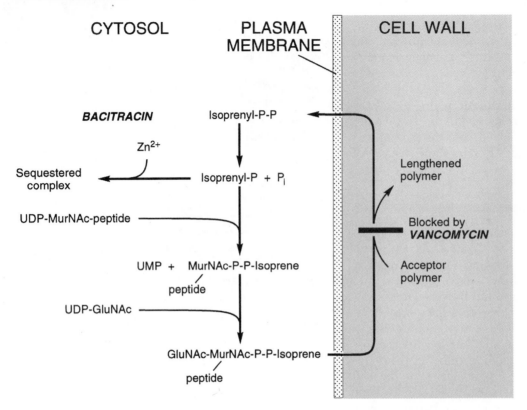

Figure 53-2. Sites of action of bacitracin and vancomycin as inhibitors of cell wall synthesis. UDP = uridine diphosphate; UMP = uridine monophosphate; MurNAc = N-acetylmuramic acid; GluNAc = N-acetylglucosamine.

that differ in different bacterial species. **Penicillins** and **cephalosporins** bind to the active site of the enzyme (in susceptible species) and prevent the formation of the cross-links.

The specificity of penicillins and cephalosporins for the transpeptidase involved in cell wall synthesis is due to the similarity of the antibiotic's three-dimensional structure to that of D-alanylalanine, which is the site on the peptidoglycan strand to which these enzymes bind. These transpeptidases are actually part of a group of proteins in bacterial cell walls called **penicillin-binding proteins (PBPs)**, which have a high affinity for penicillins and cephalosporins. The degree to which the binding of β-lactams to other penicillin-binding proteins contributes to their antibacterial activity is unknown but is probably very important for the action against Gram-negative organisms. One such penicillin-binding protein cross-links lipoprotein to peptidoglycan in the wall of Gram-negative bacilli. In addition, penicillins and cephalosporins have been reported to activate an endogenous autolytic system in some bacteria which initiates cell lysis and death.

PENICILLINS

The penicillins are the most diverse and probably the most important group of antibiotics used for the treatment of infection. In 1928 Alexander Fleming fortuitously isolated penicillin from a sample of the mold *Penicillium notatum* which was growing in his laboratory. However, it was not introduced into clinical medicine until 1941, when Florey, Chain, and associates devised suitable methods for large-scale culture of the mold and extraction of the penicillin. Since its original production, extensive chemical manipulation of the natural product has been carried out, resulting in a large number of natural and semisynthetic congeners with diverse pharmacokinetic characteristics and altered spectra of activity.

Chemistry

The basic structure of penicillin consists of a nucleus (6-aminopenicillanic acid, 6-APA) and side-chains

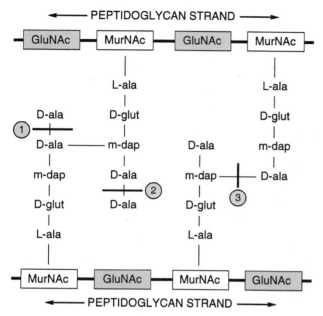

Figure 53-3. Sites of action of cross-linking and unlinking enzymes in *E. coli* cell wall synthesis. (1) Transpeptidase cleaves terminal D-ala and connects remaining D-ala to *m*-dap in peptide side-chain on adjacent peptidoglycan strand. (2) Carboxypeptidase cleaves terminal D-ala from side-chain of second strand, preventing further cross-linkage at that site. (3) Endopeptidase splits cross-link, providing site for transverse wall formation before dividing bacteria separate. Penicillins and cephalosporins prevent transpeptidation (see text). D-ala = D-alanine; L-ala = L-alanine; D-glut = D-glutamate; *m*-dap = *m*-diaminopimelate; GluNAc = *N*-acetylglucosamine; MurNAc = *N*-acetylmuramic acid.

(acyl groups in amide linkage with 6-APA). The 6-APA nucleus has a thiazolidine ring connected to a β-lactam ring (Fig. 53-4). In the natural penicillin, penicillin G, the R group is benzyl; in the semisynthetic penicillins other R groups are substituted for the benzyl group (Fig. 53-5).

These agents contain a **β-lactam ring** that is chemically unstable (and therefore reactive) because of ring strain (i.e., the normal bond angle for carbon atoms is 109–120° but is forced by the ring to be 90°). The chemical reactivity of the β-lactam ring, which confers antibacterial activity by ring opening and covalent bonding to the target enzyme, is also responsible for *instability in an acid medium* (Fig. 53-6). The R group has a major effect on acid stability; an electron-withdrawing atom close to the β-lactam, such as the oxygen in penicillin V or the nitrogen in ampicillin, confers relative acid stability.

Cloxacillin and dicloxacillin are also relatively resistant to acid hydrolysis because of the electron-withdrawing effect of the heterocyclic ring.

The R group also controls susceptibility of the molecule to the **penicillinases,** produced by most *S. aureus* and some other bacteria, which hydrolyze the β-lactam ring and inactivate penicillins, causing the microorganisms to be resistant to the action of these antibiotics. Large, bulky groups, such as those found in methicillin, prevent binding and, therefore, inactivation by these enzymes. Other penicillins that are resistant to penicillinase are oxacillin, cloxacillin, dicloxacillin, and nafcillin. Unfortunately, these bulky groups decrease binding to the transpeptidases and other penicillin-binding proteins that is responsible for the activity of penicillins; and, in general, penicillinase-resistant penicillins are less active than penicillin G against organisms that do not produce penicillinase (see Fig. 53-5 and Table 53-1).

While most of the clinically significant microbial resistance to β-lactam antibiotics is due to bacterial β-lactamase activity, a new type of nonenzymatic penicillin resistance has been described in which one or more of the penicillin-binding proteins in the bacterial cell membrane are changed by mutation, rendering them less sensitive targets for penicillins. These resistant bacteria require several-thousandfold increases in minimal inhibitory concentration (MIC) values for the β-lactam antibiotics, and the newly resistant bacteria emerge as a significant fraction of the respective pathogenic flora. For example, some strains of staphylococcus (called methicillin-resistant) possess an altered penicillin-binding protein. This protein has decreased affinity for methicillin and confers resistance to that antibiotic.

Penicillin can also be reacted, via its free carboxyl group, with amines such as **procaine** and **benzathine** to form salts that have a low solubility. These salts are given by intramuscular injection and slowly

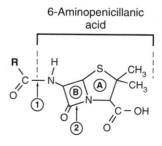

Figure 53-4. Structure of penicillin nucleus: A = thiazolidine ring; B = β-lactam ring. Sites of penicillinase action: (1) = amidase; (2) = β-lactamase.

R SIDE CHAIN	CHEMICAL NAME	NONPROPRIETARY NAME	PROPRIETARY NAMES
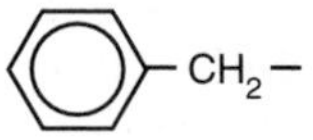	Benzyl penicillin	Penicillin G	Megacillin, others
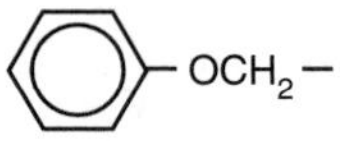	Phenoxymethyl penicillin	Penicillin V	Pen-Vee, others
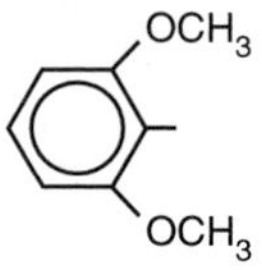	Dimethoxyphenyl penicillin	Methicillin	Staphcillin
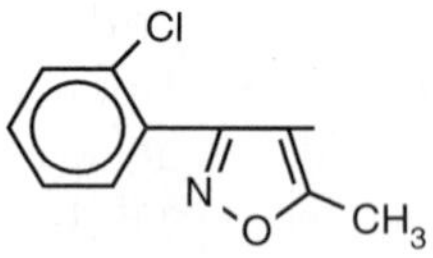	5-Methyl-3-o-chloro-phenyl-4-isoxazolyl penicillin	Cloxacillin	Orbenin
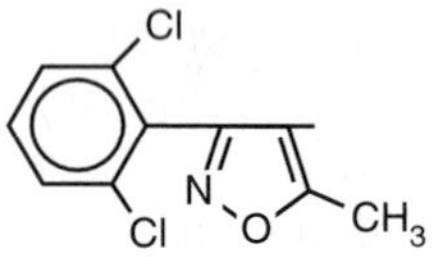	5-Methyl-3-(2,6-dichloro-phenyl)-4-isoxazolyl penicillin	Dicloxacillin	Dynapen
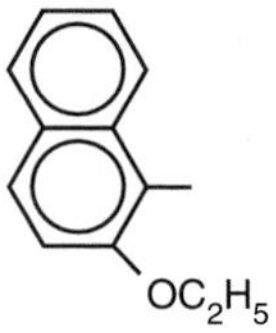	2-Ethoxy-1-naphthyl penicillin	Nafcillin	Unipen
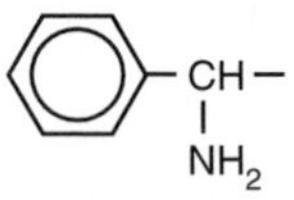	α-Aminobenzyl penicillin	Ampicillin	Ampicin, Penbritin, others
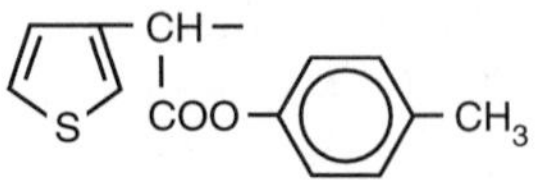	α-p-Cresylcarbonyl-3-thienylmethyl penicillin	Ticarcillin	Ticar
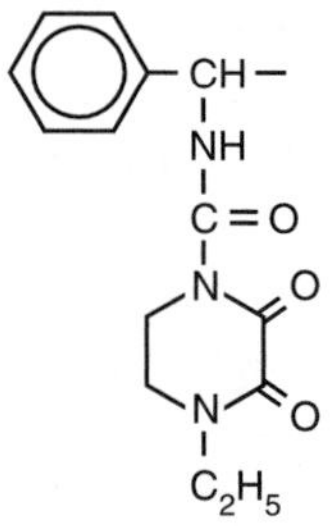	α-[(4-Ethyl-2,3-dioxo-1-piperazinyl)-carbonyl-amino] benzyl penicillin	Piperacillin	Pipracil

Figure 53-5. Chemical structures of R side-chains and names of various penicillins.

release penicillin to provide a sustained level of antibiotic. A single injection of benzathine penicillin provides therapeutic levels for almost 1 month and measurable levels for about 3 months.

Bacterial Susceptibility

The penicillins can be divided into three groups on the basis of their antibacterial spectra. These groups

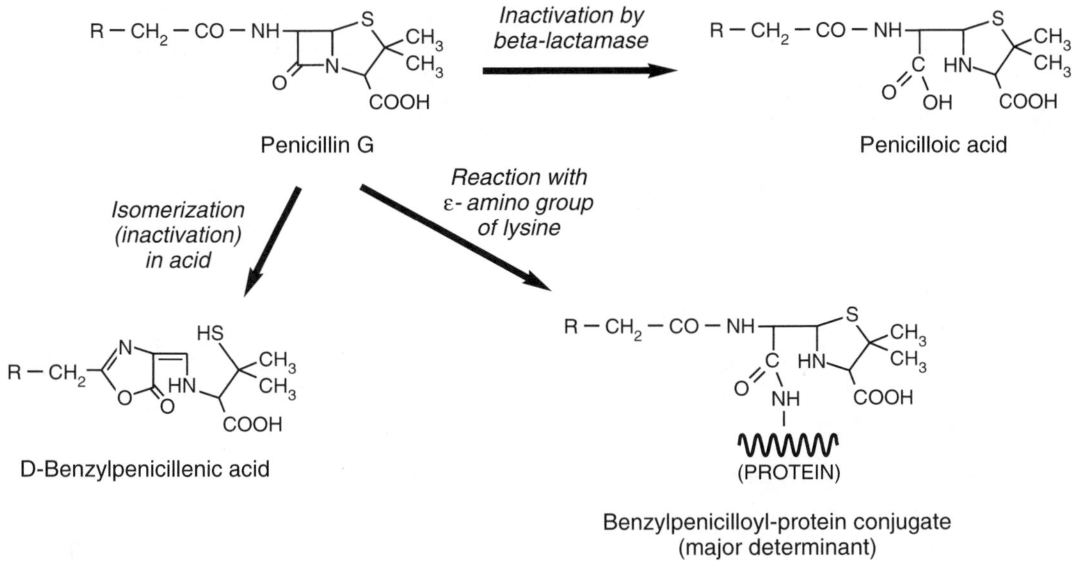

Figure 53-6. Inactivation of penicillin by β-lactamase, by acid, and reaction with protein to form the major determinant causing penicillin hypersensitivity reactions.

are: narrow spectrum, β-lactamase sensitive; broad spectrum, β-lactamase sensitive; and β-lactamase resistant.

The antibacterial activity of penicillins representative of each of these groups is outlined in Table 53-1. The attainable serum concentrations of these antibiotics that can be related to the MICs are discussed below.

Narrow-spectrum, β-lactamase-sensitive penicillins

Penicillin G is the prototype of this group. The oral formulation representing this group is phenoxymethyl penicillin (**penicillin V**). As outlined in Table 53-1, penicillin G is very active against many Gram-positive bacteria, both aerobes and anaerobes, with the exception of penicillinase-producing *S. aureus*. Unfortunately the majority of *S. aureus* strains encountered in clinical practice are now penicillinase producers. Penicillin G is also very active against the Gram-negative anaerobes with the exception of β-lactamase-producing strains of *Bacteroides fragilis*. However, this antibiotic is not active against enteric Gram-negative organisms such as *Escherichia coli*, and hence the designation of narrow-spectrum. Although penicillin is very active against *Neisseria* species, many strains of *N. gonorrhoeae* are now resistant and this drug is no longer considered the drug of choice for gonorrhea in some metropolitan areas.

The basis for the lack of activity of penicillin G against Gram-negative enteric organisms lies in the nature of the cell wall. Although Gram-negative organisms also have a cell wall composed of peptidoglycan and its synthetic enzymes, these organisms are surrounded by an additional membrane of lipopolysaccharide and a capsule, which are relatively impermeable to penicillin. Furthermore, Gram-negative organisms have β-lactamases in the periplasmic space that contribute to the failure of penicillin to reach its site of action.

Broad-spectrum, β-lactamase-sensitive penicillins

Modification of the R group (e.g., adding an amino group to make **ampicillin** and **amoxicillin**) leads to activity against some enteric Gram-negative organisms. As described earlier, this also increases stability to acid and does not significantly decrease activity against Gram-positive organisms, nor does it prevent hydrolysis by penicillinases. These agents also have increased activity against *Enterococcus* species and *Haemophilus* species, although the emergence of penicillinase-producing *Haemophilus* species has made these agents inappropriate as the sole therapy for severe infections due to *Haemophilus*.

Adding a carboxyl group (i.e., **carbenicillin** and **ticarcillin**) markedly increases activity against *Pseudomonas* but decreases activity against Gram-

Table 53-1 Median MICs (in μg/mL) of Some Penicillins

Bacteria	Penicillin G	Cloxacillin	Ampicillin	Ticarcillin	Piperacillin
Gram-positive					
Staphylococcus aureus, penicillinase (−)	0.03	0.25	0.05	1.25	0.8
Staphylococcus aureus, penicillinase (+)	25 – >800	0.5	125.0	25.0	25.0
Streptococcus group A	0.007	0.1	0.05	0.5	0.05
Streptococcus viridans	0.01	—	0.012	0.2	1.2
Enterococcus faecalis	2.0	25.0	0.38	34.0	4.0
Streptococcus pneumoniae	0.015	0.5	0.05	0.25	0.05
Listeria	0.1	—	0.1	2.5	1.25
Clostridium	0.06	—	0.05	0.5	—
Gram-negative					
Neisseria meningitidis	0.05	0.5	0.02	0.1	0.05
Neisseria gonorrhoeae	0.06	1.0	0.125	0.1	0.05
Haemophilus influenzae	0.16	—	0.05	0.5	0.25
Salmonella sp.	5.0	>250	2.0	4.0	4.0
Shigella	16.0	>250	6.0	—	—
Klebsiella	50.0	>250	50.0	50.0	4.0
Escherichia coli	64.0	>250	5.0	5.0	2.0
Pseudomonas aeruginosa	>400	>250	>400	25.0	10.0
Proteus mirabilis	32.0	>250	1.25	1.25	1.25
Bacteroides fragilis	32.0	—	25.0	37.5	—
Other *Bacteroides*	0.12	—	6.2	2.0	—

positive organisms. The newer ureidopenicillins (az-locillin, mezlocillin, and piperacillin) have even greater activity against *Pseudomonas* and other Gram-negative organisms and also have significant activity against *Klebsiella*.

These β-lactamase-sensitive antibiotics can be made resistant to β-lactamase by combination with β-lactamase inhibitors such as clavulanic acid, as discussed later.

β-Lactamase-resistant penicillins

Cloxacillin is the representative of this group (Table 53-1). Other members include methicillin, oxacillin, nafcillin, and dicloxacillin. The principal bacteriological advantage of this group of antibiotics is their high degree of activity against the penicillinase-producing staphylococci. They are, however, much less active than penicillin G against the other Gram-positive bacteria and are totally inactive against Gram-negative enteric organisms. Some strains of *S. aureus* have developed resistance to these agents through a different mechanism. As mentioned pre-

viously, these bacteria have penicillin-binding proteins that have a much lower affinity for penicillins.

Pharmacokinetics

The degree of absorption of the various penicillin preparations from the gastrointestinal tract is variable and most dependent on their relative susceptibility to acid hydrolysis in the stomach (see Fig. 53-6). Penicillin V, ampicillin, cloxacillin, dicloxacillin, and oxacillin, which are quite acid-stable, are well absorbed. Penicillin G, methicillin, nafcillin, carbenicillin, ticarcillin, and piperacillin are more acid-labile and hence are poorly absorbed. These latter penicillins are, therefore, preferably administered parenterally. Of this group, only penicillin G is available in an oral formulation. Serum concentrations of the penicillins after representative doses are outlined in Table 53-2.

The volumes of distribution for the penicillins range from 0.1 to 0.3 L/kg. Their degree of protein binding is quite variable, as noted in Table 53-2. The penicillins spread widely throughout the body and enter all body fluids. Concentrations in brain and

Table 53-2 Serum Concentrations and Protein Binding of Different Penicillins

Agent	Dosage (mg and Route)		Serum Concentration (μg/mL)	Protein Bound (% at Therapeutic Concentrations)
Ampicillin	1000	IV	40	20
	500	PO	4–6	—
Cloxacillin	500	PO	8	95
Dicloxacillin	250	PO	8	95
Methicillin	1000	IV	20–40	35–40
Nafcillin	15/kg	IV	20–40	90–95
Oxacillin	1000	IV	40	90
	500	PO	4	—
Penicillin G	~670	IV	10	65
	500	PO	2	—
Penicillin G procaine	800	IM	3	—
Penicillin G benzathine	800	IM	0.1	—
Penicillin V	250	PO	2–3	80
Carbenicillin	5000	IV	200–300	50
Ticarcillin	3000	IV	150–200	50

cerebrospinal fluid (CSF), however, vary depending upon the specific penicillin under consideration and on the degree of meningeal inflammation, which increases permeability of the blood–brain barrier, present at time of dosing. The approximate concentrations attained in the CSF during treatment for meningitis are 25–30% of serum concentrations with penicillin G, ampicillin, carbenicillin, and ticarcillin. Methicillin, oxacillin, cloxacillin, and nafcillin, however, penetrate the CSF poorly.

The penicillins are not significantly biotransformed but are administered, distributed, and excreted in a biologically active form. Free penicillins are rapidly eliminated in the urine, with serum half-lives of less than 1 hour. They are mainly excreted by glomerular filtration and renal tubular secretion. In addition, there is significant excretion of nafcillin, oxacillin, and the ureidopenicillins in the bile. Renal tubular secretion takes place through the organic anion transport system and can be blocked, and the action of the penicillins prolonged, by probenecid. Probenecid may also increase serum concentrations by blocking distribution into tissues. In theory at least, therapeutic efficacy might be compromised by this action.

Adverse Reactions

Penicillins are of very low toxicity. Their specificity of action as antibiotics is such that they have little effect on mammalian cells. However, all penicillins have the potential to cause hypersensitivity reactions, neurotoxicity, nephrotoxicity, and hematological toxicity.

Hypersensitivity reactions are the major type of toxicity seen with penicillin, and they occur in about 5% of patients. The most serious of these occur immediately after exposure (in less than 30 minutes) and are mediated by IgE (anaphylaxis). The incidence of anaphylaxis is about 0.01% of treatment courses. The mechanism of these reactions also involves the chemical reactivity of the β-lactam ring. Penicillins are a classic example of haptens (i.e., small molecules that are not immunogenic but bind to larger molecules, making them immunogenic) and react with the ϵ-amino group of lysine in proteins to make them immunogenic (see Fig. 53-6). This is the so-called major determinant because it is the major reaction leading to protein conjugates that can lead to a hypersensitivity reaction. There are also minor determinants composed mainly of penicilloic and penilloic acids. Although these determinants are quantitatively minor and are less commonly responsible for hypersensitivity reactions, a high percentage of the life-threatening immediate hypersensitivity reactions (i.e., anaphylaxis) is due to the minor determinants.

Accelerated reactions (occurring within 1–48 hours) are usually manifested by rash and sometimes by fever. Delayed reactions (beginning more than 48 hours after exposure) can consist of skin reactions or other systemic reactions such as nephritis or serum sickness. In addition to these reactions, ampicillin and amoxicillin are commonly associated with a characteristic nonurticarial maculopapular rash. The mechanism of this rash is not understood, but it is not an "allergic reaction." It usually starts 3–4 days after the onset of therapy. For reasons not understood, this reaction is much more frequent in patients with viral infections, especially mononucleosis, or when penicillin is taken together with allopurinol.

In deciding on therapy for a patient with a history of **penicillin allergy** several facts should be kept in mind. The vast majority of patients who have been labeled as having a penicillin allergy will not have a reaction if given penicillin. This can be because the patient really was never allergic to penicillin and the adverse event was due to some other factor. Examples of such factors include a viral infection causing a rash, for which antibiotic was inappropriately prescribed; some other drug or allergen to which the patient was exposed at the same time; or, in cases that had occurred many years before, it may have been due to impurities in earlier preparations of penicillin. Other patients may have had a nonallergic reaction such as an ampicillin rash, or incorrectly refer to other types of adverse reactions, such as nausea, vomiting, or diarrhea, as an allergy. The other possibility is that the patient did have an allergic reaction to a penicillin but has lost the sensitivity to penicillin. Most patients who have had an allergic reaction to penicillin will lose their sensitivity after a period of about 2 years. Despite this fact, *the possible consequences make a past history of a severe reaction to a penicillin a contraindication to its use unless skin testing (which includes the minor determinant) indicates that the patient is not now allergic to penicillin.*

Alternatively, if the infection is life-threatening and can be adequately treated only with a penicillin (e.g., bacterial endocarditis), a program of **desensitization** is indicated. Unfortunately, there is not a good correlation between the nature of the penicillin reaction history and the probability of a severe adverse reaction on reexposure; therefore, most physicians would *elect to use an alternative antibiotic* irrespective of the nature of the past history of penicillin allergy. Although adequate skin testing would solve most of these problems, the minor determinant is unstable and is not commercially available; therefore, penicillin skin testing that includes the minor determinants is, at present, available in only a few centers.

Convulsions and other forms of **encephalopathy** may occur when extremely high doses of a penicillin have been prescribed. These reactions are more likely to occur in patients with renal insufficiency, a condition that predisposes to high serum concentrations of the penicillin. In addition, renal failure can lead to the accumulation of organic anions, which, like probenecid, inhibit the active anion transport system that pumps penicillin out of the CSF. These reactions are most closely related to the concentration of the penicillin in the CSF and have occurred more frequently in patients with meningeal inflammation.

Interstitial nephritis can occur during the course of therapy with any penicillin, although it is most frequently associated with the administration of methicillin. Hypokalemia may be a side effect of high-dose parenteral penicillin therapy because the penicillins act as nonreabsorbable anions.

Coombs' test-positive **hemolytic anemia** may occur with excessive doses, or on an allergic basis, with any of the penicillins. **Neutropenia,** which is reversible upon discontinuing the drug, is also seen in some patients, especially those receiving methicillin, nafcillin, or cloxacillin. **Decreased platelet aggregation** has been noted at high concentrations of most penicillins but has been most marked with carbenicillin and ticarcillin. This may predispose to bleeding diathesis.

Drug Interactions

High concentrations of penicillins bind to and inactivate aminoglycoside antibiotics (see Chapter 55) in vitro and in vivo. Therefore, penicillins and aminoglycosides should not be mixed in intravenous infusions, and when administered to the same patient their infusions should be separated in time.

Penicillins and bacteriostatic drugs are often antagonistic in vitro, especially if the bacteria are exposed to the bacteriostatic agents first. The only in vivo example of this antagonism is the poorer outcome of *Streptococcus pneumoniae* meningitis if treated with both penicillin and tetracycline than if treated with penicillin alone.

Probenecid, indomethacin, sulfinpyrazone, and high-dose aspirin (>3 g/day) can block the tubular secretion of penicillins and may lead to prolonged high serum levels. Probenecid may also block the active transport of penicillin out of the CSF and thereby potentially lead to neurotoxicity as described above.

Dosage Regimens and Routes of Administration

Penicillins may be administered by the oral, intramuscular, or intravenous route. The choice of dosage, route, and regimen is dependent upon the specific agent, the infecting pathogen, and the seriousness and site of infection. The approximate daily dose of the penicillins that can be administered orally (penicillin V, ampicillin, cloxacillin, and oxacillin) ranges from 20 to 30 mg/kg. This amount is usually divided into four equal doses. The approximate daily dose of the penicillins that can be administered intravenously or intramuscularly (as in the treatment of serious infections requiring high blood levels of the antibiotic) is between 50 and 200 mg/kg for ampicillin, cloxacillin, methicillin, nafcillin, and oxacillin; 300 mg/kg for ticarcillin; 400–500 mg/kg for carbenicillin; and 100,000–200,000 IU/kg for aqueous benzyl penicillin G. (Penicillin G is prescribed in international units, 1 unit being equivalent to 0.6 μg.) The parenteral penicillins are usually administered in four to six equal doses per day. The longer-acting penicillin G preparations (procaine and benzathine) are administered as a single daily dose or as a single weekly to monthly dose, respectively. The approximate unit dose for these penicillins is 1.2 million units.

It must be emphasized that those are only broad guidelines. Considerable variation is observed among clinicians and institutions, even for similar indications.

Therapeutic Applications

The penicillins belong to perhaps the most frequently prescribed class of antimicrobial agents.

Penicillins G and V are used for a variety of mild-to-severe infections proved or presumed to be caused by sensitive organisms. Examples of mild infections for which oral penicillin V would be indicated include pharyngitis and skin and soft-tissue infections caused by group A streptococcus. Moderate-to-severe infections treated with parenteral penicillin G include streptococcal pneumonia, meningitis caused by *S. pneumoniae* and *Neisseria meningitidis*, gonorrhea, and syphilis, to name a few. However, the increasing incidence of penicillinase-producing *N. gonorrhoeae* has resulted in the replacement of penicillin by ceftriaxone for empirical (i.e., in the absence of bacterial diagnosis or sensitivity testing) treatment of gonorrhea. There are increasing reports from many parts of the world of strains of *S. pneumoniae* that have developed resistance to penicillin. In these areas,

vancomycin or a third-generation cephalosporin is used to treat infections caused by these organisms.

Ampicillin is used to treat mild-to-severe Gram-negative urinary tract infections.

Carbenicillin and ticarcillin are used almost exclusively for *Pseudomonas* infections of the urinary tract, lung, and blood.

Cloxacillin, oxacillin, nafcillin, and methicillin are used almost exclusively for infections caused by staphylococci, including skin and soft-tissue infections, pneumonia, osteomyelitis, endocarditis, and septicemia.

CEPHALOSPORINS

Cephalosporium acremonium, the first source of the cephalosporins, was isolated from the sea near a sewer outlet off the Sardinian coast. Crude filtrates from cultures of this fungus inhibited the growth of *S. aureus* in vitro and cured staphylococcal infections in humans.

Since the original isolation of *Cephalosporium acremonium* and the identification of its active product, cephalosporin C, many semisynthetic derivatives and structurally related analogs have been developed. The newer derivatives possess an increasing spectrum of activity and diverse pharmacokinetic characteristics.

Chemistry

The nucleus of cephalosporin C (7-aminocephalosporanic acid, Fig. 53-7), which formed the basis for all early cephalosporins, is closely related but not identical to the penicillin nucleus, 6-aminopenicil-

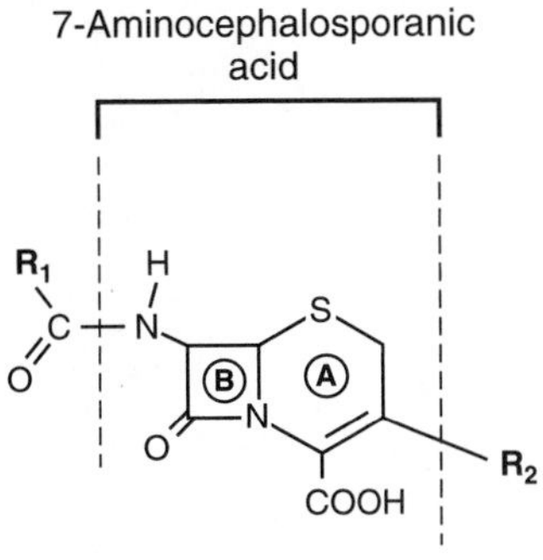

Figure 53-7. Structure of 7-aminocephalosporanic acid, the parent structure of cephalosporins, which are made by substitutions at R_1 and R_2. A = dihydrothiazide ring; B = β-lactam ring.

lanic acid. It also contains a β-lactam ring, the chemical reactivity of which is responsible for the antibacterial activity, acid instability, susceptibility to β-lactamase hydrolysis, and the hypersensitivity reactions to the cephalosporins. The diversity of the cephalosporins is based on the R_1 and R_2 substituents placed on the parent structure (see Fig. 53-7). As with penicillin, the presence of electron-withdrawing substituents on R_1 near the ring increases the stability in acid.

Bacterial Susceptibility

The evolution of cephalosporins and diversity of their properties have led to their division into three "generations." The original agents are referred to as first-generation cephalosporins and the most recently introduced are referred to as third-generation cephalosporins. (Fourth-generation cephalosporins are currently being studied.) In general, with each new generation, the activity against Gram-negative organisms increases while that against Gram-positive organisms decreases. A list of representative cephalosporins from each generation is provided in Table 53-3. In the following account, the details of only one or two representative agents from each generation are discussed, unless important differences exist for other members. The antibacterial activity of cephalosporins representative of each of the three generations is outlined in Table 53-4. The attainable serum concentrations of these antibiotics that can be related to the MICs are discussed below.

Resistance to the first-generation cephalosporins can be mediated by plasmid-encoded β-lactamase enzymes. These are typically found in certain strains of the enterobacteriaceae, including *Escherichia coli* and *Klebsiella*, and resistance is mediated by an enzyme called TEM. Resistance to third-generation cephalosporins may be due to either plasmid- or chromosome-mediated β-lactamase enzymes. Plasmid-mediated resistance is very uncommon, but it has been described in strains of *E. coli* and *Klebsiella* in which mutations have occurred in the amino acid structure of the TEM β-lactamase enzyme. Resistance is more commonly seen in certain strains of *Pseudomonas*, *Serratia*, and *Enterobacter* in which high levels of chromosome-mediated β-lactamase activity is expressed.

First generation cephalosporins

The prototype of this group of cephalosporins is **cephalothin**, which has a low oral bioavailability because of instability in acid. The acid-stable orally administered representative of this group is **cephalexin**. As outlined in Table 53-4, this antibiotic is

Table 53-3 Generations of Cephalosporins

	First	Second	Third
Compounds for parenteral use	Cephalothin *Keflin*	Cefamandole *Mandol*	Cefotaxime *Claforan*
	Cefazolin *Ancef, Kefzol*	Cefoxitin *Mefoxin*	Cefoperazone *Cefobid*
	Cephaloridine *Ceflorin*	Cefuroxime *Ceftin*	Ceftazidime *Captaz, Tazidime*
		Cefotetan *Cefotan*	Ceftizoxime *Cefizox*
			Ceftriaxone *Rocephin*
Compounds for oral use	Cephalexin *Keflex*	Cefaclor *Ceclor*	Cefixime *Suprax*
	Cephaloglycin *Kefglycin*	Cefuroxime axetil *Ceftin*	
	Cephradine *Cefradex*		
	Cefadroxil *Duricef*		

Table 53-4 Median MICs (in µg/mL) of Some Cephalosporins

Bacteria	Cephalothin	Cefamandole	Cefoxitin	Cefotaxime
Gram-positive				
Staphylococcus aureus, penicillinase (−)	0.2	0.25	3.1	2.0
Staphylococcus aureus, penicillinase (+)	0.4	0.5	3.1	2.0
Streptococcus group A	0.1	0.06	0.4	0.01
Streptococcus viridans	—	0.5	1.6	0.125
Enterococcus faecalis	50.0	32.0	100.0	>128
Streptococcus pneumoniae	0.1	0.25	3.12	0.03
Listeria	4.0	6.0	25.0	25.0
Clostridium	0.4	0.12	1.0	0.25
Gram-negative				
Neisseria meningitidis	0.5	<0.125	0.12	0.004
Neisseria gonorrhoeae	3.1	<0.125	0.12	0.015
Haemophilus influenzae	6.3	0.5	8.0	0.03
Salmonella sp.	2.0	1.0	2.0	0.25
Shigella	125.0	2.0	25.0	0.25
Klebsiella	10.0	1.0	12.5	0.25
Escherichia coli	20.0	0.5	8.0	0.25
Pseudomonas aeruginosa	>200	>125	>400	16.0
Proteus mirabilis	10.0	1.0	6.3	0.1
Bacteroides fragilis	<25	64.0	16.0	8.0
Other *Bacteroides*	12.5	1.0	1.0	—

very active against staphylococci, pneumococci, and streptococci except enterococci. Activity against aerobic and anaerobic Gram-negative organisms is limited, whereas there is good activity against *Clostridia* species and many of the other Gram-positive anaerobes. **Cefazolin,** another member of this generation, has somewhat more activity against aerobic Gram-negatives, especially against *E. coli* and *Klebsiella* species.

Second-generation cephalosporins

Cefuroxime, cefoxitin, and **cefotetan** are three representative members of this group. Their Gram-positive spectrum is similar to that of the first-generation cephalosporins, but they possess increased activity against Gram-negative organisms. They are, however, inactive against *Pseudomonas* species. The principal advantage of cefuroxime is its activity against *H. influenzae* and its ability to penetrate the CNS, whereas that of cefoxitin and cefotetan is their broadened activity against anaerobic organisms. Strictly speaking, cefoxitin is not a cephalosporin derivative but rather a cephamycin, a fermentation product of *Streptomyces*. **Cefaclor** and **cefuroxime axetil** are

the prototype oral preparations of this group, with similar activity.

Third-generation cephalosporins

Cefotaxime, ceftriaxone, and **ceftazidime** represent this rapidly increasing group of antibiotics. This generation retains most of the activity of the first two generations against Gram-positive bacteria but possesses in addition a remarkable amount of activity against Gram-negatives. Ceftazidime also has activity against many isolates of *Pseudomonas*. **Cefixime** is an oral agent belonging to this group. Although it has activity against the Enterobacteriaceae, the antibacterial activity is inferior to that of the intravenous members of this group.

Pharmacokinetics

Parenterally administered cephalosporins must be given by that route because they are poorly absorbed from the gastrointestinal tract. Those for oral administration, however, are almost completely absorbed, and serum concentrations are similar to those obtained after equivalent doses of the parenteral preparations. Serum concentrations of some of the cephalosporins after representative doses are outlined in Table 53-5.

The apparent volumes of distribution for the cephalosporins range from 0.1 to 0.4 L/kg and their degree of plasma protein binding at therapeutic concentrations ranges from 17 to 90% (see Table 53-5). The cephalosporins distribute widely throughout the body. The first- and second-generation derivatives (except cefuroxime), however, do not penetrate well into the CSF even in the presence of meningitis and, hence, must never be used to treat this infection. At least three of the third-generation cephalosporins (cefotaxime, ceftazidime, and ceftriaxone) do penetrate into the CSF to a sufficient degree (10–30%) to be the drugs of choice in the treatment of Gram-negative meningitis.

In general, the cephalosporins are not extensively biotransformed, but are distributed and excreted principally in a biologically active form. The primary route of excretion for most of the cephalosporins is renal (60–100%), although there are exceptions. Ceftriaxone is excreted through both the biliary and urinary tracts. Both glomerular filtration and tubular secretion are involved in the excretion of cephalosporins, although with some (e.g., cephaloridine, ceftriaxone, and ceftazidime) the amount of drug undergoing tubular secretion is negligible.

The elimination half-lives of the cephalosporins range from 0.5 to 8 hours depending on the specific agent, as noted in Table 53-5.

Adverse Reactions

As with most antibiotics, the full spectrum of hyper-sensitivity reactions including rash, hives, fever, eosinophilia, serum sickness, and anaphylaxis may occur. It is estimated that primary allergic reactions to the cephalosporins are seen in approximately 5% of cases. Reversible neutropenia and thrombocytopenia, both of which may have an allergic basis, have been observed occasionally.

The incidence of allergic reactions to the cephalosporins is increased in patients known to be allergic to penicillins. The precise frequency of such cross-reactions is, however, unclear; estimates have varied from 5 to 16%. Whether or not these reactions are due to cross-sensitivity is unknown because the sensitivity to penicillin was not confirmed by skin testing and, in addition, it may be that patients with a sensitivity to penicillin have a higher incidence of reactivity to immunologically unrelated drugs. It is generally held, however, that *all cephalosporins probably should be avoided in patients with a clear past history of anaphylaxis or immediate-type hypersensitivity to any of the penicillins*. It is reasonable, however, to consider their use in patients with a less severe type of reaction to the penicillins, if they are otherwise the agents of choice against a particular infection.

Adverse reactions related to the route of administration are also common with the cephalosporins. These reactions include pain after intramuscular injection, phlebitis with intravenous administration, and minor gastrointestinal complaints with oral preparations.

Table 53-5 Serum Concentrations, Half-Lives, and Protein Binding of Different Cephalosporins

Drug	Dosage (mg and Route)		Serum Concentration (μg/mL)	Protein Bound (% at Therapeutic Concentration)	Half-Life (hours)
Cephalothin	1000	IV	40–60	60–70	0.5
Cefazolin	1000	IV	90–120	85	1.5
Cephalexin	500	PO	15–20	low	0.5–1.0
Cefoxitin	1000	IV	60–80	70	1.0
Cefamandole	1000	IV	60–80	70	1.0
Cefaclor	200	PO	6	—	0.5
Cefotaxime	1000	IV	41	40	1.1
Ceftriaxone	1000	IV	145	90	8.0
Cefoperazone	1000	IV	125	90	2.0
Ceftazidime	1000	IV	83	17	1.8

Therapy with the cephalosporins may lead to the development of a positive direct Coombs' reaction, although it is not commonly associated with hemolytic anemia. The incidence of positive Coombs' test is approximately 3%.

Some of the cephalosporins (e.g., cephaloridine) have been withdrawn from use because of **dose-related nephrotoxicity**, probably resulting from proximal tubular damage. Interstitial nephritis has been described with some of the other cephalosporins (e.g., cephalothin); however, the risk of nephrotoxicity with currently available cephalosporins is very low.

The third-generation cephalosporins have also been associated with transient elevations of aspartate aminotransferase and alanine aminotransferase levels, reversible elevation of the blood urea nitrogen, and disturbances of vitamin K-dependent clotting function. This latter reaction is seen with cefamandole, cefotetan, and cefoperazone, which contain a methylthiotetrazole (MTT) ring. The MTT group competitively inhibits vitamin K-dependent carboxylase that is responsible for converting clotting factors II, VII, IX, and X to their active forms. The MTT group may also inhibit vitamin K–2,3-epoxide reductase that converts inactive vitamin K to its active form. This same structure also inhibits aldehyde dehydrogenase and can lead to a disulfiram-like reaction when the patient drinks alcohol (see Chapter 26).

Drug Interactions

Although it was once believed that cephalosporins enhanced the nephrotoxicity of aminoglycosides, more recent studies have found no evidence for such an interaction.

Cephalosporins may produce a "false-positive" glycosuric reaction with Clinitest.

Uricosuric agents such as probenecid may decrease the clearance of some cephalosporins by blocking renal tubular secretion.

Dosage Regimens and Routes of Administration

Cephalosporins may be administered by the oral, intramuscular, or intravenous route, depending on the specific agent and the therapeutic indications (see Table 53-3). In general, however, the intramuscular route is avoided, as these agents tend to cause pain upon injection. The approximate daily dose of the cephalosporins that can be administered orally ranges from 25 to 50 mg/kg. This amount is usually divided into two to four equal doses. The approximate daily dose of the cephalosporins that are administered intravenously is 50–200 mg/kg. This amount is usually divided into two to six equal doses depending on the half-life of the individual agents (see Table 53-5). Agents with the longest half-lives (e.g., ceftriaxone) may be administered every 24 hours, whereas those with short half-lives (e.g., cephalothin) must usually be administered every 4–6 hours.

As emphasized with the penicillins, these are only broad dosing guidelines, and considerable variation is common in clinical practice.

Therapeutic Applications

The therapeutic applications of the cephalosporins are different for each of the three generations and, therefore, each will be considered separately.

First-generation cephalosporins are rarely the antibiotics of first choice; however, they are useful for infections caused by penicillin-resistant staphylococci, *Klebsiella* species, and urinary tract infections resistant to penicillins and sulfonamides. This group of antibiotics, particularly cefazolin, is also useful for short-term perioperative prophylaxis for selected operations carrying a high risk of infections caused by Gram-positive organisms, but where Gram-negative organisms cannot be ruled out. They may also be useful in patients with a history of minor penicillin allergy but should not be administered to patients who have had immediate or accelerated penicillin reactions.

The broadened spectrum of activity of **second-generation cephalosporins** increases their range of potential therapeutic applications, although they also are rarely the antibiotic of first choice. The activity of cefuroxime against Gram-positive cocci as well as against β-lactamase-producing *H. influenzae* makes it a theoretically attractive agent for infections that might be caused by one or more of these organisms. It is particularly useful in pediatric infections, including otitis media and pneumonia.

Cefoxitin and cefotetan, with their effectiveness against anaerobic and Gram-negative organisms, are potentially useful single agents for the treatment of pelvic infections or peritonitis and for short-term perioperative prophylaxis for pelvic or abdominal operations.

The most important indication for the **third-generation cephalosporins** is in the treatment of meningitis caused by Gram-negative aerobes. Although they have not replaced aminoglycosides, the third-generation cephalosporins can sometimes be used instead of the more toxic combination of a penicillin and an aminoglycoside. Their indications also include the treatment of hospital-acquired Gram-negative aerobic infections or those otherwise rendered resistant to multiple antibiotics, empirical treatment in neutropenic patients, and some intraabdominal infections. Single-dose ceftriaxone is effective for the treatment of gonorrhea, even when the organism is resistant to penicillin.

β-LACTAMASE INHIBITORS

The resistance of many bacteria to penicillins is due to their production of β-lactamase; therefore, the coadministration of an agent that inhibits β-lactamase would extend the antibacterial spectrum of the penicillins. Examples of such agents are clavulanic acid, sulbactam, and tazobactam. These compounds act as "suicide" inhibitors by irreversibly binding to the bacterial β-lactamases which would otherwise inactivate the penicillins.

Clavulanic acid (Fig. 53-8) is a naturally occurring β-lactam isolated from *Streptomyces clavuligerus*. Sulbactam and tazobactam are semisynthetic penicillanic acid sulfones. None of these agents has significant antibacterial activity when used alone, and they are used solely to extend the activity of penicillins or cephalosporins. Current examples of such combinations are amoxicillin–clavulanic acid, ticarcillin–clavulanic acid, ampicillin–sulbactam, piperacillin–clavulanic acid, and piperacillin–tazobactam. The β-lactamase inhibitors have pharmacokinetic parameters similar to those of penicillin; their major route of elimination is renal. Their half-lives are about 1 hour but are increased in neonates and the elderly. Unlike the penicillins, however, their half-lives are not increased by probenecid.

The combination of amoxicillin–clavulanic acid is useful for the oral treatment of otitis media, sinusitis, and infections of the lower respiratory tract caused by β-lactamase-producing strains of pathogens. The combination of ticarcillin–clavulanic acid increases the activity of ticarcillin against β-lactamase-producing strains of *S. aureus*, *H. influenzae*, *N. gonorrhoeae*, *E. coli*, *Klebsiella*, and *B. fragilis*. The combination of ampicillin–sulbactam has broad-spectrum activity in the treatment of infections caused by β-lactamase-producing strains of *H. influenzae*, *Branhamella catarrhalis*, *Neisseria*, many anaerobes, *E. coli*, *Proteus*, *Klebsiella*, *S. aureus*, and *S. epidermidis*. The combination of piperacillin–tazobactam increases the activity of piperacillin against β-lactamase-producing strains of *E. coli*, *Klebsiella*, *Bacteroides*, and *Haemophilus*.

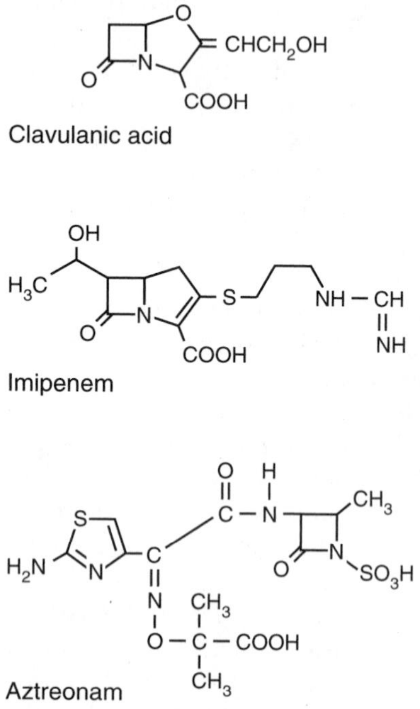

CARBAPENEMS

Imipenem is the first of a new class of β-lactam antibiotics, the carbapenems (Fig. 53-8). It is a more stable derivative of the natural product, thienamycin. Imipenem is inactivated by a dehydropeptidase in the brush border of the kidney, and therefore it is given in combination with an inhibitor of this enzyme, cilastatin, which increases tissue and urinary levels of active drug.

Bacterial Susceptibility

Imipenem has the broadest spectrum of all antibacterial agents that are presently available for clinical use. It is active against most Gram-positive and Gram-negative bacteria, including anaerobes; however, methicillin-resistant staphylococci are usually resistant to imipenem, and it is not active against *Chlamydia* and *Mycoplasma*. Although it is active against *Legionella* in vitro, it may not be useful clinically because *Legionella* are intracellular organisms. It is active against most anaerobes, including *B. fragilis*, but has low activity against *C. difficile*.

Figure 53-8. Structures of other β-lactams.

Imipenem is active against *P. aeruginosa*, but resistant strains have already emerged. When resistance appears, it is usually due to a modification of the cell wall that prevents penetration of the drug. Less commonly, resistance results from modification of penicillin-binding proteins or from the induction of β-lactamases that are capable of inactivating the β-lactam ring of imipenem. Imipenem is a potent inducer of cephalosporinases, which do not hydrolyze imipenem itself, but do hydrolyse a broad range of other β-lactam antibiotics; therefore, it is irrational to combine imipenem with other β-lactam antibiotics.

Pharmacokinetics

Imipenem is administered intravenously. Its clearance is renal, and cilastatin increases the proportion of the drug that is cleared intact from 20 to 70%. The average half-life is 1 hour. Penetration of the CNS is variable, but because imipenem can cause seizures, it is not usually used for the treatment of meningitis.

Adverse Reactions

The most common adverse reactions are pain at the site of infusion, nausea and vomiting, and diarrhea. In one study a rash or drug fever occurred in 2.7% and seizures in 1.5% of patients. When seizures occur, they are usually observed in patients with CNS abnormalities or with renal failure. The degree of cross-reactivity between imipenem and penicillins has not been accurately determined, but imipenem should not be used in patients with a clear history of an anaphylactic reaction to penicillin.

Therapeutic Applications

Its broad spectrum of activity makes it most useful for severe infections with mixed bacterial flora. The number of well-controlled studies comparing imipenem to other therapy is limited, and for many indications, such as intraabdominal infections, pneumonia, and empirical therapy of febrile patients with cancer and neutropenia, imipenem is probably not significantly better than conventional therapy, although it may have fewer side effects. In order to slow the emergence of resistant bacteria, its use should be limited to those infections for which less broad-spectrum (and less costly) agents cannot be used.

Dosage and Routes of Administration

Imipenem is only available for intravenous administration in combination with cilastatin (Primaxin). The dose depends on the susceptibility of the organism and the type of infection being treated; however, the usual daily dose for patients with normal renal function is 2 g divided into four doses. For patients with glomerular filtration rates less than 30 mL/min, the dose should be decreased by 50%.

MONOBACTAMS

As the name suggests, the monobactams have a β-lactam ring, which, unlike that of penicillins and cephalosporins, is not fused to a second ring. The first of the monobactams to be marketed, **aztreonam** (Azactam, Fig. 53-8), contains a sulfonic acid group attached to the N of the β-lactam ring, which activates the β-lactam ring but also limits oral absorption. Aztreonam is therefore used only parenterally, usually by intramuscular injection. This agent is not universally available.

Bacterial Susceptibility

Although the mechanism of action of the monobactams is similar to that of other β-lactams, aztreonam does not bind to the penicillin-binding proteins of Gram-positive bacteria or anaerobic organisms; therefore, activity is limited to aerobic Gram-negative organisms. Aztreonam is not hydrolyzed by most β-lactamases but it is destroyed by those that hydrolyze cefotaxime or ceftazidime. It is active against most Enterobacteriaceae and all isolates of *N. gonorrhoeae*, *N. meningitidis*, and *H. influenzae*. Although it has activity against *P. aeruginosa* and *Enterobacter* species, some strains may be resistant.

Therapeutic Applications

Except for its lack of activity against Gram-positive organisms, aztreonam has a spectrum of activity similar to that of the aminoglycosides. It has been demonstrated to be effective in the treatment of urinary tract infections due to Enterobacteriaceae, *P. aeruginosa*, and *Providencia*, some of which were resistant to penicillins, first- and second-generation cephalosporins, and aminoglycosides. It has also been used to treat urinary tract, pelvic and peritoneal infections, pneumonia, and osteomyelitis, either as a single agent or in combination with other drugs.

Dosage can range from 0.5–1.0 g every 8–12 hours to as much as 2 g every 6–8 hours in life-threatening infections.

Pharmacokinetics

Aztreonam is almost completely absorbed from injection sites and distributes into virtually all body fluids. After an intravenous dose of 2 g, aztreonam reaches CSF concentrations of 2 μg/mL at 1 hour and 3.2 μg/mL at 4 hours. Its plasma half-life is 1.5–2 hours, and elimination is mainly by excretion in the urine by both glomerular filtration and tubular secretion. Dosage may therefore have to be reduced if renal function is impaired.

Adverse Reactions

Aztreonam is usually well tolerated, and the pattern of adverse effects is similar to that of other β-lactam antibiotics. Despite having a β-lactam ring, aztreonam shows little cross-reactivity to antibodies against penicillins and cephalosporins and has been used safely in some patients with positive skin test reactions against penicillin.

VANCOMYCIN

Vancomycin (Vancocin) was isolated from *Streptomyces orientalis*, an actinomycete found in soil samples from Indonesia and India. It was purified and characterized in 1956. The agent is not chemically related to any of the antimicrobial agents in present use. It is an unusual glycopeptide containing a chlorinated polyphenyl ether and has a molecular weight of about 1500 Da.

Bacterial Susceptibility

The primary activity of vancomycin is against Gram-positive bacteria. The importance of this agent has increased with the emergence of organisms resistant to the antistaphylococcal penicillins and with better purification techniques that have reduced its toxicity. The vast majority of staphylococcal species including penicillinase-negative and -positive strains, and streptococcal species including enterococci, are killed by less than 1.6 μg/mL of this antibiotic. Gram-positive bacilli including *Clostridia* species are also very sensitive to vancomycin. Gram-negative bacteria are invariably resistant. Recently, strains of enterococci resistant to this agent have been reported.

This is of great concern, as there are now no effective antibiotics available to treat these strains.

Pharmacokinetics

Vancomycin is not absorbed from the gastrointestinal tract. A single intravenous dose of 10 mg/kg in adults produces serum concentrations of 20–30 μg/mL at 1–2 hours after the infusion.

The volume of distribution of vancomycin is 0.5–0.9 L/kg. It is less than 10% protein-bound. It appears in various body fluids, and 20–30% is detectable in the cerebrospinal fluid when the meninges are inflamed.

Vancomycin is normally not biotransformed in the body. It is excreted by the kidneys, and about 80–90% of a dose can be recovered from the urine during the first 24 hours. Its serum half-life is 6–9 hours.

Adverse Reactions

Hearing loss has been associated with sustained high serum concentrations of vancomycin in excess of 60–80 μg/mL. Nephrotoxicity is rare at recommended doses. The early reports of this complication may have been due to an impurity in the formulation. Both ototoxicity and nephrotoxicity are more common when the drug is used together with an aminoglycoside. A "red man" syndrome is manifested as flushing and a maculopapular rash on face, neck, trunk, and extremities during, or shortly after, intravenous administration. It is believed to be caused by histamine release and may lead to hypotension, tachycardia, shock, and cardiac arrest. This syndrome is most likely to occur if vancomycin is administered rapidly as an intravenous bolus; therefore, the dose should be infused over a period of 45–60 minutes.

Drug Interactions

Cholestyramine can bind vancomycin *if the two drugs are administered together orally*. Heparin also binds to vancomycin and inactivates it if the two are mixed in the same intravenous line. The ototoxicity of vancomycin may be increased by coadministration with aminoglycosides.

Dosage and Routes of Administration

Because vancomycin is not absorbed from the gastrointestinal tract, it should be administered orally only if high concentrations in the intestine are desired (see below). The recommended daily intravenous dose is 20–30 mg/kg divided into two or three doses.

Therapeutic Applications

The primary clinical use of vancomycin is in the treatment of severe staphylococcal and streptococcal (including enterococcal) infections in patients who are allergic to penicillin. In addition, some recently isolated multiply-resistant staphylococci and *S. pneumoniae* are sensitive only to this antibiotic.

Vancomycin is administered orally in the treatment of antibiotic-associated pseudomembranous colitis. This illness is caused by the toxin produced by *Clostridium difficile*.

BACITRACIN

In contrast to the penicillins and cephalosporins, which act on the *outside* of microbial cells, inhibit transpeptidation and cross-linking of peptidoglycan strands, and thus interfere with bacterial cell wall synthesis in susceptible microorganisms, bacitracin acts *intracellularly* by binding to, and rendering unusable, the isoprenyl phosphate lipid carrier responsible for transport of cell wall precursors from the bacterial cytoplasm to the exterior of the cell membrane (see Fig. 53-2). Bacitracin therefore lacks the high degree of selective antibacterial toxicity of the majority of antibiotics classified as cell wall inhibitors and is capable of also causing damage to susceptible mammalian cells.

Because of an unacceptably high degree of nephrotoxicity when administered systemically, the use of bacitracin in anti-infective therapy is confined to topical administration in the form of ophthalmic and topical skin ointments and as a powder for specialized topical applications, from which it cannot be absorbed.

Bacitracin inhibits a variety of Gram-positive cocci and bacilli and some *Neisseria* and *Haemophilus* species. Because of its limitations in treating superficial skin infections when used alone, it is available for topical use in mixtures with neomycin and/or polymyxin. Its other main clinical use is in the eradication of nasal carriage of *S. aureus*.

Hypersensitivity reactions to bacitracin are very rare.

CYCLOSERINE

Cycloserine (Seromycin), an antibiotic isolated from *Streptomyces orchidaceus*, interferes with the *intracellular* synthesis of glycopeptides that are required, after transfer to the outside, for the construction of bacterial cell walls. As noted at the beginning of this chapter, it inhibits the conversion of L-alanine to D-alanine and the linking of two D-molecules (see Fig. 53-3).

The antibiotic has marked in vitro inhibitory activity against *Mycobacterium tuberculosis*, without cross-resistance between cycloserine and other antitubercular agents. Resistance develops, however, because of bacterial enzyme adaptation and altered pathways in cell wall synthesis.

Cycloserine is well absorbed after oral administration, is well tolerated by the GI tract, and is distributed widely in tissues, body fluids, and the CSF. About two-thirds of a dose is excreted unchanged in the urine, and the remainder is biotransformed to unknown metabolites. Peak plasma concentrations of the drug are reached in about 3–4 hours, with a plasma half-life of about 10 hours. The usual adult dose of cycloserine is 250 mg twice a day, which is associated with a negligible risk of toxicity.

Adverse reactions are seen most commonly as the consequence of the drug's considerable CNS toxicity, such as excitement, aggression, confusion, depression, hyperreflexia, and focal or tonic-clonic seizures. This CNS toxicity can be minimized by limiting peak plasma concentrations to less than 30 μg/mL. A history of epilepsy, severe depression, or severe anxiety is a contraindication to the use of cycloserine.

Cycloserine is considered a second-line antitubercular drug, useful for retreatment or in the presence of microbial resistance to other drugs, and it must always be given in combination with other effective drugs, as outlined in Chapter 56. Although its use had decreased, it is increasing again for the management of infections caused by multiple-drug-resistant strains of *M. tuberculosis* (MDRTb) encountered in prisons and hospitals in some parts of the United States.

ISONIAZID (INH)

Isoniazid (Fig. 53-9) was discovered in 1952. It is the hydrazide of isonicotinic acid and has proved to

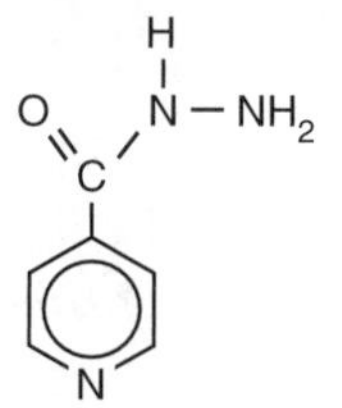

Figure 53-9. Structural formula of isoniazid.

be the most useful antimicrobial agent for the treatment and prophylaxis of tuberculosis.

INH is bactericidal against actively replicating *M. tuberculosis* and bacteriostatic against nonreplicating organisms. Resting organisms resume multiplication when drug contact is ended. The minimal tuberculostatic concentration is 0.025–0.05 μg/mL.

Among the variety of proposed mechanisms of action, there is strong evidence that the primary action of INH is inhibition of oxygen-dependent synthetic pathways of mycolic acid, an important and unique constituent of mycobacterial cell walls. The inhibition of mycolic acid synthesis by INH produces very rapid effects on mycobacteria (in 60–90 minutes), whereas the inhibition of DNA synthesis is slow (10–12 hours). The effects on mycolic acid synthesis are obtained with the lowest effective concentration of isoniazid, and they are seen in INH-sensitive mycobacteria, but not in INH-resistant strains.

Pharmacokinetics

Isoniazid is readily absorbed after oral administration. Peak plasma levels of 1–5 μg/mL are attained 1–2 hours after an oral dose of 5 mg/kg.

The volume of distribution of INH is approximately 0.6 L/kg. It is poorly protein-bound, diffuses readily into all body fluids and cells, and is present, in varying concentrations, in all body organs. Cerebrospinal fluid penetration is variable, but CSF concentrations may be nearly equal to those in serum. Isoniazid penetrates well into the caseous material in the central parts of the tubercles from which the disease gets its name. Infected tissues retain the drug for long periods of time in quantities well above those required for tuberculostasis.

The main method of inactivation of the drug is acetylation in the liver by an enzyme, *N*-acetyltransferase, which converts INH to acetylisoniazid. This in turn is partly hydrolyzed to isonicotinic acid and acetylhydrazine. Nonacetylated INH is excreted in the urine in its unchanged form or as its hydrazone

conjugates. The rate of INH acetylation is genetically controlled. The amount of INH acetylation metabolites in the urine reflects the acetylator status of the patient. About 90% of Orientals are rapid acetylators compared to about 45% of Caucasians and Negroes (see Chapter 12).

Approximately 70% of administered INH is excreted via the kidneys, but most of this is in an inactive form. Slow acetylators excrete about ten times more active INH in the urine than do rapid acetylators. The half-life of INH is 0.5–1.5 hours in rapid acetylators compared with 2–3 hours in slow acetylators.

Adverse Reactions

Neurotoxicity and hepatotoxicity are the two most important side effects of INH. The incidence of neurotoxicity is higher in slow acetylators, but acetylator phenotype probably has no bearing on the incidence of hepatotoxicity. It was once thought that patients of the rapid acetylator phenotype had the highest risk of hepatotoxicity because the mechanism appears to involve an acetylhydrazine intermediate; however, although acetylhydrazine is formed more rapidly in rapid acetylators, it is also converted rapidly to nontoxic diacetylhydrazine.

Neurotoxic manifestations, including psychosis, confusion, convulsions, and coma, may occur with overdosage. Peripheral neuropathy may occur at therapeutic doses, but it is more common with larger doses than smaller ones and in older or malnourished patients with pyridoxine deficiency. The administration of pyridoxine prevents this toxicity.

Hepatotoxicity is an age-related occurrence more prevalent in patients over 35 years of age. Hepatitis may progress to hepatocellular necrosis with jaundice if the drug is not discontinued. Alcoholics are more prone to this liver injury. An early asymptomatic transient rise in serum transaminases is noted in about 20% of INH recipients, but this does not, in itself, necessitate discontinuance of INH.

A significant number of INH recipients develop antinuclear antibodies, and some develop a lupus-like syndrome. This is reversible with discontinuation of the drug. The incidence of this adverse reaction is probably higher in slow acetylators.

Drug Interactions

Aluminum hydroxide or other antacids may interfere with the absorption of INH. Also, isoniazid may inhibit the cytochrome P450-mediated metabolism of phenytoin or anticoagulants, thereby causing excessively high serum concentrations and related toxicity of these drugs.

Dosage Regimen, Route of Administration, and Therapeutic Applications

Isoniazid is usually administered orally as a single daily dose of 5–10 mg/kg. If pyridoxine is given concomitantly, its dose is 10 mg for every 100 mg of INH.

Isoniazid is a first-line tuberculocidal drug. It is used in combination with various other antituberculous drugs for the treatment of all types of tuberculosis. Isoniazid is also used as a prophylactic agent in persons infected with *M. tuberculosis* but who do not have active disease. Isoniazid prophylaxis (300 mg/day for 6–12 months) is recommended for persons with positive tuberculin skin test, without evidence of active disease, who (1) are under 35 years of age, (2) have demonstrated TB skin test conversion, (3) have household contacts of active cases of pulmonary TB, (4) are over 35 years of age with an increased risk of reactivation, especially those with silicosis, immunosuppression, dialysis, or gastrectomy, (5) are coinfected with HIV, or (6) have old fibrotic scars on chest X-ray. If the person is thought to be infected with an INH-resistant strain, either INH plus rifampin or rifampin alone (see Chapter 56) can be considered.

It is important to remember that approximately one in 10^6 tubercle bacilli is resistant to isoniazid and one cavitary lesion usually contains 10^7–10^9 bacilli; therefore, combination therapy (e.g., isoniazid and rifampin) must be used to treat active disease to prevent the emergence of a resistant infection. This is in contrast to prophylactic therapy in patients with a positive TB skin test, where there are only a few dormant tubercle bacilli present and treatment with isoniazid as a single agent is appropriate.

ETHAMBUTOL

Ethambutol (Myambutol) was discovered in 1961 when randomly selected compounds were being tested for antituberculous activity. It is a relatively simple molecule, consisting of two residues of aminobutanol connected by an ethylene bridge. Ethambutol is bacteriostatic against *Mycobacterium tuberculosis*, with in vitro activity against about 75% of strains at a concentration of 1 μg/mL.

Ethambutol does inhibit RNA synthesis, but it simultaneously inhibits the transfer of mycolic acid into cell walls of mycobacteria. Ethambutol was also shown to break the "exclusion barrier" in cell walls, thus enabling other drugs to penetrate into cells.

Pharmacokinetics

Ethambutol is well absorbed after oral administration. Peak serum concentrations of approximately 5 μg/mL are attained about 4 hours after a 15 mg/kg dose.

The apparent volume of distribution of ethambutol approximates 1.5 L/kg. It is 20–30% protein-bound in plasma. There are no data available on its distribution to various body tissues. However, it is known that levels equal to 25–50% of the serum concentration are attained in the CSF when the meninges are inflamed.

Between 8% and 15% of absorbed ethambutol is converted to various inactive metabolites, which are excreted in the urine together with approximately 80% of absorbed drug in its active unchanged form. About 20% of an oral dose is unabsorbed and excreted unchanged in the feces.

Adverse Reactions

The most important adverse reaction to ethambutol is a **reversible retrobulbar neuropathy**, which results in defective red-green vision and eventual field constriction or blindness. The incidence of this reaction increases with increasing doses, reaching approximately 5% of patients at 25–50 mg/kg/day. Patients should have baseline visual acuity tests and then be monitored regularly every 4–6 weeks. They should be instructed to report optic symptoms promptly.

Dosage Regimen, Route of Administration, and Therapeutic Applications

Ethambutol is administered orally as a single daily dose of 15–25 mg/kg. Its main use is in combination with other antimicrobial agents to treat infections caused by *M. tuberculosis*. It is also increasingly used in combination with other agents to treat *M. avium intracellulare* infections in patients with AIDS.

SUGGESTED READING

Cunha BA. Vancomycin. Med Clin North Am 1995; 79:817–832.

Klein NC, Cunha BA. Third-generation cephalosporins. Med Clin North Am 1995; 79:705–720.

Nagarajan R. Antibacterial activities and modes of action of vancomycin and related glycopeptides. Antimicrob Agents Chemother 1991; 35:605–609.

Neu HC. Beta-lactam antibiotics: structural relationships affecting in vitro activity and pharmacologic properties. Rev Infect Dis 1986; 8(Suppl 3):S237–S259.

Neu HC. The crisis in antibiotic resistance. Science 1992; 257:1064–1072.

Norrby SR. Carbapenems. Med Clin North Am 1995; 79:745–760.

Rastogi N, David HL. Mode of action of antituberculous drugs and mechanisms of drug resistance in *Mycobacterium tuberculosis.* Res Microbiol 1993; 144:133–143.

Sahm DF, Kissinger J, Gilmore US, et al. In vitro susceptibility studies of vancomycin-resistant *Enterococcus faecalis.* Antimicrob Agents Chemother 1989; 33(9):1588–1591.

Sensacovic JW, Smith LG. Beta-lactamase inhibitor combinations. Med Clin North Am 1995; 79:695–704.

Swanson DS, Starke JR. Drug-resistant tuberculosis in pediatrics. Pediatr Clin North Am 1995; 42:553–582.

Tan JS, File TM. Antipseudomonal penicillins. Med Clin North Am 1995; 79:679–694.

Tomasz A. Penicillin-binding proteins and the antibacterial effectiveness of beta-lactam antibiotics. Rev Infect Dis 1986; 8(Suppl 3):S260–S278.

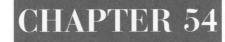

CHAPTER 54

Antimicrobial and Antifungal Agents That Act on Cell Membranes

J. UETRECHT AND S.L. WALMSLEY

CASE HISTORY

A 35-year-old gay man who was HIV-infected and had a CD4 count of 150×10^6/L saw his physician because of the complaint of dry mouth and sore throat. Clinical examination showed that he had developed oral thrush (candidiasis), which was successfully treated with "swish and swallow" nystatin, 500,000 IU three times daily for 7 days. Six months later he had a recurrent episode of thrush, which responded to similar treatment.

Three months later the patient saw his physician with complaints of retrosternal discomfort on swallowing. Endoscopy confirmed the diagnosis of esophageal candidiasis. The patient was therefore treated with oral ketoconazole, 200 mg/day for a period of 2 weeks, and showed improvement. Because the patient tolerated the drug well, it was decided to continue oral ketoconazole, 200 mg/day, as secondary prophylaxis.

One year later, the patient came to the Emergency Room with a 5-day history of bifrontal headache, fever, and chills. The headache increased when he bent over or coughed, and he had vomited on four occasions. On physical examination he looked unwell and had a temperature of 39°C. There were no focal neurological deficits and there was no neck stiffness. A lumbar puncture was performed and India ink examination of the cerebrospinal fluid showed budding yeast cells that were confirmed on culture as *Cryptococcus neoformans*. A cryptococcal antigen

test of the CSF was reported positive with a titer of 1:5096. The patient was admitted and was treated with intravenous amphotericin B at a dose of 1 mg/kg/day. After 2 weeks, he had improved significantly and treatment was changed to oral fluconazole at a dose of 400 mg/day. After a total of 6 weeks of treatment, the lumbar puncture was repeated and the CSF cultures for cryptococcus were reported negative. Therefore, the dose of fluconazole was decreased to 200 mg/day, which was continued indefinitely as secondary prophylaxis against cryptococcus.

MECHANISMS OF ACTION

Cytoplasmic membranes maintain the intracellular contents, both by controlling passive diffusion and by providing the mechanisms of active transport. Human and microbial cell membranes are similar in that they both possess lipid and protein structural elements. However, bacterial lipids are primarily phospholipids, and fungi contain sterols. These differences in lipid composition give rise to differences in sensitivity of human, bacterial and fungal cell membranes to the actions of relatively selective detergent compounds.

Polymyxins and **colistin** are large cyclic polypeptides with amino and carboxyl groups providing a polar face and hydrocarbon chains providing a nonpolar face. Thus they act as cationic detergents, reacting with the phosphate groups of cell envelope phospholipids. Disorganization of the cytoplasmic

677

membrane follows, with leakage of the intracellular contents and cell death. Unfortunately, these agents can affect mammalian cell membranes in the same way, especially in the renal tubule where they are concentrated after excretion. Therefore they are used mainly topically, for superficial infections, but they can also be used for certain systemic infections if other, less toxic, antibiotics have failed.

Amphotericin B (Fig. 54-1) and **nystatin** have an analogous action on fungal cell membranes. Both of these antifungal agents have multiple conjugated double bonds (i.e., they are "polyenes," see Fig. 54-1), which cause them to interact preferentially with ergosterol, the main sterol in certain fungal cell membranes, rather than with the cholesterol of mammalian cell membranes. They produce hydrophilic channels through the fungal membrane, permitting leakage of essential cell contents including potassium.

The **imidazoles,** such as miconazole and clotrimazole, also exploit the requirement for ergosterol in the fungal cell membrane. These drugs inhibit the specific cytochrome P450 that demethylates lanosterol, the precursor of ergosterol. This leads to an accumulation of 14-α-methylsterols and reduced concentrations of ergosterol, a sterol necessary for a normal fungal cell membrane. A related class of drugs with a triazole ring instead of an imidazole ring (and therefore called **triazoles**) have the same antifungal spectrum and mechanism of action as the imidazoles but have less effect on human steroid metabolism. Examples of this class are **fluconazole** and **itraconazole.**

The **allylamines,** a new class of synthetic antifungal drugs, also inhibit the synthesis of ergosterol; in this case the target enzyme is squalene epoxidase. This inhibition not only leads to a decrease in ergosterol, but also a buildup of squalene, which is toxic to the cell. The major drug in this class at the present time is **terbinafine,** which has a minimum inhibitory concentration (MIC) of 0.001–0.01 μg/mL for *Trichophyton rubrum*, a common fungal pathogen in skin, hair, and nails. The squalene pathway is also involved in the synthesis of cholesterol in mammalian cells, and the basis for the selective toxicity is that terbinafine is 10,000 times more active against the fungal enzyme than the mammalian enzyme.

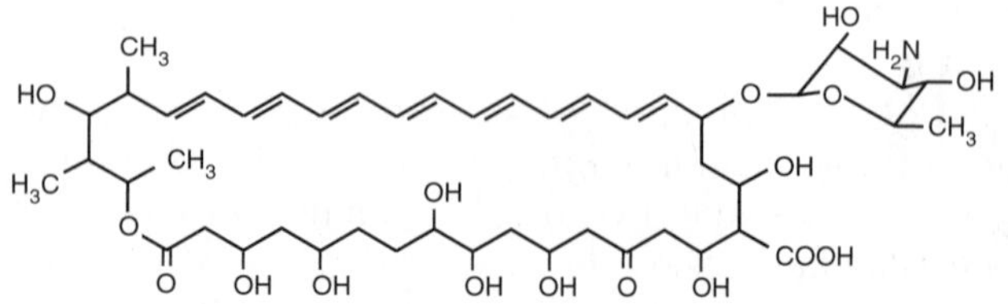

POLYMYXINS AND COLISTIN

The polymyxins were discovered as antimicrobial agents in 1947. Polymyxin is a generic term for a group of closely related antibiotic substances (polymyxins A, B, C, D, and E, relatively simple basic polypeptides with molecular weights of about 1000 Da) elaborated by various strains of an aerobic spore-forming rod, *Bacillus polymyxa*, which is found in soil. Polymyxin B (Polysporin), in the form of its sulfate, is the least toxic to humans. Colistin (Methacolymycin) is identical to polymyxin E but is supplied as the sulfomethyl derivative (methane sulfonate).

Bacterial Susceptibility

The activity of the polymyxins is related to a detergent action on the bacterial cell membrane, resulting in lysis of the organisms even in hypertonic media. This action is restricted to Gram-negative bacteria. *Enterobacter, Escherichia, Haemophilus, Klebsiella, Pasteurella, Salmonella, Shigella,* and *Vibrio* are sensitive to concentrations of 0.02–2 μg/mL. Most strains of *Pseudomonas aeruginosa* are inhibited by less than 4 μg/mL. Most strains of *Proteus* and some *Neisseria* are resistant to the drug. In general, the antibacterial activity of colistin is inferior to that of the methane sulfonate derivatives.

Adverse Reactions

The same detergent action that is responsible for the bactericidal effect can also be exerted on mammalian cell membranes, especially in the renal tubule where the drug is concentrated during excretion. Neurotoxicity and nephrotoxicity are the major severe adverse effects of these drugs.

Drug Interactions

Neuromuscular blockade from muscle relaxants or general anesthetics may be potentiated by the neurotoxic effects of these drugs.

Figure 54-1. Structural formula of amphotericin B.

Dosages and Routes of Administration

Polymyxin B is administered intramuscularly at a dose of 25,000–40,000 units/kg/day divided into two or three doses (10,000 units = 1 mg).

Colistin is administered intramuscularly or intravenously at a dose of 3–5 mg/kg/day divided into two or three doses.

The polymyxins are also available in numerous topical preparations such as creams, ointments, solutions, sprays, and eye drops. They are usually combined in these preparations with other antibiotics such as neomycin and bacitracin (see Chapters 53 and 55).

Therapeutic Applications

At the present time, the parenteral preparations of these agents have fallen into disuse clinically because of the availability of more efficacious, less toxic substances. The topical preparations of polymyxin B, however, are widely used because of its excellent activity against Gram-negative organisms, its lack of absorption, and, hence, its lack of toxicity when applied superficially. Oral colistin has been used successfully as part of an oral decontamination regimen to prevent systemic infections in patients with acute leukemia and chemotherapy-induced neutropenia.

NYSTATIN

Nystatin (Mycostatin, Nilstat) is an antifungal antibiotic that was isolated from *Streptomyces noursei* in 1950. It belongs to the group of polyene antibiotics. Its large, conjugated double-bond ring system is linked to an amino acid sugar, mycosamine.

Fungal Susceptibility

Nystatin is fungicidal against *Candida, Cryptococcus, Histoplasma, Blastomyces, Trichophyton, Epidermophyton,* and *Microsporum audouini* in vitro at concentrations ranging from 1.5 to 6.5 μg/mL.

Pharmacokinetics

Nystatin is too toxic for parenteral administration; it is therefore used only for the treatment of superficial mycotic infections. For these reasons the pharmacokinetics and toxic effects of parenteral nystatin need not be described. Very little, if any, nystatin is absorbed after topical or oral administration of pharmacological doses.

Adverse Reactions

There are virtually no side effects related to the topical use of nystatin. The drug may cause irritation or allergic reactions when applied to skin or mucous membranes. Nausea and diarrhea may occur following the administration of large doses orally.

Dosage Regimens and Routes of Administration

Many preparations of this drug (1 mg = 3500 units) are available, including oral tablets (500,000 units), oral suspension (100,000 units/mL), and vaginal tablets (100,000 units). Vaginal and skin creams are also available containing nystatin either alone or in combination with other antimicrobials (e.g., bacitracin, neomycin, polymyxin B) or anti-inflammatory agents (principally steroids). Usually one tablet (orally or vaginally) or 5 mL of the suspension (swished in the mouth and swallowed) is administered two to four times a day. Topical application is usually made two or three times a day.

Therapeutic Applications

Nystatin is used almost exclusively for the treatment of mucosal or cutaneous candidal infections, including oral and vaginal candidiasis. However, some instances of oral candidiasis, especially those appearing as superinfections during the use of an antimicrobial agent, or in patients with advanced HIV infection, may fail to respond.

AMPHOTERICIN B

Amphotericin is an antifungal compound that was isolated from *Streptomyces nodosus* in 1956. It exists in two forms, A and B: The latter, being more active, is used clinically. Amphotericin B (Fungizone) is another polyene antibiotic; the basic moiety is amino-desoxyhexose, an aminomethyl pentose. It is closely related chemically to nystatin.

Fungal Susceptibility

Candida species, *Histoplasma capsulatum, Cryptococcus neoformans, Coccidioides immitis, Rhodotorula, Blastomyces dermatitidis, Paracoccidioides brasiliensis, Sporotrichum schenckii, Aspergillus,*

Cladosporium species, *Phialophora* species, *Mucor*, and *Rhizopus* are usually killed by less than 1.0 μg/mL of amphotericin B. The drug acts by binding to ergosterol in the fungal cell membrane, leading to formation of channels through which potassium, other ions, and essential metabolites are lost, a mechanism of action that is identical to that postulated for nystatin.

Pharmacokinetics

As would be expected from its structure (it is a large hydrophobic molecule; Fig. 54-1), amphotericin B is poorly absorbed from the gastrointestinal tract. The intravenous injection of 0.5–1 mg/kg yields peak plasma concentrations of 1.5–2 μg/mL.

Data on the distribution of amphotericin B in both humans and animals are very limited. It is very lipophilic and it apparently distributes to cholesterol-containing membranes. This gives it a large volume of distribution of approximately 4 L/kg. In serum, desoxycholine separates from amphotericin B, and more than 95% of the latter binds to plasma proteins, primarily β-lipoprotein, presumably on cholesterol moieties. The drug leaves the circulation promptly. Amphotericin B is stored in the liver and other organs, and it reenters the circulation slowly. Only small quantities enter the CSF.

The primary route of elimination of amphotericin B is unclear. Most of the drug is degraded, and only a small amount is excreted in urine and bile. Only 2–5% of a given dose is excreted in biologically active form in the urine. Blood levels are not influenced by renal or hepatic function or by hemodialysis.

The elimination of this agent is biphasic with an initial half-life of 24 hours, followed by a terminal half-life of 15 days, reflecting slow release from the large peripheral compartment.

Adverse Reactions

The main adverse reactions to amphotericin B are those that occur during intravenous infusions, or later as renal and hematological toxicity.

Infusion reactions include fever, chills, headache, anorexia, nausea, vomiting, and thrombophlebitis. These reactions may be due to deoxycholate used to form a colloidal solution of the drug, or to the colloidal solution itself. They may be ameliorated by analgesics, antiemetics, antipyretics, heparin (to prevent thrombophlebitis), or hydrocortisone.

Nephrotoxicity is a common and most important side effect of amphotericin B. Impairment of renal function and nephrotoxic reactions often limit the total amount of drug that can be administered. Early manifestations caused by the disruption of renal tubular cell membranes include hypokalemia, hypomagnesemia, and renal tubular acidosis. The degree of hypokalemia is often great enough to require potassium replacement. This drug also causes progressive impairment of renal function that is probably mediated by ischemia induced by renal artery spasm. This is manifested by rises in blood urea and serum creatinine, decrease in creatinine clearance, and the appearance of red and white blood cells, albumin, and casts in the urine. Such renal damage is usually reversible; however, permanent impairment and irreversible renal failure can occur and appear to be related to the total dose of drug used. Some degree of renal impairment has been demonstrated in 40% of adults who have received more than 4 g of amphotericin B. Recent evidence suggests that progression of amphotericin-induced nephrotoxicity may be limited by sodium loading to prevent proximal tubular uptake of the drug.

Hematological toxicity includes a normochromic, normocytic anemia that may be associated with amphotericin B therapy. This is usually reversible and may be related to suppression of erythropoietin. Thrombocytopenia has also been noted occasionally.

Drug Interactions

Caution must be taken to monitor for hypokalemia in patients receiving digitalis preparations. Any drug that is renally excreted may accumulate as a consequence of the renal damage seen in most patients receiving amphotericin B. For example, the toxicity of 5-fluorocytosine (see Chapter 56), which is commonly administered with amphotericin B, may be augmented.

Dosage Regimens and Routes of Administration

Amphotericin B is administered intravenously, although it is occasionally used topically, intraperitoneally, intrathecally, or by direct instillation into the bladder. There is no universal agreement on the method of intravenous administration. It is, however, common practice to treat fungal infections on the basis of a total dose of amphotericin B. That is, anywhere between 200 mg and 3–4 g of amphotericin B will be administered to treat a specific infection. The total amount of the dose will depend upon the specific infecting organism, the host, the site of infection, and the anticipated and observed responses to the treatment. In general, a daily dose of 0.5–1 mg/kg will be administered for as many days as it takes to attain the desired total dose. Some prefer to give this on alternate days, using a similar unit dose. Amphotericin B is the only anti-infective agent that is administered on the basis of a total cumulative dose rather than on the basis of a daily dose administered for a specified period of time. The rationale for this method of administration is not entirely clear.

Therapeutic Applications

Parenteral amphotericin B is used for proven or highly suspected systemic fungal infections caused by susceptible organisms. The major infections treated with this drug in North America are disseminated candidiasis, aspergillosis, coccidioidomycosis, histoplasmosis, mucormycosis, blastomycosis, and cryptococcosis. The topical formulations of amphotericin B are useful for the treatment of cutaneous or mucosal candidiasis. Intraperitoneal amphotericin B has been used successfully for the treatment of fungal peritonitis. Because of poor distribution to the CSF, it is frequently combined with 5-fluorocytosine to treat fungal infections of the central nervous system (e.g., cryptococcal meningitis). Bladder instillation has been used to treat lower urinary tract infections (cystitis) caused by *Candida*.

There are three amphotericin B formulations in current investigational use. These include amphotericin B colloidal dispersion (ABCD), amphotericin B lipid complex (ABLC), and liposomal amphotericin B. These three formulations are less nephrotoxic than amphotericin B, and higher daily doses can be administered. Clinical efficacy superior to that of amphotericin B has not been demonstrated. Some hospitals have attempted to mix amphotericin B with intralipid, a parenteral fat emulsion. However, serum amphotericin B concentrations were lower, as the drug aggregated in the fat emulsion.

TOPICAL IMIDAZOLE ANTIFUNGAL AGENTS

The topical imidazole antifungal agents are synthetic compounds that bind to the heme of the fungal cytochrome P450 and inhibit ergosterol synthesis. Two major drugs in this class are **miconazole** (Micatin, Monistat) and **clotrimazole** (Canesten, Myclo), but there are a number of others with similar properties, such as **oxiconazole** (Oxistat), **econa-**zole (Ecostatin), and **bifonazole** (Mycospor). They are lipophilic compounds with low water solubility at neutral pH, but the imidazole ring is ionized under acidic conditions and this greatly increases water solubility.

Fungal Susceptibility

These agents have a broad spectrum of activity including *Epidermophyton*, *Microsporum*, and *Trichophyton* species; *Pityrosporon orbiculare*; and *Candida albicans*. They can be either fungistatic or fungicidal, depending on the concentration.

Adverse Reactions

Topical imidazoles seldom lead to adverse reactions although they can cause erythema, stinging, blistering, pruritus, and even urticaria at the site of application.

Therapeutic Applications

The topical imidazoles are used to treat superficial fungal infections of the feet, perineum, nails, vagina, and mouth. In general, they are very effective and represent the treatment of choice for such infections. One consideration in the treatment of fungal infections of the nails is that penetration of topical agents into the nails is poor.

SYSTEMIC IMIDAZOLE ANTIFUNGAL AGENTS

Ketoconazole (Nizoral, Fig. 54-2) is an imidazole used for systemic antifungal therapy.

Fungal Susceptibility

Ketoconazole is usually active at levels of less than 0.5 μg/mL against *C. immitis*, *C. neoformans*, and

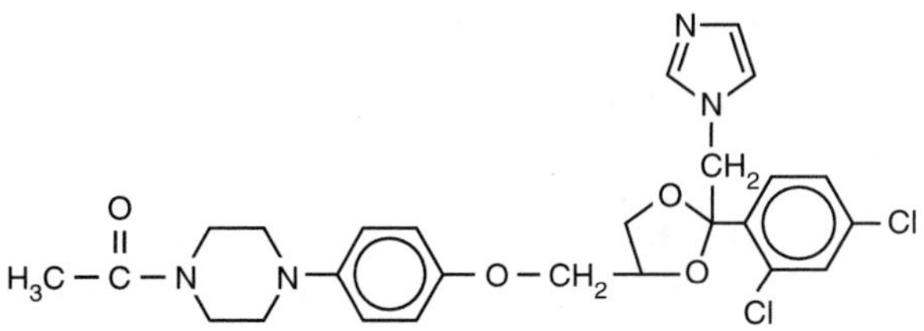

Figure 54-2. Structural formula of ketoconazole.

H. capsulatum. Activity against *Candida, Aspergillus,* and *Sporothrix* usually requires levels from 6 to more than 100 μg/mL.

Pharmacokinetics

Absorption of ketoconazole after oral administration is good; however, an acidic environment is necessary for dissolution of the drug, and absorption is markedly decreased by antacids and histamine H_2-receptor blockers, or in patients with achlorhydria. Rifampin causes a substantial lowering of ketoconazole blood levels, probably by accelerating its biotransformation. The drug is highly protein-bound (90%). Distribution is limited and the level reached in the CNS is very low.

Elimination of ketoconazole is primarily by hepatic biotransformation. The kinetics of ketoconazole appear to be dose-dependent; the half-life increases from 90 minutes after a 200-mg dose to almost 4 hours after an 800-mg dose. This implies the participation of more than one enzymatic pathway, with different kinetic parameters.

Adverse Reactions

The most common side effects of ketoconazole are nausea and vomiting. Mild, asymptomatic elevation of transaminases is observed in 5–10% of patients, and serious **hepatotoxicity** occurs with an incidence of approximately one in 15,000.

Although ketoconazole has some selectivity for the cytochrome P450 that is involved in the synthesis of ergosterol, it also inhibits the metabolism of several other drugs by hepatic cytochrome P450 in a manner similar to that of cimetidine (also an imidazole); and it also inhibits the testicular synthesis of androgens. This is the probable mechanism for the observed association of ketoconazole with gynecomastia in some patients. Cyclosporine drug levels should be monitored during combined therapy with ketoconazole, because these levels usually increase, causing nephrotoxicity.

Dosage and Route of Administration

Ketoconazole is available in 200-mg tablets for oral administration. The usual dose is 200–400 mg a day. In cases of achlorhydria, the drug may be dissolved in dilute hydrochloric acid and sipped through a straw to avoid contact with the teeth. Alternatively, patients are advised to take the drug with a cola drink or orange juice.

Therapeutic Applications

Ketoconazole is used most commonly to treat oral or esophageal candidiasis that is resistant to nystatin. It is also used in the treatment and prophylaxis of vaginal candidiasis. Clinically resistant strains of *Candida* have been noted in patients with HIV. The drug is effective in the treatment of nonmeningeal histoplasmosis involving the lungs, bones, skin or soft tissue, and disseminated disease, but it is less effective than itraconazole (see below). It is effective in nonmeningeal cryptococcal disease, but penetration of the CNS is not sufficient for the treatment of cryptococcal meningitis. It is also useful in the treatment of paracoccidioidomycosis, blastomycosis, and certain dermatomycoses. Its major limitation is its slow onset of action; therefore amphotericin B is usually the drug of choice in severe, acute fungal infections, especially in immunocompromised hosts.

TRIAZOLE ANTIFUNGAL AGENTS

Pharmacokinetics

Absorption of fluconazole (Diflucan, Fig. 54-3) is very good; oral bioavailability is greater than 90%. Oral absorption is not decreased in patients taking histamine H_2-blocking agents. The average half-life is 30 hours. Distribution is to total body water, and the major route of elimination is renal, about 80% of the administered dose appearing in the urine as unchanged drug. Only 11% of serum fluconazole is protein-bound. Concentrations in the CSF are approximately 70% of simultaneous blood levels, whether or not the meninges are inflamed. Rifampin lowers fluconazole blood levels by about 25%.

Itraconazole (Sporanox) is an analog of ketoconazole and its oral absorption is also increased by gastric acidity. The peak blood levels are lower than those of ketoconazole, but tissue levels are higher. The major route of elimination is hepatic biotransformation, and the drug is highly protein bound (99%).

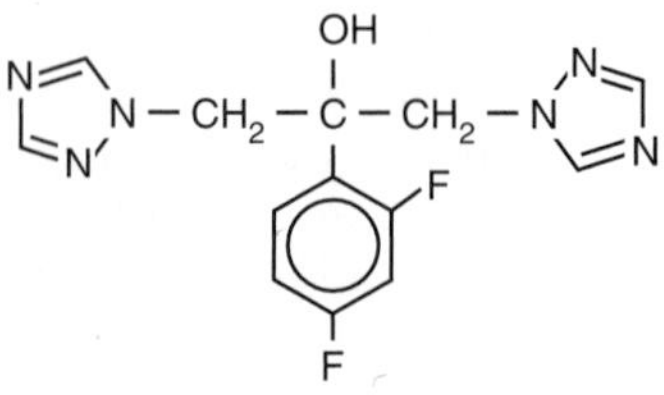

Figure 54-3. Structural formula of fluconazole.

Adverse Reactions

The two most common adverse effects associated with fluconazole appear to be an increase in serum transaminase levels, and skin rashes. Nausea, vomiting, abdominal pain, and diarrhea occur in less than 2% of patients. Hepatic necrosis has been observed but appears to be uncommon. Dose-related nausea and vomiting can complicate itraconazole use. Unlike ketoconazole, itraconazole does not suppress adrenal or testicular function.

Therapeutic Applications

Fluconazole is currently available in 50-, 100-, and 150-mg tablets and as an intravenous formulation. The drug is used in the management of oral and esophageal candidiasis in patients who are unresponsive to nystatin or ketoconazole, or in patients who do not have the gastric acidity required for absorption of ketoconazole. A single dose of 150 mg is as effective as topical therapy of vulvovaginal candidiasis. Because of enhanced CNS penetration, fluconazole is also used in the treatment of cryptococcal meningitis. In general, treatment is initiated with amphotericin B but may be completed with fluconazole. It is very useful for the long-term maintenance therapy of cryptococcal meningitis in patients with AIDS. There are increasing reports in the literature of cases of oral thrush clinically resistant to fluconazole. These are described almost exclusively in patients with advanced HIV infection on long-term use of the drug.

Fluconazole has recently been demonstrated to be equivalent to amphotericin B in the management of systemic candidiasis in nonneutropenic hosts. It has also been shown to be effective in the treatment of *Candida* endophthalmitis.

Fluconazole as prophylactic therapy has been shown to lower the incidence of superficial, deep, and systemic fungal infections (primarily candidiasis) in recipients of bone marrow transplants. An effect on survival has not been demonstrated. Although used prophylactically in febrile neutropenic patients, it has only been shown to decrease the incidence of superficial candidal infections (not invasive fungal infections) in this patient population.

Fluconazole has emerged as the drug of choice of coccidioidal meningitis.

Itraconazole has recently been released for clinical use. It is marketed as a 100-mg capsule. An oral suspension in cyclodextrin is under clinical trial. This may have the advantage of increased local effect. An intravenous formulation is under development.

Itraconazole is useful for the treatment of candidiasis. It has excellent activity against histoplasmosis, sporotrichosis, and blastomycosis, where it has become the drug of choice. There are increasing reports that it is active in invasive aspergillus infections, but its activity in relation to amphotericin B remains uncertain. It appears to be very useful as long-term maintenance therapy against histoplasmosis in AIDS.

Drug Interactions

Simultaneous ingestion with antacids and buffered didanosine (ddI; see Chapter 58) decreases absorption. Rifampin, phenytoin, and carbamazepine decrease itraconazole levels. Itraconazole increases blood levels of cyclosporine, digoxin, terfenadine, astemizole, and loratidine. The last three can lead to torsade de pointes.

Dosage and Route of Administration

Fluconazole is available for both intravenous and oral administration and the dosage is the same for both routes. For oral candidiasis the usual dose is 100 mg/day, but for more serious infections the usual dose is 200–400 mg/day as a single dose. For serious infections a loading dose of double the normal daily dose is recommended. In patients with impaired renal function the daily dose should be decreased. Resistant isolates are increasingly recognized, especially in HIV patients on long-term therapy.

Itraconazole is available for oral administration. The usual dose is 200 mg/day for oral and esophageal candidiasis. For more serious infections a dose of 400 mg/day is used.

ALLYLAMINE ANTIFUNGAL AGENTS

Fungal Susceptibility

Although the present allylamines have some activity against yeasts, they are fungistatic and require doses that are 100-fold higher than those required for activity against dermatophytes; therefore, at the present time their use is limited to the treatment of dermatophyte infections.

Pharmacokinetics

The first antifungal allylamine to be developed was **naftifine** (Naftin). It is available as a topical cream.

Terbinafine (Lamisil) (Fig. 54-4) is available in an oral dosage form. Its bioavailability after oral administration is approximately 70%. It is found in the stratum corneum as early as 24 hours after administration but requires from 3 to 18 weeks to reach therapeutic levels in the nails. After steady state has been achieved, therapeutic levels of terbinafine remain in the skin for 2–3 weeks after administration of the drug is stopped. Terbinafine is extensively biotransformed by cytochrome P450 to at least 15 metabolites. Dosage of terbinafine should be altered when given with other drugs that either induce or inhibit cytochrome P450, and also in the presence of renal failure.

Therapeutic Applications

The allylamines promise to be very effective for the treatment of difficult dermatophyte infections, especially those involving the nails.

SUGGESTED READING

Como JA, Dismukes WE. Oral azole drugs as systemic antifungal therapy. N Engl J Med 1994; 330:263–272.

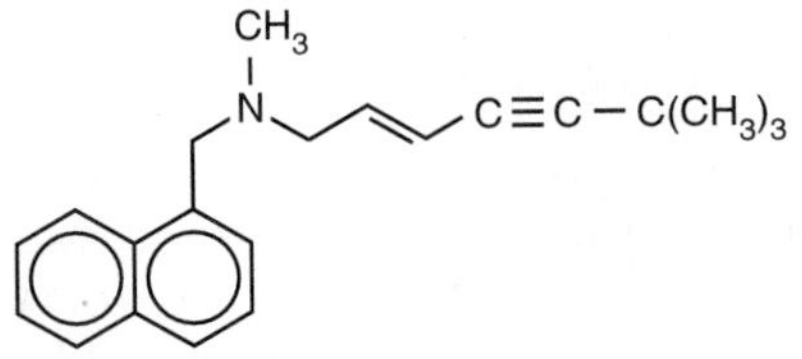

Figure 54-4. Structural formula of terbinafine.

DeMuri GP, Hostetter MK. Resistance to antifungal agents. Pediatr Clin North Am 1995; 42:665–686.

Dismukes WE, Bradsher RW Jr, Cloud GC, et al. NIAID and the Mycoses Study Group. Itraconazole therapy for blastomycosis and histoplasmosis. Am J Med 1992; 93:489–497.

Elewski BE. Mechanisms of action of systemic antifungal agents (Review). J Am Acad Dermatol 1993; 28:S28–S34.

Ernest JM. Topical antifungal agents (Review). Obstet Gynecol Clin North Am 1992; 19:587–607.

Fielding RM. Liposomal drug delivery. Advantages and limitations from a clinical pharmacokinetic and therapeutic perspective. Clin Pharmacokinet 1993; 21:1155–1164.

Sharkey PK, Rinaldi MG, Dunn JF, et al. High dose itraconazole in the treatment of severe mycoses. Antimicrob Agents Chemother 1991; 36:707–713.

Terrell C, Hermans PE. Antifungal agents used for deep-seated mycotic infections. Mayo Clin Proc 1987; 62:1116–1128.

CHAPTER 55

Antimicrobial Agents That Affect the Synthesis of Cellular Proteins

J. UETRECHT AND S.L. WALMSLEY

CASE HISTORY

A 30-year-old man presented to the Sexually Transmitted Diseases Clinic with a 4-day history of dysuria and purulent urethral discharge. He had a new sexual partner, a girl he had met in a bar about 1 week before the onset of the symptoms, and knew little about her health. Contrary to his usual practice, he had decided not to wear a condom.

A Gram stain of the urethral swab showed Gram-negative intracellular diplococci, and a diagnosis of gonorrhea was made. As the incidence of β-lactamase-producing gonorrhea in the area served by this clinic was more than 10%, and because of the patient's history of penicillin allergy, he was treated with a single intramuscular injection of 1 g spectinomycin. As was the policy of the clinic, it was also recommended that he receive treatment against *Chlamydia trachomatis*, and oral doxycycline, 100 mg twice a day for 7 days, was prescribed for him. When the patient went to get this prescription, he mentioned to the pharmacist that he had been under considerable stress recently, and that he was taking antacids. The pharmacist was concerned about the potential for diminished absorption of doxycycline by antacids and called the physician. The doxycycline prescription was changed to azithromycin, 1 g per os. The patient returned to the clinic 1 week after treatment. All symptoms had resolved and follow-up cultures were negative. He remained well.

About 2 years later, while on a camping trip, he developed periumbilical abdominal pain and fever. The pain became more intense and radiated into the lower quadrant over the next few hours. He returned to the city for medical attention. On the trip back, the pain became even more intense, he was diaphoretic, and he complained of lightheadedness. On arrival in the Emergency Room, a diagnosis of acute appendicitis was made, and he was operated on within the hour.

Before surgery he was given 500 mg metronidazole and 80 mg gentamicin intravenously as antibiotic prophylaxis. During surgery it was found that the appendix had ruptured and that there was fecal soiling of the abdominal cavity. He was treated post-operatively with intravenous clindamycin, 600 mg every 8 hours, and with intravenous gentamicin, 400 mg once per day, to cover bowel organisms. He made a successful and uneventful recovery.

BACTERIAL PROTEIN SYNTHESIS

Protein synthesis occurs through translation of the genetic information coded in mRNA. This process takes place on the ribonucleoprotein particles, the ribosomes, and it consists of three stages: initiation, elongation, and termination (shown schematically in Figure 55-1).

In general, the functional unit of bacterial protein synthesis is the 70S ribosome, which consists of two subunits: 30S and 50S. The mRNA attaches to the 30S subunit, and the anticodon of aminoacyl-tRNA

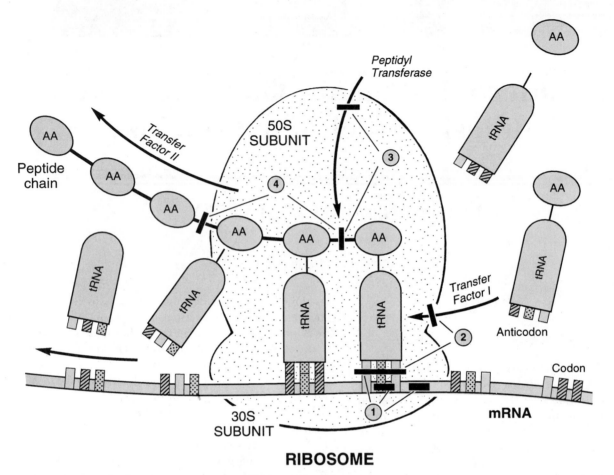

PROTEIN- BINDING (Peptidyl) SITE ("P" Site)

AA-tRNA BINDING SITE ("A" Site)

RIBOSOME

Figure 55-1. Schematic representation of basic elements and steps of bacterial protein synthesis and sites of action of antibiotics that inhibit synthesis. *Principal mechanisms of action:* (1) Aminoglycosides bind to 30S subunit, block initiation, block tRNA binding, distort codons of mRNA, and cause misreading of the genetic code. (2) Tetracy-clines block "A" site binding (tRNA to mRNA); they also chelate essential cations. (3) Chloramphenicol inhibits peptidyl transferase and prevents peptide bond formation. (4) Macrolides block translocation and prevent peptide chain extension. (See text for additional details.)

is matched to the codon on the mRNA. The amino-acyl group attached to the tRNA is bound to the 50S subunit, where peptide bond formation occurs. One of the proteins making up the 50S subunit is peptidyl transferase.

Initiation, i.e., formation of the 70S ribosome, involves various initiation factors by means of which a 30S subunit combines with mRNA and tRNA, and then with a 50S subunit, to complete the 70S ribosome. The tRNA, initially bound to the "A" (aminoacyl) site of the ribosome, is translocated to the "P" (peptidyl) site, freeing the "A" site for addi-tional tRNA.

The elongation stage is essentially a response to a "request" by the codons of mRNA for additional aminoacyl-tRNA, which is first bound to the "A" site and then translocated to the "P" site. Various elongation factors are involved in this process, which is repeated until the message is read and the protein is completed.

Termination of the peptide chain occurs when a terminating codon is reached and the completed chain is discharged from the ribosome. Various ter-mination factors are involved in the release of com-pleted protein. The 50S and 30S subunits dissociate and join a pool of free subunits before recombining with a new messenger.

MECHANISMS OF INHIBITOR ACTION

Several antibiotics inhibit protein synthesis by interfering with translation. They bind to ribosomes and prevent normal peptide chain formation at one or more of several points, which include peptide bond formation, translocation, and movement of the ribosomes along mRNA. The basis for selective toxicity to bacteria with relatively low toxicity to mammalian cells is that, with the exception of the tetracyclines and chloramphenicol, these agents do not bind to mammalian ribosomes. (Chloramphenicol inhibits mammalian mitochondrial protein synthesis in bone marrow precursor cells.) The structure of the mammalian ribosome is different from that of bacteria. Mammalian ribosomes are 80S and are not easily split into subunits.

Aminoglycosides bind tightly to the 30S subunit of the bacterial ribosome and inhibit protein synthesis at several points by blocking the normal activity of the initiation complex, interfering with tRNA attachment, and distorting the triplet codon of mRNA so that the message is misread and faulty proteins are formed. **Spectinomycin,** like the aminoglycosides, binds to the 30S ribosomal subunit, thereby inhibiting protein synthesis. It does not, however, cause misreading of the genetic code.

Tetracyclines also bind to the 30S subunit and block the binding of tRNA to mRNA. They also bind to mammalian ribosomes, but susceptible bacteria concentrate the tetracyclines and, therefore, the drugs can be used at a concentration that will kill bacteria but have little toxicity to mammalian cells. In addition, these agents chelate cations that are essential for protein synthesis, especially magnesium.

Chloramphenicol, clindamycin, erythromycin, and newer macrolides bind to the 50S subunit. Chloramphenicol prevents peptide bond formation by inhibiting the responsible enzyme, peptidyl transferase, which is also located on the 50S subunit. Clindamycin and erythromycin prevent chain extension of growing peptides on the ribosomes and also block translocation or progression to the next codon on mRNA.

It would be expected that agents that inhibit protein synthesis would inhibit bacterial growth and therefore be bacteriostatic rather than bactericidal. Although some of these agents can be bactericidal at high concentrations, this rule of thumb is generally true; however, one exception is the aminoglycosides, which are generally bactericidal. This has led some to speculate that they are active by another mechanism in addition to their action on protein synthesis.

AMINOGLYCOSIDES

The aminoglycoside group of antibiotics includes a large number of structurally related compounds all derived from different species of *Streptomyces.* **Streptomycin** was the first of this group to be discovered (1943), by means of a systematic examination of soil fungi. Subsequently, **neomycin** (1949), **kanamycin** (1957), **gentamicin** (1964), and **tobramycin** (1971) were discovered. Semisynthetic derivatives of these agents, including **amikacin** (1975) and **netilmicin** (1976), were then produced. The main impetus for the original search for these compounds was the lack of significant activity of the penicillins against Gram-negative organisms. The aminoglycoside class of antibiotics remains today one of our most important weapons against Gram-negative pathogens.

Chemistry

The members of this group of antibiotics are characterized by the presence of amino sugars glycosidically linked to aminocyclitols (hence the name "aminoglycoside"; Fig. 55-2).

The pharmacokinetics, adverse reactions, and drug interactions of all systemically used aminoglycosides are very similar, mainly because of their common physicochemical characteristics. The dosages, regimens, routes of administration, and therapeutic applications do differ somewhat, and these aspects must therefore be considered separately for each agent.

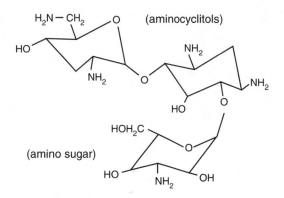

Figure 55-2. Structural formula of tobramycin, a representative aminoglycoside.

Bacterial Susceptibility

The aminoglycosides are active primarily against the Gram-negative aerobes and a limited number of Gram-positive aerobes (e.g., staphylococci). Just as their structure precludes adequate oral absorption or distribution into the CNS, it also makes simple diffusion of the aminoglycosides into bacteria insufficient for antibacterial activity. However, the aminoglycosides are taken up very efficiently by aerobic bacteria by an active transport mechanism linked to the oxidative phosphorylation system of these organisms. For the same reason, the aminoglycosides are inactive against anaerobic bacteria, which do not possess this system. They are also less active in anaerobic environments which inhibit oxidative phosphorylation. Acidic environments protonate the basic aminoglycosides and decrease their uptake. Streptomycin is also quite active against bovine and human mycobacteria (MIC $\sim$ 0.5 μg/mL). Streptomycin, neomycin, and kanamycin are not active against Pseudomonas aeruginosa, but the other four aminoglycoside agents have varying degrees of activity against this organism (Table 55-1). Tobramycin is the most active against the majority of P. aeruginosa isolates and netilmicin is the least active of the four. Other differences in the activity of the four most commonly used aminoglycosides against a variety of microorganisms can also be seen in Table 55-1. For instance, gentamicin is the most active against Serratia marcescens.

An important aspect of activity against Gram-negative aerobes is that increasing resistance has developed in some hospitals and other enclosed environments after extensive use of aminoglycosides. However, problems with resistance to these agents are far less frequent than those observed with the new cephalosporins and quinolones. Resistance results from either chromosomal mutations or plasmid-mediated R-factors that induce the bacteria to produce enzymes that can inactivate some or all of the aminoglycosides. These enzymes cause aminoglycoside inactivation by acetylation, adenylation, or phosphorylation of specific amino or alcohol groups that are necessary for activity (see Fig. 55-2). Of the aminoglycosides represented in Table 55-1, gentamicin is susceptible to the largest number of these enzymes (nine of 12) and amikacin is susceptible to the smallest number (one of 12). It is thus not surprising that the development of resistance appears to be most common with gentamicin and least common with amikacin. When widespread resistance develops to one of the aminoglycosides being used in a particular hospital it is often beneficial to change to another aminoglycoside (to which the bacteria are still sensitive) for some period of time.

There are well-documented cases of endocarditis due to enterococci with a high level of resistance to aminoglycosides. Resistance results from disruption of the synergistic bactericidal interaction between cell-wall–active antibiotics and aminoglycosides. Enterococci are intrinsically resistant to low concentrations of aminoglycoside (4–250 μg/mL) because of their anaerobic metabolism. Strains with MICs of

Table 55-1 Median MICs (in μg/mL) of Aminoglycosides

Bacteria	Gentamicin	Tobramycin	Amikacin	Netilmicin
Gram-positive				
Staphylococcus aureus	0.39	0.5	1.8	0.5
Streptococcus group A	6.3	>25.0	>200	4.0
Streptococcus viridans	4.0	—	>40	—
Enterococcus faecalis	25.0	25.0	>80	16.0
Gram-negative				
Haemophilus influenzae	1.0	0.8	5.0	1.0
Salmonella	0.78	0.4	0.8	0.4
Shigella	0.78	0.8	4.0	0.8
Klebsiella	1.0	1.5	3.0	1.0
Escherichia coli	3.2	2.0	2.0	0.7
Pseudomonas aeruginosa	4.0	1.6	6.0	8.0
Proteus mirabilis	1.0	1.0	2.0	1.0
Serratia marcescens	1.0	3.0	4.0	3.0

2000 μg/mL or more are defined as showing high-level resistance (HLR). HLR is mediated by modifying enzymes.

Pharmacokinetics

Very little of a dose of any of the aminoglycosides is absorbed from the gastrointestinal tract even after oral administration of large doses. They are, however, rapidly absorbed after intramuscular injection and they can also be given intravenously. The concentrations of the various aminoglycosides obtained after specified doses are outlined in Table 55-2. Neomycin is not included in this table as it is too toxic to use systemically.

The apparent volume of distribution of the aminoglycosides ranges from 0.25 to 0.7 L/kg. In general, it is lower in adults and higher in infants. The drugs are not highly protein-bound (less than 30%). They are distributed in all the extracellular fluids but do not generally attain sufficiently high concentrations in the CSF after parenteral administration to be of therapeutic benefit to patients with meningitis. The main site of uptake of the aminoglycosides is the kidney, which accounts for approximately 40% of the total antibiotic in the body. The cortex accumulates approximately 85% of this load, and the resulting concentrations are more than 100 times greater than serum concentrations.

The aminoglycosides are not significantly biotransformed by body tissues but rather are eliminated unchanged, primarily by the kidneys by glomerular filtration. The complete dose is usually not excreted during the first 1–2 days of therapy, but thereafter, over a prolonged period, nearly 100% elimination by this route occurs. The serum elimination half-life of these agents in normal adults ranges from 1.5 to 2.5 hours.

Table 55-2 Pharmacokinetics of Aminoglycosides

Agent	Unit Dose	Usual Serum Concentration (μg/mL)	Half-Life (hours)
Streptomycin	500 mg	15–20	2.5
Kanamycin	7.5 mg/kg	25	2.0
Gentamicin	1.5 mg/kg	5–7	2.4
Tobramycin	2.0 mg/kg	6–8	2.0
Amikacin	7.5 mg/kg	15–30	1.5–2.0
Netilmicin	1.0 mg/kg	3.5–5.0	2.0–2.5

Adverse Reactions

The most important toxicities of the aminoglycosides are those affecting the inner ear and the kidneys.

Ototoxicity may be primarily vestibular or primarily cochlear (in both cases associated with ablation of hair cells). The agents most likely to cause **vestibular toxicity** are streptomycin and gentamicin. The most severe vestibular reactions were noted when streptomycin was used in high doses. Nearly 75% of patients who were given 2 g of streptomycin daily for 60–120 days manifested some vestibular disturbance, whereas reduction of the dose to 1 g daily decreased this incidence to approximately 25%. Inflammation of the meninges also appeared to predispose to ototoxicity, and repeated intrathecal injections of the drug caused earlier and more severe damage than did administration by other routes. The incidence of vestibular symptoms with gentamicin therapy is approximately 2%. This ranges from slight vertigo to an acute Ménière's syndrome. Damage is usually permanent, but patients may diminish their symptoms through adaptation.

The agents most likely to cause **cochlear toxicity** are neomycin, kanamycin, amikacin, and tobramycin. The cochlear toxicity of neomycin is so severe that the systemic use of this agent is precluded. Irreversible deafness will occur from just 1–2 weeks of daily intramuscular therapy using 0.5–1 g. The frequency of hearing loss with tobramycin and amikacin is low, but it may occur without any warning and may be irreversible.

Risk factors that seem to predispose to ototoxicity include increased serum concentrations, prolonged use, advanced age, preexisting renal disease or hearing loss, and the concomitant administration of other ototoxic drugs (e.g., furosemide, ethacrynic acid; see Chapter 41).

The accumulation of the aminoglycosides in the proximal tubules of the renal cortex predisposes to the development of **nephrotoxicity**. Early manifestations of nephrotoxicity include proteinuria, hypokalemia, glycosuria, alkalosis, hypomagnesemia, and hypocalcemia. The usual course is a nonoliguric renal failure that progresses gradually. This nephrotoxicity is dose-related and generally reversible. Its incidence may increase with the concomitant administration of cisplatin, furosemide, ethacrynic acid, or cephalothin, and it is potentiated by volume depletion.

Another adverse reaction to the aminoglycosides is a competitive type of **neuromuscular blockade** (blocking potency of the aminoglycosides is less than

1% that of *d*-tubocurarine), which occurs most frequently after intraperitoneal administration. Hypersensitivity reactions to the aminoglycosides are infrequent, although a contact dermatitis is the most common side effect of topically applied neomycin. This usually occurs after prolonged use and is unlikely to be noted with short-term treatment.

Over the years, considerable research has led to a better understanding of the pharmacokinetics and pharmacodynamics of aminoglycosides, ensuring the achievement of therapeutic concentrations to optimize antibacterial activity and lessen their toxicity. Consequently, many hospitals have now adopted once-daily dosing schedules for administration of aminoglycosides.

The aminoglycosides demonstrate a property known as concentration-dependent killing. Clinical studies have demonstrated that achievement of high peak-serum concentrations relative to the MIC of the infecting microorganism is a major determinant of the clinical response. This can best be obtained by once-daily administration. In addition, aminoglycosides demonstrate a property known as the postantibiotic effect. This is defined as a period of time after complete removal of the antibiotic during which there is no growth of the organism. Therefore, despite the 12-hour period after which there are no detectable serum concentrations when aminoglycosides are given once daily, therapeutic efficacy is not compromised consequent to this postantibiotic effect. The once-daily dosage schedule is also theoretically associated with lesser toxicity. The uptake and accumulation of aminoglycosides into renal cortical tissue demonstrate saturable kinetics, making peak concentrations irrelevant. Less frequent dosing does allow for serum concentrations to fall below the threshold for binding to tissue receptors and allows back-diffusion of the aminoglycosides from the renal cortex and inner ear. Numerous published studies have shown equivalent outcomes between once and multiple daily dosing of aminoglycosides with no excess of toxicity, but with considerable cost savings and elimination of the need for therapeutic drug-level monitoring.

Drug Interactions

The β-lactam ring of penicillins and cephalosporins reacts with the amino group of aminoglycosides and inactivates them; therefore, penicillins and cephalosporins should not be mixed in the same bottle with aminoglycosides. Inactivation can also occur in vivo,

but this is of little clinical significance with the possible exception of patients with renal failure, in whom the concentration of penicillin can be very high. In such instances, the administration of the β-lactam and the aminoglycoside on a staggered schedule will minimize this interaction.

There is also a positive interaction between aminoglycosides and β-lactams as well as other agents, such as vancomycin, which inhibit cell wall synthesis, because these agents increase the uptake of aminoglycosides into bacteria, especially Gram-positive bacteria. This is especially important for the treatment of bacterial endocarditis and *P. aeruginosa* infections.

Other nephrotoxic agents, such as amphotericin B, may increase the risk of renal toxicity.

Dosage Regimens, Routes of Administration, and Therapeutic Applications

Streptomycin

Adults are usually treated with 15 mg/kg/day intramuscularly, in one or two doses. The drug may be given only once or twice weekly in the initial treatment of tuberculosis. This is used uncommonly today as first-line initial treatment of tuberculosis, except in multiple-drug-resistant strains, because of its toxicity by this route and the availability of more acceptable therapeutic alternatives.

Neomycin (Mycifradin, Myciguent, Neobiotic)

The drug may be used topically in combination with other antibiotics (to prevent the emergence of resistant bacteria) in the treatment of superficial staphylococcal or Gram-negative infections. Oral neomycin is also used to reduce the quantity of intestinal flora in patients with hepatic failure. Bladder irrigation with neomycin is used in the prevention or treatment of urinary tract sepsis in patients with indwelling urethral catheters or in those who have just undergone a urological procedure (e.g., cystoscopy).

Gentamicin (Cidomycin, Garamycin), tobramycin (Nebcin, Tobrex), amikacin (Amikin), and netilmicin (Netromycin)

The usual dosages and regimens of these four aminoglycosides are outlined in Table 55-3. (As stated earlier, however, there may be a move to once-a-day administration rather than the fractional doses

Table 55-3 Dosages and Regimens of Aminoglycosides

Agent	Usual Daily Total Dose (mg/kg)	Usual Number of Fractional Doses per Day
Gentamicin	4.5–5.0	3
Tobramycin	5.0–7.5	3
Amikacin	15–20	2–3
Netilmicin	4.5–6.0	3

described in this table.) They are administered by the intravenous, and rarely by the intramuscular, route. Occasionally in the treatment of cephalosporin-resistant Gram-negative meningitis and other CNS infections these aminoglycosides are also administered by the intrathecal or intraventricular route. Topical formulations (e.g., ointments, ear drops, eye drops) are also available.

The most important indications for using one of these aminoglycosides are Gram-negative infections, including infections of blood, bones and joints, intraabdominal and pelvic cavities, soft tissue and wounds, and the urinary tract. These drugs are also invaluable in the empirical treatment of neutropenic febrile hosts who are at great risk of Gram-negative septicemia. They also act in synergy with the penicillins or cephalosporins against numerous bacteria (see Drug Interactions above). This is particularly important in the treatment of serious enterococcal infections. The choice among the four aminoglycosides is influenced by several factors including the resistance pattern of organisms within the institution, the familiarity of the clinicians with the individual antibiotics, and the cost of each agent to the patient.

SPECTINOMYCIN

Spectinomycin (Trobicin) is an antibiotic produced by *Streptomyces spectabilis*. The drug is an aminocyclitol. It is active against a number of Gram-negative bacterial species but is inferior to other drugs. Its most important activity is that against *N. gonorrhoeae*, which it inhibits at concentrations of 7–20 μg/mL.

Absorption, distribution, and excretion of spectinomycin are similar to those of the aminoglycosides. A single dose of 2 g produces peak plasma concentrations of 100 μg/mL at 1 hour.

Local discomfort after intramuscular injection is the most common adverse reaction. The risk of oto- and nephrotoxicity is low because the drug is administered as a single injection in a dose of 35 mg/kg (up to 2 g). It is used exclusively for the treatment of gonorrhea suspected or proven to be due to a penicillin-resistant strain, where ceftriaxone or quinolones cannot be used.

TETRACYCLINES

The development of tetracycline antibiotics was the result of systematic screening of soil samples from many parts of the world. The first tetracycline, chlortetracycline, was introduced in 1948. The most recent tetracycline congener is minocycline (introduced in 1972).

Chemistry

The tetracyclines are all derivatives of the polycyclic substance naphthacenecarboxamide (Fig. 55-3). There are a number of these agents, including **tetracycline** (Achromycin, Tetracyn), **chlortetracycline** (Aureomycin), **oxytetracycline** (Terramycin), **demeclocycline** (Declomycin), **rolitetracycline** (Reverin), **methacycline** (Rondomycin), **doxycycline** (Vibramycin), and **minocycline** (Minocin). Of these, the three most commonly used are tetracycline, doxycycline, and minocycline.

Bacterial Susceptibility

The tetracyclines are active against a broad spectrum of bacteria. Susceptible strains include a wide range of Gram-positive and Gram-negative bacteria, *Mycoplasma*, *Rickettsia*, and *Chlamydia*. They are also very active against *Treponema pallidum*. The median MICs for three commonly used tetracyclines against representative organisms are shown in Table 55-4. Minocycline is generally the most active of the tetracyclines, especially against *S. aureus*. When resistance develops, it is usually due to bacterial membrane transport proteins that prevent the accumulation of tetracyclines by decreasing the influx and increasing the ability of the bacteria to export antibiotics. Such proteins are coded for by plasmids, which can be transferred between bacteria and usually result in resistance to all tetracyclines.

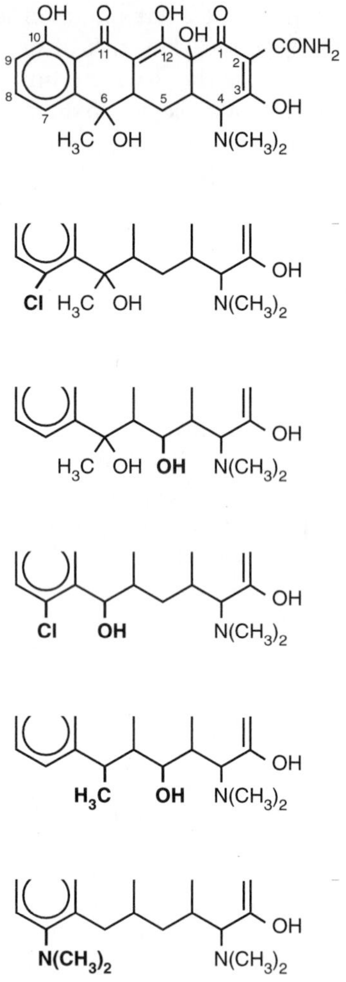

Figure 55-3. Structural formulae of tetracyclines.

Pharmacokinetics

All tetracyclines are absorbed adequately but incompletely after an oral dose. Absorption is most active in the stomach and upper small intestine and is greater in the fasting state. With the exception of minocycline and doxycycline, which do not have a hydroxyl group in the 6 position (see Fig. 55-3), the tetracyclines are unstable in the acid environment of the stomach, and this contributes to their incomplete oral bioavailability.

Tetracyclines are effective chelating agents against various cations, with which they form poorly soluble complexes. Accordingly, absorption from the intestinal tract is impaired by milk and milk products, which contain Ca^{2+}, and by the coadministration of aluminum hydroxide gels or calcium, magnesium, or iron salts. After a 250 mg oral dose of tetracycline to an average-sized adult, the serum concentrations are 2–3 μg/mL. After a 100-mg oral dose of doxycycline or minocycline, serum concentrations are 1–2 μg/mL.

The volumes of distribution of the tetracyclines range from 0.4 L/kg for minocycline to 1–2 L/kg for doxycycline and tetracycline. Their protein binding ranges from 60% (tetracycline) to 80–95% (doxycycline). Tetracyclines are widely distributed, especially the highly lipid-soluble compounds minocycline and doxycycline. They enter the CSF quite freely, attaining concentrations 10–50% of those in the serum, but they are seldom used for meningitis because of better alternative agents. Because of chelation of tissue calcium deposits, the drugs become markedly bound to bones, teeth, and neoplasms, in which they cause yellow fluorescence.

The main mode of elimination of most of the tetracyclines is renal glomerular filtration, but they are also eliminated to a greater or lesser extent via the biliary route. For most of the tetracyclines, 20–60% of the administered dose is found in the urine in unchanged form. Minocycline is recoverable in the urine and feces in significantly lower amounts than the other tetracyclines, and it appears to be biotransformed to a considerable degree. Doxycycline is excreted primarily in the feces (90%) as an inactive metabolite or perhaps as a chelate. The half-lives of these drugs range from 6 hours (tetracycline) to 24 hours (doxycycline).

Adverse Reactions

Hypersensitivity reactions to the tetracyclines are rare. **Gastrointestinal disturbances** (nausea, vomiting, and diarrhea) are common, and pseudomembranous colitis has been described.

Photosensitivity reactions may be caused by any of the tetracyclines but are most frequent with doxycycline.

Tooth and bone deposition of these agents represents the most important side effect of the tetracyclines in pediatrics and is the reason these agents are **contraindicated in children** and, because they cross the placenta, during fetal development. The depositions are in the calcifying areas of teeth and bones, and they may discolor both deciduous and permanent teeth. Tetracycline deposition in bone may result in temporary cessation of bone growth. This latter effect is reversible when the drug is discontinued.

Hepatotoxicity is an uncommon but serious adverse reaction, which has been described primarily after the intravenous administration of large doses of tetracycline to pregnant women. This reaction has

Table 55-4 Median MICs (in μg/mL) of Tetracyclines

Bacteria	Tetracycline	Doxycycline	Minocycline
Gram-positive			
Staphylococcus aureus	3.19	1.6	0.78
Streptococcus group A	0.78	0.39	0.39
Streptococcus viridans	3.1	0.39	0.39
Enterococcus faecalis	>100	>100	>100
Streptococcus pneumoniae	0.8	0.2	0.2
Gram-negative			
Neisseria meningitidis	0.8	1.6	1.6
Neisseria gonorrhoeae	0.78	0.39	0.39
Haemophilus influenzae	1.6	1.6	1.6
Shigella	100.0	100.0	100.0
Klebsiella	50.0	50.0	25.0
Escherichia coli	12.5	12.5	6.3
Pseudomonas aeruginosa	200.0	100.0	200.0
Proteus mirabilis	>100	>100	>100
Serratia	200.0	50.0	25.0
Bacteroides fragilis	12.5	—	—
Other *Bacteroides*	0.25	—	—
Others			
Mycoplasma pneumoniae	1.6	1.6	1.6
Treponema pallidum	0.4	0.1	—
Chlamydia	2.0	2.0	2.0

usually been fatal. The liver shows extensive fatty infiltration at autopsy.

Outdated tetracycline products have resulted in a "Fanconi-like" syndrome (renal tubular abnormalities), with acidosis, nephrosis, and aminoaciduria. Tetracyclines may also cause further increases in BUN and serum creatinine in patients with renal failure. These biochemical changes, as well as tetracycline-induced azotemia, have been attributed to an antianabolic effect of the drugs.

Benign increase of the intracranial pressure (pseudotumor cerebri) has been observed as a side effect of tetracycline therapy. It is reversible upon discontinuation of the medication.

Manifestations of neurotoxicity are observed frequently and almost exclusively with minocycline. Dizziness, weakness, ataxia, and vertigo appear within the first few days of therapy.

Drug Interactions

Antacids containing the divalent cations Ca^{2+}, Al^{3+}, or Mg^{2+}, and iron salts used in the treatment of anemia, can bind these antibiotics and may result in diminished absorption of the tetracyclines from the intestinal tract when administered concomitantly.

Diuretics, presumably acting by volume depletion, may aggravate the increases in BUN observed with the tetracyclines.

Dosage Regimens and Routes of Administration

Tetracycline is usually administered orally at a daily dose of 25–50 mg/kg divided into four equal doses. Minocycline is usually administered orally in a daily dose of 4 mg/kg divided into two equal doses. The daily dose of doxycycline is 5 mg/kg, administered in two doses orally.

Therapeutic Applications

Possible clinical indications for the tetracyclines include acute exacerbations of chronic bronchitis, *Mycoplasma* pneumonia, gonorrhea and syphilis in penicillin-allergic patients, early Lyme disease, Q fever, psittacosis, brucellosis, rickettsial infections, and lymphogranuloma venereum. Minocycline has a therapeutic advantage over the other tetracyclines in the treatment of *Nocardia* infections. Doxycycline and minocycline are unique among the tetracyclines in that they do not accumulate in renal insufficiency. Doxycycline can therefore be used in the rare situation in which a tetracycline is the drug of choice in a patient with renal insufficiency. It may also be the drug of choice for genital tract infection with *Chlamydia* or *Mycoplasma*.

CHLORAMPHENICOL

Chloramphenicol (Chloromycetin) was first isolated in 1947 from *Streptomyces venezuelae*, an organism found in a soil sample from Venezuela. After the structural formula of this antimicrobial agent was determined, it was prepared synthetically.

Chemistry

Chloramphenicol is a lipid-soluble compound lacking acidic and basic groups that could form salts. It is unique among natural compounds in that it contains a nitrobenzene moiety, which can be *reduced* by cytochrome P450 (see Chapter 4). Of the four stereoisomers of the propanediol moiety, only the D-threo isomer has antibacterial activity (Fig. 55-4).

Bacterial Susceptibility

Most aerobic bacteria except *P. aeruginosa*, practically all anaerobes, and the majority of clinically important types of *Mycoplasma*, *Chlamydia*, and *Rickettsia* are susceptible to chloramphenicol at concentrations achievable in the serum. MICs of chloramphenicol against representative bacteria are outlined in Table 55-5.

Although chloramphenicol is bacteriostatic against most organisms, it is bactericidal in vitro against most strains of *Haemophilus influenzae*, *Streptococcus pneumoniae*, and *Neisseria meningitidis*. The mechanism of this bacterial killing action is not known.

The principal mechanisms of acquired resistance to chloramphenicol are the production of a bacterial

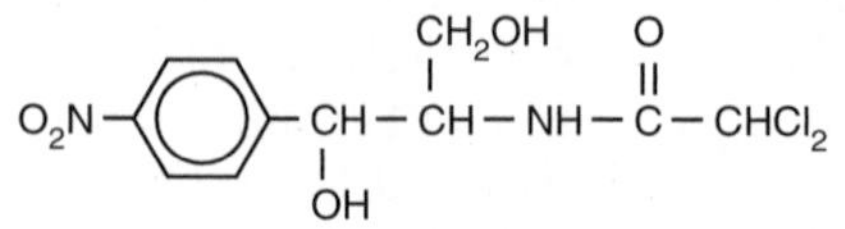

Figure 55-4. Structural formula of chloramphenicol.

Table 55-5 MIC Ranges (in μg/mL) of Chloramphenicol

Gram-positive bacteria	
Staphylococcus aureus	1.0–5.0
Streptococcus group A	0.3–6.0
Streptococcus viridans	0.6–2.5
Enterococcus faecalis	6.3– >100
Streptococcus pneumoniae	0.06–12.5
Gram-negative bacteria	
Neisseria meningitidis	0.78–6.25
Neisseria gonorrhoeae	0.78–6.3
Haemophilus influenzae	0.2–3.5
Salmonella	0.75–5.0
Shigella	2.5–6.0
Klebsiella	0.5–25.0
Escherichia coli	3.0–50.0
Pseudomonas aeruginosa	8.0–1000
Proteus mirabilis	3.0–25.0
Serratia marcescens	2.5–5.0
Bacteroides fragilis	0.5–16.0
Other *Bacteroides*	0.1–16.0

acetyltransferase that inactivates the drug and the loss of permeability of the bacterial cell wall to chloramphenicol.

Pharmacokinetics

Chloramphenicol is rapidly and completely absorbed from the intestinal tract. It is generally administered as the tasteless palmitate, which must be hydrolyzed to free active base in the intestinal lumen before absorption can occur. The peak serum concentration is approximately the same as that attained after a similar dose given intravenously, but the peak is not reached until 2 hours after an oral dose.

After an intravenous dose of 500 mg of the succinate form administered to an adult, rapid hydrolysis to the free drug results in serum concentrations of 6–10 μg/mL.

The apparent volume of distribution of chloramphenicol is approximately 0.9 L/kg. It is 50–60% protein-bound. It diffuses into most body fluids and tissues, and unlike many other antibiotics, chloramphenicol penetrates well into the CSF even in the absence of meningitis. In the presence of meningitis, CSF concentrations often reach 70–80% of serum levels; brain tissue concentrations exceed those in the serum.

Chloramphenicol is converted in the liver to a highly water-soluble monoglucuronide, which has no biological activity. Impaired liver function might reduce the rate of conjugation to glucuronic acid (see Chapter 4) and correspondingly increase serum concentrations of active drug.

About 90% of chloramphenicol is excreted in the urine, but only 5–10% of this is in the unchanged active form. Active chloramphenicol is excreted only by glomerular filtration, but the inactive derivatives (glucuronic acid conjugates) are also eliminated by tubular secretion. Only a small amount of chloramphenicol (2–3%) is excreted in bile, mostly in the inactive form, and less than 1% appears in the feces. The serum half-life of chloramphenicol is approximately 3 hours.

Adverse Reactions

The most feared complication of chloramphenicol therapy is **aplastic anemia.** It occurs in approximately one in 40,000 patients treated with this drug. The mechanism is unclear but appears to be related to the presence of the nitro group, because the analog in which the nitro group is replaced with a methylsulfone group has not been associated with aplastic anemia.

A second type of hematopoietic depression is dose-related. Serum concentrations in excess of 20–25 μg/mL invariably result in reduced iron utilization by the bone marrow, and vacuolization of erythroblasts, megakaryocytes, and leukocyte precursors. Anemia, thrombocytopenia, and leukopenia result. This type of **marrow toxicity,** apparently due to inhibition of mitochondrial protein synthesis in bone marrow precursor cells, is reversible and responds to discontinuance of the drug.

A toxic reaction to chloramphenicol observed almost exclusively in neonates is the **gray baby syndrome** (see Chapters 4 and 65). This is a form of circulatory collapse associated with excessive serum concentrations of unconjugated chloramphenicol maintained for several days because of immaturity of the glucuronyl transferase system in the liver of the neonate.

Drug Interactions

Chloramphenicol may inhibit cytochrome P450-mediated metabolism of phenytoin, oral hypoglycemic agents, and oral anticoagulants, with resultant phenytoin toxicity, hypoglycemia, or hemorrhage, respectively.

Some drugs such as phenobarbital can induce liver microsomal enzymes and, hence, increase the total body clearance of chloramphenicol, resulting in reduced serum concentrations of the drug. Acetaminophen, on the contrary, can prolong the half-life of chloramphenicol and lead to drug accumulation, perhaps because of reduction of its rate of biotransformation by glucuronidation.

Dosage Regimens and Routes of Administration

The drug can be administered by the oral or intravenous route. The recommended dose by either route is the same, 50–100 mg/kg/day divided into four doses. Significant dose reductions are necessary in neonates (see above). Marked variations in individual patient kinetics necessitate the monitoring of serum concentrations and appropriate adjustments in dosage.

Therapeutic Applications

Chloramphenicol is active against most strains of bacteria that commonly cause meningitis, including *H. influenzae, N. meningitidis, and S. pneumoniae.* It is also active against *Salmonella,* including *S. typhi,* rickettsiae, and almost all anaerobic bacteria that would be found in abscesses. However, the risk of aplastic anemia and the availability of new alternatives have resulted in the replacement of chloramphenicol by other drugs for most indications. Some remaining indications are bacterial meningitis or brain abscesses in patients with a history of a severe hypersensitivity reaction to penicillins and cephalosporins, or in cases of penicillin-resistant pneumococcal meningitis, and also rickettsial infections, such as Rocky Mountain spotted fever, typhus, or Q fever in children or pregnant women for whom tetracyclines would be contraindicated.

CLINDAMYCIN

Lincomycin, the parent compound of clindamycin, was isolated from the fermentation products of a soil streptomycete found in Lincoln, Nebraska, and called *Streptomyces lincolnensis.* Clindamycin is the 7-chloro-7-deoxy derivative of lincomycin. This family of agents is referred to as the lincosamides.

Bacterial Susceptibility

The antibacterial activity of the lincosamides is very similar to that of erythromycin (see below). Clindamycin is generally more active than lincomycin.

These agents generally show activity against Gram-positive organisms except the enterococci, but are inactive against Gram-negative aerobes with the exception of *H. influenzae*. They are also active against anaerobic bacteria, notably the cocci and Gram-negative rods. MICs against representative bacteria are given in Table 55–6.

Pharmacokinetics

Clindamycin hydrochloride (Dalacin C) is well absorbed from the gastrointestinal tract; a dose of 300 mg produces peak serum concentrations of 4–5 μg/mL, 1–2 hours after administration. The ester, clindamycin palmitate hydrochloride, is available as a suspension. This compound must be hydrolyzed in vivo to the active base, but serum levels attained with it are nearly the same as those with clindamycin capsules.

The intramuscular and intravenous preparation is a 2-phosphate derivative. It, too, must be converted in vivo to its active form. Peak serum concentrations are higher after intravenous administration. After a 300-mg intramuscular dose the mean peak concentration is 4–5 μg/mL. After a similar intravenous dose the mean peak concentration is 14–15 μg/mL.

The apparent volume of distribution of clindamycin is 0.6–0.75 L/kg. It is 90–95% protein bound. It is widely distributed in the body and does not appear to be concentrated in any particular organ. Penetration into bone and across the inflamed meninges into the CSF is moderate, the concentrations reaching approximately 40% of those in serum.

After the administered compound is converted to active drug in the serum, biotransformation takes place primarily in the liver. Two metabolic derivatives are a dimethyl and a sulfoxide form. The former is more active, and the latter is less active, than the base.

The main organ of clindamycin elimination is the liver, and only 8–28% of the drug is excreted in the urine. Thus, hepatic insufficiency has a more profound effect on clindamycin kinetics than does renal insufficiency. The half-life of clindamycin is normally 2–4 hours.

Adverse Reactions

Gastrointestinal disturbances represent the most important group of adverse reactions to clindamycin. Diarrhea, which is self-limited and subsides with discontinuance of therapy, occurs in up to 30% of cases. It may be associated with nausea, vomiting, and/or abdominal cramps. A more significant gastrointestinal side effect is pseudomembranous colitis. This was first described in association with clindamycin, but almost every antibiotic has now given rise to cases of it. It is caused by overgrowth of toxin-producing *Clostridium difficile* in the feces. The observed variation in incidence reflects the inconsistent presence of *C. difficile* in stools of patients in different locations and institutions.

Minor abnormalities of liver function tests occur with clindamycin use. No significant drug interactions have been reported.

Dosage Regimens and Routes of Administration

The usual recommended oral dose of clindamycin is 10–25 mg/kg/day, administered in four equal doses. The intravenous or intramuscular daily dose is 10–40 mg/kg, divided into two to four equal doses.

Therapeutic Applications

Clindamycin is primarily useful in the treatment of a variety of anaerobic infections, including those

Table 55-6 Median MICs (in μg/mL) of Clindamycin and Erythromycin

Bacteria	Clindamycin	Erythromycin
Gram-positive		
Staphylococcus aureus	0.1	0.5
Streptococcus group A	0.04	0.04
Streptococcus viridans	0.02	0.5
Enterococcus faecalis	100.0	1.5
Streptococcus pneumoniae	0.01	0.1
Gram-negative		
Neisseria meningitidis	12.5	0.78
Neisseria gonorrhoeae	3.1	0.94
Haemophilus influenzae	12.5	2.5
Salmonella	>100	>100
Shigella	>100	>100
Klebsiella	>100	>100
Escherichia coli	>100	>100
Pseudomonas aeruginosa	>100	>100
Proteus mirabilis	>100	>100
Serratia marcescens	>100	>100
Bacteroides fragilis	0.1	1.6
Other *Bacteroides*	0.1	1.0

caused by *B. fragilis*. Some examples of anaerobic infections that have been successfully treated with clindamycin, either alone or in combination with other antimicrobial agents, include intraabdominal and pelvic infections, aspiration pneumonia, anaerobic pleuropulmonary infections, infected decubitus ulcers, diabetic foot infections, and periodontal disease. Unfortunately the incidence of resistance among *B. fragilis* is increasing; estimates as high as 19% have been reported recently.

Clindamycin is a useful antibiotic in a variety of staphylococcal and streptococcal infections as an alternative to penicillin, and it has recently been recommended for patients with structural heart defects who require prophylactic antibiotic therapy but are allergic to penicillin and intolerant to erythromycin. It is also used topically as an effective treatment for acne vulgaris.

Other newer uses that are being explored include combination with primaquine for the treatment of *Pneumocystis* pneumonia; in combination with pyrimethamine for the treatment of toxoplasmosis; and in combination with quinine for the treatment of chloroquine-resistant *P. falciparum* malaria (see Chapter 57).

MACROLIDES

Erythromycin (E-Mycin, Erythromid) was discovered in 1952 in the metabolic products of a strain of *Streptomyces erythreus*, originally obtained from a soil sample collected in the Philippine Archipelago. It is a macrolide antibiotic, so named because it contains a many-membered lactone ring to which are attached deoxy sugars.

New macrolides are being developed. One such erythromycin analog, **clarithromycin** (Biaxin), is 6-methoxyerythromycin. Clarithromycin and **azithromycin** (Zithromax) have recently been marketed and others, such as roxithromycin, are under investigation. They have significant advantages over erythromycin, including less frequent dosing, less GI toxicity, and higher tissue levels; but they are also much more expensive. They have increased in vitro activity against many of the respiratory pathogens including *H. influenzae*, *Legionella*, *C. pneumoniae*, and *Moraxella*.

Bacterial Susceptibility

The antibacterial activity of **erythromycin** is very similar to that of clindamycin (see above). The agent is mainly active against Gram-positive aerobes. It is generally inactive against Gram-negative aerobes with the exceptions of *Neisseria* species, *Haemophilus*, *Bordetella*, *Campylobacter*, and *Legionella*. The Gram-negative anaerobes are not reliably sensitive. Erythromycin is also active against *Rickettsia*, *M. pneumoniae*, *Ureaplasma*, and *Chlamydia*. MICs against representative bacteria are shown in Table 55–6.

Clarithromycin is two to four times more active than erythromycin against most strains of *Staphylococcus* and *Streptococcus*, but cross-resistance with erythromycin has been observed. Clarithromycin also appears to have increased activity against *Haemophilus influenzae* and good activity in vitro against *Branhamella*, *Legionella*, *Mycoplasma*, and *Chlamydia*.

Development of resistance against the macrolides is uncommon, but it may develop by

1. Alteration in the single 50S ribosomal protein of the receptor
2. Plasmid-mediated alteration (i.e., methylation of adenine moiety) in the 50S ribosomal RNA
3. Enzymatic inactivation
4. Decreased cell envelope permeability

Pharmacokinetics

Erythromycin base is adequately absorbed from the gastrointestinal tract, although its activity is destroyed by gastric juice, and food in the stomach delays its absorption. These problems are overcome by enclosing the drug in acid-resistant capsules or by administering a stearate derivative. Another derivative, erythromycin estolate, is less susceptible to acid than the base, and food does not appreciably alter its absorption. Peak serum concentrations of erythromycin range from 0.5 to 1 μg/mL after a 500-mg oral dose of erythromycin base or stearate. Peak serum concentrations are two to four times higher when an equivalent dose of the estolate preparation is given. After intravenous administration of 500 mg of erythromycin, serum concentrations are approximately 5 μg/mL.

The volume of distribution of erythromycin is approximately 0.7 L/kg, and it is 70–75% protein-bound. It is distributed throughout the body water and tends to be retained longer in the liver and spleen than in the blood. Only very low levels are attained in the CSF even in the presence of inflamed meninges.

Only a small amount of erythromycin is excreted

in its original form. It is presumed that the remainder is demethylated or otherwise degraded. Excretion occurs in both the urine and the bile, but only a fraction of the dose can be accounted for in this way. The half-life of erythromycin is approximately 1.5 hours.

Adverse Reactions

Gastrointestinal side effects, including nausea, vomiting, diarrhea, and abdominal cramps, are frequent after oral erythromycin and represent a major limitation to its use. The incidence of gastrointestinal side effects associated with clarithromycin or azithromycin is much lower than that with erythromycin, and patients who are unable to tolerate erythromycin can usually tolerate the newer macrolides.

Hepatotoxicity, which has been documented with the estolate and other erythromycin preparations (although considerably less frequently), is felt to be due to the propionyl ester linkage. Manifestations may include jaundice, fever, pruritus, rash, increased liver size, and eosinophilia. Liver histology reveals a hypersensitivity cholestasis with or without necrosis. This adverse reaction generally resolves when the antibiotic is discontinued.

Thrombophlebitis is a common side effect after intravenous administration. Ototoxicity, manifested as tinnitus and transient deafness, is a rare adverse reaction that has occurred more frequently after intravenous than after oral administration. Rashes are not uncommon in association with erythromycin use, but significant allergic reactions are rare.

Drug Interactions

Erythromycin has been found to inhibit some isozymes of cytochrome P450, especially CYP3A4. Thus, the use of erythromycin has led to increases in theophylline and cyclosporine concentrations. It was recently shown that the concomitant use of erythromycin and terfenadine or astemizole leads to elevated levels of their active metabolites. In some patients this appears to be associated with a prolongation of the Q-T interval and cardiac arrhythmias. Inhibition of the metabolism of other drugs is likely, but evidence for other interactions will require further trials.

Dosage Regimens and Routes of Administration

The usual recommended oral dose of erythromycin ranges from 20 to 50 mg/kg/day, divided into two to four equal doses. The daily intravenous dose is the same, usually administered in two doses.

Therapeutic Applications

Erythromycin is useful in the treatment of staphylococcal, streptococcal, and pneumococcal infections in patients who cannot tolerate penicillins. Additional indications for erythromycin therapy include the treatment of *Mycoplasma* infections *(M. pneumoniae* and *Ureaplasma)*, the eradication of *Bordetella pertussis* and *diphtheriae* from the nasopharynx, *Chlamydia* infections, the treatment of Legionnaire's disease, the treatment of gonorrhea or syphilis during pregnancy, and the eradication of *Campylobacter* from the stools of patients with *Campylobacter* gastroenteritis.

Clarithromycin and azithromycin are useful as alternatives to erythromycin in patients who have a gastrointestinal intolerance to erythromycin, or in serious infections where they are more active. They may be particularly useful in community-acquired pneumonia. They are currently being evaluated in the treatment and prevention of disseminated *Mycobacterium avium* infections in patients with AIDS.

SUGGESTED READING

Barradell LB, Plosker GL, McTavish D. Clarithromycin: a review of its pharmacological properties and therapeutic use in *Mycobacterium avium-intracellulare* complex infection in patients with acquired immune deficiency syndrome (Review). Drugs 1993; 46:289–312.

Brittain DC. Erythromycin. Med Clin North Am 1987; 71:1147–1154.

Davey P. Clinical use of the aminoglycosides in the 1990's. Rev Med Microbiol 1991; 2:22–30.

Gilbert DW. Once daily aminoglycoside therapy. Antimicrob Agents Chemother 1991; 35:399–405.

Klein NC, Cunha BA. Tetracyclines. Med Clin North Am 1995; 79:789–802.

Leclercq R, Dutka-Malen S, Brisson-Noel A, et al. Resistance of enterococci to aminoglycosides and glycopeptides (Review). Clin Infect Dis 1992; 15:495–501.

Lortholary O, Tod M, Cohen Y, Petitjean O. Aminoglycosides. Med Clin North Am 1995; 79:761–788.

Schlossberg D. Azithromycin and clarithromycin. Med Clin North Am 1995; 79:803–815.

Shaw KJ, Rather PN, Hare RS, Miller GH. Molecular genetics of aminoglycoside resistance genes and familial relationships of the aminoglycoside-modifying enzymes (Review). Microbiol Rev 1993; 57:138–163.

Smilack JD, Wilson WR, Cockerill FR. Tetracyclines, chloramphenicol, erythromycin, clindamycin, and metronidazole. Mayo Clin Proc 1991; 66:1270–1280.

Whitman MS, Tunkil AR. Azithromycin and clarithromycin: overview and comparison with erythromycin. Infect Control Hosp Epidemiol 1992; 12:357–368.

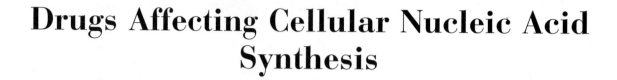

CHAPTER 56

Drugs Affecting Cellular Nucleic Acid Synthesis

J. UETRECHT AND S.L. WALMSLEY

CASE HISTORY

A 36-year-old male immigrant from Sri Lanka saw his physician after a 3-week history of cough, hemoptysis, fever, and weight loss of about 5 kg. A chest X-ray revealed a right upper lobe infiltrate with cavity. A sputum smear was positive for acid-fast bacilli, and *Mycobacterium tuberculosis* was later confirmed on culture. He was started on treatment with isoniazid 300 mg/day, rifampin 600 mg/day, ethambutol 25 mg/kg/day, and pyrazinamide 25 mg/kg/day. His wife and children were also seen by the physician and were given isoniazid prophylaxis at a dose of 300 mg/day (wife) and 10 mg/kg/day (children) when their skin tests were found to be positive. On culture, the patient's infecting microorganisms were found to be sensitive to all first-line antituberculous drugs.

Ethambutol and pyrazinamide were discontinued after 2 months of treatment. Isoniazid and rifampin were continued for another 4 months. His signs and symptoms resolved completely and his chest X-ray improved.

After full recovery from this bout of tuberculosis, he visited his homeland for a period of one month. Three days before his return to North America, he developed fever and bloody diarrhea, which was quite severe during the flight home. He immediately saw his family physician, who collected a stool specimen. Because he had a fever of 39°C and continued bloody diarrhea, the physician started him empiri-

cally on oral ciprofloxacin at a dose of 500 mg twice daily. The physician received a report that *Shigella* was isolated from the stool samples, whereupon ciprofloxacin was continued for a period of seven days. All signs and symptoms of the disease resolved.

Bacterial replication, like that of all living cells, requires replication of the DNA and RNA that contain and transfer the genetic codes for the synthesis of all constituents of the cell. Compounds that inhibit the replication of bacterial nucleic acids but are sufficiently selective to have little or no effect on mammalian nucleic acids are potentially useful in treating infectious diseases. Inhibition of nucleic acid replication by these compounds may be either direct or indirect.

DIRECT INHIBITORS OF NUCLEIC ACID REPLICATION

Rifampin (antibiotic), and perhaps griseofulvin (antifungal), inhibit the replication of nucleic acids directly. **Rifampin** acts by inhibiting bacterial RNA polymerase, which is concerned with RNA replication. Human DNA-dependent RNA polymerase, however, is resistant to rifampin. **Nalidixic acid** and the newer **fluoroquinolones** inhibit the enzymatic activities of bacterial DNA gyrase (DNA topoisomerase), which is responsible for introducing superhelical twists into closed double-stranded DNA. The DNA gyrase produces breaks in the DNA strands, supercoiling occurs by the passage of another strand of DNA through the break, and then the break is resealed. The superhelical twists are necessary to allow packaging of the DNA within the bacterial nucleus. DNA topoisomerase is necessary in DNA replication, repair, and genetic recombination. Binding of a quinolone to the DNA gyrase results in an inhibition of the rejoining reaction after a breaking reaction has occurred. It has been proposed that **griseofulvin** exerts its antifungal activity by inhibiting fungal DNA production. Griseofulvin also binds to microtubular protein and inhibits mitosis. It is also toxic to mammalian cells, and the basis for useful selective toxicity appears to involve the selective distribution of the drug to keratinized cells, especially those that are diseased.

5-Fluorocytosine is also thought to inhibit the replication of nucleic acids directly, by acting as a fluorine analog of the normal body constituent cytosine. It appears that this drug enters susceptible yeast cells and is deaminated by cytosine deaminase to the antimetabolite 5-fluorouracil. 5-Fluorouracil is converted through several steps to 5-fluorodeoxyuridylic acid monophosphate, a noncompetitive inhibitor of thymidylate synthetase. This interferes with DNA synthesis. Conversion of flucytosine to 5-fluorouracil within the body occurs to a sufficient degree to be a possible explanation for its toxicity to bone marrow and the gastrointestinal tract (mucositis).

INDIRECT INHIBITORS OF NUCLEIC ACID REPLICATION

Sulfonamides, sulfones, probably **para-aminosalicylic acid,** and the diaminopyrimidines (**trimethoprim** and **pyrimethamine**) inhibit the replication of nucleic acids more remotely by interfering with the synthesis of folic acid by microbial cells. Folic acid functions as a coenzyme for transfer of one-carbon units from one molecule to another, a step necessary for the synthesis of thymidine and the other nucleosides. Mammals require preformed folic acid (it is a vitamin for them; see Chapter 49). In contrast, bacteria cannot use preformed folic acid, which cannot enter the bacterial cell; instead, they must synthesize it intracellularly from para-aminobenzoic acid (PABA). Sulfonamides act by competitively inhibiting the incorporation of PABA into folic acid. The presence of an extraneous source of PABA

(e.g., pus, blood, tissue exudates) can decrease the effectiveness of the sulfonamides as competitive binders. Trimethoprim is a dihydrofolate reductase inhibitor. It potentiates the activity of sulfonamides by sequential inhibition of folinic acid synthesis (Fig. 56-1). The resulting depletion of folic or tetrahydrofolic acid within the bacterial or parasitic cells inhibits the formation of coenzymes necessary for the synthesis of purines, pyrimidines, and other substances required for growth and reproduction. Although this does not usually result in cell death, the sulfonamides and related compounds are selectively toxic to bacteria. Pyrimethamine is more active than trimethoprim in inhibiting the dihydrofolate reductases of *Plasmodium* species and *Toxoplasma gondii*, whereas trimethoprim is more active against bacteria. Both drugs can inhibit mammalian dihydrofolate reductase at high concentrations. Trimetrexate is a lipid-soluble dihydrofolate reductase inhibitor with activity against *T. gondii* and *Pneumocystis carinii*. (Methotrexate, which binds to *human* as well as microbial dihydrofolate reductase, is used as an antimetabolite in the treatment of some neoplastic diseases, severe psoriasis, and rheumatoid arthritis. See Chapter 60.)

ANTIFUNGAL AGENTS

Griseofulvin (Fulvicin, Grisovin)

Griseofulvin was isolated from *Penicillium griseofulvium* in 1939, but was not used clinically as an antifungal agent until nearly 20 years later.

It inhibits the growth in vitro of various species of *Microsporum*, *Epidermophyton*, and *Trichophyton*. Minimum inhibitory concentrations against sensitive fungi range from 0.18 to 0.42 μg/mL.

Pharmacokinetics

Griseofulvin is reasonably well absorbed from the intestinal tract, although there is considerable variability and fluctuation in serum concentration in the same subject, or in different individuals receiving the same dose. A serum concentration of 1–2 μg/mL is attained about 4 hours after a 1-g dose. Concentrations are enhanced approximately twofold if the drug is taken after a fatty meal rather than fasting.

The volume of distribution and degree of protein binding of this drug are unknown, but some of it is carried in the circulation to the skin, hair, and nails,

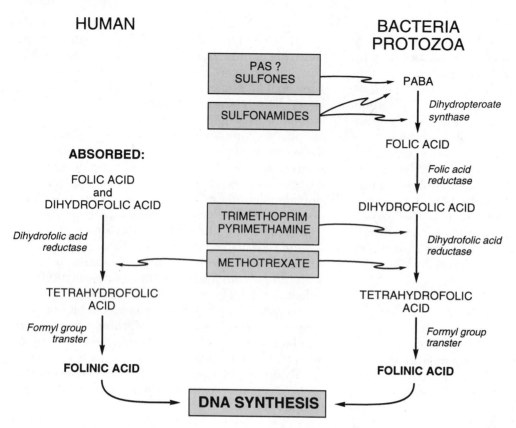

Figure 56-1. Sites of action of sulfonamides and inhibitors of dihydrofolic acid reductase (trimethoprim in bacteria, pyrimethamine in protozoa, methotrexate in all species including human). Because it binds to *human* dihydrofolate reductase, methotrexate is used as an antineoplastic drug of the antimetabolite class. (See Chapter 60 for structure and mechanism of action.)

where it is concentrated by selective binding to keratin.

Most of the absorbed drug is inactivated in the liver by dealkylation. This inactivation may be enhanced by barbiturates through induction of drug-biotransforming enzymes. The inactive metabolite of griseofulvin is excreted in the urine. A considerable proportion of an oral dose, which is unabsorbed, appears unchanged in the feces. The plasma half-life is 10–20 hours.

Adverse reactions

Nausea, vomiting, diarrhea, headache, fatigue, and mental confusion may all occur with griseofulvin therapy but are uncommon.

Drug interactions

The coadministration of barbiturates may increase the rate of biotransformation of griseofulvin, resulting in reduced serum concentrations.

Griseofulvin itself may induce liver microsomal enzymes and may increase the biotransformation of warfarin, thus diminishing the anticoagulant effect of the latter.

Therapeutic applications

Griseofulvin is effective in the systemic treatment of dermatophyte infections caused by *Microsporum, Trichophyton,* and *Epidermophyton.* It is primarily useful in infections of the scalp, hands, feet, and nails that are refractory to topical therapy.

5-Fluorocytosine (5-FC, Flucytosine) (Ancobon)

5-Fluorocytosine was synthesized in 1957 as a cytosine antimetabolite for the treatment of leukemia. It was found to be ineffective for this purpose but was noted in 1964 to possess selective antifungal activity.

Fungal susceptibility

The drug inhibits *Cryptococcus neoformans* and *Candida albicans* in concentrations of 0.46–3.9 μg/mL and kills them at concentrations of 3.9–15.6 μg/mL. Other fungi that are sensitive to this drug include the non-*albicans* species of *Candida* and *Torulopsis glabrata*. *Aspergillus* species are variably sensitive with MIC ranges of 0.48–500 μg/mL.

Drug resistance arising during therapy is frequent and rapid, usually profound, and accompanied by clinical deterioration. Fungal mechanisms for resistance include loss of deaminase (for conversion of 5-FC to 5-fluorouracil) and decreased permeability. 5-FC is usually used in combination with amphotericin B because of this problem.

Pharmacokinetics

Flucytosine is well absorbed following oral administration. Peak serum concentrations of approximately 45 μg/mL are attained 2–6 hours after a 2-g dose.

The volume of distribution of 5-FC is 0.6–0.7 L/kg. It is approximately 10% protein-bound. It is well distributed in body fluids and tissues, and during the treatment of fungal meningitis it attains concentrations in the CSF that are 50–100% of those in the serum.

A small amount of 5-FC is converted to 5-fluorouracil, and approximately 90% of 5-FC is excreted unchanged via the kidney by glomerular filtration. It must be used cautiously in patients with impaired renal function. Unabsorbed 5-FC, usually less than 10%, is excreted unchanged in the feces. Its plasma half-life is 3–4 hours, which may increase to more than 100 hours in the presence of renal disease.

Adverse reactions

Dose-dependent hematological toxicity with thrombocytopenia and/or granulocytopenia is common and is dose-limiting. Agranulocytosis and aplastic anemia have also been reported. Nausea and vomiting are frequent. Given the high incidence of adverse reactions, it is imperative that the dosage recommendations be followed carefully, especially in patients receiving concurrent amphotericin B, and serum levels should be monitored.

Dosage, route of administration, and therapeutic applications

Flucytosine is administered orally every 6 hours to provide a total daily dose of 50–150 mg/kg. It is

most useful in the treatment of cutaneous and mucocutaneous candidiasis, *Candida* urinary tract infections, and in combination with amphotericin B in the treatment of cryptococcal meningitis. It may also play a therapeutic role as a synergistic agent in other systemic fungal infections caused by sensitive organisms.

ANTITUBERCULOUS DRUGS

(See also Chapter 53: Cycloserine, Isoniazid, Ethambutol.)

Rifampin (Rifadin, Rimactane)

Rifampin is a complex macrocyclic antibiotic produced by *Streptomyces mediterranei*, which was first isolated in 1959.

Bacterial susceptibility

The drug is active against a wide range of Gram-positive and Gram-negative organisms (Table 56-1). However, resistance, which may emerge rapidly when it is used alone, limits its widespread use. Its strongest antibacterial attribute is its activity against the majority of *Mycobacterium tuberculosis* strains (MIC = 0.5 μg/mL or less).

Table 56-1 Median MICs (in μg/mL) of Rifampin

Gram-positive bacteria	
Staphylococcus aureus	0.001
Streptococcus group A	0.04
Streptococcus viridans	0.05
Enterococcus faecalis	4.0
Streptococcus pneumoniae	0.05
Gram-negative bacteria	
Neisseria meningitidis	0.016
Neisseria gonorrhoeae	0.2
Haemophilus influenzae	0.5
Klebsiella	10.0
Escherichia coli	5.3
Pseudomonas aeruginosa	20.0
Proteus mirabilis	3.9
Serratia	64.0
Bacteroides fragilis	0.26
Other *Bacteroides*	0.1
Mycobacterium tuberculosis	0.5

Pharmacokinetics

Rifampin is well absorbed from the intestinal tract. The peak concentration of 8 $\mu g/mL$ is reached approximately 2 hours after a 600-mg oral dose. Serum concentrations are lower if the drug is taken immediately after food.

The volume of distribution of rifampin is approximately 1.6 L/kg. It is 60–90% protein-bound. Rifampin penetrates well into most tissues and fluids including lungs, liver, pleural and ascitic fluid, bone, tears, saliva, and the CSF whether or not the meninges are inflamed. Concentrations in the CSF during therapy for tuberculous meningitis usually exceed 50% of serum concentrations.

Rifampin is deacetylated in the liver, and it must also be inactivated elsewhere in the body to some extent, because a proportion of the dose remains undetected in excretion studies.

Adverse reactions

The major serious adverse reaction associated with the use of rifampin is liver disease. The type of injury is usually obstructive and jaundice occurs in 0.6% of treated patients; however, hepatocellular disease with an increase in transaminases can also occur. The use of high doses, or interruption and reinstatement of therapy, can lead to what appear to be immune-mediated reactions. Such reactions can consist of hemolytic anemia and thrombocytopenia, acute renal failure, a syndrome of fever, chills, myalgia and arthralgia, and even hepatorenal syndrome. Rifampin has been reported to cause immune suppression, but the significance of this effect is unknown. Patients should be warned that rifampin leads to an orange-pink coloration of tears, urine, and sweat and can stain soft contact lenses.

Drug interactions

Rifampin is a potent inducer of cytochrome P450 and can decrease the levels of many other drugs. This can lead to break-through bleeding and pregnancy in women using birth control pills.

Therapeutic applications

The major indication for rifampin is the treatment of mycobacteria infections, especially tuberculosis. Despite its high activity, it should always be used in combination with at least one other agent for the treatment of active tuberculosis to decrease the emer-

gence of resistant strains (see isoniazid, Chapter 53). Rifampin is also the antibiotic of choice for the chemoprophylaxis of contacts of patients with meningococcal or *H. influenzae* meningitis. Rifampin is often used in combination with cloxacillin in the treatment of serious *S. aureus* infections. It is effective against intracellular organisms. Its penetration into nasal-pharyngeal secretions also allows its use in the eradication of *S. aureus* nasal carriage.

Pyrazinamide (Tebrazid)

Pyrazinamide is a synthetic analog of nicotinamide. Its mode of action on tubercle bacilli is not known. The drug is bactericidal at acid pH, like that existing intracellularly in phagolysosomes, but replicating microorganisms become rapidly resistant to it when it is used alone. Metabolically inactive tubercle bacilli are resistant, rendering the drug inappropriate for long-term therapy. It may be used as an antitubercular drug only together with other agents in multiple-drug treatment schedules.

Pharmacokinetics

Pyrazinamide is well absorbed after oral administration. It is widely distributed, it readily penetrates cells and diffuses into cavities, and it enters the CSF when the meninges are inflamed. The drug is biotransformed in the liver to pyrazinoic acid and then to 5-hydroxypyrazinoic acid, which is excreted by renal glomerular filtration. The half-life is about 6 hours.

Adverse reactions

Pyrazinamide at high doses (40–50 mg/kg/day) causes hepatotoxicity, which has resulted in fatal hepatic necrosis in some instances. Therefore the drug is currently used at much lower dosage, but it still requires monitoring for hepatotoxicity during the entire period of therapy. Since pyrazinamide inhibits urate excretion, episodes of hyperuricemia are frequently observed, as well as occasional nausea, vomiting, fever, polymyalgia, and malaise.

Dosage regimens and therapeutic application

Pyrazinamide is an important drug for short-term (4–6 months) multiple-drug therapy, primarily in areas with high primary resistance to antitubercular agents. The daily dosage is 20–35 mg/kg orally, divided into three or four equally spaced doses, not to exceed 3 g per day regardless of the patient's weight.

Para-Aminosalicylic Acid (PAS) (Nemasol)

Over 50 years ago, it was determined that benzoic and salicylic acids increased the oxygen consumption of tubercle bacilli. It was speculated that similar compounds played a role in the normal metabolism of *M. tuberculosis*, and it was theorized that structurally altered analogs might have an opposite effect. This led to the discovery of PAS, a drug that is chemically closely related to salicylic acid and that probably acts as a competitive antagonist of *p*-aminobenzoic acid.

Thus, PAS inhibits folate synthesis, but also mycobactin synthesis. Mycobactin is a "siderophore," and its inhibition reduces the uptake of iron by mycobacteria.

Pharmacokinetics

PAS is well absorbed from the intestinal tract. Maximum serum concentrations of 50–150 μg/mL are attained 1–2 hours after a 2-g dose. The drug is 50–60% protein-bound. It is distributed throughout the total body water and reaches concentrations in the pleural fluid and in caseous tissues approximately equal to those in the circulation. It does not yield effective CSF concentrations, possibly because it is actively transported out of the CSF.

PAS is biotransformed in the liver mainly by acetylation. Over 80% of the drug is excreted in the urine by glomerular filtration and tubular secretion. Only 14–33% of the total dose is excreted in the urine as the active unchanged drug. The remainder is excreted as metabolites such as acetyl-*p*-aminosalicylic acid, *p*-aminosalicyluric acid, and other conjugated amines. The half-life of PAS is less than 1 hour.

Adverse reactions

Nausea, vomiting, anorexia, abdominal cramps, and diarrhea occur to some extent in nearly all patients. These may be reduced by taking the drug with meals or by the concomitant administration of antacids.

Drug interactions

Para-aminosalicylic acid may enhance the effect of anticoagulants and inhibit the biotransformation of acetylsalicylic acid, thereby allowing toxic amounts to accumulate. Probenecid may inhibit tubular secretion of PAS, and PAS may impair the absorption of rifampin.

Dosage regimen, route of administration, and therapeutic applications

The usual daily dose of PAS is 200–300 mg/kg administered orally, divided into two or three doses. This drug is used as a second or third agent, in combination with other more effective agents, in the treatment of infections caused by *M. tuberculosis*. More recently, it has been used in combination with second-line antitubercular drugs in the treatment of multiple-drug-resistant tuberculosis.

QUINOLONE ANTIBACTERIAL AGENTS

The prototype drug is **nalidixic acid** (NegGram), an old drug with limited use as a urinary antiseptic. The development of **fluoroquinolones** has greatly extended the antibacterial spectrum and usefulness of these agents. Three examples of the fluoroquinolones are **norfloxacin** (Noroxin), **ciprofloxacin** (Cipro), and **ofloxacin** (Floxin).

Bacterial Susceptibility

Although nalidixic acid has a broad spectrum of activity against Gram-negative organisms, its activity is weak, resistance emerges rapidly, and it is inactive against all Gram-positive organisms.

Nalidixic acid (Fig. 56-2) is bacteriostatic. Addition of a fluorine and removal of the ethyl side-group yields norfloxacin. The fluoroquinolones show activity against Gram-positive organisms and increased activity against Gram-negative organisms. The fluoroquinolones also are bactericidal. Their spectrum of activity includes *Staphylococcus aureus* (including methicillin-resistant strains), most streptococci, enterococci, and most other Gram-negative enteric organisms, *H. influenzae*, and *Neisseria gonorrhoeae*. Addition of a piperazine ring, as in ciprofloxacin, increases fluoroquinolone activity against *Pseudomonas*.

There are many new analogs under development in attempts to improve the activity against Gram-positive, anaerobic, and pseudomonal organisms. There has been a rapid emergence of resistant strains in a short period of time since the introduction of these drugs, which may seriously limit their continued usefulness. For example, in one prospective study

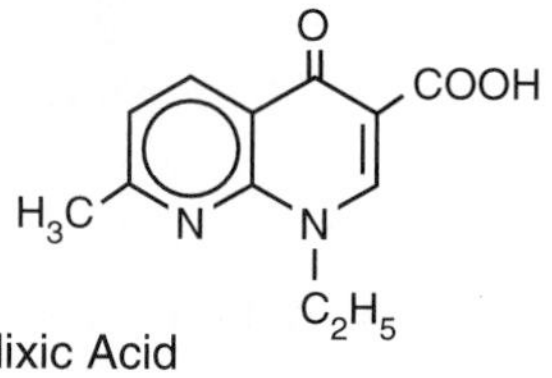

Nalidixic Acid

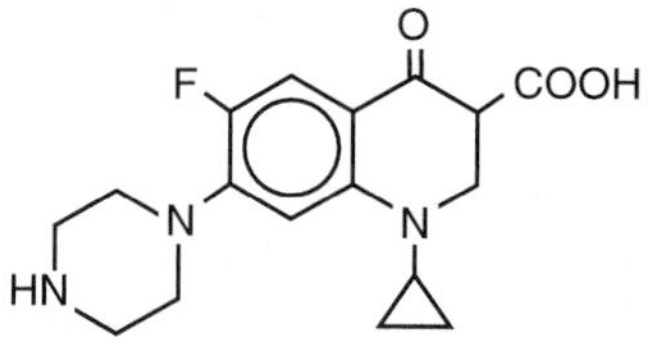

Ciprofloxacin

Figure 56-2. Structural formulae of nalidixic acid and ciprofloxacin.

the incidence of resistance of methicillin-resistant strains of *S. aureus* to ciprofloxacin increased from zero to 79% in just 1 year. The rate of development of resistance among *P. aeruginosa* and mycobacteria is also about 1000 times faster than that of most other bacteria. The development of such resistance is probably due to changes in the outer membrane proteins that lead to decreased permeability to the drug and/or alteration in DNA gyrase.

Pharmacokinetics

The fluoroquinolones are well absorbed when given orally; they are available for both oral and parenteral administration. They penetrate well into most body fluids. However, the activity of norfloxacin is relatively low and it does not achieve adequate concentrations in serum or tissues to treat most systemic infections; its use is limited to infections of the urinary tract. The half-lives of norfloxacin and ciprofloxacin are about 4 hours, and these agents need to be administered only every 8–12 hours. Elimination is about half by renal excretion and half by biotransformation, and the dose may need to be adjusted in renal and hepatic failure.

Adverse Reactions

Severe adverse reactions are uncommon with the fluoroquinolones. The most common side effects are gastrointestinal symptoms. CNS symptoms, includ-

ing headache, confusion, and hallucinations are infrequent, and seizures have been reported but are rare. Rashes and other allergic reactions, including anaphylaxis, have also been observed. The fluoroquinolones cause damage to developing cartilage in animals, and although there is no evidence that this also occurs in humans, these agents are not recommended for use in children or in pregnant or nursing women. Although laboratory abnormalities such as increased transaminases and leukopenia have been reported, these abnormalities appear to be reversible.

Drug Interactions

When coadministered with aluminum-, magnesium-, and to a lesser degree calcium-containing antacids, the quinolones have markedly reduced bioavailability, presumably due to the formation of cation–quinolone complexes. Some quinolones inhibit hepatic microsomal enzymes involved in theophylline and caffeine metabolism. This can result in decreased theophylline clearance and toxicity. This is a greater problem with ciprofloxacin than with ofloxacin.

Therapeutic Applications

A major indication for the fluoroquinolones is the treatment of urinary tract infections and chronic prostatitis involving organisms, such as *P. aeruginosa*, that are resistant to other oral agents. They are also used as second-line therapy in complicated urinary tract infections or in patients who are allergic to sulfonamides. Another important indication is the treatment of chronic osteomyelitis and diabetic foot infections caused by Gram-negative organisms, and these agents have allowed many such infections to be treated at home rather than in hospital; in contrast, the only other antibiotics effective for this indication require frequent intravenous administration. Likewise, the use of fluoroquinolones for the treatment of pneumonia in patients with cystic fibrosis, commonly caused by *P. aeruginosa*, has allowed many patients to be treated at home. However, given their poor activity against *Streptococcus pneumoniae*, they should not be used in the treatment of most community-acquired pneumonia. Other uses for the fluoroquinolones include the empirical treatment of bacterial diarrhea, including travellers' diarrhea; the treatment of invasive external otitis; treatment of gonorrhea, including penicillin-resistant strains; treatment, in combination with other agents, of disseminated *Mycobacterium avium-intracellulare* infections in AIDS patients; prophylaxis in some patients at high risk of Gram-negative infections, such as cancer patients receiving chemotherapy; and for the outpatient management of diabetic foot infections. Given their activity against Gram-negative organisms, they are frequently used as step-down therapy for patients with nosocomial pneumonia. As with imipenem, it is important to avoid the indiscriminate use of these agents in order to slow the development of resistant strains of bacteria.

Dosage and Routes of Administration

Norfloxacin and ofloxacin are given orally while ciprofloxacin is available in both oral and intravenous dosage forms. The recommended daily dose of ciprofloxacin for urinary tract infections is 500 mg divided into two doses, but for more severe infections doses of up to 1.5 g/day are given. The recommended daily dose of norfloxacin for urinary tract infections is 800 mg, while that of ofloxacin is 400–800 mg, both divided into two doses.

ANTIFOLS

Sulfonamides

Sulfonamides were the first group of synthetic antibacterial compounds for systemic use, based on Ehrlich's concepts of selective toxicity as outlined in Chapter 52. The original studies of the clinical effectiveness of Prontosil were reported by Domagk in 1935. At first, the claims pertained only to infections caused by hemolytic streptococci, but soon, with modifications of the molecule, activity against a wider range of bacteria was demonstrated.

Chemistry

All sulfonamides are amides of *p*-aminobenzene–sulfonic acid (sulfanilamide, Fig. 56-3). Three basic features necessary for antibacterial action are (1) a benzene ring with a sulfonic acid group, (2) an amide nitrogen on the sulfonic acid, and (3) a free amino group in the para position. The activity of the sulfonamides is also dependent on a negative charge on the amide nitrogen such that it mimics the carboxylate anion of *p*-aminobenzoic acid. The free amino group in the para position represents the primary site of sulfonamide degradation.

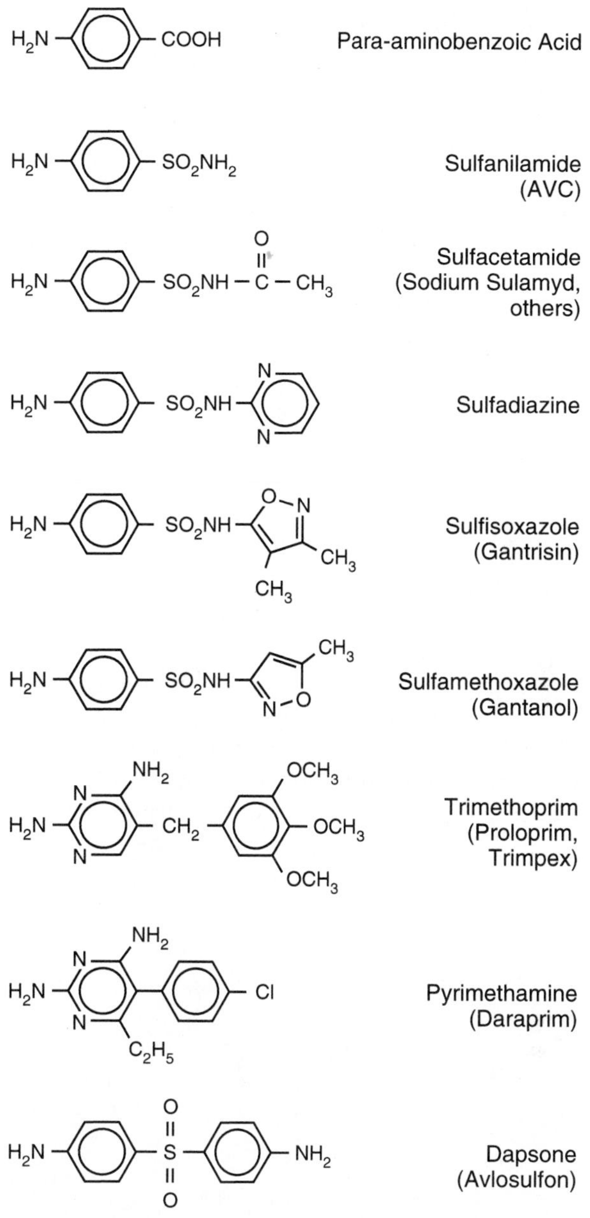

Figure 56-3. Structural formulae of para-aminobenzoic acid, some sulfonamides, trimethoprim, pyrimethamine, and dapsone.

Bacterial susceptibility

The sulfonamides originally had a wide range of activity, but this range has been seriously compromised by acquired bacterial resistance. Resistance is usually due to either microbial overproduction of PABA or structural changes in the dihydropteroate synthase enzyme. Resistance may also be mediated by plasmids. This form of resistance has increased in recent years, often in combination with trimethoprim resistance.

Gram-positive bacteria that are usually sensitive to sulfonamides include group A streptococci, *Streptococcus viridans*, some *Streptococcus pneumoniae*, and *Nocardia*. Staphylococci are variably sensitive and *Enterococcus faecalis* is resistant. The most sensitive Gram-negative species are the *Neisseria*, many enterobacteria, *H. influenzae*, and *Bordetella pertussis*. Some representative bacteria and their median MICs are outlined in Table 56-2. Sulfonamides are also active against *Chlamydia*, *Toxoplasma*, and some *Plasmodium* species.

Pharmacokinetics

The sulfonamides are often classified on the basis of their pharmacokinetics, specifically on the basis of their half-lives. Hence, there are short-acting, medium-acting, long-acting, and ultra-long-acting forms. There are also those that are poorly absorbed from the intestinal tract. Only a few sulfonamides remain in use today, notably sulfadiazine, sulfisoxazole, and sulfamethoxazole. These drugs are described below as a group, using sulfisoxazole (a widely used short-acting sulfonamide) as a representative. Where important differences exist between various agents, they are specifically noted below.

All sulfonamides (excepting sulfaguanidine and the other poorly absorbable derivatives) are well absorbed after oral administration. Serum concentrations vary somewhat between the sulfonamides. The peak concentrations of sulfisoxazole after a 1-g dose range from 50 to 100 μg/mL. Intravenously injectable sulfonamides attain high plasma concentrations extremely well.

The sulfonamides are generally well distributed throughout the body, including the CSF. There is some variation in this distribution between individual agents. For instance, CSF concentrations of sulfisoxazole are approximately 30% of those in the serum, whereas the CSF concentrations of sulfadiazine are about 50% of serum concentrations. The volume of distribution of the sulfonamides is small, that of sulfisoxazole being 0.16–0.2 L/kg. Protein binding is very variable amongst these agents, ranging from 20% for some of the short-acting forms to over 90% for the long-acting drugs.

A percentage of the absorbed sulfonamide is acetylated (at the para-amino group) in the liver to inactive conjugates. Individual acetylating capacity is variable in a manner analogous to that for INH. Some sulfonamides also undergo glucuronide conjugation to inactive metabolites in the liver.

Free and conjugated sulfonamides are excreted via the kidneys by both glomerular filtration and tubular secretion. The long-acting forms, which are more extensively protein-bound, undergo more complete tubular reabsorption and hence have prolonged half-lives. Since the sulfonamides and their metabolites are weak acids, their clearance is increased in alkaline urine. Minimal amounts of sulfonamides are excreted in the bile. Half-lives of the sulfonamides range from 2 hours to as much as 200 hours, depending on the individual agent. The half-life of sulfisoxazole is 5–6 hours.

Table 56-2 Median MICs (in μg/mL) of Sulfonamides and Trimethoprim

Bacteria	Sulfonamides*	Trimethoprim
Gram-positive		
Staphylococcus aureus	50.0	0.2
Streptococcus group A	12.5	0.4
Streptococcus viridans	8.0	0.25
Enterococcus faecalis	100.0	1.0
Streptococcus pneumoniae	32.0	1.0
Gram-negative		
Neisseria meningitidis	5.0	8.0
Neisseria gonorrhoeae	4.0	12.0
Haemophilus influenzae	0.5	0.12
Salmonella	10.0	0.4
Shigella	4.0	0.4
Klebsiella	16.0	0.5
Escherichia coli	8.0	0.2
Pseudomonas aeruginosa	25.0	>100
Nocardia	12.5	>100

*Variations between individual sulfonamides occur.

Adverse reactions

Hypersensitivity reactions ranging from a mild rash to severe Stevens-Johnson syndrome may occur. The latter reaction is an extreme form of erythema multiforme, characterized by bulla formation in the mouth, pharynx, anogenital region, and conjunctivae. Though rare, it produces serious morbidity when it does occur. It is more common in children, especially with long-acting sulfonamides. The incidence of adverse reactions in patients with AIDS who receive sulfonamides, usually given as co-trimoxazole for the treatment of *Pneumocystis carinii* pneumonitis (PCP), is about 50% (or about 100 times higher than in other patients). These reactions usually consist of a rash and fever with variable involvement of other organs such as the liver, kidneys, or bone marrow. The basis for this increased risk of an adverse reaction to sulfonamides in patients with AIDS is unknown.

Hematological toxicity may also occur with sulfonamide use. Reactions include agranulocytosis, which is usually reversible on discontinuance of the drug, and hemolytic anemia in patients with G-6-PD deficiency. Aplastic anemia has also been described as a rare complication.

In the neonate, sulfonamides are contraindicated because they may displace bilirubin from protein binding sites and hence predispose these patients to the development of jaundice and even kernicterus (see Chapter 68).

Renal damage was common with older forms of sulfonamides that were poorly water-soluble. Patients developed crystalluria, which led to obstruction and hematuria. However, this reaction is rare with the more soluble congeners in use today. Nevertheless, renal damage on the basis of hypersensitivity may still be observed.

Drug interactions

Sulfonamides may augment the action of oral hypoglycemic agents by displacing them from plasma proteins. Transient accentuation of hypoprothrombinemia may be observed when sulfonamides are given together with oral anticoagulants because of displacement of the anticoagulant from protein binding sites and also perhaps because of inhibition of their biotransformation. Sulfonamides may also interfere with the biotransformation of phenytoin, with resultant increase in serum concentrations of that drug.

Dosage regimens and routes of administration

The usual daily dose of sulfisoxazole is 120–150 mg/kg orally, divided into four to six doses, and that of sulfamethoxazole is 50–60 mg/kg orally, divided into two equal doses.

Therapeutic applications

Common clinical uses of the sulfonamides include the treatment of acute, uncomplicated urinary tract infections, either alone or in combination with trimethoprim (co-trimoxazole, co-trimazine); *Nocardia* infections including those in the lung and central nervous system; *Toxoplasma* infections (in combination with pyrimethamine); and chloroquine-resistant *Plasmodium falciparum* malaria (in combination with pyrimethamine).

Trimethoprim (Proloprim)

This drug, a 2,4-diaminopyrimidine, was first synthesized in 1956 as a result of a planned systematic study. It was designed at first as an antibacterial agent, but it was subsequently found to have valuable antiparasitic activity also.

Bacterial susceptibility

Trimethoprim has an antibacterial spectrum similar to that of the sulfonamides, although it is more active than the sulfonamides against most bacterial species with the exception of *Neisseria*, *Brucella*, and *Nocardia*. The enterococci, which are resistant to the sulfonamides, are sensitive to trimethoprim, as are malaria parasites (see Chapter 57). The comparative activities of trimethoprim and the sulfonamides are shown in Table 56-2. As may be expected from its mechanism of action (see Fig. 56-1), trimethoprim is synergistic with sulfonamides against many bacterial species.

Pharmacokinetics

Trimethoprim is well absorbed from the gastrointestinal tract. A peak serum concentration of about 2 μg/mL is attained 1–2 hours after a 160-mg oral dose.

After absorption, trimethoprim is rapidly distributed in the body, and tissue concentrations often exceed serum concentrations except in the brain, skin, and fat. Its apparent volume of distribution is greater than total body water. Trimethoprim is 42–46% protein-bound.

A substantial proportion of trimethoprim is converted in the liver to at least five inactive metabolites, all of which are excreted in the urine. The amount of active (unchanged) drug excreted by this route during a 24-hour period ranges from 42 to 75% of an administered dose. A small amount of trimethoprim is excreted via the bile. The serum half-life is about 13 hours.

Adverse reactions

Trimethoprim may cause nausea and diarrhea, especially at high doses. On rare occasions trimethoprim may also be associated with various blood dyscrasias, including agranulocytosis, thrombocytopenia, and anemia. Inhibition of folate synthesis leading to anemia is a problem only in patients who are already folate-deficient and who are receiving large doses of the drug. This anemia is reversible with the administration of folates, preferably folinic acid, and these measures do not interfere with the antibacterial/antiparasitic effects of the drug. Trimethoprim may inhibit creatinine secretion and thus increase the serum creatinine concentration. Adverse reactions are more common when trimethoprim is administered in combination with a sulfonamide (e.g., sulfamethoxazole). The incidence of serious toxicity from this combination is especially high (about 50%) in patients with AIDS (see Sulfonamides above). The mechanism of this interaction is unknown.

Dosage regimens and routes of administration

Trimethoprim is most commonly administered in a **fixed 1:5 ratio with sulfamethoxazole (co-trimoxazole,** Bactrim, Septra) **or sulfadiazine (co-trimazine,** Coptin). The usual dose of the trimethoprim contained in these combinations ranges from 5 to 20 mg/kg/day, with the specific dose determined by the infecting organism and the severity of the infection. The combinations may be administered orally or intravenously, divided into two to four equal doses. An oral preparation of trimethoprim alone is also available. Its usual daily dose is 4 mg/kg, divided into two equal doses.

Therapeutic applications

The combination of trimethoprim with a sulfonamide (e.g., co-trimoxazole) is used extensively for the treatment of a variety of infections including urinary tract infections, prostatitis, exacerbations of chronic bronchitis and pneumonia, sinusitis, otitis media, traveller's diarrhea *(Shigella, Salmonella,* enterotoxic *E. coli)*, brucellosis, nocardiasis, and *Pneumocystis carinii* pneumonitis (PCP). Septicemia, pneumonia, and meningitis caused by multiple-resistant Gram-negative aerobes (e.g., *Serratia marcescens, Pseudomonas cepacia, Stenotrophomonas maltophilia)* have also been treated successfully with this combination, as are some atypical mycobacterial species *(M. marinum, M. kansasi).* In addition, the combination of agents is often used prophylactically in patients with recurrent urinary tract infections, in immunocompromised patients at risk for PCP, and in

neutropenic hosts to reduce the incidence of serious bacterial infections.

Trimethoprim alone may be used for the treatment and prevention of urinary tract infections. Trimethoprim (15 mg/kg divided into four equal doses) is used in combination with dapsone (100 mg/day) for the treatment of mild to moderate PCP in patients with HIV who are allergic to co-trimoxazole.

Pyrimethamine (Daraprim)

This drug, which was first synthesized in 1951, is very similar to trimethoprim, also being a 2,4-diaminopyrimidine (see Fig. 56-3). It is more specific than trimethoprim in its activity against protozoal dihydrofolate reductase and is therefore useful in the treatment of protozoal infections. It is primarily active against *P. falciparum* and *Toxoplasma gondii* with lesser activity against other *Plasmodium species.*

Pharmacokinetics

Pyrimethamine is completely and regularly absorbed from the intestinal tract. Blood concentrations are prolonged and urinary excretion may persist for 30 days or more after ingestion of the last dose. Between 20 and 30% is excreted unchanged in the urine. The half-life is approximately 36 hours.

Adverse reactions

Pyrimethamine can inhibit mammalian dihydrofolate reductase more strongly than trimethoprim does; it is therefore more toxic. **Gastrointestinal** disturbances are common, and **hematological** toxic effects such as megaloblastic anemia, leukopenia, and thrombocytopenia may occur if daily doses are administered without the concomitant administration of folinic acid.

Dosage regimens, route of administration, and therapeutic applications

The drug is administered orally in one daily dose or divided into two equal doses. The total daily dose is 0.5–1 mg/kg, up to a maximum of 25 mg/day. The drug is given daily for the treatment of toxoplasmosis or malaria and every second week for the prophylaxis of malaria. See Chapter 57 for its specific use (also in combination with a sulfonamide) in *P. falciparum* malaria.

Sulfones

The major sulfones used clinically are **dapsone (DDS)** (Avlosulfon) and its water-soluble derivative **sulfoxone sodium** (Diasone). Their mechanism of action is probably identical to that of the sulfonamides. Dapsone was first used against streptococcal infections but is now used for the treatment of leprosy, dermatitis herpetiformis, malaria, and *Pneumocystis carinii* pneumonitis.

Pharmacokinetics

Dapsone is slowly but almost completely absorbed from the gastrointestinal tract. Absorption of sulfoxone is less, but it causes less gastric distress. Sulfoxone is hydrolyzed to dapsone, which is the active agent. Distribution to most tissues is very good and the drug can accumulate in the skin, muscle, liver, and kidney. The major pathways of biotransformation involve *N*-acetylation and *N*-oxidation, which are reversible, and *N*-glucuronidation and *N*-sulfation, which lead to urinary excretion.

Adverse reactions

The sulfones are aromatic amines, and their most common untoward effect, which occurs in most patients (especially those with erythrocytic glucose-6-phosphate dehydrogenase deficiency) who are treated with 200–300 mg/day, is hemolysis of varying degree. Methemoglobinemia is also common, but is not affected by G-6-PD deficiency. Anorexia, nausea, and vomiting can limit the use of dapsone, and sulfoxone is often better tolerated. An infectious mononucleosis-like syndrome occurs occasionally and can be fatal.

Therapeutic applications

Dapsone is the primary drug used in the treatment of **leprosy.** The emergence of resistant strains has forced the search for alternate drugs. As mentioned earlier, dapsone can also be used in the treatment of chloroquine-resistant malaria and dermatitis herpetiformis. Dapsone is also used in combination with trimethoprim for treatment and prophylaxis of *Pneumocystis carinii* infection.

SUGGESTED READING

Cockerill FR, Edson FS. Trimethoprim-sulfamethoxazole. Mayo Clin Proc 1991; 66:1260–1269.

Hooper DC, Wolfson JS. Fluoroquinolone antimicrobial agents. N Engl J Med 1991; 324:384–394.

Sanders EW. Oral ofloxacin: a critical review of the new drug applications. Clin Infect Dis 1992; 14:539–554.

Suh B, Lorber B. Quinolones. Med Clin North Am 1995; 79:869–894.

Van Scoy RE, Wilkowske CJ. Antituberculosis agents. Mayo Clin Proc 1992; 67:179–187.

Walker RC, Wright AJ. The fluoroquinolones. Mayo Clin Proc 1991; 66:1249–1259.

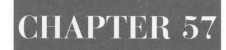

CHAPTER 57

Chemotherapy of Common Parasitic Infections

J.S. KEYSTONE

CASE HISTORY

A 30-year-old African-Canadian woman visited her physician because of fever, chills, aching muscles, and headache 2 weeks after having returned from a 3-month visit to her birthplace in Nigeria. She had taken no precautions against insect bites while in Africa, nor had she taken malaria chemoprophylaxis. At the time of that office visit her blood films showed many ring forms of *Plasmodium falciparum* malaria and a moderately high (5%) parasitemia.

Believing it to be the correct action, the physician prescribed chloroquine for treatment, but the patient refused, explaining that she is "allergic" to the drug. She said that during her childhood in Africa she had developed marked itching whenever chloroquine was given to her.

The physician thereupon consulted a tropical disease expert who explained that chloroquine is inappropriate therapy because chloroquine-resistant *P. falciparum* malaria is widespread in Africa. In addition, up to 45% of black Africans develop pruritus with chloroquine treatment as a result of a drug metabolite that is deposited in the skin; in other words, the patient suffered no "allergy" to the drug. Since the reaction does not seem to occur with quinine, the expert recommended quinine as the drug of choice for this patient.

A discussion of drug dosage ensued, and the consultant recommended an oral loading dose (twice the maintenance dose of 600 mg) of quinine sulfate because of the patient's high parasitemia. The consul-

tant explained that, by administering a loading dose, steady-state plasma levels of the drug would be reached within hours, whereas initiating therapy with a maintenance dose (quinine $t\frac{1}{2}$ = 16 hours) would delay the attainment of steady-state levels for 2–3 days.

Twenty-four hours after the start of treatment the patient complained of headache, severe ringing in the ears, mild hearing loss, and diarrhea. In a panic, the attending physician called the consultant who explained that these symptoms, known as "cinchonism," are to be expected with quinine, a cinchona alkaloid, that they will occur in most patients, and that they will resolve after the drug is discontinued. However, when the attending physician mentioned that the patient was somewhat confused, diaphoretic, and had tachycardia, the consultant suggested that the patient's blood sugar be assessed immediately by glucometer. The patient's blood sugar was 2.1 mmol/L. After the patient's condition was stabilized with an intravenous bolus of glucose, the consultant explained that hypoglycemia is an important and frequent complication of severe malaria, particularly when quinine is used for treatment, since the drug is known to cause insulin to be released from the pancreas.

Three months later the patient had a recurrence of fever and headache, at which time a diagnosis of *Plasmodium ovale* malaria was made. This bout of malaria can be explained by the fact that the previous therapy for *P. falciparum* malaria did not eradicate dormant hepatic forms (hypnozoites) of *P. ovale*. Quinine and adjuvant drugs such as tetracycline and pyrimethamine/sulfadoxine are blood schizonticides that act on developing parasites within red blood cells. They have little effect on the liver (exoerythrocytic) phase of the plasmodial life cycle.

The patient was treated with quinine again (because of her unwillingness to take chloroquine), followed by a course of primaquine, 15 mg per day. Four days into this latter therapy she complained of fatigue and noticed a reddish-colored urine. A clinical diagnosis of drug-induced hemolysis was made, presumably due to the oxidant effects of primaquine. The diagnosis was confirmed when the patient's glucose-6-phosphate dehydrogenase (G-6-PD) level was found to be low.

For organisms not covered in this section, the reader is referred to standard parasitology textbooks and the Medical Letter Handbook.

On a global basis parasitic infections are the leading cause of chronic illness and contribute directly or indirectly to the deaths of millions of children annually in the developing world. However, it is important to understand that the majority of infected individuals are asymptomatic, either because the parasite has a low degree of virulence, or because the parasite load is too low to cause tissue damage, or because the host has the ability to control the infection. Consequently, the clinician must first decide whether or not a parasitic infection requires treatment before a therapeutic agent is even considered.

Antiparasitic drugs (Table 57-1) are directed against two major groups of parasites: (1) protozoa, which constitute the single-celled organisms, and (2) metazoa, the multicelled creatures or worms. Metazoa include the flatworms (cestodes and trematodes) and roundworms (nematodes). With few exceptions, drugs that act against intestinal parasites are usually ineffective against tissue-dwelling or blood parasites and vice versa.

PROTOZOAN INFECTIONS

INTESTINAL AND VAGINAL PROTOZOA

Amebiasis

Strictly speaking, amebiasis refers to an infection by the intestinal protozoan *Entamoeba histolytica*, which has the ability to invade tissue. Since standard laboratory techniques cannot distinguish pathogenic from nonpathogenic strains, all isolates should be considered to be potentially pathogenic and therefore should be eradicated. There are many other amebae that are harmless commensals not requiring treatment. These include *Endolimax nana*, *Entamoeba coli*, *Entamoeba hartmanni*, and *Iodamoeba bütschlii*.

In the large bowel *E. histolytica* is found in two forms: cyst and trophozoite. The motile trophozoite is the vegetative form that maintains the infection by replication. Under an unknown stimulus, trophozoites, which normally live as commensals, may invade the intestinal mucosa and give rise to amebic colitis. Hematogenous spread to liver, lung, or brain may result in the formation of an amebic abscess. Under adverse conditions, trophozoites develop a protective covering and transform themselves into cysts. Cysts are transmitted by the fecal–oral route via flies, fingers, food (and water), or fornication.

Amebicides can be divided clinically into two groups: those acting in the intestinal lumen, and those acting in the tissue.

Agents acting in the lumen

These agents act directly on organisms in the lumen of the bowel. They are often poorly absorbed from the intestine and are used primarily for eradicating the infection at that site. These drugs cannot eradicate trophozoites that have invaded the intestinal wall and beyond. They include halogenated quinolines, macrolides, and diloxanide furoate. In asymptomatic (or minimally symptomatic) persons passing cysts or trophozoites, in whom tissue invasion presumably has not occurred, a lumen-active agent is all that is required. For symptomatic invasive amebiasis (intestinal or extraintestinal) a tissue-active drug *plus* one that acts in the lumen are needed.

Halogenated hydroxyquinoline derivatives: **Iodoquinol** (Yodoxin). This organic iodine compound is the only lumen-active agent of this group marketed in the United States and Canada. In addition to eradicating *E. histolytica*, iodoquinol is effective in some patients with *Dientamoeba fragilis*, *Balantidium coli*, and *Blastocystis hominis*. It functions by inactivating enzymes or halogenating proteins of the protozoan. The drug is absorbed moderately well from the intestine, and extensively biotransformed. Less than 10% of an oral dose is recovered in the urine, largely as glucuronides and ethanol sulfates.

Table 57-1 Antiparasitic Drug Doses

Infection		Drug	Adult Dosage	Pediatric Dosage
Amebiasis				
(*Entamoeba histolytica*		(Lumen-active agents)		
1. Asymptomatic or		Iodoquinol*	650 mg tid×20 d	30–40 mg/kg/d in 3 doses × 20 d
minimal symptoms	or			20 mg/kg/d in 3 doses × 10 d
		Diloxanide furoate	500 mg tid×10 d	
	or	Paromomycin	25–30 mg/kg/d×10 d	Same as adult
2. Moderate to severe		Metronidazole	750 mg tid×5–10 d	
disease or amebic		**plus**		35–50 mg/kg/d in
abscess		lumen-active agent	(as above)	3 doses×5–10 d
Ascariasis		Mebendazole	100 mg bid×3 d	Same as adult
(*Ascaris lumbricoides,*	or	Pyrantel pamoate*	11 mg/kg once (max 1g)	Same as adult
roundworm)	or	Albendazole	400 mg once	Same as adult
Clonorchiasis				
(*Clonorchis sinensis*)		Praziquantel	25 mg/kg tid×1 d	Same as adult
			15% cream topically	
Cutaneous larva migrans			bid×5 d, or 25 mg/kg bid	
(creeping eruption)		Thiabendazole	orally (max 3 g)×2 d	Same as adult
Cysticercosis		Albendazole*	15 mg/kg/d in 2 doses×30 d	Same as adult
(*Cysticercus cellulosae*)	or	Praziquantel	50 mg/kg/d in 3 doses×14 d	Same as adult
Dientamebiasis				30–40 mg/kg/d in 3 doses×20 d
(*Dientamoeba fragilis*)		Iodoquinol*	650 mg tid×20 d	
	or			40 mg/kg/d in 4 doses×10 d
		Tetracycline	500 mg qid×10 d	(max 2g/d)
	or	Paromomycin	25–30 mg/kg/d×10 d	Same as adult
Diphyllobothrium latum				11–34 kg: 1 g once
(fish tapeworm)		Niclosamide*	2 g chewed once	>34 kg: 1.5 g once
	or	Praziquantel	10–20 mg/kg once	Same as adult
Echinococcosis				
(*E. granulosus,*				
hydatid disease)		Albendazole	400 mg bid×3–6 mo	15 mg/kg/d×3–6 mo
Enterobiasis		Pyrantel pamoate*	11 mg/kg once (max 1 g); repeat after 2 wk	Same as adult
(*Enterobius vermicularis,*				
	or		100 mg once; repeat after	
pinworm)		Mebendazole*	2 wk	Same as adult
	or		5 mg/kg (max 250 mg)	
		Pyrvinium pamoate	once; repeat after 2 wk	Same as adult
	or		65 mg/kg (max 2.5 g)×7 d;	
		Piperazine citrate	repeat after 2 wk	Same as adult
Fascioliasis				
(*Fasciola hepatica,*			30–50 mg/kg on alternate	
sheep liver fluke)		Bithionol	days×10–15 doses	Same as adult
				<25 kg: 35 mg/kg/d once×3 d
Giardiasis				>25 kg: 50 mg/kg/d
(*Giardia intestinalis*)		Metronidazole*	2 g once×3 d	once×3 d
	or			15 mg/kg/d in
			250 mg tid×5–7 d	3 doses×5–7 d

Table 57-1 *Continued*

Infection		Drug	Adult Dosage	Pediatric Dosage
Giardiasis (Cont.)	**or**	Quinacrine	100 mg tid×7 d	6 mg/kg/d in 3 doses×7 d
	or	Furazolidone	100 mg qid×10 d	6 mg/kg/d in 4 doses×10 d
Hookworm *(Ancylostoma duodenale, Necator americanus)*	**or** **or**	Mebendazole* Pyrantel pamoate Albendazole	100 mg bid×3 d 11 mg/kg (max 1g)×3 d 400 mg once	Same as adult Same as adult Same as adult
Hymenolepiasis *(Hymenolepis nana,* dwarf tapeworm)		Niclosamide	2 g chewed once; then 1 g/d×5 d	11–34 kg: 1 g once; then 0.5 g/d×5 d >34 kg: 1.5 g once; then 1 g/d×5 d >40 kg: same as adult
	or	Praziquantel*	25 mg/kg once	Same as adult
Isosporiasis *(Isospora belli)*		Co-trimoxazole (trimethoprim-sulfamethoxazole)	TMP 160 mg & SMX 800 mg qid×10 d; then bid×3 wk	Same as adult
Malaria treatment *(P. falciparum, P. vivax, P. ovale, P. malariae)*				
1. All except chloroquine-resistant *P. falciparum* **Plus** for *P. vivax* & *P. ovale*		Chloroquine phosphate Primaquine	1 g(salt) stat; 500 mg in 6 h; then 500 mg/d×2 d 15 mg(base)/d×14 d	10 mg/kg (max 500 mg); then 5 mg/kg in 6 h; then 5 mg/kg d×2 d 0.3 mg base/kg/d ×14 d
2. Chloroquine-resistant *P. falciparum*				
Oral		Quinine sulfate* **plus**	600 mg tid×3 d	25 mg/kg/d in 3 doses×3 d
		(a) Pyrimethamine-sulfadoxine	3 tabs once	<1 yr: 1/4 tab 1–3 yr: 1/2 tab 4–8 yr: 1 tab 9–14 yr: 2 tab
	or	(b) Tetracycline*	250 mg qid×7 d	20 mg/kg/d in 4 doses×7 d
	or	(c) Clindamycin Mefloquine alone	900 mg tid×3 d 1250 mg once	20–40 mg/kg/d in 3 doses×3 d 25 mg/kg once
	or **or**	Halofantrine alone	500 mg q6h×3 over 12 hrs; repeat in 1 wk	8 mg/kg×3 over 12 hrs; repeat in 1 wk
Parenteral		Quinidine gluconate	10 mg(salt)/kg(max 600 mg) in N/saline over 1 h; then 0.02 mg/kg/min by infusion for 3 d max	Same as adult
	or	Quinine dihydrochloride	20 mg(salt)/kg in 10 mL/kg 5% D/W over 4 h; then 10 mg/kg over 2–4 h q8h (max 1800 mg/d) until oral therapy can be given	

Table 57-1 *Continued*

Infection		Drug	Adult Dosage	Pediatric Dosage
Malaria prevention 1. Chloroquine-sensitive areas		Chloroquine	500 mg(salt)/wk; start 1 wk before & continue for 4 wk after last exposure	8.3 mg(salt)/kg once/ wk as for adults (max 500 mg/d)
2. Chloroquine-resistant areas		Mefloquine*	250 mg/wk for 4 wks after last exposure	15–19 kg: 1/4 tab 20–30 kg: 1/2 tab 31–45 kg: 3/4 tab >45 kg: 1 tab
	or	Doxycycline	100 mg daily & for 4 wk after last exposure	>8 yr: 1 mg/kg/d (max 100 mg)
	or	Chloroquine **plus**	(as above)	
		Pyrimethamine-sulfadoxine	Carry 3 tabs for self-treatment of a febrile illness when medical care not available	<1 yr: 1/4 tab 1–3 yr: 1/2 tab 4–8 yr: 1 tab 9–14 yr: 2 tab
	or	Chloroquine **plus**	(as above)	
		Chloroguanide	200 mg daily & for 4 wk after last exposure	<2 yr: 50 mg 2–6 yr: 100 mg 7–10 yr: 150 mg
Paragonimiasis (*Paragonimus westermanni*, lung fluke)		Praziquantel	25 mg/kg tid×2 d	Same as adult
Pneumocystosis		Co-trimoxazole* (trimethoprim-sulfamethoxazole)	TMP 15–20 mg/kg/d & SMX 75–100 mg/kg/d, oral or IV in 3 or 4 doses×14–21 d	Same as adult
	or	Pentamidine	3–4 mg/kg IV qd×14–21 d	Same as adult
Schistosomiasis				
(*S. haematobium*)		Praziquantel	40 mg/kg/d in 2 doses×1 d	Same as adult
(*S. japonicum*)		Praziquantel	60 mg/kg/d in 3 doses×1 d	Same as adult
(*S. mansoni*)		Praziquantel	40 mg/kg/d in 2 doses×1 d	Same as adult
Strongyloidiasis (*Strongyloides stercoralis*)		Thiabendazole	50 mg/kg/d in 2 doses (max 3 g/d)×2 d	Same as adult
	or	Ivermectin	200 μg/kg/d×1–2 d	Same as adult
	or	Albendazole	400 mg bid×3–7 d	Same as adult
Toxoplasmosis (*Toxoplasma gondii*)		Pyrimethamine* **plus**	25–100 mg/d×3–4 wk	2 mg/kg/d×3 d, then 1 mg/kg/d (max 25 mg/d ×4 wk
		Sulfadiazine	1–2 g qid×3–4 wk	100–200 mg/kg/d ×3–4 wk
	or	Spiramycin alone	3–4 g/d×3–4 wk	50–100 mg/kg/d ×3–4 wk
Trichomoniasis (*Trichomonas vaginalis*)		Metronidazole	2 g once, or 250 mg tid orally×7 d	15 mg/kg/d orally in 3 doses×7 d
Trichuriasis (*Trichuris trichiura*, whipworm)		Mebendazole*	100 mg bid×3 d	Same as adult
	or	Albendazole	400 mg once	Same as adult

*Drug of choice.

Occasional adverse reactions include GI upset, rash, and thyroid gland enlargement. Rarely, iodoquinol produces subacute myelo-optic neuropathy when larger-than-recommended doses are given. The drug is contraindicated in patients who are hypersensitive to iodine.

Diloxanide furoate (Furamide). This safe and highly effective lumen-active agent for treatment of asymptomatic amebiasis is classified as an emergency drug in the United States and Canada, available from the Centers for Disease Control Drug Service, Atlanta, Georgia, and by authorization of the Bureau of Human Prescription Drugs, Health Canada, Ottawa. Diloxanide is rapidly absorbed and its ester linkage is largely hydrolyzed in the intestine. Peak blood levels are reached in 1 hour. The elimination half-life is approximately 6 hours; the major portion is excreted in the urine as glucuronide. The mechanism of action of diloxanide is unknown.

Toxicity is rare. Excessive flatulence is the most frequent side effect. GI upset and allergic reactions are uncommon.

Paromomycin (Humatin). Antibiotic amebicides are transiently effective for invasive amebiasis. When they are used alone, relapses are frequent. Antibiotics such as paromomycin and tetracyclines are adjunct therapy, especially useful for symptomatic relief of severe amebic dysentery. Although its primary role is as a luminal amebicide, it has some tissue activity. Therefore it is an alternative to metronidazole in mild-to-moderate intestinal amebiasis and can be used to eliminate cyst passage. Paromomycin also has variable efficacy in giardiasis and cryptosporidiosis (see below). Some of the therapeutic action of paromomycin in intestinal amebiasis occurs by modifying the intestinal bacterial flora, thereby depriving amoebae of nutrient and rendering the intestinal medium less favorable to parasite multiplication and invasion. It has greater amebicidal activity than tetracycline. Paromomycin is poorly absorbed from the intact gastrointestinal tract.

GI upset is the most frequently reported adverse reaction. Rash, headache, and vertigo occur occasionally.

Agents acting in the tissues

These substances act directly on organisms that have invaded tissues. Therefore, unlike those acting in the lumen, they must be well absorbed and reach high concentrations in tissue, and be sufficiently nontoxic to permit systemic use. Metronidazole has now replaced emetine, its less toxic analog dehydroemetine, and chloroquine as treatment for invasive amebiasis.

Metronidazole (Flagyl). This agent has been considered the drug of choice for the treatment of vaginitis caused by *Trichomonas vaginalis*, and it is also effective against the protozoan *Giardia intestinalis*, *Blastocystis hominis*, *Dientamoeba fragilis*, and some anaerobic bacteria such as *Bacteroides fragilis*. Although metronidazole has been promoted as being efficacious against all stages of amebiasis *(E. histolytica)*, it appears to be poorly effective in the lumen but an excellent agent in tissues. Metronidazole is currently the drug of choice for invasive amebiasis; it should be combined with a lumen-active agent. A parenteral form of the drug is now available.

Metronidazole is a nitroimidazole compound with a mode of action that is common to all nitroaromatics. The drug is reduced by enzymes present in susceptible anaerobic microorganisms, giving rise to reactive metabolites. These intermediates are oxidized by molecular O_2 to generate superoxide anions that in turn damage the parasite by producing toxic ionizing OH radicals that cause peroxidation of lipids and DNA in the parasite.

Absorption of metronidazole is rapid and complete. After a single oral dose, peak plasma concentrations are reached within 0.5–3 hours; the serum half-life is 7 hours. The drug is poorly protein-bound and therefore penetrates tissue readily, including the brain and CSF; it also crosses the placenta. Most of the drug is excreted by the kidney, about 20% unchanged and the remainder as a variety of metabolites formed by sidechain oxidation and glucuronide conjugation.

Common adverse effects include dark urine (probably due to a metabolite of the drug), nausea, vomiting, diarrhea, headache, and a metallic taste in the mouth. Rarely, seizures and reversible peripheral neuropathy have been reported. Alcohol should not be consumed during treatment with metronidazole because of a possible disulfiram-like reaction (see Chapter 26).

Recently, concern has been expressed about the ability of metronidazole to cause cancer and birth defects in experimental animals as well as gene mutations in bacteria. In high and prolonged dosage, the drug is carcinogenic in mice. Although it has been regarded by some clinicians as potentially dangerous in humans, there are no data to support this claim. The drug should not be used for trivial indications.

Giardiasis

This is an infection of the small bowel with the flagellated protozoan *Giardia intestinalis* (previously called *Giardia lamblia*). The parasite resides in the upper part of the small intestine and exists in two forms, trophozoite and cyst. The latter is the infective stage of the parasite. The trophozoite, with its ventral sucking disk, is responsible for the damage to the upper small bowel. Water-borne epidemics have occurred as well as person-to-person transmission by the fecal–oral route. Invasion beyond the bowel lumen does not occur. Only symptomatic infections or asymptomatic food handlers require treatment.

Metronidazole. This is the drug of choice for the treatment of giardiasis (see Amebiasis above).

Quinacrine (mepacrine HCl; Atabrine*).* Quinacrine is less effective than metronidazole for the treatment of giardiasis and potentially has more adverse effects. Thus, in giardiasis, quinacrine is an alternative for patients who should not receive or who do not tolerate metronidazole. It is presently unavailable in North America because the manufacturer has chosen to discontinue production of the drug due to a shortage of raw materials.

Quinacrine is well absorbed and widely distributed in tissues, where it is largely bound and therefore excreted slowly for prolonged periods. Nausea and vomiting are the most common adverse effects. Prolonged administration stains the skin yellow. Up to 2% of adults receiving quinacrine have developed drug-induced psychosis. Aplastic anemia, exfoliative dermatitis, and acute hepatic necrosis are rare.

Furazolidone (Furoxone). This drug is the only liquid preparation available that is easy to administer and is well tolerated by children. The drug is marketed in the United States. It is no longer marketed in Canada but is available as an emergency drug from the Bureau of Human Prescription Drugs, Health Canada, Ottawa.

Paromomycin. This drug has limited efficacy, approximately 50% cure rate, against *G. intestinalis*. It is poorly absorbed and therefore is safe in pregnancy (see Amebiasis). Recent studies suggest that it has limited efficacy against cryptosporidiosis in AIDS patients.

Trichomoniasis

Vaginal infections with *Trichomonas vaginalis* are common during the reproductive years. Trichomonads may persist in the urethra and periurethral glands of both sexes. Therefore, both partners should be treated to prevent recurrence of infection.

Metronidazole, the drug of choice, can be administered orally or vaginally.

Dientameba fragilis

D. fragilis is a large-bowel flagellate which only recently has been shown to be a potential human pathogen. It is likely transmitted in pinworm eggs and therefore is frequently seen in daycare nursery children and institutionalized persons. For symptomatic individuals the treatment of choice is **iodoquinol.** Alternatively, **tetracycline, paromomycin,** or high-dose **metronidazole** may be used. Asymptomatic infections do not require treatment.

Blastocystis hominis

It is not yet clear whether this large-bowel protozoan has the ability to produce gastrointestinal symptoms in infected humans. Limited clinical experience suggests that therapy with **iodoquinol,** high-dose **metronidazole,** or **paromomycin** results in a 60–70% cure rate. Treatment should be reserved for symptomatic individuals.

Isosporiasis

Isosporiasis, caused by the coccidian parasite *Isospora belli*, is endemic in developing countries and has been seen in institutionalized patients. It is now recognized as an important opportunistic infection of the small bowel, causing chronic diarrhea in AIDS patients.

Trimethoprim–sulfamethoxazole (co-trimoxazole) or **pyrimethamine plus sulfadiazine** (see Toxoplasmosis) is recommended therapy for this infection. High-dose pyrimethamine alone has also been shown to be effective. Although metronidazole and furazolidone have been reported to be effective, they should be relegated to second-line therapy.

Cryptosporidiosis

Cryptosporidium parvum is an important ubiquitous coccidian protozoan pathogen in both immunocompetent and immunosuppressed patients. In AIDS patients the organism produces a chronic, unrelenting, watery diarrhea associated with weight loss and malabsorption. In hosts with normal immunity, *Cryptosporidium* causes self-limited watery diarrhea, particularly in children. No effective therapy has been found. Spiramycin (see Toxoplasmosis) and paromomycin (see Amebiasis) appear to have some antiparasitic activity, but the clinical response to these drugs has been disappointing.

Microsporidiosis

Enterocytozoon bieneusi and *Septata intestinalis* are two intestinal microsporidia, small intracellular protozoa that have recently been shown to be a common cause of diarrhea in AIDS patients; other species may cause hepatitis, myositis, peritonitis, and keratopathy. At this time there is no known treatment for the parasite, although albendazole (see Intestinal Helminth Infections) appears to be beneficial against *S. intestinalis* only.

BLOOD AND TISSUE PROTOZOA

Toxoplasmosis

Toxoplasma gondii, an obligate intracellular protozoan, causes a ubiquitous infection that is transmitted congenitally or orally through ingestion of tissue cysts in poorly cooked meat or through oocysts in cat feces. Clinical disease includes congenital toxoplasmosis, ocular toxoplasmosis, a mononucleosis-like picture in immunocompetent hosts, and CNS disease in immunocompromised hosts, especially AIDS patients. Agents used for the treatment of toxoplasma diseases include pyrimethamine/sulfadiazine, spiramycin, and clindamycin. Therapy is generally not given for the lymphadenopathic form in immunocompetent hosts unless symptoms are particularly severe or persistent.

Pyrimethamine–sulfadiazine. The effect of this drug combination is synergistic; it acts by sequential blockage of two consecutive steps in the formation of folinic acid from *p*-aminobenzoic acid (PABA) by the parasite. Sulfadiazine prevents the parasite from utilizing PABA to synthesize folic acid; pyrimethamine inhibits dihydrofolate reductase, thereby preventing formation of tetrahydrofolic acid (folinic

acid) (see also Chapter 56). This combination is the most effective therapy presently available for treatment of toxoplasmosis.

Both drugs are well absorbed. Peak plasma concentrations are reached in 1.5–8 hours for pyrimethamine and in 2–4 hours for sulfadiazine. The elimination half-life for pyrimethamine and sulfadiazine is 50–100 hours and 10–12 hours, respectively. Both drugs are excreted primarily by the kidney.

Frequent adverse reactions include myelosuppression and thrombocytopenia, headache, GI upset, bad taste in the mouth, and rash (especially in AIDS patients). Convulsions and shock have been reported rarely. In order to minimize the marrow-suppressant effects of these antifols, folinic acid is administered concurrently. Since the parasite cannot utilize exogenous folinic acid, but must synthesize its own, the addition of folinic acid (as citrovorum factor) does not reduce the efficacy of the pyrimethamine/sulfadiazine combination.

In patients with AIDS, toxoplasmosis is one of the most important opportunistic infections causing CNS disease. Since the cyst form of the parasite is not susceptible to drug therapy, relapses after treatment occur in 80% or more of patients unless maintenance therapy with low doses of pyrimethamine and sulfadiazine is carried on indefinitely.

Spiramycin (Rovamycine). This macrolide antibiotic has been used successfully for the therapy of acutely infected pregnant women to prevent congenital infection. For other indications it is less effective than the pyrimethamine/sulfadiazine combination. It is stable in gastric HCl and well absorbed from the intestine. Adverse effects include gastrointestinal disturbances and occasional allergic cutaneous reactions.

Clindamycin (Dalacin, Cleocin). Like spiramycin, clindamycin is a macrolide antibiotic (see Chapter 55) with activity against *T. gondii*. The drug is concentrated in the choroid of the eye and has been used for ocular toxoplasmosis with favorable results. Clindamycin has also been used with pyrimethamine for the treatment of toxoplasmic encephalitis in AIDS patients who have sulfonamide sensitivity. However, the response in this clinical setting may be due to pyrimethamine alone.

Adverse reactions include diarrhea (especially *C. difficile* colitis) hepatotoxicity, hypersensitivity reactions, and myelosuppression.

Systemic corticosteroids. Corticosteroids are used as adjunct therapy for chorioretinitis and occasionally for cerebral toxoplasmosis to reduce cerebral edema. They should be administered with antiparasitic agents and preferably in brief courses.

Pneumocystosis

Pneumocystis pneumonia (PCP) is caused by an organism of uncertain taxonomic status, *Pneumocystis carinii*. It is one of the most frequent opportunistic infections in persons with AIDS and is occasionally seen in other immunosuppressed patients.

The management of pneumocystosis includes **treatment** of the primary infection and **chemoprophylaxis** thereafter in those who remain immunocompromised. Drugs used for the treatment and prophylaxis of PCP include co-trimoxazole (trimethoprim–sulfamethoxazole; TMP-SMX), pentamidine isethionate, dapsone (diaminodiphenylsulfone, DDS), and clindamycin plus primaquine. Generally, co-trimoxazole, trimethoprim plus dapsone, and pentamidine are considered first-line therapy. Most authorities recommend co-trimoxazole over pentamidine because it was shown to have less frequent adverse effects. Corticosteroids are an important adjunct for therapy of severe forms of PCP.

Co-trimoxazole (trimethoprim–sulfamethoxazole; TMP-SMX; see also Chapter 56). This drug combination is a broad-spectrum antimicrobial agent that (like pyrimethamine-sulfadiazine) acts by interfering with the synthesis of tetrahydrofolic acid. Trimethoprim, a diaminopyrimidine, inhibits dihydrofolate reductase, while sulfamethoxazole, a sulfonamide, inhibits the incorporation of p-aminobenzoic acid into dihydrofolate. The optimal ratio of concentrations of trimethoprim to sulfamethoxazole for antimicrobial synergy is 1:20. This ratio is achieved in the serum by using a combination of 1:5 (TMP:SMX) for both treatment and prophylaxis of PCP.

Co-trimoxazole may be administered orally or intravenously. In healthy individuals absorption from the GI tract is excellent. TMP and SMX are predominantly excreted in the urine and have an elimination half-life of 10–11 hours. Most of the TMP is excreted as the unchanged drug, but about 80% of the SMX is excreted as the N-acetylated compound.

The incidence of adverse reactions is 65% in patients with AIDS, but only 12% in those with other immunosuppressive disorders. The most common adverse reactions are leukopenia, allergic rash, hyponatremia, nausea and vomiting, fever, elevated hepatic enzymes, azotemia, anemia, and thrombocytopenia. Less frequent adverse reactions include Stevens-Johnson syndrome and toxic epidermal necrolysis.

Trimethoprim–dapsone. This drug combination has been shown to be as effective as co-trimoxazole for the treatment and prevention of PCP. The advantage of substituting dapsone for sulfamethoxazole is the lower incidence of toxic effects, particularly allergic rash.

The mechanism of action of this combination is identical to that of co-trimoxazole.

Once-daily dosage of dapsone is adequate, as the serum half-life is approximately 24 hours. Dapsone is acetylated, and the bulk of the metabolites are excreted in the urine.

The major toxicity of dapsone for patients with AIDS has been anemia, skin rash, granulocytopenia, and increased transaminase levels. Dapsone has been associated with dose-dependent hemolysis and methemoglobinemia, which are more severe in patients with G-6-PD deficiency. Anorexia, nausea, and vomiting occur infrequently.

Pentamidine (Pentacarinat, Pentam 300). This aromatic diamidine is administered parenterally for treatment of PCP and by aerosol for chemoprophylaxis. Its mechanism of action is not known with certainty, but there is some evidence that it binds selectively to the DNA of *P. carinii*, and also that it inhibits the Ca^{2+} pump activity in the membrane. Pentamidine has a terminal half-life of 9 hours and is eliminated by renal excretion. The drug should be administered when the patient is in the recumbent position to avoid orthostatic hypotension.

Pentamidine is N-hydroxylated by hepatic cytochrome P450 and excreted in the urine by active tubular secretion.

Adverse reactions to pentamidine occur in 40–80% of patients with PCP regardless of the cause of immunosuppression. Frequent adverse reactions include hypotension, renal insufficiency, ECG abnormalities, drug fever, hypersensitivity reactions and rash, leukopenia, neutropenia, anemia, thrombocytopenia, and hypocalcemia. Blood sugar irregularities are due to the direct cytotoxic action of the drug on β cells of the pancreas, causing release of insulin and consequent hypoglycemia. Infrequently, hyperglycemia may ensue due to insulin-dependent diabetes from β-cell destruction.

Nebulized pentamidine inhalation has been most

widely used for prophylaxis of PCP. About 5% of the dose is retained in the lung. High concentrations of the drug can be delivered to the alveoli, the site of infection. It has been reported that pentamidine inhibits release of inflammatory mediators from alveolar macrophages and may thus decrease lung damage. Pentamidine is also an effective *N*-methyl-D-aspartate (NMDA) receptor antagonist (see Chapter 20) and may therefore possibly protect against Ca^{2+}-mediated brain damage in patients with PCP. Little of the aerosolized drug is absorbed systemically, but leukopenia and hypoglycemia have occasionally been associated with this mode of administration. Toxicity is limited primarily to bronchospasm, which can be managed with inhaled β-adrenoceptor agonists, and occasional spontaneous pneumothorax. One of the drawbacks of nebulized pentamidine is the reoccurrence of infection in the upper lobes where drug concentrations are lowest, and extrapulmonary disease.

Malaria

Malaria parasites are blood protozoa of the genus *Plasmodium*. Four species infect humans: *Plasmodium falciparum* (malignant tertian malaria), *Plasmodium vivax* (benign tertian malaria), *Plasmodium malariae* (quartan malaria), and *Plasmodium ovale* (ovale tertian malaria).

The **plasmodial life cycle** begins when sporozoites are inoculated into humans from the salivary glands of a feeding female *Anopheles* mosquito. The organisms multiply in the liver and form tissue schizonts (**exoerythrocytic stage**). When liver schizonts rupture, merozoites are released into the bloodstream. In *P. vivax* and *P. ovale* malaria only, some merozoites, now called hypnozoites, may lie dormant in the liver and later cause a relapse of malaria. This stage is not present in *P. falciparum* and *P. malariae*, which have a single passage through the liver. In all species, merozoites released from the liver invade red cells and develop through a trophozoite into a schizont stage (**erythrocytic stage**). When the red cell schizont ruptures, most of the released merozoites invade new red cells. Some merozoites develop into male and female gametocytes that do not multiply; subsequently they are ingested by a feeding mosquito. Mating of these gametocytes in the mosquito gut leads to sporozoite production and a completion of the malaria cycle (Fig. 57-1).

The modern classification of antimalarial drugs is based on the stage of the *Plasmodium* life cycle upon which the drugs act:

1. Tissue schizonticides: Primaquine acts in the liver on hypnozoites of *P. vivax* and *P. ovale* and has some activity against red cell schizonts. In addition to acting as blood schizonticides, chloroguanide (proguanil) and pyrimethamine act on the liver phase of *P. falciparum* only. These latter two drugs are known as "causal" prophylactics since they prevent symptoms of malaria from occurring by inhibiting the exoerythrocytic phase.

2. Blood schizonticides: Quinine, quinidine, chloroquine, mefloquine, halofantrine, chloroguanide, pyrimethamine, primaquine, sulfonamides, sulfones, clindamycin, tetracycline, atovaquone, and artemisinin derivatives (artesunate, artemether) act in the blood on the erythrocytic phase of all four species of malaria. When one of these drugs is used to prevent malaria it is known as a "suppressive" agent because it suppresses the symptoms of malaria by eradicating parasites in the circulation.

Tissue schizonticides

Primaquine. The drug is an 8-aminoquinoline that destroys the exoerythrocytic (hepatic) forms of malaria. Also, it is highly gametocytocidal and has some schizonticidal activity. Primaquine is not usually used as a prophylactic agent but rather to eradicate dormant hypnozoites of *P. vivax* and *P. ovale* after a blood schizonticide (such as chloroquine) has been used to arrest the clinical attack of malaria. However, the drug may be used prophylactically and to prevent late relapses of *P. vivax* in those who return from areas where the infection is highly endemic. *Plasmodium ovale* is sufficiently rare to make prophylactic use of primaquine unnecessary. The mechanism of action of primaquine is unknown but it appears to exert its effects through a metabolite. *Plasmodium vivax* resistance to primaquine occurs in about one-third of those infected with the Chesson strain in Southeast Asia and Oceania.

Primaquine is rapidly and completely absorbed, extensively distributed, and converted to carboxyprimaquine. Less than 5% of the administered dose is found in the urine.

The most serious adverse effect of primaquine is intravascular hemolysis manifested as acute hemolytic anemia in those with glucose-6-phosphate dehydrogenase (G-6-PD) deficiency. Ethnic groups in which G-6-PD deficiency is found include Mediterraneans, African-Americans and -Canadians, Asians, and Orientals (see also Chapter 12). Primaquine may cause GI upset, headache and, rarely, leukopenia and agranulocytosis. Primaquine may also induce

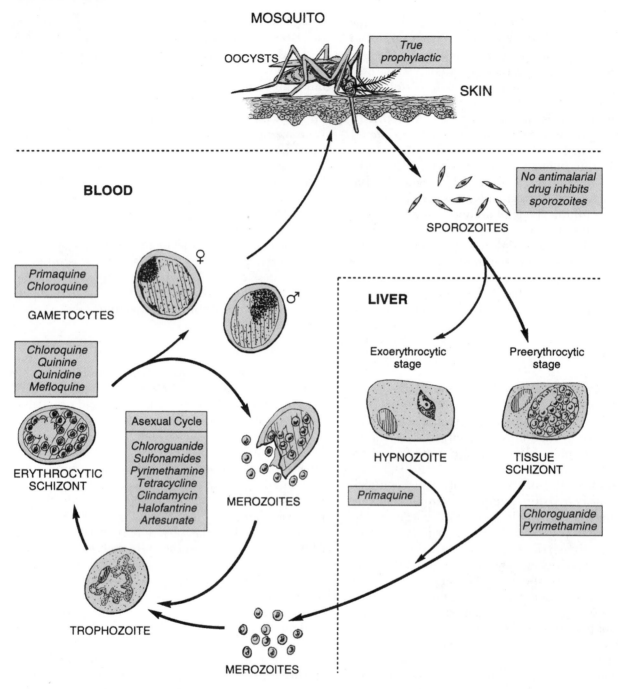

Figure 57-1. Life cycle of malaria parasites in humans and sites of action of antimalarial drugs. Omitted for simplicity is the phase of development of sporozoites in *Anopheles* mosquitoes, which consists of the ingestion of gametocytes in a blood meal, their fusion and production of motile zygotes in the mosquito stomach, formation of oocysts on the outer stomach wall, and release of sporozoites from oocysts into salivary glands, from which they are injected into the bloodstream of humans during a mosquito bite.

hemolysis in individuals with other defects of glucose metabolism and certain hemoglobinopathies.

Chloroguanide (Proguanil; Paludrine). This biguanide breaks down to its active metabolite, cycloguanil. The latter is a dihydrofolate reductase inhibitor that prevents the conversion of dihydrofolic acid to tetrahydrofolic acid (folinic acid). Chloroguanide is used for suppression but not for curative treatment of malaria. Because of widespread resistance to the drug, it is usually combined with another antimalarial such as chloroquine, sulfamethoxazole, or recently, atovaquone. Chloroguanide should not be given with primaquine as it inhibits the degradation of the latter.

Absorption is slow; peak plasma levels are reached within 3 hours. Approximately half of the drug is excreted in the urine, about 60% as unchanged drug and the rest as a metabolite.

Chloroguanide is well tolerated and safe in pregnant women. Gastrointestinal upset and mouth ulcers are common but mild side effects.

Pyrimethamine (Daraprim). This diaminopyrimidine compound blocks the dihydrofolate reductase enzyme required for folinic acid synthesis. Because parasites readily develop resistance to the drug, it is now rarely used alone to prevent malaria but is combined synergistically with a sulfonamide such as sulfadoxine to treat and occasionally prevent chloroquine-resistant *P. falciparum* (CRPF) malaria.

The hazards from small, suppressive, antimalarial doses of pyrimethamine are minimal. Prolonged administration may produce toxicity in the form of bone marrow suppression. Because pyrimethamine has antifolate activity and is teratogenic in animals, it should be used with caution in pregnancy.

Blood schizonticides

Quinine and Quinidine. These cinchona alkaloids are rapid-acting blood schizonticides. They are optical isomers with qualitatively but not quantitatively identical pharmacological actions. Although quinidine appears to have greater efficacy against malaria, it is potentially more toxic. Both drugs are quinoline-containing antimalarials (as are chloroquine and amodiaquine), which are weak bases that accumulate within the digestive vacuole of the malaria parasite. Current evidence suggests that these drugs specifically inhibit the malarial parasite enzyme, heme polymerase, which converts the breakdown products of hemoglobin into a nontoxic malarial pigment, hemozoin. Inhibition of this enzyme leads to the accumulation of soluble ferric heme that is highly toxic to the parasite membrane.

Because of their short half-lives and side effects these drugs are used only for *treatment* of malaria, not for *prophylaxis*, and they are rarely employed alone because of drug resistance. Quinine is given orally or intravenously while quinidine is administered only intravenously.

Quinine is well absorbed, widely distributed, and metabolized primarily in the liver. The elimination half-life is approximately 11 hours. In antimalarial doses, quinine sulfate frequently causes mild-to-moderate cinchonism (tinnitus, headache, decreased hearing, blurred vision, nausea and vomiting), but symptoms seldom necessitate cessation of treatment. Less common problems with both drugs include allergic reactions, hemolysis, thrombocytopenia, and agranulocytosis. Hypoglycemia has been associated with treatment of severe malaria because these drugs cause insulin to be released from the pancreas. When used intravenously they must be administered slowly to prevent arrhythmias and hypotension. Electrocardiographic monitoring should accompany parenteral quinidine use, and glucose monitoring is mandatory for both drugs, especially when the parenteral forms are used.

Chloroquine (Aralen). Chloroquine phosphate (sulfate or hydrochloride salt) is a 4-aminoquinoline that is effective against the erythrocytic phase of *P. malariae* and *P. ovale* and, except for some strains in Southeast Asia and Latin America, it is very effective for *P. vivax.* However, chloroquine-resistant *P. falciparum* malaria is present everywhere in the world except in Central America, Haiti, and North Africa. Therefore, the use of chloroquine for treatment and prevention of malaria has diminished considerably. The mechanism of chloroquine resistance relates to the ability of parasitized cells to concentrate the drug in their food vacuoles. Drug-resistant strains of *P. falciparum* cause efflux of the drug from infected erythrocytes by an active transport mechanism that is inhibited by calcium-channel blockers.

The mechanism of action of chloroquine in malaria is similar to that of quinine. Chloroquine can be administered orally, intramuscularly, subcutaneously, and intravenously. Chloroquine is rapidly and completely absorbed and has a very large volume of distribution. The drug is concentrated in the liver and in the cornea and retina of the eye. The plasma half-life is 6–12 days. About 30% of the drug is metabolized in the liver; excretion is primarily by renal pathways.

Adverse reactions are dose-related and include

GI upset, pruritus, headache, and CNS stimulation. Pruritus, seen primarily in blacks of African origin, is not an allergic reaction. Permanent retinopathy is associated with prolonged daily use of chloroquine (such as in rheumatic diseases), but not when the drug is used weekly for malaria suppression. Acute overdosage (with as few as 10 tablets in adults) can lead to circulatory failure, respiratory and cardiac arrest, and death. Chloroquine can safely be used during pregnancy for treatment and prevention of malaria.

Pyrimethamine–sulfadoxine (Fansidar). A combination of pyrimethamine and sulfadoxine has been used for both suppression and treatment of malaria. However, because of fatal cutaneous reactions to this drug combination (toxic epidermal necrolysis, Stevens-Johnson syndrome, and erythema multiforme) during chemosuppression, the drug is now reserved for treatment of malaria or self-treatment of presumptive malaria in a febrile traveller. Resistant *P. falciparum* malaria is widespread in parts of Africa and Southeast Asia, Oceania, and the Amazon area of Brazil.

With the exception of the long (200 hours) half-life of sulfadoxine, the mechanism of action, adverse effects, and pharmacokinetics of pyrimethamine–sulfadoxine are similar to those of the pyrimethamine–sulfadiazine combination used for the treatment of toxoplasmosis (see above).

Mefloquine (Lariam). This is a quinoline methanol derivative that is used primarily for the prevention of chloroquine-resistant *P. falciparum* malaria. Mefloquine appears to act in the same way as chloroquine. It is less often used for treatment of malaria because of the increased frequency of serious neuropsychiatric reactions associated with higher dosage. The drug is well absorbed, partly biotransformed in the liver, and excreted mainly in feces. It has a long (1–4 weeks) terminal half-life.

Adverse events such as gastrointestinal upset, dizziness, headache, and sleep disturbances occur with the same frequency as when chloroquine is used for chemosuppression. Although confusion, psychosis, and convulsions have been reported rarely with both chemosuppression and treatment, these side effects are much more likely to occur with treatment. Mefloquine-resistant *P. falciparum* malaria has already been documented by in vitro studies in many countries. The drug is no longer effective in multidrug-resistant areas of Thailand.

Halofantrine (Halfan). This is a new phenanthrene methanol derivative that is very effective for the treatment of drug-resistant malaria. Its wide variability of absorption has made it unacceptable as a chemosuppressant. Side effects include GI upset, pruritus, cough, and cardiotoxicity (QTc prolongation). A significant number of treatment failures have been documented in Thailand, suggesting the possibility of cross-resistance with mefloquine. Anecdotal reports of sudden death, likely from cardiac conduction disturbance, have recently appeared, prompting the manufacturer to recommend that the drug not be administered *with* food, *to* those with conduction abnormalities, or *with* drugs known to affect cardiac conduction.

Artesunate. This drug is a new oral and intravenous derivative of ginghaosu, an antimalarial derived from the ancient Chinese herb *Artemisia annua*. It is a very rapid-acting schizonticide that clears parasitemia and symptoms of malaria considerably faster than any other compound. However, because recrudescences are common when the drug is used alone, it is often combined with other antimalarials such as mefloquine or doxycycline. In the few published clinical studies artesunate appears to be very well tolerated. Its rapid action on the early blood-stage trophozoite makes it an ideal drug for the treatment of severe *P. falciparum* infections.

Atovaquone (Mepron). A new hydroxynaphthoquinone derivative, atovaquone, is a rapid-acting blood schizonticide in the final stages of testing before being submitted for licensing. The site and mode of action of this drug are distinct from those of other antimalarial blood schizonticides. Atovaquone appears to block pyrimidine synthesis by acting as an antagonist to ubiquinone, thus leading to inhibition of cell replication. When it is used alone for treatment of *P. falciparum* malaria, recrudescence is common. Current studies are focusing on the combination of atovaquone with proguanil or tetracycline as a way to prevent drug resistance.

Antibiotics. Tetracycline, doxycycline, and clindamycin are slow-acting blood schizonticides that are combined with quinine to treat drug-resistant *P. falciparum* malaria. In addition, doxycycline is currently a most effective chemosuppressant, even along the Thai–Myanmar and Cambodian borders where multidrug-resistant strains of *P. falciparum* are endemic.

Malaria treatment

Chloroquine is the drug of choice for treatment of *P. malariae*, *P. ovale*, most strains of *P. vivax*, and a few strains of *P. falciparum*. In the management of *P. vivax* and *P. ovale*, chloroquine or other blood schizonticides must be followed by a course of primaquine, which will eradicate hepatic hypnozoites, thereby ensuring that relapse will not occur.

Mefloquine, quinine in combination with tetracycline or clindamycin, halofantrine alone, artesunate followed by mefloquine, and atovaquone plus proguanil are all effective treatments of drug-resistant *P. falciparum* malaria. However, as of this writing, the latter three treatment options are not yet available in the United States or Canada. In many areas of the world quinine plus pyrimethamine–sulfadoxine, or pyrimethamine–sulfadoxine alone, have been successfully used to treat drug-resistant *P. falciparum* malaria; the former is preferred when nonimmune patients are being treated. Mefloquine alone is not generally recommended for treatment of malaria because of the relatively high incidence of severe neuropsychiatric reactions associated with treatment doses of this drug.

Malaria chemosuppression (chemoprophylaxis)

Since no drug kills sporozoites, the traditional term "malaria chemoprophylaxis" is a misnomer. A better term is "malaria chemosuppression." Most antimalarials act beyond the liver on the erythrocytic phase by suppressing the parasitemia and hence the symptoms of malaria. If chemosuppression is continued beyond the liver stages of *P. falciparum* and *P. malariae*, i.e., for 4 weeks after exposure to malaria, a "suppressive cure" of these species will result and no late recrudescence will occur. The additional weeks of prophylaxis will not cure *P. ovale* and *P. vivax* malaria, because these parasites may lie dormant in the liver and relapse at a later date. Only a tissue schizonticide, such as primaquine, will provide a "radical cure" of these latter infections.

Chloroquine is the drug of choice for suppression of all species of malaria, except in areas where resistant *P. falciparum* and *P. vivax* strains occur.

Malaria chemosuppression for chloroquine-resistant areas of the world has become a very complex and controversial subject among those responsible for making recommendations. At present, there is no uniformity of opinion concerning optimal regimens for this purpose. To make matters worse, the World Health Organization recently declared that "no available chemoprophylaxis regimen will guarantee protection against malaria."

Mefloquine has become the drug of choice for prevention of chloroquine-resistant *P. falciparum* malaria throughout the world, except along the Thai–Myanmar and Thai–Cambodian borders where multidrug resistance is high. In Thailand, daily doxycycline is currently the suppressant of choice. In areas of Asia where drug resistance is low, some authorities recommend that travellers use weekly chloroquine and carry a single treatment dose (three tablets) of pyrimethamine–sulfadoxine for self-administration whenever fever develops in a situation where medical care is unavailable. Regardless of which chemosuppressive regimen is used, travellers must take personal-protection measures against mosquito bites (e.g. insect repellents, bed nets, screened accommodation) and seek medical attention at the first sign of fever while in a malarious area or within 1 year of departure from one. Pregnant women are advised not to travel to mefloquine-resistant areas due to the lack of safe and effective alternatives to mefloquine.

INTESTINAL HELMINTH INFECTIONS

Intestinal helminths (Table 57-2) are found in the lumen of the large or small bowel where they frequently attach themselves to the intestinal mucosa. Unlike protozoa, helminths do not usually multiply in the human host. This means that the worm burden (i.e., the total number of worms in the individual's gastrointestinal tract) may increase only when the patient is reexposed to infective eggs or larvae. Since human morbidity from helminth infections is directly proportional to worm burden, it follows that reduction in worm burden, without a parasitological cure, may produce an acceptable therapeutic result.

Disease outside of the intestine can occur from the systemic dissemination of eggs or larvae of certain worm species. **Hydatid disease** arises from the ingestion of tapeworm eggs *(Echinococcus granulosus* and *Echinococcus multilocularis)* from feces of dogs and related species. In the infected individual, larvae migrate from the intestine into the portal circulation and travel mostly to the liver or lungs (occasionally to kidneys, bone, and brain), where they form hydatid cysts of increasing size that can rupture and become the source of new cysts. **Cysticercosis** arises from the ingestion of eggs of the pork tapeworm *(Taenia solium)*. These eggs develop into larval cysticercus forms in the brain, eye, and muscles, producing inflammation and cystic lesions.

Table 57-2 Drugs Used in the Treatment of Selected Helminth Infections*

Drug	Roundworm	Hookworm	Pinworm	Whipworm	Threadworm	Tapeworm	Flukes
Albendazole	+	+	+	+	+	+	
Mebendazole	+	+	+	+			
Niclosamide						+	
Piperazine citrate	+		+				
Praziquantel						+	+
Pyrantel pamoate	+	+	+				
Pyrvinium pamoate			+				
Thiabendazadole					+		

*Key:
Roundworm: *Ascaris lumbricoides*
Hookworm: *Ancylostoma duodenale; Necator americanus*
Pinworm: *Enterobius (Oxyuris) vermicularis*
Whipworm: *Trichuris trichiura*
Threadworm: *Strongyloides stercoralis*
Tapeworm: *Taenia saginata; Taenia solium; Diphyllobothrium latum; Hymenolepis nana*
Flukes: *Schistosoma* species; *Fasciolopsis buski; Paragonimus* species; *Clonorchis sinensis*
The symbol (+) means effective use of these drugs in specific helminth infections.

Mebendazole (Vermox)

This drug is a broad-spectrum benzimidazole anthelminthic. It is the drug of choice for trichuriasis and is effective for ascariasis, hookworm, and enterobiasis. For the management of invasive parasites (such as trichinosis, toxocariasis, and hydatid disease) it has been replaced by **albendazole,** since the latter is better absorbed and gives higher tissue levels.

By inhibiting glucose uptake into susceptible parasites, mebendazole causes a decrease in ATP production and death of the organism. The drug is poorly absorbed (<10%) from the gastrointestinal tract. Bioavailability is very low (<5%) because of very high first-pass elimination. The elimination half-life of mebendazole ranges from 3 to 9 hours. Unchanged drug and its major metabolites are excreted in the urine.

Mebendazole is an extremely safe drug which only rarely causes mild GI upset, pruritus, and skin rash. Since it has been shown to be teratogenic in rats, mebendazole should not be used in pregnancy.

Pyrantel Pamoate (Combantrin, Antiminth)

This is a drug of choice for ascariasis, hookworm, and enterobiasis; it is ineffective in trichuriasis and strongyloidiasis. Pyrantel acts as a depolarizing neuromuscular blocking agent that paralyzes worms, which subsequently "lose their grip" on the bowel mucosa and are expelled in the feces.

Pyrantel is poorly and incompletely absorbed from the GI tract; most of an oral dose is excreted unchanged in the feces. The drug is well tolerated except for infrequent, mild gastrointestinal upset.

Piperazine Citrate (Entacyl)

Piperazine is an alternative drug for the treatment of ascariasis and enterobiasis, frequently used in the developing world. (Pyrantel and mebendazole are preferred for both infections.) The drug exerts its action by inducing flaccid paralysis of the worm, thereby causing it to detach from the intestinal mucosa.

Piperazine is well absorbed from the small intestine. Approximately two-thirds of a dose is eliminated unchanged in the urine within 24 hours. It is a relatively safe drug that occasionally produces GI upset, urticaria, and dizziness. It may reduce seizure threshold and is therefore contraindicated in patients with epilepsy.

Pyrvinium Pamoate *(Vanquin)*

This salt of a cyanine dye has largely been replaced by pyrantel and mebendazole for the treatment of enterobiasis. The drug acts by inhibiting glucose uptake by the parasite.

Pyrvinium is poorly and incompletely absorbed from the GI tract and hence is one of the few anthelmintics considered to be safe in pregnancy. Mild GI upset is uncommon. Because it is a dye, it colors the stool orange and may stain the patient's underwear and bed sheets.

Thiabendazole *(Mintezol)*

This is a drug of choice for treatment of strongyloidiasis. When used topically, thiabendazole is also a treatment of choice for cutaneous larva migrans caused by dog or cat hookworms. Variable success has been shown in the treatment of toxocariasis (visceral larva migrans) and trichinosis.

Thiabendazole prevents polymerization of tubulin in adult nematodes, blocking microtubule assembly and thus interfering with microtubule-dependent transport processes such as protein secretion and glucose transport.

The drug is well absorbed, quickly biotransformed in the liver to a 5-hydroxy derivative, conjugated to glucuronide, and excreted in the urine within 24 hours.

Adverse reactions are seen in most patients and consist of anorexia, nausea, vomiting, dizziness, drowsiness, headache, and lethargy. Hypotension, seizures, syncope, and severe cutaneous allergic reactions are rare. Thiabendazole interferes with the metabolism of xanthine derivatives such as theophylline. Because of its toxicity, thiabendazole should be replaced by safer anthelmintics (such as albendazole) when they are available.

Albendazole *(Zentel)*

This is one of the most potent and broad-spectrum benzimidazole anthelmintics. It is effective against adult and larval forms of many nematodes and cestodes. Like mebendazole, the drug acts by interfering with parasite uptake of glucose with subsequent depletion of glycogen and ATP stores.

At present, albendazole is available only by emergency drug release in Canada and is investigational in the United States. Albendazole is highly effective in single oral dose against ascarids, hookworms (including those that cause cutaneous larva migrans), pinworms, and whipworms. It is somewhat less effec-

tive for adult tapeworm infections. However, because it is much better absorbed than mebendazole, it is effective for the treatment of larval cestode infections such as hydatid disease and cysticercosis. Recent data suggest that it is effective against filaria larvae (microfilaria), Loa loa adults, and may be effective against *Giardia intestinalis.*

Approximately 50% of a dose of albendazole is absorbed compared to less than 10% for mebendazole. The drug is rapidly converted to its active metabolite, albendazole sulfoxide, and then excreted in the urine. The elimination half-life of the metabolite is approximately 8 hours.

Short, 1–3-day courses are well tolerated; GI upset and dizziness occur infrequently. Prolonged courses of therapy used for larval cestode infections have occasionally caused reversible hepatotoxicity, neutropenia, and alopecia.

Niclosamide *(Yomesan, Niclocide)*

This agent is a drug of choice for intestinal tapeworm infections such as *T. saginata, T. solium, D. latum,* and *D. caninum.* Although it may be used to treat *H. nana,* the dwarf tapeworm, praziquantel (see below) is preferable because a single-dose regimen is effective. Niclosamide is not effective against larval cestodes. Inhibition of oxidative phosphorylation in cestode mitochondria is the proposed mechanism of action.

Since very little niclosamide is absorbed from the GI tract, side effects are infrequent. Mild abdominal pain, nausea, and malaise occur in up to 10% of treatments.

Praziquantel *(Biltricide)*

This pyrazino-isoquinoline compound has a broad spectrum of activity against trematodes (flukes) and cestodes (tapeworms). It is the drug of choice for all species of schistosomiasis, clonorchiasis, opisthorchiasis, paragonimiasis, and fasciolopsiasis *(F. buski).* It has only limited efficacy against fascioliasis *(F. hepatica).* Praziquantel is as effective as niclosamide for the treatment of taeniasis *(T. saginata, T. solium),* diphyllobothriasis *(D. latum),* and hymenolepiasis *(H. nana).* Also, praziquantel is very effective in the treatment of cysticercosis and in the eradication of echinococcal protoscolices that have leaked from a ruptured cyst.

Praziquantel is readily absorbed, rapidly biotransformed in the liver by first-pass hydroxylation, and largely excreted in the urine. The unchanged drug has a serum half-life of approximately 1 hour with a terminal elimination half-life of 3–10 hours. Although the clinical significance is uncertain, corticosteroids and anticonvulsants have been shown to decrease serum levels of the drug markedly.

Praziquantel increases the permeability of the worm's cell membrane to calcium ions, causing spastic paralysis of its musculature and dislodgement of worms from sites of attachment. Subsequently, disintegration of the worm tegument takes place with lysis of the parasite.

Dizziness, headache, malaise, drowsiness, abdominal pain, and nausea are common, particularly when larger doses are used. Vomiting, urticaria, and mild-to-moderate increases in hepatic transaminases occur less frequently.

SUGGESTED READING

Addiss DG, Juranek DD, Spencer HC. Treatment of children with asymptomatic and nondiarrheal Giardia infection. Pediatr Infect Dis J 1991; 10:843–846.

Anon. Chapter 3. Antiprozoal drugs in AMA drug evaluations. AMA 1990; 3:1–39.

Anon. Chapter 4. Anthelmintics in AMA drug evaluations. AMA 1990; 4:1–27.

Anon. Drugs for parasitic infections. Med Lett Drugs Ther 1995; 37:99–108.

Aucott JN, Ravdin JI. Amebiasis and nonpathogenic intestinal protozoa. In: Maguire JH, Keystone JS, eds. Parasitic diseases. Infect Clin North Am 1993; 7:467–486.

Cook GC. Anthelmintic agents: some recent developments and their clinical application. Postgrad Med J 1991; 67:16–22.

Davidson RA. Issues in clinical parasitology: the treatment of Giardiasis. Am J Gastroenterol 1984; 79:256–261.

Hoffman SL. Diagnosis, treatment and prevention of malaria. In: Wolfe M, ed. Travel medicine. Med Clin North Am 1992; 76:1327–1355.

Irusen EM, Jackson TFHG, Simjre AE. Asymptomatic intestinal colonization by pathogenic *E. histolytica* in amebic liver abscess: prevalence, response to therapy and pathogenic potential. Clin Infect Dis 1992; 145:889–893.

McCabe R, Chirugi V. Issues in toxoplasmosis. In: Maguire JH, Keystone JS, eds. Parasitic diseases. Infect Clin North Am 1993; 7:587–604.

Schwartz IK. Prevention of malaria. In: Gardner P, ed. Health issues of international travelers. Infect Clin North Am 1992; 6:313–331.

White NJ. The treatment of malaria. N Engl J Med 1996; 335:800–806.

CHAPTER 58

Antiviral Agents

S.L. WALMSLEY

CASE HISTORY

A 38-year-old gay man known to be HIV-infected had been treated with oral acyclovir 200 mg three times daily as suppressive treatment for recurrent perianal herpes simplex infections. He was well in all other respects. When he developed oral thrush (candidiasis), he approached his physician about treatment. This opportunistic candidal infection was treated with nystatin, 500,000 IU three times daily, using the "swish and swallow" technique. A blood test showed a low CD4 count of 200×10^6/L, and it was decided that he should take zidovudine (AZT) at a dose of 200 mg three times daily and didanosine (ddI) 200 mg twice daily, as combination antiretroviral therapy. This caused an initial increase in his CD4 count, but it gradually declined over the next 2 years, although he remained clinically well.

Two years after the candidal infection and the start of AZT and ddI therapy, he noticed a purplish lesion on the tip of his nose, and more lesions developed over his thorax and extremities during the next 3 months. The lesions, which the patient could mask quite well with cosmetics, were diagnosed as Kaposi's sarcoma, and he was started on therapy with subcutaneous α-interferon. This drug, however, had to be discontinued after 2 weeks because of side effects characterized by flu-like symptoms, malaise, and myalgia, which occurred with each injection and interfered significantly with his quality of life.

One year later, his CD4 count had decreased to 30×10^6/L and he complained of floaters in his visual field. A diagnosis of cytomegalovirus (CMV) retinitis

in one of his eyes was made, and he was started on induction therapy with intravenous ganciclovir, 5 mg/kg twice daily, via a Hickman line inserted for long-term therapy. AZT therapy was discontinued because of the patient's low hemoglobin (98 g/L) and neutrophil count (1200×10^6/L); it was felt that the combined marrow-suppressant effects of AZT and ganciclovir would be too great. Ritonavir (Norvir) at a dose of 600 mg twice daily was substituted for AZT. Acyclovir was discontinued because ganciclovir at a maintenance dose of 5 mg/kg/day provided adequate control of the herpes simplex infections.

After 6 months on ganciclovir maintenance therapy he developed CMV retinitis in the other eye. This caused concern about resistance to ganciclovir, and therapy was changed to intravenous foscarnet at an induction dose of 90 mg/kg twice daily. This brought the CMV infection under control within a month, after which the patient could continue with intravenous foscarnet maintenance therapy at a dose of 90 mg/kg/day.

The history of human antiviral chemotherapy is relatively short; the first agent was licenced for clinical use in North America within the past three decades. Despite drug developments, the major approach to the control of viral infections is through prevention. This includes prophylactic treatment in high-risk populations (e.g., recipients of organ transplants) and programs of vaccination.

A number of viral pathogens remain major therapeutic problems not only in the normal host but more significantly in those whose immunity has been compromised by underlying disease or its therapy.

The development of antiviral agents has been slow relative to that of other antiinfective agents because their effectiveness is closely related to cellular metabolism, and much had to be learned in this field before effective drugs could be devised. It was long believed that viral replication was so closely coupled with normal host cellular metabolism that antiviral therapy would not be possible without seriously compromising the host. Extensive research has increased our understanding of viral metabolism, especially those aspects of viral genome replication that are different from host cell replication. This has led to the development of antivirals that are selective for the virus and inhibit virus-specific events or, preferentially, inhibit virus-directed macromolecular synthesis. As these agents inhibit specific events in viral replication, most have a restricted spectrum of activity.

Despite these advances, few of the many antiviral drugs developed to date have had a sufficiently high ratio of therapeutic value to toxicity in animal models to warrant proceeding to clinical trials in humans. Even fewer have shown sufficient clinical benefit to achieve licensing.

The current epidemic of human immunodeficiency virus (HIV) infections has had an enormous impact on the field of virology. Infection with this virus has become a major public health problem world-wide since its recognition in 1981. It has posed a serious challenge to researchers concerned with developing viral vaccines and antiviral drugs. Many researchers have turned their efforts toward this problem, and although a solution to the epidemic is not yet in sight, remarkable advances have been made in our understanding of viruses, their replicative mechanisms, and potential targets for antiviral drugs and vaccines.

Chemotherapeutic agents for viral infections can be classified into one of three major groups:

1. Agents that directly inactivate intact viruses (virucidal)
2. Agents that inhibit viral replication at the cellular level (antiviral)
3. Agents that augment or modify the host's response to infection (immunomodulating)

The mechanisms of action of antivirals currently available for clinical use include (1) the prevention of viral penetration and/or uncoating, (2) the selective inhibition of enzymes specific for viral genome replication, and (3) the shutting off of viral mRNA trans-

lation (e.g., interferon). Immune modulating agents are also available for some viral infections (see Chapter 61). Virucidal drugs are usually too toxic for clinical use.

There are many variables that may influence the outcome of antiviral chemotherapy. These include:

- Type of the underlying disease and immune competence of the host
- Age of the patient
- Stage of the illness at the time of initiation of treatment
- Dosage of the antiviral agent utilized
- Ability of the virus to remain latent within its host
- Ability of the virus to penetrate the central nervous system
- Ability of the virus to change genetically over time
- Development of resistance by the virus to the inhibitory action of the drug

In clinical trials of antiviral agents, it is important that these variables be carefully considered during data analysis. It is also important to recognize that viral infections often follow an unpredictable course; some viral infections may improve even if the patient is treated with a placebo. For these reasons it is imperative that any trial of antiviral chemotherapy be double blind and placebo-controlled until an agent with clinical efficacy is identified. As most agents are inhibitory in their activity, viral infections may relapse when the compound is removed, especially when the host's immune function remains compromised as in human immunodeficiency virus infections, transplants, etc.

Antiviral drugs act at various points in the viral replication cycle, the key steps of which are shown in Figure 58-1. Given these various steps in viral replication, it is possible to search for new drugs that will cause a block at some point in the replication cycle. Thus, there are agents that:

- Interfere with virus attachment to host cell receptors, penetration, and uncoating
- Inhibit virion-associated enzymes such as reverse transcriptase
- Inhibit transcription of the parental genome
- Inhibit translation processes of viral mRNA
- Interfere with viral regulatory proteins
- Interfere with viral protein glycosylation
- Interfere with viral assembly
- Interfere with release of virus from cell membranes

The agents discussed in this chapter are limited to those that are currently, or will soon be, available for clinical use (Table 58-1).

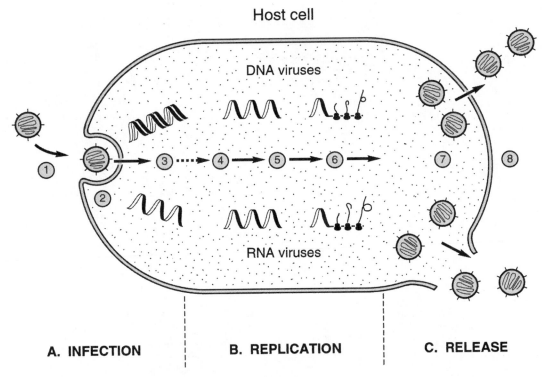

Host cell

DNA viruses

RNA viruses

A. INFECTION　　**B. REPLICATION**　　**C. RELEASE**

Figure 58-1. Basic strategy (key steps) of viral replication.
A. Infection: (1) Adsorption of virion to host cell plasma membrane receptors. (2) Entry of virion into host cell (akin to phagocytosis). (3) Uncoating of virion (i.e., removal of protein capsid, exposure of viral nucleic acids to initiate replication).
B. Replication: (4) Viral DNA-dependent RNA polymerases (DNA viruses) and RNA-dependent RNA polymerases (RNA viruses) catalyze the synthesis of mRNAs for production of viral structural and nonstructural proteins. (5) Viral genome may integrate into host chromosome. (6) Modification of viral proteins by glycosylation and cleavage.
C. Release: (7) Assembly of virions. (8) Slow leakage from host cell (budding), or cell rupture.

The use of combinations of antiviral agents with different mechanisms (or sites) of action is an active area of research. This is being investigated as a means to increase the antiviral activity, decrease drug toxicity, and prevent the development of resistant viruses.

DRUGS

Amantadine

This antiviral agent is a stable tricyclic amine that has been chemically synthesized and has a peculiar cage-like structure (Fig. 58-2). It increases the dopaminergic activity in the striatum and was initially used in the treatment of Parkinson's disease (see Chapter 21).

Antiviral mode of action

This is not fully known, but it is thought to interfere with the uncoating and nucleic acid release of certain RNA viruses. In vitro it is active against certain myxoviruses (type A influenza), a paramyxovirus (Sendai virus), and a toga virus (rubella).

Pharmacokinetics

Amantadine (as the hydrochloride, Symmetrel) is slowly but probably completely absorbed by the oral route. It is available in capsule, tablet, and syrup forms. It has a long half-life of approximately 15 hours and is almost entirely recoverable unmetabolized in the urine. Plasma half-life increases in the elderly and in patients with impaired renal function, and doses are adjusted accordingly.

Table 58-1 Characteristics of Antiviral Agents

Drug	Mechanism of Action	Clinical Indications	Main Adverse Effects
Amantadine and rimantadine	Interference with uncoating of the virus	Prophylaxis and treatment of influenza A	Confusion, insomnia, anxiety
Trifluorothymidine (Trifluridine)	Competitively inhibits the incorporation of natural nucleotide into viral DNA	Topical treatment of herpetic keratitis and herpetic skin ulcerations	Burning and irritation upon instillation
Adenine arabinoside (vidarabine, ara-A)	Competitive inhibition of viral DNA polymerase	Herpes simplex encephalitis; herpes of the newborn; herpes infections in immunocompromised hosts; genital herpes; varicella-zoster in immunocompromised hosts; herpes keratitis	Gastrointestinal upset; CNS toxicity
Acycloguanosine (Acyclovir)	Inhibition of viral DNA polymerase	As for adenine arabinoside; drug of choice	Transient increases in BUN and creatinine; thrombophlebitis
Ribavirin	Suppression of biosynthesis of guanosine-5'-monophosphate; blocks capping of viral mRNA	Influenza A and B; respiratory syncytial virus and paramyxovirus bronchiolitis and pneumonia	Macrocytic anemia; conjunctival injection; embryolethal in some animal species
Ganciclovir (DHPG)	Inhibits DNA polymerase, thereby inhibiting DNA synthesis and terminating chain elongation	Serious cytomegalovirus (CMV) infections in compromised hosts	Bone marrow suppression; liver toxicity; hallucinations
Foscarnet (PFA)	Inhibits DNA polymerase	CMV retinitis in compromised hosts	Transient increases in creatinine; anemia; nausea; tremor; genital ulcers
Zidovudine (AZT)	Inhibits reverse transcriptase; chain terminator of DNA synthesis	Selected patients with AIDS and ARC	Anemia; leukopenia; neutropenia; ↓ vitamin B_{12}; myositis
Didanosine (ddI)	Inhibits reverse transcriptase	Patients with HIV who are intolerant or nonresponsive to AZT	Peripheral neuropathy; pancreatitis; diarrhea
Zalcitabine (ddC)	Inhibits reverse transcriptase	Patients with HIV who are intolerant or nonresponsive to AZT; in combination with AZT in early HIV infection	Peripheral neuropathy; pancreatitis; aphthous stomatitis
Interferons	Activation of an endoribonuclease and phosphorylation of a peptide initiation factor	Herpes keratitis; rhinovirus prophylaxis and treatment; varicella-zoster infection in immunocompromised hosts	Headache; somnolence; gastrointestinal upset

Resistance

Resistance to amantadine is readily achieved in the laboratory. It develops from mutations in the matrix proteins of the virus. Drug-resistant strains have been isolated from treated and untreated patients, but more studies are needed to assess the clinical importance of such strains.

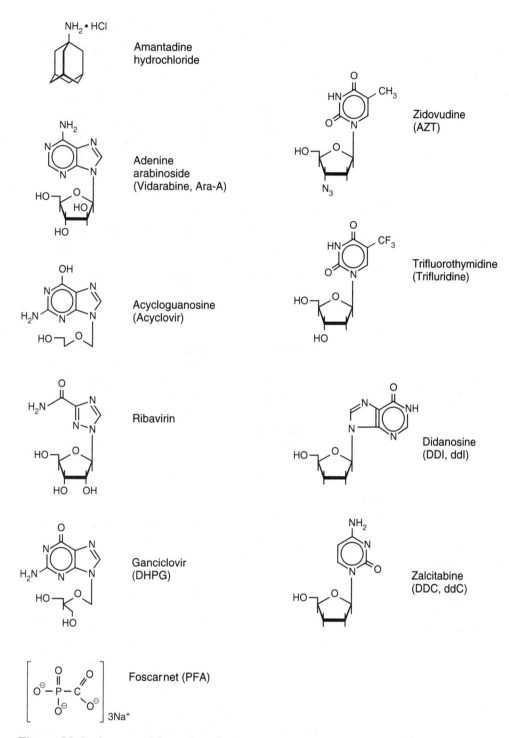

Figure 58-2. Structural formulae of some antiviral agents.

Adverse reactions and toxicity

These include difficulty in thinking, confusion, light-headedness, hallucinations, anxiety, insomnia, and a reduced seizure threshold. The approximate incidence of these primarily CNS manifestations is 3–7%. Very often they may occur within 48 hours of initiating therapy but they are usually reversible despite continuation of the drug. The other major side effects are gastrointestinal, including nausea and lack of appetite. Amantadine has been found to be embryotoxic and teratogenic in animals.

Clinical indications

Amantadine at a dose of 200 mg per day is currently used in chemoprophylaxis and therapy of influenza A virus infections. In persons 65 years of age or older, the dose is decreased to 100 mg. It is compatible with influenza vaccine and may be used in combination therapy under epidemic conditions. As a chemoprophylactic agent, the drug has been found to reduce the incidence of clinical illness by 50–100% (in persons at high risk, e.g., patients with chronic respiratory or cardiovascular disease). As a chemotherapeutic agent against influenza A virus infections, amantadine produces a diminution of fever in 50% of patients and a reduction in illness duration by 1–2 days if it is administered within the first 2–3 days of the onset of illness. It also reduces viral shedding. It does not appear to be useful in the treatment or prophylaxis of influenza B.

Rimantadine

This antiviral agent is a structural analog of amantadine with an identical mechanism of action. Its activity against influenza A virus in vitro is four to eight times that of amantadine. It has also been found to be more efficacious against influenza A virus infections in animals. Until recently, its use has been primarily in the former Soviet Union. A clinical trial of its usefulness as a prophylactic agent against influenza A infections in humans, conducted in the United States, revealed that it is *not* more efficacious than amantadine but that it produces considerably fewer CNS side effects. This quality of rimantadine may soon make it the preferred agent. Gastrointestinal effects, however, are reported frequently. In contrast to amantadine, rimantadine is extensively metabolized with less than 15% excreted unchanged in the urine and approximately 20% as a hydroxylated metabolite. Its half-life averages 24–36 hours.

Trifluorothymidine (Trifluridine)

Mechanism of action

Trifluridine (Viroptic) is a thymidine analog (see Fig. 58-2). It is phosphorylated by cellular thymidine kinase to a monophosphate, which is further phosphorylated by cellular enzymes. The triphosphate is incorporated into DNA by competitively inhibiting the incorporation of the natural nucleotide. Viral DNA polymerase has a higher affinity for trifluridine triphosphate than does the DNA polymerase of uninfected cells. Trifluridine is active against herpes simplex viruses, including some acyclovir-resistant strains.

Adverse reactions and toxicity

The drug is limited to topical usage, primarily ocular. Patients may experience burning on instillation, eyelid edema or irritation, and blurring of vision. Allergic reactions occur infrequently.

Clinical indications

Trifluridine is used primarily for the treatment of primary keratoconjunctivitis and recurrent epithelial keratitis due to herpes simplex virus. It has also been shown to be effective in the management of some chronic cutaneous ulcerations secondary to herpes simplex virus in HIV-infected patients with acyclovir-resistant strains.

The drug is given by drops onto the cornea and continued for 7 days after reepithelialization has occurred. It should not be given for more than 3 weeks.

Resistance of herpes simplex virus type II to trifluridine has been produced in vitro, and these strains are able to produce infection in vivo.

Adenine Arabinoside (Ara-A, Vidarabine)

This agent (see Fig. 58-2) was first introduced as an anticancer drug in 1960. Its antiviral activity was noted in 1964.

Mechanism of action

Vidarabine is a nucleoside derivative of adenine deoxyriboside that inhibits DNA synthesis by competitive inhibition of DNA polymerase. Vidarabine is phosphorylated by cellular enzymes to the triphosphate derivative. The principal metabolite is hypoxanthine arabinoside, a compound with 30–50 times less antiviral activity. It is primarily active against the DNA viruses, including members of the herpes group viruses and pox viruses.

Pharmacokinetics

When vidarabine (Vira-A) is administered by intravenous infusion, it is very rapidly deaminated to a hypoxanthine derivative. It may also be converted by phosphorylation to various phosphate nucleotides. The drug requires large administration volumes because of poor solubility (≤ 0.5 mg/mL). When given intravenously at a dose of 1 mg/kg, plasma levels of 1–2 μg/mL have been achieved, with a plasma half-life of 1.5–3 hours. After an intramuscular injection of 1 mg/kg, the peak serum concentration is only 0.2–0.3 μg/mL, but the half-life is prolonged to 10–16 hours. The differences in half-life are probably caused by protracted absorption from the intramuscular site. Most of the drug is excreted in the urine as an arahypoxanthine derivative. A dosage reduction of 25% has been recommended for patients with severe renal insufficiency.

Adverse reactions and toxicity

The most important side effects are gastrointestinal upset consisting of anorexia, nausea, vomiting, weight loss, and diarrhea. Less commonly, but more importantly, CNS toxicities including tremors, ataxia, paresthesias, dizziness, hallucinations, confusion, and even psychosis may occur. These CNS side effects are most common in patients with reduced renal function. Another problem with vidarabine therapy relates to its poor solubility, which necessitates a large fluid volume for administration of the drug. In patients being treated for encephalitis, this large fluid volume is relatively contraindicated. Other adverse reactions include skin rashes, weight loss, leukopenia, thrombocytopenia, anemia, megaloblastosis, and increased levels of aspartate transferase (AST, synonymous with SGOT). This drug has been shown to be mutagenic, teratogenic, and oncogenic in animal models.

Clinical indications

Current clinical indications for vidarabine therapy include its topical administration to patients with herpetic keratitis, and its systemic administration to patients with herpes encephalitis, or to neonates with disseminated herpes infection. Controlled clinical trials in these latter two groups of patients have demonstrated a reduction in mortality from approximately 70% to approximately 40%. Vidarabine has also been successfully employed for the treatment of varicella infections in hosts with compromised immunity,

resulting in more rapid healing of the vesicular lesions and reduction in pain, as well as a reduced incidence of dissemination to internal organs.

Vidarabine has been largely replaced by acyclovir for serious herpes simplex and herpes varicella-zoster infections, because studies have shown increased efficacy and decreased toxicity of the latter. Vidarabine has been disappointing in the treatment of cytomegalovirus (CMV) infections in compromised hosts.

Acycloguanosine (Acyclovir)

Mechanism of action

This antiviral agent is a guanine derivative with an acyclic side chain (see Fig. 58-2). As a nucleoside derivative, it has a mechanism of action similar to that of vidarabine, but it displays a unique selectivity in action. It appears to be selectively taken up by virus-infected cells and converted to its monophosphate form by a virus-specific thymidine kinase. This monophosphate form is then converted to the active triphosphate form by cellular enzymes. The triphosphate form interferes with viral replication by inhibiting viral DNA polymerase. Acyclovir is much more active against the viral DNA polymerase than it is against cellular DNA polymerase. It may also be incorporated into the viral DNA and act as a chain terminator for viral DNA synthesis. The spectrum of activity in vitro includes members of the herpes group of DNA viruses. It is most active against herpes simplex viruses and the varicella-zoster virus, and it is less active against cytomegalovirus and Epstein-Barr virus.

Resistance

Alterations or deficiency in the viral thymidine kinase or alterations in viral DNA polymerase can cause acyclovir resistance in vitro. Most clinically significant isolates have been thymidine-kinase-deficient mutants usually isolated from immunocompromised patients on long-term or multiple treatment courses. These viruses have led to progressive mucocutaneous infections in these patients, particularly those infected by the human immunodeficiency virus.

Pharmacokinetics

Acyclovir (Zovirax) is available in topical, oral, and intravenous preparations. The topical preparation consists of 5% acyclovir in polyethylene glycol ointment. Oral acyclovir is slowly and incompletely absorbed from the gastrointestinal tract with only 15–30% oral bioavailability. With multidose administration, steady-state concentrations (0.6–1.6 μg/mL) are reached within 24–48 hours. Peak serum concentrations of 20 to more than 100 μmol/L are achieved following a 1-hour infusion of acyclovir of 2.5–15 mg/kg. The terminal half-life is 2–3 hours in adults with normal renal function. (Acyclovir prodrugs with increased absorption and provision of blood levels comparable to intravenous dosing are currently being studied.)

The excretion of acyclovir is primarily via the kidneys by both glomerular filtration and tubular secretion. There is minimal transformation of the drug in vivo. Dosage must be reduced in patients with renal insufficiency.

Adverse reactions and toxicity

The topical and oral formulations of acyclovir are relatively free of side effects. The intravenous formulation can result in transient and reversible increases in BUN and creatinine in approximately 5–10% of treatments, and local reactions consisting of thrombophlebitis or bullae formation have been noted in approximately 3% of patients.

Neurological symptoms including lethargy, agitation, tremor, disorientation, and paresthesia have been noted after intravenous infusion in approximately 1% of patients, especially after bone marrow transplantation or in those with renal failure. Psychiatric symptoms including depersonalization, hallucinations, and hyperactivity have also been observed. Complicating illnesses and concomitant drug use may be contributing factors. These adverse reactions are reversible when acyclovir is discontinued.

Clinical indications

Extensive clinical evaluation has established acyclovir as the treatment of choice in many types of herpes simplex and varicella-zoster viral infections. The most important clinical use of **topical acyclovir** is for herpes genitalis infections. The drug has been found to be most effective in those patients suffering from their first episode of this infection. In such patients, topical application results in rapid decrease in viral shedding, reduced symptomatology, and prompt healing of lesions, but it is less effective than oral or intravenous therapy. The drug is less effective in patients suffering from recurrent episodes of genital herpes. Topical acyclovir has also been

found to be of benefit in the treatment of mucocutaneous herpes infections in patients with compromised immunity, but oral therapy is generally preferred. A liquid formulation of topical acyclovir is effective in the treatment of herpetic keratitis infections.

Oral acyclovir at a dose of 200 mg five times per day is effective in the treatment of first-episode genital herpes simplex infection. Effects include decreased duration of viral shedding, decreased time to healing, and decreased duration of constitutional symptoms. Use of the drug does not alter the time to first recurrence. Oral acyclovir is associated with antiviral activity and, in some trials, with statistically significant but modest clinical effects with recurrent genital herpes simplex infection. Several placebo-controlled studies have shown that chronic suppressive treatment with oral acyclovir (200 mg three times per day) will reduce by up to 80% recurrences of genital herpes. Treatment should be interrupted every 12 months to reassess the need for continued suppression.

Similarly, long-term suppressive oral acyclovir may decrease recurrences of mucocutaneous herpes simplex infections in compromised hosts, such as transplant recipients and patients with acquired immunodeficiency syndrome (AIDS). Oral administration of acyclovir in high dose (800 mg five times per day) accelerates the rate of cutaneous healing from varicella-zoster if given within 72 hours of the onset of the rash.

Clinical trials have also shown that high-dose acyclovir can lead to more rapid healing of varicella (chickenpox) in children if given less than 24 hours of onset. Although the results were statistically significant, the clinical benefits are limited and the role of acyclovir in immunocompetent (i.e., not compromised) children is controversial.

Intravenous acyclovir (like the oral formulation) is effective in the treatment of first-episode genital herpes simplex infections in immunocompetent patients. Effects are less dramatic in recurrent episodes. It is also effective in the prevention and treatment of mucocutaneous herpes simplex infections in the compromised host. The usual dose is 5 mg/kg three times per day.

Localized and disseminated infections due to varicella-zoster in immunocompetent as well as immunocompromised hosts respond to intravenous therapy. There is no dramatic effect on the incidence or the duration of postherpetic neuralgia. In the compromised host, visceral dissemination of varicella-zoster herpes is decreased by treatment with acyclovir.

Two large randomized trials of acyclovir and vidarabine in the treatment of herpes simplex encephalitis demonstrated increased survival and decreased morbidity in patients treated with acyclovir. This is now considered the drug of choice in the treatment of herpes simplex encephalitis. The dose is 12.4 mg/kg every 8 hours.

Studies comparing vidarabine and acyclovir in the treatment of neonatal herpes simplex infection show the two drugs to be equally efficacious.

Acyclovir is of no benefit in the treatment of severe cytomegalovirus (CMV) infections in transplant recipients. The drug has been found to be useful as a prophylactic agent when used in high dose in renal and bone marrow transplant patients to decrease the frequency of symptomatic CMV infections.

Ribavirin

This agent, 1-β-D-ribofuranosyl-1,2,4-triazole-3-carboxamide (Virazole; see Fig. 58-2), a guanosine analog, was synthesized in 1972 as part of a major program to search for a compound with broad-spectrum antiviral activity. In vitro it inhibits a wide range of DNA and RNA viruses including myxoviruses, paramyxoviruses, arena, corona, bunya, RNA tumor, herpes, and pox viruses. In contrast, rotavirus, poliomyelitis, hepatitis B virus, and CMV seem relatively insensitive to inhibition by the drug.

Mechanism of action

The mechanism of action is uncertain but relates to the alteration of cellular nucleotide pools and viral mRNA formation. Mechanisms proposed include (1) decrease in intracellular GTP, (2) inhibition of 5'-cap formation of mRNA, and (3) inhibition of the initiation and elongation of viral mRNAs through effects on RNA polymerase.

Pharmacokinetics

After oral administration in humans, bioavailability averages 45%. The estimated serum half-life is 9 hours. Peak plasma levels of 1–3 μg/mL occur at 1–2 hours. Tenfold-higher peak plasma levels occur following intravenous administration. Aerosol administration of the lyophilized agent by means of a small-particle aerosol generator delivering an estimated 0.8 mg/kg/hr achieves drug levels in respiratory secretions of 50–200 μg/mL, the actual concentration depending on ventilation and lung pathology.

The half-life in tracheal secretions is 1–2 hours. The drug is biotransformed and secreted in the urine.

Adverse reactions and toxicity

Aerosolized ribavirin is well tolerated except for mild conjunctival irritation, rash, and transient wheezing in some patients. (When used in conjunction with mechanical ventilation, in-line filters, modified circuits, and frequent monitoring are required to prevent plugging of the valves or tubing with precipitates.)

After oral administration, reversible increases in serum bilirubin, iron, and uric acid have been observed. The drug was found to be teratogenic and embryotoxic in small mammals during the first trimester. Prolonged use in animals has also caused macrocytic anemia.

Clinical indications

Ribavirin by aerosol is effective in the treatment of lower respiratory tract infections (bronchiolitis and pneumonia) by the respiratory syncytial virus (RSV) in infants and young children with congenital heart disease, pulmonary disease, or immune deficiency. Infants treated with ribavirin showed a significantly faster improvement in their illness severity score. However, no differences were noted in viral shedding.

Opinion varies about the overall clinical value, indications for use, and optimal length of treatment in RSV infections.

Other indications for ribavirin aerosols are respiratory infections secondary to influenza A and influenza B. Treated groups improve statistically more rapidly than controls; however, the clinical improvements are minimal. The drug cannot be used prophylactically for these infections.

In Sierra Leone, intravenous ribavirin was used for the treatment of Lassa fever. Mortality rates decreased significantly when treatment was initiated within the first 6 days of illness. Oral ribavirin was less effective.

Data on the use of ribavirin in HIV infection are conflicting and inconclusive.

9-(1,3-Dihydroxy-2-Propoxymethyl) Guanine (DHPG, Ganciclovir)

This acyclic nucleoside analog of guanine (Cytovene; see Fig. 58-2) has in vitro activity against all herpes virus strains, but its unique characteristic is its potent inhibition of CMV replication.

Mechanism of action

The drug is an inhibitor of viral DNA synthesis. Intracellular ganciclovir is phosphorylated to its monophosphate derivative by infection-induced kinases. Ganciclovir di- and triphosphate are formed by cellular enzymes. Ganciclovir triphosphate is a competitive inhibitor of dGTP incorporation into DNA and preferentially inhibits viral DNA polymerase. The drug incorporates into growing viral DNA and inhibits chain elongation.

Resistance

Herpes simplex virus strains resistant to ganciclovir because of DNA polymerase mutations have been demonstrated in the laboratory. Ganciclovir-resistant strains of herpes and cytomegalovirus have also been isolated from immune-compromised hosts.

Pharmacokinetics

The oral bioavailability is very low (less than 5%), and therefore the drug is usually given intravenously. Prodrugs that are converted to ganciclovir and have greater bioavailability are currently under development. Peak plasma concentrations average 8–11 μg/mL. Cerebrospinal fluid levels average 25–70% of those in plasma. The elimination half-life averages 3–4 hours in patients with normal renal function. It is excreted unchanged in the urine, and dose reduction is necessary in patients with renal insufficiency.

Adverse reactions and toxicity

The most common (and typically dose-limiting) adverse events have been anemia, neutropenia, and thrombocytopenia occurring in up to 40% of treated patients. Central nervous system side effects, including headache, behavioral changes, psychosis, convulsions, and coma, have been described in 5–15%. Rash, fever, abnormal liver function tests, nausea, and vomiting have also been reported. Ganciclovir is teratogenic in rabbits and mutagenic in a number of different systems.

Clinical indications

The drug is used in the treatment and prophylaxis of serious cytomegalovirus infections in immunocom-

promised hosts. In patients with AIDS, ganciclovir has been used successfully in the suppression of CMV retinitis. Approximately 80–90% of patients will respond to treatment. The dose used for induction therapy is 5 mg/kg twice daily, usually for 2–3 weeks. Long-term maintenance therapy (5 mg/kg/day) is required as relapse will occur after 1–2 months off the drug. An oral formulation with $t_{1/2} = 6.3$ hours has been licensed for use in the maintenance therapy of HIV patients and is equivalent to the intravenous preparation used for this purpose. Relapses, however, occur despite long-term maintenance therapy and may be related to inadequate drug concentrations in the eye or resistant strains. Intraocular drug administration by intravitreal injection and slow-release intraocular implants are being evaluated.

Ganciclovir has also been found useful (clinical response up to 65%) in the management of other cytomegalovirus syndromes in patients with HIV, including esophagitis, colitis, cholangitis, and pneumonia. The role of long-term maintenance therapy is controversial for these infections.

In bone marrow transplant patients, virological responses but no decrease in mortality have been observed during treatment of cytomegalovirus pneumonia. Increased survival has been reported when ganciclovir is used in combination with anti-CMV immune globulin.

Ganciclovir has been found useful in the prophylaxis of CMV infections and disease in transplant recipients. However, the optimal dose, duration, and appropriate selection of patients have not been determined.

A recent randomized placebo-controlled study has demonstrated efficacy of oral ganciclovir as prophylaxis against CMV infection in HIV patients at risk.

Foscarnet (PFA)

Trisodium phosphoformate hexahydrate (see Fig. 58-2) is an inorganic pyrophosphate analog that inhibits herpes viruses, DNA polymerase, and retroviral reverse transcriptase. It is active in vitro against most herpes viruses, including cytomegalovirus and herpes simplex virus.

Pharmacokinetics

It is usually given by the intravenous route as a bolus followed by either continuous or intermittent infusions of 90 mg/kg. The plasma half-life averages 3–6 hours. Foscarnet penetrates the cerebrospinal fluid and the eye. The drug is excreted by the kidneys and dosages must be adjusted in renal failure.

Adverse reactions and toxicity

The major toxicity is renal insufficiency. It has been associated with malaise, nausea, vomiting, fatigue, and headache. Tremors, seizures, irritability, and hallucinations have been associated with increased serum concentrations. Local phlebitis, hypo- or hypercalcemia, hyperphosphatemia, and abnormal liver function tests may develop. Neutropenia has been reported infrequently. In a small number of patients, painful oral and genital ulcers have been described following the intravenous infusion of this drug. Nephrogenic diabetes insipidus is an uncommon complication.

Clinical indications

Foscarnet (Foscavir) has been used primarily to treat CMV infections in HIV-infected patients. In cytomegalovirus retinitis, clinical responses appear to be similar in frequency to those observed with ganciclovir and may be associated with small survival benefit. The problem of relapse after discontinuation of therapy is similar to that observed with ganciclovir so that long-term maintenance therapy is required. Resistant strains have been described, probably resulting from mutations in the viral polymerase gene.

Foscarnet also appears to be a useful agent in the treatment of acyclovir- and ganciclovir-resistant strains of herpes simplex virus and cytomegalovirus.

ANTIRETROVIRAL DRUGS

The human immunodeficiency virus (HIV) infects the CD4 T lymphocytes, resulting in progressive deterioration of the cell-mediated immune system. As the CD4 count declines, patients are at increasing risk of opportunistic infections and malignancies complicating their viral infection and resulting in AIDS. HIV is a chronic disease; patients survive an average of 8–10 years. No cure is presently available. However, numerous antiretroviral drugs have been developed to slow the progressive immunological deterioration, increase CD4 cell counts, decrease HIV viral loads, and eventually delay complications and prolong survival. Unfortunately, resistance can develop to all of these drugs, as a result of mutations at different points in the reverse transcriptase enzyme or other enzymes involved in viral replication.

3'-Azido-3'-Dideoxythymidine (AZT, Zidovudine)

A deoxynucleoside analog structurally related to thymidine, this drug (see Fig. 58-2) was synthesized more than 20 years ago; however, no therapeutic application was found until recently. This was the first agent shown to be effective in the management of HIV-1 infections and was approved for use in 1987.

Pharmacokinetics

The drug is well absorbed orally with 65% bioavailability, and it penetrates the central nervous system. Plasma protein binding is only 30%. Peak plasma concentrations of 5 μmol/L are achieved with intravenous doses of 2.5 mg/kg or oral doses of 5 mg/kg. Its half-life is approximately 1–1.5 hours. The determination of intracellular levels is difficult, but they are probably a more reliable indicator of the drug's antiviral activity.

Biotransformation is primarily hepatic (glucuronidation) with subsequent renal excretion. The drug undergoes extensive first-pass metabolism to an inactive metabolite. After oral administration 65–75% of the drug is recovered as a metabolite in the urine, 8–15% as parent compound, and the remaining 15–20% is excreted by extrarenal mechanisms.

The dose needs to be decreased in patients with severe hepatic or renal dysfunction.

Adverse reactions and toxicity

The major adverse effects include reversible anemia and leukopenia. Macrocytosis is a common finding but does not usually require treatment. Significant frequencies of nausea, headache, insomnia, and myalgias are reported. These symptoms occasionally require dosage adjustment or may resolve spontaneously despite continuation of the drug. Myositis with elevation of CPK and proximal muscle weakness have been reported. Nail pigmentation may occur in dark-skinned patients.

Clinical indications

In patients with AIDS or symptomatic AIDS-related complex (ARC), AZT (Retrovir) has been found to increase survival and decrease the risk of development of HIV-related opportunistic infections. In patients with HIV infection and lesser degrees of immunosuppression (CD4 count less than 500×10^6/L), AZT has been found to prolong the time to the development of an opportunistic infection. The effect of early treatment on survival and the optimal time to initiate treatment remain controversial.

More recent studies have shown that AZT in combination with protease inhibitors, or with other reverse transcriptase inhibitors such as ddI, ddC, and 3TC, can produce greater benefits than AZT alone, with respect to virus levels, immune system function, and clinical condition.

AZT was found effective in the treatment of HIV-associated neurological disease; it is also the preferred treatment for HIV-related thrombocytopenia.

AZT, when given by mouth to women 14–34 weeks pregnant with CD4 counts more than 200×10^6/L during their pregnancy, and as an intravenous preparation during delivery and as an oral suspension to newborns for the first 6 weeks, can lower the rate of maternal–fetal transmission from 25% to 8%.

The minimal effective dose for long-term treatment is undefined. However, a low dose (500–600 mg per day) is as effective as a higher one (1200 mg per day) and is associated with reduced toxicity.

Resistance

In vitro resistance to AZT has been found in a significant number of patients receiving treatment for more than 6 months, especially in those with more advanced immunosuppression and higher viral loads. Resistance occurs by mutations at various sites on the reverse transcriptase enzyme. The clinical significance of AZT resistance remains undefined, but patients may benefit from a change to, or addition of, a different antiretroviral agent.

2'3'-Dideoxyinosine (ddI, DDI, Didanosine)

This purine nucleoside analog (see Fig. 58-2) interferes with the HIV replicative cycle by competitive inhibition of the reverse transcriptase. It is converted to an active triphosphate form.

Pharmacokinetics

The plasma half-life is approximately 1 hour. The active metabolite ddATP has a longer intracellular half-life, thereby allowing less frequent administration. It is acid-labile and therefore must be buffered for oral use. The drug is currently available as a chewable tablet, with average bioavailability of 43%.

Unfortunately, many patients find the taste unpleasant. The dosage is 100–300 mg twice a day based on body weight.

Adverse reactions and toxicity

The main dose-limiting toxicity includes peripheral neuropathy and pancreatitis. Peripheral neuropathy usually resolves in 3–5 weeks when the drug is discontinued. Fatal pancreatitis has been reported. Other symptoms include diarrhea, dry mouth, headache, insomnia, irritability, and seizures. Hyperuricemia is commonly seen but is rarely clinically important. Hypokalemia, hypomagnesemia, and hypocalcemia have been described.

Clinical indications

ddI (Videx) is an alternative antiretroviral agent for patients with advanced HIV infection who are either intolerant or unresponsive to AZT. It is also useful in combination with other reverse transcriptase inhibitors such as AZT, 3TC, and D4T. A number of phase I and II studies have shown benefit from the drug by increases in weight, decrease in clinical symptoms, and a stabilization of the CD4 count. In one trial, ddI was found to be more effective than AZT in slowing the progression of HIV infection in persons with CD4 counts less than 300×10^6/L who had been treated for more than 16 weeks with AZT.

2'3'-Dideoxycytidine (ddC, DDC, Zalcitabine)

The drug is a pyrimidine nucleoside analog (see Fig. 58–2). It is phosphorylated by cellular kinases to an active triphosphate form and is incorporated into DNA by the DNA polymerase of the virus, resulting in the termination of chain elongation.

Pharmacokinetics

The oral bioavailability of the drug is 87%. The plasma half-life is 0.34 hour and the intracellular half-life is 2.6 hours.

Adverse reactions and toxicity

The major dose-limiting toxicity is peripheral neuropathy, especially in patients on higher doses and with more advanced infection. Pancreatitis has also been reported. Aphthous stomatitis with fever, malaise, and esophageal ulcerations can occur.

Clinical indications

ddC (Hivid) is used in patients with advanced HIV infections who are either unable to tolerate, or whose disease progresses despite, AZT and ddI. The usual dose is 0.75 mg three times per day. The drug has also been shown in small studies to be effective in combination with AZT or saquinavir in HIV infections and a CD4 count of less than 300×10^6/L. Phase I and II trials have shown improvement in surrogate markers of HIV infections, including P24 antigen and CD4 count. The drug appears to be less effective than AZT as a first-line treatment in patients with advanced HIV disease.

3TC (2'deoxy-3'-thiacytidine, *Lamivudine*)

This is a dideoxypyrimidine analog that inhibits the HIV reverse transcriptase. The negative enantiomer has greater activity and less toxicity than the positive enantiomer and was selected for clinical testing and use. 3TC has activity against a wide range of retroviruses including strains of HIV that are resistant to AZT. It is also synergistic with AZT in vitro and in vivo.

Pharmacokinetics

The mean oral bioavailability of 3TC is 80% and the mean plasma half-life is approximately 2–4 hours.

Adverse reactions

The drug is generally well tolerated. Neutropenia and mild and transient episodes of diarrhea, headache, fatigue, nausea, and abdominal pain are the most frequent adverse events reported. Rare cases of pancreatitis have occurred.

Clinical indications

3TC is used in combination with AZT for patients with HIV infection who have not been treated previously with antiretroviral agents. The combination has a superior virological (decreased HIV plasma loads) and immunological (increased CD4 lymphocyte counts) effect compared to either drug used alone. For patients already treated with AZT, the addition of 3TC gives better short-term virological and immunological effects than addition of ddC. Addition of 3TC to monotherapy or combination therapy with nucleoside analogs also improves survival.

Resistance

Resistance to 3TC results from a mutation in the HIV reverse transcriptase gene that is selected when 3TC is present.

D4T (2',3'-didehydro-2',3'-dideoxythymidine, *Stavudine*)

This is a nucleoside reverse transcriptase inhibitor closely related to AZT. It must be phosphorylated in order to compete with endogenous 2'-deoxynucleoside-5'-triphosphate for binding to the reverse transcriptase and to thus prevent elongation of the viral DNA intermediates.

Pharmacokinetics

D4T is rapidly absorbed with an overall mean bioavailability of 91%. At peak plasma concentrations of 1.2–4.2 mg/L, CSF concentrations range from 0.08 to 0.4 mg/L. The mean plasma half-life is 1–1.6 hours. Approximately 40% is excreted unchanged in the urine. Because of the prolonged half-life of the triphosphate metabolite, fewer daily doses are required than for the other reverse transcriptase inhibitors.

Adverse reactions

The major limiting toxicities are peripheral neuropathy and pancreatitis, which are dose-related. Other adverse events reported include headache, asthenia, GI disturbance, and raised liver enzyme levels.

Clinical indications

D4T is typically used as a component of combination antiretroviral therapy, often as a substitute for AZT in patients intolerant of that medication. In vitro, AZT inhibits the intracellular phosphorylation of D4T. Combination of the two drugs may therefore be therapeutically undesirable.

Resistance

Resistance to D4T has been associated with a mutation at codon 75 of reverse transcriptase.

HIV PROTEASE INHIBITORS

This is a new class of antiretroviral drugs with potent activity against HIV. The major enzymatic and structural proteins of the virus are synthesized as a polyprotein that must be cleaved into the individual proteins by a viral aspartic protease. This protease is essential for the release of infectious virus.

The protease inhibitors are selective inhibitors of this protease. Three agents are currently licensed for clinical use in the United States and Canada and others are under development.

Saquinavir mesylate (Invirase)

Pharmacokinetics

The compound has a low oral bioavailability of about 4% due to a combination of incomplete absorption (30%) and extensive first-pass metabolism. The extent of absorption is substantially increased following food. A gel capsule with increased bioavailability is under study. The half-life of the drug is 1.1–1.9 hours. Protein binding is approximately 98% and therefore CSF penetration is low. There is extensive hepatic clearance, but only 4% is cleared by the kidney.

Drug interactions

Saquinavir is metabolized by CYP3A4. Drugs that inhibit this isoenzyme (such as ketoconazole) cause an increase in the plasma concentrations of saquinavir. In contrast, drugs such as rifampin that induce the CYP3A4 isoenzyme can significantly decrease saquinavir plasma concentrations by up to 80%. Saquinavir itself can inhibit the biotransformation of other drug substrates of CYP3A4 such as the antihistamines terfenadine and astemizole (see Chapter 33).

Adverse reactions

The majority of adverse reactions are mild. The most frequently reported reactions involve the gastrointestinal tract. They include diarrhea, abdominal discomfort, and nausea.

Resistance

Mutations of the HIV protease enzyme appear to develop in the presence of saquinavir and lead to phenotypic resistance.

Clinical indications

Saquinavir is indicated in combination with reverse transcriptase inhibitors for the treatment of HIV infection. Studies have shown superior virological, immunological, and survival benefits when combination therapy is used.

Ritonavir (Norvir)

Pharmacokinetics

The oral bioavailability of the drug is approximately 80–90% and the half-life is 3–4 hours. These two factors allow for twice daily dosing schedules. The drug is 99% protein-bound and does not penetrate well into the central nervous system. The drug induces its own metabolism so that plasma levels (and adverse events) are greatest during the first few days of treatment. To decrease the toxic effects, the drug dose is initially low and is increased gradually.

Drug interactions

Ritonavir is metabolized by cytochrome P450 isoenzymes and therefore interacts with other medications that either inhibit or induce these isoenzymes.

Adverse events

Adverse events are very common (85–100% of patients), especially during the first weeks of treatment, and include nausea, vomiting, diarrhea, headaches, asthenia, circumoral paresthesia, and increased plasma transaminase levels.

Resistance

Long-term therapy with ritonavir is associated with the emergence of multiple mutations in the HIV protease at codons 10, 54, 63, 71, 82, and 84. Phenotypic resistance is detected in the majority of patients at 1 year. Resistance to ritonavir is usually accompanied by cross-resistance to indinavir.

Clinical indications

A recent clinical trial showed that the use of ritonavir as "salvage therapy" in patients with advanced HIV disease and CD4 counts less than 50×10^6/L, either as monotherapy or in combination with reverse transcriptase inhibitors, resulted in significant virological and immunological effects as well as survival gains. Ritonavir is being studied as combination therapy with reverse transcriptase inhibitors and with saquinavir in earlier-stage HIV disease.

Indinavir (Crixivan)

Pharmacokinetics

Indinavir is well absorbed orally. Absorption can be reduced to 78% when administered with a standard meal high in calories, fat, and protein. It has a relatively short half-life of 1.8 hours. It is approximately 60% protein-bound. Less than 20% of indinavir is excreted in the urine.

Adverse reactions

Indinavir is usually well tolerated. Nephrolithiasis has been reported in 4% of patients receiving this drug. In general, these stones are not associated with renal dysfunction and resolve with hydration and temporary interruption of therapy. Asymptomatic elevation of the indirect bilirubin level is found in about 10% of patients. In less than 1% this is associated with elevations of ALT or AST. A minority of patients develop rash, dry skin, taste disturbances, and drug interactions. Indinavir should not be administered concurrently with terfenadine, triazolam, cisapride, astemizole, midazolam, or other substrates of CYP3A4.

Resistance

Resistance to indinavir is correlated with the accumulation of mutations in the viral genome, at various sites of the HIV protease enzyme, involving at least 11 different amino acid residue positions. No single substitution produces measurable resistance, which requires the coexpression of multiple substitutions. In general, the greater the number of substitutions, the higher the level of resistance. Substitutions appear to accumulate sequentially through successive viral replications.

HIV isolates with reduced susceptibility to indinavir show varying degrees of cross-resistance to ritonavir, saquinavir, and other HIV protease inhibitors. Concomitant use of indinavir with a nucleotide analog may lessen the chance of development of resistance to both agents.

Clinical indications

Indinavir is indicated in combination with reverse transcriptase inhibitors for the treatment of HIV infection. Combination therapy yields superior virological and immunological results.

MEDIATORS OF IMMUNE RESPONSE

Some viral infections can be treated by modification of the body's natural immune responses. The organization and functions of the immune system are described in detail in Chapter 61. Readers who are not familiar with this topic are advised to review Chapter 61 before reading the following sections.

Interferon (IFN)

The interferons are a family of **host-range-specific** glycoproteins (e.g., bovine IFN is not cross-protective for humans). These agents have become recognized as potent cytokines that are associated with complex antiviral, immunomodulatory, and antiproliferative activity. They are synthesized by host cells in response to various inducers. The human interferons are divided into three classes as follows:

1. **Leukocyte IFN (α-IFN,** Alferon, Intron, Roferon, Wellferon) is produced when null lymphocytes, B lymphocytes, and macrophages are stimulated by viruses, bacteria, foreign cells, and mitogens for B lymphocytes.
2. **Fibroblast IFN (β-IFN)** is produced in fibroblasts, epithelial cells, myeloblasts, lymphoblasts, and T lymphocytes when stimulated by viruses, polynucleotides, and inhibitors of RNA and protein synthesis.
3. **Immune IFN (γ-IFN,** Actimmune) is produced in T lymphocytes when stimulated by foreign antigens, mitogens for T lymphocytes, galactose oxidase, and calcium ionophores.

More recently, interferons have been produced by means of recombinant DNA technology, thereby providing adequate quantities of pure interferon for clinical trials.

The interferons have a range of biological and biochemical effects. These include:

- Antiviral action
- Immunoregulatory action
- Antitumor action
- Cell growth inhibition
- Macrophage activation
- Enhancement of cytotoxicity of lymphocytes
- Induction of new cellular proteins
- Alteration of initiation factor eIF-2
- Induction of 2,5-oligoadenylic synthetase and activation of endonuclease activated by 2′,5′-oligoadenylic acid

The interferon system is the earliest-appearing host defense against viral infection, coming into operation within a few hours of infection. As the virus infection subsides and the titer of virus declines, there is a corresponding drop in the level of interferon. Several other lines of evidence strongly suggest a causal relationship between the interferon system and natural recovery from many viral infections of humans and animals. In addition, there is increasing evidence that interferon may inhibit the growth of some tumors. Numerous trials are currently being carried out to determine the effects of the various interferons in the treatment of a variety of neoplasms, and as immunosuppressants.

Mechanisms of action

Interferons can be induced by active and inactive viruses, double-stranded RNA, and a number of other compounds. They tend to be species-specific.

A wide range of viruses are sensitive to the antiviral effects of interferon, although considerable differences exist for different viruses and assay systems. Interferons are not directly antiviral but cause biochemical changes in exposed cells that lead to viral resistance. Depending upon the viruses and cell type, interferon antiviral effects are mediated through inhibition of viral penetration or uncoating, synthesis or processing of mRNA, translation of viral proteins, or viral assembly and release. For most viruses, the primary step inhibited by interferon is protein synthesis. The interferon produced is released into the extracellular fluid and binds to specific cell receptors. This initiates a series of events leading to the production of two enzymes, protein kinase and 2,5-oligoadenylate synthetase. Protein kinase inhibits the formation of the initiation complex for protein syn-

thesis, and 2,5-oligoadenylate synthetase activates a cellular endonuclease that degrades viral mRNA. Consequently viral protein synthesis is inhibited at two stages.

Pharmacokinetics

The pharmacokinetics of interferons are not well characterized. Doses of interferon given every 12 hours provide relatively steady serum levels. Maximum levels in blood following intramuscular injection are achieved in 5–8 hours. Interferon does not penetrate well into the CSF.

Orally administered doses do not result in detectable serum levels and are not used clinically. After intramuscular or subcutaneous injection, plasma levels are dose-related.

Adverse reactions and toxicity

Both purified natural and recombinant interferons cause dose-related toxicity that limits their clinical use. A systemic dose of 1×10^6 IU/day is generally well tolerated, but with prolonged systemic administration, an influenza-like syndrome of fever, chills, headaches, myalgias, nausea, vomiting, and diarrhea frequently occurs. Major toxicities that limit parenteral use are bone marrow suppression, mental confusion, behavioral changes, fatigue, myalgias, and cardiotoxicity. Local reactions consist of tenderness and erythema at the injection site. Intranasal administration is associated with mucosal friability, ulceration, and dryness.

Clinical use

Extensive testing has been done with various formulations and routes of administration to assess the possible value of interferons in the prevention and treatment of various viral infections. Clinical use has been limited by the lack of potency and the high incidence of adverse reactions.

Topical administration (nasal sprays) has been studied most extensively in the prophylaxis and treatment of rhinovirus infections. Although trials have shown some response, the clinical significance is debatable.

Condyloma acuminatum has responded to various interferon preparations administered topically, subcutaneously, or directly into the lesion. Efficacy has been demonstrated in patients in whom previous conventional therapies had failed, but side effects frequently preclude long-term use.

Chronic hepatitis B viral infections have shown responsiveness to the parenteral administration of recombinant α-IFN, which is associated with a loss of DNA polymerase activity. Optimal dosage schedules and possible effects on long-term sequelae remain uncertain.

SUGGESTED READING

Collier AC, Coombs RW, Schoenfeld DA, et al. Treatment of human immunodeficiency virus infection with saquinavir, zidovudine and zalcitabine. N Engl J Med 1996; 334:1011–1017.

Connor EM, Sperling RS, Gelber R, et al. Reduction of maternal-infant transmission of human immunodeficiency virus type I with zidovudine treatment. N Engl J Med 1994; 331:1173–1181.

Danner SA, Carr A, Leonard JM, et al. A short-term study of the safety, pharmacokinetics, and efficacy of ritonavir, an inhibitor of HIV-1 protease. N Engl J Med 1995; 333:1528–1539.

Dolin R, Reichman RC, Madore HP, et al. A controlled trial of amantadine and rimantadine in the prophylaxis of influenza A infection. N Engl J Med 1982; 307:580–584.

Drew WL, Ives D, Lalezari JP, et al. Oral ganciclovir as maintenance treatment for cytomegalovirus retinitis in patients with AIDS. N Engl J Med 1995; 333:615–620.

Erice A, Balfour HH. Resistance of human immunodeficiency virus type 1 to antiretroviral agents: a review. CID 1994; 18:149–156.

Eron JJ, Benoit SL, Jemsek J, et al. Treatment with lamivudine, zidovudine or both in HIV-positive patients with 200 to 500 CD4+ cells per cubic millimeter. N Engl J Med 1995; 333:1662–1669.

Hall C. Ribavirin: beginning the blitz on respiratory viruses? Pediatr Infect Dis 1985; 4:668–671.

Hayden FG, Albrecht JK, Kaiser, et al. Prevention of natural colds by contact prophylaxis with intranasal alpha-2 interferon. N Engl J Med 1986; 314:71–75.

Korenman J, Baker B, Waggoner J. Long-term remission of chronic hepatitis B after alpha-interferon therapy. Ann Intern Med 1991; 114:629–634.

McCormick JB, King IJ, Webb PA, et al. Lassa fever: effective therapy with ribavirin. N Engl J Med 1986; 314:20–26.

McLeod G, Hammer S. Zidovudine: five years later. Ann Intern Med 1992; 117:487–501.

Meng TC, Fischl MA, Boota AM, et al. Combination therapy with zidovudine and dideoxycytidine in patients with advanced human immunodeficiency virus infection. Ann Intern Med 1992; 116(1):12–20.

Roberts NA. Drug-resistance patterns of saquinavir and other HIV proteinase inhibitors. AIDS 1995; 9(2):S27–S32.

Rozencweig M, McLaun C, Beltangady M, et al. Overview of phase 1 trials of 2′3′-dideoxyinosine (ddI) conducted on adult patients. Rev Infect Dis 1990; 12:5570–5575.

Safrin S, Crumpacher C, Chatis P, et al. A controlled trial comparing foscarnet with vidarabine for acyclovir-resistant mucocutaneous herpes simplex in the acquired immunodeficiency syndrome. N Engl J Med 1991; 325(8):551–555.

Stein DS, Fish DG, Bilello JA, et al. A 24-week open-label phase I/II evaluation of the HIV protease inhibitor MK-639 (indinavir). AIDS 1996; 10:485–492.

CHAPTER 59

Antiseptics, Disinfectants, and Sterilization

E.L. FORD-JONES

Foul odors were first associated with disease long before bacteria were discovered, and many empirical attempts were made to minimize these odors and the suppuration of wounds by application of chemicals. As long ago as 450 B.C. a sort of chemical disinfection was practiced, as it was noted that water stored in copper or silver vessels was less likely to acquire a foul odor and taste than that stored in pottery vessels. At the time of Hippocrates, wine and vinegar were used in wound dressings. In 1847, the importance of hand decontamination in surgery and obstetrics was first appreciated when Semmelweis reduced the mortality rate of puerperal sepsis in an obstetrical unit from about 12% to less than 2% by requiring each student to wash his hands in chlorinated lime before performing examinations. Shortly after this, Pasteur introduced the concept of sterilization of surgical instruments by heat, and Lister began to use phenol to kill bacteria on instruments, dressings, and other operating materials and to spray carbolic acid over the wounds during an operation to kill bacteria before they could enter the wound. Such concepts, however, remained generally unpopular until the turn of the century.

Currently, 5–10% of adults entering hospital acquire an infection that was neither present nor incubating on admission to hospital and is therefore considered nosocomial (from the Latin *nosocomium* = hospital). Prevention of nosocomial infections depends in part on the effective use of antiseptics, disinfectants, and sterilization procedures, combined with other measures to limit transmission of infection. In accredited North American hospitals, Infection Control Committees composed of physicians, surgeons, pharmacists, nurses, and Central Sterile Supply staff, among others, are responsible for infection control activities. Each physician must understand the processes, their limitations, and methods of monitoring effectiveness. The major definitions follow.

Antiseptics are chemicals that are applied to living tissue to destroy bacteria or limit their growth.

Disinfectants are agents or processes applied to inanimate objects to destroy bacteria except spore forms. Their main purpose is to eliminate the hazards of infection. Depending on the agent or process, mycobacteria, viruses, and fungi may also be eliminated.

Sterilization is the physical or chemical process of destroying all microorganisms including spore forms.

Germicides are agents that destroy pathogenic microorganisms, but not necessarily spore forms, mycobacteria, viruses, or fungi, and are used on both living tissue and inanimate objects.

A **fungicide** is an agent that destroys fungi.

A **sporidicide** is an agent that destroys spores.

A **virucide** is an agent that destroys viruses.

Sanitizers are agents that reduce the number of bacterial contaminants to a safe level, to meet public health requirements.

PRINCIPLES OF INFECTION CONTROL

Antiseptics

There are few situations in which antiseptics are of proven therapeutic value. They are mainly used in prophylaxis, and they are applied topically because of toxicity that would make systemic administration unacceptable. Systemic absorption through broken skin, or permeable skin as in the infant of less than 32 weeks gestation, may result in toxicity. The following properties are desirable for antiseptics:

- Potency and selectivity for the organism(s) concerned
- Low surface tension for ease of spread
- Retention of potency in the presence of inflammatory exudates
- Rapid and sustained action
- Absence of toxicity to skin or tissue and noninterference with mechanisms of healing and tissue repair
- Nonallergenicity
- Lack of systemic absorption
- Pleasant aesthetic qualities (odor, color, lack of staining)
- Low cost

Disinfectants

The properties listed above for antiseptics are equally desirable for disinfectants, and in addition, the disinfectants should be noncorrosive and otherwise nondamaging to instruments and materials. It is, however, of greatest importance to consider the purpose for which the disinfectant is used. Sterilization or thorough cleaning may be more appropriate, and disposable equipment may be more economical. Three categories of risk to the patient should be considered (high, intermediate or occasional, and low), which determine the stringency of asepsis required:

High risk: Equipment in contact with broken skin, mucous membranes, vascular system, or sterile body cavity where any form of microorganism could be harmful, e.g., surgical instruments, urinary catheters, parenteral fluids.
Intermediate or occasional risk: Equipment in contact with mucous membranes and some nonintact skin where pathogenic organisms such as nonlipid-containing viruses, tubercle bacilli, and fungi could be harmful, e.g., respiratory and ophthalmic equipment.
Low risk: Equipment *not* in close contact with the patient's mucous membranes, nonintact skin, sterile cavities, or vascular system, and where only significant numbers of bacterial pathogens would be harmful. Cleaning is usually adequate, e.g., walls, ceilings, mattresses.

Sterilization

Once a decision is made that all forms of microbial life, including spore forms, must be killed, the method is selected on the basis of the ability of the material to withstand the process. Steam under pressure (autoclaving) is most widely used, and other gaseous or chemical methods are chosen only if equipment will not withstand autoclaving. Because ethylene oxide gas sterilization is more complex and expensive, it is restricted to objects that might be damaged by heat or excessive moisture. All objects processed in this way require special aeration to remove toxic residues of ethylene oxide. Flash sterilization must be used judiciously and is not recommended for implantable items.

Factors Influencing the Efficacy of Antimicrobial Agents or Processes

The organism

The differences in response of microorganisms to chemical and physical agents are very great, bacterial endospores being most resistant, followed by tubercle bacilli, fungal spores, small or nonlipid viruses, vegetative fungi, medium-sized or lipid viruses, and vegetative bacterial cells. There is no evidence that the hepatitis viruses are unusually resistant. Among the vegetative bacteria, those with the highest lipid content, the Gram-negative organisms, are the most resistant. "Naturally occurring" organisms found in the hospital environment are often more resistant than those subcultured in the microbial laboratory, and this may reflect variations in temperature, pH, humidity, and growth factors present.

The agent

Intrinsic or in-use **contamination** of many antiseptics and disinfectants, including benzalkonium chloride, chlorhexidine, hexachlorophene, iodophors, and phenolics, has been described following interaction with organic material or when they have been dispensed into unsterile containers.

Inactivation on contact with certain materials may occur, as in the case of benzalkonium chloride and cotton fibers.

Degree of dilution for use must be appropriate.

Duration of contact must be adequate. (Only incineration works immediately!)

Mechanical cleaning

Good physical cleaning must precede any disinfection or sterilization process. Organic material will protect bacteria from penetration by the agent or directly inactivate certain agents. In a recent outbreak of *Serratia* species septicemia associated with a contaminated endoscope, the instrument had been gas-"sterilized" but not properly cleaned first.

Evaluation of Antimicrobial Activity

Sterilization

This process is easy to monitor with well-recognized techniques, and this is the most reliable means of eliminating microbial life. Quantitative assurance of true sterilization is achieved through the challenge of a sterilizing process with 10^6 dried bacterial endospores, sterilization being defined as the state in which the probability of one spore surviving is $1:10^6$ or lower.

Disinfectants

Disinfectant tests have not been standardized. Many factors must be considered, such as choice of test organism, preparation of cell suspensions, neutralization of the disinfectant residues in subculture, and determination of the end point. There is some agreement over the need for three levels of testing, **in vitro, in vivo** (tests carried out in the lab under conditions simulating real life situations), and **in use,** but methodology and results vary widely. Evaluation of disinfection procedures is thus less reliable than that of sterilization processes.

Antiseptics

Although it might seem most reasonable to assess the value of antiseptics by measuring how effectively they reduce wound infections, as Semmelweis did, there are many variables in these situations, and antiseptics are therefore assessed on their ability to reduce numbers of resident and transient bacteria on the skin. Methods include culture of handwashing samples, bacterial counts in used gloves, contact plates, and skin biopsies. There is no satisfactory standard method for in vitro kinetic study of virucidal activity of antiseptics.

MECHANISMS AND SITES OF ACTION

Figure 59-1 and Table 59-1 show the main targets for antibacterial agents or processes.

RESISTANCE

Intrinsic Resistance

Gram-negative bacteria and mycobateria are generally associated with a greater resistance to antiseptics and disinfectants, probably because of the unique character of their cell walls, which contain polysaccharide and lipid, leading to exclusion of agents that could otherwise act on intracellular targets.

Plasmid-Mediated Resistance

Bacteria occasionally contain small, autonomously replicating cytoplasmic DNA strands called plasmids, which may contain genes for antibiotic resistance (see also Chapter 52). Such plasmids may determine resistance to mercury and organomercurials, cadmium, arsenic, and hexachlorophene, either by detoxification and removal of the agent from the bacterial cell or by alteration of permeability of the cell surface. This resistance is often linked to plasmids that specify resistance to antibiotics.

Resistance of Bacterial Spores

The mechanism of resistance of spores to heat and chemicals is unknown, and a variety of different factors are probably important.

AGENTS

Table 59-1 summarizes the cellular targets for non-antibiotic antimicrobial compounds.

Alcohols

Isopropyl and ethyl alcohol are effective in killing vegetative bacteria and mycobacteria but are not sporidicidal. The presence of water is essential for the activity of the alcohols, and the most effective alcohol concentrations are 60–70%. Concentrations less than 30% are ineffective. Coloring agents may be added to differentiate the alcohols from water or saline and prevent errors through inadvertent admin-

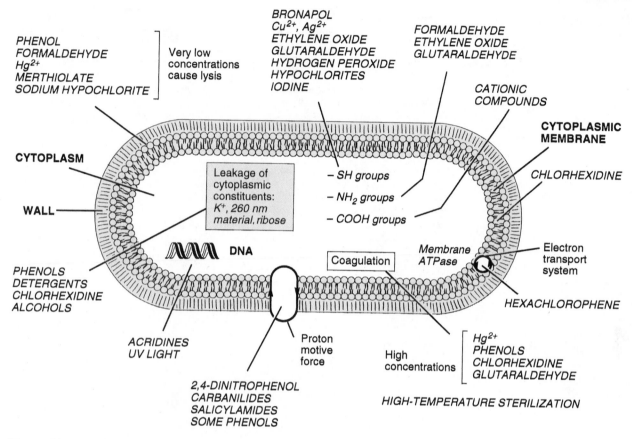

Figure 59-1. Diagram showing the main targets for nonantibiotic antibacterial agents. (Modified from Russell, Hugo & Ayliffe, 1982.)

istration. They are corrosive and an antirust agent (0.1% sodium nitrite) must be added when they are used on metals. Killing requires between 1 and 30 minutes exposure to alcohol, depending on the organisms being attacked. A disadvantage is the failure of alcohol to exert any persistent effect.

Aldehydes

Glutaraldehyde is effective against bacteria, fungi and their respective spores, many viruses, and probably mycobacteria. It is supplied for disinfecting purposes as a 2% alkalinized solution. It is a popular high-level disinfectant and sterilizing agent because of its broad spectrum of activity, effectiveness in the presence of organic material, and noncorrosive qualities. It has, however, an irritating odor and the toxicity of the vapor to the user is largely unstudied. It must be removed with sterile water rinses before use of the disinfected object.

Formaldehyde has been a popular disinfectant in both liquid and gaseous states, but because inhala-

tion of vapor may pose a carcinogenic risk to humans, its use is generally limited to the disinfection of dialysis equipment.

Antimicrobial Dyes

Triphenylmethane dyes are basic dyes that include crystal violet, brilliant green, and malachite green. They are used as local antiseptics because of their activity against Gram-positive bacteria and some fungi.

Biguanides

Chlorhexidine has a wide spectrum of antibacterial activity against Gram-positive and Gram-negative organisms, although it is not sporidicidal, virucidal, or fungicidal, or active against mycobacteria. It is an N^1,N^5-substituted biguanide that is available as a dihydrochloride, diacetate, and most commonly, gluconate. Its activity is reduced in the presence of organic matter, soap, and other anionic compounds,

Table 59-1 Cellular Targets for Nonantibiotic Antibacterial Agents*

Nonantibiotic Antimicrobial Agent	Target or Reaction Attacked											
	CW	AMP	ETC	AT	ETG	AGMP	GC	R	NA	TG	AG	HRC
Acridine dyes									+			
Alcohols						+						
Anilides (TCS, TCC)		+				+						
Bronopol					+					+		
Chlorhexidine				+		+	+++					
Copper salts					+		+++			+		
Ethylene oxide				+	+					+	+	+
Formaldehyde	+										++	
Glutaraldehyde					+		++			+	+	+
Hexachlorophene		+	+				+++					
Hydrogen peroxide					+			+		+		
Hypochlorites, chlorine releasers	+				+					+	+	+
Iodine					+					+		
Mercury salts, organic mercurials	+				+		+++	+				
Phenols	+	+				++	+++					
β-Propiolactone					+					+	+	+
Quaternary ammonium compounds						+	+++					
Silver salts					+		+++			+		
Sulfur dioxide, sulfites					+						+	
Ultraviolet radiation									+			

*Crosses, indicating activity, demonstrate the multiple actions of most compounds. Activity is nearly always concentration-dependent, and the number of crosses indicates the order of concentration at which the effect is elicited (*i.e.,* + = low concentration, + + + = high concentration). A cross in only one target column indicates the only known site of action of that agent. Note the range of reactions, varying specificity, and probable efficacy. CW = cell wall; AMP = action on membrane potentials; ETC = electron transport chain; AT = adenosine triphosphatase; ETG = enzymes with thiol groups; AGMP = action on general membrane permeability; GC = general coagulation; R = ribosomes; NA = nucleic acids; TG = thiol groups; AG = amino groups; HRC = highly reactive compounds.

but at a 2–4% concentration it remains most popular because of its immediate and persistent effect in reducing bacterial counts. Administration directly into the middle ear may cause deafness, but the agent is otherwise nontoxic.

Chelating Agents

EDTA (ethylenediamine tetraacetic acid; edetate) may potentiate the activity of many antibacterial agents against many types of Gram-negative bacteria, but not Gram-positive bacteria. EDTA causes an increase in the permeability of the outer envelope of Gram-negative cells. It is used as a stabilizing agent in certain injections and eye-drop preparations.

Iodine

Iodine compounds are generally active against bacteria and other spores, yeasts, and viruses. Surface-active carrier agents such as polyvinylpyrrolidone (povidone) solubilize iodine as micellar aggregates to form iodophors (iodine carriers); the concentration of free iodine is responsible for the antimicrobial activity. Below a certain critical micelle concentration, at which the free iodine is slowly liberated, the iodine is simply in aqueous solution, not free, and is therefore inactive.

Iodophors produce less pain, staining, and irritation than tincture of iodine and are also nonallergenic. Severe metabolic acidosis and iodism occur when the agent is applied to large surfaces such as burns or peritoneal cavities. Transient biochemical evidence of hypothyroidism occurs when it is routinely used in babies of less than 37 weeks of gestational age.

Chlorine

Hypochlorites are effective against bacteria and many spore forms and viruses, although possibly not mycobacteria. The stability in solution is dependent on chlorine concentration, pH, presence of organic matter, and light. Chlorinated soda solution (Dakin's solution) contains 0.5–0.55% (5000–5500 ppm) available chlorine. Sodium hypochlorite solution (Javex) is a 6% solution that is used in a 1:20 dilution containing about 1000 ppm available chlorine.

Heavy Metal Derivatives (Silver, Mercury)

Silver nitrate has strong activity against staphylococcal and Gram-negative organisms. Silver sulfadiazine has excellent activity against Gram-negative organisms. Combination of silver oxide or nitrate with a high-molecular-weight polymer results in slow release of silver ions and reduces their protein precipitant effect.

Mercurochrome is only of historical interest and of no proven value as a skin antiseptic. Other organic mercury preparations, such as thimerosal (Merthiolate) and nitromersol (Metaphen), are also of very little value for disinfecting skin because they are only bacteriostatic.

Organic and Inorganic Acids

Both aromatic and aliphatic compounds are used. Salicylic, undecylenic, and benzoic acids are used in the topical treatment of fungal infections of the skin.

Phenols and Their Derivatives

Phenols have a wide spectrum of activity depending on para-substitutions of an alkyl chain up to six carbon atoms in length, halogenation, and nitration.

Cresols are ortho-, meta-, and paramethyl phenols, three to 10 times more active than phenol yet without increased toxicity.

Phenols with higher boiling points (up to 310°C) have decreased water solubility, cause less tissue trauma, have increased bactericidal activity, but are more readily inactivated by organic materials. As previously mentioned, thorough mechanical cleaning must precede any disinfection. These less toxic and more bactericidal derivatives of phenol are used today. Because of their association with hepatic disease in neonates, they are not used in the pediatric setting.

Hexachlorophene has good activity against Gram-positive organisms but is generally bacteriostatic rather than bactericidal. It is a chlorinated bisphenol compound. Repeated bathing of premature infants in hexachlorophene has been associated with vacuolar encephalopathy of the brainstem reticular formation. People who use the agent regularly, such as some operating room personnel, have detectable blood levels of it.

Surface-Active Agents

Depending on the predominance of the hydrophobic and hydrophilic group and, more specifically, ionization of the hydrophilic group, surface-active agents are classified as anionic, cationic, and nonionic. Cationic agents have strong bactericidal but weak detergent properties. Quaternary ammonium compounds are most commonly used and are active against Gram-positive organisms and, at higher concentrations, Gram-negative organisms. Because of the ease with which they may become contaminated, in the very rare instances in which they are still used as antiseptics, they should be dispensed in single-use containers. The practice of adding to a partially filled container ("topping up") should be discouraged.

THERAPEUTIC USES

Disinfectants

Noninvasive devices, surfaces (walls, floors), and equipment such as beds and blood pressure cuffs constitute a lower source of infection than invasive devices and can probably be managed by good housekeeping techniques, separation of clean and dirty areas, and common sense in handling of equipment.

In contrast, inadequately sterilized or disinfected invasive devices such as intravascular cannulae, urinary catheters, endoscopes, bronchoscopes, and respirator components present a major risk. Epidemic and endemic disease in association with these devices continues to be reported.

The therapeutic uses of disinfectants are best summarized in the chart produced by the Centers for Disease Control (CDC), Atlanta, Georgia, and shown here as Table 59-2. Specific guidelines for certain disciplines such as dentistry and ophthalmol-

Table 59-2 Methods of Sterilization and Disinfection

	Sterilization		Disinfection High-Level	Disinfection Low-Level
Object	Will enter tissue or vascular system, or blood will flow through the object		Will come in contact with mucous membranes but not enter tissue or vascular system	Will not come in contact with mucous membranes or skin that is not intact
Item Classification	Critical		Semicritical	Noncritical
	Procedure (See Key)	Exposure Time (hours)	Procedure (Exposure Time at least 30 min)*	Procedure (Exposure Time at least 10 min)
Smooth, hard surface	A	mr	C	J
	B	mr	D	L
	C	10	E	M
	D	18	F	N
	E	6	G	P
			H	
			I	
			J	
Rubber tubing and catheters†	A	mr	C	
	B	mr	E	
	E	6	F	
			H	
			I	
Polyethylene tubing and catheters†‡	A	mr	C	
	B	mr	D	
	C	10	E	
	D	18	F	
	E	6	H	
			I	
			J	
Lensed instruments	B	mr	C	
	C	10	E	
	E	6		
Thermometers (oral and rectal)§	B	mr	K	
	C	10		
	D	18		
	E	6		
Hinged instruments	A	mr	C	
	B	mr		
	C	10		
	E	6		

KEY TO TABLE 59-2

A Heat sterilization including steam or hot air, following mr.

B Ethylene oxide gas, following mr.

C Glutaraldehyde (2% aqueous solution—suitable data are not available to permit an adequate assessment of the comparative effectiveness of dilutions of 2% glutaraldehyde for high-level disinfection of in-use patient-care equipment).

D Formaldehyde (8%) – alcohol (70%) solution (corrosion inhibitor needed if formulated in hospital).

E 6% stabilized hydrogen peroxide (will corrode copper, zinc, and brass).

F Wet pasteurization at 75°C for 30 minutes after detergent cleaning.

G Sodium hypochlorite (1000 ppm available chlorine) (will corrode metal instruments).

H Phenolic solutions (3% aqueous solution of concentrate).

I Iodophor (500 ppm available iodine).

J Ethyl or isopropyl alcohol (70–90%).

K Ethyl alcohol (70–90%).

L Sodium hypochlorite (100 ppm available chlorine).

M Phenolic germicidal detergent solution (1% aqueous solution of concentrate).

N Iodophor germicidal detergent (100 ppm available iodine).

P Quaternary ammonium germicidal detergent solution (2% aqueous solution of concentrate).

mr Manufacturer's recommendations.

*The recommended exposure time for high-level disinfection, 30 minutes, is primarily based on an unpublished CDC study involving disinfection of used respiratory therapy equipment with 2% glutaraldehyde. This time and concentration may differ from those approved by the Environmental Protection Agency (U.S. agency that regulates disinfectant usage) for use on product labels. EPA-approved times are based on results from manufacturers' studies that are infrequently verified by EPA.

†Tubing must be completely filled for disinfection.

‡Thermostability should be investigated when indicated.

§Do not mix rectal and oral thermometers at any stage of handling or processing.

Modified from Centers for Disease Control. Isolation techniques for use in hospitals. 2nd ed. Washington, DC; U.S. Government Printing Office, 1975 (DHEW publication No. (CDC) 78-8314).

ogy are available (e.g., human immunodeficiency virus [HIV] is easily inactivated by simple and readily available physical and chemical agents including 1:10 dilution of bleach, alcohol, and heat [56°C for 10 minutes]).

Antiseptics

The distinction between pathogens and nonpathogens is becoming increasingly difficult as coagulase-negative staphylococci assume greater importance. Aerobic staphylococci, micrococci, and diphtheroids are distributed all over the body, with greater numbers in the axillae, groin, face, and under the nails; 20% are in the depths of the skin. Other organisms are thought not to survive in the skin because of the effects of drying, production of fatty acids by diphtheroids, and formation of bacteriocins by coagulase-negative cocci. Important pathogens such as *Salmonella* and *Pseudomonas* colonize the skin transiently, but also for longer periods of time where contamination is high, as in the intensive care unit. Regardless of the agent used, vigorous mechanical cleaning is essential.

Antiseptics and operative sites

As with surgical handwashing, chlorhexidine or povidone-iodine will satisfactorily reduce bacterial counts if applied for 2–5 minutes. The best results have been shown when the antiseptic is applied by vigorous mechanical activity by the gloved hand, as opposed to rubbing on with gauze or spraying.

Antiseptics in the bath or shower

A preoperative chlorhexidine or hexachlorophene bath or shower of the patient has been shown to reduce bacterial counts and infection rates.

Elimination of bacterial spores by antiseptics

While the number of spores in a wound may be reduced by soaking with a compress of 10% aqueous povidone-iodine for 15–30 minutes, systemic penicillin prophylaxis is necessary in cases where gas gangrene and tetanus are potential hazards because of the presence of *Clostridium tetani* and *perfringens* spores.

Antisepsis of the nares

In personnel who are carrying an epidemic strain of *Staphylococcus aureus* that has been associated with disease in patients, creams containing neomycin in combination with chlorhexidine or other antimicrobial agents may reduce or remove the organism, provided that treatment is continued for 14 days or longer. Systemic (oral) antibiotics may also be required, because eradication of nasal colonization by staphylococci can be very difficult.

Antiseptics and mucous membranes

Solutions of 1% or more chlorhexidine, as well as iodine, potassium iodide, or an iodophor, will all give a reduction in the number of potential pathogens.

Antiseptics at vascular catheter sites

Although topical iodophors are widely used at catheter sites, there is insufficient evidence to suggest that it is necessary. Their use may be associated with a decrease in *Candida*, enterococcal, and Gram-negative infections, but the results are not statistically significant and staphylococcal infections may continue to occur. Use of strict aseptic technique during insertion of such intravenous catheters, followed by appropriate aseptic technique in maintaining the dressing, are the most important aspects of care of intravenous lines.

Urinary antiseptics

In the noncatheterized patient, increasing numbers of adverse reactions to nitrofurantoin, particularly in older patients, have led to a need to reevaluate the role of this drug in the prevention and treatment of urinary tract infections.

In the catheterized patient, prophylactic continuous irrigations in closed catheter systems are unnecessary. Aseptic insertion and maintenance, specifically minimizing disconnections of the catheter, connecting tube, and bag, are most important.

Umbilical cord prophylaxis

Triple Dye (crystal violet, brilliant green, and malachite green) has long been used for the prevention of staphylococcal disease, although silver sulfadiazine has a greater effect against group B streptococci. No need has been demonstrated for anything other than application of 70% isopropyl alcohol to a moist cord.

Prevention of gonococcal conjunctivitis

One percent silver nitrate instilled in the eyes of the newborn at birth is considered adequate to prevent gonococcal conjunctivitis, although there are other topical antimicrobials, such as erythromycin, which may be more appropriate in view of the increasing recognition of chlamydial disease.

Antiseptics in wounds

Most antiseptics have been used in the treatment of wounds at one time or another, but the removal of foreign or necrotic material and improvement of the blood supply are of greater importance than any direct antibacterial agents. Of the debriding agents, sodium hypochlorite (Dakin's solution) and hydrogen peroxide are most effective. The systemic absorption of other agents such as silver nitrate, hexachlorophene, or an iodophor may result in undesirable side effects. In addition, hexachlorophene and other agents may be harmful to cartilage, synovia, and other soft tissues.

Antiseptics in burn patients

In contrast to wounds, burns benefit from the application of topical therapy. This is because of the large amount of nonviable tissue present. Serious subcutaneous infection subjacent to the burn wound is the single most important factor leading to burn death, and massive colonization of the wound is the source of potential invasion. The criteria for diagnosis of burn wound infection include a bacterial count of greater than 10^5 organisms per gram of tissue and histological evidence of bacterial invasion of subjacent viable tissue. Topical therapy reduces the number of bacteria below the critical level necessary for invasion.

Mafenide (Sulfamylon) was initially used in the therapy of burns but later abandoned when pain and respiratory alkalosis associated with carbonic anhydrase inhibition occurred.

The use of silver nitrate also has been abandoned. The silver, on contact with tissue, is precipitated as silver chloride, thereby limiting penetration beyond the surface tissue, and its successful use requires constant debridement. In addition, staining of clothing and linen, and electrolyte dilution from the absorption of large amounts of distilled water from the dressing, are problems.

Silver sulfadiazine combines the wide spectrum of activity of the silver ion and the antibacterial effect of the sulfonamide and is not inactivated by wound exudate or p-aminobenzoic acid. The release of sulfadiazine is slow enough to obviate toxicity.

Gauze impregnated with framycetin sulfate (Sofra-tulle) is used in the management of burns in outpatients.

HANDWASHING

Handwashing is the most important single procedure in preventing the spread of nosocomial (hospital-acquired) infections.

Skin flora can be categorized as either resident or transient; resident flora survive and multiply on the skin and can be repeatedly cultured, while transient flora usually survive on the skin less than 24 hours, can be removed by detergents, and can be killed or inhibited by antiseptics. They are usually of low virulence and are implicated in infections only when surgery or other invasive procedures allow them to enter deep tissues. Transient flora, often found on the hands, can be acquired from colonized or infected patients and are frequently implicated in nosocomial infections.

The purpose of routine handwashing is simply to remove transient flora. In outbreaks of Gram-negative infections, a large percentage of hand cultures from physicians and nurses will yield the organism. Rhinovirus has been recovered from the hands of 40% of persons with rhinovirus infections and from as many as 90% by repeated sampling. The purpose of antiseptic handwashing is to reliably eliminate virulent microorganisms with which the hands are possibly contaminated, and to reduce the number of permanent bacteria.

Routine Handwashing Requirements and Techniques

Between patient contacts (other than those as brief as taking a blood pressure or shaking hands, which do not require hand washing), a vigorous washing with chlorhexidine 2% for 15 seconds is adequate. Hands should be rinsed and then dried with a paper towel, and the towel should then be used to turn off the faucet. A 2-minute "surgical wash" should antecede invasive procedures.

Because rings and cracked nail polish make microorganisms on the hand difficult to remove, personnel who take care of patients should be discouraged from wearing rings or nail polish while on duty; a single band is permissible. Wrist watches should not be placed in a way that prevents thorough washing and should not be worn while giving direct patient care.

Because dermatitis may predispose to carriage of pathogenic organisms, efforts should be made to prevent it. Single-use packages of hand lotion are available. Multiple-use bottles should not be employed, because experience has shown that they have sometimes become contaminated.

Surgical Handwashing

Because perforations occur in approximately 25% of gloves worn by a surgical team, the hands must be scrubbed thoroughly before the gloves are put on. A 2-minute scrub with chlorhexidine or povidone-iodine is recommended and will reduce bacterial counts by 70–85% after one application and by 99% if used six times over a 2-day period.

Although chlorhexidine, hexachlorophene, and povidone-iodine all have a residual effect, chlorhexidine seems preferable because it is unaffected by the presence of blood on the skin. During a 3-hour operation, for example, there may even be a further fall in bacterial counts from that determined after the initial application.

SUGGESTED READING

Ayliffe GAJ. The effect of antibacterial agents on the flora of the skin. J Hosp Infect 1980; 1:111–124.

Buehler JW, Finton RJ, Goodman RA, et al. Epidemic keratoconjunctivitis. Report of an outbreak in ophthalmology practice and recommendations for prevention. Infect Control 1984; 5:390–394.

Dineen P. Local antiseptics. In: Modell W, ed. Drugs of choice 1980–1981. St. Louis: CV Mosby, 1980.

Favero MS. Strategies for disinfection and sterilization of endoscopes: the gap between basic principles and actual practice. Infect Control Hosp Epidemiol 1991; 12:279–281.

Ford-Jones EL. Antiseptics. In: Koren G, Prober CG, Gold R, eds. Antimicrobial therapy in infants and children. New York: Marcel Dekker, 1988:483–514.

Goldmann D, Larsen E. Handwashing and nosocomial infections. N Engl J Med 1992; 327:120–122.

Hospital Infections Branch: Atlanta, Georgia, USA: Centers for Disease Control Publications, 1981–1982, 1985.

Ibid.: Recommended infection-control practices for dentistry. Centers for Disease Control Publications, 1986; 35:237–242.

Kaul AF, Jewett JF. Agents and techniques for disinfection of the skin. Surg Gynecol Obstet 1981; 152:677–685.

Maki DG, Hassemer CA. Flash sterilization: carefully measured haste. Infect Control 1987; 8:307–310.

Russell AD, Hugo WB, Ayliffe GAJ. Principles and practice of disinfection, preservation and sterilization. Oxford: Blackwell, 1982.

Rutala WA. APIC guideline for selection and use of disinfectants. Am J Infect Control 1990; 18:99–114.

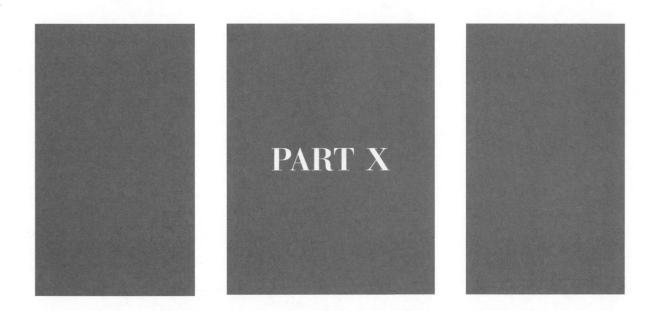

PART X

ANTINEOPLASTIC CHEMOTHERAPY, IMMUNOPHARMACOLOGY

CHAPTER 60

Antineoplastic Drugs

M.J. MOORE AND G.J. GOLDENBERG

CASE HISTORY

In January 1988, a 55-year-old woman noted dimpling in the upper outer quadrant of her left breast. Her family physician palpated a firm fixed mass in this area, measuring about 3 cm in diameter, and mammogram revealed calcifications suspicious of malignancy. Open biopsy showed infiltrating ductal carcinoma with vascular invasion and tumor extending to the resection margins. In March 1988 the patient underwent simple left mastectomy and axillary node dissection. Pathological examination showed an infiltrating ductal carcinoma of nuclear grade III, clear resection margins, and involvement of six of 11 axillary lymph nodes. The tumor was strongly positive for estrogen and progesterone receptors (380 and 250 fmol/mg of cytosolic protein, respectively).

A chest film, serum calcium, liver function tests, ultrasound examination of the liver, and bone scan were all negative for metastases. However, the lymph node involvement and the microscopic findings suggested a high risk of recurrence, and the patient was started on tamoxifen 20 mg daily. She tolerated the tamoxifen and remained well and asymptomatic until February 1992, when she complained of severe pain in the left chest wall and right hip. Physical examination revealed tenderness at both sites. A bone scan showed metastases in several ribs, the vertebral bodies of T-6, T-8, L-2, and L-3, the pelvis and the right femur. X-rays demonstrated osteolytic lesions at these sites and a pathological fracture of one rib. Tamoxifen was discontinued, a course of radiother-

apy was administered to the right femur to prevent a pathological fracture, and the patient was started on megestrol acetate 160 mg daily in March 1992. The pain grew worse and more widespread. In July 1992 megestrol was discontinued and therapy with aminoglutethimide was initiated. The pain became progressively worse and by September 1992 the patient developed dyspnea and cough. A chest film showed lymphangitic spread, and hormonal therapy was abandoned.

On September 20, 1992, a course of combination chemotherapy with cyclophosphamide, methotrexate, and 5-fluorouracil (CMF) was initiated. The patient also received antiemetic therapy with dexamethasone 10 mg IV, prochlorperazine 10 mg orally, and lorazepam 1 mg sublingually. The cycle of chemotherapy was repeated at 28-day intervals. After three cycles, the patient developed alopecia requiring a hairpiece. The pain and other symptoms subsided, and follow-up X-rays confirmed the improvement in the lungs as well as the bony lesions. The patient progressed well on this regimen except for leukopenia that necessitated an increase of the intercycle interval to 35 days.

She remained well until August 1994 when she became confused and dyspneic, and complained of thirst, polydipsia, and polyuria. Chest X-ray showed a large pleural effusion on the right. The serum calcium and alkaline phosphatase were both elevated. Two liters of blood-tinged fluid was removed by thoracocentesis, with dramatic improvement in respiration, but the pleural fluid showed clumps of carcinoma cells, and X-rays revealed new skeletal metastases. The hypercalcemia responded promptly to intravenous corticosteroids. Systemic therapy was changed from CMF to intravenous doxorubicin, given at 3-week intervals. Once again the patient responded well to therapy and all signs and symptoms improved. She remained stable until July 1995, when doxorubicin was discontinued because of the risk of serious cardiotoxicity.

Therapy with paclitaxel was initiated, together with dexamethasone and diphenhydramine orally to reduce the risk of an allergic reaction. Subsequent cycles were given at 3-week intervals. Other than one episode of infection related to neutropenia, the patient was well until February 1996, when she developed a severe headache, confusion, sleepiness, bilateral blurring of the optic discs, engorgement of the retinal veins, and pyramidal tract signs on the right side. Magnetic resonance imaging (MRI) of the brain revealed two intracranial lesions in the left frontoparietal area, with surrounding edema and midline shift. A diagnosis of cerebral metastases was made, and intracranial radiotherapy was given, together with IV dexamethasone to reduce cerebral edema. The patient's neurological status improved promptly, but the improvement was not sustained. The patient's symptoms reappeared in March and rapidly grew worse; she died on April 15, 1996.

Neoplasia is characterized by uncontrolled proliferation of transformed cells at the expense of the host. Cancers spread by invasion of the surrounding tissues and by metastasizing to distant sites. Tumors may be very heterogeneous with respect to karyotype, morphology, immunogenicity, rate of growth, ability to metastasize, and responsiveness to antineoplastic drugs. Although surgery and radiation can often cure or control tumors locally, many patients eventually succumb because of distant metastases. Most present treatments for systemic disease employ cytotoxic or hormonal agents, or both. More recently, some immunological agents have been introduced (see Chapter 61). In patients with cancer, antineoplastic drugs are used to eradicate established metastases, to prevent disease recurrence after local treatment (adjuvant therapy), or to decrease tumor size prior to local treatment (neoadjuvant therapy).

PRINCIPLES OF CANCER CHEMOTHERAPY

1. A "clonogenic" cell is one that has the potential for unlimited replication. A single clonogenic malignant cell can give rise to sufficient progeny to kill the host. The effectiveness of chemotherapy depends on its ability to eliminate *all* clonogenic cells.

2. The cell kill caused by antineoplastic drugs follows first-order kinetics, i.e., in each successive time period a constant percentage or fraction rather than a constant number of cells is killed by a given therapeutic intervention. For example, a patient with cancer might harbor 10^{12} malignant cells (about 1 kg). A drug treatment that kills 99.99% of these cells would reduce the tumor mass to about 100 mg (i.e., a complete clinical remission). However, 10^8 malignant cells would survive, and any remaining clonogenic cells would cause a recurrence of the disease.

3. Some cancer chemotherapeutic agents have steep dose-response curves. Cancer treatments are generally given at the highest tolerable dosage, and in some cases the dose is increased further by using marrow transplantation to overcome toxic effects.

4. Tumor cells may grow in body compartments (e.g., the central nervous system) to which chemotherapeutic agents have limited or no access. Local drug administration (e.g., intrathecal) can be effective in eradicating malignant cells in such sites.

5. Most antineoplastic drugs have a low therapeutic index and are not specific for cancer cells. Many normal body tissues such as bone marrow, gonads, oral mucosa, or hair follicles may be damaged also.

6. Doses and schedules of drug administration that can be used to achieve tumor cell kill are limited by normal tissue tolerance. High-dose intermittent schedules are believed to be more effective than schedules employing low-dose daily administration. These intermittent schedules allow time for recovery of normal host tissues between drug treatment cycles.

7. Several drugs used together (combination chemotherapy) are more effective than drugs used individually. Ideally each drug in the combination has a different mechanism of action, is effective as a single agent, and has qualitatively different toxicities, so all can be given at or near their individual maximum tolerated doses.

8. Theoretically, it would be best to start treatment early when the number of cancer cells is small, when many of these cells may still be in cycle (see below), and when there is a low probability of resistant cells. This principle has led to the development of **adjuvant chemotherapy,** defined as the administration of drugs to patients who have no evidence of disease by currently available methods of study but who are at high risk of developing recurrent cancer according to current knowledge. It is assumed that such patients have small numbers of cancer cells and a low probability of resistant cells. This approach has been quite useful in the treatment of breast and colorectal cancers. In the case described, the use of tamoxifen after surgery was adjuvant therapy, while the remaining therapies were used in the presence of demonstrated metastatic disease.

9. Combined-modality treatments involving surgery, radiotherapy, and chemotherapy are now used commonly. Such an approach is particularly successful in the treatment of childhood cancers.

CLASSIFICATION OF ANTINEOPLASTIC DRUGS

Antineoplastic drugs were formerly classified on the basis of where they act in the cell cycle. Drugs were classed as cell-cycle-independent if they affected cells in any phase of the cycle, including resting cells; cell-cycle-dependent if they affected only cells actively cycling at the time of exposure to drugs; and phase-dependent if they acted mainly on cells in one specific phase of the cycle. However, there were too many exceptions to this classification and, in general, all such agents are more active against cells that are actively cycling.

A more useful means of classifying these drugs is on the basis of their mechanism of action and derivation (Fig. 60-1). Six classes can be designated, as illustrated in Table 60-1. In the following sections, representative drugs from each class are discussed, and the more common clinically useful agents are summarized. Practical considerations for drug administration are outlined in Table 60-2. Some indications of the therapeutic uses of antineoplastic drugs are given in each section.

Table 60-1 Classification of Antineoplastic Agents According to Mechanisms of Action or Derivation

Alkylating and DNA-binding agents
  Nitrogen mustard
  Melphalan
  Cyclophosphamide & ifosfamide
  Chlorambucil
  Busulphan
  Nitrosoureas
  Cisplatin & Carboplatin
  Dacarbazine (DTIC)
  Procarbazine
  Mitomycin C

Antimetabolites
  Methotrexate
  5-Fluorouracil
  Cytosine arabinoside (Ara-C), Gemcitabine
  6-Mercaptopurine, 6-thioguanine
  Fludarabine, 2-chlorodeoxyadenosine

Antibiotics
  Actinomycin D
  Doxorubicin, daunorubicin, & epirubicin
  Mitoxantrone
  Bleomycin

Natural plant derivatives
  Vincristine
  Vinblastine
  Vinorelbine
  Etoposide (VP-16)
  Teniposide (VM-26)
  Paclitaxel & docetaxel
  Camptothecin derivatives

Miscellaneous
  L-Asparaginase
  Hydroxyurea

Hormones
  Glucocorticoids
  Tamoxifen
  Progestational agents
  Aminoglutethimide
  GnRH agonists
  Antiandrogens

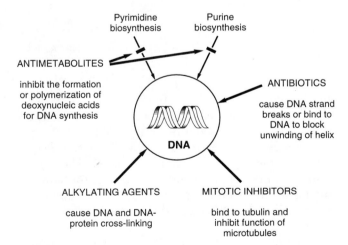

Figure 60-1. Mechanisms of action of major groups of antineoplastic drugs.

Table 60-2 Doses, Routes of Administration, Schedules, Elimination, and Toxicities of Common Antineoplastic Agents

Drug	Route of Administration	Dose* (mg/m²)	Frequency†	Major Route of Elimination‡	Commonly Encountered Toxicities
Melphalan	Oral	9	Daily×4 q 4–6 wk	Renal	Leukopenia, thrombocytopenia, mild nausea, vomiting
Cyclophosphamide	Intravenous Oral	500–3500 150	q 3 wk Daily×14	Biotransformation	Leukopenia, thrombocytopenia, nausea, vomiting, cystitis, alopecia
BCNU (carmustine)	Intravenous	225	q 6 wk	Biotransformation	Leukopenia, thrombocytopenia, nausea, vomiting, alopecia
CCNU (lomustine)	Oral	100–150	q 6 wk	Biotransformation	Leukopenia, thrombocytopenia
Cisplatin	Intravenous	50–125	q 3 wk	Renal	Nausea, vomiting, mild myelosuppression, renal failure
Methotrexate	Intravenous	30–60	q 2–4 wk	Renal	Leukopenia, thrombocytopenia, mucositis, skin rash
5-Fluorouracil	Intravenous	350–600	Daily×5 or weekly	Biotransformation	Leukopenia, thrombocytopenia, diarrhea, mucositis
Ara-C	Intravenous infusion	100	5–10 days	Biotransformation	Myelosuppression, mucositis, neurotoxicity
6-Mercaptopurine	Oral	100	Daily×5	Biotransformation	Myelosuppression, cholestasis
Doxorubicin	Intravenous	75	q 3 wk	Biotransformation	Myelosuppression, nausea, vomiting, alopecia, cardiomyopathy
Bleomycin	Intravenous Intramuscular Subcutaneous	10–15	Weekly	Renal	Skin and pulmonary fibrosis, fever, allergic reactions
Vincristine	Intravenous	1.4	Weekly	Biotransformation	Neuropathy, SIADH
Vinblastine	Intravenous	6	q 1–2 wk	Biotransformation	Mucositis, myelosuppression
Etoposide (VP-16)	Intravenous	100–120	Daily×3	Biotransformation	Myelosuppression, neuropathy

*Dose as a single agent.
†Frequency when given as a single agent.
‡"Renal" means renal excretion of unchanged drug. "Biotransformation" includes both hepatic and extrahepatic reactions; the metabolites may be excreted in the urine and bile.

DRUG RESISTANCE

A major limitation of cancer chemotherapy is the problem of drug resistance, which can be either intrinsic or acquired. *Intrinsic resistance* refers to those tumors that are resistant from the beginning, failing to respond to the initial course of chemotherapy (e.g., cancer of the pancreas, squamous cell cancer of the lung). *Acquired resistance* refers to those tumors that are responsive or sensitive to initial therapy but develop resistance on repeated exposure

to the same drugs (e.g., breast cancer, cancer of the ovary, lymphomas). The case of breast cancer presented for this chapter responded well to the antiestrogen tamoxifen for 4 years, but the disease later became resistant to that same agent. The patient also responded subsequently to cyclophosphamide–methotrexate–5-fluorouracil (CMF) for almost 2 years only to relapse again because of drug resistance.

Resistance to antineoplastic agents may be multifactorial, including one or more of the following mechanisms:

1. Decreased drug influx, e.g., decreased carrier-mediated transport of methotrexate into resistant cells.
2. Increased drug efflux, e.g., increased expression of P-glycoprotein, a drug extrusion pump on the cell membrane that pumps drugs such as doxorubicin out of resistant cells.
3. Decrease of the effective intracellular drug concentration due to increased drug biotransformation. For example, elevated levels of glutathione or increased expression of glutathione *S*-transferase reduces the intracellular concentration of antineoplastic agents (e.g., cyclophosphamide) that is available to react with DNA, RNA, and protein.
4. Decreased levels of drug activating enzymes, e.g., the microsomal cytochrome P450 system that converts cyclophosphamide from an inactive precursor into an active alkylating agent.
5. Increase of target enzyme, e.g., overexpression of the gene for dihydrofolate reductase in methotrexate-resistant cells, or for thymidylate synthase in cells resistant to 5-fluorouracil.
6. Decrease of an enzyme mediating the cytocidal activity, e.g., down-regulation of DNA topoisomerase II in cells resistant to doxorubicin or etoposide.
7. Increase of DNA repair enzymes, e.g., in cells resistant to ionizing radiation and/or alkylating agents such as cyclophosphamide.

Each of these mechanisms probably contributed to the manifestations of drug resistance observed in the patient described in the Case History.

ALKYLATING AGENTS

Alkylating agents are chemically diverse drugs that act through the covalent bonding of alkyl groups (e.g., CH_2Cl^-) to intracellular macromolecules. These agents are classified as monofunctional (one reactive group) or bifunctional (two reactive groups). Bifunctional alkylating agents can form cross-links between biological molecules and are the most clinically useful type. Alkylating agents were the first agents for treating malignant disease and are now used in many of the combination chemotherapy regimens. The prototypic alkylating agents are nitrogen mustard and its derivatives melphalan, chlorambucil, cyclophosphamide, and ifosfamide (Fig. 60-2). Structurally they contain chloroethyl groups ($CH_2CH_2Cl^-$) which, on separation of the chloride

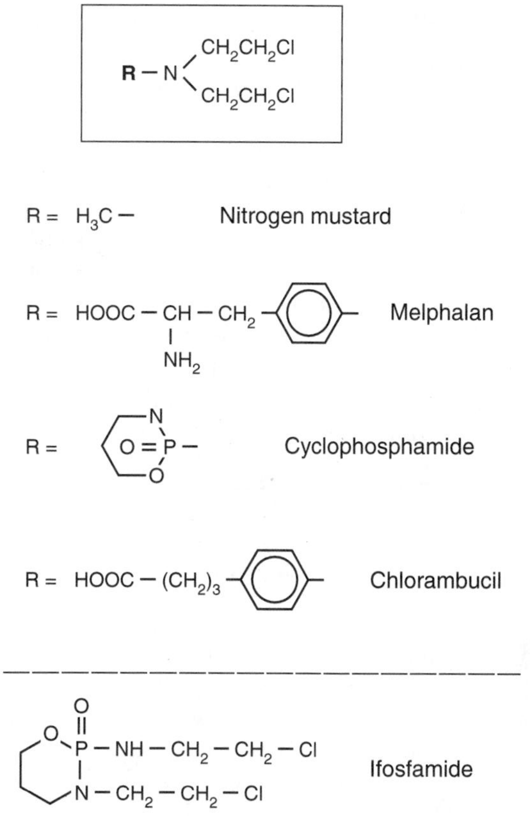

Figure 60-2. Structural formulae of mustard alkylating agents.

ions, form highly reactive carbonium ions crucial to the mechanism of action of these compounds.

The most important targets are pyrimidine and purine bases in DNA. Each chloroethyl group binds covalently to a N, C, or O atom in a target molecule. The mustard thus forms a bridge between two target sites, resulting in cross-links within single DNA strands, between two strands of DNA, or between strands of DNA and nucleoproteins. These reactions either inhibit separation or result in abnormal separation of DNA during cell division, and this leads to subsequent cell death.

Alkylating agents have many effects in common. The dose-limiting toxicity is myelosuppression (a reduction in the production of white blood cells and platelets). Neutropenia (a neutrophil count below $2000/\mu L$) appears about 10 days after drug administration, and the lowest or nadir blood counts are seen at around 15 days. Recovery to baseline levels usually occurs by 21–28 days; this can be delayed with melphalan and the nitrosoureas. Nausea and vomiting are common but short-lived (usually less than 24 hours after administration). Alopecia (loss of hair) is frequent with cyclophosphamide and ifosfamide and occurs after two to four courses of treatment.

Effects on the host's genetic material may cause serious side effects in long-term survivors. These drugs can induce amenorrhea in women and oligospermia in men. The degree and duration of these side effects depend on the duration of drug treatment and the patient's age at the time of treatment. Second malignances in patients receiving long-term treatment with alkylating agents, and birth defects in infants of women inadvertently treated with these drugs during pregnancy, reflect the mutagenic effect of these drugs (see Chapters 69 and 70).

Nitrogen Mustard

Nitrogen mustard (mechlorethamine; Mustargen) was the first anticancer drug introduced into clinical practice. Its discovery was based on observations of reductions in white blood cells and lymph nodes seen in men exposed to mustard gas (sulfur mustard), a chemically similar compound. Nitrogen mustard was useful in the treatment of Hodgkin's disease and non-Hodgkin's lymphomas. It is unstable, reacting with water and other nucleophiles within a few minutes of preparation. It also can cause severe tissue necrosis if extravasation outside the intravenous injection site occurs. Analogs of nitrogen mustard that are more active and chemically more stable have largely replaced it in clinical use.

Melphalan

Melphalan (L-phenylalanine mustard; Alkeran) is an alkylating agent that is taken up into the cell via active transport systems for naturally occurring amino acids located in cell membranes. It is administered primarily by mouth, but higher doses can be given intravenously. About 50% of an administered dose is absorbed, but there is marked interpatient variability in bioavailability. The major clinical uses for this agent are in the treatment of myeloma. It is also active against ovarian cancer and breast cancer but its use in these diseases has been mostly replaced by cisplatin (ovarian cancer) and cyclophosphamide (breast cancer). Common doses, frequency of administration, and route of elimination are summarized in Table 60-2.

Cyclophosphamide

Cyclophosphamide (Cytoxan) is the most commonly used alkylating agent. It is inactive until transformed to alkylating metabolites by hepatic microsomal mixed-function oxidases. It can be given orally or intravenously. Metabolites are excreted primarily in the urine and may irritate the bladder mucosa, resulting in a chemical cystitis. This complication is prevented by adequate hydration, which decreases the concentration of metabolites in the urine. In patients receiving high doses, cystitis can be prevented by using mesna (sodium 2-mercaptoethane sulfonate), which conjugates with the metabolite in urine. Cyclophosphamide is given in a wide range of doses ranging from 150 mg/day orally in immunological diseases and breast cancer, up to 3500 mg/day as part of marrow ablation regimens prior to allogeneic transplantations. It is active against leukemia, lymphomas, lung cancer, and sarcomas. As demonstrated in the Case History, it is one of the most useful drugs in the treatment of breast cancer. Cyclophosphamide dosages and schedule of administration are listed in Table 60-2.

Ifosfamide (Ifex) is a structurally related compound that also requires metabolic activation in the liver, by a pathway different from that of cyclophosphamide. As a result, higher doses are required and the side-effect profile is somewhat different. Ifosfamide does have a role in the treatment of soft-tissue sarcomas and germ-cell tumors.

Nitrosoureas

The drugs in this group, which includes BCNU (carmustine; BiCNU) and CCNU (lomustine; CeeNU) are nonmustard alkylating agents (Fig. 60-3). One major difference between these drugs and other alkylating agents is their lipophilic character, which enables a significant fraction of these drugs to cross the blood–brain barrier and act against tumors in the CNS. Whereas most alkylating agents cause leukocyte nadirs about 10 days after administration, and recovery by day 21–28, the nitrosoureas cause two nadirs, one occurring at about day 10 and a second about day 28, with recovery by about day 42. Therefore, these agents are given at intervals of 6–8 weeks instead of 3–4 weeks as for other alkylating agents. Pulmonary toxicity (interstitial pneumonitis) can occur with chronic use. The nitrosureas now have a very limited role in the treatment of cancers.

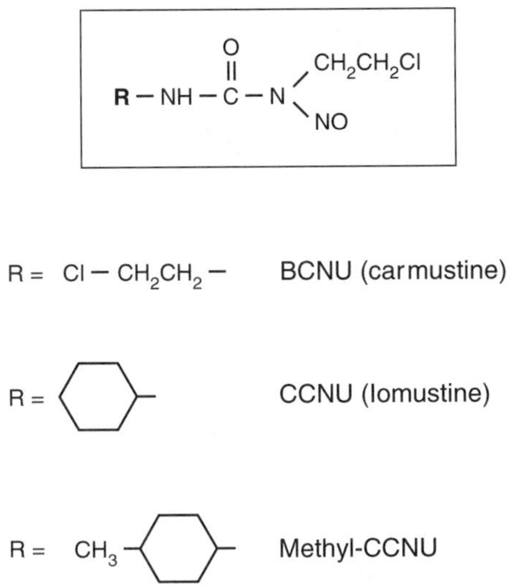

R = Cl — CH₂CH₂ — BCNU (carmustine)

R = ⬡— CCNU (lomustine)

R = CH₃—⬡— Methyl-CCNU

Figure 60-3. Structural formulae of nitrosoureas.

Dacarbazine

Dacarbazine (DTIC) was originally synthesized as an antimetabolite to inhibit purine biosynthesis. It is believed to function through formation of a metabolite with alkylating properties. The drug is used mainly for treatment of sarcomas, Hodgkin's disease, and melanoma. It causes nausea and vomiting in a high proportion of patients, and the dose-limiting toxicity is myelosuppression.

Cisplatin

Cisplatin (*cis*-diamminedichloroplatinum; Platinol) is a platinum coordination complex with two chlorine leaving groups in the *cis* position (Fig. 60-4). While not a classical alkylating agent, it has cytotoxic effects that correlate with its DNA cross-linking activ-

Cisplatin

Carboplatin

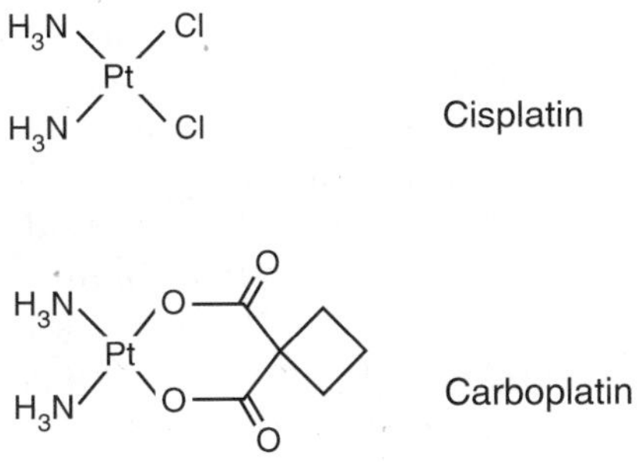

Figure 60-4. Structural formulae of cisplatin and carboplatin.

ity, as is seen with the nitrogen mustards. Cisplatin is given intravenously and binds avidly to proteins; a lesser proportion is excreted unchanged by the kidneys. The major toxicities of this drug differ somewhat from those of the mustards. Nausea and vomiting are severe and almost universal. 5-Hydroxytryptamine analogs such as **ondansetron** are the most useful agents in controlling this problem. Nephrotoxicity with progressively declining creatinine clearance is dose-limiting but may be prevented in part by adequate hydration and mannitol-induced diuresis. Renal tubular damage may result in magnesium wasting with associated hypomagnesemia.

Multiple courses of cisplatin may cause ototoxicity manifested by high-frequency hearing loss and neurotoxicity manifested by a sensory peripheral neuropathy. There is no known strategy to circumvent these problems. They are more common in patients with preexisting hearing or neurological problems and will limit the number of cisplatin cycles that can be given. Myelosuppression is less of a problem than with the mustards. Cisplatin is one of the most useful antineoplastic agents. It is the drug of choice for the treatment of testicular tumors, and cisplatin-based combinations can cure the majority of patients with advanced disease. It is also first-line therapy for lung, bladder, ovarian, and head and neck cancer and is second-line therapy for malignant lymphomas. It is relatively inactive against breast cancer.

Carboplatin

Due to the severity of cisplatin toxicity, attempts were made to develop analogs with the same cytotoxic activity but lesser side effects. Many analogs have been tested, but the only one that is commonly used is carboplatin (Paraplatin).

Carboplatin [*cis*-diammino(1,1-cyclobutanedicarboxylato) platinum (II)] is a compound structurally related to cisplatin (Fig. 60-4), but with a dicarboxylate chelate ligand replacing the two chlorine atoms. The presence of the dicarboxylate group renders carboplatin more stable and thus less reactive with proteins and DNA. The antitumor activity in vivo is comparable to that of cisplatin but the spectrum of toxicity differs. Nausea and vomiting, neurotoxicity, nephrotoxicity, and ototoxicity are less severe, while myelosuppression (particularly thrombocytopenia) is dose-limiting. Carboplatin is primarily excreted by the kidneys, and dosage reductions are required in the presence of renal dysfunction. Despite its more favorable toxicity profile, carboplatin has not replaced cisplatin in clinical practice, except perhaps in ovarian cancer. It is less active than cisplatin against testicular, bladder, and lung cancers. In addition, because its primary toxicity is myelosuppression, it can be a poor substitute for cisplatin in combination regimens with other myelosuppressive agents.

Mitomycin C

Mitomycin C (Mutamycin) is derived from a *Streptomyces* species and requires activation to an alkylating metabolite by reductive metabolism. The drug is more active against hypoxic than against aerobic cells in tissue culture, but it has not been shown to have preferential toxicity for hypoxic cells in vivo. It causes a delayed and rather unpredictable myelosuppression. More seriously, the drug can produce a hemolytic-uremic syndrome that is usually fatal and is probably due to small-vessel endothelial damage. Another potentially lethal effect is interstitial lung disease that progresses to pulmonary fibrosis. The availability of equally active drugs with lower toxicities limits the clinical utility of mitomycin C.

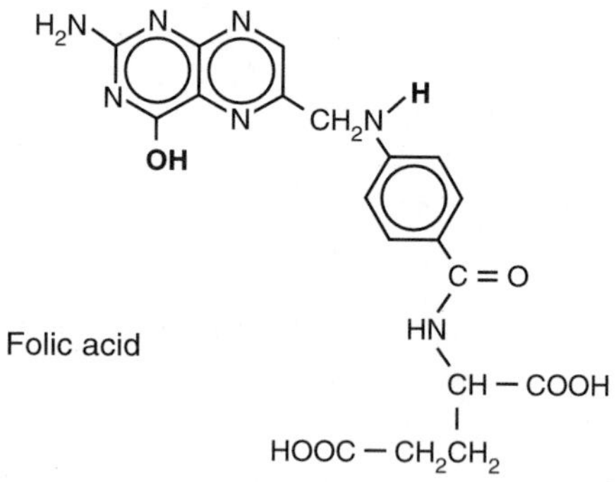

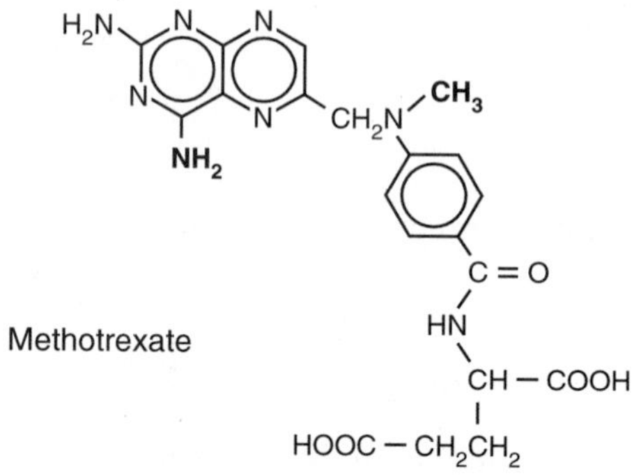

ANTIMETABOLITES

Antimetabolites are synthetic drugs that act as inhibitors of critical biochemical pathways in the formation of DNA, or as abnormal substitutes for naturally occurring nucleic acid bases, resulting in the formation of abnormal DNA. These agents tend to be cycle-dependent. As they affect rapidly dividing cells, the most common toxicities are seen in the gastrointestinal mucosa (stomatitis and diarrhea) and the bone marrow (neutropenia and thrombocytopenia).

Methotrexate

Methotrexate (4-amino-N^{10}-methylpteroylglutamic acid, also known as amethopterin; Rheumatrex, Folex) is a folic acid analog (Fig. 60-5) that competes with dihydrofolate (a naturally occurring folate) for binding to the enzyme dihydrofolate reductase (DHFR) (see also Fig. 56-1). This leads to inhibition of tetrahydrofolate synthesis and a decrease in intracellular reduced folates. Reduced folates play a central role in one-carbon fragment transfer reactions that are necessary in DNA and purine biosynthesis. Therefore competitive inhibition of DHFR by methotrexate results in decreased purine biosynthesis, a

Figure 60-5. Structural formulae of folic acid and methotrexate.

cessation of DNA synthesis, and cell death. Leucovorin (folinic acid), the end-product of the dihydrofolate reductase reaction, may overcome the effect of inhibition of this pathway if given within 48 hours of methotrexate administration.

Methotrexate can be given orally, intravenously, or intrathecally (directly into the cerebrospinal fluid). It can cross membranes slowly and accumulate in body cavities and spaces such as pleural effusions, from which it will slowly redistribute. This release from "third space" fluid collections can lead to excessive toxicity, and drainage of such collections prior to methotrexate administration is required. The parent compound and its hepatic metabolites are excreted by the kidney, and dose adjustment is necessary in the presence of renal dysfunction. Acetylsalicylic acid, nonsteroidal anti-inflammatory agents, and sulfonamides can displace methotrexate from its binding sites on albumin and lead to increased toxicity.

"High-dose" methotrexate treatment, ranging from about 200 mg/m^2 to 20 g/m^2, has also been used. With this treatment a high urine output must be maintained, and the urine must be kept alkaline in order to minimize the likelihood of drug precipitation in the renal tubules. Leucovorin must be given

24–48 hours after such doses of methotrexate, to "rescue" normal tissues from drug toxicity. Otherwise, such high doses of methotrexate would be lethal.

The major clinical uses of methotrexate are in the systemic treatment of leukemia, lymphoma, choriocarcinoma, and bladder and breast cancer. Methotrexate can be given intrathecally for meningeal leukemia or meningeal carcinomatosis. This will result in higher concentrations of methotrexate in the CSF than can be achieved by conventional doses given intravenously. The major forms of toxicity are myelosuppression and mucositis.

5-Fluorouracil

5-Fluorouracil (5-FU) (Adrucil and others) is a fluorinated pyrimidine derivative, originally synthesized in 1957, that functions as an antimetabolite (Fig. 60-6). 5-FU remains today as one of the most widely used anticancer drugs, with activity against gastrointestinal adenocarcinomas and cancers of the breast, esophagus, and head and neck. It is the only currently available anticancer drug with activity against colorectal cancer, the second leading cause of cancer deaths in North America.

The primary mechanism of 5-FU cytotoxicity is inhibition of thymidylate synthase (TS) through the generation of the intracellular nucleotide 5-fluorodeoxyuridine monophosphate (FdUMP), which binds to TS and prevents formation of dTMP. The ability of 5-FU to inhibit TS can be enhanced in the presence of reduced folates such as leucovorin that stabilize the binding of FdUMP to TS and allow for a more sustained inhibition of dTMP formation. 5-FU in combination with leucovorin is the standard treatment for patients with metastatic colorectal cancer. Toxic effects of 5-FU include stomatitis, diarrhea, skin rash, and myelosuppression. The toxicity profile differs somewhat, depending on whether 5-FU is given by repeated daily doses, once weekly, or by chronic intravenous infusion.

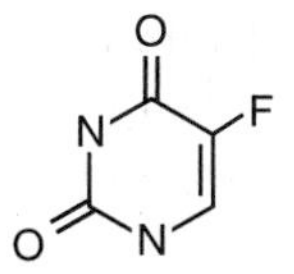

Cytosine Arabinoside (Ara-C, Cytarabine)

Ara-C (Cytosar) is an arabinose nucleoside that differs from physiological nucleosides by the presence of a β-OH group in the 2-position of the sugar (Fig. 60-7). It acts as an analog of a naturally occurring nucleoside, deoxycytidine, and is phosphorylated to ara-cytosine triphosphate (ara-CTP). Ara-CTP is a competitive inhibitor of DNA polymerase, an enzyme necessary for DNA synthesis and repair. By binding

Figure 60-6. Structural formula of 5-fluorouracil.

to this enzyme, it arrests DNA synthesis and replicating cells die. Therefore, this agent is more effective against cycling cells. (A related compound, adenine arabinoside [ara-A, vidarabine], is primarily active in blocking viral DNA synthesis, which makes it a useful drug to treat herpetic infections [see Chapter 58].)

The drug is given intravenously, either by frequent injections or by continuous infusion, since it is rapidly degraded ($t_{1/2}$ = 7–20 min) by the enzyme cytidine deaminase found in blood. The parent compound and its inactive metabolite, uracil arabinoside, are excreted in the urine. Myelosuppression is the major dose-limiting toxicity, but gastrointestinal toxicity is also common. Central nervous system toxicity, with abnormal behavior and mentation, occurs uncommonly.

This agent is used primarily for the treatment of acute leukemia and may be given intrathecally for meningeal infiltration by leukemia.

Gemcitabine

Gemcitabine (2′,2′-difluorodeoxycytidine) is a cytosine analog with structural similarities to cytosine arabinoside. Unlike ara-C, gemcitabine has significant activity against a variety of solid tumor cell lines. Similarly to ara-C, gemcitabine requires intracellular activation to its triphosphate derivative, which is incorporated into DNA and then inhibits

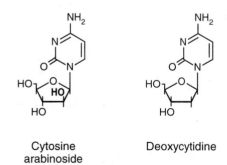

Figure 60-7. Structural formulae of cytosine arabinoside and deoxycytidine.

DNA replication. In clinical studies, gemcitabine is active against non–small-cell lung cancer and cancers of the pancreas, breast, and bladder. The major toxicity is myelosuppression.

6-Mercaptopurine (6-MP)

6-MP (Purinethol) is a thiopurine analog of hypoxanthine, a naturally occurring purine base. It is transformed intracellularly to ribonucleotide forms. These may be incorporated into RNA or DNA or act at several enzymatic steps of purine biosynthesis to inhibit purine formation. 6-MP is usually given orally and its reported bioavailability is about 50%. The drug is degraded by xanthine oxidase to 6-thiouric acid, which is devoid of antitumour activity. Allopurinol, used for the treatment of hyperuricemia, may inhibit the degradation of 6-MP and thereby increase its toxicity. The major toxicity of 6-MP is myelosuppression. It is used clinically in the treatment of acute leukemia, particularly in children.

Other Purine Antimetabolites

Analogs of adenine and adenosine are the most recent of the DNA base analogs to be introduced into clinical practice. **Fludarabine** (Fludara) is an adenosine derivative that is resistant to deamination by adenosine deaminase (ADA). Fludarabine is active mainly against tumors with low proportions of actively cycling cells (low-grade lymphomas, chronic lymphocytic leukemia, and hairy cell leukemia). Its mechanism of cytotoxicity against these tumors is not well understood; it may involve activation of programmed cell death (apoptosis) following DNA and RNA damage. The major toxicities are myelosuppression and immunosuppression; other toxic effects are mild or infrequent.

2-Chlorodeoxyadenosine (2CdA) is a more potent fluorinated adenosine derivative. Its spectrum of activity and toxicity profile are similar to those of fludarabine.

Deoxycoformycin is an inhibitor of ADA that has demonstrated activity against hairy cell leukemia and some other indolent lymphomas. It is not clear why an accumulation of adenine nucleosides would be cytotoxic, but it may lead to a secondary inhibition of DNA synthesis. The dosages required to maximally inhibit ADA lead to significant toxicity. However, "hairy cell" leukemias have low ADA activity and the dose of deoxycoformycin required to treat this disease is therefore lower and has minimal toxicity.

ANTITUMOR ANTIBIOTICS

Antitumor antibiotics, like their antimicrobial counterparts, are fermentation products derived from fungal cultures. Their mechanisms of action differ, and there are specific toxicities characteristic of each drug.

Actinomycin D

Actinomycin D (dactinomycin; Cosmegen) is produced by a fungus of the *Streptomyces* class. It acts by intercalating between base pairs of DNA; it thus inhibits synthesis of RNA at low drug concentrations, and of both RNA and DNA at higher drug concentrations. Like doxorubicin and daunorubicin (see below), it also interacts with DNA topoisomerase II to produce DNA strand breaks. Dose-limiting toxicity is myelosuppression; other side effects include ulceration of the oral mucosa and gastrointestinal tract. Actinomycin D is used primarily in pediatric oncology in the treatment of Wilms' tumor, Ewing's sarcoma, and embryonal rhabdomyosarcoma.

Doxorubicin, Daunorubicin, and Epirubicin

Doxorubicin (Adriamycin) and daunorubicin (Cerubidine) are antibiotics produced by the fungus *Streptomyces peucetius*. These drugs are anthracyclines with a tetracyclic ring structure and an unusual sugar, daunosamine, attached by a glycosidic linkage (Fig. 60-8); their chemical structure differs by a

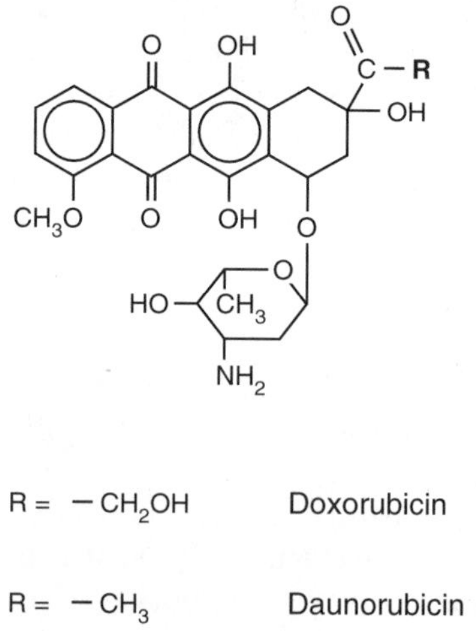

R = —CH₂OH   Doxorubicin

R = —CH₃   Daunorubicin

Figure 60-8. Structural formulae of anthracyclines.

single hydroxyl group at position 14. Their mechanism of cytocidal action is complex. A major effect involves interaction with the nuclear enzyme DNA topoisomerase II to inhibit the religating activity of this enzyme, thereby causing DNA double-strand breaks and cell death. Other actions include DNA intercalation leading to partial unwinding of the DNA helix, and free radical formation by oxidation-reduction of the quinone-hydroquinone group.

Doxorubicin has an initial plasma half-life of 10–15 minutes and a terminal half-life of 25–30 hours. It is distributed widely in body tissues and is approximately 75–80% protein-bound in plasma. The liver is the main site of biotransformation and elimination of the drug. Therefore, patients with hepatic dysfunction may need their doses adjusted.

Doxorubicin is one of the most useful antineoplastic drugs available for the treatment of lymphoma, breast cancer, lung cancer, and sarcomas. In the breast cancer case presented for this chapter, a good partial if not a complete remission was induced by using doxorubicin as second-line chemotherapy.

Major acute adverse effects include myelosuppression, alopecia, local tissue necrosis (if extravasation occurs during intravenous administration), and ulceration of the oral mucosa. A major long-term toxicity is cardiomyopathy. In the case history, therapy with doxorubicin was discontinued when the cumulative dose of doxorubicin approached the toxic threshold of 450 mg/m^2.

Daunorubicin is used in the treatment of acute leukemia in children and adults. Its toxic effects are similar to those of doxorubicin, except that it is much less cardiotoxic.

Epirubicin (Pharmorubicin) is also a close structural analog of doxorubicin, differing only in the position of the hydroxyl group on the daunosamine sugar. The clinical activity and toxicity are similar to those of doxorubicin, but the drug may be somewhat less cardiotoxic.

Mitoxantrone

Mitoxantrone (Novantrone) is a synthetic drug with a tricyclic structure; it intercalates between DNA bases and inhibits DNA topoisomerase II, thereby causing DNA double-strand breaks and cell death. Mitoxantrone is used clinically in the treatment of breast cancer and acute myeloblastic leukemia. It causes less nausea, vomiting, and alopecia than doxorubicin and is also less cardiotoxic.

Bleomycin

Bleomycin (Blenoxane) consists of a mixture of antibiotic peptides with the predominant component being the A2 peptide (Fig. 60-9). Bleomycin produces DNA strand breaks through a complex sequence of reactions involving the binding of a bleomycin–ferrous iron complex to DNA. It is useful in the treatment of head and neck, testicular, and lung cancers, as well as lymphomas. It has little myelosuppressive activity but may cause fever, chills, rigors, hyperpigmentation, and skin thickening. Anaphylactoid reactions have been reported rarely with the administration of this agent. Its dose-limiting toxicity is the development of an interstitial pulmonary fibrosis.

PLANT DERIVATIVES

This group of drugs is represented by the vinca alkaloids, the epipodophyllotoxins, the taxanes, and camptothecin and its analogs, all of which are extracted from plants.

Vinca Alkaloids

The commonly used vinca alkaloids are **vincristine** (Oncovin, Vincasar) and **vinblastine** (Velban). They are derived from the periwinkle plant, *Vinca rosea*. Vinca alkaloids are structurally similar compounds consisting of two multiringed subunits, vindoline and catharanthine (Fig. 60-10).

The vinca alkaloids bind to tubulin and thus inhibit spindle formation, resulting in metaphase ar-

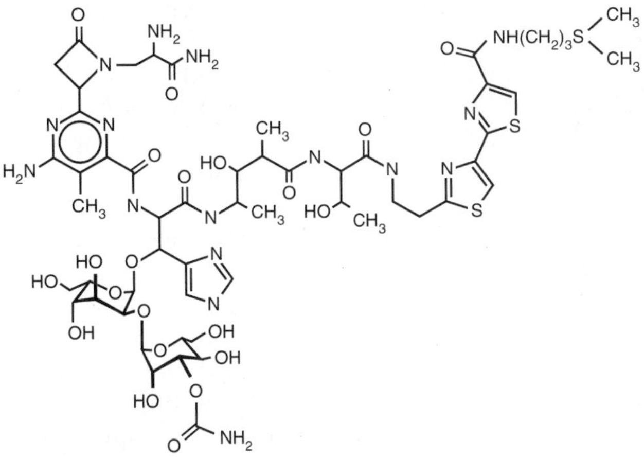

Figure 60-9. Structural formula of bleomycin A2.

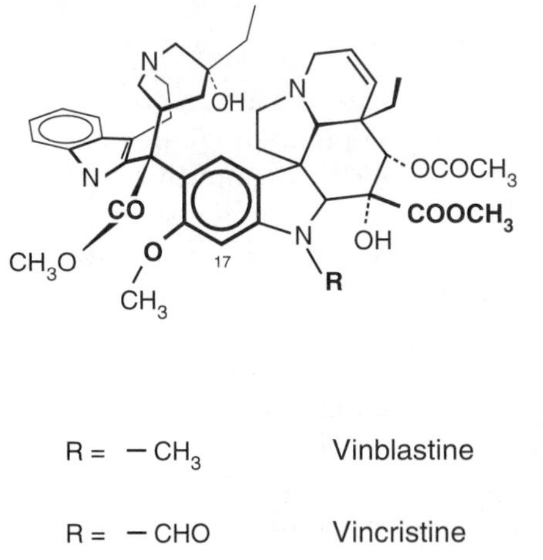

R = —CH$_3$ Vinblastine

R = —CHO   Vincristine

Figure 60-10. Structural formulae of vinca alkaloids.

rest of cells undergoing mitosis. The pharmacokinetics of vincristine and vinblastine are somewhat different because of the side-chain substitutions. Both drugs are given intravenously. Vincristine clearance is rapid, with a terminal half-life of 2–3 hours, while vinblastine is eliminated more slowly (terminal $t_{1/2}$ of 20 hours). Both drugs are eliminated by hepatic biotransformation. They are useful in the treatment of lymphomas, breast cancer, testicular cancer, and sarcomas, usually as part of a combination chemotherapy protocol. Their major toxicities are different: Neuropathy is the main dose-limiting toxicity for vincristine, and myelosuppression for vinblastine. Vincristine can also cause a syndrome of inappropriate ADH secretion (SIADH).

Vinorelbine (Navelbine) is a novel vinca alkaloid that also appears to inhibit mitosis at metaphase by interacting with tubulin. It differs structurally from the other vinca alkaloids in having a modified catharanthine subunit. Like the other vinca alkaloids, vinorelbine is administered intravenously. Its plasma clearance is triphasic, consisting of a rapid initial phase due to distribution to peripheral compartments, an intermediate component representing drug metabolism, and a slow tertiary phase of drug efflux from those compartments. Clinically, the drug has been used as a single agent or in combination to treat patients with advanced non–small-cell lung cancer. It has also been used to treat patients with metastatic breast cancer who have not responded to first-line chemotherapy including anthracyclines. For example, the case described in this chapter could have been treated with vinorelbine rather than paclitaxel after having received CMF and doxorubicin.

Etoposide (VP-16) and Teniposide (VM-26)

VP-16 (etoposide; VePesid) and VM-26 (teniposide; Vumon) are semisynthetic glycosidic derivatives of podophyllotoxin (Fig. 60-11), which is an antineoplastic agent derived from the mandrake plant. Podophyllotoxins bind to tubulin, but their cytocidal activity is mainly mediated by DNA topoisomerase II. The epipodophyllotoxins inhibit religating activity of this enzyme, leading to increased DNA double-strand break formation and cell death. Unlike doxorubicin, VP-16 and VM-26 do not intercalate between DNA bases. Resistance to these drugs is correlated with decreased activity of DNA topoisomerase II, as well as overexpression of P-glycoprotein that promotes increased drug efflux.

VP-16 is usually given intravenously, although it can be given orally with approximately 50% absorption of the dose. After intravenous administration, disposition of VP-16 from plasma follows a two-compartment model with initial and terminal elimination half-lives of approximately 3 and 15 hours, respectively. About 45% of administered drug is excreted unchanged in the urine and an additional 15% in the feces. Its dose-limiting toxicity is myelosuppression. Both VP-16 and VM-26 are used in treating testicular and lung cancer and lymphomas.

Paclitaxel

Paclitaxel (Taxol) is a diterpene plant alkaloid derived from the bark of the Pacific yew tree *(Taxus brevifolia)*. The tree, which grows in the shadow of large pine and spruce in old-growth forests, is relatively rare, and the drug is costly. Paclitaxel consists

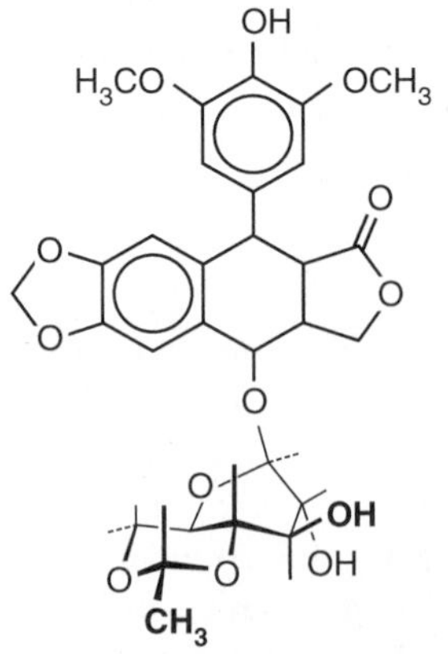

Figure 60-11. Structural formula of etoposide (4-dimethylepipodophyllotoxin ethylidene; VP-16).

of a complex 15-membered taxane ring structure with an ester side-chain that is essential for antitumor activity. The mechanism of cytocidal action involves binding to microtubule polymers and preventing their depolymerization. This is essentially opposite to the action of the vinca alkaloids (see above).

Paclitaxel is administered intravenously and demonstrates a biphasic plasma clearance profile. The initial rapid phase is due to distribution to the peripheral compartment and the slower second phase represents slow efflux from that compartment. Toxic effects that have been observed are bone marrow toxicity, hypersensitivity reactions, hypotension, nausea and vomiting, diarrhea, alopecia, peripheral neuropathy, myalgia, and arthralgia. Corticosteroids are given 6 and 12 hours prior to the paclitaxel, together with an H_1 antihistamine and an H_2 antagonist (such as cimetidine or ranitidine), in order to reduce the risk of hypersensitivity reactions.

Paclitaxel has significant antitumor activity against cancer of the ovary and breast. It has also been used in combination with cisplatin or carboplatin as a second- or third-line treatment for patients with breast cancer.

Docetaxel

Docetaxel (Taxotere) is a close structural analog of paclitaxel, differing structurally in the composition of the side-chain. It is more soluble than paclitaxel and has a slightly different toxicity profile. It appears to have similar activity to paclitaxel although a definitive comparison of the efficacy of the two agents has not been undertaken.

Camptothecin Derivatives

Camptothecin, a heterocyclic alkaloid, was isolated from the stem wood of *Camptotheca acuminata*, a tree indigenous to northern China. Although the drug had demonstrable antitumor activity, clinical use was terminated because of severe and unacceptable bladder toxicity. Structure–activity studies established that close structural analogs, such as 9-amino-camptothecin or a 10-hydroxy derivative (topotecan), had increased antitumor activity.

Camptothecin and its analogs act by inhibiting the enzyme DNA topoisomerase I. Under physiological conditions the enzyme produces transient single-strand breaks in DNA, binds covalently to the 3'-phosphoryl end of DNA at the break site, facilitates passage of an intact DNA strand through the break site, and religates the cleaved DNA. In the presence of camptothecin or analogs, the drug forms a ternary complex with the enzyme and DNA, shifting the reaction equilibrium markedly in the direction of DNA cleavage. Down-regulation of DNA topoisomerase I, the putative target of these drugs, has been reported in drug-resistant cells.

Topotecan is administered intravenously and has a biphasic plasma clearance pattern. The drug has been used in the treatment of patients with non–small-cell lung cancer, cancer of the ovary and cancer of the esophagus. The major toxic effect is myelosuppression; other side effects include alopecia, mild diarrhea, and elevation of liver enzymes.

CPT-11, another analog, has been used clinically in the treatment of patients with cancer of the ovary, colorectal cancer, small-cell lung cancer, untreated non–small-cell lung cancer, and non-Hodgkin's lymphoma. Pharmacokinetic studies of CPT-11 demonstrate a triphasic plasma clearance curve. The major side effects are leukopenia and diarrhea. Neither topotecan nor CPT-11 causes bladder toxicity, which was the reason the parent compound camptothecin was withdrawn from clinical use.

MISCELLANEOUS AGENTS

L-Asparaginase

The use of the enzyme L-asparaginase (Elspar, Kidrolase, Oncaspar) is the result of one of the few successful attempts to identify some factor or trait unique to the cancer cell that might be exploited for diagnostic or therapeutic purposes. Certain leukemic cells are deficient in the enzyme L-asparagine synthetase and therefore are dependent upon an extracellular supply of the amino acid L-asparagine. If that supply is depleted by administration of L-asparaginase, those leukemic cells lacking L-asparagine synthetase suffer marked inhibition of protein synthesis and cannot survive. This treatment has proven useful in approximately 50% of cases of childhood acute lymphoblastic leukemia (ALL). The enzyme is used along with other antineoplastic agents to induce (but not maintain) remissions. Resistance occurs as a result of up-regulation of the expression of the gene for L-asparagine synthetase in cells exposed to L-asparaginase.

L-asparaginase is usually administered intravenously. Two major side effects are hypersensitivity reactions and protein depletion. The enzyme is derived from *E. coli* or *Erwinia carotovora* and is thus a foreign protein in humans; after repeated courses of treatment, hypersensitivity reactions such as urticaria, angioneurotic edema, bronchospasm, and hypotension may be observed. Inhibition of protein synthesis leads to depletion of anticoagulant factors such as protein C, protein S, antithrombin III, and plasminogen and may result in thrombosis of major vessels. Other toxic effects that have been observed are nausea, vomiting, chills, and acute pancreatitis.

Hydroxyurea

Hydroxyurea is a derivative of urea that is used primarily to rapidly reduce high white blood cell counts in patients with chronic granulocytic leukemia (CGL). Its mechanism of action is inhibition of the enzyme ribonucleotide reductase, thereby depleting intracellular nucleotide pools and causing an accumulation of cells in late G_1 and early S phase of the cycle. Hydroxyurea is rapidly absorbed after oral administration. The drug has been used to maintain patients with CGL in remission, especially those who have developed resistance to the alkylating agent busulfan.

HORMONES

Some synthetic hormone analogs or antagonists are used in the treatment of hormone-dependent malignancies, most notably breast and prostatic cancers. More details of their mechanism of action, pharmacokinetics, and toxicity are described in Chapters 49 and 51.

Glucocorticoids

These agents have useful roles in the treatment of many cancers, either for their antitumor effect or for treatment of complications related to malignancy. **Prednisone** is often combined with other drugs in the treatment of leukemia, myeloma, lymphomas, and breast cancer. Glucocorticoids are also useful for treating patients with brain edema and hypercalcemia, as illustrated in the Case History.

Hormones for the Treatment of Breast Cancer

Many breast cancers grow more rapidly in the presence of female hormones. Whether a breast cancer will respond to hormonal therapy can often be predicted by the measurement of estrogen and progesterone receptors in the tumor tissue, as was done in the illustrative case. The hormonal treatments for breast

cancer include antiestrogens (tamoxifen), progestational agents (megestrol acetate), or inhibitors of estrogen production (aminoglutethimide). For tumors that are positive for hormone receptors, a hormonal treatment would generally be used before any chemotherapy (as in the Case History), because there is a higher chance of success and the toxicities are generally less severe.

Tamoxifen

Tamoxifen (Nolvadex and others; Fig. 60-12) is a nonsteroidal antiestrogen analog of clomiphene. Although tamoxifen can bind to the cellular estrogen receptor, when the tamoxifen–receptor complex is translocated to the nucleus it inhibits DNA and RNA synthesis instead of inducing synthesis as estrogens usually do. This is probably due to successful competition of this complex for estrogen-receptor nuclear binding sites. Approximately 70% of breast cancers positive for estrogen and progesterone receptors will respond to tamoxifen. Tamoxifen also alters prostaglandin production and decreases circulating levels of prolactin, LH, and FSH.

The drug is given orally and undergoes extensive hepatic biotransformation. The two major metabolites, 4-hydroxytamoxifen and desmethyltamoxifen, have long half-lives and also have antiestrogen activity. Conjugates are excreted in the bile and undergo extensive enterohepatic recirculation. Toxicity is generally mild, consisting chiefly of nausea and menopausal symptoms, but the drug can produce a transient flare-up of pain and other symptoms arising from the breast cancer and metastases. Retinopathy has been reported in patients on long-term treatment with very high doses. Other antiestrogens are under development.

Progestational agents

It is not clear how these drugs act to suppress breast cancer, but **medroxyprogesterone** and **megestrol**

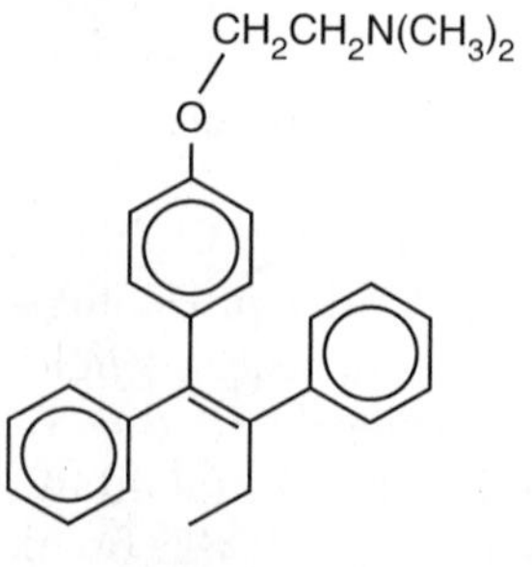

Figure 60-12. Structural formula of tamoxifen.

are both known to be active against hormone-sensitive cancers. They are usually second-line agents after tamoxifen because of a less favorable toxicity profile that includes weight gain and thromboembolism.

Aminoglutethimide

Aminoglutethimide (Cytadren) is an inhibitor of aromatase, an important enzyme in the conversion of androgens to estrogens in extraadrenal tissue. It also inhibits steroidogenesis by blocking conversion of cholesterol to pregnenolone. These two actions, if combined with administration of enough hydrocortisone to prevent ACTH secretion, can depress plasma and urinary estradiol to levels observed in patients who have undergone surgical adrenalectomy. This antiestrogenic effect is useful in managing metastatic breast cancer. The drug undergoes extensive hepatic biotransformation. It also inhibits thyroxine synthesis, but in most cases there is a compensatory increase in TSH that maintains a euthyroid state, and thyroid replacement therapy is seldom necessary. Inhibition of steroidogenesis may be great enough that the patient requires supplementary mineralocorticoid. The major side effects are skin rash, lethargy, drowsiness, and mild nausea. A number of other specific aromatase inhibitors with less toxicity are currently being developed.

Hormones for the Treatment of Prostate Cancer

Most prostate cancer cells are stimulated by androgens. It was discovered over 50 years ago that the removal of male hormones by surgical castration could lead to regression of advanced prostate cancer. More recently, a variety of pharmacological approaches have been developed, based either on inhibition of androgen production or on blockade of androgen action (antiandrogens). Androgen synthesis occurs mainly in the testis, but a small proportion (5–10%) occurs in the adrenal gland. To achieve nearly complete androgen blockade, an inhibitor of testicular androgen production is combined with an antiandrogen. The agents used are described below.

Gonadotropin-releasing-hormone agonists

Gonadotropin-releasing hormone (GnRH) is a hypothalamic polypeptide that binds to receptors in the pituitary gland and stimulates the production of luteinizing hormone (LH) and follicle-stimulating hormone (FSH) (see also Chapter 49). In the male, LH stimulates testosterone production and secretion.

Normal secretion is pulsatile; with continuous GnRH secretion there is an immediate increase in LH and FSH secretion followed by complete inhibition of their release. Various synthetic GnRH analogs cause a biochemical castration by binding very strongly to the receptor and suppressing the pituitary–gonadal axis. These analogs are given parenterally or intranasally; monthly depot formulations are also available. The commercial preparations include **leuprolide** (Lupron), **buserelin** (Suprefact), and **goserelin** (Zoladex); all provide results equivalent to an orchiectomy and differ mainly in the route of administration.

Estrogens

High doses of estrogens will also inhibit androgen production by feedback inhibition of LH release. The preparation most commonly used has been **diethylstilbestrol.** The use of estrogens has fallen out of favor because of a concern about excessive cardiovascular side effects.

Antiandrogens

Flutamide (Euflex, Eulexin) and **nilutamide** (Anandron) are nonsteroidal agents that block effects of dihydrotestosterone (DHT) at the androgen receptor. The side effects are primarily related to androgen deficiency. A compensatory increase in testosterone secretion may partially overcome the effects of these drugs. Antiandrogens are not appropriate as single agents in the therapy of prostate cancer but are most effective in combination with an inhibitor of androgen production.

Cyproterone (Androcur) is a steroidal antiandrogen that also blocks DHT at the androgen receptor. It does have antigonadotrophic effects as well; It produces feedback inhibition of GnRH release so that no compensatory increase in testosterone secretion occurs. It is thus suitable for single-agent therapy of prostate cancer.

DEVELOPMENT OF NEW CANCER TREATMENTS

Currently available chemotherapy can cure testicular cancer, Hodgkin's disease, non-Hodgkin's lymphoma, choriocarcinoma, and many childhood cancers. Although some of the common solid tumors can be cured by adjuvant chemotherapy, most are relatively resistant. The development of new drugs and strategies to improve the results of cancer chemotherapy is a major priority.

The screening of naturally occurring and synthetic compounds is one strategy of drug development. New compounds are screened for activity against human and animal tumor cell lines in vitro. The most promising agents are tested further to identify the maximally tolerated dose in mice and other species. Other new agents are developed as specific inhibitors of pathways known to be important in cancer growth and metastasis. Initial testing of new anticancer drugs in humans is often performed in cancer patients when no other treatment is available or when conventional therapy has been unsuccessful. In analogy to the universal drug development and testing rules described in Chapter 75, these studies are referred to as phase I or dose-finding trials. The starting dose, based on body surface area; is usually equivalent to one-tenth of the maximally tolerated dose in the mouse. If this produces no major toxicity, the dose may be escalated by 25–100% in the next group of patients. This process continues until the maximally tolerated dose (MTD) is determined. Once the MTD has been ascertained, phase II studies are conducted. These involve patients with cancer of a specific type or site who meet defined eligibility criteria. A drug dose slightly less than the MTD is used. Assessment of antitumor efficacy is the major purpose. If the drug shows activity (usually defined as reduction in the size of measurable lesions) in more than 20% of patients, further studies are performed. These might include studies of combination therapy with other active drugs, or comparisons with the best available current therapy, in randomized phase III studies.

SUGGESTED READING

Calabresi P, Clark J. Pharmacology of antineoplastic agents. In: Calabresi P, Schein PS, eds. Medical oncology. 2nd ed. New York: McGraw Hill, 1993.

Chabner BA. Anticancer drugs. In: DeVita VT, Hellman S, Rosenberg SA, eds. Cancer, principles and practice of oncology. 4th ed. Philadelphia: Lippincott, 1993:325–417.

Chabner BA, Collins J, eds. Cancer chemotherapy: principles and practice. Philadelphia: Lippincott, 1990.

DeVita VT. Principles of chemotherapy. In: DeVita VT, Hellman S, Rosenberg SA, eds. Cancer, principles and practice of oncology. 4th ed. Philadelphia: Lippincott, 1993:276–292.

Donehower RD, Abeloff MD. Chemotherapy. In: Abeloff MD, Armitage J, eds. Clinical oncology. New York: Churchill Livingstone, 1995:210–218.

Erlichman C. Pharmacology of anticancer drugs. In: Tannock I, Hill R, eds. The basic science of oncology. New York: McGraw Hill, 1992:317–337.

Fleming IR, Cooper MR. In: American Cancer Society textbook of clinical oncology. Atlanta: American Cancer Society, 1995:110–134.

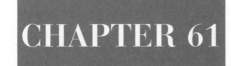

CHAPTER 61

Immune System Organization, Modulation, and Pharmacology

J.W. SEMPLE AND J.M. BRANDWEIN

CASE HISTORY

A 26-year-old woman came to her physician with a 2-week history of easy bruising and a rash on her legs. She had also had several nosebleeds over the past week and had noticed gum bleeding when brushing her teeth. In addition, her last menstrual period 2 weeks ago had been heavier than usual. There was no hematuria, melena, or visible blood in the stools. She was otherwise in good health and was on no medications. She had not had a recent illness, and the past medical history and family history were unremarkable.

On examination she appeared well, with no pallor or jaundice. Vital signs were normal. Conjunctivae and fundi were normal. There was slight oozing from her gums and several petechial lesions were noted on her hard palate. There was no lymphadenopathy. Respiratory, cardiovascular, and abdominal examinations were normal; the liver and spleen were not enlarged. A number of ecchymoses were noted on her extremities, and numerous petechiae were present on both lower legs. The musculoskeletal and neurological examinations were normal.

A complete blood count (CBC) revealed RBC = 4.6×10^{12}/L, WBC = 5.4×10^9/L with normal differential, hemoglobin = 125 g/L, platelets = 8×10^9/L. The blood film confirmed the presence of marked thrombocytopenia with large platelets present. RBC and WBC morphology were normal. Prothrombin and partial thromboplastin times were nor-

mal. A bone marrow aspiration was normal with numerous megakaryocytes present.

A diagnosis of *immune thrombocytopenic purpura* was made. The patient was started on prednisone 80 mg PO daily and was advised to avoid products containing aspirin (ASA). After 5 days the platelet count rose to 20×10^9/L and no new bruising or bleeding was noted. The platelet count rose steadily thereafter and 2 weeks later was normal at 240×10^9/L. The prednisone was gradually tapered off over the ensuing 6 weeks and then discontinued, with careful monitoring of the platelet count, which remained normal.

After treatment had been initiated, further investigations were performed to search for an etiology for the immune thrombocytopenia. Antinuclear antibody, rheumatoid factor, and HIV serology were negative. Abdominal ultrasound was normal, showing no lymphadenopathy and normal spleen size.

Six months after the cessation of prednisone, routine follow-up showed that the platelet count had dropped to 70×10^9/L. She was asymptomatic and had no evidence of bleeding by history or physical examination. No treatment was initiated. She was advised to have her blood counts monitored regularly, but she did not return for follow-up.

Three months later the patient came to the Emergency Room with a 1-week history of bruising and petechiae. This time she had also had several episodes of melena over the previous 12 hours and was feeling increasingly weak. On examination, she appeared pale, blood pressure was 120/80 mmHg with a postural drop of 15 mmHg, and pulse was

110/min. She again had extensive petechiae and ecchymoses on her skin. Stool was grossly black and was confirmed to be positive for blood.

Her CBC revealed RBC $= 2.8 \times 10^{12}$/L, WBC $= 5.0 \times 10^9$/L, hemoglobin $= 80$ g/L, platelets $= 3 \times 10^9$/L. The blood film again showed marked thrombocytopenia as well as red cell polychromasia.

The patient was admitted to hospital, cross-matched, and transfused with two units of packed red cells. She was also started on intravenous IgG 1 g/kg daily for 2 days. The morning after admission her hemoglobin had increased to 100 g/L, and her vital signs had stabilized. Within 2 days her platelet count had increased to 70×10^9/L and her melena had stopped. Her platelet count peaked at 250×10^9/L after 1 week and subsequently dropped to 50×10^9/L over the ensuing 2 weeks. She was restarted on prednisone, vaccinated against pneumococcus, and referred for splenectomy, which was performed 10 days later. Following splenectomy, the platelet count increased to 300×10^9/L and has remained in the normal range on follow-up.

Immunopharmacology is a relatively new discipline that deals with the control (enhancement or suppression) of the immune response by chemical and/or biological mediators. The ultimate goal is to identify molecules that act on specific individual components of the immune system (preferably in an antigen-specific manner) to enhance or block the action of those particular components: the modern equivalent of Ehrlich's "magic bullet."

The generation of an immune response to a foreign antigen or antigens (e.g., a microorganism or transplanted organ) is a complex biological process involving the interaction of many cell types and their secreted products (Fig. 61-1). In general, initiation of the response occurs when the antigen, e.g., a cellular protein, first interacts with an antigen-presenting cell (APC), i.e., a cell that is positive for major histocompatibility complex (MHC) class II; this can be a macrophage, dendritic cell, or B cell within a lymph node. The MHC is a series of genes located on chromosome 6 in humans and codes for cell surface glycoproteins responsible for immune recognition. Class I MHC molecules are found on virtually all cell types (with the exception of red blood cells in humans). Class II molecules are more narrowly restricted in their expression on APC. Once the APC interacts with antigen and internalizes it, the cell can then "process" the antigen by proteolysis into smaller antigenic peptides and present them on its membrane, in association with class II molecules encoded by the MHC, to antigen-specific T-helper (Th) cells.

Th cells in turn become activated by signals passed via their T-cell-receptor (TcR) complex, proliferate, and secrete cytokines such as interleukin-2 (IL-2). These events subsequently stimulate antigen-specific B cells to produce and secrete antibodies, which can ultimately either destroy the antigen or enhance its removal by the reticuloendothelial system.

Th cells are the critical cell type that will determine whether antibodies are produced against the foreign antigen. They finely control the response by activating other regulatory cells or by secreting various regulatory agents, e.g., T-suppressor cells or cytokines, respectively. Any defect in, or abnormal activation of, antigen-specific Th cells can thus alter the magnitude of the immune response. Furthermore, modulation of the components of T-cell recognition—i.e., the trimolecular complex of antigen, TcR, and MHC—is a potential avenue of immunotherapy.

During an immune response, CD4-positive T-helper (Th) cells can be subdivided into Th0, Th1, or Th2 cells depending on the cytokines they secrete. In humans, Th0 cells are thought to be less differentiated than Th1 and Th2 cells, since they can secrete most or all of the cytokines made by either cell type, particularly IL-2 and IL-10. Th1 activation usually results in the secretion of IL-2 and immune interferon (IFN-γ), whereas Th2 cells secrete IL-4, IL-5, IL-6, and IL-10 when activated. Th1 and Th2 cells respond differentially to different APC; the site of exposure of the antigen and the physical nature of the antigen will influence which CD4-positive T cell predominates in a given immune response. Th1 responses generally mediate delayed-type hypersensitivity (DTH) reactions, whereas Th2 responses generally mediate superior humoral immune responses, particularly IgE responses. It is becoming apparent that these Th responses critically influence immune reactivity, and modulation of these cell types through cytokine networks is a promising approach to immunopharmacology.

Immune-system modulators are of two general types: (1) immunosuppressants, which usually suppress the immune response in a nonspecific manner and are used to minimize the effects of autoimmune diseases or rejection of organ transplants; and (2) biological response modifiers or immunopotentiators, which can enhance the immune response and may be used in the treatment of conditions in which the immune response is depressed, such as cancer. Figure

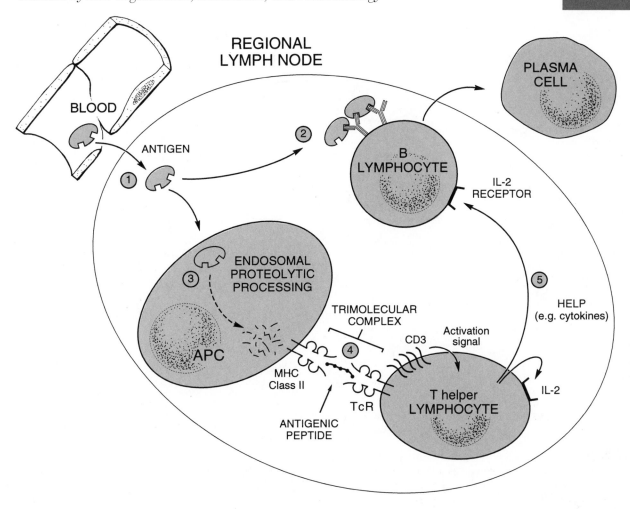

Figure 61-1. The generation of a humoral immune response. (1) Antigen passes from the circulation into a regional lymph node. (2) B lymphocytes (with antigen-specific surface immunoglobulin) recognize the antigen and become "primed" for T-cell help (i.e., they increase the surface expression of IL-2 receptors). (3) Antigen is taken up (either by phagocytosis of a cell or by fluid-phase pinocytosis of a soluble protein) by an antigen-presenting cell (APC) and processed by proteolysis within an endosomal compartment. (4) Antigenic peptides are reexpressed on the surface of the APC, within the antigen binding groove of major histocompatibility complex (MHC) class II molecules. This complex can then be recognized by T-helper (Th) cells via their T-cell receptor (TcR); Th cells become activated as a result. (5) Th-cell activation causes secretion of cytokines (e.g., IL-2), which stimulate the antigen-primed B cells to differentiate into plasma cells and secrete antibodies. Abbreviations listed under Figure 61-2.

61-2 is a simplified diagram showing components of the immune system and sites of action of some of the immune-system modulators that are used as immunopharmacological agents.

IMMUNOSUPPRESSANTS

Many immunosuppressive drugs in use today are also classed as antineoplastic agents, but the therapeutic plan differs for the two applications. For example, those cytotoxic agents that act primarily against proliferating cells can act against both the proliferating cancer cells and normal immune cells. Cancer cell proliferation, however, is generally random while immune cell proliferation is usually "synchronized" in a burst of mitotic division after introduction of antigen. Therefore, when drugs are used at the time of a transplant or during treatment of an autoimmune disease, a large portion of the proliferating immune precursor cells can be destroyed by an initial high dose of immunosuppressant, and long-term im-

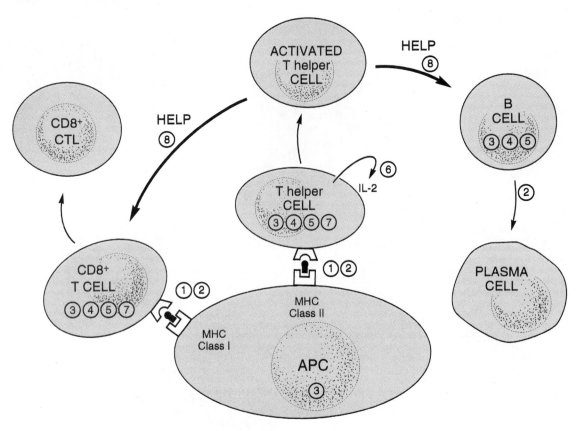

Figure 61-2. Sites of action of some of the modulators that are used as immunopharmacological agents. *Specific modulation:* (1) Agents that can act on the trimolecular complex (e.g., anti-MHC or TcR antibodies, suppressive peptides). These agents are still used only experimentally. (2) IVIg (anti-idiotypic antibodies). IVIg may be more appropriately classed as nonspecific, because it can affect all B cells; however, specific anti-idiotypes (for a B-cell clone) have been experimentally induced. *Nonspecific modulation:* (3) Prednisone. (4) Azathioprine. (5) Cyclophosphamide. (6) Cyclosporine. (7) Antithymocyte globulin. (8) Cytokines. Abbreviations (including those in Fig. 61-1): APC = antigen-presenting cell; CD = cluster determinant; CTL = cytotoxic T lymphocyte; IL-2 = interleukin-2; MHC = major histocompatibility complex; TcR = T-cell receptor. HELP (heavy arrows) can be in the form of cytokines, cell contact, etc. Light arrows represent differentiation pathways.

mune suppression is maintained with a low-dose daily schedule thereafter. When the same drugs are used against cancer (see Chapter 60), they are given in high-dose pulses every 3–6 weeks in order to allow immune rebound between treatments.

Immunosuppressant therapy from the 1960s to the present has consisted of combinations of various drugs such as corticosteroids and azathioprine to produce maximal immunosuppression while keeping adverse side effects to a minimum. Recently, a new wave of immunosuppressant therapy characterized by the selective regulation of defined subpopulations of lymphocytes has been used with such drugs as the cyclosporines and FK506. The future of immunosuppressant therapy will be the induction of antigen-

specific depression of autoimmunity and allograft reactivity.

Prednisone

The corticosteroids were the first group of agents recognized as having lympholytic properties. Corticosteroids inhibit the generation of arachidonic acid, thus preventing the production of various inflammatory mediators (e.g., prostaglandins) by the cyclooxygenase and lipoxygenase metabolic pathways (see Chapter 31). Prednisone, the most commonly used immunosuppressant, can reduce the size and lymphoid cell content of the lymph nodes and the spleen, although it has no toxic effect on proliferating myeloid or erythroid stem cells in the bone marrow.

Prednisone suppresses the inflammatory response of cell-mediated immunity and may also directly suppress antibody synthesis. It is cytotoxic to certain subsets of T cells, and some of its diverse effects may be due to lysis of either suppressor or helper T cells. Continuous administration of prednisone increases the fractional catabolic rate of IgG, thus lowering the concentration of specific antibodies.

The corticosteroids also offset some effects of the immune response by reducing tissue injury from inflammation and edema. Prednisone is used in a wide variety of clinical conditions in which the immunosuppressant properties of the drug account for its beneficial effects. These include autoimmune disorders (e.g., autoimmune hemolytic anemia, autoimmune thrombocytopenic purpura, systemic lupus erythematosus) and organ transplantation (e.g., kidney, bone marrow). Other uses and adverse effects are described in Chapter 51.

Azathioprine

Until the development of cyclosporine A, azathioprine (Imuran) was the drug most often used for immunosuppression in relation to organ transplantation. It is now used as a second immunosuppressant therapy in specific situations where corticosteroids have been found to have no beneficial effects (e.g., in one-third of patients with autoimmune thrombocytopenic purpura). Azathioprine is a precursor of mercaptopurine, which is the active molecule. Mercaptopurine, a structural analog or antimetabolite of hypoxanthine, interferes with nucleic acid metabolism (purine synthesis) during the wave of lymphoid cell proliferation that follows antigen stimulation, and it is especially effective against T cells. Its toxic effects are primarily bone marrow depression and possible reactivation of viral hepatitis (see Chapter 60).

Cyclophosphamide

The alkylating agent cyclophosphamide is an antineoplastic drug that is also a potent immunosuppressant used chiefly in patients who do not tolerate azathioprine. It is a modified nitrogen mustard that destroys proliferating lymphoid cells but that also alkylates some resting cells, rupturing the DNA double helix and inducing lethal mutations. Cyclophosphamide (Cytoxan) was originally designed as an inactive nitrogen mustard precursor that would be converted to the active alkylating form at its site of action. Its adverse effects are those of the nitrogen mustards (see Chapter 60).

Cyclosporine

This cyclic polypeptide is produced by the fungus *Tolypocladium inflatum* and has profound immunosuppressive effects on cell-mediated cytolysis in graft–host reactions and on delayed-type hypersensitivity. It has a remarkably specific affinity for T lymphocytes. With its introduction in 1983, organ survival rates have improved significantly. Although its therapeutic effects are palliative rather than curative, one of its great advantages is that the use of steroids can be greatly reduced or, in certain diseases, eliminated totally.

Cyclosporine A (Sandimmune) does not interfere with hematopoiesis, including the maturation of lymphoid stem cell precursors. Only when mature immunocompetent T cells have received an activation signal from antigen-presenting cells does cyclosporine block the ensuing cellular activation. The precise mechanism of action is still unclear. Cyclosporine blocks the activity of cyclophilin, a peptidyl-prolyl *cis-trans* isomerase that catalyzes protein unfolding. It has been postulated that through this mechanism, transcription of interleukin-2 (IL-2) and its receptor are blocked. Cyclosporine A can also suppress immune interferon (IFN-γ) and other macrophage growth factors, resulting in a decrease of interleukin-1.

Studies of the clinical pharmacology of the drug indicate a very large variation in bioavailability (ranging from 5 to 90%), large amounts bound to erythrocytes and plasma proteins, and extensive biotransformation. The major route of elimination is biliary.

A major adverse effect of the agent is nephrotoxicity, which can be potentiated when the drug is administered together with amphotericin B, aminoglycosides, and co-trimoxazole. Other side effects such as elevated serum bilirubin, alkaline phosphatase, and transaminases; neurotoxicity; and a risk of lymphomas have been reported.

FK506 is a newly developed macrolide derived from the fungus *Streptomyces tsukubaensis*. In general, FK506 is more potent than cyclosporine in a number of experimental models of transplantation and autoimmunity. However, the two compounds have a similar spectrum of activity.

Antithymocyte Globulin

The concentrated IgG fraction of plasma from hyper-immune rabbits immunized with human thymic lymphocytes (rabbit antithymocyte serum, or RATS) is primarily used today in patients undergoing kidney transplants. It reduces the number of T cells in the thymus-dependent areas of the spleen and lymph nodes and thus reduces the immune response. Since the human recipient can make an immune response against the rabbit IgG, RATS is usually administered with other immunosuppressants such as azathioprine. Common adverse reactions include fever, chills, leukopenia, and skin reactions.

Intravenous γ-Globulin (IVIg)

IVIg (Iveegam) is concentrated γ-globulin from normal human plasma. It thus represents a wide spectrum of naturally expressed antibodies, including IgG autoantibodies. IVIg has been shown to be effective in down-regulating the immune response in a number of autoimmune diseases that are mediated primarily by autoantibodies (e.g., myasthenia gravis, chronic inflammatory demyelinating polyneuropathy, autoimmune thrombocytopenia, rheumatoid arthritis). For example, there are numerous reports that IVIg, given at a dose of 400 mg/kg for 5 days or 1 g/kg for 1 day, results in a significant rise in platelet counts in patients with autoimmune thrombocytopenic purpura. Its mechanism of action is still unknown; however, two working theories have been suggested and there is experimental evidence which supports both: (1) The crystallizable fragment (Fc) portions of the concentrated IgG molecules bind to Fc receptors on phagocytic cells and competitively inhibit the binding of autoantibody-opsonized particles or cells. (2) Naturally occurring anti-idiotypic antibodies (i.e., reactive with the antigen-binding portion of antibodies) within the IVIg preparation directly bind to autoantibodies and/or B cells and inhibit their function.

Monoclonal Antibodies

An alternative means of nonspecific immunosuppression has recently been developed with the use of monoclonal antibodies against individual leukocyte surface antigens, including CD3 (total T cells), CD4 (T-helper cells), and various T-cell activation markers (IL-2 receptor, CD25). In animal models, these agents have been shown to be effective in suppressing the immune response, probably via their ability to block the specific function of the cell surface molecules. Anti-CD3 in conjunction with cyclosporine has been used to produce immunosuppression in renal transplant recipients.

Future Considerations for Immunosuppressants

All the current immunosuppressant therapeutic strategies in autoimmune diseases and transplantation are aimed at inhibiting the emergence of pathological clones of lymphocytes. Unfortunately, they are generally nonspecific, in that the total immune response is affected, and therefore the treatments eventually have to be discontinued. Antigen-specific therapies that would inhibit only the clones responsible for the disease are still at an experimental stage. The majority of these therapies are aimed at the trimolecular complex: MHC + peptide + T-cell receptor. Treatment with monoclonal antibodies specific for class II MHC molecules, blocking the function of the MHC with immunosuppressive competitor peptides, and idiotype-specific suppression are all examples of potential antigen-specific immunosuppression.

IMMUNOPOTENTIATION

Immunopotentiation can be defined as a process which directly or indirectly enhances immune functions. It can be classed as specific or nonspecific, and each of these classes can be subdivided into active, passive, or adaptive events. Table 61-1 summarizes

Table 61-1 Classification of Immunopotentiation Mechanisms

Specific mechanisms	
Active:	Vaccination
Passive:	Rabbit antithymocyte serum (RATS) therapy
Adoptive:	Tumor-infiltrating lymphocytes; sensitized lymphocytes
Nonspecific mechanisms	
Active:	Cytokines; synthetic chemicals
Passive:	Intravenous γ-globulin (IVIg) therapy; plasmapheresis
Adoptive:	Lymphokine-activated killer (LAK) cell therapy

the classification scheme of immunopotentiation mechanisms.

Levamisole

This drug is an anthelmintic agent that has been shown to potentiate immune responses in animals and humans. It is an imidazole derivative and is thought to act by inhibiting the production of a substance by T-suppressor cells that has immunosuppressive properties. A major side effect of this drug is arthralgia.

Cytokines

Cytokines are soluble molecules secreted by a wide variety of cell types and are primarily concerned with cellular communication. Within the immune system, this communication is in the form of either activation events or suppressive events. The major cytokines associated with the immune system are the interferons and the interleukins. In addition, there are a number of specific factors which also play an important role in modulating the immune response (e.g., colony-stimulating factors, tumor necrosis factor, transforming growth factors).

Interferons (IFN) are a group of glycoproteins first identified as compounds that inhibit intracellular viral replication (see Chapter 58). Currently there are three major classes: α, β, and γ.

Interferons have been produced by stimulation of a variety of cell types including lymphocytes, fibroblasts, and epithelial cells. As with many cytokines, they are now available through recombinant DNA technology. The α- and γ-interferons are derived primarily from human lymphoblasts, and β-interferon from human fibroblasts. γ-Interferon is also referred to as immune interferon.

α-Interferon can modulate antibody responses by directly inhibiting B lymphocytes, and it enhances natural killer cell activity. Currently, it is approved for use in hairy cell leukemia. It has been found in the serum of patients with a variety of autoimmune diseases and in AIDS, and it is now being shown to be an effective treatment in certain autoimmune diseases, e.g., autoimmune thrombocytopenic purpura. β-Interferon is derived primarily from fibroblasts and causes a number of in vivo effects including stimulation of expression of class I and class II HLA molecules and stimulation of natural killer activity. β-Interferon has recently been approved for the treatment of relapsing forms of multiple sclerosis, although its mechanism of action in this illness is not yet known. The biological activity of γ-interferon is highly species-specific. It is a potent activator of macrophage tumoricidal activity. Its interaction with other lymphokines can be either antagonism (IL-4) or synergism (IFN-α and -β).

Adverse effects have included fever, chills, hypotension, paresthesias, and altered mental state. Neutropenia and elevated serum transaminases are commonly observed.

Interleukins (IL) are small polypeptide hormones that are primarily associated with the immune system. They are produced by lymphocytes and have multiple effects on the immune response. Their fine control is essential for adequate regulation of the immune response.

In humans, probably the most important interleukin responsible for the stimulation of both humoral and cellular immunity is IL-2. Originally termed T-cell growth factor, it is produced primarily by T cells but acts on all lymphoid cells. Its major effects are the activation of T cells, B cells, and macrophages and the stimulation of secretion of other interleukins to further modulate the immune response. It has potent antitumor effects against metastatic melanoma and renal cell cancer. IL-2 has also been used as an ex vivo stimulus of lymphokine-activated killer (LAK) cells and tumor-infiltrating lymphocytes (TIL), which have been shown to be potentially therapeutic against certain tumors (e.g., lymphomas).

Various autoimmune diseases, including multiple sclerosis, rheumatoid arthritis, and systemic lupus erythematosus, have been found to be associated with increased serum levels of IL-2. Hypersecretion of endogenous IL-2 may lead to autoaggression by a number of mechanisms such as bypassing the need for T-cell costimulation, up-regulating costimulatory CD80 molecules on B cells, or by the induction of other cytokines such as IFN-γ and IL-10. Thus, therapies that can regulate the production of IL-2 may have potential benefits in treating some autoimmune disorders.

SUGGESTED READING

Paul WE, ed. Fundamental immunology. 3rd ed. New York: Raven Press, 1993.

St. Georgiev V, Yamaguchi H, eds. Immunomodulating drugs. Ann NY Acad Sci 1993; vol 685.

Sigal NH, Dumont F. Cyclosporine A, FK-506, and rapamycin: pharmacologic probes of lymphocyte signal transduction. Ann Rev Immunol 1992; 10:519–560.

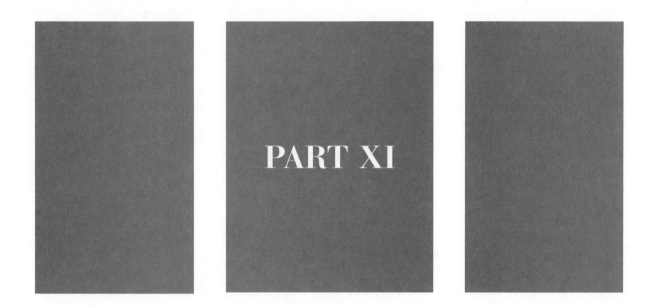

SPECIAL TOPICS OF PHARMACOLOGY

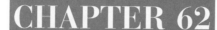

CHAPTER 62

Sources of Individual Variation in Drug Response

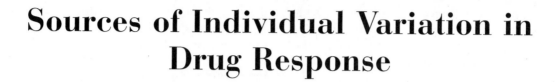

H. KALANT

In all textbooks of pharmacology, medicine, and therapeutics, recommended dosages of drugs are given in absolute amounts (e.g., 10 mg three times daily) or, less frequently, in amounts relative to body weight (e.g., 1 mg/kg). Such dosages represent a combination of statistical statement and value judgement because they are based on extensive clinical observations indicating that the recommended dosage will, in *most* patients, on *most* occasions, produce the desired therapeutic effect with an *acceptably low* risk of toxicity.

Like all statistical statements, dosage recommendations represent mean values and imply that some individuals will require more than the mean and some will require less. This chapter deals with the following basic question: If an accepted normal dosage of a drug is prescribed, why do some patients show either too much or too little response? The answer to this question is really a composite of the answer to four subsidiary questions:

1. Was the prescribed dosage actually taken by the patient? This is dealt with below under the heading of **Compliance.**

2. If it was taken as prescribed, was it properly absorbed and delivered to the systemic circulation? This is considered under **Bioavailability.**

3. If absorbed and delivered to the circulation, was the drug distributed normally in the body, in such a way as to achieve the intended concentration and duration at the site(s) of action? This is examined under sources of **Pharmacokinetic Variation.**

4. If the drug was distributed in the expected way, did the target tissue(s) respond to it in the usual manner? This is considered under sources of **Pharmacodynamic Variation.**

COMPLIANCE

Most patients probably do intend to follow their physicians' instructions concerning prescribed medication, because most prescriptions are filled promptly. One study showed that 97% of the prescriptions written by physicians were filled within 5 days. If the patients did not intend to take the drugs, it is unlikely that they would go to the trouble and expense of having the prescriptions filled at a pharmacy. However, other studies have found that actual compliance with the physician's instructions is very variable; for *short-term preventive* medication (i.e., medication intended to prevent the development of symptoms rather than to treat existing ones) the compliance rate was found to be about 80%. For *long-term preventive* medication (e.g., for the treatment of asymptomatic hypertension) compliance was only 40%.

In efforts to examine the causes of such low compliance, investigators have assessed the possible contributions of many individual factors that might conceivably affect the patient's understanding of the physician's instructions and the willingness or determination to follow them. A variety of **demographic factors** such as age, sex, socioeconomic level, educational level, and ethnic background do not appear to exert any statistically significant effect on the degree of compliance. There is also no significant correlation with the **specific disease** for which the medication is prescribed, except for some psychiatric illnesses, such as schizophrenia, in which the disease itself may interfere with the patient's attention to, or comprehension of, the physician's explanations, or may give rise to negative responses, apathy, or inertia. In such cases, responsibility for ensuring that the prescribed dosage schedule is followed should probably be assigned to a family member, friend, or guardian of the patient.

The degree of **complexity** and **inconvenience** of the treatment schedule can have an important effect in decreasing compliance. The larger the number of different drugs the patient must take, the poorer is the compliance, especially if the various drugs are to be taken at different times of the day and different numbers of times each day. This may be one reason for the marketing of pharmaceutical mixtures, in which a single tablet or capsule contains fixed proportions of two or more drugs that are frequently prescribed together for patients with certain illnesses. Among the very numerous examples are mixtures of a thiazide diuretic with a hypotensive agent (for hypertension), of an atropine-like anticholinergic agent with a sedative (for peptic ulcer), of an NSAID with an H_2-receptor blocker or prostaglandin E_1 (for rheumatoid arthritis), and of a glucocorticoid with a β-adrenergic agonist (for bronchial asthma). It is possible that compliance is improved by such mixtures, since only a single dosage instruction has to be remembered. However, the serious disadvantage is the loss of therapeutic flexibility, since the dosages of the individual constituents of the mixture cannot be separately adjusted according to the patient's needs and responses.

In contrast, several factors contribute significantly to improved compliance. One is the **continuity and ease of contact with the physician.** The longer the patient has known and trusted the physician, and the greater the convenience of and promptness in scheduling follow-up visits, the better is the physician's opportunity to remind the patient about the importance of the drugs and to strengthen the patient's motivation to use them. Closely related to this factor is the **patient's perception of the seriousness of the disease** and of the importance and efficacy of the drug therapy, both of which tend to improve compliance. In contrast, medications or treatment schedules with a high incidence of unpleasant side effects generally give rise to poor compliance.

An illustrative case: Noncompliance is a problem of particular importance for patients with chronic diseases that require lifetime drug therapy, such as grand mal epilepsy, diabetes mellitus, and arterial hypertension. On the one hand, high blood pressure per se does not cause obvious and troublesome symptoms in the majority of patients. On the other hand, the adverse effects of antihypertensive drugs may cause some patients to feel miserable. It is not surprising, therefore, that patients who feel quite fit frequently fail to comply with physicians' recommendations to take drugs that aim to prevent the occurrence of cerebral, cardiac, or renal consequences of hypertension at some unknown time in the future. Unfortunately, physicians only rarely obtain exact information on how accurately patients follow their prescriptions. In most cases, measurement of blood or urine levels of antihypertensive drugs is neither feasible nor practical to detect noncompliant patients.

A study at a large steel factory in Hamilton, Ontario (*Lancet* 1975; I:1205–1207 and *Lancet* 1976; I:1265–1268) on improvement of compliance in hypertension brought interesting results. Of 230 hypertensive employees, 38 were identified as noncompliant with instructions on medication. Twenty of these were placed on an experimental protocol for 6 months. Even when these men were given better opportunities to see the doctor, for instance during working hours, or when they received instruction about the nature of hypertension, most of them remained noncompliant, and their blood pressure remained elevated. However, when the patients were taught to measure their own blood pressures, asked to chart their own pressure readings and pill taking, and taught how to tailor pill taking to their daily habits, and when these maneuvers were reinforced with supervision every 2 weeks, the compliance increased by 21% and the control of their blood pressures improved significantly (Fig. 62-1). This study demonstrated that compliance with medication instructions can be improved in hypertensive patients by the use of proper methods.

Important measures to assure compliance in long-term antihypertensive therapy include simplified dosage schedules, use of long-acting rather than short-acting drugs, choosing drugs with minimal side effects, and assuring continuous supervision of the patient. In addition, patients should be thoroughly familiarized with the importance of taking prescribed drugs regularly in order to prevent the serious consequences of high blood pressure. The physician can help to monitor compliance by asking patients to bring their medication bottles with them when they come for checkups. Comparison of the number of

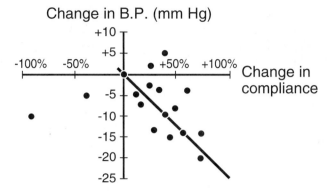

Figure 62-1. Effect of improved compliance, due to combined strategies, on improvement in blood pressure. (From Haynes et al. 1976.)

tablets or capsules prescribed and the number remaining will help to identify patients who are not taking the drugs regularly. *Such principles are not specific for antihypertensive therapy, but apply equally to medications used in long-term treatment of other diseases.*

BIOAVAILABILITY

The concept of bioavailability, methods of measuring it, and the clinical significance of bioavailability are all covered in detail in Chapter 5. Therefore the topic is mentioned only briefly here, as one potentially important source of variation in drug response.

As described in Chapter 5, the term "bioavailability" refers to the fraction of an administered dose (by any route other than intravenous) that is absorbed and reaches the systemic circulation. It is most commonly measured by determining the area under the concentration–time curve after that dose and expressing it as a percentage of the corresponding area after intravenous injection of the same dose. This percentage can be reduced, for the same preparation of the same drug, by a variety of physiological and pathological factors in the gastrointestinal tract and liver. For example, hypermotility, diarrhea, steatorrhea, biliary obstruction, reduced gastrointestinal blood flow, and induction of hepatic drug uptake and biotransformation (see Chapter 4) can all reduce the fraction of an oral dose that finally reaches the systemic circulation, and hence reduce the drug effect. In contrast, liver disease, especially in cases that produce intrahepatic or extrahepatic shunts (see Chapter 46), may result in an unusually large frac-

tion of the dose reaching the circulation and producing an unexpectedly large effect.

Independently of the patient, however, bioavailability may vary because of differences in the formulation of the tablet, capsule, or other preparation, leading to differences in the rate and completeness of release of the active drug into solution in the gastrointestinal fluids. Dissolution is a necessary first step before the drug can be absorbed. If it does not occur rapidly enough, the undissolved part of the dose may be lost in the feces. For this reason, an overly compact tablet may show lower bioavailability than the same dose of the same drug given as a solution (Fig 62-2). Different companies marketing the same drug may use different tablet formulations, which may differ significantly in disintegration rate and uniformity. "Brand name" drugs are often better formulated than so-called "generic" drugs, giving better and more uniform bioavailability. However, this is not always the case (Fig. 62-3), and the physician must be aware of potential differences of this type when evaluating different products in clinical practice.

PHARMACOKINETIC VARIATION

Apart from variations in drug absorption and bioavailability mentioned above, other important pharmacokinetic factors contributing to variation in drug response are differences in drug distribution, biotransformation, and elimination. Some of the main sources of **variation in drug biotransformation** are reviewed in Chapter 4. Genetically determined

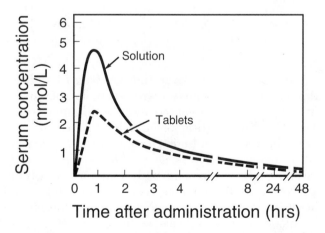

Figure 62-2. Time course of serum digoxin concentration after oral administration of 0.75 mg as an aqueous solution and as tablets.

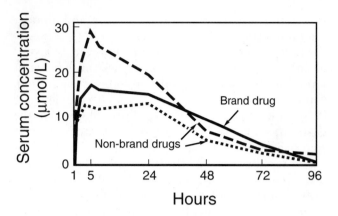

Figure 62-3. Bioavailability of different preparations of phenytoin following oral administration of 500-mg doses.

alterations in biotransformation are discussed in Chapter 12. The effects of liver disease on drug biotransformation and elimination are covered in some detail in Chapter 46.

The potential magnitude of these variations is illustrated by the following examples:

- In a group of geriatric inpatients, the mean plasma half-life of antipyrine was 45% greater and that of phenylbutazone was 29% greater than in young controls (i.e., impaired hepatic biotransformation).
- Absorption of a 400-mg oral dose of mecillinam was only slightly reduced in a group of elderly subjects (65 or more years old) compared to a group of young adults, but the elimination half-life was markedly prolonged (4 hours versus 0.9 hour), and the urinary drug levels were correspondingly lower in the elderly (i.e., impaired renal excretion).
- The plasma levels of phenacetin after a standard dose were markedly lower in regular smokers than in nonsmokers (i.e., induction of biotransforming enzymes) (Table 62-1).

The main causes of variation in **drug distribution** are those associated with early infancy (see Chapter 65) and advanced age (see Chapter 66). However, drug distribution may be affected at any age by differences in **body composition.** It is generally recognized that dosage for adults should take account of body size and body build. Obviously a large person will need more drug than a small person to achieve the same desired drug concentration in the blood or tissues. This is the basis for giving dosages in relative values such as mg/kg. However, the modifying factor of the percentage of body fat must be taken into account. Many differences of

drug response between men and women are due to differences in body composition, especially in percentage of body fat. An obese person will require a smaller dose of a highly water-soluble drug than a lean person *of the same total body weight* in order to avoid excessively high drug concentration in the body water, including the plasma water. Conversely, the obese person will probably require more of a lipid-soluble drug than the lean person to achieve the same plasma level, but the large store of drug in body fat may result in greatly prolonged drug action.

Drug distribution may also be modified by disease processes. For example, normally the blood–brain barrier may prevent the passage of penicillin and various other antibiotics into the central nervous system. In the presence of inflammatory conditions (meningitis) the permeability of the blood–brain barrier is increased, and these antibiotics may pass much more readily. This improves their therapeutic value, but may also increase the risk of seizures or other toxic effects in the brain. In contrast, when an inflammatory process gives rise to a localized abscess or other walled-off infection (e.g., empyema), systemic antibiotic therapy may be ineffective because the drug will not be distributed into the abscess or other cavity in which the bacteria are growing. For this reason, surgical drainage may be required, together with local application of the antibiotic directly into the affected site.

VARIATION IN REQUIRED DOSAGE IN CHILDREN

A special case of pharmacokinetic variation as a source of variation in drug response is encountered in relation to dosage in children of different ages. As noted above, body composition can account for substantial variation in the drug concentration pro-

Table 62-1 Plasma Levels of Phenacetin (μg/mL) in Cigarette Smokers and Nonsmokers at Various Intervals After the Oral Administration of 900 mg of Phenacetin

	Hours After Phenacetin Administration			
	1	*2*	*3.5*	*5*
Nonsmokers	0.81	2.24	0.39	0.12
Smokers	0.33	0.48	0.09	0.02

duced by a given dose. However, the required dose for a given individual is usually more strictly proportional to **body surface area** than to body weight. The discrepancy is not large for adults, but is important for babies and small children, whose surface-to-mass ratio is considerably higher than that of adults. The relationship is described by the equation: $S \ (cm^2) = W^{0.425} \ (kg) \times H^{0.725} \ (cm) \times 71.8$, but this is obviously impractical for calculating dosages in a physician's office or a patient's home. Therefore, simplified approximations have been made for calculating **children's doses** on the basis of age or surface area.

Calculation of children's dose by age (Young's rule):

$$Age/(age+12) = \text{fraction of adult dose to be given to child}$$

Calculation of children's dose by body surface area:

$$(1.5 \times \text{weight in kg}) + 10 = \text{percentage of adult dose to be given to child}$$

Each of these calculations is based on some standard of comparison. Young's rule makes the assumption that a 12-year-old, weighing 35–40 kg, should receive one-half of an adult dose. The surface area rule is based on the assumption that the average adult has about 65 kg of metabolically active mass and a corresponding surface area of about 1.7 m². Table 62-2 illustrates the relative doses calculated by these two methods. The younger the child, the more clearly superior is the surface area method of calculation.

PHARMACODYNAMIC VARIATION

Variations in drug response are probably less frequently attributable to changes in responsiveness of the target tissue than to the causes discussed in the preceding sections. Nevertheless, there are some important instances. Examples of **genetically determined abnormalities** of tissue response to drugs, such as malignant hyperthermia and warfarin insensitivity, are described in Chapter 12.

Other changes in tissue response can be caused by **disease processes.** For example, hyperthyroidism is frequently associated with an increased number of β-adrenoceptors, leading to increased sensitivity to the cardiovascular and other effects of norepinephrine and related catecholamines.

Sometimes **drug interactions** will alter pharmacodynamic sensitivity to one or more of the drugs concerned (Chapter 64). Patients with chronic left ventricular failure, for example, may be given a diuretic as well as a cardiac glycoside. Improvement in cardiac output by the cardiac glycoside increases renal blood flow and may therefore improve the urinary response to the diuretic. Conversely, if the diuretic then causes excessive loss of K^+ in the urine, the hypokalemia will increase myocardial sensitivity

Table 62-2 Some Comparisons of Age, Weight, and Surface Area, and Relative Doses for Children

Age	Weight (kg)	Approximate Surface Area m²	Approximate Surface Area Percent of Adult Area	Relative Drug Dose as Percent of Adult Dose* By Young's Rule	Relative Drug Dose as Percent of Adult Dose* By Body Surface Rule
Newborn	3	0.2	12	0	15
3 months	6	0.3	18	2	19
1 year	10	0.45	26	8	25
6 years	20	0.8	47	33	40
9 years	30	1.0	59	43	55
12 years	40	1.3	76	50	70
14 years	50	1.5	88	54	85
24 years (adult)	65–70	1.7	100	100	100

*For this purpose, the "adult dose" referred to is the average dose in mg for a 65–70 kg person of normal body build.

to the digitalis glycoside and increase the risk of arrhythmia (see Chapter 36).

Previous drug history can also affect target tissue sensitivity. This is perhaps seen most clearly in relation to central nervous system depressants such as alcohol (Chapter 26), benzodiazepines and other sedatives and anxiolytics (Chapter 27), and opioid analgesics (Chapter 23). Prolonged or high-dose use of these drugs usually leads to changes in receptor number or sensitivity or to other compensatory functional changes offsetting the drug effects, and giving rise to **tolerance** (Chapter 72). This not only decreases the response to the drug itself, but may also lead to **cross-tolerance,** i.e., decreased response to other drugs with similar effects. A well-recognized example is the decreased sensitivity to general anesthetics that is frequently encountered in alcoholics.

CONCLUSIONS

Every aspect of drug absorption, distribution, action, and elimination is subject to greater or lesser degrees of variability, from an infinite range of causes. It is impossible to catalog all the sources of variation in this chapter. The physician prescribing drugs must be aware of their importance and be prepared to modify the dosage in individual patients in the light of the most probable factors operating in any given case.

SUGGESTED READING

Haynes RB, Sackett DL, Gibson ES, et al. Improvement of medication compliance in uncontrolled hypertension. Lancet 1976; I:1265–1268.

Sackett DL, Haynes RB, Gibson ES, et al. Randomized clinical trial of strategies for improving medication compliance in primary hypertension. Lancet 1975; I:1205–1207.

Schmidt D, Leppik IE, eds. Compliance in epilepsy. Epilepsy Res, Suppl. 1. Amsterdam: Elsevier, 1988.

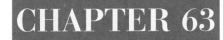

CHAPTER 63

Adverse Drug Reactions

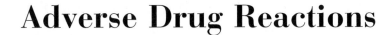

C.A. NARANJO, N.H. SHEAR, AND U. BUSTO

IDENTIFYING ADVERSE REACTIONS TO DRUGS

Epidemiological Approach

All drugs have the potential to cause deleterious effects. Before a drug can be approved for general use, it must be carefully studied in several thousand patients. While some adverse effects are detected in such premarketing studies, some serious but relatively infrequent types of toxicity may become apparent only when the drug is used in a large population of patients over long periods of time. Consequently, the early detection and assessment of adverse drug reactions has become increasingly important.

From the time that humans first used different substances as medicines, toxic effects were observed. Reference to toxicity of drugs is found in the writings of several famous physicians of ancient times. For example, Hippocrates (460–377 B.C.) instructed his students and fellow physicians that they should "above all, do no harm"; this was obviously a reference to the potential hazards associated with remedies of that time. The balance between beneficial and toxic effects of drugs has been a continuing concern as medicine has progressed. Occasionally, wise laymen, such as Voltaire in his work *Le Medecin Malgré Lui*, have expressed doubts about the proper use of drugs by physicians. ("They poured drugs of which they knew little into bodies of which they knew less.") However, interest in the detection and prevention of serious drug toxicity reached a peak after the occurrence of the thalidomide disaster in 1961.

In that year there was a sudden outbreak of births of babies suffering from deformities known as phocomelia or micromelia. Astute physicians suspected that the development of these abnormalities was associated with the use of a new and presumably safe hypnotic, thalidomide, by the mothers of these babies during the first trimester of pregnancy when the forelimb buds were forming and developing (see also Chapters 65 and 70). Case-control studies established that thalidomide was indeed the factor responsible for the malformation. All these events led to a reassessment of the methodology and regulations applied to the testing of the safety of drugs. As a consequence, more stringent legislation was implemented in several countries in order to improve the possibility of detecting serious toxicity before drugs were administered to humans.

In recent years, new knowledge has been acquired concerning the diagnosis, assessment, mechanism, treatment, and prevention of adverse drug reactions. This chapter is a brief review of the most relevant knowledge and procedures.

Clinical Approach

Patients may develop unwanted symptoms during drug therapy. This is called an adverse drug event (ADE). If the ADE is believed to be caused by the drug therapy, then the reaction is called an adverse drug reaction (ADR). The clinical management of a patient with an ADE includes four steps:

• Diagnosis of the reaction
• Differential diagnosis of the reaction
• Drug history

- Determination of the probability that the drug caused the reaction

Each of these steps is critical for the optimal management of an ADR and will be discussed in greater detail.

DEFINITIONS, MECHANISMS, AND CLASSIFICATION

An adverse drug reaction (ADR) is any noxious, unintended, and undesired effect of a drug that is observed at doses usually administered therapeutically in humans. This definition excludes cases of drug overdose, drug abuse, or therapeutic errors.

The severity of ADRs is usually classified as mild, moderate, severe, or lethal. These terms are defined as follows.

Mild: No antidote, therapy, or prolongation of hospitalization is necessary.
Moderate: Requires a change in drug therapy, although not necessarily discontinuation of the offending drug. It may prolong hospitalization and require specific treatment.
Severe: Potentially life-threatening, requires discontinuation of the drug and specific treatment of the adverse reaction.
Lethal: Directly or indirectly contributes to the death of the patient.

The adequate assessment and classification of ADRs requires a knowledge of the mechanisms by which they are produced. Adverse drug reactions are the result of an interaction between the characteristics of the administered drug and some inherent or acquired characteristics of the patient that determine the individual pattern of response to drugs. Thus, there are some reactions that are determined principally by the drug (physicochemical and pharmacokinetic characteristics, formulation, dose, rate and route of administration), others that are determined chiefly by the patient's characteristics (genetic, physiological, or pathological), and others in which both drug and patient variables are important.

ADRs can be **dose-related** (e.g., CNS depression by sedative hypnotics). These reactions are the most common (about 95% of cases). In these cases the frequency and severity of the ADRs are directly proportional to the administered dose and therefore can be prevented and/or treated by adjusting the dosage to the patient's needs and tolerance. In some of these cases, impairment of drug elimination by renal disease (for drugs such as digoxin, predominantly excreted by the kidney) or liver dysfunction (for drugs eliminated after biotransformation in the liver) can contribute to the development of toxicity. The ADR can represent an extension of the usual pharmacological effects of the drugs or an unusual toxicity caused by the drug and/or its metabolites. These reactions are usually predictable from animal toxicological studies.

Other ADRs are **not dose-related.** These reactions are uncommon (less than 5% of cases) and are due to an increased susceptibility of the patient. The ADR is usually manifested as a qualitative change in the patient's response to drugs, and it may be caused by a pharmacogenetic variant (see Chapter 12) or an acquired drug allergy. Most reactions with a pharmacogenetic basis are detected only after the patient is exposed to the drug and therefore are difficult to prevent on first administration. An example of genetically determined toxicity is the polyneuropathy caused by isoniazid, a drug that is mainly biotransformed by acetylation. Within populations, there tends to be a clear separation of individuals into groups of slow or rapid acetylators on the basis of differences in the activity of liver N-acetyltransferase (NAT2). The neuropathic effects from isoniazid are more common in slow acetylators. Most such pharmacogenetic reactions can be prevented by avoiding readministration of the drug to the affected individuals.

The identification of a reaction as dose-related or not dose-related allows practical decisions concerning the treatment of an individual patient and/or the prevention of ADRs. The main features of these reactions are summarized in Table 63-1.

Allergic or hypersensitivity immunological reactions have been classified into four main clinical types: 1—anaphylactic; 2—cytotoxic; 3—immune-complex-mediated; and 4—cell-mediated.

Type 1 or immediate hypersensitivity reactions involve interaction of the allergen (the drug) with IgE antibody on the surface of basophils and mast cells, resulting in the release of chemical mediators such as histamine, slow-reacting substances of anaphylaxis, kinins, and prostaglandins that lead to capillary dilatation, contraction of smooth muscle, and edema. A type 1 reaction may be limited to cutaneous weals and flares, but it can also result in life-threatening systemic anaphylaxis (characterized by shock and bronchoconstriction), asthma, or laryngeal angioneurotic edema. Anaphylactic reactions

Table 63-1 Adverse Drug Reactions (ADRs)

	Dose-Related ADR	*Not Dose-Related ADR*
Nature of abnormality	Quantitative	Qualitative
Incidence	High	Low
Is ADR predictable?	Yes	No
In the presence of liver and/or kidney dysfunction	Increased toxicity, depending on the main route(s) of elimination of the drug in question	Not affected
Prevention	Adjustment of dose	Avoid drug administration
Treatment	Adjustment of dose	Discontinue drug administration
Mortality	Usually low	Usually high

may occur after the injection of penicillin and other antimicrobials. For example, many drugs and biological response modifiers can cause urticaria and angioedema. For most the mechanism is unknown but not related to IgE. Up to 25% of asthmatic patients may demonstrate intolerance to acetylsalicylic acid (ASA), which may cause severe bronchospasms, a pharmacological reaction that is not due to IgE.

Type 2 reactions are complement-fixing reactions between antigen and antibody on a cell surface (e.g., RBC, WBC, platelets), leading to lysis of the cell. Drugs are usually haptens, binding to a protein on the cell surface to constitute a complete antigen against which a specific antibody is formed. Subsequent antigen–antibody reactions with complement fixation may lead to hemolytic anemia (e.g., after methyldopa, chlorpromazine), agranulocytosis (e.g., after amidopyrine, cephalothin, sulfonamides), or thrombocytopenic purpura (e.g., after ASA, quinidine, phenytoin).

Type 3 hypersensitivity reactions (toxic immune-complex reactions) occur when antigen–antibody complexes deposit on target tissue cells. Complement is then activated and causes tissue destruction by releasing lysosomal enzymes. This mechanism may cause glomerulonephritis, collagen diseases, and vasculitic skin eruptions. The classic adverse reaction associated with immune complex formation is the serum sickness reaction. This is a syndrome of fever, arthralgia/arthritis, a rash consisting of an exanthem and purpura, and nephritis. This is due to foreign proteins used in therapy, such as antithymocyte glob-

ulin for immune suppression. Drugs may cause a reaction that has been confused with serum sickness but is very different. The serum sickness-like reaction (SSLR) is defined as the triad of fever, arthralgia/arthritis, and an exanthematous or urticarial rash, but this is not associated with immune complexes, and renal disease is very rare. The drug most commonly associated with this reaction is the antibiotic cefaclor. Other drugs commonly implicated in these reactions are penicillins, sulfonamides, erythromycin, hydralazine, and nitrofurantoin.

Cell-mediated **type 4** allergic reactions arise from a direct interaction between an allergen (the drug) and sensitized lymphocytes, resulting in the release of lymphokines (see Chapter 61). Most cases of eczematous and contact dermatitis are cell-mediated allergic reactions. Common causes are topical antihistamines, para-aminobenzoic acid compounds, and mercury derivatives. A delayed hypersensitivity reaction syndrome (HSR) is believed to be initiated by the formation of reactive metabolites of the drug and the initiation of a type 4 response to the metabolite acting as a hapten. HSR is a syndrome of fever, rash (exanthem, erythema multiforme, Stevens-Johnson syndrome, or toxic epidermal necrolysis) and internal organ involvement. The most common internal manifestations are hepatitis, nephritis, agranulocytosis, and thrombocytopenia. Drugs that are commonly implicated are aromatic anticonvulsants (phenytoin, phenobarbital, carbamazepine, and lamotrigine; see Chapter 22), sulfonamides, allopurinol, and nonsteroidal anti-inflammatory agents.

EPIDEMIOLOGY OF ADVERSE DRUG REACTIONS

Drug Monitoring Methods

Drug monitoring is the systematic collection, recording, and assessment of information on adverse drug reactions. This information is collected to allow the early identification of severe ADRs, to determine the possible causal association of drugs and adverse events, to establish the frequency of ADRs, and to identify the factors predisposing to their development.

Estimation of the frequency of adverse reactions to a drug depends on the reliable identification of the number of subjects presenting the adverse event (numerator) and the accurate estimate of the number of subjects exposed to the drug (denominator). The determination of these two numbers is generally difficult because the denominator is usually unavailable, and the numerator can be over- or underestimated. Information on adverse drug reactions is collected using several methods that are briefly described below.

Spontaneous communication to national drug monitoring centers

Since the thalidomide disaster of the 1960s, several countries have established national drug monitoring centers to collect information on ADRs. These agencies encourage physicians and other health personnel to report any clinical event suspected of being an ADR. The system has met with varying success. The most active drug monitoring centers are located in the United Kingdom and Sweden, and they periodically report their findings. This system mostly collects information on the number of cases of ADRs, but it is not designed to yield information on the number of prescriptions for various drugs. Another disadvantage is that the collection of information is highly dependent on the motivation of physicians to report the events. Therefore, underreporting is common. However, these systems have obviously contributed to an early recognition of severe reactions, and thus they are still operative in various countries. In the United States, the Food and Drug Administration has a Drug Monitoring Center to which physicians can report information on suspected ADRs. The corresponding monitoring agency in Canada is in the Health Protection Branch, Health and Welfare Canada. The monitoring agencies in many countries are united in an international network, reporting data regularly to a World Health Organization Collaborating Center in Uppsala, Sweden.

Cohort studies

Another procedure frequently used has been the systematic collection of prospective information on drug therapy and adverse events in subjects with a particular characteristic (patient-oriented) or receiving a particular drug (drug-oriented). This system allows the collection of information on both the number of subjects with ADRs and the number of subjects receiving the drug. This procedure has been applied mostly to medical patients in teaching hospitals. The best-known example is the Boston Collaborative Drug Surveillance Program. In this and similar programs, information on the demographic and clinical characteristics of patients, the drugs administered to them, and the suspected ADRs is collected by trained nurse or pharmacist monitors. The data are subsequently analyzed to establish the drugs most commonly inducing ADRs, the frequency of different types of ADR, and the factors predisposing to them. These procedures have provided information about the clinical use of, and adverse reactions to, the most commonly prescribed drugs. They have also been used to determine the clinical toxicity of drugs in subjects with special characteristics, for example, those suffering from renal or liver dysfunction. However, these data have obvious shortcomings, the most important being that the information has been collected exclusively on medical inpatients in university centers, making extrapolation of results to other populations difficult.

More recently, the postmarketing surveillance of a cohort of subjects receiving a new drug has gained popularity. These studies begin immediately after a new drug has been marketed, and the drug's performance is closely monitored during months or years when widespread use may result in the discovery of rare side effects or previously unknown drug interactions. Cohort studies are expensive and difficult to perform because large populations must be studied if the incidence of uncommon but severe ADRs is to be determined.

Case-control studies

These studies are retrospective but useful for suggesting cause–effect relationships between drugs and adverse events. In the case of a suspected ADR, the relative use of the suspected drug is compared in subjects with the presumed drug-induced illness and in a matched control group without the illness. If the illness really is associated with the drug, those showing the adverse event will have had a greater exposure to the drug. This procedure was employed to discover the link between thalidomide and phocomelia. In his classic letter to *Lancet*, McBride reported that "Congenital abnormalities are present in approximately 1.5% of babies. I have observed that the incidence of severe abnormalities in babies of women who were given the drug thalidomide . . . during pregnancy . . . (was) almost 20%." This method is very efficient when the undesirable event is clinically unique. However, when the adverse event is a common clinical occurrence such as jaundice, ulcer, or depression, it may be difficult to suspect that it is an ADR, and the event may be attributed to causes other than the drug. This is why so many adverse effects (e.g., ASA-induced bleeding) remained unrecognized for a long time. The most obvious limitation of this procedure is that it is retrospective; therefore, it is difficult to confirm the validity of the history of drug exposure. However, in spite of this problem it is a very useful method for generating hypotheses about possible drug-induced illness.

Frequency of ADRs

The reported overall incidence of ADRs in different studies varies widely from 1% or less to approximately 30%. This disparity is a reflection of the different methodologies used to detect and report the ADRs, the different populations surveyed, the different prescribing habits in various countries, and the inclusion or exclusion of mild reactions. However, most prospective studies show that the incidence of ADRs in hospitalized patients (excluding the mild ones) is between 10% and 20%. Admission to hospital due to an ADR is relatively common; a recent review of published studies indicated that in highly developed industrialized countries, between 0.2 and 21% (median, 5%) of patients are admitted to a hospital because of an ADR (e.g., digitalis intoxication). About 10–20% of ADRs occurring in hospitalized patients are severe. Drug-induced deaths occur in 0.5–0.9% of medical inpatients.

The drugs most commonly causing ADRs vary from one study to another. This reflects the differences in the populations surveyed and in the methods employed for collecting the data. Most studies have been conducted in hospitalized medical patients. In

such patients, most reactions are caused by cardiac glycosides, diuretics, antimicrobials, anticoagulants, and nonsteroidal anti-inflammatory agents.

Risk Factors Associated with ADRs

There are few well-conducted studies of factors that predispose to ADRs. However, epidemiological studies in hospitalized patients have identified some of these factors, and laboratory-based investigations of systemic hypersensitivity reactions (HSR) due to pharmacogenetic defects have helped to identify individual differences in drug metabolism.

Age

Most studies show that older subjects (over 60 years of age) are more susceptible to ADRs. For example, it has been consistently shown that, compared to younger subjects, older patients are more likely to bleed during heparin treatment, are more sensitive to potent analgesics, are at a higher risk of developing digitalis toxicity, and are more likely to develop potassium depletion during diuretic therapy. Impaired drug elimination and increased receptor sensitivity to drugs have been proposed as likely mechanisms responsible for this increased susceptibility to ADRs. However, older patients usually have concomitant diseases and receive more drugs than younger patients; both of these factors are associated with higher incidence of ADRs. The newborn, particularly when premature, is also more sensitive to some ADRs, probably as a consequence of incomplete development of enzymes involved in the biotransformation of drugs. The increased toxicity of chloramphenicol in the newborn may be explained by this mechanism (see also Chapters 4, 55, and 65).

Gender

Women are more likely than men to develop ADRs, especially drug-induced gastrointestinal symptoms. Women also appear to be more susceptible to the toxic effects of digoxin. In the over-60 age group, women are more likely than men to show bleeding induced by heparin.

Other factors

Patients on multiple-drug therapy have an increased probability of developing ADRs. This may be due merely to the additive risk of ADR when receiving several drugs, or to increased opportunity for drug–drug interactions.

A patient history of "allergic disorders" is a good predictor of ADRs including those that are *not* allergic in nature. The predisposition to hypersensitivity reactions may be inherited, and close relatives may be at an increased risk (e.g., for idiosyncratic reactions to sulfonamides and anticonvulsants). Patients who have previously presented an ADR are also more likely to develop a new adverse reaction. The disease state of the patient can also influence the susceptibility to ADRs. For example, impaired renal function predisposes patients to adverse reactions to those drugs that are mainly excreted by the kidneys. Hepatic dysfunction has a similar effect in relation to drugs that are inactivated in the liver. However, few drug monitoring studies have conclusively documented these relationships.

Important Adverse Reactions Detected Since the Thalidomide Reports

A summary of the most important ADRs identified since the occurrence of the thalidomide-induced congenital abnormalities, together with the drug monitoring methods that contributed to their discovery, is shown in Table 63-2. It is of interest to note that a simple and relatively inexpensive procedure, the spontaneous reporting system (case reports), has allowed the identification of half of these reactions.

CLINICAL ASSESSMENT AND MANAGEMENT OF INDIVIDUAL CASES OF ADRs

A major problem in the evaluation of an adverse event in a particular patient is to establish whether there is a causal association between the untoward clinical event and the suspected drug. This can be particularly difficult because the manifestations of ADRs are not unique to that drug. The suspected drug is often administered together with other drugs, and frequently the features of the adverse clinical event cannot be distinguished from the symptoms of the underlying disease.

The four-step approach described at the beginning of this chapter helps in the evaluation of adverse events. The correct *diagnosis* is essential before further assessment should be done. If the diagnosis is an entity that is never caused by a drug, obviously the drug is unlikely to be the cause of this specific event. The diagnostic possibilities for drug reactions include almost every known disease, and some specific drug-related syndromes including the serum-sickness-like reaction (SSLR), hypersensitivity syndrome (HSR), and many rare conditions, such as the dermatological fixed drug eruption. The *differential diagnosis* is important to give a perspective on all the possible causes of the reaction. Thus an exanthematous rash could be due to an infection as well as the drug. This diagnostic list is important to ensure that important causes are looked at in a comprehen-

Table 63-2 Ten Important Adverse Drug Reactions Detected Since the Occurrence of Thalidomide-Induced Reactions

Adverse Drug Reaction	Drug	Method of Discovery
Oculomucocutaneous syndrome	Practolol	Spontaneous communication (i.e., case reports)
Thromboembolism	Oral contraceptives	Case-control study
Nephropathy	Analgesics (especially phenacetin)	Case reports
Lactic acidosis	Phenformin	Cohort study
Deaths from asthma	Sympathomimetic aerosols	Case-control study
Subacute myelo-optic neuropathy	Clioquinol	Case reports
Vaginal cancer (in daughters)	Diethylstilbestrol (maternal)	Case-control study
Aplastic anemia	Chloramphenicol	Case reports
Jaundice	Halothane	Case reports
Retroperitoneal fibrosis	Methysergide	Cohort study

Data from Venning, 1983.

sive manner. The list of *drugs* that the patient has been exposed to is not always easy to obtain. The list should include nonprescription medication, herbal, and traditional treatments, as well as the prescribed drugs.

Conventionally, the **degree of probability** that an adverse event is associated with the administration of a particular drug has been classified as definite, probable, possible, or doubtful, as follows.

Definite: A reaction that (1) follows a reasonable temporal sequence after administration of the drug, or in which the drug level has been measured in body fluids or tissues; (2) follows a known pattern of response to the suspected drug; (3) is confirmed by improvement on removal of the drug and by reappearance on rechallenge; and (4) cannot be explained by the known characteristics of the patient's disease.

Probable: A reaction that (1) follows a reasonable temporal sequence after drug administration; (2) follows a known response pattern; (3) is confirmed on suspension of the drug ("dechallenge") but not on rechallenge; and (4) cannot be explained by the known characteristics of the patient's disease.

Possible: A reaction that (1) follows a reasonable temporal sequence; (2) may or may not follow a known response pattern; but (3) *could* be explained by the known characteristics of the patient's clinical state.

Doubtful: The event is more likely related to factors other than the suspected drug.

However, physicians often disagree on their assessment of the probability of ADRs. In an attempt to standardize the assessment of causality of ADRs, several algorithms of varying complexity have been developed. A simple method, the Adverse Drug Reaction Probability Scale (APS), is valid and reliable in a variety of clinical situations. The APS is a short questionnaire (Table 63-3) that systematically analyzes the various components described here that must be assessed to establish a causal association between drug(s) and adverse events. Each question can be answered positive (yes), negative (no), or unknown/inapplicable (do not know) and is scored accordingly. The probability of the ADR is given by the total score, which can range from −4 (a drug-unrelated event) to +13 (a definitely drug-related event). The use of such procedures for assessing cases of ADRs observed in daily practice, as well as those reported in medical journals, should be encouraged.

Recently, a Bayesian Adverse Reaction Diagnostic Instrument (BARDI) has been developed. This method considers the assessment of the causality of ADRs as a special case of conditional probability. The application of this methodology to clinical practice has been simplified by the development of a microcomputer-based program.

DISCOVERY OF ADVERSE EVENTS INDUCED BY NEW DRUGS IN HUMANS

The toxicity of new drugs is assessed in animal and human studies as prescribed by law, and described in Chapter 75. Nevertheless, toxicological studies in animals do not always predict the toxicity in humans. In addition, the possibility of discovering ADRs in clinical trials that are designed primarily to assess the efficacy and safety of new drugs depends on a variety of factors of which the most important are (1) the relative frequency of drug-related and drug-unrelated events; (2) the mechanism of the drug toxicity (i.e., dose-related or not dose-related reactions); (3) the number of subjects exposed to the drug; and (4) the methodology used for detecting ADRs. Since the contribution and limitations generated by these various factors are often ignored, it is appropriate to analyze briefly how they may influence the discovery of drug-induced illness.

Relative Frequency of Drug-Related and Drug-Unrelated Events

The manifestations of ADRs are usually nonspecific and the contribution of the drug must be distinguished from other possible etiologies. Accordingly, the discovery of an ADR depends on the relative magnitudes of two risks: the added risk of illness experienced by the users of a drug and the baseline risk in the absence of the drug. In the event that the drug-induced illness is frequent and severe, it is usually recognized very early during clinical use of the drug, and the identification is mostly based on well-documented case reports in medical journals and/or from national drug monitoring centers. In contrast, when the drug-induced illness is less common, prospective investigations of cohorts of patients receiving the drug and retrospective case-control studies are indicated.

Mechanism of Drug-Induced Toxicity

The probability of discovery of an ADR may be determined by its mechanism. As described before, ADRs can be dose-related and dose-unrelated. Since

Table 63-3 Adverse Drug Reactions Probability Scale[a]

	Yes	No	Do Not Know	Score
Are there previous *conclusive* reports on this reaction?	+1	−0	0	
Did the adverse event appear after the suspected drug was administered?	+2	−1	0	
Did the adverse reaction improve when the drug was discontinued, or a *specific* antagonist was administered?	+1	−0	0	
Did the adverse reaction reappear when the drug was readministered?	+2	−1	0	
Are there alternative causes (other than the drug) that could on their own have caused the reaction?	−1	+2	0	
Did the reaction appear when a placebo was given?	−1	+1	0	
Was the drug detected in the blood (or other fluids) in concentrations known to be toxic?	+1	−0	0	
Was the reaction more severe when the dose was increased, or less severe when the dose was decreased?	+1	−0	0	
Did the patient have a similar reaction to the same or similar drugs in *any* previous exposure?	+1	−0	0	
Was the adverse event confirmed by any objective evidence?	+1	−0	0	
			Total score:	

[a]To assess the adverse drug reaction, the questions are answered by inserting the pertinent score for each. The total score (which can range from −4 to +13) indicates the increasing probability of an observed event being drug-related.
After Naranjo *et al.* 1981.

dose-related ADRs are the most common, they are easier to detect in the early phases of human studies. In addition, animal studies are usually good predictors of the toxicity that must be ascertained in humans. In contrast, dose-unrelated ADRs (drug allergy and pharmacogenetically based reactions) are peculiar to a group of subjects with very discrete genetic or immunological characteristics. Therefore, these reactions are detected only when the new drug is administered to individuals with such characteristics. These reactions are rarely detected in early clinical trials and generally are not predictable from toxicological studies in animals.

Sample Size Required for Detecting Drug-Induced Disease

Clinical trials are usually short-term studies conducted in a few hundred patients before the drug is marketed. Therefore, only the most common acute

dose-related ADRs are detected in the premarketing phase. A dramatic example of the limitation imposed by this factor is the case of the antipsychotic drug clozapine. Clozapine was introduced in Finland in 1975 when only about 200 subjects had been previously treated. Within the first 6 months of drug use, 17 cases of serious hematological reactions (10 cases of agranulocytosis and seven of neutropenia) were reported to the Finnish national drug monitoring center from among about 3200 users, indicating that the risk of developing agranulocytosis or severe granulocytopenia during clozapine treatment was at least 0.6–0.7% in Finland. (For unexplained reasons, this frequency was 21 times higher than in other countries.) Because of these reactions, the drug was withdrawn from the market. Interestingly, clozapine has been reintroduced for the treatment of schizophrenia resistant to other medications. Recently, other drugs have been discontinued because of inadequate safety (e.g., benoxaprofen). A new quinolone antibacterial agent, temafloxacin, was withdrawn from the market only 15 weeks after being made available for clinical use in the United States because postmarketing monitoring showed it to have much more frequent and more serious ADRs than the related drugs ciprofloxacin, norfloxacin, and ofloxacin. These examples illustrate the importance of the close postmarketing monitoring of any new drug, irrespective of the safety shown in clinical trials. It also indicates the important role of physicians in evaluating the toxicity of newly introduced drugs by voluntarily reporting ADRs to national drug monitoring agencies. No currently available method for detecting ADRs could have predicted such reactions; only the administration of the drug to a sufficient number of subjects resulted in the discovery.

Methods for Assessing ADRs

Methods for collecting information on ADRs in clinical trials are varied and consist of unstructured and structured interviews, physiological and physical examinations, and laboratory tests. The procedures most commonly used are the unstructured interview, designed to eliminate the risk of suggestion of reactions to the patient, and a standardized list of symptoms (checklist). The frequency of symptoms elicited by these scales during treatment with the test drug is compared with symptoms observed during treatment with a placebo. Those symptoms most commonly observed with the test drug are suspected of being ADRs. However, since the clinical manifestations of ADRs are usually nonspecific, the detected associations may be difficult to interpret. Therefore, despite the above-mentioned scales, a more definite assessment of individual cases of suspected ADRs is possible only by using the procedures for assessing causality mentioned above.

The discovery of ADRs also depends on the frequency of assessments and the validity, reliability, and sensitivity of the tests employed. Theoretically, if frequent assessments are performed with a sensitive method, all ADRs should be detected. In practice, no such procedure exists. However, the systematic recording of all adverse events occurring during a drug trial greatly improves the chances of detecting ADRs.

CONCLUSIONS

The discovery and evaluation of ADRs depends on information collected in the preclinical and clinical studies. The most common dose-related acute ADRs are usually detected before a drug is marketed. However, uncommon ADRs or manifestations of chronic toxicity may become apparent only after the drug has been used in a large number of subjects for long periods of time. A more definite assessment of individual cases of ADRs should include the use of the APS or similar methods. Because knowledge about the clinical toxicity of a new drug will always be incomplete at the time of marketing, further investigation of the frequency and determinants of ADRs must be pursued in the postmarketing phase.

SUGGESTED READING

Bakke OM, Wardell WM, Lasagna L. Drug discontinuations in the United Kingdom and the United States, 1974 to 1983: issues of safety. Clin Pharmacol Ther 1984; 35:559–567.

Bernstein JA. Nonimmunologic adverse drug reactions. How to recognize and categorize some common reactions. Postgrad Med 1995; 98:120–122, 125–126.

Davey P, McDonald T. Postmarketing surveillance of quinolones, 1990 to 1992. Drugs 1993; 45(Suppl 3):46–53.

Davies DM. Textbook of adverse drug reactions. 3rd ed. London: Oxford University Press, 1985.

Dukes MNG, ed. Meyler's side effects of drugs, vol. 10. Amsterdam: Excerpta Medica, 1984.

Einarson TR. Drug-related hospital admissions. Ann Pharmacother 1993; 27:832–840.

Fletcher AP. Drug safety tests and subsequent clinical experience. J R Soc Med 1978; 71:693–696.

Jankel CA, Fitterman LK. Epidemiology of drug-drug interactions as a cause of hospital admissions. Drug Safety 1993; 9:51–59.

Jick H. The discovery of drug-induced illness. N Engl J Med 1977; 296:481–485.

Lane DA, Kramer MS, Hutchinson TA, et al. The causality assessment of adverse drug reactions using the Bayesian approach. Pharm Med 1987; 2:265–283.

Naranjo CA. A clinical pharmacologic perspective on the detection and assessment of adverse drug reactions. Drug Info J 1986; 20:387–393.

Naranjo CA, Busto U, Janecek E, et al. An intensive drug monitoring study suggesting possible clinical irrelevance of impaired drug disposition in liver disease. Br J Clin Pharmacol 1983; 15:451–458.

Naranjo CA, Busto U, Sellers EM, et al. A method for estimating the probability of adverse drug reactions. Clin Pharmacol Ther 1981; 30:239–245.

Naranjo CA, Shear NH, Lanctôt KL. Advances in the diagnosis of adverse drug reactions. J Clin Pharmacol 1992; 32:897–904.

Recchia A, Shear NH. Organization and functioning of an adverse drug reaction clinic. J Clin Pharmacol 1994; 34:68–79.

Rieder MJ. Mechanisms of unpredicatable adverse drug reactions. Drug Safety 1994; 11:196–212.

Shear NH, Spielberg SP. Anticonvulsant hypersensitivity syndrome: In vitro assessment of risk. J Clin Invest 1988; 82:1826–1832.

Shear NH, Spielberg SP, Grant DM, et al. Differences in metabolism of sulfonamides predisposing to idiosyncratic toxicity. Ann Intern Med 1986; 105:179–184.

Tsong Y. False alarm rates of statistical methods used in determining increased frequency of reports on adverse drug reaction. J Biopharmaceut Stat 1992; 2:9–30.

Venning GR. Identification of adverse reactions to new drugs. I. What have been the important adverse reactions since thalidomide? Br Med J 1983; 286:199–202.

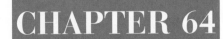

CHAPTER 64

Drug Interactions

E.M. SELLERS AND M.K. ROMACH

CASE HISTORY

A 63-year-old man who had been receiving medication for major depression boarded Air Canada flight #007, which departed Toronto at 1930 hours and arrived at London Heathrow at 0730 hours. Upon arrival, the cabin crew were shocked to discover an unrousable passenger in seat 83A. His passport indicated that he was 63 years old. A search of his carry-on bag revealed three prescription containers. One was for nefazodone for depression, indicating that the patient had been taking the medication regularly for 1 month. The second was a 6-month supply of ketoconazole for a fungal infection. The label of the third container indicated that it had contained three tablets of triazolam 0.125 mg for "transient insomnia" and was dated the day of departure. One tablet of triazolam remained.

The simultaneous use of several therapeutic agents has become commonplace. At some time during their stay in a general hospital most patients receive more than five drugs concurrently. On medical services the median number of drugs administered to patients during one hospitalization is 10–13, and many patients receive 20 or more drugs. Concomitant prescription of several drugs for ambulatory patients is the rule in many diseases. Furthermore, such patients commonly consume analgesics, cold remedies, and other drugs that are available without prescription. Finally, there is universal exposure to bioactive for-

eign chemicals in the form of food additives, insecticides, cleaning agents, cosmetics, and inhalants.

Unfortunately, it is an exceptional drug that does only "its own thing" in the body. One drug may change the effect of another by altering its metabolic fate or by enhancing or opposing its activity at the site of action. The latter type of interaction is more predictable and more generally appreciated, particularly when it is related to the expected pharmacological actions of the drugs. There is nothing surprising about the ability of propranolol to alter the actions of isoproterenol, nor in the interactions between insulin and glucagon. Metabolic interactions between drugs are generally more subtle and are fully predictable only when the processes of absorption, distribution, binding, biotransformation, and excretion of each drug are thoroughly understood. Since this is seldom the case, the frequency of unexpected, adverse, and sometimes serious drug interactions has grown with the increasing use of potent drugs.

CLASSIFICATION OF DRUG INTERACTIONS

Consequence

The consequence of drug interactions can be:

1. Beneficial (enhancement of therapeutic effectiveness, diminution of toxicity) or
2. Adverse (diminution of therapeutic effectiveness, enhancement of toxicity) (Table 64-1)

The tactics of optimal, modern drug therapy often rely on the wise combination of drugs with complementary modes of action in order to reduce toxic-

Table 64-1 Classification of Drug Interactions

Consequence
  Beneficial or adverse

Site
  External or internal

Mechanism
  Pharmacodynamic
  Pharmacokinetic
  Physiological

ity or enhance therapeutic efficacy. Several examples are shown in Table 64-2.

However, unintentional interactions frequently lead to increased toxicity. Table 64-3 illustrates the mutual enhancement of CNS-depressing effects of barbiturates and ethanol.

Site of Interaction

External

Not surprisingly, there are many physicochemical incompatibles when drugs are mixed in intravenous infusion vials or syringes. Precipitation or inactivation may occur. In general, it is better not to mix drugs together in the same solution. Hospital pharmacies can usually provide a full listing of intravenous incompatibilities when this information is needed.

Internal

This can be a body site or system (e.g., GI tract, liver) or the site of drug action (e.g., cell membrane, receptor sites, DNA, RNA, or intermediary metabolism). With respect to interactions at drug receptors, much of pharmacology is in fact the study of drug interactions! For example:

Cholinergic receptors: Hexamethonium competitively blocks the depolarizing action of carbachol at nicotinic synapses in ganglia; some antibiotics (e.g., kanamycin, gentamicin) potentiate the depolarizing block produced by succinylcholine at the neuromuscular junction; atropine competitively blocks pilocarpine at muscarinic receptors (see Chapters 15, 19, and 55).

Adrenergic receptors: Phentolamine, phenothiazines, and phenoxybenzamine block norepineph-

Table 64-2 Examples of Drug–Drug Interactions and their Consequences

Therapeutic Efficacy	*Toxicity*
Enhanced	
Combination drug therapy in cancer, hypertension, angina pectoris, infection, etc.	CNS depressants + ethanol (see Table 64-3)
Diminished	
Quinidine decreases codeine analgesia by inhibiting the metabolism of codeine to morphine	Vasodilator + β-blocker Naloxone + opiates Thiazides + potassium Carbidopa + L-dopa

rine action on α-adrenoceptors in blood vessels. Metoprolol blocks β_1 (cardiac)-adrenoceptor agonists such as isoproterenol (see Chapters 17 and 28).

Other receptors: Morphine-induced respiratory depression is reversed by the opioid antagonist naloxone (see Chapter 23).

Mechanism

Pharmacodynamic interaction

This term refers to drug-induced changes in the effects of other drugs and needs to be distinguished from interactions based on changes in disposition (i.e., "pharmacokinetic" interaction). The barbiturate–ethanol interaction shown in Table 64-3 is a pharmacodynamic interaction. The term **physiological interaction,** which may be encountered in some publications, refers to drug actions that are exerted at or on different sites or systems (e.g., heart and

Table 64-3 Concentrations of Barbiturate and Ethanol in Blood Associated with Death in Various Groups of Overdose Patients

Mean *barbiturate* concentration in blood (mg/L)	
Death from barbiturate alone	3.67
Death from barbiturate + ethanol	2.55
Mean *ethanol* concentration in blood (mg/L)	
Death from ethanol alone	6500
Death from ethanol + barbiturate	1750

peripheral resistance vessels) but have the net effect of augmenting or offsetting each other. For example, the antihypertensive agent hydralazine decreases total peripheral resistance; β-blockers can block the reflex tachycardia induced by the fall in peripheral resistance and thereby augment the antihypertensive effects of hydralazine. After reading this book, one should be able to think of many other examples.

With respect to quantitating the magnitude of pharmacodynamic drug interactions, several descriptive terms are encountered.

- **Additive:** The consequence *(C)* of an interaction is the simple sum of the separate effects of each drug *(A* and *B):* $C = A + B.$
- **Supra-additive:** $C > A + B.$
- **Infra-additive:** $C < A + B.$
  These terms, though used, have very limited usefulness because they are only correct for a particular drug effect at a specified dose (more accurately, concentration), at a specified point in time, under specified conditions. These terms say nothing about mechanisms of interaction.

Pharmacokinetic interaction

Pharmacokinetic interactions are changes in the pharmacokinetics of one drug that are induced by another drug. Table 64-4 classifies pharmacokinetic interactions, which are taken up in detail in the remainder of this chapter.

PHARMACOKINETIC INTERACTIONS

Gastrointestinal Absorption

Physicochemical interactions

The following five examples illustrate physicochemical interactions that may affect absorption of a drug from the stomach or small intestine (Fig. 64-1).

- Changes in gastrointestinal pH by one drug—e.g., an H_2-receptor antagonist such as cimetidine, or antacids—that affect the ionization of another drug (see Chapter 44).
- Chelation, e.g., of Ca^{2+} or Fe^{3+} by tetracycline (see Chapter 55).
- Exchange resin binding, e.g., binding of warfarin and other drugs by cholestyramine (see Chapter 39).
- Adsorption. Activated charcoal (AC) adsorbs many drugs. This observation is used therapeutically in drug poisonings by giving patients activated charcoal (approximately 1.5 g/kg) mixed in water. Typically a 10:1 ratio of AC to drug is desired in order to maximize gastrointestinal sequestration of the ingested drug and minimize systemic absorption (see Chapter 74).

Table 64-4 Pharmacokinetic Interactions

Absorption
  Physicochemical interaction
  Altered gastrointestinal motility
  Change in bacterial flora
  Mucosal damage

Distribution
  Blood flow
  Serum binding
  Tissue binding
  Active transport at site of action

Biotransformation
  Hepatic
  Other sites (e.g., lung, kidney, brain)

Excretion
  Renal
  Biliary
  Other sites

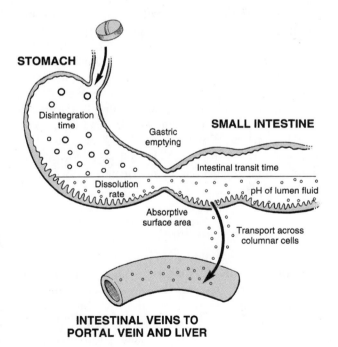

Figure 64-1. Factors involved in gastrointestinal drug interactions.

- Dissolution of the therapeutic agent in nonabsorbable material present in the GI tract, e.g., fat-soluble vitamins that become dissolved in mineral oil taken as a laxative (see Chapter 67).

Changes in gastrointestinal motility

Changes in gastrointestinal motility affect the rate and/or the completeness of drug absorption (i.e., the absolute bioavailability). It is important to realize that absorption may be complete in spite of being slowed, since absorption of some substances occurs along the whole gastrointestinal tract. The importance of interactions brought about through changes in GI motility depends on the rate of onset of action of the drug that is affected, and its therapeutic index.

Increased gastric emptying and intestinal motility. Metoclopramide increases the rate of gastric emptying, and hence might result in earlier and higher peak concentrations for drugs rapidly absorbed from the upper small intestine (see Chapter 14). Cathartics increase intestinal motility and might decrease the completeness of absorption of drugs by moving a medication to the colon, where absorption for some drugs is poor (see Chapter 45).

Decreased gastric emptying and intestinal motility. All opioid analgesics and drugs with anticholinergic activity decrease the rate of gastric emptying and intestinal motility (e.g., codeine, morphine, atropine, loperamide; see Chapters 15 and 23). A decreased rate of gastric emptying will be associated with slower absorption, lower peak drug concentrations, and later times of peak concentration.

Figure 64-2 summarizes the results of a study to determine the effects of opioids (pentazocine, meperidine, heroin) on drug absorption. Acetaminophen was used as the test drug. Note that metoclopramide did not reverse the decreased gastric emptying caused by the opioids.

Changes in bacterial flora

Bowel bacteria may play an important role in synthesizing the vitamin K that is essential for normal clotting function, or may reactivate some inactive drug metabolites, excreted via the bile, by deconjugating them. Hence, chronically administered broad-spectrum antibiotics may interact indirectly with these drugs by modifying or eliminating intestinal flora (see Chapters 55 and 56).

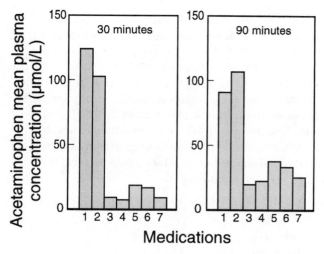

Figure 64-2. Mean plasma acetaminophen concentrations (standard error omitted for clarity) in 46 women in labor and 10 women postpartum at 30 and 90 minutes after a single oral dose of 1.5 g, with and without administration of opioid analgesics alone or in combination with metoclopramide. *Medications:* 1 = no opioids; 2 = postpartum; 3 = pentazocine; 4 = meperidine; 5 = meperidine/metoclopramide; 6 = heroin; 7 = heroin/metoclopramide. (Modified from Prescott LF, Nimmo WS, Heading RC. "Drug Absorption Interactions." In: Grahame-Smith DG, ed. Drug interactions. Baltimore: University Park Press, 1977:45–51.)

Drug-induced changes in mucosal function

Drugs with specific gastrointestinal toxicity (e.g., colchicine) may damage the GI mucosa or block active transport (see Chapter 45). This action can, in theory, result in interactions with other drugs.

Distribution

Blood flow

Since organ uptake and clearance of drug are ultimately dependent on blood flow, it is not surprising that some drug interactions involve alterations in blood flow. For example, β-blockers and some antiarrhythmics may produce an important decrease in cardiac output. This in turn can reduce hepatic blood flow and hepatic clearance of drugs with high extraction ratios, such as lidocaine (see Chapter 7).

Tissue uptake, extraction, or binding

Drug localization in tissues is usually nonspecific. Many drugs localize in tissues at sites that have nothing to do with the desired therapeutic action of the drug (e.g., digoxin in skeletal muscle). Tissue binding of these drugs serves as a potentially large store from which they can be displaced by other drugs.

The strategic placement of the liver between the small intestine and the systemic circulation can permit important drug interactions. Recall that F (bioavailability) $= 1 - E$ (extraction ratio). Drugs that interfere with hepatic uptake, biotransformation, intracellular binding, or biliary excretion of other drugs may markedly increase the systemic bioavailability of those with high first-pass effect during the absorptive phase. For example, ethanol, administered 1 hour before amitriptyline, causes a doubling of amitriptyline concentrations during the absorptive phase of this antidepressant (Fig. 64-3). Cimetidine has similar effects on the uptake of propranolol.

Serum protein binding

Many drugs are highly bound to serum proteins, especially to albumin. Such highly bound drugs may be displaced by other highly bound drugs administered concurrently. For example, warfarin is displaced by trichloroacetic acid (a metabolite of chloral hydrate), and thus increased anticoagulation may occur. Bilirubin is displaced by some sulfonamides, and kernicterus may result (see Chapter 56).

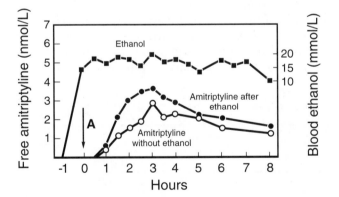

Figure 64-3. Mean plasma concentrations of free amitriptyline (nmol/L) and ethanol (mmol/L) for five subjects. Ethanol was administered as an oral loading dose of 0.9 g/kg lean body weight, followed by approximately 0.1 g/kg every half-hour to maintain blood ethanol levels at 15–20 mmol/L. Amitriptyline 25 mg (A) was administered at time zero, with and without a preceding dose of ethanol. (Modified from Dorian P, et al. "Amitriptyline and Ethanol: Pharmacokinetic and Pharmacodynamic Interaction." *Eur J Clin Pharmacol* 1983; 25:325–331.)

When a displacing drug is added to therapy, it can in theory cause the immediate appearance of toxicity or otherwise altered response (Fig. 64-4, Table 64-5). Even a small amount of displacement of a highly plasma-bound drug causes a large relative increase in the free active fraction of the drug in the serum (Fig. 64-4; in the case illustrated, displacement of 18% *of the bound drug* causes a 100% increase in free concentration). However, the displaced drug does not remain confined in the circulation but redistributes throughout the body. After such redistribution the increase in free drug concentration in serum and extracellular fluid depends mainly on the apparent volume of distribution for the free drug. If the distribution volume for the free drug is large, the increase in free drug concentration will be small and probably pharmacologically unimportant.

Other processes also act to buffer the consequences of the acute changes in free concentration after partial displacement of the drug from albumin. An increase in the concentration of unbound drug in the serum also makes more drug available for glomerular filtration or hepatic biotransformation. For drugs exclusively eliminated by the liver, this displacement results in a greater elimination of the free drug (via first-order Michaelis–Menten kinetics), which may be reflected temporarily in slight shortening of the serum half-life of total drug. At the new steady state, the total drug concentration in the serum is lower than before displacement, the serum half-life of total drug is the same, and the free drug concentration in the serum is a higher fraction of the total. Clearance of free drug will be the same as before displacement, but clearance calculated on the basis of total drug will be apparently greater.

For drugs that are removed from the circulation by high-capacity or high-affinity uptake mechanisms in kidney or liver, displacement from albumin may decrease the rate at which drug is delivered to these sites of elimination. Thus, displacement of such drugs from albumin can, in theory, increase both their total and free concentrations (see Chapter 7).

Clinically important pharmacokinetic interaction due to displacement from plasma proteins will occur only when (1) administration of the displacing drug is started in high doses during chronic therapy with the displaced drug; (2) the volume of distribution of displaced drug is small; and (3) the response to the drug occurs faster than redistribution or enhanced elimination. Maximum potentiation occurs shortly after addition of the displacing drug and reaches a maximum fairly quickly. The potentiation is usually transient.

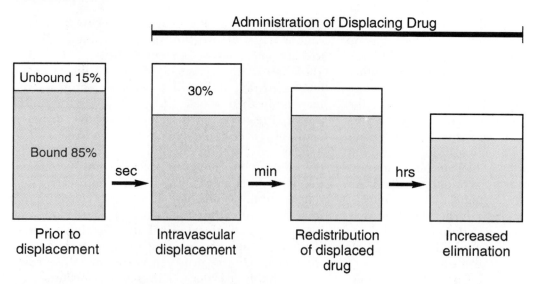

Figure 64-4. Sequence of changes in plasma drug concentrations during displacement interactions.

Because the free drug level is the determinant of the pharmacological effect, changes in *total* steady-state levels may not predict a change in pharmacological effect observed clinically during concurrent therapy with an interacting drug. For example, inhibition of biotransformation of warfarin, coupled with its displacement from plasma proteins, could result in "normal" steady-state *total* drug concentration in the plasma, yet free concentrations would be markedly elevated and result in a prolonged prothrombin time (see Chapter 42).

Active transport at site of action

A number of complex interactions involve alterations in regulation of neurotransmitters. A classical example of such an interaction is summarized in Figure 64-5.

Tricyclic antidepressants block the uptake of norepinephrine, thus increasing the postsynaptic concentration of active neurotransmitter. Guanethidine decreases the release of norepinephrine, and with chronic guanethidine treatment one can expect the postsynaptic norepinephrine receptors to be "supersensitive," in compensation for the chronically low transmitter level (see Chapters 16–18). Thus, when the low synaptic level of norepinephrine during guanethidine treatment is somewhat increased by administration of desipramine it results in a significant rise in blood pressure. Desipramine decreases the pressor activity of tyramine infusions but increases the pressor action of norepinephrine. Interactions involving

Table 64-5 Potential Consequences of Drug Displacement from Plasma Proteins

	Immediately After Displacement*	At Steady State
Free drug fraction in serum	Increased	Increased
Free drug concentration in serum	Increased	Unchanged
Total drug concentration in serum	Unchanged	Decreased
Pharmacological activity	Increased	Unchanged
Glomerular filtration	Increased	Unchanged
Tubular secretion	Variable	Unchanged
Diffusion into liver cells	Increased	Unchanged
Active hepatic uptake	Variable	Unchanged

*All changes are compared to those concentrations and effects immediately prior to displacement. This phase may last only a short time, because redistribution starts to occur immediately (see also Fig. 64-4).

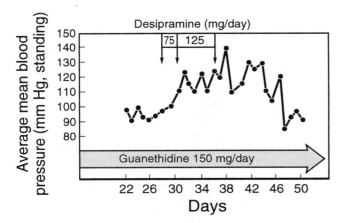

Figure 64-5. Antagonism of guanethidine by desipramine. Guanethidine was given in increasing doses until the blood pressure was controlled with 150 mg daily. Desipramine was administered as indicated.

antihypertensives and tricyclic antidepressants, L-dopa, phenothiazines, direct- and indirect-acting sympathomimetics, and amphetamine analogs often have a similar basis.

Biotransformation

Many drugs are metabolized by cytochrome P450 enzymes, principally in the liver. These enzymes exist in specific isoforms that display catalytic selectivity for particular drugs (see Chapter 4 for classification and nomenclature). Table 64-6 partially summarizes drugs that are known substrates and inhibitors for particular cytochromes. The utility of this type of formulation is that one can anticipate that cytochrome-selective inhibitors will result in inhibition of the biotransformation of a substrate metabolized by the same cytochrome. The fact that inhibition can be demonstrated in vitro does not necessarily mean that clinically important interactions will occur. However, the possibility of such an interaction should raise one's index of clinical caution. The likelihood of clinically significant interactions depends on the potency of the inhibitor, the proportion of metabolism of the affected drug that is catalyzed by a particular cytochrome, and the relative concentrations of the substrate drug and inhibitor drug.

Enzyme induction

Stimulation of microsomal enzyme activity by drugs and other chemicals is an important clinical problem. Hundreds of drugs including analgesics, anticonvul-

sants, oral hypoglycemics, sedatives, and tranquilizers stimulate the biotransformation of either themselves or other drugs (see Chapter 4).

Enzyme induction:

- Increases the rate of hepatic biotransformation of drug
- Increases the rate of production of metabolites
- Increases hepatic drug clearance
- Decreases serum drug half-life
- Decreases serum total and free drug concentrations
- Decreases pharmacological effects if the metabolites are inactive

Drugs and xenobiotics that induce major increases of drug-biotransforming enzymes in the human include phenobarbital, rifampin, tobacco smoke constituents, and ethanol (chronic).

With barbiturates, approximately 4–7 days is required before any clinically significant effect occurs, but enzyme induction may take 2–4 weeks to disappear after barbiturate administration ends. This period of offset of induction can be important. For example, phenobarbital enhances the biotransformation of the anticoagulant warfarin, and higher doses of warfarin will be needed to achieve satisfactory anticoagulation if phenobarbital is given concurrently. If the phenobarbital is discontinued and the warfarin dose is not adjusted, bleeding may result (Fig. 64-6).

The antibiotic rifampin is another potent enzyme inducer. Concurrent administration with oral contraceptives can result in contraceptive failure because of increased biotransformation of the steroid. Similar

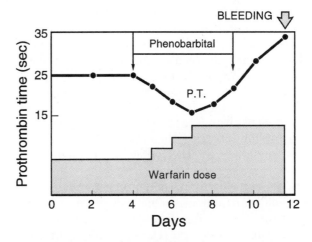

Figure 64-6. Clinical consequences of enhancement of warfarin biotransformation by phenobarbital. P.T. = prothrombin time.

increases in biotransformation during rifampin therapy have been shown with prednisone, oral anticoagulants, and some hypoglycemics.

Enzyme inhibition

Inhibition of microsomal enzymes:

- Decreases the rate of hepatic biotransformation of drug
- Decreases the rate of production of metabolites
- Decreases total clearance
- Increases serum drug half-life
- Increases serum total and free drug concentrations
- Increases pharmacological effects if the metabolites are inactive

Clinically important inhibitors of drug biotransformation include acute ethanol exposure, chloramphenicol and some other antibiotics, cimetidine, disulfiram, and propoxyphene.

Acute ethanol exposure inhibits numerous biotransformations mediated by the cytochrome P450 system, including demethylation and hydroxylation of diazepam, chlordiazepoxide, propranolol, amitriptyline, propoxyphene, and others. As with other inhibitors, conjugation reactions seem to be spared.

Cimetidine (a histamine H_2-receptor blocker used to reduce gastric acid secretion; see Chapter 44) is a potent inhibitor of the cytochrome P450 system and has been reported to inhibit the biotransformation of acetaminophen, β-blockers, chlordiazepoxide, diazepam, digitoxin, ethanol, imipramine, phenytoin, quinidine, theophylline, and warfarin. Since cimetidine also decreases hepatic blood flow, more than one mechanism may be present. Another widely used H_2-receptor blocker, ranitidine (see Chapter 44), has lesser effects on drug biotransformations.

Disulfiram inhibits the mitochondrial enzyme acetaldehyde dehydrogenase and causes acetaldehyde accumulation after consumption of alcohol. This is the cause of the disulfiram–alcohol reaction and is the theoretical basis for use of the drug in the treatment of alcoholism (see Chapter 26). However, disulfiram also inhibits several microsomal enzymatic processes, including hydroxylation and demethylation, but not conjugation.

Some clinically important drug interactions that are usually attributed to changed albumin binding of one or both drugs can actually involve other mechanisms as well. For example, phenylbutazone can displace both warfarin isomers from plasma albumin in vivo and in vitro and invariably and importantly enhances the hypoprothrombinemia of patients on anticoagulant therapy with warfarin. In addition, however, phenylbutazone inhibits the biotransformation of the S-isomer of warfarin (by inhibiting CYP2C9) while stimulating the elimination of the R-isomer. Since the S-isomer is five times as potent as the R-isomer, potentiation of warfarin-induced hypoprothrombinemia occurs. Another example is sulfaphenazole, which displaces the oral hypoglycemic drug tolbutamide from albumin but also reduces its rate of hepatic oxidation, thereby preventing the compensatory increase in inactivation that usually occurs after displacement interactions. Both effects undoubtedly play a role in the potentiation of tolbutamide-induced hypoglycemia by sulfaphenazole. *In general, inhibition of drug biotransformation is the clinically most important mechanism of pharmacokinetic interactions.*

A recently discovered interaction, based on inhibition of specific cytochrome P450 enzymes, occurs when *grapefruit juice* is drunk by patients under treatment with certain medications. Grapefruit juice, whether fresh or frozen, contains a bioflavonoid, naringen, that is biotransformed in human liver to naringenin. This product appears to be an inhibitor of CYP3A4, CYP1A2, and CYP2A6, and reduces the first-pass hepatic metabolism of a number of drugs that are substrates for these enzymes, including several calcium-channel blockers (felodipine, nifedipine, nimodipine, and verapamil), cyclosporine, terfenadine, midazolam, and caffeine. As a result, the oral bioavailability of these drugs, as reflected by their plasma levels and the area under the concentration–time curves, is increased when the drugs are taken after drinking grapefruit juice. The clinical importance of this interaction is currently being studied.

Excretion

Theoretically, drug interactions may alter the rates of elimination of drugs by any of the excretory routes (urine, feces, bile, sweat, tears, and lungs). However, the only drug interactions of this type that have received careful study are those involving renal excretion. The following major types have been observed:

1. Glomerular filtration of drugs is increased by displacement from albumin.
2. Tubular reabsorption of filtered drugs is decreased by:
   - Diuretics (in some instances)
   - Urine alkalinizers (e.g., $NaHCO_3$, acetazolamide) for weakly acidic drugs such as salicylates and barbiturates

- Urine acidifiers (e.g., ascorbic acid, NH_4Cl) for weak amines such as amphetamines, methadone, quinidine, and procainamide
3. Tubular secretion of drugs is decreased by competition for active transport systems (e.g., historically the action of probenecid to block tubular secretion of penicillin G was important when penicillin G was in short supply during World War II), so their half-life in the body is prolonged.

In recent years, interactions at the renal tubular site have been recognized as important and more frequent than previously thought. For example, cimetidine was studied in six healthy volunteers by comparing the single-dose pharmacokinetics of oral procainamide before and during a daily dose of cimetidine. The area under the procainamide plasma-concentration/time curve was increased by cimetidine by an average of 35%, from 27.0 ± 0.3 μg/mL/hr to 36.5 ± 3.4 μg/mL/hr. The elimination half-life increased from a harmonic mean of 2.92 hours to 3.68 hours. The renal clearance of procainamide was reduced by cimetidine from 347 ± 46 mL/min to 196 ± 11 mL/min. The area under the plasma-concentration/time curve for *N*-acetyl-procainamide (NAPA, the active metabolite of procainamide) was increased by a mean of 25% by cimetidine because of a significant reduction in renal clearance from 258 ± 60 mL/min to 197 ± 59 mL/min. The data suggest that cimetidine inhibits the tubular secretion of both procainamide and *N*-acetylprocainamide. Such a renal interaction is important not only for basic drugs that are cleared by the kidney but also for metabolites of basic drugs and endogenous substances that require active transport into the lumen of the proximal tubule of the kidney for their elimination.

Digoxin (a cardiac glycoside used to treat heart failure; see Chapter 36) provides another example of interactions involving renal excretion of drugs. Digoxin concentration rises almost twofold when the antiarrhythmic drug quinidine is given concurrently and this increase is associated with clinically important toxicity. Subsequent studies have shown similar effects with verapamil and amiodarone. Detailed studies suggest that the basis of this interaction is a

Table 64-6 Selected Substrates and Inhibitors of Specific Cytochromes P450*

Cytochrome Isoform	Substrate	Inhibitor
1A2	Caffeine	Oral contraceptives
2C9	Warfarin	Sulfaphenazole Phenylbutazone
2C19	Mephenytoin Diazepam	Mephenytoin
2D6	Codeine Dextromethorphan Imipramine Neuroleptics Propranolol Verapamil and many others; mainly cardiovascular and psychotropic drugs	Quinidine Fluoxetine and other selective serotonin reuptake inhibitors used in treating depression Neuroleptics
3A4/5	Benzodiazepines: Alprazolam, Diazepam, Midazolam, Triazolam and others Alfentanil Codeine Dextromethorphan Terfenadine and many others	Erythromycin Ketoconazole Nefazodone Troleandomycin
2E1	Carcinogens Ethanol	Chlormethiazole? Disulfiram?

*This table can be used to anticipate some potential clinical interactions between drugs that are substrates and those that are inhibitors.

fall (34%) in renal clearance of digoxin without a change in glomerular filtration, a decrease (32%) in V_d, and a fall (36%) in total body clearance. Half-life does not change greatly. Other studies suggest that quinidine may displace digoxin from tissue binding sites. The importance of renal tubular transport systems for bases and neutral compounds has become clinically apparent.

CONCLUDING EXERCISE

From Table 64-6, select one clinically used drug which is a substrate for CYP3A4/5 and one inhibitor of the same enzyme, and see if any clinically important interactions have been reported. The case history at the beginning of this chapter is an example of the type of interaction one may find reported. Ketoconazole and nefazodone are CYP3A inhibitors that can increase the area under the concentration–time curve of triazolam. Often the duration, timing, and order of dose ingestion are important. Could the circumstances in the described case be changed so that the medications implicated could be taken safely together?

SUGGESTED READING

Doering W. Quinidine-digoxin interaction. N Engl J Med 1979; 301:400–404.

Newton DJ, Wang RW, Lu AYH. Cytochrome P450 inhibitors: evaluation of specificities in the in vitro metabolism of therapeutic agents by human liver microsomes. Drug Metab Dispos 1995;23:154–158.

Rizack MA, ed. Medical Letter Handbook on adverse drug interactions (1996 update). New Rochelle, NY: The Medical Letter, 1996.

Ross EM. Pharmacodynamics: mechanisms of drug action and the relationship between drug concentration and effect. In: Hardman JG, Limbird LE, et al., eds. Goodman and Gilman's the pharmacological basis of therapeutics. 9th ed. New York: McGraw Hill, 1996:29–41.

Somogyi A, McLean A, Heinzow B. Cimetidine-procainamide pharmacokinetic interaction in man: evidence of competition for tubular secretion of basic drugs. Eur J Clin Pharmacol 1983; 25:339–345.

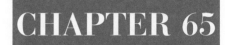

CHAPTER 65

Perinatal Pharmacology

L.A. MAGEE AND G. KOREN

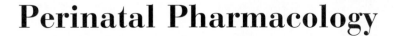

CASE HISTORY

Mrs. M. is a 25-year-old woman with a history of epilepsy since childhood, who has come for pre-pregnancy counseling. Her only medication is phenytoin 300 mg daily. Her last plasma phenytoin concentration was 45 μmol/L (normal 40-80 μmol/L), and her last seizure was 2 years ago.

The patient has been told by another physician that carbamazepine is considered by many to be the drug of choice for epilepsy in pregnancy, given (1) the approximate 1% risk of neural-tube defects that can be detected by prenatal diagnosis, (2) the known teratogenicity of phenytoin, which may *not* be detected antenatally, and (3) the evidence that phenytoin may also have neurotoxic effects on the developing central nervous system. However, she is also aware that changing from one anticonvulsant to another puts her at risk of seizure recurrence. She does not want to lose her driver's license, and she wishes to remain on phenytoin throughout pregnancy. Mrs. M.'s only other medication is a prenatal vitamin preparation that contains 0.8 mg/day of folic acid. She is otherwise well.

If she remains on phenytoin throughout pregnancy, what are the implications of such a decision with respect to maternal pharmacokinetics, risk of teratogenicity, and the feasibility of breastfeeding while on therapy?

Progressive physiological changes occur throughout pregnancy in the mother that affect maternal phar-macokinetics and pharmacodynamics. At the same time, there are many developmental changes in phar-macokinetics and pharmacodynamics that take place in the perinate (i.e., the fetus after 12 weeks of gestation and the newborn up until 28 days of life). These changes occur along a continuum and are inextricably linked to maternal pharmacology by the uteroplacental circulation (for the fetus), and the breast milk (for the neonate). Perinatal pharmacology and toxicology therefore involve consideration of all the interactions among mother, fetus, and new-born, as illustrated in part in Figure 65-1. An under-standing of the general principles, and their applica-tion to the individual mother–child pair, is a prerequisite for safe and appropriate drug therapy at this unique time in human life.

RISK ASSESSMENT

Maternal drug ingestion occurs in 40–90% of preg-nancies. While some agents are unnecessary or avoid-able, others are critical to the physical and psycho-logical well-being of the mother, upon which the fetus, and subsequently the neonate, rely. It is not acceptable to deny beneficial drug therapy to the pregnant woman, since the vast majority of drugs used in pregnancy are not harmful to the fetus or neonate.

The potential fetal risks of drugs used in gesta-tional pharmacotherapy are assessed by mandatory reproductive toxicology studies in animals during the premarketing phase of drug development. However, interspecies differences in genetics, drug disposition, and embryology, as well as the large doses of drugs administered to animals, give these studies limited

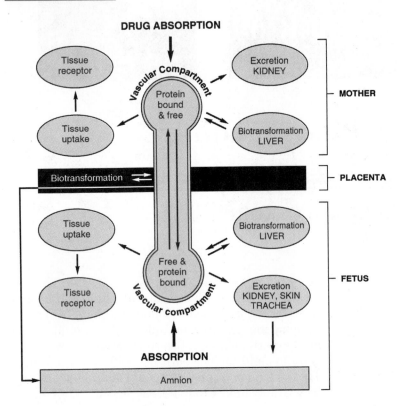

Figure 65-1. Drug distribution and disposition in mother and fetus in utero.

negative and positive predictive values with respect to possible harm to the human fetus. As it is obviously unethical to administer agents to pregnant women solely to assess fetal effects, postmarketing surveillance of inadvertent or unavoidable drug exposures during human pregnancy is a critical step in information gathering.

Postmarketing research on gestational pharmacotherapeutic agents is voluntarily conducted by drug manufacturers in North America. However, such information is often incomplete and potentially biased; women whose babies have malformations are more likely to report drug exposures than are women whose babies are normal. In addition, the data are not readily accessible and are not usually included in product monographs. These generally contain disclaimers advising that therapy with the drug in question is not recommended during pregnancy, or that the risks have not been assessed, but that if the drug is used, the 'potential benefits must outweigh the potential risks.' Such vague statements may be made even when a significant body of literature exists about a drug's *safety*, and they do nothing to dispel the misconception that all drug exposures during pregnancy are somehow teratogenic or fetotoxic. The

situation is made worse by the frequent failure to recognize or acknowledge that (1) other factors, such as maternal disease, can adversely affect pregnancy outcome and thereby confound the interpretation of adverse drug effects, and that (2) all women, regardless of illness or drug therapy, have a baseline risk for spontaneous abortion (in excess of 10–15%), major birth defects (1–3%), and other adverse outcomes.

GENERAL OVERVIEW

There is currently somewhat sparse evidence for pregnancy-induced alterations in maternal receptor sensitivity, but some changes do occur, such as alterations in uterine contractile responses and increase in the hepatotoxicity of some agents (e.g., tetracyclines). Physiologically induced modifications in pharmacokinetics are thought to be responsible for other changes in maternal drug effects and in control of maternal disease, which may indirectly affect fetal well-being. For example, fetal hypoxemia can result from maternal generalized convulsions, especially if they are prolonged. Drug action on uterine muscle or uteroplacental vasculature may also indirectly affect the fetus.

Direct fetal effects occur only when agents reach the fetal circulation, and the extent to which they do so depends on maternal drug disposition, placental drug transfer, and fetal drug disposition. Given that fetal exposure occurs, the nature of the agent and the timing of exposure relative to conception will determine the potential adverse outcomes. If the drug is administered at term, the infant may be born with drug in its systemic circulation, and neonatal pharmacodynamics and pharmacokinetics will determine whether neonatal health problems occur. This chapter considers collectively all of the aforementioned factors as part of an integrated approach to gestational pharmacotherapy.

Maternal Pharmacokinetics

Drugs known to have low systemic absorption (e.g., some topical preparations that are not administered for systemic disease) do not reach the maternal systemic circulation and cannot directly or indirectly affect the fetus. There are no clinically important changes in absorption of orally administered drugs during pregnancy, despite decreases in gastric emptying rate and gut motility. However, in hyperemesis gravidarum, persistent severe vomiting may make oral administration unreliable and may require the drugs to be given parenterally.

The substantial increases in total body water (by as much as 8 liters) and plasma volume (by 50%) that occur during the average normal pregnancy may increase the distribution of drugs into water compartments. Decreases in plasma albumin (by 5–10 g/L) and reduced binding to plasma albumin (through competition with endogenous ligands such as free fatty acids) may increase the free drug fraction; the same may occur for basic drugs that bind to α_1-acid glycoprotein. This reduction in protein binding may increase the amount of free drug available for maternal clearance, but also for placental transfer into the fetus (e.g., **salicylates**).

Metabolizing systems may be stimulated by elevated levels of progesterone in pregnancy. Although wide interpatient variability in metabolic rate has made it difficult to discern pregnancy-induced changes in biotransformation, drugs such as **phenytoin** and **metoprolol,** for which clearance is limited by intrinsic hepatic metabolism (see Chapter 7), have been found to exhibit shorter elimination half-lives during pregnancy. However, the hepatic clearance of most agents is not modified, as their transformation is limited primarily by hepatic blood flow, which is unchanged in pregnancy. Agents cleared primarily or exclusively by the kidney may also exhibit shorter elimination half-lives due to increases of up to 50% in renal blood flow and glomerular filtration rate.

Pregnancy-induced changes in maternal pharmacokinetics are likely to be of greatest importance for drugs with small volumes of distribution or high protein binding. If serum drug concentrations are closely correlated with maternal drug effects, and if the therapeutic index is low, the problem can be magnified. Anticonvulsants such as **phenytoin** and **carbamazepine** are excellent examples. Serum concentrations of both drugs decrease during pregnancy because of increases in plasma volume, free fraction, and intrinsic hepatic clearance. As a result there may be increased seizure activity. **Ampicillin** is another drug exhibiting lower serum concentrations in pregnancy, due to increases in distribution volume, free fraction, and renal clearance. However, because of its high therapeutic index this drug is usually administered to patients in high doses that produce plasma and tissue concentrations well above the minimum therapeutic levels. Therefore, a good therapeutic effect can usually still be achieved in pregnant women, despite the reduced serum concentrations. **Lithium** is an example of a drug that is eliminated almost entirely by glomerular filtration; increased renal clearance during pregnancy may cause reductions in serum concentration and a resulting decrease in therapeutic effect.

In the end, what is important is the knowledge that pregnancy-induced alterations in drug disposition *may* occur, and the application of this knowledge to the clinical status of the *individual patient*. As with all drug therapy, changes in drug concentration should be interpreted in light of the patient's clinical status.

Placental Drug Transfer

Most drugs cross the placenta. However, the degree of transfer is dependent upon characteristics of the placenta, the drug, and fetal blood pH (Table 65-1).

The placenta

Aside from thickness and surface area of the placental epithelial barrier, the most important determinant of the rate of drug transfer may be uteroplacental blood flow. Transit may be very rapid, especially for highly lipid-soluble agents. For example, nitrous oxide attains concentrations in the fetus that are 80%

Table 65-1 Factors Determining Placental Drug Transfer

Placental characteristics
  Placental blood flow
  Placental transport mechanisms
  Placental metabolism

Drug characteristics (favoring transfer)
  Not bound to plasma proteins
  High lipid solubility
  Low molecular weight
  Weakly basic

Fetal blood pH (lower than maternal by 0.1–0.15 pH unit)

of maternal levels within 3 minutes of induction of maternal anesthesia. The mechanisms by which placental perfusion is regulated are complex and poorly understood. It is known that the placenta is not innervated and that local production of autacoids may be important for regulation of blood flow. It is also known that the uteroplacental vasculature may be directly affected by drugs with effects on the cardiovascular system (such as antihypertensive agents, or vasoconstrictors such as cocaine), even if the agents themselves do not cross the placenta.

The most important mode of placental transport is passive diffusion along a concentration gradient, although some agents also cross by means of specialized transport mechanisms. The placenta has drug-biotransforming systems capable of oxidation, reduction, hydrolysis, and conjugation. For example, placental metabolism of most corticosteroids is known to decrease their transfer to the fetus; it is the lower degree of placental metabolism of betamethasone that has led to its use for promotion of fetal lung maturity. For most agents at steady state, the contribution of placental biotransformation is thought to be small relative to maternal metabolism. However, placental enzymatic activity may theoretically be of clinical importance when a drug is administered rapidly (e.g., a bolus of cocaine).

The drug

It is free *(unbound)* drug that equilibrates across the placenta. The fetal:maternal ratio of free drug is usually close to unity, even if the ratio of total drug is not. Exceptions may occur in the case of drugs that are subject to ion trapping in the fetus (see following section). As the placenta, like other biologi-

cal membranes, contains lipid barriers to drug diffusion, it follows that lipid-soluble, nonionized drugs generally cross most readily. The placenta is impermeable to drugs with molecular weights of more than 1000 Da, but most drugs have molecular weights less than 600 Da and cross easily (e.g., penicillins, aminoglycosides). Within the range of 100–1000 Da, both molecular weight and lipid solubility are important factors in placental transfer. Many drugs are relatively unbound, nonionized, lipid-soluble molecules of rather low molecular weight and can therefore cross the placenta readily. This fact has enabled physicians to administer drugs to the mother in order to treat fetuses suffering from such conditions as cardiac arrhythmia and heart failure.

Standard heparin and low-molecular-weight heparins are notable exceptions, having mean molecular weights of 15,000 and 5000 Da, respectively; consequently these agents do not cross the placenta. From the fetal point of view, they represent superior alternatives to the known teratogenicity of warfarin when the mother requires anticoagulant therapy. However, even low-dose heparin given for a few months may in some cases cause maternal osteoporosis and vertebral crush fractures. This fact illustrates the weighing of risks and benefits that must be done when pharmacotherapy is prescribed for pregnant patients.

Fetal blood pH

Fetal blood pH is slightly more acidic (by 0.1 to 0.15 pH units) than the maternal pH; as a result, ionization and ultimate trapping of weakly basic drugs (e.g., lidocaine or procainamide) in the fetal circulation may occur. Fetal acidosis, such as that associated with maternal cardiac arrhythmia and hypotension, will magnify such pH differences and result in more ion trapping. Intracellular accumulation of weak acids may also occur because of the greater pH gradient between the intracellular and extracellular compartments in the fetus. Such accumulation, especially in the central nervous system, is an important factor in the fetal toxicity of **salicylates.**

Fetal Drug Disposition

The fetus is not simply a passive bystander during maternal drug therapy. Rather, drugs delivered into the fetal bloodstream are subject to fetal pharmacokinetics that may be altered by peculiarities of the fetal circulation.

Amniotic fluid is a potential source of drug acting

on the fetus, in addition to that delivered through the uteroplacental circulation. Agents that are excreted by the fetal kidney into the amniotic fluid may be swallowed by the fetus and reabsorbed from the gastrointestinal tract, thus creating what is termed the 'enterorenal cycle.' This also provides a route for fetal therapy, such as the injection of thyroid hormone into the amniotic fluid for the treatment in utero of fetal hypothyroidism. Drug absorption may also occur directly across the fetal respiratory epithelium or through unkeratinized fetal skin. After keratinization has taken place at 24–26 weeks, the skin is an unlikely transfer site other than for very-lipid-soluble, low-molecular-weight compounds (e.g., carbon dioxide).

The affinity of fetal plasma albumin and other proteins for drugs may sometimes be higher (e.g., salicylates) but is usually lower (e.g., phenytoin) than that of maternal proteins. Protein binding may also change as a function of the gestational age.

Although the placenta is the main organ involved in fetal drug clearance, both fetal renal clearance (glomerular filtration and tubular secretion) and fetal hepatic biotransformation do occur. Drugs that are cleared by the liver may show increased bioavailability and decreased clearance in the fetus, because a substantial proportion (15–40%) of portal venous blood bypasses the fetal liver via the ductus venosus for up to 20 weeks of gestation. Biotransformation (at least at steady state) occurs primarily in the mother, although enzymatic systems necessary for drug transformation are present and functional to varying degrees early in gestation. In general, parent drugs are metabolized in the fetus to more polar compounds, just as they are after birth, and the polar metabolites are less likely than nonpolar compounds to transfer back into the maternal circulation.

One of the proposed mechanisms for **thalidomide**-induced birth defects (see Chapters 63 and 70) was the fetal production of a toxic intermediate metabolite. Fetal biotransformation may play a particularly important role in the metabolism of parent compounds to reactive intermediates and the clearance of drugs in non–steady-state conditions, such as maternal **acetaminophen overdose**. *Acetaminophen overdose is the most common poisoning in pregnancy.* Hepatic toxicity results from the formation, by hepatic cytochrome P450 activity, of the highly reactive intermediate *N*-acetyl-benzoquinoneimine, which is normally excreted as a urinary sulfate or glucuronide. In an overdose, detoxification occurs by conjugation with glutathione, which becomes depleted when stores reach 70% of normal. The specific antidote is *N*-acetylcysteine (NAC), which acts as a glutathione precursor (see also Chapters 4, 46, and 74).

Acetaminophen is known to cross the placenta. Metabolic studies using human fetal hepatocytes at 18–23 weeks of gestation demonstrated low levels of cytochrome P450 activity (about 10% of normal adult levels). This would be protective for the fetus, because only low levels of the toxic metabolite are produced. However, cytochrome P450 activity was found to increase linearly with advancing gestational age, suggesting that fetal risk may be higher when maternal acetaminophen overdose occurs later in pregnancy. These findings give rise to concern because the same metabolic studies failed to demonstrate the presence in fetal hepatocytes of the glucuronidation mechanism necessary to conjugate the harmful acetaminophen metabolite. There are several reports of stillbirth attributed to fetal hepatic necrosis following acetaminophen overdose in the third trimester. However, NAC has recently been shown to cross the human placenta and achieve fetal levels in the range of those present in maternal blood; therefore NAC may protect the fetus when given to the mother.

TIMING OF EXPOSURE

Early Exposures: Teratogenicity

Maternal drug therapy during pregnancy must be understood in the context of the development of the embryo. From conception until day 14, damage to the embryo may result in its death (in which case the woman may not even know that she was pregnant), or complete repair and recovery may occur. For obvious reasons, this is termed the 'all-or-none' phenomenon.

Drug exposure during days 14 through 60 after conception (i.e., the time of major organogenesis) may result in fetal death (i.e., spontaneous abortion) or in structural malformations or functional changes. The compounds that produce them are called 'teratogens.' With the exception of the brain and eye, which both develop throughout gestation, organogenesis is complete by the end of the first trimester. Each organ exhibits a sensitive period during which major malformations are more likely to occur, although exposures prior to complete organ formation can potentially affect tissue development. This must be considered in the interpretation of the link between a drug exposure and an associated adverse effect. If a causal relationship seems feasible on the basis of embryological principles, one then looks at the consistency of defects described in the available case reports. Most teratogens produce not one particular abnormality, but, rather, constellations of abnormalities (termed syndromes), particularly after exposure during a specific ('critical') period of gestation (see also Chapter 70).

In contrast, exposures after day 60 following conception do not result in major structural malformations unless there is a substantial disruption of vascular supply. Instead, such exposures have the potential to impair fetal growth or function, especially that of the central nervous system. Such effects may extend into infancy and childhood, and are discussed below under Later Exposures: Fetotoxicity.

It is remarkable that, given the rapidly expanding number of therapeutic agents, relatively few drugs have been found to be human teratogens (see Table 65-2). In fact, various authors have estimated that only 1% of malformations can be attributed to drug, chemical, or physical exposures during pregnancy, whereas 65–70% remain completely unexplained and are thought to have multifactorial causes (which *may* include some effect of a drug or drugs).

Table 65-2 Recognized Human Teratogens/Fetotoxins *

Drugs
  Alcohol
  ACE inhibitors
  Anticonvulsants
  Carbon monoxide
  Chemotherapeutic (antineoplastic) agents
  Coumarins
  Diethylstilbestrol
  Lithium
  Retinoids
  Streptomycin
  Tetracyclines
  Thalidomide

Physical exposure
  Heat
  High-dose radiation

Infections
  Cytomegalovirus
  Parvovirus B19
  Rubella
  Syphilis
  Toxoplasmosis
  Varicella

* In addition to various maternal diseases and maternal nutrition.

Isotretinoin (Accutane), a vitamin A congener, is the drug with the highest human teratogenic potential on the market today. It has most of the characteristics that have been described as factors in the development and expression of teratogenicity and fetotoxicity. Isotretinoin crosses the human placenta, and in premarketing animal studies it has produced malformations in 38% of exposed fetuses. The knowledge gained from these studies helped to avoid a catastrophe on the scale of that caused by thalidomide. However, case reports of inadvertent exposures during human pregnancy have confirmed that the drug has powerful teratogenic effects on the human embryo similar to those seen in the animal studies. The interaction between the drug and the unique genetic makeup of the fetus is probably responsible for the fact that about 38% rather than 100% of exposed fetuses have had major birth defects. Isotretinoin, and its major metabolite 4-oxo-isotretinoin, produce a classic retinoid embryopathy characterized particularly by central nervous system and craniofacial abnormalities and agenesis and/or stenosis of the external ear canal.

The drug is thought to act by binding to a nuclear receptor, thereby affecting transcription of developmental control genes that play a role in the differentiation and migration of cranial neural crest cells. The critical period for birth defects to occur is 2–5 weeks postconception, although there is also a high rate of spontaneous abortions. Exposure later in pregnancy can in some cases present a risk for neurobehavioral deficits, given the fact that the brain develops throughout gestation. Vitamin A consumption during pregnancy is encouraged at the recommended daily allowance of 1 mg; however, isotretinoin is prescribed at a much higher dose, about 40 mg/day, which clearly contributes to its dose-dependent teratogenic-fetotoxic potential (see also Chapter 67).

Later Exposures: Fetotoxicity

The principles of teratogenicity apply equally to exposures later in pregnancy. These have the capacity to produce nonspecific fetal effects, such as the growth restriction associated with β-blocker therapy and with cigarette smoking. However, effects may also be specific to a particular target organ, depending on the pharmacodynamics of the drugs as well as the sensitivity and maturity of the fetal organ in question. For example, **angiotensin converting enzyme (ACE) inhibitors** are contraindicated in pregnancy because they have been associated with fetal renal failure; the fetal kidney appears to be more dependent on angiotensin II-mediated renal perfusion than the adult kidney, which is usually adversely affected only in the presence of bilateral renal artery stenosis. **Propylthiouracil** may produce fetal hypothyroidism in up to 15% of exposed fetuses, but this will occur only after exposures to propylthiouracil that occur at a gestational age of more than 12–14 weeks when the fetal thyroid begins to concentrate iodide. **Tetracyclines** chelate calcium ions and are deposited in developing teeth, producing discoloration; this occurs only with exposures to tetracyclines after 16–20 weeks gestation, when the deciduous teeth begin to calcify.

It must be remembered that fetotoxic effects may not become manifest until later in life. There are far fewer examples of such effects, as adequate long-term follow-up has been conducted for few medications. Transplacental carcinogenesis has been described in animals, although development of vaginal carcinoma in young women exposed in utero to **diethylstilbestrol (DES)** represents the only established example in humans.

Behavioral teratogenesis has also been well described in animals. Of particular concern are the effects of psychotropic or other agents that affect neurotransmitter activity, as this may be important for regulating cell proliferation. An adverse effect of phenytoin, but not of carbamazepine, on neurobehavioral development has recently been demonstrated. This is also a good example of how developmental effects can be confounded by other factors, such as maternal epilepsy, socioeconomic factors, and parenting skills.

NEONATAL PHARMACOLOGY

The neonate may carry a drug burden from three potential sources: in utero exposure, direct administration after birth, and ingested breast milk. The half-life of drugs may be very prolonged. Renal function is immature at birth; renal plasma flow and glomerular filtration rate (GFR) are only 30–40% of adult values (especially in preterm babies born before 34 weeks of gestation). Although GFR increases rapidly thereafter, the development of tubular secretion lags behind, and functional maturity is not achieved until 1 year of age. Hepatic biotransformation can be quite variable in terms of the pathways involved and their enzymatic activity. The best-known example of this is the neonatal jaundice due to immaturity of the hepatic mechanism for glucuronidation of bilirubin. It should be noted, however, that more active pathways may compensate for deficiencies in an enzymatic pathway by which a drug is commonly metabolized; a good example is the increased sulfation of the intermediate metabolite of acetaminophen in neonates as compared to adults. The potential problems created by low drug clearance rate are magnified if the drug has a long elimination half-life to begin with, and if the neonate is more sensitive to the known pharmacological and toxicological effects of the drug.

Drug Burden at Birth

After birth, the neonate must eliminate drugs entirely on its own, without the aid of maternal or placental clearance. Neonates may be forced to clear drugs that they would not normally receive. Psychotropic drugs are examples. **Tricyclic antidepressants** administered to the mother during late pregnancy are slowly biotransformed by the newborn and may produce irritability, tremor, muscle spasms, seizures, and urinary retention within a few hours after birth. Neonatal sedation may follow administration of high doses (>30 mg) of **diazepam** during labor because the drug has a long half-life and an active metabolite (desmethyldiazepam). Use of shorter-acting benzodiazepines (e.g., lorazepam) having inactive metabolites may pose less of a risk, although sedation of the neonate has still been described.

Drug-withdrawal reactions after birth may also be a problem following long-term drug exposure in utero. The opioid withdrawal syndrome (manifested by irritability, tremor, increased tonus, tachypnea, convulsions, and high-pitched cry) usually occurs within 24 hours of delivery, although signs may be delayed if **methadone,** which has a considerably longer half-life than **morphine** or **heroin,** is used. High doses of other opioids, such as **codeine** at >50 mg/day, may also be associated with this reversible neonatal syndrome.

Drug Exposure Through Breastfeeding

The health benefits of breastfeeding have been recognized to include decreased neonatal morbidity and mortality. Given that over 90% of infants world-wide are breast-fed at birth, and a high percentage of women receive at least one drug in the postpartum period, it follows that nursing infants have a high chance of being exposed to medications through ingestion of breast milk.

Whether a drug is excreted in milk depends on its movement from the maternal circulation into the alveolar acini of the mammary glands, and then into the breast milk. Only free drug will pass into milk, and drugs with high protein binding (e.g., warfarin) are therefore less likely candidates for transfer. Given the relatively high fat content of milk, transfer is also facilitated by high lipid solubility (e.g., amiodarone) and low molecular weight. High pK_a (i.e., basic drugs) also increases the likelihood of transfer, because the lower pH of breast milk (pH 6.9–7.2) compared to maternal plasma (pH 7.4) increases ionization of basic drugs in the milk, and they cannot then easily transfer back into maternal plasma.

The estimated drug dose received by a nursing infant, as a fraction of the maternal dose, can be calculated from the following formula:

$$\text{Dose per feed} = \frac{C_{max} \times 30 \text{ mL/kg/feed}}{\text{Maternal (dose/weight)}}$$

where C_{max} = maximum drug concentration in the breast milk, and 30 mL/kg/feed is the estimated infant milk consumption per feed. Other formulae are also available, based on the milk:plasma ratio of drug. However, isolated ratios of drug concentration can be misleading, because the average daily amount of drug ingested by the infant may be small and of no potential harm.

To determine drug safety during lactation, the dose per feed (there are usually five feedings per day in a newborn) is related to a therapeutic dose of that drug for an infant. By convention, it is assumed that if the neonate receives less than 10% of the therapeutic dose (expressed in mg/kg), then dose-dependent adverse effects are unlikely. For most drugs, the amount consumed by nursing infants is less than 5% of the maternal dose (in mg/kg) and has no appreciable effect on the infant. A number of good reference sources are available from which one may estimate drug excretion into breast milk.

Even if the estimated dose of drug ingested by the nursing infant is small, it is still important to monitor the breast-fed infant for unwanted drug effects. Many factors other than dose can come into play. For example, neonates may be more sensitive to the CNS effects of narcotics and sedatives because of immaturity of the blood–brain barrier. Drug-induced idiosyncratic adverse reactions may also occur. Also, the neonate may fail to clear the drug adequately, a point that is well illustrated by atenolol. **Atenolol** is renally excreted, and there have been reports of adverse reactions, predictable from the known pharmacology of the drug and based on prolonged drug half-life in the neonate. Drug effects

may also be potentially harmful to the infant during the early period of growth and development for reasons not yet known. For example, the American Academy of Pediatrics lists a group of agents 'whose effect on nursing infants is unknown but may be of concern.' This statement was based mostly on psychotropic drug activity, for which clinically demonstrable short-term adverse effects have not been reported in nursing infants.

BIOLOGICAL MARKERS OF DRUG EXPOSURE

Biological markers of fetal drug exposure can be tested in amniotic fluid, meconium, neonatal urine, and/or neonatal hair. Each provides different information and is therefore of different clinical usefulness.

Least useful are amniotic fluid and neonatal urine. Amniotic fluid may be obtained before delivery by amniocentesis, or it may be collected at the time of delivery. Not only is collection often complicated, but the measured drug levels may not reflect drug originating in the fetal circulation. Agents may be present due to fetal urine production, as well as from diffusion across the chorioallantoic membranes. Neonatal urine reflects only very recent drug exposure at term, which may be useful if neonatal drug withdrawal is a concern, as with opioids. However, meconium and hair offer distinct advantages, because they act as stable matrices for drugs and their metabolites, and they are easy to obtain.

Meconium is fetal stool formed from the 12th to 16th week of gestation onward that is passed within the first few days of life. It contains drug from both swallowed amniotic fluid and biliary excretion. Positive assays may reflect early fetal drug exposure. In contrast, terminal fetal hair grows during the third trimester and reflects drug exposure throughout this later period. Hair growth occurs at a rate of approximately 1 cm per month, and drugs are incorporated into the shaft of the hair, from which they can be extracted and assayed. Fetal hair with which the infant is born is not lost until 5–6 months after birth, so there is a large window during which fetal drug exposure can be assessed. Concomitant maternal hair analysis also affords the opportunity to ascertain more exactly the timing of exposure, given that maternal hair also grows at a fairly constant rate of 1.0–1.5 cm per month. Therefore, hair analysis offers distinct advantages over other biological markers of fetal drug exposure.

Biological markers have been used primarily to investigate fetal exposure to drugs of abuse. Cocaine (and its active metabolite benzoylecgonine) and nicotine (and its major metabolite cotinine) are notable examples. However, experience has shown that no single screening test is sufficiently sensitive to pick up all drug-exposed fetuses, even when maternal reports of respective drug exposure are available as indicators. This may reflect differences in placental processes for bolus versus chronic drug administrations. Thus, until these relationships can be defined more precisely, negative results for biological markers of fetal drug exposure must be interpreted with caution.

ANSWER TO QUESTION IN CASE HISTORY

During late pregnancy the phenytoin concentrations in the mother's serum are likely to decrease because of increased body weight, distribution volume, and clearance rate. She may need more drug. The mother should be made aware of the risk of fetal hydantoin syndrome, including facial and bony changes, and of an increased risk of developmental delay. Excretion of phenytoin into breast milk is minimal, and the infant can be safely breast-fed.

SUGGESTED READING

Beeley L. Adverse effects of drugs in the first trimester of pregnancy. Clin Obstet Gynaecol 1986; 13(2):177–195.

Beeley L. Adverse effects of drugs in later pregnancy. Clin Obstet Gynaecol 1986; 13(2):197–214.

Bennett PN, Matheson I, Dukes NMG, eds. Drugs and human lactation. Amsterdam: Elsevier Science, 1988.

Brent RL. The complexities of solving the problem of human malformations. Clin Perinatol 1986; 13(3):491–503.

Briggs GG, Freeman RK, Yaffe SJ. Drugs in pregnancy and lactation. 4th ed. Baltimore: Williams and Wilkins, 1990.

Committee on Drugs, American Academy of Pediatrics. The transfer of drugs and other chemicals into human milk. Pediatrics 1994; 93:137–150.

Cunningham AS, Jelliffe DB, Jelliffe EFP. Breast-feeding and health in the 1980's. A global epidemiologic review. J Pediatr 1991; 118:659–666.

Cupit GC, Rotmensch HH. Principles of drug therapy. In: Gleicher N, Elkayam U, Galbraith RM, Gall SA, Sarto GE, Sibai BM, eds. Principles and practices of medical therapy in pregnancy. 2nd ed. Connecticut: Appleton & Lange, 1992: 68–78.

Dam M, Christiansen J, Munck O, Mygind KI. Antiepileptic drugs: metabolism in pregnancy. Clin Pharmacokinet 1979; 4:53–62.

Jelovsek FR, Mattison DR, Chen JJ. Prediction of risk for human developmental toxicity: how important are animal studies for hazard identification? Obstet Gynecol 1989; 74(4):624–636.

Johnson D, Schwartz H, Forman R, et al. Assessment of in utero exposure to cocaine: radioimmunoassay testing for benzoylecgonine in meconium, neonatal hair and maternal hair. Can J Clin Pharmacol 1994; 1(2):83–86.

Kauffman RE. Drug therapeutics in the infant and child. In: Yaffe SJ, Aranda JV, eds. Pediatric pharmacology; therapeutic principles in practice. Philadelphia: WB Saunders, 1992: 212–219.

Koren G, ed. Maternal-fetal toxicology; a clinician's guide. 2nd ed. New York: Marcel Dekker, 1994.

Krauer B, Krauer F. Drug kinetics in pregnancy. In: Gibaldi M, Prescott L, eds. Handbook of clinical pharmacokinetics, section II. New York: ADIS, 1983: 1–17.

Lammer EJ, Chen DT, Hoar RM, et al. Retinoic acid embryopathy. N Engl J Med 1985; 313:837–841.

Morselli PL. Clinical pharmacology of the perinatal period and early infancy. Clin Pharmacokinet 1989; 17(Suppl 1):13–28.

Mucklow JC. The fate of drugs in pregnancy. Clin Obstet Gynaecol 1986; 13(2):161–175.

Schimmel MS, Eidelman AJ, Wilschanski MA, et al. Toxic effects of atenolol consumed during breast feeding. J Pediatr 1989; 114:476–478.

Schou M, Amidsen A, Steenstrup DR. Lithium and pregnancy. II: Hazards to women given lithium during pregnancy and delivery. Br Med J 1973; 2:137–138.

Szeto H. Kinetics of drug transfer to the fetus. Clin Obstet Gynecol 1993; 36(2):246–254.

Whitelaw AGL, Cummings AJ, McFadyen IR. Effect of maternal lorazepam on the neonate. Br Med J 1981; 282:1106.

Wilson JT. Determinants and consequences of drug excretion in breast milk. Drug Metab Rev 1983; 14:619–652.

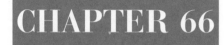

CHAPTER 66

Geriatric Clinical Pharmacology

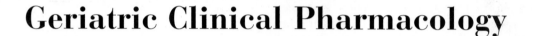

D.S. SITAR

CASE HISTORY

A community-dwelling 75-year-old woman has mild congestive heart failure controlled with a single daily dose of furosemide (40 mg). Recently she has had trouble sleeping, and her physician prescribed diazepam (5 mg) to treat this condition. On the second evening after starting to take the diazepam, she awoke with urinary urgency and fell on her way to the bathroom. The patient self-medicated with ibuprofen (400 mg every 6 hours) for relief of the pain resulting from the fall. She became more confused; her heart failure worsened; and she now appears in the Emergency Room of her community hospital for assessment.

Pharmacological Issues

- Benzodiazepines in the elderly
- Self-medication
- Choice of analgesic
- Drug interactions
- Prostaglandins and renal function

In the industrialized countries, 12% of the population was older than 65 in 1990. This cohort of the population probably will increase more rapidly than any other age group over the next several years. In fact, the largest increase in population over the next 20 years is projected to be of persons older than 85 years. Operating definitions of the elderly have divided them arbitrarily into two groups, the "young-old," 65–84 years, and the "old-old," >85 years. Much of our most recent knowledge with respect to pharmacological issues in aging is based on studies in the young-old cohort.

The prevalence of disease increases substantially as persons age, and they utilize a greater fraction of their own resources and those of society in an effort to maintain acceptable health status. Drug therapy is an important tool in this effort. Most often, diseases of the elderly are chronic and multiple, and polypharmacy is a major factor in the high incidence of adverse drug reactions, which increase with patient age (Table 66-1; see also Chapter 63).

Together with the increase in disease prevalence, the elderly have less effective homeostatic responses to the multitude of functional disturbances they suffer. As we age, physiological responses become more heterogeneous, reflecting the variable rate of declining organ and tissue function. Thus, the predictability of patient response to drug therapy becomes less certain. Suboptimal drug therapy often stems from disease progression, increased adverse drug reactions, defective compliance due to the complication of timing of doses of many drugs with differing dose schedules, and the inevitable attempt by the patient to self-medicate with "over-the-counter" drugs purchased without prior consultation with physicians or other health care professionals.

The problem of drug-related adverse patient events (DRAPEs) has been known for many years, but its prevalence remains the same despite the

Table 66-1 Age and Adverse Drug Reactions	
Age of Patients (Years)	*Incidence (%)*
10–19	3.1
20–29	3.0
30–39	5.7
40–49	7.5
50–59	8.1
60–69	10.7
70–79	21.3
80–89	18.6

After Hurwitz N. *Br Med J* 1969; 1:536–539.

greater knowledge and educational effort of the last twenty years. This finding has led to an increasing acceptance of the need to individualize drug doses for older patients.

In North America, the Boston Collaborative Drug Surveillance Program has provided valuable information on the incidence of adverse drug reactions with increasing age. It must be remembered, however, that this type of information is useful in alerting the physician to a potential problem with a particular drug or drug group in the elderly, but it does not tell us the mechanism(s) underlying these observations. Although the observation has been attributed to increasing frailty with older age, most studies which have examined specifically the effect of age have failed to demonstrate such an association (Fig. 66-1). The mechanisms remain to be determined by more detailed examination of the problem in the affected patient group.

However, it is universally accepted that the number of drugs prescribed and the number of diseases diagnosed correlate much better with the incidence of observed adverse drug reactions than the age (Fig. 66-2). Since these last two predictive factors are not independent variables, it is likely that the increased prevalence of chronic diseases in the older patient population is the most important determinant of increased adverse drug reactions observed (Fig. 66-3).

Both pharmacokinetic and pharmacodynamic explanations are possible for the apparently altered responses of the older patients to drug therapy. It is most likely that both processes contribute. Without an understanding of the effects of aging on both these processes, a rational approach to drug treatment of older patients is not possible. A more detailed examination of the evidence for potential and demon-

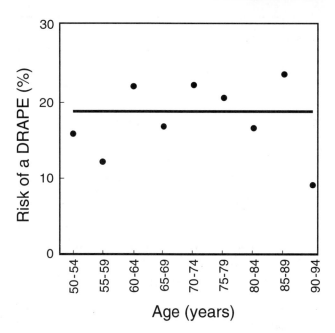

Figure 66-1. Relationship between DRAPE (drug-related adverse patient event) risk at admission and age. The line shows the mean rate of 19% of a group of 863 eligible admissions. (After Grymonpre et al. 1988.)

strated contributions of aging to alteration in pharmacokinetics and pharmacodynamics is presented here.

PHARMACOKINETIC CHANGES IN THE ELDERLY

For the following discussion, it is useful to recall some of the fundamental pharmacokinetic equations. For this short summary, only the model-independent relationships are presented:

$$(1) \quad Cl_p = \text{dose/AUC} = V_d \times \lambda$$

$$(2) \quad V_d = Cl_p/\lambda$$

$$(3) \quad t_{1/2} = 0.693/\lambda = 0.693 \times V_d/Cl_p$$

where Cl_p = plasma (serum) clearance, AUC = area under the plasma (serum) concentration versus time curve, V_d = apparent volume of distribution, λ = the terminal disposition rate constant, and $t_{1/2}$ represents the half-life corresponding to the terminal disposition rate constant.

Earlier investigators inferred, from observed alterations of $t_{1/2}$, that the elderly handled drugs differ-

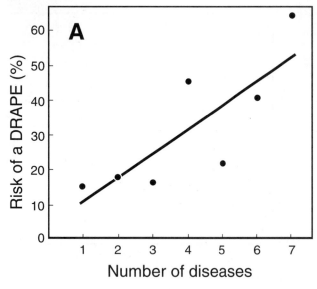

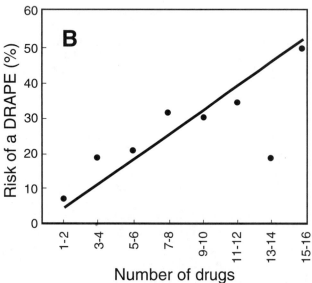

Figure 66-2. Relationship of DRAPE risk to the number of diseases before admission (panel A: $r = 0.81$; $P = <0.026$) and to the number of prescribed drugs used (panel B: $r = 0.77$; $P = <0.001$). (After Grymonpre et al. 1988.)

Although the overall effect observed may be a decrease in the rate of drug elimination, without knowledge of the V_d it is impossible to determine whether the observation is related to altered drug distribution, impaired elimination capability by the responsible organ(s), or a combination of both.

The reader is referred to Chapter 5 for a more detailed discussion of pharmacokinetic relationships.

Physiological Changes with Increasing Age

Body composition

The proportion of fat as a fraction of total body weight is a function of several variables, including height, weight, gender, age, diet, and physical activity. Generally, women have a higher proportion of total body weight as fat than men do. In both sexes the proportion of total body weight as fat increases with age. The increment in fat content in the body is generally localized to the middle and upper body regions. In women, there appears to be a postmenopausal acceleration of this trend. In the elderly, a considerable fraction of body fat tends to accumulate

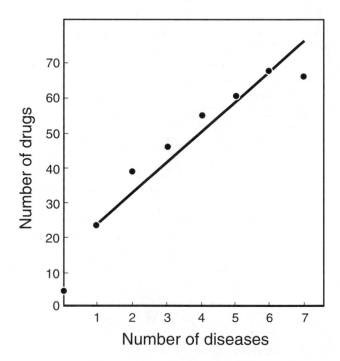

Figure 66-3. Relationship between the number of prescribed drugs used before admission and the number of diseases ($r = 0.52$; $P = <0.001$). (After Grymonpre et al. 1988.)

ently from the young. The problem with this simplistic approach is that $t_{1/2}$ is a hybrid of V_d and Cl_p (equation 3). Thus, if V_d changes, then $t_{1/2}$ does not necessarily reflect the ability of the body to eliminate the drug (Cl_p). The mechanism could in fact be the inability of the drug to reach the clearance site. However, Cl_p represents the ability of an elimination site to act on that fraction of the drug dose to which it is exposed without reference to the concurrent presence of additional drug molecules at remote sites.

within organs rather than being localized as adipose tissue. Recent studies suggest a maximum age for fat accumulation around the sixth decade of life, with a plateau phase, and a subsequent reduction in the amount and proportion of body fat in the old-old population. Thus it can be anticipated that distribution of drugs will be affected by this altered accumulation and distribution profile of body fat.

Body water content is generally accepted as a measure of fat-free mass. For all ages, the proportion of body weight attributed to water is less in women than in men. Body water as a percentage of total body weight generally declines with increasing age. In women, for example, it decreases from about 56% at age 20 to about 45% at age 70. This trend continues until approximately age 80, when the percentage of water begins to increase again. This decline in body water begins in middle age in men. It is less rapid in women until about the sixth decade, when it accelerates. At the same time, the fraction of muscle per unit of body weight decreases with increasing age in both sexes.

If dosage is based on total body weight, drugs that are localized to lean tissue (generally hydrophilic drugs, i.e., those with lower lipid:water partition coefficient) will achieve a higher plasma concentration for the same mg/kg dose in older patients, while there will be increased tissue sequestration of more lipophilic drugs (higher lipid:water partition coefficient) and a lower circulating drug concentration.

The profile of plasma proteins in the circulation also changes with age. Serum albumin concentration decreases with increasing age, although it remains within the normal range unless it is affected by clinically important pathology. Reduced serum albumin concentration could result in an increased circulating free fraction of acidic drugs which bind to it, e.g., nonsteroidal anti-inflammatory drugs. However, serum α_1-acid glycoprotein concentration increases with age. The lability of this glycoprotein makes it difficult to determine whether its concentration contributes to the altered pharmacological response to basic drugs that bind to it, e.g., tricyclic antidepressants. This change in protein profile may have important consequences for drugs that are highly protein-bound, but studies of this issue have been restricted mostly to drugs that are highly bound to albumin.

Organ function

Organ function tends to change with time, usually in the direction of decreased functional reserve with increasing age. Thus, the glomerular filtration rate of the kidney, as reflected by creatinine clearance, decreases in the majority of older patients. However, serum creatinine concentration may not be elevated even in the presence of clinically important renal impairment because of the decrease in serum creatinine concentration resulting from decreased muscle mass. In about one-third of apparently healthy community-dwelling elderly persons, renal function remains high and stable even in old age.

Liver size as a fraction of body weight decreases with increasing age. Although liver blood flow per unit of organ weight may not be significantly different in older persons, the decrease in mass results in decreased total hepatic blood flow and decreased rates of elimination of many drugs from the body, especially those that are lipophilic and have a high hepatic extraction ratio.

Cardiac output is also lower in older patients, but it is unclear to what degree this is due to a more sedentary lifestyle, to progressive tissue degeneration due to aging, or to disease. There is often a redistribution of cardiac output to maintain optimum blood flow to critical organs. Thus, perfusion of sites of drug elimination from the body is often compromised in cardiac failure. Also, the baroreceptor reflex is decreased in older patients, resulting in their increased susceptibility to orthostatic hypotension.

Decline in the function of other organs is also more prevalent with increasing age, and often forms the basis of the need for drug therapy, e.g., hypothyroidism and type II diabetes. Some representative changes in body composition and function are presented in Table 66-2.

Consequences for Drug Disposition

Absorption

Various data indicate that gastric acid secretion decreases, gastric emptying time increases, and the surface area of the upper intestinal tract is reduced with increasing age. Also, cardiac output may be lower and blood flow to the gastrointestinal tract may be reduced in the elderly patient. Although these observations provide a theoretical basis for predicting altered drug absorption in the aged, few examples exist to indicate that it is an important practical problem. Nevertheless, the possibility must be considered when multiple drugs are ingested concurrently, especially when their pharmacology includes modification of gastrointestinal physiological func-

Table 66-2 Average Changes in Body Composition and Function (Males and Females)

	Change From Age 20 to Age 80 (%)
Body fat/total body weight	+35
Plasma volume	−8
Plasma albumin	−10
Plasma globulin	−10
Total body water	−17
Extracellular fluid (from age 20 to age 65)	−40
Conduction velocity	−20
Cardiac index	−40
Cardiac output	−30 to −40
Vital capacity	−60
Glomerular filtration rate	−50
Splanchnic and renal blood flow	−40

pam, will have a lower circulating concentration for an equivalent dose due to distribution into the increased fat of the older patient. Although the elderly are capable of biotransforming diazepam to an extent similar to that in younger patients (Fig. 66-5), delivery to the liver is decreased, and the drug persists longer in the body at levels which exert a CNS-depressant effect. Although the plasma $t_{1/2}$ of diazepam approximates chronological age in adults (Fig. 66-6), this is not due to decreasing ability of the body to metabolize diazepam as much as to increased tissue sequestration (Fig. 66-7).

Another example of an important quantitative difference in tissue sequestration in the elderly is provided by digoxin. This drug is highly concentrated in muscle tissue. Since the proportion of muscle in the body invariably declines with increasing age, the circulating concentration of digoxin will be higher than expected for a given mg/kg dose. Although this is not the sole determining factor in dose estimation for digoxin, it is an important one that is often overlooked.

tion. Drug absorption from the skin of older patients also has not been shown to be a clinically important problem related to the aging process.

The reductions in surface area of the upper intestinal tract and in liver size with advancing age are given as reasonable hypotheses to explain reduced presystemic drug elimination and increased bioavailability of drugs that are normally subject to extensive elimination by this process, e.g., morphine and propranolol (Fig. 66-4). Although these postulated mechanisms seem reasonable, more research is required to confirm their contribution to the observed increase in bioavailability in some elderly patients.

Tissue distribution

The changes in body composition with increasing age, described previously, have important clinical consequences with respect to the choice of drug and dose optimization in the elderly patient. Thus, relatively hydrophilic drugs, e.g., alcohol and morphine, will achieve higher concentrations in blood for the same weight-adjusted dose. The perception that the elderly are more sensitive to these CNS-depressant drugs is likely to be explained, at least in part, by increased delivery to the brain due to the reduced V_d.

However, relatively lipophilic drugs, e.g., diaze-

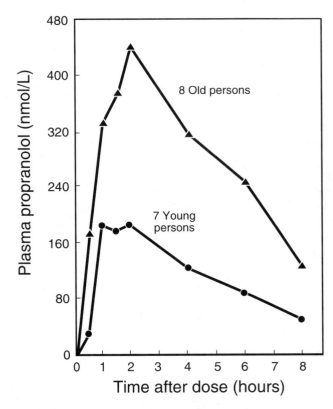

Figure 66-4. Mean plasma propranolol concentrations in two different age groups, following a single oral dose of 40 mg. Differences between age groups are statistically significant. (After Castleden & George 1979.)

Protein binding

The decrease in plasma albumin and increase in α_1-acid glycoprotein have implications for acidic and basic drugs that bind to them. Thus, the decrease in plasma albumin is implicated in the increased toxicity of acetylsalicylic acid in older patients at an equivalent total plasma concentration of salicylic acid. It is possible that increased binding of some basic drugs by α_1-acid glycoprotein could cause the total drug concentration to be misleading, since only the free drug concentration is believed to determine the intensity of pharmacological activity. This might be an important contributing factor for variable responses to tricyclic antidepressant drugs in the elderly, but the possibility remains virtually unexplored. However, it can be reasonably assumed that drugs that have a small V_d and are extensively bound to plasma proteins are likely to alter the pharmacological response of concurrently ingested drugs with similar protein-binding properties, usually to the detriment of the patient. An informative example is provided by the interaction of tolbutamide and salicylates. In this instance the salicylic acid displaces tolbutamide from its protein binding sites, thus increasing the hypoglycemic effect of tolbutamide. Although tolbutamide will also displace salicylate from its protein binding sites, the clinical consequences for the pharmacology of salicylate are not usually considered.

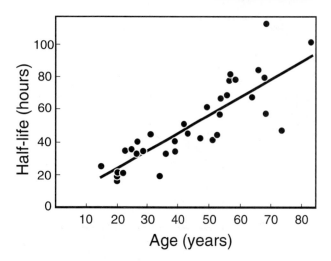

Figure 66-6. Correlation of diazepam $t_{1/2}$ (β-phase) and age. Each symbol refers to an individual study. (After Klotz et al. 1975.)

Drug biotransformation

In vitro studies with human liver microsomes have failed to demonstrate a consistent decrement in intrinsic drug biotransformation capability with increasing age. However, results from in vivo studies are less clear. Most of the available evidence suggests that drug biotransformation decreases with increasing age primarily in males, and this effect is seen with phase I reactions (oxidation, reduction, and hydrolysis). Interpretation of studies published to date is confounded by environmental influences that have a profound effect on interpatient variability in drug biotransformation. Evidence for a decrease in phase II reactions (conjugation) with increasing age is much less compelling and is generally believed not to be an important consideration in altered drug biotransformation in geriatric patients.

Reduced liver blood flow due to reduced organ size remains an important confounding factor in interpreting the mechanism(s) contributing to observations of decreased drug clearance in the geriatric patient.

There is reasonable evidence that the inductive effect of some commonly prescribed drugs (e.g., rifampicin) on the phase I reactions of other drugs is suppressed in older patients. However, there is also evidence that the multiple forms of tissue cytochromes P450 are not uniformly suppressed with increasing age. Thus, the inducing effect of smoking on theophylline biotransformation is not blunted in elderly males. Alteration of dose in an older patient

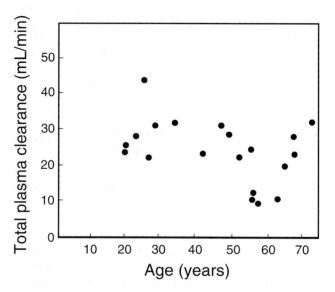

Figure 66-5. Relationship of total plasma clearance of diazepam with age. Each symbol represents a single normal individual. (After Klotz et al. 1975.)

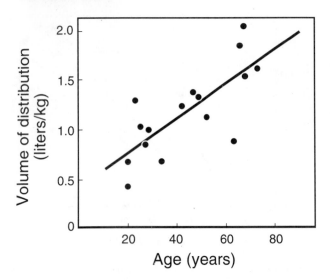

Figure 66-7. Correlation of volumes of distribution of diazepam and age. Each symbol refers to an individual study. (After Klotz et al. 1975.)

concurrently ingesting a known inducer of drug biotransformation often will differ from that required in younger patients.

In the older patient, multiple drug ingestion is more likely to result in toxicity due to inhibition of biotransformation. The increased frequency of this phenomenon in older patients is undoubtedly related, at least in part, to the competition for the available mechanisms of elimination among the drugs used concurrently to treat their chronic disease states. It is likely that influenza virus infection, which can produce a relatively nonspecific depression of the cytochromes P450, could also be an important contributing mechanism of increased drug toxicity in the elderly.

Diet is also a potentially confounding factor in altering drug biotransformation. The rate of biotransformation is depressed with high carbohydrate and stimulated with high protein diets. Diminishing affluence in the older patient cohort makes it more likely that carbohydrates constitute an increasing fraction of their total caloric intake, and contribute to the decrease of drug biotransformation rate.

Excretion

Although renal function does not inevitably decline with increasing age, it is clear that most older patients have decreased renal function compared to younger patients. Thus, drugs that depend on renal elimination of a substantial fraction of the dose (e.g., aman-

tadine, digoxin, procainamide) will have to be prescribed in smaller doses or at greater time intervals. It should be remembered also that a "normal" serum creatinine concentration in an older patient actually reflects impaired renal function, since creatinine production is reduced because there is a decreased muscle mass. If it is not possible to determine creatinine clearance directly, renal function may be estimated from the widely accepted algorithm of Cockroft and Gault:

$$Cl_{creatinine}\ [mL/min] = \frac{(140-age)\times weight\ [kg]}{0.8145\times C_{p,creatinine}\ [\mu mol/L]}$$

in which $C_{p,creatinine}$ is the concentration of creatinine in the plasma. Values for creatinine clearance in women should be multiplied by 0.85. It cannot be overemphasized that this relationship provides only an approximation of renal function in the older patient and that direct determination of plasma concentrations for drugs with narrow therapeutic indices is recommended when available. Alternatively, consideration should be given to the possibility of drug therapy with an agent having a higher therapeutic index.

The increasing incidence of incontinence in the elderly often is addressed by decreasing their fluid intake. Together with the decreased homeostatic response to dehydration, there is decreased urine formation and an increased drug concentration in the bladder, which is able to diffuse back into the body down a concentration gradient. Both processes may contribute to a decreased rate of drug excretion by the kidney. Also, this situation leads to an increased possibility of crystalluria due to precipitation of poorly soluble drugs and metabolites, e.g., acetylated sulfonamides, in the smaller urine volume.

PHARMACODYNAMIC CHANGES IN THE ELDERLY

Much less is known about altered pharmacodynamics as a function of increasing age, but some important examples have become better appreciated recently.

There has been considerable controversy regarding the mechanisms contributing to the observed increase in the response to CNS-depressant drugs in the elderly. Alteration in pharmacokinetic disposition has been convincingly demonstrated for some drugs, e.g., ethanol and benzodiazepines, but pharmacodynamic changes have been more difficult to prove.

The suggestion of increased neuronal sensitivity to drugs such as alfentanil, fentanyl, and nitrazepam is based on changes in the observed effect relative to concurrently measured drug concentrations in plasma. However, these data are based on the unproved assumption of an unchanged equilibrium between drug concentration in plasma and that in the brain.

There is more convincing evidence that older persons are less responsive to β-adrenoceptor agonists, especially of the β_1-receptor type. This finding suggests the possibility of a blunted response to β-blocker drug therapy in older patients. However, the therapeutic implications of this interaction have not yet been clearly defined by definitive studies in the patient population at risk.

There is an increasing incidence of abnormal glucose tolerance tests in older persons. This is conventionally attributed to an altered insulin response rather than to a deficiency of the hormone. Recent studies implicate a postreceptor defect. Since exercise is known to improve tissue utilization of glucose, it may be that part of this observed insulin resistance could be explained by the increasingly sedentary lifestyle of older people.

REPRESENTATIVE DRUG CLASSES FOR PHARMACOTHERAPY OF DISEASES IN ELDERLY PATIENTS

Analgesics

Chronic pain occurs commonly in older patients, and it is often poorly managed. Recent studies have indicated that acetaminophen in analgesic doses is just as effective as equivalent analgesic or anti-inflammatory doses of nonsteroidal anti-inflammatory drugs (NSAIDs) in the treatment of osteoarthritis. Thus, the question arises as to whether acetaminophen might be a safer treatment in those patients with reduced creatinine clearance when renal prostaglandin synthesis is an important factor in maintaining residual tubular function.

In those patients with rheumatoid arthritis and impaired renal function, consideration may be given to the use of the NSAID sulindac, since the kidney converts the active sulfide metabolite back to the prodrug sulindac in the majority of patients. However, its use does not guarantee protection of renal prostaglandin synthesis. Concurrent use of diuretics increases the kidney's susceptibility to inhibitors of prostaglandin synthesis and to renal impairment by NSAIDs. However, the interaction is reversible on cessation of therapy with the offending analgesic if renal ischemia has not induced acute tubular necrosis.

Recent studies, which have shown that acetaminophen but not acetylsalicylic acid raises pain threshold, suggest that use of these two analgesics together to improve pain control may eliminate the need to switch to an opioid analgesic. Also, there is evidence to show that caffeine improves the analgesic efficacy of nonopioid drugs. Thus, alternatives exist to opioid analgesics if the mechanism of pain is amenable to these agents.

For management of severe pain, morphine remains the opioid agent of choice. The relatively recent appreciation that morphine-6-glucuronide contributes substantially to the analgesic response raises the question of optimal dose schedules in older patients with decreased renal function. It must be emphasized that sufficient analgesic doses at regular intervals represent the optimal use of this drug class. Rationing of doses until severe pain has returned will usually result in the requirement of larger doses with concomitantly increased respiratory depression and decreased mental acuity. Meperidine should be used with extreme caution in these patients, since the likelihood of accumulation of the proconvulsant metabolite normeperidine is substantially increased.

Cardiovascular Drugs

Among all drug groups, cardiovascular drugs are the most commonly prescribed for older patients. Although the use of these drugs is often life-saving, many of them have a low therapeutic index, and large interpatient variability is to be expected.

Most diuretics are prone to cause electrolyte disturbances in geriatric patients. Although hypokalemia is recalled more often as an undesirable side effect, the negative effect on body calcium stores is often forgotten. In the elderly female patient with osteoporosis, chronic use of diuretics may increase susceptibility to fractures. In this situation, use of hydrochlorothiazide is least likely to disturb calcium homeostasis. However, long-acting diuretics may increase the risk of episodes of incontinence and thus limit the social activities of geriatric patients. Although the benefit of treatment of hypertension with diuretics and other cardiovascular drugs has been demonstrated convincingly in elderly patients, their increased susceptibility to orthostatic hypotension usually will limit the choice and dose of drug that may be considered for this purpose.

Oral anticoagulants often produce morbid events in elderly patients. Although some controversy exists about the proposed mechanisms contributing to the exaggerated responsiveness, the probable causes include concurrent ingestion of other drugs that impair coagulation (e.g., NSAIDs), reduced receptor sensitivity to and increased clearance of vitamin K, and decreased availability of other clotting factors. Thus, lower warfarin doses usually will suffice in this patient group. Dose should be guided by the plasma prothrombin time.

Digoxin dose is commonly a problem in the older patient. By itself, dose adjustment must take into consideration the decreased muscle mass and renal function. Also, quinidine and calcium-channel blockers increase plasma digoxin concentration when added to the therapeutic regimen. Depletion of body stores of potassium by diuretics is likely to increase digoxin toxicity.

Psychotropic Drugs

Benzodiazepines are rather commonly prescribed for older patients. Lipophilic benzodiazepines persist for a much longer time in the elderly. Thus, the body burden with chronic ingestion is likely to be much greater than in younger patients. The susceptibility to cognitive impairment is substantial and may compromise the ability of the patient to maintain an independent lifestyle. Because of altered drug disposition in the elderly, there is an increasing belief that the more lipophilic benzodiazepines (e.g., diazepam and flurazepam) are contraindicated in older patients. If prescription of a benzodiazepine is considered necessary, serious consideration should be given to the use of a congener with lower lipophilicity that is biotransformed primarily by conjugation, e.g., oxazepam.

Antidepressant drugs, particularly of the tricyclic type (e.g., amitriptyline and imipramine), are much more likely to cause side effects in older patients. Prominent among the side effects are postural hypotension, anticholinergic activity that can cause or aggravate urinary retention and impair gastrointestinal motility, and sedation.

All CNS-depressant drugs increase the risk of cognitive impairment, falls, and hip fractures. The consequent morbidity and mortality from these side effects should weigh heavily in the decision to prescribe these drugs and the expected benefit:risk ratio.

ADVERSE DRUG REACTIONS AND PATIENT COMPLIANCE

There is ample evidence that appropriately prescribed drug therapy for elderly patients can assist in maintaining an improved quality of life in an independent setting. However, an older patient who has an undesirable experience with a prescribed drug may be reluctant to comply with instructions to continue its use. Because the patient may not wish to offend the physician, this problem may not be communicated between them and the result may be a misinterpretation of the outcome of the prescribed treatment. It has been estimated that up to half of elderly patients are noncompliant with prescribed drug therapy. Thus it is incumbent on the prescriber to simplify dose regimens and communicate effectively the importance of compliance with prescribed therapy in order that outcome is correctly attributed.

Although there has been emphasis on consideration of prescribing habits by the physician as a major contributing factor to drug-related adverse patient events (DRAPEs), the problem of concurrent ingestion of over-the-counter drugs as a confounding factor has been relatively ignored. Older patients commonly ingest multiple vitamins in order to maintain their health. Often, these vitamin preparations contain significant amounts of iron. Recently it has been demonstrated that iron can interact with drugs containing phenolic groups and thus decrease their bioavailability. Important examples of this interaction include iron and α-methyldopa and iron and carbidopa. In the case of α-methyldopa, there is a loss in control of hypertension due to erratic drug absorption. In the case of carbidopa, interaction with concurrent iron ingestion is likely to be reflected by more erratic control of the rigidity and tremor of Parkinson's disease.

SUMMARY OF ISSUES FOR CONSIDERATION IN GERIATRIC DRUG THERAPY

1. Is drug therapy really necessary? Is it possible that the symptoms are due to concurrently prescribed agents or self-medication with over-the-counter drugs? Are alternate treatments with acceptable outcome available to the patient?

2. What are the goals of drug therapy?

3. What other drugs, both prescribed and over-the-counter, is the patient taking which might alter the physician's choice of agent? Is the benefit:risk ratio better for an alternate drug in this pharmacological category in older patients, e.g., a short-acting diuretic in preference to a long-acting one?

4. Is the dose schedule likely to confuse the patient with respect to concurrently ingested drugs? What about the drug formulation and its packaging? Is it convenient for the patient? Will the patient remember the instructions? Does the patient understand the consequences of noncompliance? Has the dose been modified to account for altered body composition and physiological response to the drug effects?

5. Has the physician waited long enough to insure that the patient is at steady-state before increasing the dose or changing the choice of drug therapy?

SUGGESTED READING

Drugs and the elderly (Proceedings of a symposium). J Chronic Dis 1983; 36:1–143.

Grymonpre RE, Mitenko PA, Sitar DS, et al. Drug associated hospital admissions in older patients. J Am Geriatr Soc 1988; 36:1092–1098.

Klotz U, Avant GR, Hoyumpa A, et al. The effects of age and liver disease on the disposition and elimination of diazepam in adult man. J Clin Invest 1975; 55:347–359.

Montamat SC, Cusack BJ, Vestal RE. Management of drug therapy in the elderly. N Engl J Med 1989; 321:303–309.

Ray WA, Griffin MR, Schaffner W, et al. Psychotropic drug use and the risk of hip fracture. N Engl J Med 1987; 316:363–369.

Schmucker DL. Aging and drug disposition. An update. Pharmacol Rev 1985; 37:133–148.

CHAPTER 67

Vitamins

M.J. BAIGENT

GENERAL CONCEPTS

The association between diet and the prevention or cure of a number of specific diseases began with the description by James Linde, in his classic *Treatise on Scurvy* in 1753, of the successful use of lime juice to treat British sailors suffering from scurvy. In the early part of this century, Hopkins and others recognized that animals could not survive on purified diets containing only carbohydrate, fat, and protein. They proposed the existence of "accessory growth factors," present in foods, that were essential for life. By this time three other diseases, beriberi, rickets, and pellagra, had been linked to diet. In 1912, Casimir Funk proposed the "vitamine" theory in which he suggested four different "vitamines," which he presumed were amines, to be essential elements in foods. This term has been retained for historical reasons, although the final "e" was dropped when it became apparent the factors were not amines.

To date, 13 vitamins have been identified as essential for human health. Vitamins are now recognized as a diverse group of organic chemicals that either cannot be synthesized in the body at all, or not in sufficient amounts to maintain normal tissue function. They must be supplied from exogenous sources, i.e., food. More recently it has been recognized that vitamins A and D function as hormones. However, the vitamin designation has been retained since a food source is still required.

Categories of Vitamins

Traditionally, the vitamins have been categorized as water- or fat-soluble on the basis of their solubility in water or fat solvents:

Water-Soluble	*Fat-Soluble*
B vitamins	Vitamins A, D, E, K
Vitamin C	

A number of other compounds normally synthesized in the body become, under some circumstances (e.g., prematurity, total parenteral feeding, genetic aberrations) "conditionally" essential, e.g. choline, carnitine. For other factors claimed to have vitamin function, there is no supportive evidence, e.g. laetrile (vitamin B_{17}), pangamic acid (vitamin B_{15}), orotic acid (vitamin B_{13}), gerovital (vitamin H_3), bioflavonoids. Promotion of this latter group of compounds as vitamins is considered fraudulent.

Nomenclature

The familiar (or alpha) nomenclature of the vitamins designates (in general) the historical order in which the function or structure of the vitamins was elucidated. In some cases (e.g., vitamins E, K, A, B_6), the familiar name is a generic descriptor of a family of chemically related compounds that have comparable biological functions; these members of the same vitamin family are termed "vitamers." Two vitamins, vitamin A and niacin, have precursor forms, β-carotene and tryptophan, respectively, which can be metabolized to the active form of the vitamin.

The official chemical nomenclature of the vitamins is established and periodically revised as appropriate by the International Union of Pure and Applied Chemists, the International Union of Biochemists, and the Committee on Nomenclature of the American Institute of Nutrition.

Recommended Intakes

Many countries, and scientific committees of international bodies such as the World Health Organization, have established recommended intakes for most of the essential nutrients (energy, protein, vitamins, minerals, and trace elements). These recommendations are revised periodically as new evidence of their physiological relevance becomes available. In formulating these recommendations, it is assumed that diets will be based on a variety of foods so that even essential nutrients for which no specific recommendations have been established will be provided. Although a consistent daily intake of the essential nutrients is preferable, it is more practical and quite adequate to ensure that the daily intake averaged over a short period of time is at the recommended level, i.e., as short as 3 days for nutrients with fast turnover rates to several weeks or months for nutrients having a slower turnover.

Recommended intakes for the essential nutrients are based on the average physiological requirements of normal healthy individuals, measured experimentally and from population studies. These requirements are the amounts that will prevent a nutrient deficiency and will allow for modest tissue stores. To these requirements is added a "safety factor," which allows for individual variability within a population. If the recommended intakes are set at two standard deviations above the average requirement, the physiological needs of 97.5% of normal individuals are met. This means that the recommended intakes are well in excess of the requirements for most normal healthy people. They are not intended to be sufficient for therapeutic purposes, however, and they do not allow for losses of nutrients during commercial and shelf storage and processing of food. Specific recommendations are given for the different age groups and sexes, and for pregnancy and lactation.

Recommended intakes for the vitamins as published by the governments of the United States and Canada, and by the World Health Organization, are presented in Tables 67-1, 67-2, and 67-3. Variations in recommendations among these three dietary standards reflect differences in interpretation of the data used to establish the values rather than differences in physiological requirements among nationalities. For vitamins not listed, a specific recommended intake has not been set.

Vitamin Deficiencies

A vitamin deficiency may be classified as a primary deficiency, i.e., an inadequate dietary intake, or as a secondary deficiency due to malabsorption, drug–nutrient interactions, or increased vitamin needs due to physiological stress or disease.

Inadequate dietary intake

In "westernized" cultures, deficiency may occur in individuals who are dieting vigorously to lose weight; among the poor who have insufficient incomes to purchase or prepare foods; in those who do not appreciate the need for, or who have lifestyles incompatible with, balanced diets (e.g., "bachelor's scurvy"); in those who respond to gastrointestinal or other symptoms by restricting their diet without medical advice; or in those who acquire restrictive or bizarre eating patterns from religious or philosophical convictions. Loss of appetite, poor dentition, and inadequate cooking facilities are common causes among the elderly. In poorly industrialized and economically depressed areas, extreme poverty and unsatisfactory food production and/or distribution are major factors. In some cultures, weaning practices often do not provide sufficient nutrients to support optimal growth and health of the young child.

Drug–nutrient interactions

A large number of therapeutic agents interfere with absorption and increase the rate of turnover of some vitamins. Addiction to, or excessive use of, common substances such as alcohol, caffeine, and nicotine also interfere with vitamin metabolism. Little is known about the specific effects of illicit drugs, as distinct from the effects of poor dietary habits in many heavy users.

Increased vitamin needs

Normal physiological processes such as growth, pregnancy, and lactation impose higher requirements for vitamins. Increased needs for some vitamins may also occur in postsurgical, burn, or trauma patients and in a number of disease processes.

There is now convincing evidence that intakes above the recommended levels of some vitamins, especially folate, are effective in reducing the incidence of neural-tube defects in infants if taken by the mother during the initial months of the pregnancy. Although the evidence is less clear-cut, there appears

Table 67-1 Recommended Dietary Allowances (RDA) for Healthy People in the United States (Daily Intake)*

Category	Age (years) or Condition	Weight (kg)	Fat-Soluble Vitamins				Water-Soluble Vitamins						
			Vitamin A (μg RE)	Vitamin D (μg)	Vitamin E (mg α-TE)	Vitamin K (μg)	Vitamin C (mg)	Thiamin (mg)	Riboflavin (mg)	Niacin (mg NE)	Vitamin B_6 (mg)	Folate (μg)	Vitamin B_{12} (μg)
Infants	0.0–0.5	6	375	7.5	3	5	30	0.3	0.4	5	0.3	25	0.3
	0.5–1.0	9	375	10	4	10	35	0.4	0.5	6	0.6	35	0.5
Children	1–3	13	400	10	6	15	40	0.7	0.8	9	1.0	50	0.7
	4–6	20	500	10	7	20	45	0.9	1.1	12	1.1	75	1.0
	7–10	28	700	10	7	30	45	1.0	1.2	13	1.4	100	1.4
Males	11–14	45	1000	10	10	45	50	1.3	1.5	17	1.7	150	2.0
	15–18	66	1000	10	10	65	60	1.5	1.8	20	2.0	200	2.0
	19–24	72	1000	10	10	70	60	1.5	1.7	19	2.0	200	2.0
	25–50	79	1000	5	10	80	60	1.5	1.7	19	2.0	200	2.0
	51+	77	1000	5	10	80	60	1.2	1.4	15	2.0	200	2.0
Females	11–14	46	800	10	8	45	50	1.1	1.3	15	1.4	150	2.0
	15–18	55	800	10	8	55	60	1.1	1.3	15	1.5	180	2.0
	19–24	58	800	10	8	60	60	1.1	1.3	15	1.6	180	2.0
	25–50	63	800	5	8	65	60	1.1	1.3	15	1.6	180	2.0
	51+	65	800	5	8	65	60	1.0	1.2	13	1.6	180	2.0
Pregnant			800	10	10	65	70	1.5	1.6	17	2.2	400	2.2
Lactating	1st 6 months		1300	10	12	65	95	1.6	1.8	20	2.1	280	2.6
	2nd 6 months		1200	10	11	65	90	1.6	1.7	20	2.1	260	2.6

*RE, TE, and NE are defined in text.

Excerpted from National Academy of Sciences, Washington DC, 1989. Recommended Dietary Allowances, 10th revised ed. Washington, DC: National Academy of Sciences, 1989.

to be an inverse relationship between the intake of a number of vitamins and the incidence of some types of cancer. The vitamins so implicated (retinol, β-carotene, vitamin E, vitamin C) are thought to exert antioxidant, and hence protective, effects upon the cells and tissues. These protective effects may require a new perspective to be taken of vitamin requirements.

Megavitamin Therapy

The basis for advocating the consumption of very large doses of vitamins is the belief that the recommended intakes are inadequate for some individuals and that greatly increasing the intake of certain vitamins will overcome symptoms purportedly due to a vitamin deficiency not previously recognized as such. In the case of the water-soluble vitamins used in some megavitamin therapies, it has been shown that intake greatly in excess of the recommended intake leads to excretion of the excess vitamin. There-

fore, provided that vitamin stores are normal, increased intake does not result in increased tissue or plasma levels. In general, it would be fair to state that megavitamin therapy is difficult to rationalize on scientific grounds; its enthusiastic acceptance in some quarters is based largely on anecdotal evidence. It is probably fortunate that compliance with some of the recommended regimens is variable and that on the whole the vitamins involved have low toxicity. Nevertheless, niacin and, more recently, pyridoxine have demonstrated toxicity. It is possible, however, that some of the observed megavitamin effects are pharmacological in nature (rather than normal physiological effects of the vitamin), and one must await the outcome of research in this area. At this time, megavitamin therapy is not a scientifically accepted medical practice.

FAT-SOLUBLE VITAMINS

Vitamin A

Structure, dietary sources, and recommended intake

Vitamin A, as the preformed vitamin, exists as all-*trans* retinol (the physiologically active form; Fig. 67-1), as long-chain fatty acyl esters of retinol (the main storage form in tissues), and as retinal (the active form in the retina). In the cells, retinol is converted to retinoic acid, also considered to be physiologically active. The *cis*-isomers have no significant vitamin activity. Vitamin A activity is also provided by β-carotene (provitamin A), which can be converted to retinol. Other members of the carotenoid group have marginal activity.

Preformed vitamin A, as retinyl esters, is found only in animal products, the major sources being liver, fish liver oils, milk and dairy products, egg yolk, and fortified margarine. β-Carotene occurs in

Table 67-2 Recommended Nutrient Intakes (RNI) for Vitamins for Canadians (Daily Rates)*

			Fat-Soluble Vitamins			Water-Soluble Vitamins					
Age	Sex	Weight (kg)	Vita-min A (RE)	Vita-min D (µg)	Vita-min E (mg)	Vitamin C (mg)	Folate (µg)	Vitamin B_{12} (µg)	Thia-min (mg)	Ribo-flavin (mg)	Niacin (NE)
Months											
0–4	Both	6.0	400	10	3	20†	25	0.3	0.3	0.3	4
5–12	Both	9.0	400	10	3	20†	40	0.4	0.4	0.5	7
Years											
1	Both	11	400	10	3	20†	40	0.5	0.5	0.6	8
2–3	Both	14	400	5	4	20†	50	0.6	0.6	0.7	9
4–6	Both	18	500	5	5	25†	70	0.8	0.7	0.9	13
7–9	M	25	700	2.5	7	25†	90	1.0	0.9	1.1	16
	F	25	700	2.5	6	25†	90	1.0	0.8	1.0	14
10–12	M	34	800	2.5	8	25†	120	1.0	1.0	1.3	18
	F	36	800	2.5	7	25†	130	1.0	0.9	1.1	16
13–15	M	50	900	2.5	9	30†	175	1.0	1.1	1.4	20
	F	48	800	2.5	7	30†	170	1.0	0.9	1.1	16
16–18	M	62	1000	2.5	10	40†	220	1.0	1.3	1.6	23
	F	53	800	2.5	7	30†	190	1.0	0.8	1.1	15
19–24	M	71	1000	2.5	10	40†	220	1.0	1.2	1.5	22
	F	58	800	2.5	7	30†	180	1.0	0.8	1.1	15
25–49	M	74	1000	2.5	9	40†	230	1.0	1.1	1.4	19
	F	59	800	2.5	6	30†	185	1.0	0.8	1.0	14
50–74	M	73	1000	5	7	40†	230	1.0	0.9	1.2	16
	F	63	800	5	6	30†	195	1.0	0.8	1.0	14
75+	M	69	1000	5	6	40†	215	1.0	0.8	1.0	14
	F	64	800	5	5	30†	200	1.0	0.8	1.0	14
Pregnancy (additional)											
1st trimester			0	2.5	2	0†	200	1.2	0.1	0.1	1
2nd trimester			0	2.5	2	10†	200	1.2	0.1	0.3	2
3rd trimester			0	2.5	2	10†	200	1.2	0.1	0.3	2
Lactation (additional)			400	2.5	3	25†	100	0.2	0.2	0.4	3

*Pyridoxine: 0.015 mg/g protein eaten.

†Smokers should increase vitamin C intake by 50%.

Excerpted from Health and Welfare Canada, Ottawa, 1990.

Table 67-3 World Health Organization Recommended Intakes for Vitamins per Day*

Age (years)	Weight (kg)	Vitamin A as RE (µg)	Vitamin D (µg)	Thiamin (mg)	Riboflavin (mg)	Niacin (mg)	Folate (µg)	Vitamin B₁₂ (µg)	Ascorbic Acid (mg)
Children									
<1	7.3	350	10.0	0.3	0.5	5.4	16–32	0.1	20
1–3	13.4	400	10.0	0.5	0.8	9.0	50	0.5	20
4–6	20.2	400	10.0	0.7	1.1	12.1	50	0.9	20
7–9	28.1	400	2.5	0.9	1.3	14.5	102	0.9	20
Male adolescents									
10–12	36.9	500	2.5	1.0	1.6	17.2	102	1.0	20
13–15	51.3	600	2.5	1.2	1.7	19.1	170	1.0	30
16–19	62.9	600	2.5	1.2	1.8	20.3	200	1.0	30
Female adolescents									
10–12	38.0	500	2.5	0.9	1.4	15.5	102	1.0	20
13–15	49.9	600	2.5	1.0	1.5	16.4	170	1.0	30
16–19	54.4	500	2.5	0.9	1.4	15.2	170	1.0	30
Adult men (moderately active)	65.0	600	2.5	1.2	1.8	19.8	200	1.0	30
Adult women (moderately active)	55.0	500	2.5	0.9	1.3	14.5	170	1.0	30
Pregnancy (later half)		600	10.0	+0.1	+0.2	+2.3	370–470	1.4	50
Lactation (first 6 months)		850	10.0	+0.2	+0.4	+3.7	270	1.3	50

*The 1988 FAO/WHO report uses "safe level of intake" in place of (but synonymous with) "recommended intakes" as the term to describe appropriate dietary intakes.

Adapted from Passmore R, Nicol BM, Rao MN. *WHO Monograph Series No. 61*, Geneva, 1974 (vitamin D, thiamin, riboflavin, niacin, vitamin C), and *Report of a Joint FAO/WHO Expert Consultation, FAO Food and Nutrition Series No. 23*, 1988 (vitamin A, folate, vitamin B₁₂).

plant foods such as green and yellow vegetables and yellow fruits.

Recommended intakes (see Tables 67-1, 67-2, and 67-3) are expressed as Retinol Equivalents (RE). In humans with a mixed diet, the activity of β-carotene is approximately one-sixth that of retinol because of incomplete absorption and inefficient conversion to retinol.

$$1 \text{ RE} = 1 \text{ µg retinol}$$
$$= 6 \text{ µg } \beta\text{-carotene}$$
$$= 12 \text{ µg other carotenes}$$

Older usage expressed the activity of vitamin A in U.S.P. units or International Units (IU). These were based upon biological activity in the vitamin A-deficient rat, and 1 IU = 0.3 µg of retinol or 0.6 µg of β-carotene. Thus,

$$1 \text{ RE} = 3.33 \text{ IU retinol}$$
$$= 10.0 \text{ IU } \beta\text{-carotene}$$

One-third to one-half of the daily intake of vitamin A in mixed diets is β-carotene. In strict vegetarian diets containing no animal foods, β-carotene is virtually the sole source of vitamin A.

Pharmacokinetics

The preformed vitamin is well absorbed from the upper intestine by a carrier-mediated process at low intakes and by diffusion at higher doses. β-Carotene is cleaved to retinol mainly in the intestinal mucosal cells during absorption, and to a lesser extent by liver and other tissues. Bile salts enhance retinol absorption and are required for the absorption of β-carotene. Both vitamin A and β-carotene are trans-

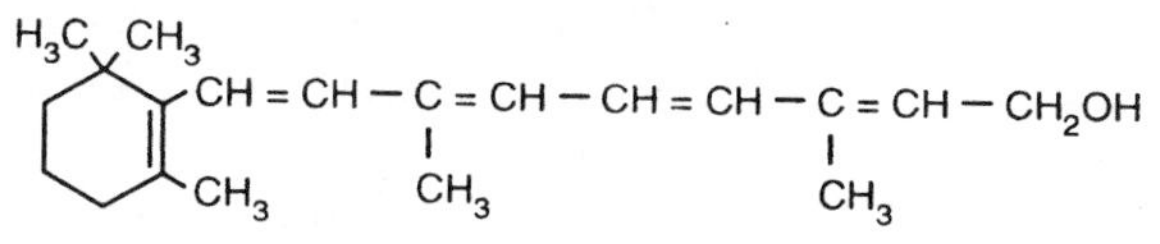

Vitamin A_1 (Retinol)

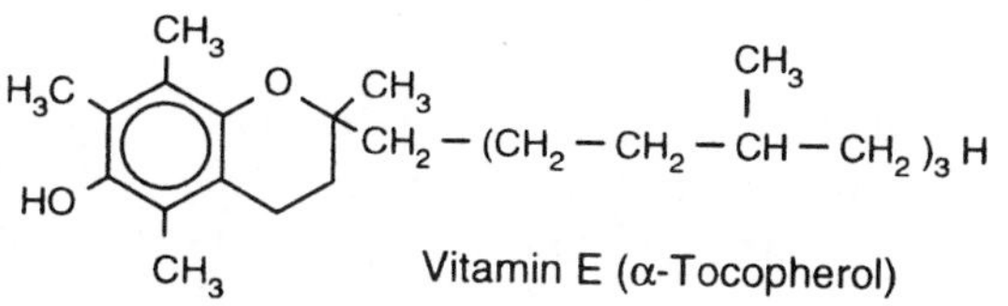

Vitamin E (α-Tocopherol)

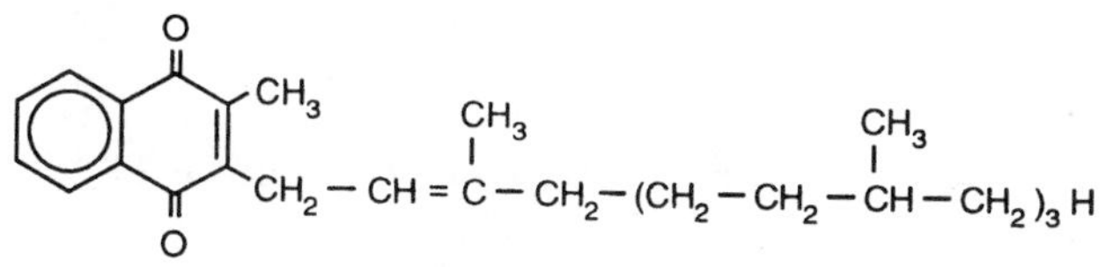

Vitamin K_1

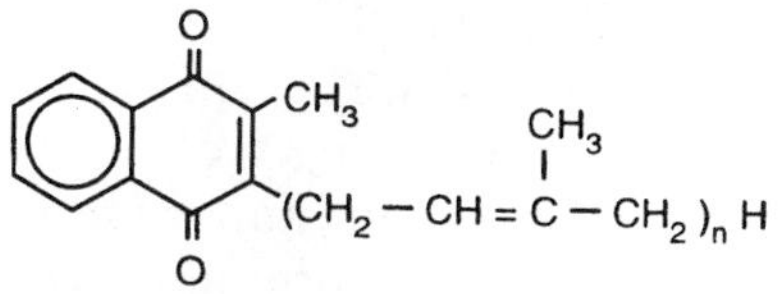

Vitamin K_2

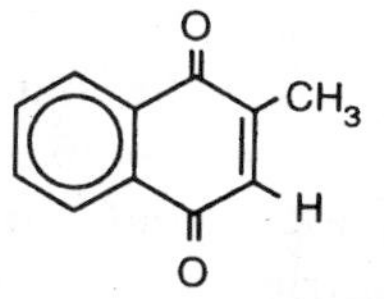

Vitamin K_3 (Menadione)

Figure 67-1. Structural formulae of the fat-soluble vitamins A, E, and K.

ported from the intestine in the chylomicra via the lymph, in a manner identical to that seen in fat absorption.

The liver is the major storage organ and it can sequester very large amounts of vitamin A as the ester. Smaller amounts are found in kidney, adipose tissue, and lung. Stored vitamin A is released from the liver into the plasma as retinol, bound to a specific retinol-binding protein, by a tightly regulated process to maintain a constant supply of retinol to the target tissues. Normal plasma retinol levels are maintained at 30–70 μg/dL (1.05–2.45 μmol/L) and are not significantly reduced even in vitamin A deficiency until depletion of liver stores is well advanced. When large amounts of vitamin A, in excess of the normal requirement, are taken in chronically, they are not excreted but are stored in the liver and can ultimately exceed the hepatic storage capacity.

Physiology

In the retina of the eye, all-*trans* retinol is converted to the aldehyde and isomerized to 11-*cis* retinal, which then combines with the protein, opsin, in the rod cells of the retina to produce rhodopsin. This compound is responsible for vision in dim light. In the cone cells, iodopsin is similarly formed and is responsible for daylight vision.

Retinol and retinoic acid, a metabolite of retinol, are required for normal cell differentiation, particularly of the mucus-secreting epithelial cells. In the absence of retinol, mucus-secreting cells are replaced by keratin-producing cells in many body tissues. This action may be exerted via the influence of retinol on gene expression in the nucleus. Retinol also serves as a carrier for mannose to effect its incorporation into cell-surface glycoproteins, which appear to serve a number of functions including that of regulation of cell differentiation. The requirement for vitamin A in normal reproduction, bone development and growth, as well as its influence on the immune system, may be allied to the general function of cell differentiation.

Deficiency

Vitamin A deficiency is most prevalent in preschool children in Southeast Asia, and parts of Africa and South America, because of poor intakes of both vitamin A and carotene. Also at risk are the newborn (especially the premature infant), since liver stores of vitamin A at birth are low. In the alcoholic individual, liver structure is affected (see Chapter 46) and storage of vitamin A is compromised. In the nonalcoholic adult, vitamin A deficiency occurs largely as a consequence of gastrointestinal abnormalities resulting in fat malabsorption. The major deficiency signs include night blindness (nyctalopia) and xerophthalmia, the latter characterized by a progressive xerosis of the conjunctiva and cornea of the eye culminating in disintegration of the cornea and extrusion of the lens, and hence irreparable blindness. There is also keratinization of other epithelial cells in the bronchorespiratory, genitourinary, and gastrointestinal tracts, and in sweat glands, leading to an increased frequency of infections in these tissues.

Therapeutic use

Supplementation is necessary only to treat frank deficiency or as a preventive measure in pregnancy, lactation, or infancy when dietary intakes are obviously inadequate. In the last case, the supplement plus usual dietary intake should not exceed the recommended intake. In areas where intake of vitamin A is chronically inadequate, prophylactic intramuscular injections of 30–120 mg retinol given every 3–6 months to infants and small children have proven effective in reducing blindness induced by vitamin A deficiency.

Vitamin A palmitate, and more recently isomers of retinoic acid, have proved effective in the treatment of various skin disorders, including acne vulgaris and psoriasis, albeit not without toxic side effects.

Toxicity

Vitamin A is highly toxic when taken in large amounts, either acutely or chronically. Hypervitaminosis A occurs most frequently as a result of over-enthusiastic supplementation of children's diets or self-medication, but it may also result from the excessive consumption of retinol-rich foodstuffs (e.g., a single serving of polar bear liver, or chronic intakes of large portions of chicken or beef liver).

Acute toxicity may result from a single dose of about 200 mg (666,000 IU) of vitamin A in adults, or half of this amount in children. Toxicity signs include headache, nausea and vomiting, increased cerebrospinal fluid pressure, blurred vision, and bulging of the fontanelle in infants. Larger doses cause extensive peeling of the skin.

Chronic toxicity may follow repeated intakes of vitamin A over long periods of time (3–6 months or more) in amounts greater than 10 times the recommended intake. There is an extensive array of symptoms that vary with the individual, the more serious including hepatotoxicity (fibrosis, cirrhosis, central vein sclerosis, portal hypertension), hypercalcemia, hyperlipemia, spontaneous abortions, and fetal malformations. Although fatalities are not common, they have occurred; for example, a death from apparent vitamin A toxicity has been reported in a newborn receiving 25 mg/day for 11 days.

In both acute and chronic toxicity, the symptoms are transient and disappear after withdrawal of the supplement. Toxic dose levels also vary considerably because of marked variation in individual sensitivity to large intakes.

Retinoic acid isomers, e.g., etretinate and isotretinoin, used in the treatment of skin disorders, cause minor side effects including dryness of mucous membranes and conjunctivitis, but more importantly are teratogenic if taken in early pregnancy.

Large intakes of β-carotene produce an orange coloration of the skin. Hypercarotenemia is a benign condition that does not result in vitamin A toxicity because of the slow conversion of β-carotene to retinol.

Vitamin D

Structure, dietary sources, and recommended intake

The vitamin exists in two major precursor forms, 7-dehydrocholesterol and ergosterol, which are converted to their vitamin forms cholecalciferol (vitamin D_3) and ergocalciferol (vitamin D_2) respectively, upon exposure to ultraviolet radiation. This photobiosynthesis of vitamin D_3, occurring in the skin upon exposure to sunlight, is of major importance in humans. The physiologically active form appears to be 1,25-dihydroxycholecalciferol or calcitriol (Fig. 67-2). Vitamin D levels are particularly high in fish liver oils. Few other natural foods contain the vitamin in significant amounts, and it has therefore been necessary to add the vitamin to some foods in countries where the amount of sunlight is inadequate. The policy governing the choice of foods that may be fortified varies in different countries. In North America milk, margarine, butter, cheese, and infant foods are fortified with vitamin D_3.

In climates where exposure to sun is year round, biosynthesis of vitamin D in the skin provides sufficient vitamin. In northern climates or in areas with heavy air pollution that occludes ultraviolet penetration, a dietary or supplemental source must be provided.

Recommended intakes are given in Tables 67-1, 67-2, and 67-3 and are expressed in micrograms vitamin D_3. As with vitamin A, older usage was in International Units; 1 IU of vitamin D_3 = 0.025 μg.

Pharmacokinetics

Both vitamins D_2 and D_3 are absorbed from the intestine, the latter more completely. As with other

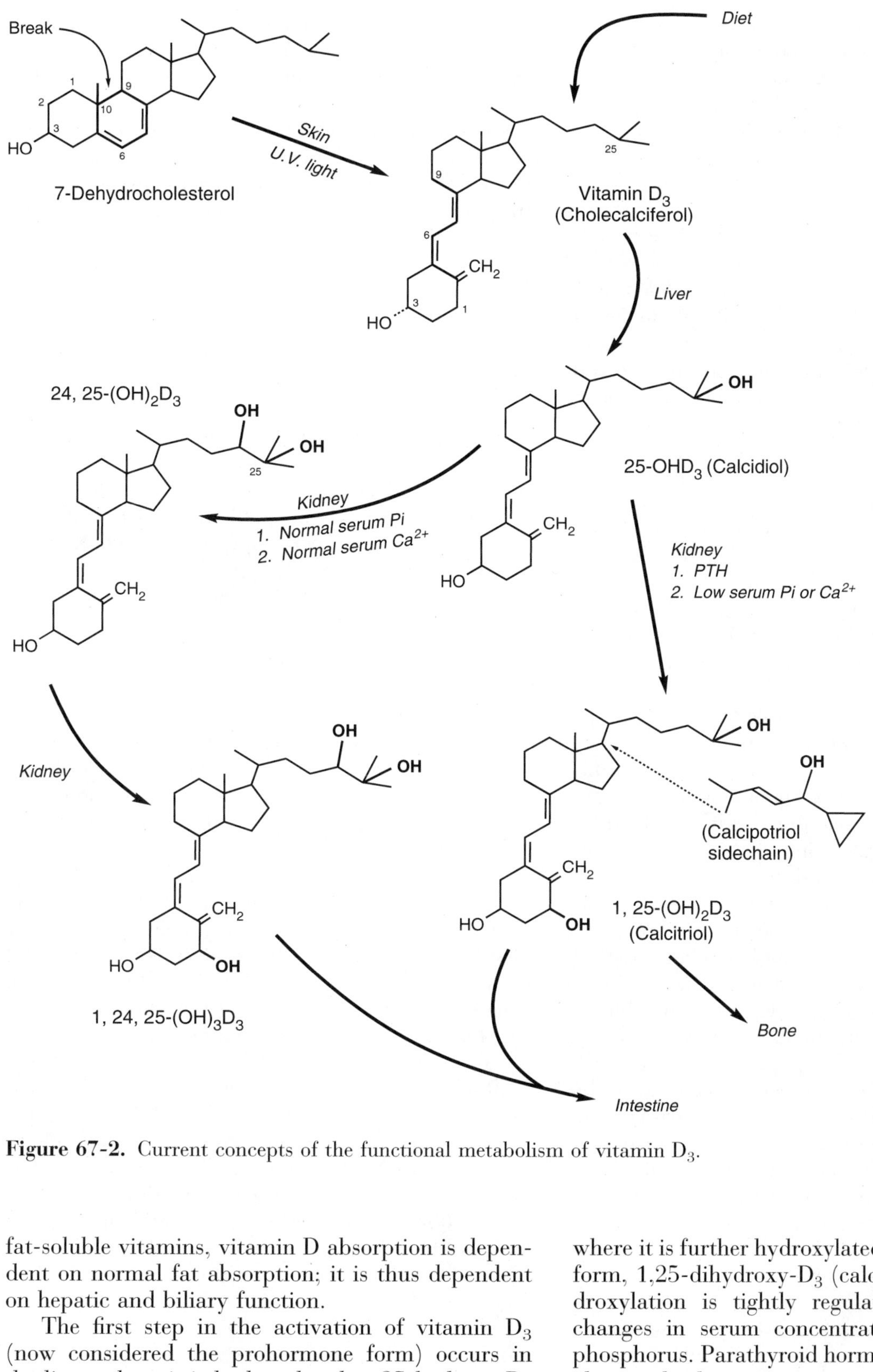

Figure 67-2. Current concepts of the functional metabolism of vitamin D_3.

fat-soluble vitamins, vitamin D absorption is dependent on normal fat absorption; it is thus dependent on hepatic and biliary function.

The first step in the activation of vitamin D_3 (now considered the prohormone form) occurs in the liver, where it is hydroxylated to 25-hydroxy-D_3 (calcidiol). From there it circulates to the kidney,

where it is further hydroxylated to its active hormone form, 1,25-dihydroxy-D_3 (calcitriol). This latter hydroxylation is tightly regulated and responds to changes in serum concentrations of calcium and phosphorus. Parathyroid hormone and calcitonin are also involved.

There is no significant storage of vitamin D in

the liver (as occurs with vitamin A). It is distributed among various tissues in the body; adipose and muscle tissue are considered the major storage sites in humans. Excretion of vitamin D and its metabolites occurs primarily in the feces with the aid of bile salts. (The details of the functional metabolism of vitamin D_3 are shown in Fig. 67-2.)

Physiology

Vitamin D has a primary role in the homeostatic regulation of serum calcium and phosphate levels through the promotion of intestinal absorption and renal reabsorption of calcium and phosphorus, and the resorption of calcium and phosphate from bone (see also Chapter 68). Maintenance of serum calcium levels permits mineralization and remodeling of bone and the maintenance of normal excitability in the central autonomic and somatic nervous systems.

Because it is produced exclusively in the kidney in response to hypocalcemia and hypophosphatemia and exerts its function on specific target tissues, vitamin D is considered to be a hormone. The finding of high-affinity receptors for 1,25-dihydroxy-D_3 in a number of tissues (e.g., pancreas, skin, muscle, brain, and hematopoietic cells) not related to calcium homeostasis suggests additional roles for vitamin D, e.g., in cell growth and differentiation.

Calcipotriol (calcipotriene), an analog of vitamin D_3 with a modified side-chain containing a 24-hydroxyl group and a cyclopropyl group formed by carbons 25, 26, and 27, binds strongly to the D_3 receptor on keratinocytes in skin but has only about 0.5% of the activity of D_3 on calcium and phosphorus metabolism. However, it is very potent in suppressing proliferation of keratinocytes and inducing normal differentiation; the mechanism is not yet known with certainty, but D_3 and calcipotriol are both able to decrease the binding of interleukin-8 to human keratinocytes and increase the expression of certain cell adhesion molecules. These properties have led to the clinical use of calcipotriol to treat psoriasis. Despite the low potency of calcipotriol in promoting calcium absorption, if excessive amounts are applied to the skin there can be enough transdermal absorption to cause hypercalcemia.

Deficiency

Vitamin D deficiency occurs mainly as a consequence of inadequate exposure to sunlight and/or dietary deficiency. It can also occur as a result of an increased requirement (e.g., multiple pregnancies, lactation) or of a deficit in the 1-hydroxylation pathway of 25-hydroxy-D_3. Deficiency results in rickets in children and osteomalacia in adults as a consequence of decreased mineralization of bone and teeth. The matrix is decalcified, so the bone is softened and may become grossly deformed. Rickets was formerly a major problem in Canada and northern regions of the United States because of insufficient sunlight during the winter but has been largely eliminated by vitamin D fortification of milk.

Therapeutic use

Rickets due to inadequate exposure to sunlight can be reversed by 10 μg vitamin D daily. Fully developed rickets and osteomalacia may require dosages of 0.1–1.0 mg vitamin D daily, depending on the etiology of the disease. Since 45–50 μg vitamin D daily can lead to hypervitaminosis D, high-potency preparations are only available by prescription.

A form of vitamin D-dependent rickets that has a genetic rather than dietary etiology will respond to 1.25–2.50 mg (50,000–100,000 IU) of vitamin D daily.

Toxicity

An excessive intake of vitamin D leading to toxicity is unlikely from natural food sources but can result from overzealous use of vitamin D supplements. For this reason, fortification of foods with vitamin D is regulated in most countries.

Symptoms of vitamin D toxicity include fatigue, headache, diarrhea, and hypercalcemia, which may lead to calcium deposition in kidney, heart, lungs, blood vessels, and skin. Hypercalcemia may also lead to an arrest of growth that cannot be fully reversed. This may be associated with irreversible effects on calcitonin production (see Chapter 68).

The amount of vitamin D that produces toxicity varies widely. Acute toxicity may occur after ingestion of 25–75 μg/kg (1000–3000 IU/kg). Chronic toxicity in adults has been seen with doses as low as 250 μg (10,000 IU) daily over several months but more commonly occurs with doses approaching 1250 μg (50,000 IU) or more over several years. Infants and children, and the elderly, may be sensitive to chronic intakes as low as 50 μg (2000 IU) per day.

Vitamin E

Structure, dietary sources, and recommended intake

Several tocopherols are known to have vitamin E activity. The highest biological activity is shown by *d*-α-tocopherol (RRR-α-tocopherol; Fig. 67-1). Animal tissues contain primarily this form. The vitamin is found mainly in plant products; the richest sources are vegetable oils and wheat germ.

Recommended intakes of vitamin E (see Tables 67-1 and 67-2) are given either as *d*-α-Tocopherol Equivalents (U.S. RDA) or in milligrams (Canadian RNI). The older terminology for vitamin E activity is the International Unit (IU): 1 IU = 1 mg *dl*-α-tocopheryl acetate (all-*rac*-α-tocopheryl acetate), the commercially synthesized form, or 1.49 mg *d*-α-tocopherol, the naturally occurring form.

Pharmacokinetics

Absorption of vitamin E, like that of other fat-soluble vitamins, depends on the integrity of fat-absorption processes in the intestine. At normal intakes, approximately 50% of dietary tocopherols are absorbed. Efficiency of absorption falls to less than 10% with pharmacological doses, e.g., 200 mg or more. Tocopherols are carried in the blood by plasma β-lipoproteins. Liver and muscle are the major storage sites. Although large amounts are also deposited in the adipose tissue, tocopherol is mobilized only very slowly from adipocytes.

Physiology

Vitamin E is an antioxidant and probably acts as a free radical scavenger in cell membranes to protect membrane polyunsaturated fatty acids from peroxidation. It appears to act in concert with other antioxidant systems in the cell, e.g., selenium-dependent glutathione peroxidase, superoxide dismutase, catalase, and ascorbic acid.

Vitamin E not located in the membranes likely serves as a protective antioxidant for other easily oxidized lipid-soluble compounds such as vitamin A.

It has also been suggested that vitamin E has a specific function as a repressor, regulating the synthesis of specific enzymes.

Deficiency

Vitamin E is accepted as an essential nutrient for humans, but although deficiency states have been clearly defined in animals, this is a subject of much debate in human health and nutrition.

Adults rarely develop a vitamin E deficiency due to poor dietary intake. However, individuals with chronic fat malabsorption or a genetic deficiency of β-lipoprotein, the plasma carrier for vitamin E, are at risk. In these individuals erythrocyte stability is diminished, resulting in decreased erythrocyte survival, although severe anemia does not usually ensue.

Premature newborns have limited tissue stores of vitamin E at birth and have intestinal malabsorption for the first few weeks of life. Decreased erythrocyte survival in these infants leads to a severe hemolytic anemia. In both children and adults, severe fat malabsorption results in a progressive neurological disorder that has been attributed to vitamin E deficiency.

In many animal species, vitamin E deficiency leads to male sterility and fetal reabsorption or abortion, muscular dystrophy, and pathological changes in cardiac and vascular smooth muscle. In humans these syndromes are not observed in vitamin E deficiency, and evidence to support the efficacy of vitamin E in treating these disorders is largely anecdotal or based on small, poorly organized clinical trials.

A number of international comparative studies indicate an inverse correlation between mean intake of α-tocopherol and incidence of coronary heart disease. However, the results of large-scale double-blind placebo-controlled studies of the effect of vitamin E supplements on the risk of coronary heart disease are still controversial.

Therapeutic use

Correction of the deficiencies noted above may require up to 300 mg vitamin E. Vitamin E in high doses (about 300 mg) also appears to be effective in treating intermittent claudication in adults and to ameliorate oxygen-induced retrolental fibroplasia in premature infants. Claims for its efficacy in treating a myriad of other conditions (the effects of aging, cardiovascular disease, sexual dysfunction, etc.) are largely unfounded.

Toxicity

Vitamin E has extremely low toxicity, producing only mild gastrointestinal upsets or fatigue in some individuals. However, it may exacerbate a vitamin K deficiency, especially in those individuals on anticoagulant therapy with coumarin compounds.

Vitamin K

Structure, dietary sources, and recommended intake

Vitamin K (Fig. 67-1) exists in two forms, one of plant origin (phylloquinone, or K_1), and the other of bacterial origin (a series of menaquinones, K_2). A number of synthetic quinones have vitamin K-like activity, of which the most important is menadione (K_3). Sources in the diet are green leafy vegetables, cheese, egg yolk, and liver.

One-half of the requirement for vitamin K may be met by intestinal bacterial synthesis. The U.S. Recommended Dietary Allowance is given in Table 67-1. Canada and FAO/WHO have not yet set a recommended intake.

Pharmacokinetics

Vitamin K is readily absorbed by the usual pathways of fat absorption, and it is therefore dependent on the presence of bile salts. There is only limited tissue storage of vitamin K, and the stores can be depleted in 10–20 days.

Physiology

Vitamin K is required for the γ-carboxylation (activation) of glutamic acid residues in a number of inactive precursors of biologically important proteins. The best known of these are prothrombin and at least seven other factors involved in the coagulation of blood (see Chapter 42).

Other vitamin K-dependent proteins have been identified, e.g., osteocalcin in bone and proteins in plasma and kidney cortex. The common feature of these proteins is their capacity to bind calcium, presumably at the γ-carboxyglutamyl sites.

Oral anticoagulants of the coumarin class (including warfarin; see Chapter 42) are vitamin K antagonists and are useful in reducing thrombus formation in patients at risk of intravascular clotting, as in ischemic heart disease, nonhemorrhagic strokes, etc. Paradoxically, vitamin K in megadose amounts has been reported to prolong the prothrombin time; a dose of 1200 IU may potentiate the anticoagulant effects of the coumarin drugs and cause bleeding.

Deficiency

Requirements are easily met in the diet and may also be met in part from synthesis by intestinal bacteria.

In adults, deficiency is usually secondary to malabsorption or the administration of a vitamin K antagonist. In deficiency there is an increased prothrombin time and a tendency to hemorrhage.

Newborn infants, particularly premature ones, are susceptible to a vitamin K deficiency, "hemorrhagic disease of the newborn." Little vitamin crosses the placenta to the fetus, and the gut is sterile for the first few days of life. Human breast milk is sterile and contains little vitamin K, placing the breast-fed infant at further risk. Therefore, vitamin K is usually administered prophylactically to the newborn.

Therapeutic use

The only rational uses of vitamin K are to increase the hepatic biosynthesis of clotting factors, especially as an antidotal agent in oral anticoagulant therapy (see Chapter 42) and in the prevention of hemorrhagic disease of the newborn.

Toxicity

Excessive doses of menadione (K_3) produce a hemolytic tendency and kernicterus in infants. It irritates mucous membranes and may depress liver function. Vitamin K_1 does not have these effects and, moreover, it is nontoxic in animals. In humans, flushing, dyspnea, and death have occurred, but these may have been due to other constituents in the pharmaceutical dosage forms of vitamin K_1 used in those cases.

WATER-SOLUBLE VITAMINS

B-Complex Vitamins

Thiamin (vitamin B_1)

Structure, dietary sources, and recommended intake. Thiamin (Fig. 67-3) consists of a pyrimidine and a thiazole moiety. It is widely distributed in foods but most contain low concentrations. The major dietary sources are yeasts (brewer's or baker's yeast), pork, beef, liver, wheat germ, whole or enriched cereals, and grains and legumes.

The vitamin is easily destroyed by heat (during cooking), in alkaline medium, and by oxidation or by sulfites added in food processing. Thiamin is also destroyed by agents occurring naturally in foods, e.g., heat-labile thiaminases (in raw fish), or heat-stable thiamin antagonists such as polyphenols in tea, ferns, and betel nut.

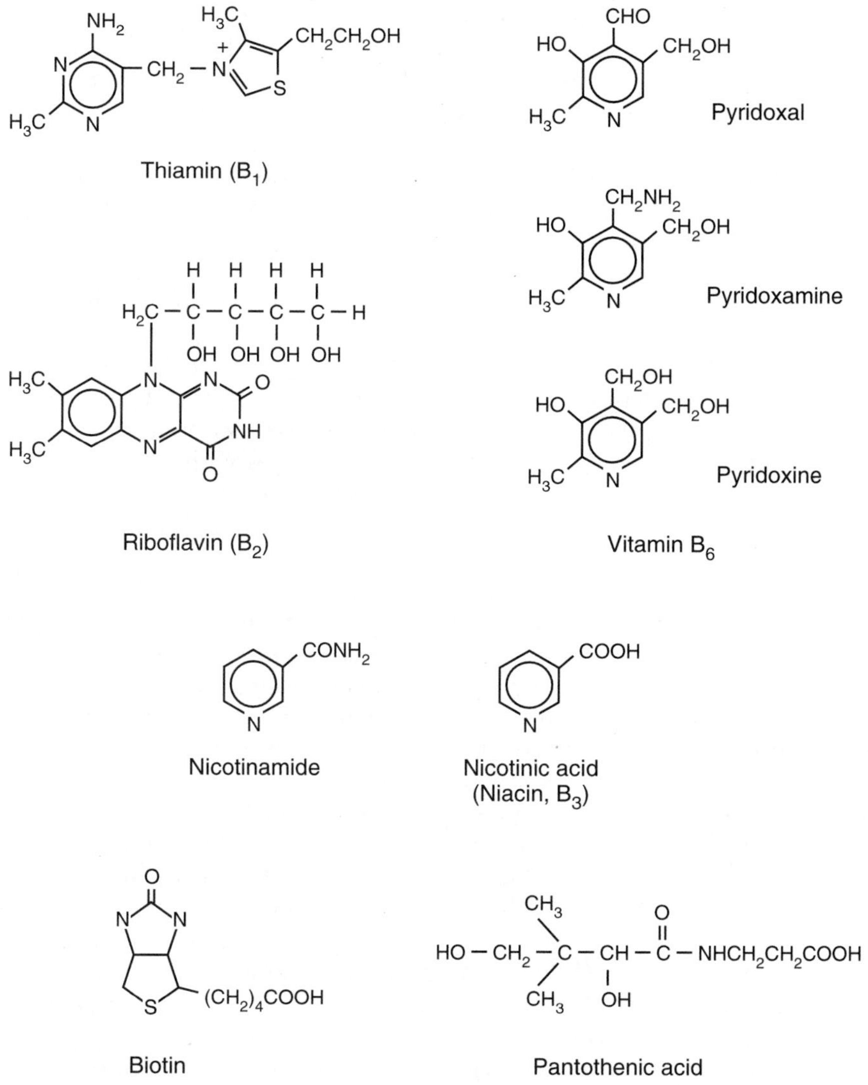

Figure 67-3. Structural formulae of the water-soluble vitamins of the B complex.

Recommended intakes (see Tables 67-1, 67-2, and 67-3) are based on energy intake. In instances of very low energy consumption, the thiamin intake should not fall below the amount required for 2000 kcal (1.0 mg/day, United States; 0.8 mg/day, Canada and WHO).

Pharmacokinetics. Thiamin is absorbed from the upper small intestine by a carrier-mediated active transport process when intakes are less than 5 mg/day (well above the recommended intake). At higher intakes, passive diffusion contributes. Absorption is significantly impaired in alcoholics and in patients with folate deficiency.

The body pool is small, about 30 mg in the adult, half of which is in skeletal muscle and the remainder in heart, liver, kidney, and brain. Excess thiamin is not stored but is excreted in the urine. In addition to free thiamin, the urine also contains a number of catabolites of thiamin that arise as a consequence of the coenzyme action of thiamin.

Physiology. Thiamin pyrophosphate functions as a coenzyme in the oxidative decarboxylation of pyruvic and α-ketoglutaric acids, and in the "transketolase" reactions of the triose phosphate pathway.

Thiamin is also required, likely as thiamin triphosphate, for nerve function in a reaction that is unrelated to its role as a coenzyme.

Deficiency. Beriberi is associated with white polished rice diets, as seen in Southeast Asia, and with highly milled wheat diets. The deficiency has become much less common because most countries now fortify foods with thiamin.

Acute deficiency (wet or cardiovascular beriberi) results from diets that are very low in thiamin and high in carbohydrates. Signs include edema, enlarged heart, ECG changes, and cardiac failure associated with increased cardiac output.

Slightly higher, but still inadequate, intakes produce a chronic deficiency (dry or neuritic beriberi), the essential feature of which is polyneuropathy with depressed peripheral nerve function, sensory disturbance, loss of reflexes and motor control, and muscle wasting.

Breast-fed infants whose mothers have a low thiamin intake are prone to infantile beriberi, which can be either acute or chronic. Cardiac failure and sudden death are seen with both forms.

In populations whose diet is not based on rice, thiamin deficiency is frequently seen in alcoholics because of a combination of poor diet and inhibition of the thiamin uptake mechanism by alcohol. It is the causal factor in three conditions often seen in alcoholics: alcoholic polyneuritis indistinguishable from dry beriberi; a thiamin-responsive cardiomyopathy; and an encephalopathy, known as the Wernicke-Korsakoff syndrome, that is characterized by impairment of memory, apathy, irritability, nystagmus, and oculomotor paralysis.

Therapeutic use. Deficiency may be treated with 15–30 mg/day of thiamin hydrochloride. Pharmacological doses of 50 mg/day are required for a few rare and poorly described thiamin-responsive inborn errors of metabolism.

Toxicity. No marked toxicity has been observed, and the very few isolated reports of alleged toxicity may have been due to individual hypersensitivity in patients receiving large amounts of thiamin intramuscularly.

Riboflavin (vitamin B₂)

Structure, dietary sources, and recommended intake. Riboflavin (Fig. 67-3) is a heterocyclic flavin linked to ribose, analogous to the nucleosides in RNA. Green leafy vegetables contain significant amounts of riboflavin; however, milk and meats are the most important contributors of riboflavin to the North American diet. The vitamin is heat-stable but is easily destroyed when exposed to light.

As with thiamin and niacin, the recommended intakes (see Tables 67-1, 67-2, and 67-3) are related to energy intake but should not fall below the amount required for 2000 kcal. (1.2 mg/day, United States and WHO; 1.0 mg/day, Canada).

Pharmacokinetics. Riboflavin is absorbed from the upper part of the ileum by a saturable active transport process. Bile salts facilitate absorption. The absorptive capacity is limited to 20–25 mg in a single dose. Riboflavin is distributed to all tissues; very little is stored.

Conversion of riboflavin to coenzymes occurs in most tissues. It is excreted in urine unchanged. Since there is little storage, urinary excretion reflects dietary intake. Excretion increases with conditions associated with tissue breakdown, such as weight loss, starvation, bed rest, and uncontrolled diabetes.

Physiology. Riboflavin phosphate (flavin mononucleotide, FMN) and flavin adenine dinucleotide (FAD) are involved as coenzymes in the metabolism of carbohydrates, fats, and proteins. In general, flavin dehydrogenases function as hydrogen carriers from specific substrates to the respiratory chain, resulting in the production of ATP (e.g., NADH dehydrogenase and succinate dehydrogenase). Other riboflavin enzymes not involved in energy metabolism include the *d*- and *l*-amino acid oxidases, pyridoxine-5-phosphate oxidase, and glutathione reductase.

Deficiency. Deficiency symptoms, which are generally nonspecific, include cheilosis (vertical fissures in the lips), angular stomatitis (cracks in the corners of the mouth), glossitis, corneal vascularization, photophobia, seborrheic dermatitis, and a normochromic, normocytic anemia. Peripheral neuropathy of the hands and feet may also develop. Overt clinical signs are seldom seen in industrialized societies; however, a "subclinical" deficiency, in which the activity of riboflavin-dependent enzymes is less than optimal, is common. This may result in subnormal growth in children.

Deficiency is usually the result of an inadequate dietary intake, especially a low consumption of milk. Phototherapy given to newborn infants with hyperbilirubinemia can result in a riboflavin deficiency due to photodestruction of tissue riboflavin.

Therapeutic use. For the treatment of deficiency, 5–10 mg orally (or intravenously) is administered along with other B-complex vitamins, since ariboflavinosis is usually associated with other B-vitamin deficiencies.

Toxicity. There is no known toxicity of riboflavin. Limited absorption, poor solubility, and urinary excretion of excess vitamin likely preclude the risk of toxicity even with megadoses.

Niacin (nicotinic acid, vitamin B₃)

Structure, dietary sources, and recommended intake. Niacin is the generic descriptor of pyridine-3-carboxylic acid (nicotinic acid) and the physiologically active amide derivative, nicotinamide (Fig. 67-3). Nicotinamide is metabolically active as a constituent of the pyridine nucleotide coenzymes NAD(H) and NADP(H). Tryptophan, an essential amino acid, can be converted to nicotinamide dinucleotide (NAD), but less than 2% of tryptophan metabolism follows this pathway. The conversion ratio of tryptophan to NAD is approximately 60:1. Therefore dietary intake of niacin is essential.

Dietary sources are meats, enriched cereals, and enriched grains. In many cereal grains, particularly corn, most of the niacin is bound in an unabsorbable form. Milk and eggs contain little niacin but are good sources of tryptophan.

Recommended intakes are expressed as Niacin Equivalents (NE) to take into account the presence of both preformed niacin and tryptophan in foods (see Tables 67-1, 67-2, and 67-3). As with thiamin and riboflavin, the niacin requirement is based on energy intake, but the intake should not fall below that required for 2000 kcal (i.e., 13 NE/day, United States and WHO; 14 NE/day, Canada).

Pharmacokinetics. At low intakes, niacin is readily absorbed from the intestine by a carrier-mediated facilitated diffusion. It is distributed to all tissues. The vitamin forms are converted to the coenzyme forms in tissues. Niacin released from the breakdown of NAD can be reused within the cells. Little niacin is excreted as such in the urine; most is transformed to methylated derivatives prior to urinary excretion.

Physiology. Niacin in its amide form is part of nicotinamide adenine dinucleotide (NAD) and nicotinamide adenine dinucleotide phosphate (NADP). These coenzymes serve as hydrogen carriers for many reactions catalyzed by dehydrogenases. NAD is required in all of the major metabolic pathways involving the oxidative catabolism of carbohydrates, fats, proteins, and alcohol to energy. NADP systems are common to biosynthetic reactions, and NADPH is required as a hydrogen donor for the cytochrome P450 system (see Chapter 4).

Deficiency. In niacin deficiency (pellagra) the tissues most affected are the skin, the gastrointestinal tract, and the nervous system. Early signs are nonspecific and include lassitude, anorexia, weakness, mild gastrointestinal disturbances, and emotional changes such as anxiety, irritability, and depression.

As the deficiency progresses, a bilateral pigmented scaly dermatitis develops on areas exposed to the sun. In the gastrointestinal tract the mucosa becomes inflamed and atrophic, which may account for a profuse watery diarrhea. Glossitis, angular stomatitis, and cheilosis are frequent. Mental changes intensify to include confusion, hallucinations, memory loss, and frank psychosis. Peripheral motor and sensory disturbances may also occur. Anemias are frequent, but they are likely due to associated deficiencies.

Therapeutic use. In the treatment of pellagra the recommended oral dose is 50 mg given up to 10 times a day, or 25 mg intravenously at least twice a day. Additional therapy with riboflavin and pyridoxine is usually carried out. The similarity between some mental signs of subclinical pellagra and those of schizophrenia led to the "megavitamin" approach to the treatment of schizophrenia using large doses of niacin (3–6 g/day) together with ascorbic acid (3–6 g/day) and pyridoxine (600–1500 mg/day). In addition to the advocates of the megavitamin school, some psychiatrists still use this regimen to satisfy patients' requests, in spite of the evidence (in the form of double-blind trials) of its ineffectiveness. Fortunately, neuroleptics are used in conjunction with megavitamin therapy. There is no valid reason to use megavitamin therapy alone for schizophrenia. Normal therapeutic doses can be used to treat both pellagra and subclinical pellagra.

Large doses of niacin (1–3 g/day) have been reported to lower serum cholesterol (see also Chapter 39). This appears to be a pharmacological effect unrelated to its role as a vitamin. Nicotinamide does not share this activity.

Toxicity. One gram or more of niacin per day produces marked peripheral vasodilatation (flushing), an effect that is not shared by nicotinamide. Doses over 3 g/day have been associated with activation of peptic ulcer, abnormal glucose tolerance, cardiac arrhythmias, and hepatotoxicity.

Nicotinamide is more toxic than nicotinic acid.

Chronic administration of 3 g/day produces effects such as heartburn, nausea, headache, fatigue, sore throat, and an inability to focus the eyes.

Vitamin B₆

Structure, dietary sources, and recommended intake. Vitamin B_6 is the preferred descriptor of three naturally occurring pyridine derivatives: pyridoxal, pyridoxamine, and pyridoxine (Fig. 67-3). They are present in low concentrations in virtually all plant and animal tissues. Recommended intakes (see Tables 67-1 and 67-2) are based on protein intake; thus, high protein intake increases the vitamin B_6 requirement.

Pharmacokinetics. It is well absorbed from the small intestine, likely by passive diffusion, although the vitamin in plant foods is in a glycosylated form of very low bioavailability.

The adult body pool of B_6 compounds is about 25 mg. The vitamin is excreted in the urine mainly as its major metabolite, 4-pyridoxic acid, along with small amounts of the three vitamin forms and their phosphates. Excretion reflects recent dietary intake.

Physiology. All three forms of vitamin B_6 are physiologically active; they are interconvertible. The major coenzyme form is pyridoxal phosphate, which functions in amino acid metabolism in many pathways including decarboxylation, deamination, transamination, transsulfuration, heme synthesis, and the conversion of tryptophan to niacin.

Deficiency. A dietary deficiency of vitamin B_6 is uncommon because of the diversity of foods containing the vitamin, although epileptiform convulsions have been observed in infants fed a milk formula in which vitamin B_6 had been destroyed during processing. Deficiency symptoms include peripheral neuritis, seborrheic dermatitis and other skin lesions, and a B_6-dependent sideroblastic anemia resembling iron deficiency anemia. Inborn errors of metabolism that respond to high doses of vitamin B_6 have also been reported.

Vitamin B_6 deficiency can occur also as a result of interaction with certain drugs. Pregnant women and those taking oral contraceptives have shown abnormalities in tryptophan metabolism suggestive of B_6 depletion which do respond to B_6 supplementation. Hydralazine, isoniazid, and penicillamine have similar effects, all of which appear to be due to inhibition of pyridoxal kinase, one of the enzymes that converts B_6 to its active form, pyridoxal phosphate.

Therapeutic use. Pyridoxine is included in all B-complex supplementation and is routinely used to prevent peripheral neuritis in patients receiving isoniazid. The efficacy of vitamin B_6 in amounts up to 200 mg/day in the treatment of sickle-cell disease, asthma, premenstrual tension, and carpal tunnel syndrome has yet to be confirmed.

Toxicity. Doses over 200 mg/day taken over prolonged periods may be toxic. Sensitivity to doses above 200–250 mg/day appears to vary among individuals. Instances of transient physiological dependence on vitamin B_6 (i.e., the need for an increased daily dose) have been reported in adults receiving 200 mg/day for a month. Therapeutic doses of 2–3 g/day for periods ranging from several months to 2–3 years have caused incapacitating peripheral sensory neuropathy, which subsided slowly after withdrawal of the supplement.

Vitamin B₁₂ (cyanocobalamin)

Structure, dietary sources, and recommended intake. A number of forms of vitamin B_{12} have biological activity (Fig. 67-4). Naturally occurring cobalamins are hydroxycobalamin and the two coenzyme forms, 5'-deoxyadenosyl cobalamin (coenzyme B_{12}) and methylcobalamin (methyl-B_{12}). Cyanocobalamin is an artefact of the isolation process of the vitamin but is used in clinical practice because of its greater availability and stability.

Vitamin B_{12} is found only in tissues of animals that have obtained the vitamin from synthesis by their intestinal flora and in foods that have been fermented by vitamin B_{12}-producing bacteria. Liver, the major storage site for the vitamin, is the richest source. Muscle meats, dairy products, eggs, and fish are significant sources.

The recommended intake is very small (see Tables 67-1, 67-2, and 67-3) and is readily available in a mixed diet. Strict vegetarians (vegans) are at risk of a deficiency, however.

Pharmacokinetics. The absorption of vitamin B_{12} is dependent on an Intrinsic Factor (IF), secreted from the gastric parietal cells, which serves to protect the vitamin as it proceeds from the stomach to receptor sites in the ileum, where it is absorbed. Upon entry into the tissue cells vitamin B_{12} is converted to its coenzyme forms. There is appreciable storage in the body; 60% of the total body pool is in the liver

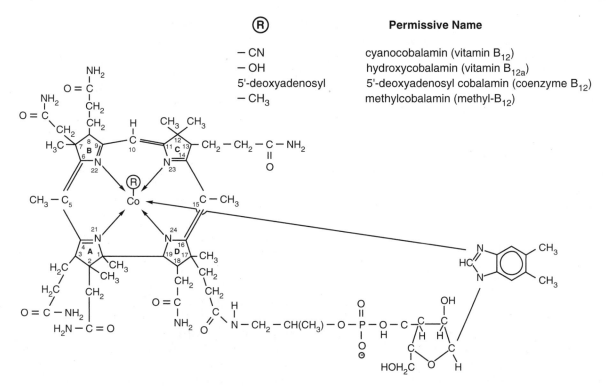

Figure 67-4. Structural formula of cobalamins.

and 30% is in the muscle. The large storage capacity and a very low turnover rate (0.1–0.2% of the body pool/day) militate against rapid depletion during dietary deprivation. An enterohepatic circulation further conserves body stores.

Physiology. Adenosylcobalamin functions in two mutase reactions that are instrumental in the degradative pathway of propionate and in the synthesis of leucine. Methylcobalamin serves as the methyl-group carrier between the donor, 5-methyl-H_4-PteGlu$_n$, and the acceptor, homocysteine, in the methylation of homocysteine to methionine. This reaction is important for the production of methionine, an important methyl-group donor, and the regeneration of H_4-PteGlu$_n$, the key functional form of folate (see Folate below).

Deficiency. A vitamin B_{12} deficiency produces a failure of cell division in all replicating cells, most notably in the intestinal mucosa and hematopoietic tissue, due to the arrested synthesis of DNA precursors. This in turn is due to a lack of folate coenzymes (see Folate below). Bone marrow shows a proliferation of erythrocyte precursors and enlarged cells or macrocytes with a shortened lifespan in the peripheral blood. This condition is termed a megaloblastic or macrocytic anemia. Disturbed maturation of buccal and intestinal mucosal cells is often present. In addition, nerve demyelination eventually occurs, beginning with the peripheral nerves and progressing eventually to the posterior and lateral columns of the spinal cord. Early peripheral demyelination responds to vitamin B_{12} treatment; however, the later CNS demyelination is irreversible.

The most common cause of vitamin B_{12} deficiency is malabsorption of the vitamin due to inadequate secretion of IF, probably a familial, immunologically based trait. The deficiency due to a lack of IF is termed "pernicious anemia" and normally affects individuals past middle age. Impaired absorption may, however, result from other causes such as pancreatic insufficiency, gastric atrophy, gastrectomy, resection of the ileum (the absorptive site for the vitamin), or diseases of the ileum (e.g., celiac or tropical sprue and ileitis). Deficiency from these causes may take 5–7 years to become evident because of the large stores of the vitamin in the body.

Absorption is also impaired by various drugs, including *p*-aminosalicylic acid (PAS), colchicine, neomycin, and the biguanides metformin and phenformin, which are used in the treatment of diabetes.

A nutritional deficiency is rare but is seen in individuals consuming a strict vegetarian (vegan) diet containing no animal products. Clinical signs take 10–20 years to develop in such cases. Several instances of a deficiency in breast-fed infants of vegan mothers have been reported.

Therapeutic use. The only therapeutic use of vitamin B_{12} (as cyanocobalamin) is the treatment of a vitamin B_{12} deficiency. Although oral administration of large doses is effective in the treatment of pernicious anemia (150 μg/day, or a single weekly dose of 1000 μg), monthly intramuscular or subcutaneous injection of 60–100 μg is the preferred treatment.

Toxicity. Preparations of cyanocobalamin are nontoxic.

Folate

Structure, dietary sources, and recommended intake. Folate (Fig. 67-5) is the generic descriptor for folic acid (pteroylmonoglutamic acid [PteGlu]) and related compounds that have biological activity. The naturally occurring and metabolically active compound is the reduced form of folic acid, 5,6,7,8-tetrahydrofolic acid (H_4-PteGlu), which is conju-

Folic acid

→ *Folic acid reductase*

7, 8 - Dihydrofolic acid

→ *Dihydrofolic acid reductase*

5,6,7,8 - Tetrahydrofolic acid

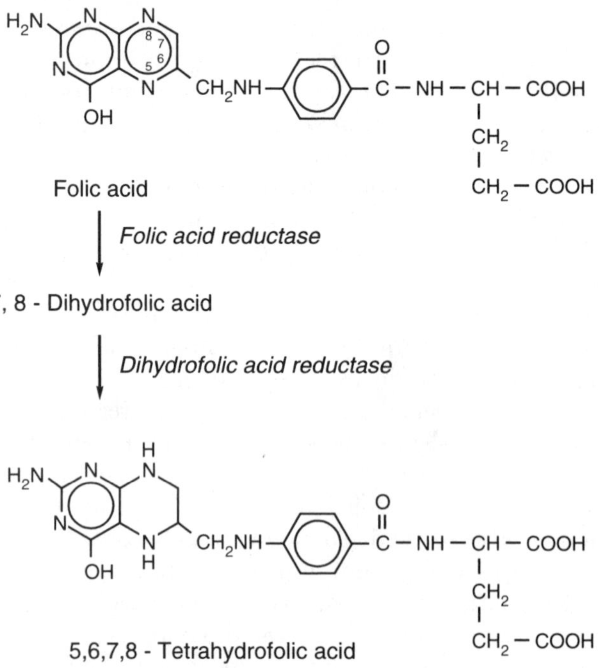

Figure 67-5. Structural formulae of folic acid and tetrahydrofolic acid (H_4-PteGlu).

gated in cells with up to eight glutamyl residues (H_4-PteGlu$_n$).

The richest dietary sources of folates are green leafy vegetables, mushrooms, and liver; however, the bioavailability of folates is variable (30–80%): It is less available from plant sources. Folates are easily oxidized and are unstable under cooking and storage conditions.

The recommended intakes (Tables 67-1, 67-2, and 67-3) assume a mixed diet including animal and plant products. The increased requirement for folate in pregnancy makes the use of a supplement a necessity for many women.

Pharmacokinetics. Dietary folates must be cleaved to the monoglutamate form by a zinc-dependent conjugase enzyme prior to absorption. The overall efficiency of absorption is about 50% (10–90%). Alcoholism or diseases that produce malabsorption interfere profoundly with absorption. Absorption is predominantly by active transport in the duodenum and jejunum. After uptake by tissue cells the monoglutamate form is conjugated with up to eight glutamyl residues. About 50% of the body pool of folate is in the liver. Small amounts of folate metabolites are excreted in the urine and bile (in feces). There is a significant conservation of folates in the body by reutilization of folates released from senescent cells and by an enterohepatic circulation of folate. Zinc depletion can interfere with folate absorption because of the dependence of the conjugase enzyme on zinc as a cofactor.

Physiology. Folate (H_4-PteGlu$_n$) functions as a coenzyme to transfer single carbon units (at the oxidation levels of methanol and formate, but not CO_2) in synthetic interconversion reactions, e.g., in the interconversions of some amino acids and in purine and pyrimidine nucleotide synthesis. This is of particular importance in the synthesis of DNA and hence in cell replication and maturation.

Deficiency. A poor intake of folate produces a folate deficiency, which results in the failure of developing cells to mature past the megaloblast phase because of a suppression of DNA synthesis. Cells with rapid turnover rates (e.g., gastrointestinal mucosa) and red blood cells are most profoundly affected, resulting in malabsorption and a megaloblastic anemia, respectively. The anemia is indistinguishable from that caused by a vitamin B_{12} deficiency. A striking clinical difference, however, is the absence of myelin degeneration and its neurological consequences.

A vitamin B_{12} deficiency may induce a secondary folate deficiency. Vitamin B_{12} is required as an intermediate methyl-group acceptor in the conversion of homocysteine to methionine. In the absence of vitamin B_{12}, this transfer is blocked and H_4-PteGlu is "trapped" in the methyl derivative form, thus blocking its ability to transfer other single-carbon units.

Chronic alcoholism, intestinal malabsorption, chronic liver disease, and vitamin C deficiency (diminished protection of folate in its reduced H_4-PteGlu form) also contribute to folate deficiency. The anticonvulsant phenytoin may produce folate deficiency in a small percentage of epileptics.

Therapeutic use. The main therapeutic use of pteroylglutamic acid is the treatment of folate deficiency. Folic acid supplements are effective in reducing the incidence of primary (0.4–0.8 mg/day) or recurring (4 mg/day) neural-tube defects in newborns if given to women with childbearing potential in the periconceptual period. Large "rescue doses" of 5-formyl-H_4-PteGlu (folinic acid or leucovorin) are used as a specific antidote for the toxic effects of antineoplastic therapy with methotrexate (see Chapter 60).

Folate is also a cofactor in the conversion of homocysteine to methionine. In patients with hyperhomocysteinemia due to genetic deficiencies in the metabolism of homocysteine, there is increased risk of premature atherosclerosis, leading to myocardial infarction and stroke. The possible value of folate supplements, to prevent these complications by reducing homocysteine levels, is currently being studied.

Toxicity. There is no established toxicity of folic acid. High intakes (5 mg/day orally) correct the megaloblastic anemia of vitamin B_{12} deficiency but may mask the concurrent development of neurological lesions. Thus the indiscriminate use of large folate supplements is unwise. The sale of over-the-counter folic acid supplements is restricted to unit doses which will produce a response only to a folate deficiency.

Biotin and pantothenic acid

These two vitamins are usually included with the B-complex vitamins. Other than the treatment of rarely occurring primary or induced deficiencies, they have no established therapeutic use. It is assumed that an adequate intake is provided in the diet. They are both virtually nontoxic. The structures are given in Figure 67-3.

Biotin. Biotin is widely distributed in the diet and may be synthesized by the bacterial flora. There are insufficient data to establish a specific recommended intake. The upper limit of usual dietary intakes of about 100 μg/day is considered adequate.

A naturally occurring deficiency is an extreme rarity. In two reported cases, large quantities of raw eggs (6–12 eggs/day) were consumed over periods of months or years. Raw egg white contains avidin, which binds biotin and renders it biologically unavailable.

Experimental deficiencies are characterized by anorexia, nausea and vomiting, and a dry scaly dermatitis.

Biotin is involved in fatty acid synthesis as the coenzyme for acetyl-CoA carboxylase and other carboxylation pathways.

Pantothenic acid. Pantothenic acid is converted to coenzyme A, which is involved in the intermediary metabolism of carbohydrates, fats, and proteins, as well as the many synthetic reactions involving acetylation.

No naturally occurring deficiency has been reported in humans. As with biotin, no recommended intake can be established; 5–7 mg/day appears to prevent signs of an experimental deficiency and is considered adequate.

Vitamin C

Structure, dietary sources, and recommended intake

Vitamin C is the generic term for L-ascorbic acid and its oxidized form dehydroascorbic acid (Fig. 67-6), both of which have vitamin C activity. The two forms are readily interconvertible. The most important dietary sources of vitamin C are citrus fruits, vegetables, and fruit drinks supplemented with ascorbic acid. Organ meats (liver, kidney, and brain) are also significant sources. However, muscle meats and milk contain very little ascorbic acid.

Vitamin C is particularly labile and is easily destroyed by exposure to air, heat, or prolonged storage.

The recommended intakes vary among countries, ranging from 30–60 mg/day (see Tables 67-1, 67-2,

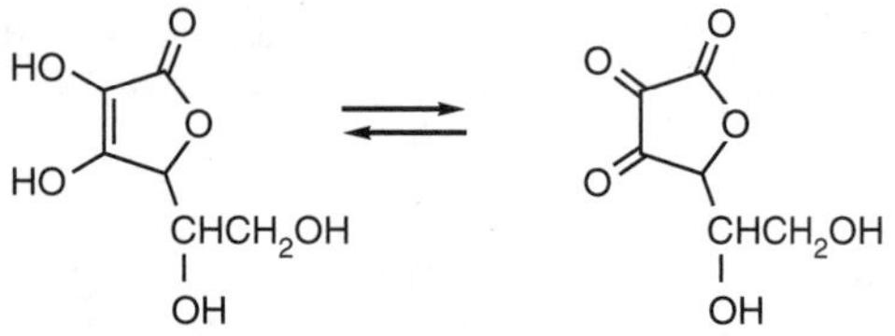

Figure 67-6. Structural formulae of ascorbic acid and its oxidation product, dehydroascorbic acid (both vitamin C).

and 67-3). A suitable intake has been disputed among experts, and recommended intakes have undergone numerous revisions.

Pharmacokinetics

Vitamin C is well absorbed from the small intestine by a saturable active transport process. The efficiency of absorption decreases with increasing intake. The vitamin is distributed in most tissues throughout the body; the adult pool is approximately 1500 mg. Excess vitamin C is not stored, and levels in leukocytes are used to estimate tissue levels. At plasma concentrations below 1.4 mg/dL (80 μmol/L), ascorbic acid is reabsorbed by the kidney; above that level ascorbic acid is actively excreted. A large number of metabolites also appear in the urine. Urinary excretion of ascorbic acid closely reflects recent dietary intake. Tissue saturation occurs when the plasma level is between 1 and 2 mg/dL (56.8 and 113.6 μmol/L); women have higher levels than men. Cigarette smoking, as well as some types of stress, may drastically lower plasma ascorbate levels. If ascorbic acid ingestion is reduced following long-term supplementation with 250 mg/day or more, the kidney continues to excrete ascorbic acid. This results in a rebound phenomenon in which plasma ascorbate may fall to scorbutic levels (especially if prior ingestion was 2 g or more per day). There is a report that after daily ingestion of 10 g of vitamin C for a week, withdrawal resulted in frank symptoms of scurvy.

Physiology

The functions of vitamin C appear to reflect its redox capacity. Thus it is involved in a number of hydroxylation reactions in which it maintains optimal enzyme activity by donating electrons, e.g., collagen synthesis (and thus wound healing and bone matrix formation), synthesis of carnitine and the neurotransmitters serotonin and norepinephrine, the metabolism of histamine and cholesterol, and the activ-

ity of detoxifying enzymes in the liver. The vitamin also enhances the absorption of nonheme iron and serves as an important mechanism to inactivate highly reactive free radicals in the tissue cells. It retards the formation in the body of nitrosamines, which are potential carcinogens. Mounting evidence links ascorbic acid to many elements of the immune system.

Deficiency

Humans, monkeys, guinea pigs, and fruit bats have lost the ability to synthesize ascorbic acid from glucose (the last enzyme in the series, L-gulonolactone oxidase, has been lost by these species). Dietary deficiency of ascorbic acid can therefore give rise, in these species, to the symptoms of scurvy, which include pathological lesions of bones, teeth, gums, skin, and blood vessels. These all appear to be due to depolymerization of connective tissue and disappearance of collagen. Death ensues if the scorbutic state is not corrected. Infantile scurvy has been a problem, and Nutrition Canada reports that there may be clinical vitamin C deficiency among the Inuit (Eskimos) and the elderly.

Therapeutic use

There is an increased requirement for ascorbic acid in tuberculosis, peptic ulcer, and other stress conditions, e.g., surgery. This can be met by ingestion of 100–200 mg per day. A transient tyrosinemia seen in some neonates has been treated with 100 mg per day. Scurvy is usually treated with 1–2 g/day until tissue saturation is attained.

Toxicity

Normal dietary levels are without toxicity. High dietary intake (in excess of 1 g/day) may cause diarrhea, and in some sensitive individuals it may promote the precipitation of cystine or oxalate stones in the urinary tract. At higher levels of ascorbate intake the possibility of rebound effects on withdrawal should be considered. There is a danger of scurvy in newborns of mothers who ingested large amounts of ascorbate during pregnancy. There are also reports of false responses to some diagnostic tests.

Megavitamin C therapy

Pauling, Stone, Szent-Györgi, and others have recommended taking 2–6 g of ascorbic acid daily for prophylaxis and therapy against the common cold, other virus infections, allergies, cancer, and aging. There have been a number of well-controlled studies on the common cold, but no good studies on other aspects of megavitamin C therapy. Its use in the treatment of these states seems to have no foundation in fact. The studies on vitamin C and the common cold demonstrate no effect on the frequency of colds, but they do indicate that some respiratory symptoms are reduced and that there is a decrease in the number of days off work. Thus, there might not be an antiviral effect, but there may be an improved response to stress. On the basis of these trials and our knowledge of the pharmacodynamics of ascorbic acid, 250 mg/day would appear to be the maximum amount required to saturate the tissues; there would appear to be no benefit obtained from taking larger daily quantities.

SUGGESTED READING

Combs GF, Jr. The vitamins, fundamental aspects in nutrition and health. San Diego: Academic Press, 1992.

Losonczy KG, Harris TB, Havlik RJ. Vitamin E and vitamin C supplement use and risk of all-cause and coronary heart disease mortality in older persons: the Established Populations for Epidemiologic Studies of the Elderly. Am J Clin Nutr 1996; 64:190–196.

Machlin LJ, ed. Handbook of vitamins. 2nd ed. New York: Marcel Dekker, 1991.

Nutrition Recommendations. The report of the Scientific Review Committee. Ottawa: Health and Welfare Canada, 1990.

Passmore R, Nicol BM, Rao MN. Handbook of human nutritional requirements. World Health Organization Monograph Series No. 61, Geneva, 1974.

Rapola JM, Virtamo J, Haukka JK et al. Effect of vitamin E and beta carotene on the incidence of angina pectoris. A randomized, double-blind, controlled trial. JAMA 1996; 275:693–698.

Recommended Dietary Allowances, 10th revised ed. Washington, DC: National Academy of Sciences, 1989.

Requirements of Vitamin A, Iron, Folate and Vitamin B_{12}. Report of a Joint FAO/WHO Expert Consultation. FAO Food and Nutrition Series No. 23, Rome, FAO, 1988.

Stephens NG, Parsons A, Schofield PM et al. Randomized controlled trial of vitamin E in patients with coronary disease: Cambridge Heart Antioxidant Study (CHAOS). Lancet 1996; 347:781–786.

CHAPTER 68

Drugs Altering Bone Metabolism

W.C. STURTRIDGE

CASE HISTORY

A 51-year-old white woman who was menopausal at age 49 was referred to a specialist in internal medicine and bone diseases by her family physician. The patient's medical history included inflammatory bowel disease (Crohn's disease) and lactose intolerance. Crohn's disease had been diagnosed at age 32 and was initially treated with prednisone (60 mg daily) for a period of approximately 6 months; the dose was then gradually tapered to a maintenance dose of 5 mg. The patient had never had to have surgical bowel resection, but two disease flare-ups required higher doses of prednisone with early tapering to maintenance levels (7.5 mg). At the time of presentation she was also on 5-aminosalicylic acid (5-ASA, Asacol). She gave no history of known fractures but spoke of two episodes of acute-onset back pain with slow resolution in each case, and residual aching pain in the lower back. Because of chronic lactose intolerance the patient had low dietary intake of calcium for many years, and only in the past 2 years had a supplement of calcium carbonate been prescribed, giving 500 mg of elemental calcium daily. She was not on any vitamin D supplement, and she received no prescription medications other than those noted above.

Physical examination findings were within normal limits, except for some tenderness on heavy percussion over the thoracolumbar spine. X-rays revealed anterior compression of the bodies of thoracic vertebra T-12 and lumbar vertebra L-1. The provisional diagnosis was osteoporosis secondary to inflammatory bowel disease with low net calcium absorption, effects of long-term treatment with a glucocorticoid, low intake of vitamin D, and postmenopausal bone loss.

Bone densitometry showed significant osteopenia in both the lumbar spine and femoral neck. Laboratory tests revealed ionized calcium levels just below the lower limit of normal, elevated alkaline phosphatase, low urinary calcium excretion, elevated intact PTH, and 25-OH vitamin D near the lower limit of the reference range.

The patient had no contraindications to hormone replacement, and after normal gynecological and breast examinations she was placed on conjugated equine estrogen (Premarin 0.625 mg) and medroxyprogesterone acetate (Provera 2.5 mg), both to be taken daily. She was changed from calcium carbonate to calcium citrate to give a daily calcium intake of approximately 1000 mg. Vitamin D, 1000 IU daily, was also begun, and she was urged to actively exercise as frequently as possible. The patient had some minimal menstrual spotting for 3 months, but she continued on hormone replacement. She had no side effects from calcium and vitamin D, and the plasma levels of ionized calcium and 25-OH vitamin D increased into the normal range. Intact PTH and alkaline phosphatase levels, and urinary calcium excretion, also became normal.

During the next 3 years of follow-up, there was a progressive increase in bone density and a resulting reduction in the risk of fracture. She has had no fractures, and the long-term prognosis is good as long as she continues the present treatment and is able to minimize the dose of glucocorticoid used to treat her inflammatory bowel disease.

Bone metabolism is part of an integrated multiorgan metabolic system that also involves the gastrointestinal tract, the kidney, and the control of extracellular concentrations of calcium and phosphorus. Extracellular fluid calcium concentration is normally controlled within very close limits through the actions of parathyroid hormone (PTH), calcitonin (CT), and vitamin D. The major effects of parathyroid hormone on calcium control were first recognized in 1908 when MacCallum and Voegtlin showed that surgical removal of the parathyroids resulted in hypocalcemia and tetany. Calcitonin was not identified as a hormone with actions on calcium and bone metabolism until after 1960, following the early research of Copp in Canada and Hirsch and Munson in the United States. Although vitamin D has long been recognized as a fat-soluble vitamin important for prevention of rickets and osteomalacia, a better understanding of its intermediary metabolism by the liver and kidney did not begin until about 1970.

A very large number of endogenous hormones and drugs may have some physiological or pharmacological actions on bone metabolism. This chapter summarizes only those with major or primary effects on bone metabolism, and in particular those agents with therapeutic applications.

PHYSIOLOGY OF BONE

Structure and Mineral Metabolism of Bone

The histological structure, metabolism, and density of bone are closely related to serum calcium concentration. Close physiological control of serum calcium within a narrow range from 2.2 to 2.6 mmol/L is maintained by secretion of PTH and CT and production of 1,25-dihydroxy-vitamin D_3. These three hormonal substances act (1) on bone to control the transfer of calcium between extra- and intracellular fluid, as well as bone resorption, formation, and mineralization; (2) on the gastrointestinal tract to regulate the absorption of calcium and phosphorus; and (3) on the renal tubule to regulate reabsorption of calcium and phosphate (Fig. 68-1).

It has been estimated that a calcium intake of about 1 g/day is required to maintain calcium balance in the normal adult. Net calcium absorption is normally about 15–45% of the oral intake when measured by isotopic calcium absorption methods. The fraction of the total calcium absorption that occurs in any specific segment of the intestine depends on the length of that segment and the transit time along it, in addition to the calcium concentration in that part of the intestinal lumen. The duodenum has the greatest capacity for transport of calcium per unit length of intestine, but the largest fraction of the total calcium absorption occurs in the ileum.

Urinary excretion of calcium ranges up to 7.5 mmol/24 hr. Many factors affect total urinary calcium excretion, including age, sex (males absorb and excrete more calcium than do females), seasonal variations, exercise, and sodium and phosphorus intake. In adults, about 100 mL of plasma water is filtered by the kidneys every minute, but only about 1% of this filtered water and less than 2% of filtered calcium are excreted in the urine. The greatest part of the filtered load of calcium is reabsorbed by the renal tubules.

If input of calcium ion from intestinal absorption and renal reabsorption is not sufficient to maintain extracellular fluid calcium concentration in the normal range, calcium can be rapidly mobilized from bone under the influence of PTH. This transfer is mediated by osteocytes and osteoblasts, and only if the deficiency is prolonged is there an increase in osteoclast-mediated bone resorption secondary to sustained increase in PTH secretion.

Ninety-nine percent of total body calcium is in the skeleton. Radioisotopic studies with ^{45}Ca and ^{47}Ca indicate that 1% of skeletal calcium is freely exchangeable with extracellular fluid. Bone metabolic activity ensures that bone is not only continuously undergoing remodeling or turnover but also that the readily exchangeable pool of calcium is maintained. The morphological unit of compact bone is the osteon, which has been defined as "an irregular, branching and anastomosing cylinder composed of a more or less centrally placed cell-containing neurovascular canal surrounded by concentric, cell-permeated lamellae of bone matrix." At one level of an osteon, the predominant cells may be osteoclasts, and bone resorption the prevailing process, while at another level of the same osteon the predominant cell type may be osteoblasts, which are forming, depositing, and mineralizing the collagen matrix of bone (Fig. 68-2).

These two processes of bone resorption and formation are normally closely coupled. As matrix formation and mineralization continue, the active osteoblasts become encircled with mineralized matrix and become osteocytes lying within lacunae. Osteocytes are capable of active bone resorption (a process known as osteolysis) and transport of mineral ions to the osteoblasts via a cytoplasmic canalicular system.

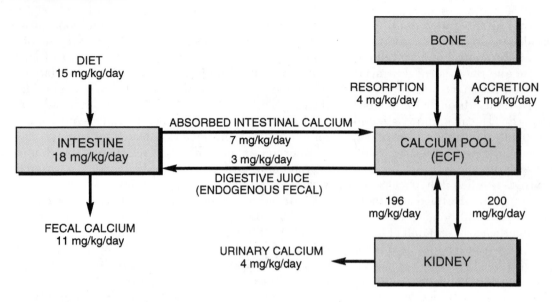

Figure 68-1. Calcium fluxes in the normal human adult who is in zero balance (on an average calcium intake).

Osteolysis rather than osteoclast-mediated resorption is probably the primary metabolic activity of bone responsible for maintaining normal extracellular fluid concentration of calcium. Osteoclasts are derived from the monocyte/macrophage system of cells of the hematopoietic system. They are important for the resorption of bone in the remodeling process, but their contribution to the normal control of calcium homeostasis is minimal.

In predominantly trabecular bone the same cellular metabolic processes of bone prevail. However, osteoclast-mediated resorption and osteoblast synthesis of bone occur on the surface of trabeculae rather than within osteons.

Recent studies of osteoblasts have indicated that the term "osteoblast" describes heterogeneous cells of a common origin, but with differentiated functions. There is increasing evidence that cells of osteoblast

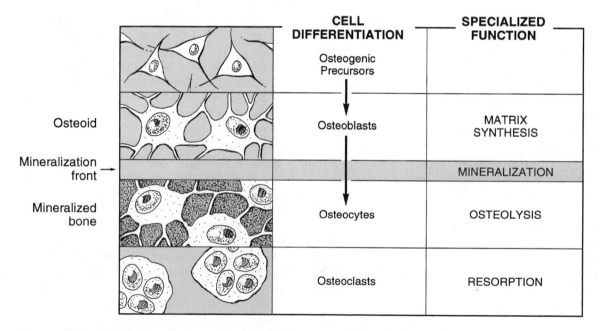

Figure 68-2. Cell differentiation and specialized functions of human bone cells.

lineage serve a central function in bone matrix turn-over, not only stimulating synthesis of new matrix but also controlling matrix resorption by osteoclasts as well.

Parathyroid Hormone (PTH)

A number of hormones play primary or secondary roles in controlling the metabolic activity of bone. PTH apparently has multiple effects on bone. It is a polypeptide composed of 84 amino acids, with a molecular weight of 9000 Da. Within the parathyroid cell, PTH is derived from larger polypeptide precursors. PTH promotes the release of calcium and phosphate into extracellular fluid, probably through stimulation of osteolysis by osteocytes. At the same time, PTH stimulates bone remodeling by increasing both resorption by osteoclasts and synthesis of bone matrix by osteoblasts. Other actions of PTH are (1) to enhance tubular reabsorption of calcium by an effect on the distal tubule; (2) to increase the excretion of inorganic phosphate by inhibiting tubular reabsorption of this ion; (3) to increase HCO_3^- excretion and decrease H^+ excretion; and (4) to stimulate production of 1,25-dihydroxy-vitamin D_3 by the kidney through stimulation of 25-hydroxy-vitamin D-1-hydroxylase, thus contributing to increased intestinal absorption of calcium and phosphate. The actions of PTH on bone are normally synergistic with those of vitamin D metabolites, but the hypocalcemia of hypoparathyroidism can be corrected by adequate therapeutic doses of vitamin D and calcium.

While parathyroid hormone is of central importance in the physiological regulation of calcium and bone metabolism, to date it has not had pharmacological significance. Recent development of synthesis of intact human PTH 1–84 by recombinant DNA techniques will likely lead to clinical testing in metabolic bone diseases such as osteoporosis. Bovine parathyroid extract and synthetic peptides of human sequence 1–34 and 1–38 are available for research purposes.

An interesting interaction occurs between PTH and thiazide diuretics (see Chapter 41). Some patients treated with thiazides show hypercalcemia as an undesired side effect. This is believed to be due to potentiation of the action of PTH and may represent an unmasking of a subclinical hyperparathyroidism. The interaction of PTH with its receptor activates an adenylyl cyclase and raises the cAMP concentration within the target cells. Thiazides inhibit phosphodiesterase, thus increasing the cAMP concentration further.

Vitamin D

Vitamin D is obtained from dietary sources or is derived from 7-dehydrocholesterol in the skin by the action of light energy in the near-ultraviolet wavelength range. The precursor is converted to the biologically active metabolite 1,25-dihydroxy-vitamin D_3 by enzymatic hydroxylations in the liver at the C-25 position and in the kidney at the C-1 position (see Chapter 67). Vitamin D enhances gastrointestinal absorption of calcium and phosphate, augments the mobilization of mineral from bone, and increases the renal reabsorption of calcium and probably of phosphate. There are nuclear receptors for 1,25-dihydroxy-vitamin D_3, but there is no evidence that an adenylyl cyclase system is involved in its actions. A direct action of vitamin D on mineralization of bone matrix has yet to be clearly demonstrated, but many authorities believe that such a physiological role exists.

Calcitonin

The physiological role of calcitonin in calcium and bone metabolism is unknown. Calcitonin is a 32-amino-acid peptide hormone with a molecular weight of 3500 Da that is produced and secreted by thyroid parafollicular cells. The acute administration of calcitonin lowers serum calcium and phosphate by inhibiting osteolysis and osteoclast activity and by decreasing renal tubular reabsorption of calcium. In sustained hypercalcitoninemia, there is a decrease in bone remodeling that is probably due to inhibition of osteoclastic activity. Calcitonin secretion is stimulated by gastrointestinal hormones such as gastrin and pancreozymin. It may be that increased calcitonin secretion during feeding, particularly of a high-calcium meal, prevents excess hypercalcemia by inhibiting calcium transport from bone into extracellular fluid and by increasing renal clearance of calcium. Significant effects of calcitonin on calcium and phosphate absorption have not been demonstrated.

Other Hormones

Other hormones also play secondary roles in the control of bone metabolism. **Thyroid hormone** certainly has an effect on metabolic activity of bone cells and calcium metabolism. In hypothyroidism, bone turnover rate is low and, as a result, parathyroid secretion is increased to maintain normal serum calcium. An increased rate of parathyroid hormone secretion results in increased production of 1,25-

dihydroxy-vitamin D_3 and increased calcium absorption. In hyperthyroidism, mobilization of mineral from bone is facilitated and PTH secretion is reduced. Although serum calcium concentration remains in the normal range, the decreased secretion of PTH results in elevated serum phosphate concentration.

Chronic administration of **adrenal steroids,** or adrenal cortical hypersecretion, leads to decreased gastrointestinal absorption of calcium, decreased synthesis of new bone matrix, and perhaps increased sensitivity of osteoclasts to PTH and decreased renal tubular reabsorption of calcium.

Sex hormones may affect the regulation of bone metabolism. When sex hormones are deficient, bone density tends to be diminished, probably due to an excessive degree of bone resorption. Androgens may be aromatized to estrogens in peripheral tissues, and receptors for estrogen in osteoblasts have been identified. There is speculation that sex hormones may also assist in the regulation of bone metabolism through increased calcitonin secretion.

Recent reports have suggested a correlation between high serum **prolactin** levels and decreased bone density. There does not appear to be a relationship between decreased bone density and plasma estrogen concentration in the presence of hyperprolactinemia. A positive correlation between elevated prolactin concentration and serum PTH has been reported, but the significance of these observations so far remains unclear. Postmenopausal bone loss is best prevented by estrogen replacement therapy, which in addition has other substantial health benefits (see Chapter 49).

AGENTS WITH PRIMARY EFFECTS ON BONE/CALCIUM METABOLISM

Table 68-1 lists various agents with primary and secondary effects on bone/calcium metabolism.

Calcium

Many vital intra- and extracellular biological processes, as well as membrane integrity and function, are dependent upon maintenance of adequate ionized calcium concentrations. Calcium salts are specific in the treatment of low calcium states. Long-term use of oral calcium dietary supplements decreases the rate of bone remodeling, thereby evening out resorption of old and formation of new bone, and it maintains positive calcium balance.

Table 68-1 Agents and Drugs Affecting Bone Metabolism

Agents with primary effects on bone/calcium metabolism
　Mineral salts: calcium, phosphate, fluoride
　Hormones: vitamin D, calcitonin
　Miscellaneous: bisphosphonates, mithramycin

Agents with secondary effects on bone/calcium metabolism
　Estrogens
　Glucocorticoids
　Thyroid hormone preparations
　Thiazide diuretics

Various salts of calcium are available for medicinal use, such as calcium chloride ($CaCl_2 \cdot 2H_2O$), calcium citrate ($Ca_3 [C_6H_5O_7]_2 \cdot 4H_2O$), calcium lactate ($[CH_3CHOHCOO]_2Ca \cdot 5H_2O$), calcium gluconate ($[CH_2OH (CHOH)_4 COO]_2Ca \cdot H_2O$), and calcium carbonate ($CaCO_3$). Calcium chloride contains 27% elemental calcium, calcium citrate 21%, calcium lactate 13%, and calcium gluconate 9%; and insoluble calcium carbonate, which is converted to soluble calcium salts in the body, contains 40% elemental calcium.

A common **adverse effect** of intravenously administered calcium chloride is irritation of veins. Oral calcium supplements may cause gastric irritation, nausea, and constipation. Calcium salts should not be taken orally at the same time as tetracycline because the absorption of tetracycline will be decreased by the formation of a calcium–tetracycline chelate (see Chapter 55). Similarly, the coadministration of fluoride or phosphates with calcium may be associated with decreased absorption due to formation of insoluble compounds in the gastrointestinal tract.

Administration of excessive calcium can lead to **hypercalcemic toxicity.** Ingestion of large quantities of calcium salts, however, is unlikely to produce hypercalcemia unless there is also administration of large amounts of vitamin D.

Therapeutic applications

Calcium gluconate and calcium chloride, 10–20 mL in a concentration of 10%, are indicated for intravenous injection in the treatment of hypocalcemic tetany. A more dilute (0.3%) solution may be infused by slow drip to provide 1 g of elemental calcium a day in the management of hypocalcemia. Calcium gluconate is preferred because it is less irritating to veins than calcium chloride. For less severe hypocalcemia, or to supplement dietary intake in osteoporosis or osteomalacia, calcium salts to provide 1–2 g elemental calcium a day are given orally.

Phosphate

Phosphate is an essential element of energy metabolism and, in addition, is essential for normal mineralization of bone matrix. It is absorbed from the gastrointestinal tract by active transport that is stimulated by vitamin D. About two-thirds of the ingested phosphate is absorbed and is balanced by an equal amount of phosphate excretion in the urine. In normal body fluids and tissues, phosphate ion has little pharmacological effect, but phosphate supplements may be required to restore normal physiological actions in states of phosphate depletion.

Effervescent tablets contain sodium acid phosphate together with potassium and sodium bicarbonate. Potassium phosphate solution for intravenous use is also available.

If large amounts of phosphate are administered orally, the unabsorbed phosphate has a marked cathartic action. Large quantities of divalent cations such as calcium or aluminum in the gastrointestinal tract will form insoluble salts and diminish phosphate absorption.

Therapeutic applications

Oral phosphate may be used in some circumstances as an adjunct in the management of hypercalcemia, where it probably decreases calcium absorption, or in hypophosphatemia. Effervescent tablets of sodium acid phosphate provide 500 mg elemental phosphorus. Four to six tablets per day are prescribed in divided doses, but in many patients diarrhea limits the amount of drug that can be tolerated. In hypercalcemic patients, intravenous injection of phosphate may precipitate soft-tissue calcification, but potassium phosphate may be given intravenously to correct severe hypophosphatemia (≤ 0.3 mmol/L). The dose required to normalize serum phosphate in adult patients with normal renal function and normal serum potassium and calcium is 9 mmol of phosphorus as KH_2PO_4 in 0.5 N saline as a continuous intravenous infusion over a 12-hour period. (The amount of potassium will be the limiting factor, because excess phosphate is excreted in the urine.)

Fluoride

Fluoride is incorporated into bone as fluhydroxyapatite, which is resistant to resorption. More importantly, however, it appears to stimulate the synthesis of new bone matrix by osteoblasts. Precisely how or why this effect occurs is as yet unknown. At the same time, fluoride appears to retard the mineralization of the newly formed matrix.

Soluble fluoride compounds such as sodium fluoride (the official fluoride preparation currently in use to affect bone metabolism) are almost completely absorbed. Fluoride is probably concentrated only in calcified tissues or sites of extraskeletal calcification. The major route of fluoride excretion is the kidney.

The only known pharmacological effects of fluoride other than on bone and teeth, where it inhibits dental caries, are **toxic effects.** Fluoride inhibits some enzyme systems, including enzymes involved in anaerobic glycolysis and tissue respiration, and it is an effective in vitro anticoagulant. It also inhibits glucose utilization by erythrocytes in vitro. However, these effects occur only at doses far in excess of those used therapeutically or prophylactically. The fluoride dose to cause death in an adult is approximately 2.5–5 g of NaF, taken in a single dose. It is estimated that the lowest acute toxic dose of water containing 1 ppm fluoride would be about 2000 L consumed at one time, if this were physically possible.

Adverse effects include gastric irritation in some patients and increased musculoskeletal pain and joint swelling of predominantly weight-bearing joints. Gastrointestinal distress is less with use of enteric-coated sodium fluoride tablets.

Therapeutic applications

Enteric-coated tablets containing 20 mg of sodium fluoride may be given one to three times daily with meals in the treatment of osteoporosis, multiple myeloma, and otospongiosis. Serum fluoride concentration must be monitored frequently to ensure adequate but nontoxic levels. Sodium fluoride, stannous fluoride, and sodium monofluorophosphate are employed in dentifrices to reduce dental caries. Fluoridation of municipal water supplies has the same objective. Pharmacological serum fluoride levels that stimulate bone matrix formation are on the order of 5–10 μmol/L; these may be attained with the daily ingestion of about 40 mg sodium fluoride (= 20 mg fluoride). Water fluoridation with the addition of 1 ppm fluoride produces lower serum fluoride levels of about 2 μmol/L.

Vitamin D

The mechanisms and sites of action of vitamin D and its pharmacological effects are outlined above, and details of its metabolism may be found in Chapter 67. In summary, vitamin D is a positive regulator of both calcium and phosphate through its actions on gut, kidney, and bone.

A large number of preparations containing vitamin D are marketed. Only four preparations need to be detailed structurally (Fig. 68-3), and the difference between them is largely in potency. However, there may be important differences in therapeutic application (see below).

Gastrointestinal absorption of orally administered vitamin D is usually adequate. Since bile is essential for vitamin D absorption, hepatobiliary disease may be associated with decreased absorption of vitamin D. Also, fat malabsorption may impair the absorption of this fat-soluble vitamin.

The only adverse or **toxic effects** of vitamin D are those related to overtreatment and development of hypercalcemia and hyperphosphatemia. Impairment of renal function due to nephrolithiasis or nephrocalcinosis, localized or generalized decreases in bone density, and gastrointestinal complaints are the most common sequelae of vitamin D toxicity.

The important **drug interactions** involving vitamin D are with anticonvulsants and glucocorticoids. Phenobarbital and other anticonvulsants either interfere with the normal hydroxylations of cholecalciferol and ergocalciferol or interfere with target-organ response. Glucocorticoids may also interfere with vitamin D metabolism and significantly inhibit the effect of 1,25-dihydroxy-vitamin D_3 on calcium absorption. Effects on bone remodeling and calcium reabsorption are probably of secondary importance.

Therapeutic applications

Vitamin D compounds are administered orally to increase calcium and phosphate absorption in diseases such as hypocalcemia, osteomalacia, osteoporosis, osteodystrophy, vitamin D deficiency, and hypophosphatemia. Doses vary considerably, depending on the indication for treatment and the preparation selected. Doses of 1.25 mg (50,000 IU) to 5 mg of ergocalciferol may be required in hypoparathy-

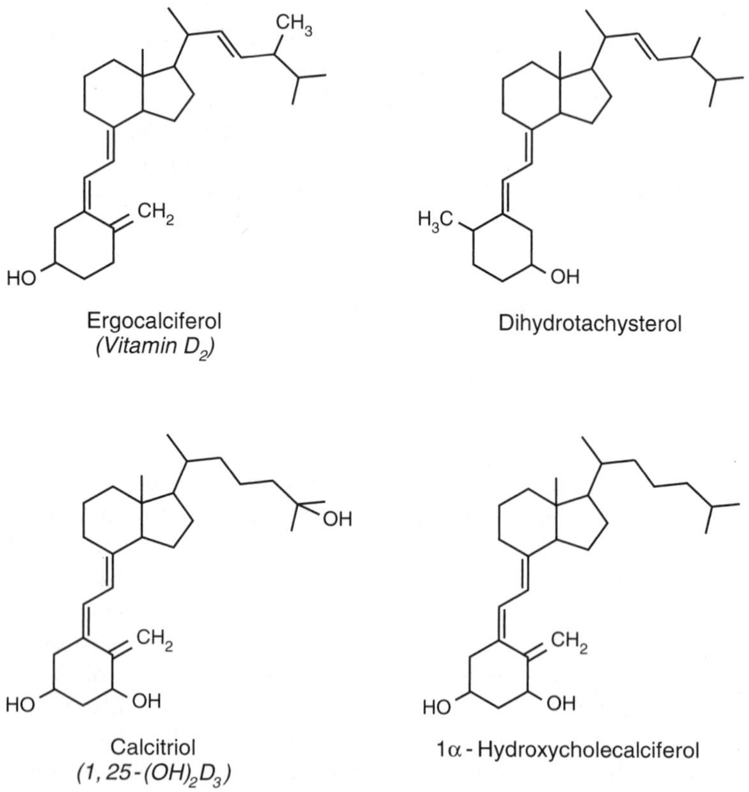

Figure 68-3. Structural formulae of clinically important vitamin D preparations and analogs.

roidism, and up to 10 mg in vitamin D-dependent rickets, whereas this latter condition may respond to 0.25–0.5 μg of calcitriol. The usual dose of calcitriol or 1α-hyroxycholecalciferol in hypoparathyroidism is 1 μg a day.

Calcitonin

The amino acid sequences of calcitonins from a number of different species have been determined, and the hormones have been characterized and synthesized. While the number of amino acids is 32 in all species, the amino acid sequence of calcitonin is quite different from one species to another, so there is little immunological cross-reactivity. The commonly used form is salmon calcitonin (Calcimar, Miacalcin).

The primary effect of calcitonin is to inhibit osteoclastic and osteocytic bone resorption or mineral transfer through a direct effect on cellular activity. Other effects of calcitonin are more variable and are more species-dependent. In humans, synthetic salmon calcitonin (Caltine) inhibits tubular reabsorption of calcium, phosphate, sodium, potassium, and magnesium. Pharmacological effects of calcitonin on intestinal absorption of calcium are still uncertain.

Calcitonin must be administered parenterally by subcutaneous or intramuscular injection. A preparation for intranasal administration has been tested in clinical trials but is not yet available for general use in North America. Absorption of calcitonin from injection sites is rapid, although it is slowed by addition of gelatin to the vehicle. In the circulation the half-life of calcitonin is on the order of 20 minutes. It is weakly and insignificantly bound to protein and is catabolized in liver and kidney.

Acute administration of calcitonin lowers serum calcium and phosphate through inhibition of bone resorption. With chronic administration, the rate of bone remodeling is decreased and the urinary excretion of calcium and hydroxyproline is diminished in spite of decreased tubular reabsorption of calcium.

Calcitonin is relatively free of adverse effects, although a small minority of patients experience nausea and flushing following its injection. Patients may become resistant to the actions of calcitonin because of antibody formation, since the preparation that is used pharmacologically is most often synthetic salmon calcitonin. Synthetic human calcitonin (Cibacalcin) is available in limited quantities for treatment of patients who have become resistant to salmon calcitonin because of antibody formation. The action

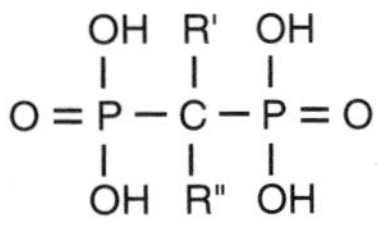

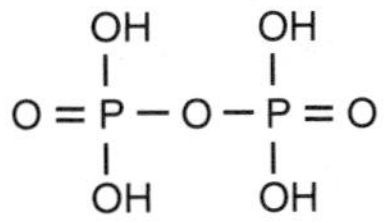

Figure 68-4. Structural formulae of bisphosphonic acid and pyrophosphoric acid. The latter is a naturally occurring inhibitor of bone mineralization.

of injected human calcitonin is not affected by high levels of anti–salmon calcitonin antibody.

Drug interactions are uncommon, but the concomitant administration of calcitonin and thiazide diuretics may be associated with potassium depletion.

Therapeutic applications

It has been stated that the three consistently established indications for the use of calcitonin are Paget's disease of bone, hypercalcemia, and osteoporosis. However, calcitonin may be effective initially in the treatment of hypercalcemia, but usually patients rapidly become refractory to it; this phenomenon most likely represents receptor down-regulation. Bone diseases with decreased bone density, such as involutional forms of osteoporosis with low bone turnover rates, are unlikely to benefit significantly from further decrease in bone turnover rate induced by calcitonin. Calcitonin is effective in diseases associated with increased skeletal remodeling, such as Paget's disease of bone. Synthetic salmon calcitonin administered subcutaneously or intramuscularly in doses of 50 to 100 IU, three times weekly, produces symptomatic relief from pain and reductions in bone remodeling and blood flow through affected areas. It has been suggested that calcitonin may decrease the spread of metastases of malignant disease in bone, with resultant decreases in bone pain and hypercalcemia. This indication for the clinical use of calcitonin needs further documentation in a well-controlled clinical study.

Bisphosphonates

The bisphosphonates are structurally similar to endogenous pyrophosphate (Fig. 68-4) and bind to the exposed mineral surface of bone at active sites of bone resorption. Based on the P-C-P structure, a large number of bisphosphonates have been synthesized. Figure 68-5 shows the structural formulae of eight bisphosphonates that were reported to have been administered to humans. These drugs have proved to be effective inhibitors of bone resorption, but their mechanism of action is uncertain. It is known that bisphosphonates alter the morphology of osteoclasts both in vitro and in vivo, and they may act as intracellular toxins.

Despite these effects on osteoclasts, bisphosphonates act almost exclusively on calcified tissues, especially bone, by virtue of their strong affinity for calcium phosphate. It appears that bisphosphonates are either incorporated into bone at sites of active bone remodeling or they are cleared rapidly in the urine.

The absorption of bisphosphonates from the small intestine is probably not more than 1–5% of an orally administered dose. Absorption is diminished when given with food, and in particular by high concentrations of calcium in the intestine. It has been estimated that 20–50% of absorbed bisphosphonate is localized in bone and the remainder excreted in the urine within 24 hours.

Studies in humans have revealed very few adverse effects with oral administration, other than mild diarrhea, nausea, and abdominal pain in relatively few cases. Etidronate, the least potent of the tested bisphosphonates as an inhibitor of resorption (Table 68-2), may inhibit bone mineralization when given in large doses or long-term treatment. No drug interactions have been reported.

Therapeutic applications

The clinical usefulness of the bisphosphonates is related to diseases and disorders of calcium and bone metabolism:

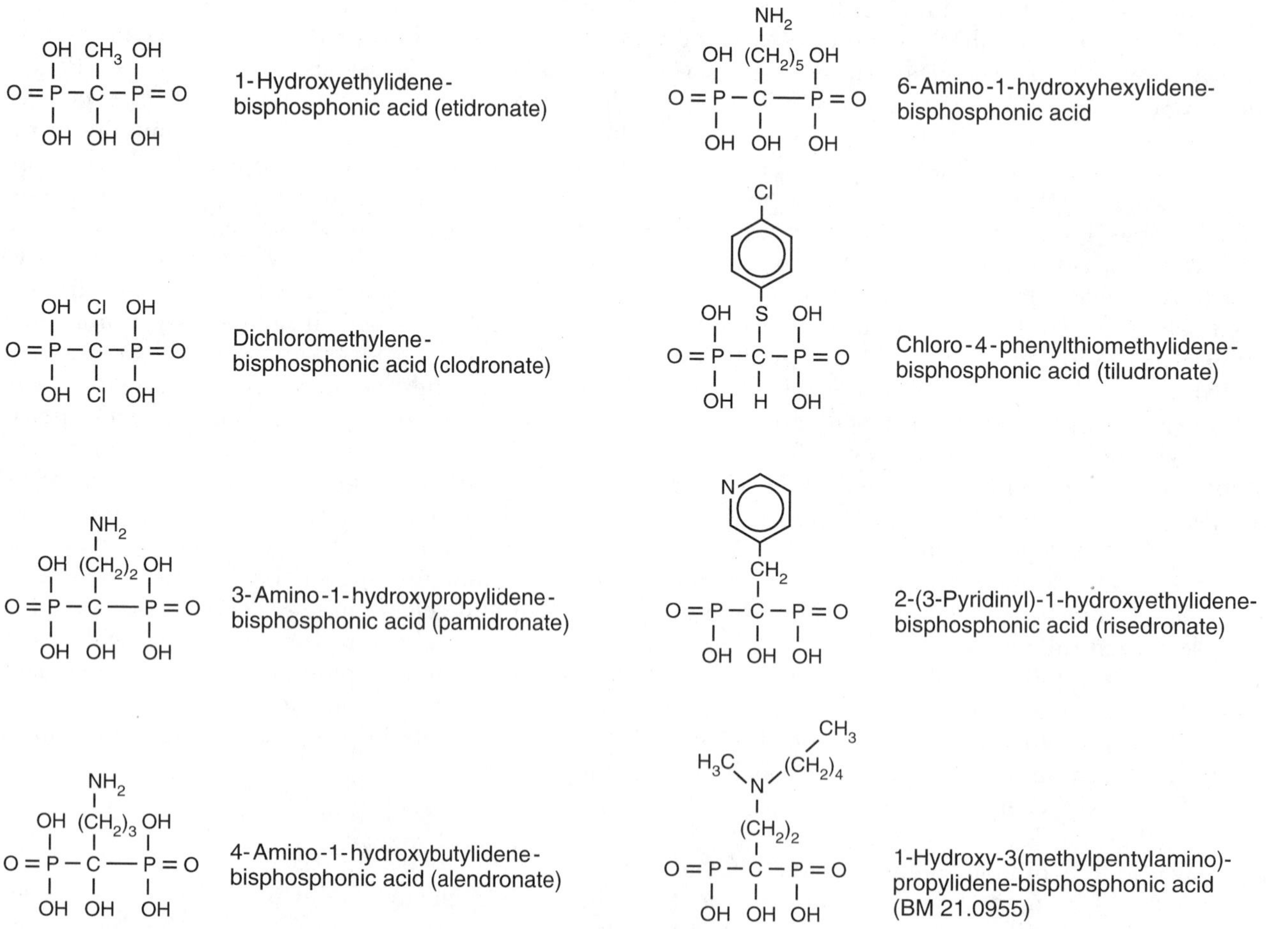

Figure 68-5. Structural formulae of bisphosphonates reported to have been administered to humans.

Table 68-2 Antiresorbing Potency of Various Bisphosphonates in Rats

Bisphosphonate	Potency
Etidronate	1
Clodronate	10
Tiludronate	10
Pamidronate	100
Alendronate	1000
Risedronate	5000
BM 210955	10,000

1. ^{99m}Tc-labeled bisphosphonates are used for diagnostic purposes in metabolic and tumor-induced bone disease.
2. The drugs inhibit soft-tissue calcification.
3. The drugs are established in the treatment of hypercalcemia, tumor osteolysis, Paget's disease, and osteoporosis.

Etidronate (Didronel), pamidronate (Aredia), and clodronate (Bonefos, Ostac) are available for prescription use. Recently, alendronate (Fosamax) has also been approved for treatment of osteoporosis in the United States and Canada, and it is likely to be approved in other countries in the near future.

Mithramycin

Mithramycin is a cytotoxic antibiotic isolated from cultures of *Streptomyces tanashiensis*. It inhibits the synthesis of RNA without affecting protein synthesis. Osteoclasts appear to be particularly sensitive to its action.

Mithramycin has to be administered intravenously and little is known about its distribution, biotransformation, or excretion. In hypercalcemic patients, low doses of mithramycin decrease bone resorption and plasma calcium concentration through a direct action on osteoclasts.

At antineoplastic doses, mithramycin is highly toxic to the liver, kidneys, and hematopoietic tissue. Severe hemorrhage may occur because of impaired synthesis of clotting factors and platelets.

Therapeutic applications

Mithramycin is useful in treating patients with hypercalcemia associated with carcinoma and increased bone resorption. For treatment of hypercalcemia or hypercalciuria associated with malignant disease, the dose has been 25 μg/kg daily for 1–3 days, diluted in 5% dextrose and water and infused intravenously over 6 hours. The effect, however, is short-lived and treatment may have to be repeated at weekly intervals. At lower doses of 10–15 μg/kg/day for 7–10 days by intravenous infusion, mithramycin may provide substantial relief of pain in Paget's disease of bone.

SUGGESTED READING

Bell NH. Vitamin D metabolism, aging, and bone loss [Editorial]. J Clin Endocrinol Metab 1995; 80:1051.

Black DM, Cummings SR, Karpf DB, et al. Randomized trial of effect of alendronate on risk of fracture in women with existing vertebral fractures. Lancet 1996; 348:1535–1541.

Favus MJ, ed. Primer on the metabolic bone diseases and disorders of mineral metabolism. 2nd ed. New York: Raven Press, 1993.

Haines CJ, Chung TKA, Leung PC, Hsu SYC, Leung DHY. Calcium supplementation and bone mineral density in postmenopausal women using estrogen replacement therapy. Bone 1995; 16:529–531.

Kanis JA, Melton LJ, Christiansen C, Johnston CC, Khaltaev N. Perspective: the diagnosis of osteoporosis. J Bone Miner Res 1994; 9:1137–1141.

Mosekilde L. Osteoporosis and exercise. Bone 1995; 17:193–195.

Prince R, Devine A, Dick I, et al. The effects of calcium supplementation (milk powder or tablets) and exercise on bone density in postmenopausal women. J Bone Miner Res 1995; 10:1068–1075.

Sturtridge WC. Osteoporosis and Paget's disease. Med North Am, May 1981:1171–1180.

Sturtridge WC, Wilson DR. Management of hypercalcemia. Drug Ther, Jan 1982:108–112.

CHAPTER 69

Chemical Carcinogenesis

A.B. OKEY AND P.A. HARPER

In North America more than one person in three will develop cancer; this can occur at any age, but the incidence and mortality for most types of cancer rise steeply with age. Cancer is the cause of death for about one person in four. What are its causes? From epidemiological studies it is estimated that 60–90% of human cancers are primarily due to environmental factors. "Environmental factors" means all nongenetic elements including not only environmental chemicals but also other contributing elements such as diet and cultural and behavioral practices that are collectively termed "lifestyle."

There is little doubt that exposure to xenobiotic (foreign) chemicals (in the form of environmental substances or drugs) is a major risk factor in the overall incidence of human cancer. About one-third of cancer deaths in North America are related to the use of cigarettes and other tobacco products. Other medical, industrial, and environmental chemicals that are strongly implicated in the human cancer problem are summarized later in this chapter.

As illustrated in Figures 69-1 and 69-2, North American mortality rates from cancer at most anatomical sites have decreased or remained relatively constant over the past 60 years. The important exception is lung cancer. In North American males, mortality from lung cancer escalated rapidly after World War II. This rise is the result of the increased frequency of cigarette smoking, a practice that became common in the male population around the time of World War I.

The lung cancer problem illustrates an important manner in which cancer differs from most other chemically induced toxic responses. That is, cancer usually appears only after a long *latent period*. Hu-

man cancers typically may not be clinically evident for as long as 10–20 years after exposure to the agent that caused the tumor. Obviously, this great time delay between exposure and cancer detection complicates identification of the responsible agent(s).

The concept of a latent period is further illustrated by cancer mortality data in North American females. Cigarette smoking did not become common in the North American female population until World War II. As shown in Figure 69-2, mortality from lung cancer in females began to increase sharply around 1960. The rise in mortality from lung cancer in females is tragically reminiscent of the escalation that began in the male population two decades earlier. Within the decade of the 1990s, lung cancer has overtaken breast cancer as the leading cause of cancer-related deaths in North American females.

CHEMICAL CARCINOGENS: DIVERSITY OF ORIGINS AND CHEMICAL STRUCTURES

"Natural" Versus "Synthetic" Carcinogens

Tables 69-1, 69-2, and 69-3 list a variety of agents that have been reported to be carcinogenic. It is important to note that these lists include both natural and synthetic chemicals. Although many of the known carcinogens are products of modern synthetic chemistry or are byproducts of industrial processes, the natural world contained carcinogens long before humans developed technologically based industrial societies.

The following are examples of naturally occurring

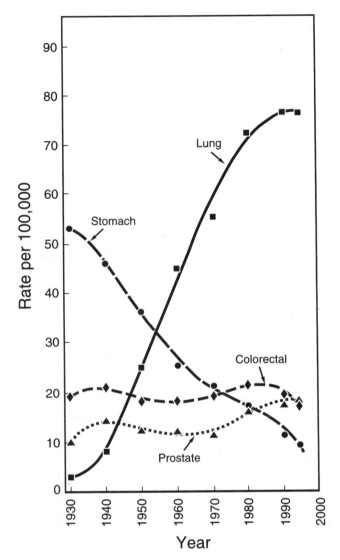

Figure 69-1. Mortality rates for selected cancer sites in males, Canada, 1931–1995. Data are redrawn from *Canadian Cancer Statistics 1995* compiled and released through the courtesy of the National Cancer Institute of Canada, with funds from the Canadian Cancer Society, Toronto, Canada, 1995. Age-standardized mortality rates from cancers at different anatomic sites are likely to be similar in the United States to those in Canada. In regard to lung cancer, cigarette consumption patterns over the past several decades have been similar in Canada, the United States, and most of western Europe (Wynder and Hoffman, 1994).

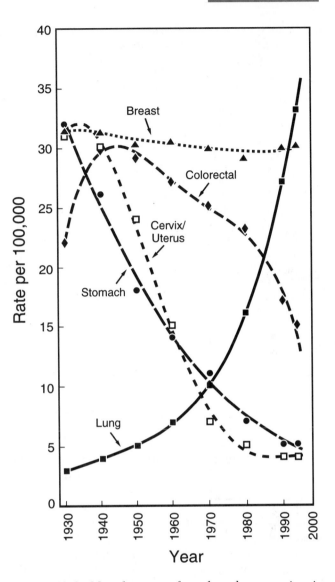

Figure 69-2. Mortality rates for selected cancer sites in females, Canada, 1931–1995. Data are redrawn from *Canadian Cancer Statistics 1995* compiled and released through the courtesy of the National Cancer Institute of Canada, with funds from the Canadian Cancer Society, Toronto, Canada 1995. Note expanded vertical scale.

carcinogens: Aflatoxin B_1, a potent liver carcinogen, is routinely formed by molds that contaminate improperly stored foodstuffs; polycyclic aromatic hydrocarbons such as benzo[a]pyrene are universally generated by partial combustion processes, including burning of wood and charcoal-cooking of food, as well as by internal combustion engines; safrole, a volatile oil from sassafras tea, is a carcinogen in mice and possibly in humans. Many other examples of naturally occurring carcinogens could be given. The point is that carcinogens are formed both by natural processes and by human activities.

Table 69-1 Some Environmental Factors and Industrial Agents Implicated in Human Carcinogenesis

Ionizing radiation
Ultraviolet radiation
Alcohol
Aromatic amines
Arsenic
Asbestos
Aflatoxins
Benzene
Benzidine
Cadmium
Carbon tetrachloride
Chromium
Soots, tars, mineral oils
Tobacco smoke
Vinyl chloride

Table 69-3 Miscellaneous Drugs Reported to be Carcinogenic

Chloramphenicol
Chloroform
Diethylstilbestrol (DES)
Metronidazole
Nitrofurantoin
Nitrofurazone
Phenacetin
Phenytoin

Prevalence of Carcinogens in the Chemical World

It is important to understand that not all chemicals have carcinogenic properties, regardless of whether they are natural products or synthetic chemicals. News reports in the popular media often give the incorrect impression that the majority of drugs and environmental chemicals cause cancer.

Table 69-4 gives some perspective on the prevalence of carcinogens among the overall spectrum of known chemicals. It can be seen that the number of *known* carcinogens is very small when compared to the number of existing chemical structures. In truth, however, the vast majority of chemicals, even those

in common use, have not been adequately tested for carcinogenicity. Thus, it is impossible to state the magnitude of total exposure to carcinogens with any degree of accuracy. The methods used to test chemicals for carcinogenicity are described later in this chapter.

Diversity of Chemical Types

It is immediately apparent, even from just the names of the agents listed in Tables 69-1, 69-2, and 69-3, that carcinogens are found in a wide variety of chemical classes. A central theme from a pharmacological perspective is that the biological activity of a compound should be related to the compound's structure. However, there are no simple structure–activity rules by which a given compound can be designated as a carcinogen (or noncarcinogen) solely by virtue of its chemical structure.

This apparent lack of structure–activity relationships perplexed early workers in the field of experimental chemical carcinogenesis. Since carcinogens occurred in a wide variety of chemical classes, it was feared that there might be a very large number of

Table 69-2 Examples of Carcinogenic Anticancer Drugs

Adriamycin
Chlorambucil
Cyclophosphamide
Doxorubicin
Mechlorethamine
Melphalan (phenylalanine mustard)
Mitomycin C
Procarbazine
Streptozotocin
Triethylene melamine (TEM)
Triethylenethiophosphoramide
Uracil mustard

Table 69-4 Cancer and Chemicals: Numerical Considerations

Total chemicals known (natural and synthetic)	>12,000,000
Chemicals in common widespread use	~60,000
Chemicals demonstrated to be carcinogenic in experimental animals	~2000
Chemicals for which there is strong evidence of carcinogenic activity in humans	~50–75

mechanisms by way of which these diverse chemical structures caused cancer. Later evidence has shown that this is not so. The scheme in Figure 69-3 provides a model that attempts to unify diverse chemical structures into a common pathway leading to cancer.

CARCINOGENESIS AS A MULTISTAGE BIOCHEMICAL AND BIOLOGICAL PROCESS

The complex diagram in Figure 69-3 provides a framework for examining the sequence of events in chemical carcinogenesis. The diagram emphasizes that cancer is the result of a progressive multistage process. The scheme in Figure 69-3 is used for reference as the particular stages in the carcinogenic process are examined below.

Direct-Acting Carcinogens

The common final target of most chemical carcinogens appears to be DNA. It is possible that certain RNA species or specific proteins also might be the critical targets, but virtually all current evidence focuses on DNA as the critical site for carcinogen action. Some drugs (such as alkylating agents used in chemotherapy of cancer) are chemically reactive in the form in which they are administered. These have the ability to bind directly to nucleophilic sites on DNA, RNA, and proteins. This ability probably is responsible both for their ability to kill cancer cells (as therapeutic agents) and for their ability to induce new tumors. (Note: Cyclophosphamide, an important alkylating agent used in cancer therapy, *does* require metabolic activation in order to exert its cytotoxic effects; see Chapter 60.)

Metabolic Activation into Ultimate Carcinogens

The term *ultimate carcinogen* refers to the chemical species that directly interacts with DNA. Most cancer-causing chemicals are not carcinogenic in the form in which they enter the body. Compounds such as polycyclic aromatic hydrocarbons (e.g., benzo[*a*]pyrene) are chemically unreactive in their parent form and cannot form covalent bonds with DNA. Enzyme systems within the organism biotransform unreactive pro- or precarcinogens into chemically reactive products that can covalently interact with nucleophilic sites on cellular macromolecules.

As Figure 69-3 suggests, metabolic activation usually requires more than one enzymatic step. Initial activation often is carried out by various species of cytochrome P450 (see Chapter 4), but activation by reductases, peroxidases, and prostaglandin synthetic pathways also is well established. Regardless of the pathway(s), the final product (ultimate carcinogen) is a reactive electrophilic species.

Some specific examples of metabolic activation pathways are given in Figures 69-4 and 69-5. Figure 69-4 outlines the biotransformation processes that result in the conversion of the procarcinogen, benzo-[*a*]pyrene (BP), into an ultimate carcinogenic form capable of covalent binding to DNA. BP has been studied more than any other carcinogen. The primary activation scheme shown in Figure 69-4 is well supported by experimental evidence, but this is not the only pathway by which BP can be activated into an ultimate carcinogen.

The first step in activation of BP is its conversion into an arene oxide, BP 7,8-oxide. This first step is catalyzed by a species of cytochrome P450 known as CYP1A1. BP 7,8-oxide then serves as a substrate for epoxide hydrolase, an enzyme that converts the oxide to a dihydrodiol by the addition of a molecule of water. The dihydrodiol is much more water-soluble than the parent compound, and it previously had been thought that the BP 7,8-oxide was effectively "detoxified" by the action of epoxide hydrolase. Further investigation, however, revealed that the dihydrodiol undergoes a second conversion by CYP1A1 to form BP 7,8-diol-9,10-epoxide. The diol epoxide is chemically reactive and capable of covalent binding to DNA; hence it is an ultimate carcinogenic form of BP.

Figure 69-5 indicates that various species of P450 enzymes also are involved in the initial activation steps for structurally diverse carcinogens such as 2-acetylaminofluorene (AAF, an aromatic amine), nitrosamines, vinyl chloride, and aflatoxins. Figure 69-5 also serves to reemphasize that metabolic activation commonly involves more than one enzymatic step before an ultimate carcinogen is formed. In the case of AAF, the initial step is formation of *N*-hydroxy-AAF catalyzed by a P450, CYP1A2. The *N*-hydroxy intermediate then may follow one of several pathways leading to formation of a sulfate ester, an acetate ester, or a nitroxide radical. All these pathways are contenders for the generation of an ultimate carcinogen. The specific pathway depends upon the tissue: Sulfotransferase activity predominates in liver, whereas acyltransferase activity predominates in nonhepatic tissues such as the mammary gland. Both liver and mammary gland are susceptible to tumor induction by AAF, implying that different ultimate carcinogens can be formed from the same parent

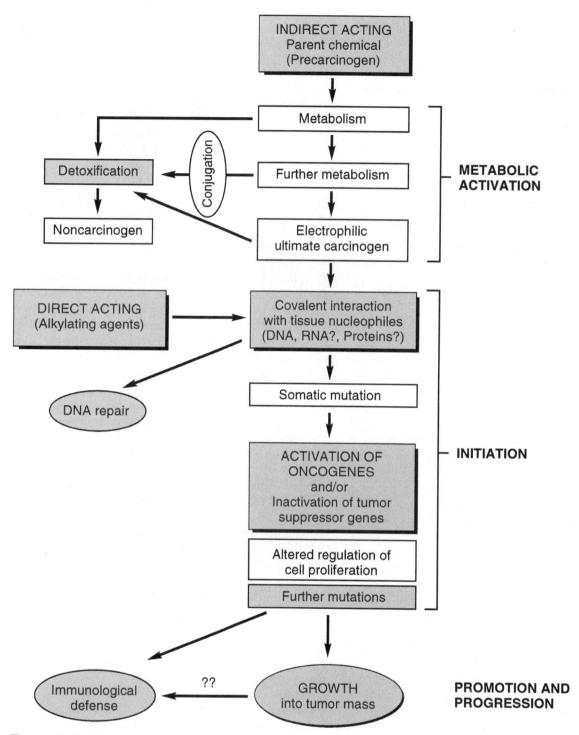

Figure 69-3. General mechanisms of chemical carcinogenesis.

compound in different tissues by different metabolic pathways. Differences in metabolic capabilities among different tissues may in part explain why some carcinogens are tissue-selective in inducing tumors.

The discussion up to this point might imply that cytochromes P450 are undesirable and are harmful to the organism. There is no question that P450 enzymes are capable of converting many classes of chemicals into reactive intermediates that are toxic

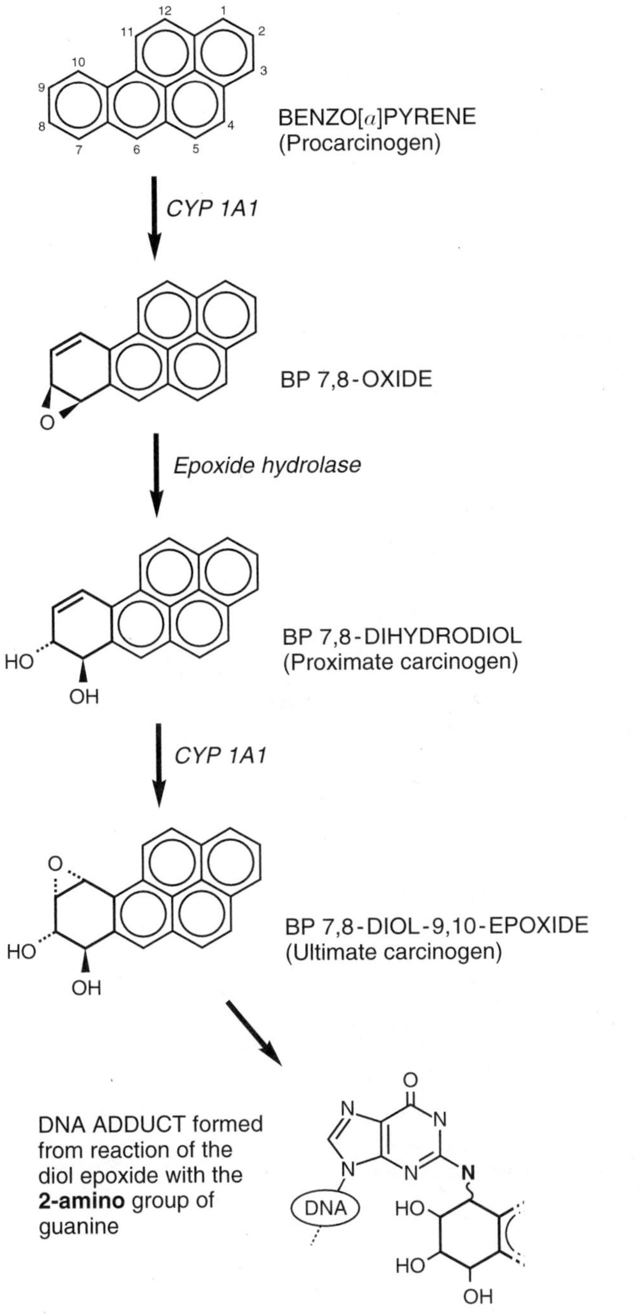

Figure 69-4. Metabolic activation of benzo[a]pyrene. Note: Only the main activation pathway is shown. Many other metabolic products can be formed from BP via several metabolic pathways involving P450 species or other enzymes.

or carcinogenic. It should be recalled, however, that P450-mediated reactions are the major pathways by which most hydrophobic drugs and environmental chemicals are converted into forms that can be conjugated and excreted (see Chapter 4).

Epoxide hydrolase also could be viewed both as a "beneficial" enzyme and as an enzyme deleterious to health. The determination of whether these enzymes are beneficial or harmful depends upon many complex factors such as dose and route of administration of their drug substrates and the efficiency with which activation pathways are coupled with conjugating enzymes. The teleological goal of P450 enzymes and epoxide hydrolase is to facilitate the elimination of xenobiotic chemicals (see Chapter 4). Conversion of some xenobiotic agents into toxic or carcinogenic metabolites could be viewed as an occasional accidental byproduct of the action of generally beneficial enzymes.

Detoxication

Metabolic activation does not invariably lead to covalent attacks on critical macromolecules such as DNA. Most cells are well equipped with mechanisms that inactivate reactive metabolites before these metabolites strike critical targets. The predominant means of "detoxication" is via conjugation with glutathione (GSH), sulfate, or glucuronides (see Chapter 4). Cells that are deficient in GSH are known to be at high risk of cell death from reactive metabolites formed in the biotransformation of many drugs (see Chapter 46). GSH-deficient cells also may be at high risk for neoplastic transformation when exposed to carcinogens. Moreover, epidemiological studies have indicated an increased risk of lung cancer in smokers with deficient glutathione S-transferase activity combined with elevated CYP1A1 activity.

In normal cells, most reactive metabolites probably are detoxified by conjugating enzymes or by reaction with noncritical protein targets. Cells at highest risk will be those that have an imbalance between the rate at which reactive metabolites are generated and the rate at which those metabolites can be conjugated and excreted.

Covalent Interaction with Tissue Nucleophiles

Much of the progress in understanding chemical carcinogenesis has been made by tracing forward the route of parent compounds from their site of application through distribution to various tissues and through specific biotransformation pathways that convert procarcinogens into ultimate carcinogens.

In several instances the chemical identity of the ultimate carcinogenic form has been determined by chemical characterization of carcinogen adducts isolated from DNA. Carcinogen adducts (bound forms)

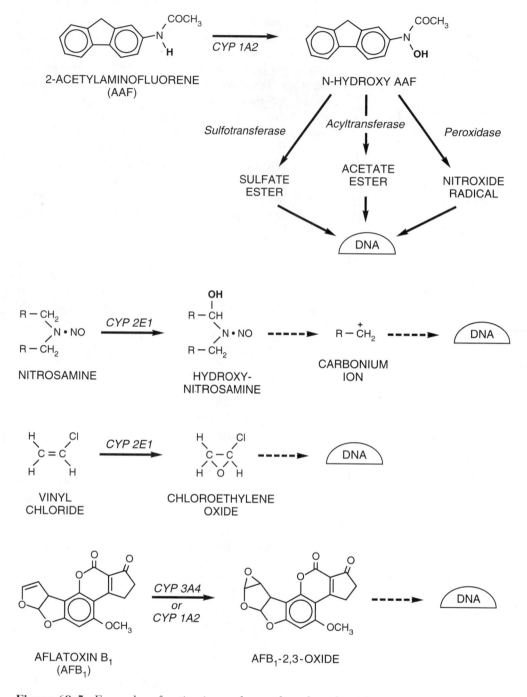

Figure 69-5. Examples of activation pathways for selected carcinogens.

have been detected on all four nitrogen bases in DNA and at several atomic sites within each base. Recent evidence indicates that major classes of chemical carcinogens, such as cigarette smoke or aflatoxins, may leave characteristic "fingerprints" consisting of specific adduct patterns on nucleotides in "hot spots" in the key genes that govern conversion of normal cells into clinical tumor. Such patterns may allow the epidemiologist to link major forms of human cancers to the causative agents.

Some chemicals appear to be carcinogenic by nongenotoxic mechanisms. These nongenotoxic agents may act via several disparate pathways including disruption of hormonal regulation of cell growth and stimulation of oxidative stress that eventually leads to DNA damage. Although the emphasis in chemical carcinogenesis usually has focused on exogenous chemicals that are foreign to the human body, endogenous processes also may contribute to DNA damage. For example, it has been proposed by Ames and colleagues that spontaneous damage to DNA from endogenous oxidants in cells may be far more abundant than the DNA damage wrought by exogenous chemicals. It is not at all clear, however, to what extent the damage to DNA from endogenous processes contributes to human cancer (see "Letters to the Editor," *Science* 1991; 252:902–904).

Initiation (Neoplastic Transformation)

Covalent binding of the ultimate carcinogen to DNA alters the genetic message. If the lesion in DNA is not recognized and repaired before cell division, the genetic lesion may be "fixed" as a mutation, which will be inherited by progeny stemming from the altered cell. This permanent alteration is the initial cellular event in the cancer process.

Not all chemically induced mutations lead to cancer. Many DNA lesions probably are lethal to the cell bearing them. In addition, DNA-repair enzymes usually operate with high efficiency. Individuals who are genetically deficient in DNA-repair enzymes exhibit an increased risk for some, but not all, forms of cancer.

Over the past several years, considerable excitement has been generated by the prospect that the primary targets of chemicals and other carcinogens might be a limited number of *oncogenes* (literally: cancer genes). As stated by Bishop (1987), "proto-oncogenes are the keyboard upon which carcinogens play." As a general model, it is proposed that the conversion of proto-oncogenes into oncogenes is a key event in the initiation of tumorigenesis (Fig. 69-3). Proto-oncogenes are normal cellular genes, most of which appear to code for cellular growth factors or growth-factor receptors, for example, *erbB*. Other important oncogenes include *myc*, *fos*, and *jun*, which act as transcription factors, and *bcl-1*, which acts as a cell-cycle kinase activator. When a proto-oncogene is damaged by a carcinogen (i.e., undergoes mutation, chromosomal translocation, etc.) the resulting oncogene drives the abnormal cell division and abnormal cell differentiation that typify neoplastic growths.

Even more important, as shown in the last few years, is inactivation of tumor-suppressor genes. One particular tumor-suppressor gene, p53, may be mu-

tated in about half of all human cancers and may be the most common genetic target in human cancer. p53 appears to play multiple roles in that it is a transcription factor that can provoke arrest of the cell cycle and also induce apoptosis ("programmed cell death"). The retinoblastoma (Rb) gene product also appears to function as a transcription factor that can alter the cell cycle, as does the tumor-suppressor gene p16.

Tumor Promotion and Promoters

In its simplest form, the multistage cancer process can be thought of as two major events: initiation (described above) and promotion.

Promotion refers to a poorly defined set of circumstances that permit initiated cells to proliferate into tumor masses. Several chemicals that are not in themselves "complete" carcinogens (i.e., do not act as initiators) are able to promote development of tumors that have been initiated by other agents. Examples of tumor promoters are listed in Table 69-5.

Generally, *initiators* are thought to be agents that are capable of forming mutagenic electrophilic metabolites as previously described. In principle, initiation can be accomplished by a single exposure to the initiating agent. The mutationally based initiation process seems essentially irreversible.

In contrast, *promoting agents* do not appear to

Table 69-5 Selected Examples of Tumor Promoters in Laboratory Animals

Mouse skin tumors
 Phorbol esters from croton oil, e.g., 12-*O*-tetradecanoyl-phorbol-13-acetate (TPA)
 Phenol
 Anthralin
 Hexadecane
 Iodoacetic acid
 Cigarette smoke condensate
 Extracts of unburned cigarettes
 Surfactants and detergents
 Benzoyl peroxide
 Abrasions or wounding

Rodent liver tumors
 Phenobarbital
 Chlorophenothane (DDT)
 Polychlorinated biphenyls (PCBs)
 2,3,7,8-Tetrachlorodibenzo-*p*-dioxin (TCDD, "dioxin")

be mutagenic; instead, they exert their effect through nongenotoxic pathways involved with selective stimulation of proliferation of the initiated cell. In order to produce tumors experimentally, the promoting agent must be given after treatment with an initiator, and the promoter must be given repeatedly over a prolonged time period. The actions of promoters appear to be reversible, at least in early stages. This simplified picture of initiation followed by promotion is giving way to an understanding that several important human tumors—for example, colon cancer—arise as a consequence of a sequential accumulation of mutations in proto-oncogenes and tumor-suppressor genes. Each mutation pushes the cell further from normal limits to proliferation and closer to the invasive and metastatic phenotype that typifies a serious clinical disease.

One hallmark of cancer cells is general instability of the genome. Human cancer cells contain high frequencies of chromosomal abnormalities as well as mutations. Damage to those genes that are responsible for maintaining stability of the genome is likely to be a key early event in the process of carcinogenesis. If these *stability genes* (including the genes governing DNA replication, DNA repair, and chromosomal segregation) are altered by mutation, the stage is set for a cascade of further mutations that may hit oncogenes and tumor-suppressor genes, thereby leading to unregulated cell growth, invasiveness, and metastasis.

DETECTION OF CARCINOGENS

Table 69-6 summarizes the major methods used at present to test chemicals for potential carcinogenic activity.

Long-Term Tests In Vivo

The ultimate "proof" that a given chemical is a human carcinogen can be obtained only by carefully designed epidemiological studies and by rigorous evaluation of clinical observations. Given the multitude of drugs and environmental agents to which humans are exposed and the long latent period between exposure and tumor appearance, it is not surprising that confirmation of carcinogenicity in humans is a protracted and difficult process.

Bioassays in laboratory animals (usually rodents) have until recently been the primary method of testing chemicals for carcinogenic potential. Rodent tests have been criticized as irrelevant to the human cancer

Table 69-6 Methods for Detection of Carcinogens

Long-term tests in vivo
 Clinical observations and epidemiology
 Bioassays in laboratory animals

Short-term screening tests

 Covalent binding of test compounds to DNA after metabolic activation in vivo or in vitro

 Tests for chromosome damage
  Chromosomal abnormalities by cytogenetic assays
  Sister chromatid exchange
  Micronucleus formation
  Sperm abnormalities

 Mutational tests
  Bacterial (Ames's *Salmonella* test)
  Mammalian cells in culture
  Other prokaryotic or eukaryotic organisms

 Neoplastic transformation of mammalian cells in culture

problem because such tests frequently employ doses that are greatly in excess of probable human exposure levels for the chemical in question. At these high doses ("maximally tolerated doses"), cytotoxic effects of the test chemical might lead to increased tumor formation via mitogenesis per se rather than by adduct-induced mutagenesis. Recent molecular epidemiology studies in humans, however, indicate that many important human cancers are associated with adduct-driven mutagenesis rather than the secondary effects of mitogenesis. Although there are legitimate concerns about the relevance of the high doses used in rodent bioassays, experience has shown that most chemicals that induce a significant frequency of tumors at high doses also induce some tumors at lower doses.

High doses are employed in animal tests for a very practical reason—namely, to increase the sensitivity of the assay. Thorough rodent bioassays for carcinogenicity of a *single chemical* typically cost in excess of $1 million and may require 2–5 years of research. High doses are used to reduce the number of animals required and the consequent cost of the assay. Usually a maximum of a few hundred animals can be studied, and it is necessary to test with doses that potentially can produce a high frequency of tumors. A chemical that caused cancer in one animal out of 1000 tested (for example, at lower doses) would not be detected as a carcinogen, yet a similar increase in cancer frequency in the North American human population would afflict more than 250,000 people.

Carcinogenic activity in rodents does not prove that a chemical will be a carcinogen in humans, but nearly all known human carcinogens are also carcinogenic in rodents. Any chemical that is a carcinogen in laboratory animals must be considered a *potential* carcinogen in humans. Specific knowledge of the exact mechanism(s) by which cancers arise is required before any discrepancies in animal testing versus human carcinogenesis can be explained.

Short-Term Screening Tests

As stated in the previous section, in vivo animal tests are the definitive method for demonstrating carcinogenic activity. Because in vivo tests are expensive and time-consuming, less-expensive short-term tests have been developed to cope with the thousands of chemicals that must be tested for potential carcinogenic activity.

Most of the screening tests are based on the premise that carcinogens act by damaging DNA and that they are therefore mutagenic. *Mutagenesis tests in bacterial systems* are much quicker and cheaper than whole-animal tests for carcinogenesis. Bacterial mutational test systems (e.g., the Ames Assay) are used in literally thousands of laboratories around the world and are especially valuable as an inexpensive screen in the development of compounds that may have market potential.

Early attempts to correlate mutagenesis in bacterial systems with carcinogenesis in animals were compromised because the necessity for host-mediated metabolic activation of procarcinogens was not yet recognized. Present-day tests employ a combined system using mammalian liver enzymes (to activate procarcinogens) and *Salmonella* bacterial strains (to detect mutations). This system has shown that approximately *90% of carcinogens are mutagenic* and that many mutagens are carcinogens.

The science of carcinogenesis has not yet developed to the stage where any single test is considered adequate as an all-encompassing screen for carcinogenic chemicals. Rather, a battery of tests is required both in vivo and in vitro.

DOSE–RESPONSE CONSIDERATIONS IN CARCINOGENESIS

In general, the carcinogenic response, like other pharmacological responses, is quantitatively related to

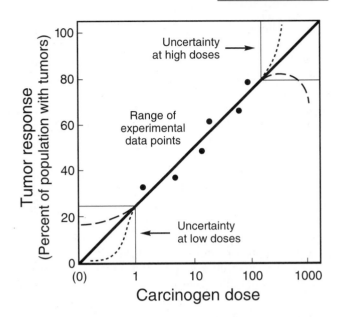

Figure 69-6. Hypothetical carcinogen dose–response curves. Uncertainty at low doses may be caused by the presence of a background of spontaneous tumors in every laboratory species (broken line).

dose (or to exposure). As illustrated in Figure 69-6, the frequency of tumors in a population increases linearly with the logarithm of the dose. This linear log-dose–response relationship has been shown experimentally to hold for several carcinogenic chemicals provided that the carcinogen doses given yield a medium level of tumor response. At very high or very low doses, linearity of the dose–response relationship is in question.

At very high doses, animals may die from toxicity before tumors have an opportunity to develop to a detectable stage.

The greatest difficulty, however, lies in *interpretation of the tumor response expected at very low doses.* Much of human exposure to potential carcinogens is of a chronic, low-dose nature. If the tumor dose-response curve is linear and originates at zero, there is no dose that will not produce a finite increase in tumor frequency. Only zero dose would yield zero increase in risk—i.e., there is no totally safe dose for carcinogens.

The other possibility is that the dose–response relationship is not linear at very low doses. This includes the possibility that a *threshold* dose may exist, below which tumor risk is not significantly elevated. Alternatively, tumors that result from exposure to the test chemical may be superimposed on a background of spontaneous tumors that are present in every laboratory species (broken line in Fig. 69-6).

To this date there has been *no satisfactory experimental definition of the nature of the dose–response curve at very low carcinogen doses.* A few large-scale experiments involving thousands of rodents have been attempted, but these still have been inadequate to define response at very low doses. Partly this is inherent in the statistical uncertainty present when any rare event is measured. Only extremely large numbers of animals would reduce this uncertainty to a level where the nature of the response itself could be determined. It also is apparent that no laboratory animal can be treated in an environment that is totally free from contamination by trace levels of other chemicals that are unwanted in the experiment. For these and other reasons, the tumor response at very low doses may never be adequately defined by animal experiments.

Various mathematical models have been constructed to attempt to predict the magnitude of tumor response at very low doses. Each model requires certain assumptions that have not all been experimentally validated. At the present time there is no conclusive answer as to whether there is a safe dose for any carcinogen. Regulatory agencies must make decisions about many potential carcinogens, often without having experimental evidence that might confirm risk at very low doses. As is true in other areas of toxicology, carcinogenic risk can be determined with greater assurance when the specific mechanism by which each agent acts is well understood.

VARIATION IN CANCER SUSCEPTIBILITY

Why does one person in three develop cancer and the other two do not? Susceptibility is determined by many factors. Chief among these is the level of exposure to potential carcinogens. But even among groups exposed to the same agents, some individuals will develop cancer and others will not. The multistage model of carcinogenesis in Figure 69-3 suggests several levels at which individuals may vary in their response to carcinogens.

DNA Repair and Immune Competence

Cells from individuals with genetically based deficiencies in DNA repair are more sensitive than normal cells to the induction of mutations by chemicals, ultraviolet light, and ionizing radiation. Several DNA-repair deficiencies have been described in humans, including Bloom's syndrome, Fanconi's anemia, ataxia-telangiectasia, and xeroderma pigmentosum. Individuals with some of these diseases are more susceptible to certain cancers than are individuals with normal DNA-repair capacity. It is not yet clear, however, whether DNA-repair deficiencies invariably lead to increased risk of chemically induced cancer. Nevertheless, very recent discoveries show that damage to genes which encode DNA-repair enzymes plays a key role in the development of such tumors as hereditary nonpolyposis colon cancer. The search for inactivation of DNA-repair genes in other forms of cancer currently is of intense interest.

The importance of the immune system as a defense against cancer is illustrated by the rise in cancer risk that occurs in patients receiving intensive immunosuppressive therapy following kidney transplantation and by the susceptibility to Kaposi's sarcoma in patients whose immune system is compromised by HIV infection.

Imbalance in Enzymes that Activate or Detoxify Chemical Carcinogens

The earliest events in the process of chemical carcinogenesis, as shown in Figure 69-3, are biotransformation reactions carried out by various carcinogen-metabolizing enzymes. In laboratory animals it can be shown that the risk of chemically induced cancer is strongly influenced by the activity of these enzymes. As noted previously, however, the relationship between enzyme activities and carcinogenesis is complex. Some enzymes (e.g., cytochromes P450 and epoxide hydrolase) function both to activate certain carcinogens and to detoxify them.

In laboratory animals it generally appears that a high level of cytochrome P450 in the *liver* protects peripheral tissues from chemical carcinogens, provided that the animal is exposed to the carcinogen by a route that permits the liver to clear the carcinogen from circulation before it is distributed throughout the body. Thus, if an animal ingests a carcinogen orally or is given an intraperitoneal injection, high hepatic P450 activities enhance first-pass clearance of carcinogen by the liver and effectively reduce the carcinogen dose that is delivered to other tissues.

In contrast, if carcinogens are applied *directly* to tissues such as the skin or lung surface, tumor risk generally rises with increased P450 activities in those tissues. In such cases metabolic activation may occur locally within the tissue (by P450 and other enzymes), but this activation is not well coupled with conjugating systems or an excretory route.

Animal experiments such as these suggest that some variation in human susceptibility to chemical carcinogens might be due to variation in levels of carcinogen-metabolizing enzymes in different individuals. It would be reasonable to hypothesize that variation in the level and activity of the many enzymes that can biotransform potential carcinogens will be one contributing factor in cancer risk. Recent advances in phenotyping and genotyping of human subjects for several carcinogen-metabolizing enzymes have made it feasible to conduct epidemiological studies on the role of these enzymes in cancer risk. As mentioned earlier, smokers who possess high activity of an activating enzyme, CYP1A1, combined with deficient activity of a conjugating enzyme, glutathione S-transferase, may have a considerably elevated risk of developing certain forms of lung cancer. A polymorphism that allows high CYP1A1 gene expression in African-American women also has been reported to substantially increase the risk of breast cancer. However, the same CYP1A1 polymorphism that appears to increase CYP1A1 enzyme activity leading to elevated lung cancer risk in Japanese men and breast cancer in African-American women does not appear to be associated with increased CYP1A1 expression in eastern Mediterranean subjects or with increased lung cancer risk in Nordic males. This example again reminds us that the process of carcinogenesis is multifactorial and that factors which elevate risk in one population might not necessarily elevate risk in another population having different genetic background or environmental circumstances.

PREVENTION OF CARCINOGENESIS/ REDUCTION OF RISK

The fact that cancer is a multiple-step process provides the opportunity for reduction in cancer frequency by intervention at several levels.

Selective Inhibition of Carcinogen Activation and Selective Enhancement of Carcinogen Detoxication

In laboratory animals it is possible to use *chemoprophylaxis to reduce cancer risk*. Chemical pretreatments can be given that inhibit activation pathways or stimulate detoxication pathways, thereby inhibiting tumor induction. For example, pretreatment of

rats with phenobarbital or even with the pesticide DDT partially protects them from induction of mammary tumors and leukemia when they are later exposed to benzo[a]pyrene. These agents appear to protect by enhancing liver P450 activities and increasing hepatic clearance of the carcinogen. Unfortunately, as previously described, phenobarbital and DDT also can promote development of liver cancer in rats treated with nitrosamines. At this time we do not have the ability to selectively switch on detoxication pathways and switch off activation pathways by chemical treatment in such a way as to confer universal protection from chemical carcinogens.

Antioxidants

Several antioxidants have been demonstrated to inhibit chemical induction of tumors in experimental animals. Such chemicals include butylated hydroxytoluene (BHT), butylated hydroxyanisole (BHA), and vitamin E. Antioxidants potentially may inhibit cancer by "scavenging" reactive metabolites before they can bind to DNA, but it is not at all clear whether this mechanism totally accounts for the anticarcinogenic action of antioxidants.

Retinoic Acid Analogs

Certain retinoic acid analogs (related to vitamin A; see Chapter 67) effectively inhibit chemically induced tumors in laboratory animals, as does the dietary constituent β-carotene. These substances now are undergoing clinical trials in persons exposed occupationally to high-risk potential carcinogens. The true value of prophylactic treatment with retinoic acid analogs will not be known for several years; preliminary studies have produced disappointing results in chemoprevention of lung cancer in certain populations. Retinoic acid must be administered continuously over a prolonged time to have effect. As with any chronic drug therapy, the possibility that the treatment itself might cause some adverse effects must be weighed against the potential benefits. For example, the estrogen antagonist tamoxifen is being studied in large-scale clinical trials to attempt to prevent development of breast cancer. This study is controversial, however, because although tamoxifen is generally considered to be relatively free of side effects, some recent studies have suggested that tamoxifen may increase the risk of uterine cancer or may form adducts with DNA.

Avoidance

Several other clinical trials have been completed or are underway to test the ability of various chemical agents to reduce cancer or precancerous lesions in human subjects. However, in view of the complexity of chemical carcinogenesis, it is not surprising that no "all-purpose anticancer pill" has yet been discovered—nor is any likely to be developed in the near future. The best method currently available for reducing cancer risk is avoiding, or reducing exposure to, known causative agents.

We can never have a completely carcinogen-free environment since carcinogens arise from both natural and human processes. We can, however, avoid high-risk situations. Elimination of cigarette smoking would reduce cancer mortality more than any other single public-health measure. It is a continual source of frustration to scientists involved in cancer research that progress in this area has taken so long to be achieved among males in a few developed countries, and that these improvements are being overshadowed by the trend to increased cigarette smoking among young females in these same countries as well as the growing market for tobacco products in the large developing nations.

SUGGESTED READING

Ames BN, Gold LS. Chemical carcinogenesis: too many rodent carcinogens. Proc Natl Acad Sci USA 1990; 87:7772–7776.

Bishop JM. The molecular genetics of cancer. Science 1987; 235:305–311.

Boyd NF. Epidemiology of cancer. In: Hill RP, Tannock I, eds. The basic science of oncology. New York: McGraw-Hill, 1992:7–22.

Castonguay A. Methods and strategies in lung cancer control. Cancer Res 1992; 52:2641s–2651s.

Cavanee WK, White RL. The genetic basis of cancer. Sci Am, March 1995:72–79.

Cohen SM, Ellwein LB. Genetic errors, cell proliferation, and carcinogenesis. Cancer Res 1991; 51:6493–6505.

Farber E. Cellular biochemistry of the stepwise development of cancer with chemicals: G.H.A. Clowes memorial lecture. Cancer Res 1984; 44:5463–5474.

Friedberg EC, Graham GC, Siede W, eds. DNA repair and mutagenesis. Washington: ASM Press, 1995.

Greenwald P, Malone WF, Cerny ME, Stern HR. Cancer prevention research trials. Adv Cancer Res 1993; 61:1–23.

Harris CC. Chemical and physical carcinogenesis: advances and perspectives for the 1990s. Cancer Res 1991; 51:5023s–5044s.

Loeb LA. Microsatellite instability: marker of a mutator phenotype in cancer. Cancer Res 1994; 54:5059–5063.

Miller JA. Research in chemical carcinogenesis with Elizabeth Miller—a trail of discovery with our associates. Drug Metab Rev 1994; 26:1–36.

Nebert DW. Role of genetics and drug metabolism in human cancer risk. Mutat Res 1991; 247:267–281.

Okey AB. Enzyme induction in the cytochrome P450 system. Pharmacol Ther 1990; 45:241–298.

Vogelstein B, Kinzler KW. Carcinogens leave fingerprints. Nature 1992; 355:209–210.

Wattenberg LW. Chemoprevention of cancer by naturally occurring and synthetic compounds. In: Wattenberg L, Lipkin M, Boone CW, Kellof GJ, eds. Cancer chemoprevention. Boca Raton: CRC Press, 1991: 19–39.

Weinstein IB. Cancer prevention: recent progress and future opportunities. Cancer Res 1991; 51:5080s–5085s.

Wynder EL, Hoffman D. Smoking and lung cancer: scientific challenges and opportunities. Cancer Res 1994; 54:5284–5295.

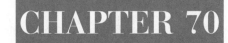

CHAPTER 70

Chemical Teratogenesis

P.G. WELLS

Teratology, or the study of congenital defects, is derived from the Greek word *teras*, meaning monster. The initiation of congenital (birth) defects is termed teratogenesis. Interest in structural abnormalities in the newborn dates back to at least 5000 B.C., when Babylonian priests had a list of 62 malformations recognizable at birth. Since the 1960s, teratology has expanded as a consequence of the recognition that mutational and functional abnormalities or anomalies result from prenatal insult, sometimes in the absence of structural defects (Fig. 70-1). There are many different causes of anomalies. This chapter is limited to teratogenesis associated with maternal exposure to drugs and environmental chemicals, which are collectively termed xenobiotics.

The study of chemical teratogenesis is relatively recent, dating from 1933, when Hale showed that maternal deprivation of vitamin A in pigs produced offspring without eyes (anophthalmia). Widespread scientific interest and public concern did not develop until 1960, when the first reports surfaced of teratogenicity associated with the sedative-hypnotic drug thalidomide (which was withdrawn from the market in 1961). The thalidomide tragedy stimulated an enormous growth in basic and applied research in this field, but we still know relatively little about how xenobiotics cause congenital anomalies and even less about how predisposing genetic and environmental factors interact in individual unborn children.

Each year in the United States about 200,000 birth defects are reported (7% of all live births). Over 560,000 infant deaths, spontaneous abortions, stillbirths, and miscarriages are estimated to be due to defective prenatal development. These figures no doubt are underestimates of the problem, since an unknown percentage of known defects are not reported and many defects, particularly functional and mutational anomalies, are not recognized. In other instances, there may be failure to recognize that the defect is associated with exposure to a drug or environmental chemical. About 20–30% of reported defects are thought to result from spontaneous genetic aberrations; 6% are clearly related to drugs and chemicals, leaving the cause unknown in over 60%. Many cases of unknown causation probably result either from unrecognized exposure to drugs and chemicals or from a complex interaction between a drug effect and genetic or environmental factors. One study found that the average woman takes 10 prescription or nonprescription drugs during her pregnancy, most of them without a physician's supervision. It has been estimated that over 125,000 women of childbearing age in the United States are exposed annually to potential chemical teratogens in their jobs, and presumably all women are exposed to some extent to the enormous array of environmental chemicals.

ASSESSMENT OF HUMAN RISK

There are a number of special problems in the detection of chemical teratogenicity and assessment of human risk that make this field of toxicology particularly difficult. Since the developmental process is complex and it takes many years to reach maturity, currently employed indices fail to detect many xenobiotic effects. In the human population, fewer than 50% of abnormalities can be detected at birth. Over 30% of early embryos are estimated to die unrecog-

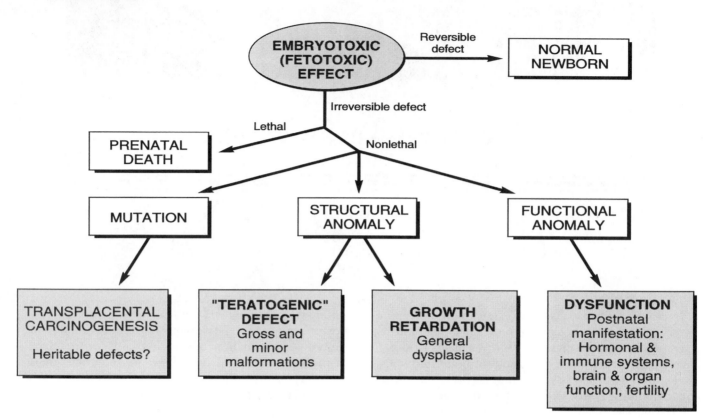

Figure 70-1. Consequences of chemical teratogenesis. (Modified from Neubert et al. 1980.)

nized; 15% of recognized pregnancies abort sponta-neously. In successful pregnancies, subtle biochemi-cal or functional defects usually go unrecognized. In other cases, the defect may be detected, but the causal role of the drug may not be identified because the defect is expressed only under conditions of ge-netic predisposition, or of certain physiological, pathological, or environmental stresses that may go unrecognized. In this case, particularly susceptible individuals will not be distinguished from the general population by epidemiological studies that cannot include sufficient detail about individual predispos-ing factors.

Most human teratological studies are restricted to the perinatal period and fail to evaluate the matu-rational process. If the children are monitored for about 5 years, the total number of defects identified during that period is more than six times greater than the number detected at birth. Some important structural defects (e.g., cardiac anomalies), subtle behavioral deficits, or mutational anomalies may not be detected until even later. For example, infants exposed in utero to the transplacental carcinogen

diethylstilbestrol did not develop vaginal adenocarci-nomas until puberty. Unfortunately, long-term fol-low-up studies are too expensive and time-consuming to be employed for all drugs. Therefore teratological evaluation often must depend upon retrospective epi-demiological studies and voluntary reporting of rare toxicities by astute physicians who have extensive records of their patients' histories.

During the clinical testing of new drugs, in studies on human volunteers and patients, pregnant women are rarely included. Therefore the fetal toxicity of most drugs can be assessed only after their use in the general population. Indeed, many drugs carry a warning that their safety during pregnancy and lactation has not been established. Once drugs are released for general use, epidemiological studies can detect potent teratogens or drug-induced anomalies that are rare in the baseline population. However, such studies are less successful in identifying weaker teratogens or drugs that are teratogenic only in pre-disposed patients. Such potential predisposing condi-tions as genetic differences, pathophysiological in-fluences, or concurrent drug use or chemical exposure seldom are discernible. Virtually never considered, especially in relation to environmental chemical teratogens, are such factors as the precise timing and magnitude of confounding influences, individual differences and gestational variations in drug disposition, and differences in specific, toxicologically critical pathways of drug elimination, bioactivation and detoxification, and associated pathways of cytoprotection and molecular repair.

To some extent, the teratological risks to humans can be reduced by preclinical studies employing in vivo animal models and in vitro tests, as discussed later. However, such methods have serious limitations. Thalidomide was found to be nonteratogenic in pregnant mice and rats but, unfortunately, in humans it proved to be an extraordinarily potent teratogen, causing embryolethality and a wide range of congenital anomalies in over 10,000 surviving children. Retrospective teratological studies have shown the teratogenic dose in mouse and rat to be about 5000 mg/kg, compared with 0.5–1 mg/kg in humans.

For all these reasons, relatively little can be stated as fact in the field of chemical teratogenesis. Teratologists disagree even about the identification of "known" human teratogens. However, Table 70-1 lists some drugs that are sufficiently potent teratogens for their effects to be recognized clearly above the spontaneous incidence of human congenital malformations. This list is not complete; if occupational and environmental chemicals and additional categories of "probable" and "suspected" human and ani-

mal teratogens were included, this list would number over 800 (Shepard, 1992).

TERATOLOGICAL PRINCIPLES

Direct Fetal Susceptibility: Critical Periods

The kinds and frequencies of anomalies caused by a teratogenic agent depend critically upon the developmental stage at the time of exposure. This so-called *critical period* is illustrated for several representative human organs in Figure 70-2. The embryonic and fetal periods represent distinct developmental stages as illustrated, but the term "fetal" will be used here to describe the entire prenatal period. The fetus is more susceptible to chemical insult than at any stage in its postnatal life because of the high rate of cellular proliferation and differentiation, functional development and growth taking place over a relatively brief period of time. For example, the DNA content of the mouse fetus is increased about one million times within the first 11 days of gestation (21-day pregnancy), and 1000 times during the first 3 days of organogenesis.

The specificity of the critical period can be illustrated by considering the formation of the palate, which involves the horizontal convergence and fusion of the two palatal shelves. In the mouse, cleft palate (failure of the palatal shelves to close) can be induced by an appropriate teratogen only when this is administered between gestational days 8 and 13. However, even this "single" process is complex. Palatal closure involves initial cellular proliferation, synthesis of intercellular substances, elevation of the two palatal shelves from a vertical to a horizontal position, midline contact and fusion of the two shelves, and finally formation of a bony plate. Thus the critical period for any organ development actually is a continuum of discrete but interdependent processes that can be affected differentially by teratogens with different mechanisms, or by the same teratogen at different times.

In the case of teratogens with different mechanisms, 6-aminonicotinamide causes cleft palates if administered at any time during palatal closure (days 8–13); dexamethasone is effective only when given around day 13; 2,4,5-trichlorophenoxyacetic acid only around day 12; and 2,3,7,8-tetrachlorodibenzo-*p*-dioxin (TCDD, dioxin) only between days 10 and 12 (Fig. 70-3). In the case of the same teratogen at different times, treatment of pregnant mice with 5-

Table 70-1 Proven or Seriously Suspected Human Teratogens *

Aminopterin †	Methylmercury
Androgens	Methotrexate †
Busulfan ‡	Phenytoin
Chlorambucil	Procarbazine ‡
Colchicine	Progestins
Cyclophosphamide ‡	Radioiodine (^{131}I)
Diethylstilbestrol (stilbestrol)	Thalidomide
Isotretinoin	Valproic acid
Mercaptopurine †	

*This list is not complete and refers primarily to drugs because of the lack of data in humans with respect to environmental chemicals.

†Antimetabolic anticancer drug.

‡Alkylating anticancer drug.

Source: Primarily from Shepard TH. In: Shirkey HC, ed. *Pediatric Therapy*, 6th ed. St. Louis: CV Mosby, 1980:94.

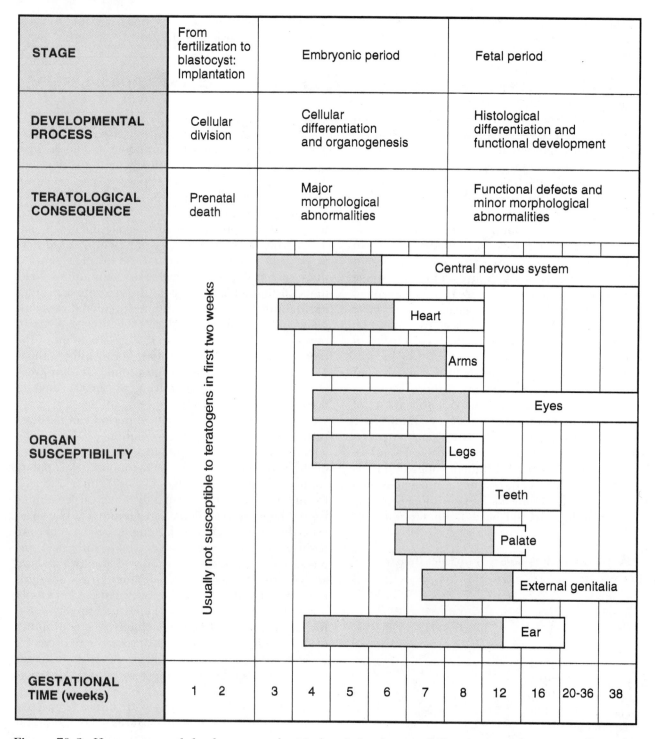

Figure 70-2. Human prenatal development and critical periods of susceptibility to teratogenic agents. Bars represent the organs, with color indicating their most susceptible period.

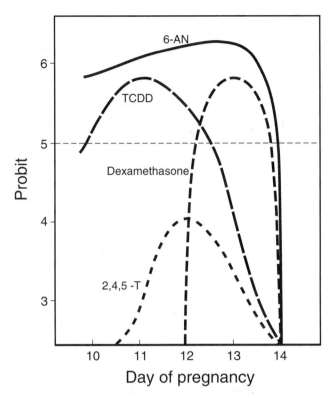

Figure 70-3. Time course of the susceptibility of NMRI mice to the induction of cleft palate by various agents. Doses given: 6-aminonicotinamide (6-AN) = 12 mg/kg; dexamethasone = 40 mg/kg; tetrachlorodibenzo-*p*-dioxin (TCDD) = 30 μg/kg; 2,4,5-trichlorophenoxyacetic acid (2,4,5-T) = 300 mg/kg. Differences in the period of maximum susceptibility suggest differences in the mode of action of the various compounds in inducing cleft palate. (From Neubert et al. 1980.)

azacytidine on gestational day 15 produces an extreme reduction in brain size, particularly in the cerebral cortex, with abnormal layering of pyramidal cells in the hippocampus and a reduced corpus striatum. Later treatment, on day 19, produces damage in more restricted areas, with dead cells observed mainly within the subependymal and external granular layers of the cerebellum.

The one critical period that often is not susceptible to the production of anomalies by teratogens is the initial development from fertilization to completion of the blastocyst. Since this stage involves little cellular differentiation, the cells have not achieved specific developmental roles, and damage at this stage often either causes the death of the embryo or has no lasting effect.

Established critical periods nevertheless are not absolute, since malformations occasionally have been demonstrated after chemical exposure during the preimplantation phase. This is particularly likely with highly lipid-soluble xenobiotics that persist in the mother, or with DNA-damaging xenobiotics that initiate molecular lesions which may lead to mutations (permanent alterations in DNA). Such mutations are retained during cell division, producing potentially teratogenic alterations in cellular function. Similarly, severe skeletal anomalies have been induced by teratogen exposure during the third trimester after the phase of organogenesis and limb formation.

Indirect Maternal Effects

In general, indirect insult to the fetus, mediated through effects on the mother, involves inadequate nutrient delivery, secondary either to maternal malnutrition or pathophysiology, or to reduced uterine blood supply to the fetus.

Maternal blood flow through the uterus to the placenta generally can be maintained at the expense of perfusion of other maternal organs; however, the homeostatic mechanisms can be overcome by high doses of drugs or endogenous substances that are vasoconstrictors (e.g., ergotamine, serotonin, bradykinin, angiotensin) or that reduce maternal cardiac function (e.g., propranolol). In humans, the consequences appear to be mainly a mild, reversible growth retardation rather than congenital malformations. In animals, treatment with vasoconstricting substances even at high doses produces resorptions (in utero death) without malformations. Thus, reduced uterine blood flow and its attendant deprivations generally do not produce measurable anomalies.

Teratogenic Consequences

As indicated in Figure 70-1, teratogenesis can be viewed according to the major outcomes—namely, fetal death or structural, mutational, or functional abnormalities.

In the early stage of cellular division before differentiation, as discussed previously, **fetal death** usually occurs in the absence of teratogenicity. During later developmental stages, often lower doses of a drug are teratogenic while higher doses cause fetal death. However, with some teratogens it is possible to induce a 100% incidence of **anomalies** such as cleft palate in the complete absence of fetal lethality (e.g., glucocorticoids in rodents), while other teratogens (possibly chloramphenicol in rodents) can induce fetal lethality without causing malformations. The latter case sometimes is difficult to establish, however, since malformed fetuses may die and be resorbed before detection. *Teratogenicity cannot be estimated reliably if fetal lethality exceeds 50%.* Since fetal death, teratogenicity, and growth retardation can be caused by different toxic mechanisms, the respective dose–response curves may be quite different, and their interrelation may vary at different times of gestation (Fig. 70-4). For example, dioxin induces about the same incidence of cleft palates (teratogenicity) in mice when given throughout gestational days 6 to 15 as throughout days 9 to 13, but fetal death is induced only when dioxin is given throughout days 6 to 15.

Chemically induced **mutations** can occur in fetal somatic cells, resulting in teratogenicity or transplacental carcinogenicity. There are few data concerning chemical mutations in fetal germ cells, and consequent hereditary disorders, in humans. Perhaps the best-known human somatic mutation involves in utero exposure to the synthetic estrogen diethylstilbestrol, as a result of which female children have developed a rare vaginal adenocarcinoma at puberty and male children developed a spectrum of structural and functional reproductive anomalies. While the correlation between mutagenicity, or DNA modifications, and carcinogenicity, or the initiation of cancer, is estimated to be between 67 and 90%, their relationship to teratogenicity is less clear. Teratogenicity is more complex than mutagenesis, and not all teratogens would be expected to be mutagens and carcinogens.

Nevertheless, mutagens can initiate six of the nine teratogenic mechanisms listed in Table 70-2. Another point common to mutagens and teratogens is that many such chemicals are enzymatically bioactivated in vivo to a reactive intermediary metabolite, as discussed in subsequent sections (see also Chapters 4 and 69). These reactive intermediates or, in a few cases, the original reactive parent chemical may bind covalently or irreversibly to essential fetal cellular macromolecules or lead to irreversible oxidation of lipids, proteins, and DNA, thereby initiating either mutagenesis or teratogenesis. Retrospective surveys of experimental studies in animals suggest a high risk of teratogenicity (80–85%) from exposure to chemicals with in vivo and/or in vitro cytogenetic activity, which refers to cellular alterations resulting from modifications in gene structure and/or expression. The relationship for carcinogenic chemicals as a subgroup is more striking; 92% also demonstrate teratogenicity. Aberrations of chromosome number can be caused by chemicals that affect microtubules and interfere with the role of spindle fibers in disjunction of chromosomes at anaphase of mitosis or meiosis; 64% of such chemicals were found to be teratogenic.

Functional anomalies are, for many teratogens, a more sensitive indication of prenatal damage than overt structural malformations. The later fetal period is most susceptible to functional teratogenesis because of the high activities of histogenesis, or specialized cellular development, and functional maturation. The earlier embryonic period of organogenesis, which has little of these activities, is relatively insensitive to functional teratogenesis. Functional teratogenicity may include permanent "imprinting" or al-

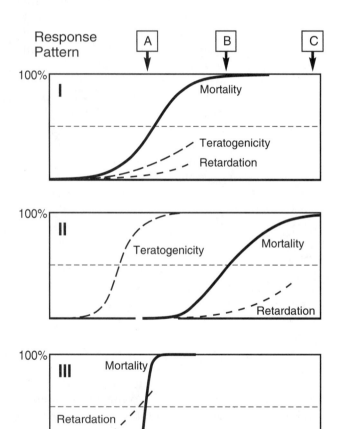

Figure 70-4. Hypothetical response pattern of an embryotoxic action. The three different effects have been evaluated separately; they may show quite different dose–response relationships. The outcome varies considerably, depending on the response pattern in early (I), mid (II), and late (III) gestation and the dose (A, B, C). (From Neubert et al. 1980.)

Table 70-2 Successive Stages in the Pathogenesis of a Developmental Defect*

Mechanisms

Initial types of change in developing cells or tissues after teratogenic insult:

Mutation (gene)

Chromosomal breaks, nondisjunction, etc.

Mitotic interference

Altered nucleic acid integrity or function

Lack of normal precursors, substrates, etc.

Altered energy sources

Changed membrane characteristics

Osmolar imbalance

Enzyme inhibition

Pathogenesis

Ultimately manifested as one or more types of abnormal embryogenesis:

Excessive or reduced cell death

Failed cell interactions

Reduced biosynthesis

Impeded morphogenetic movement

Mechanical disruption of tissues

Common pathways

Too few cells or cell products to effect local morphogenesis or functional maturation

Other imbalances in growth and differentiation

Final defect

---

*Initiation of one or more mechanisms by the teratogenic cause from the environment leads to changes in the development system that become manifested as one or more types of abnormal embryogenesis. This in turn leads into pathways that seem often to be characterized by too few cells or cell products to effect morphogenesis or functional maturation, but the suggestion that this is a single common pathway for all developmental defects is conjecture.

Source: Wilson JG (1977).

teration of discrete biochemical pathways; changes in organ function such as in the lungs or ears; and system deficits such as in the central nervous system (dysfunction and learning disabilities), the hormonal or immune systems, sexual function and fertility, and life expectancy. Since detection of such functional anomalies often requires decades of follow-up and is labor-intensive as well as costly, few human data are available in this field.

Examples in humans include behavioral anomalies (low intelligence quotients and learning disabilities) in children exposed in utero to ethyl alcohol or to phenytoin, and possibly to high doses of acetylsalicylic acid (aspirin). Examples in experimental animals include a permanently induced cytochrome P450 enzyme system in the offspring of pregnant mice treated with phenobarbital and the postnatal reduction in pulmonary oxygen consumption and respiratory rate in neonatal pups exposed in utero to excess vitamin A. Functional teratology can be produced over a wider gestational range than structural teratology, even up to the time of birth, as in the case of the developing central nervous system. Thus the traditional view of the first trimester of human pregnancy as the period of greatest teratological susceptibility can no longer be considered accurate.

Cellular Mechanisms

The basic biological mechanisms related to the early events in teratogenicity are listed in Table 70-2. Any given teratogen often initiates several mechanisms and, conversely, any given mechanism may be initiated by a variety of causes separate from, or complementary to, the effects of the potential chemical teratogen.

Pathogenesis is characterized by the appearance of demonstrable cellular and tissue damage. Increased cellular death is the most frequent sign of abnormal development, and the teratogenic process often, but not inevitably, involves some degree of focal cellular necrosis. Failure of either proper amount or sequence of cellular interaction and reduced biosynthesis of essential macromolecules such as DNA, RNA, proteins, and mucopolysaccharides can be important steps in teratogenesis. Impairment of morphogenetic movement, i.e., of the migration or translocation of cells or groups of cells, is involved notably in neuronal maldevelopment. Finally, tissues can be traumatized mechanically by invasion of foreign materials or abnormal accumulation of tissue fluids or blood, resulting in anomalous development.

Genetic and Environmental Modulation

The genetic and environmental factors modulating teratological susceptibility are poorly understood, and in many cases likely involve a complex interdependence. For most teratogens, it is not known whether the genetic predisposition or resistance is mediated via a pharmacological mechanism, as discussed later, or via a biological response mechanism. One example of the latter case may be the difference in susceptibility of various strains of mice to the induction of cleft palates. The inbred A/J mouse has a spontaneous incidence of cleft palates and is more susceptible than outbred mouse strains to induction of cleft palates by the anticonvulsant drug phenytoin.

The palatal shelves of the relatively resistant outbred mice are oriented on a horizontal plane toward each other to start with, whereas the palatal shelves of the susceptible A/J mouse remain vertical and distant from each other until late in the closure period, thus being potentially more susceptible to developmental interferences. Other cases remain unexplained, such as resistance to thalidomide teratogenicity in rats and mice compared with exquisite susceptibility in humans and to a lesser extent in rabbits. Conversely, the susceptibility of rodents and resistance of humans to salicylate teratogenicity also is unexplained, as are a multitude of other species and strain differences in teratological susceptibility.

Environmental determinants of teratological susceptibility are equally poorly recognized and understood. Stress and nutritional deficiency by themselves can increase the incidence of cleft palates in rodents and likely can potentiate the teratogenicity of many chemicals. Ambient temperature also can be important, as demonstrated in the case of 6-aminonicotinamide, a teratogenic chemical that also blocks temperature regulation in animals. In studies at room temperature, 6-aminonicotinamide produced a fall in maternal body temperature and the offspring were normal, while in studies conducted at 36°C with this chemical, normal maternal body temperature was maintained and there was a substantial increase in teratological anomalies. In animals, a growing number of drugs and chemicals with or without their own intrinsic teratogenic activity have been shown to modulate the fetal damage produced by known teratogenic agents, but in most cases the underlying mechanisms are not known.

PHARMACOLOGICAL PRINCIPLES

Placental Transfer and Fetal Chemical Disposition

Once believed to be a protective barrier isolating the fetus from harmful external influences, the placenta now is known to be more akin to a sieve, permitting ready access to the fetus of chemicals with a molecular weight under 600 Da, while excluding only the largest (molecular weight above 1000 Da) or most highly charged molecules such as heparin. Fetal blood concentrations of many chemicals are equivalent to maternal concentrations, and even some charged quaternary ammonium compounds can cross the placenta in limited quantities, possibly facilitated by a placental active transport process (see also Chapter 65).

Fetal factors such as a blood pH that is 0.1–0.15 unit below that of the mother, and occasional differences in plasma protein binding of chemicals, are theoretically important in determining chemical concentrations in fetal blood and tissues, but such factors have not been shown to have a remarkable influence on chemical teratogenicity. For complete reviews of fetal drug disposition, see Waddell and Marlowe (in Juchau, 1981).

Fetal Chemical Biotransformation

The principles of drug biotransformation are covered in Chapter 4, as well as in a number of reviews in specific reference to chemical teratogenesis (see reading list at the end of this chapter). In general, most enzymatic pathways of drug biotransformation are at a much lower level of activity in the fetus than in adults. In animals, this activity for the most part is low or negligible until birth. In the human fetal liver, enzymatic activity for most cytochromes P450 may be measurable as early as 6 weeks, but at midgestation it is only 20–40% of that in adults, with considerable interindividual variation. A few P450 isoenzymes, such as P450 3A7 (CYP3A7), have higher activity, and recent evidence indicates at least one fetal P450 (CYP1B1) that has high activity in the fetus and low activity postnatally. In nonhuman primates that have midgestational P450 activities similar to those in humans, activity increases fourfold from 10 days before to 10 days after birth. P450 activity in fetal animals cannot be induced substantially by chemicals such as phenobarbital and 3-methylcholanthrene until about 3 days before birth, although dioxin is an effective inducer of CYP1A1, a P450 isoenzyme reflected by aryl hydrocarbon hydroxylase (AHH) activity, earlier in gestation. In human fetuses, enzymatic induction appears to occur much earlier, although still less than in adults.

The developmental activity for a number of important enzymes is shown in Figure 70-5. Within any one class of enzyme, the developmental activity for a specific isoenzyme and its substrates may vary considerably, as with the cytochromes P450 (Fig. 70-5A). One of the groups of UDP-glucuronosyltransferases demonstrates high activity during the third trimester and perinatal period and declines rapidly thereafter; the other transferase group devel-

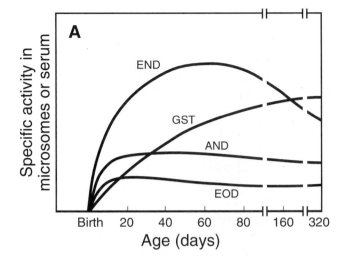

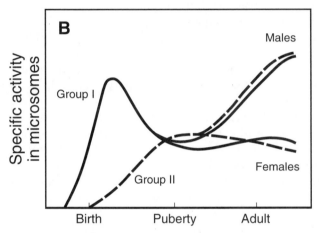

Figure 70-5. Developmental changes in activities of selected drug biotransformation enzymes in the rat. A. Hepatic cytochromes P450 and serum glutathione *S*-transferase (AND = aminopyrine *N*-demethylase; END = ethylmorphine *N*-demethylase; EOD = ethoxycoumarin *O*-demethylase; GST = serum glutathione *S*-transferase). B. Glucuronidation of group I and group II substrates in males and females.

ops after birth (Fig. 70-5B). However, sulfotransferase activity in early fetal life can be equivalent to adult levels, although this pathway is capacity-limited for chemicals. The fetus also has significant activities of prostaglandin H synthase (PHS) and lipoxygenases, which may play a role in chemical teratogenesis as discussed later. In general, however, the fetus is deficient in enzymatic activities for chemical biotransformation and thus often is unable to eliminate chemicals and detoxify reactive intermediates. In addition, the fetus is deficient in most of the

enzymes that protect tissues from xenobiotic-initiated oxidative stress, as discussed later.

Teratogenic Specificity

The concept of "critical period" (previously discussed) can be restated here as **phase specificity.** Teratogens will cause markedly different anomalies depending on the phase of fetal development. For example, methylnitrosourea is a transplacental carcinogen in rats only if administered on gestational day 20, whereas earlier administration will cause a spectrum of structural and functional anomalies. This late susceptibility to carcinogenicity may be due to a requirement for a sufficiently developed fetal enzymatic system for bioactivation of the chemical to a carcinogenic reactive intermediate within the fetus, although other factors such as increased placental transport of a maternally produced reactive intermediate or processes involved in carcinogenic promotion cannot be excluded.

Drug specificity is closely linked to phase specificity. Many teratogens interfere with intermediary processes that occur only during discrete phases in development. These *specific teratogens* cause a limited number of anomalies or a characteristic syndrome of malformations. A partial exception to the principle of drug specificity is a limited group of general or *universal teratogens* that interfere with fundamental processes such as nucleic acid metabolism or protein synthesis that occur throughout the stages of cellular division and differentiation. Universal teratogens would include the cytotoxic anticancer drugs, such as cytosine arabinoside and 6-mercaptopurine. However, even the so-called universal teratogens may demonstrate a certain degree of specificity, as shown in Figure 70-6. Treatment of pregnant mice with 6-aminonicotinamide produces more limb defects when given on gestational day 9 than on day 10, while cytosine arabinoside is teratogenic on both days, if not more so on day 10. Furthermore, 6-aminonicotinamide preferentially affects the hindlimbs, while cytosine arabinoside affects both the forelimbs and hindlimbs.

Dose specificity also can affect both the type and the frequency of anomalies. For example, low doses of a number of teratogens given to pregnant mice on gestational day 10 cause polydactyly (i.e., extra phalanges or digits), medium doses of the same teratogens reduce the length of phalanges and long bones without causing polydactyly, and high doses cause amelia (i.e., the absence of entire limbs). In

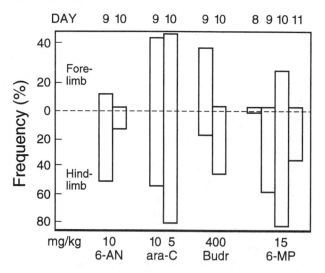

Figure 70-6. Frequency of limb abnormalities produced by various agents applied at different stages of pregnancy in NMRI mice, showing the great variability with different chemicals. 6-AN = 6-aminonicotinamide; ara-C = cytosine arabinoside; Budr = 5′-bromouracil deoxyriboside; 6-MP = 6-mercaptopurine. (From Neubert et al. 1980.)

this case the malformation is more dependent upon the dose of the teratogen than on its mechanism of action. The lowest dose is thought to act by causing limited focal necrosis in the apical region of the developing limb bud, which responds with a compensatory overproduction of phalangeal cells, leading to polydactyly.

Chemical Mechanisms

Chemical mechanisms of teratogenesis can be classified into two general categories: (1) those related to the classical, reversible interaction of a chemical or its active metabolite(s) with a receptor and (2) those involving highly reactive chemicals or their respective reactive intermediary metabolites, which can irreversibly alter essential cellular macromolecules.

The specific, reversible interaction of drugs with their receptors generally is responsible for the intended therapeutic effects of the drugs, as well as many of their side effects. Fetal toxicity caused by such an interaction is due to exaggeration of the pharmacological activity for which the drug is used therapeutically. However, fetal toxicity caused by the irreversible interaction of a reactive intermediate with fetal tissues in most cases is unrelated to the pharmacological mechanism by which the drug exerts its therapeutic effect. There are exceptions, however, such as the antineoplastic alkylating drugs,

whose therapeutic effect of destroying neoplastic cells is based on their covalent binding to DNA, which also is responsible for their teratogenicity. In the case of environmental chemicals that have no therapeutic purpose, the discrimination is based only upon reversible binding to a receptor as opposed to the irreversible interaction of a reactive intermediate with tissues.

Receptor-Mediated Mechanisms

Since fetal toxicity occurring via these mechanisms generally but not always represents an exaggerated therapeutic response, the toxicological sequelae (including teratogenic effects) usually are predictable and proportional to fetal and maternal blood chemical concentrations, if not to the dose assimilated. The principles underlying such mechanisms are discussed in Chapter 63; this discussion will be limited to teratogenesis.

The induction of cleft palates and limb anomalies in rodents by high doses of corticosteroids is an instructive example. This does not constitute an exaggerated therapeutic response, but it is an exaggeration of the physiological role of endogenous corticosteroids in palatal development and is dependent upon reversible binding of the corticosteroid to its receptor. In general, the amount of glucocorticoid administered to pregnant mice and taken up by the fetus correlates with the degree of inhibition of DNA and protein synthesis and with teratogenic susceptibility. The A/J strain of mice, which is highly susceptible to glucocorticoid teratogenicity, has the same endogenous maternal and fetal concentrations of corticosterone as the C57BL/6J strain, which is resistant. However, A/J mouse facial mesenchymal cells have two to three times more cytoplasmic glucocorticoid receptors than those from C57BL/6J mice, and this is reflected in an increased inhibition of growth and DNA synthesis in A/J compared with C57BL/6J mice.

The teratogenicity of opioid analgesic drugs likely constitutes another example of a receptor-mediated mechanism, since the incidence of most anomalies in animals can be reduced by pretreatment with opioid antagonists (see Wells, 1988).

Reactive Intermediate-Mediated Mechanisms

Drugs that themselves are not teratogenic ("proteratogens") can be enzymatically converted, or bioactivated, to two types of teratogenic reactive intermediates: electrophiles and free radicals. Teratological susceptibility to such proteratogens depends upon the balance of competing pathways of elimination, bioactivation, detoxification, cytoprotection, and repair (Fig. 70-7).

For **electrophiles,** a representative scheme for the enzymatic formation (bioactivation) of a potentially toxic, electrophilic reactive intermediary metabolite (often an epoxide) and its various detoxification pathways is presented in Figure 70-8. This type of bioactivation is only one of several kinds reviewed in detail in some of the works cited. Glutathione *S*-transferases and epoxide hydrolases are critical enzymes for the direct detoxification of reactive intermediary metabolites. In a limited number of cases, however, these so-called detoxifying enzymes can be involved in the subsequent formation of an even more reactive and toxic intermediary metabolite. UDP-glucuronosyltransferases and similar transferase enzymes, while not directly involved in detoxifying reactive intermediates, can be quantitatively major pathways of drug elimination, thereby preventing much of a chemical from being metabolized via a bioactivating pathway.

Under normal conditions, a reactive intermediate is evanescent—it is immediately detoxified and excreted. However, if bioactivation exceeds detoxifica-

tion, the highly reactive electrophilic site on the chemical intermediate will bind covalently to nucleophilic sites on essential fetal cellular macromolecules. If fetal repair mechanisms are inadequate, covalent binding of the chemical is thought to initiate a process, as yet poorly understood, that ends in cellular death or functional alterations. In a few cases, such as the antineoplastic alkylating drugs, the parent compound is sufficiently reactive to bind covalently without need for bioactivation. Chemicals believed to be bioactivated to a teratogenic electrophilic reactive intermediate include cyclophosphamide, thalidomide, phenytoin, and benzo[*a*]pyrene, although other mechanisms may be involved in their teratogenic effects.

With some chemicals, bioactivation or certain detoxifying pathways may constitute a quantitatively minor route of metabolism and yet have major teratological importance. For example, while only about 5–10% of the reactive arene oxide intermediate of phenytoin is hydroxylated and thereby detoxified by epoxide hydrolase, specific inhibition of this enzyme will dramatically increase the teratogenicity of phenytoin. Accumulating evidence suggests that the bioactivation of many if not most proteratogens occurs

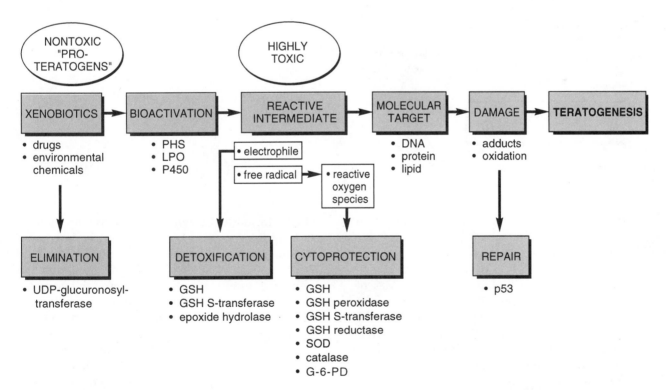

Figure 70-7. A postulated molecular and biochemical framework for understanding chemical teratogenesis and individual predisposition. PHS = prostaglandin H synthase; LPO = lipoxygenase; GSH = glutathione; SOD = superoxide dismutase; G-6-PD = glucose-6-phosphate dehydrogenase. (From Winn and Wells 1995.)

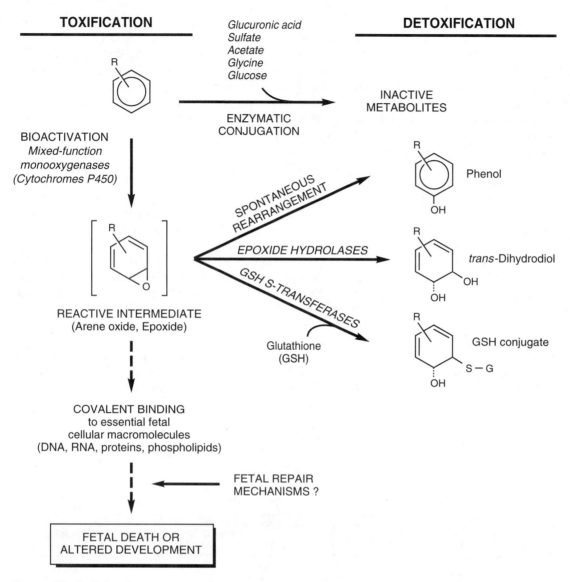

Figure 70-8. Role of proteratogen bioactivation and detoxification of electrophilic reactive intermediates in chemical teratogenesis.

within the fetus or its associated tissues, rather than in maternal tissues, from which a highly unstable reactive intermediate would have to be transported across several membranes and over a considerable distance to the fetus. In humans, fetal activities of P450 isoenzymes, while generally relatively low, nevertheless may be sufficiently high for teratologically relevant bioactivation. In rodents, fetal P450 activities are substantially lower and are less likely to contribute substantially to bioactivation. Alternatively, activities of other potential bioactivating enzymes such as prostaglandin H synthase (PHS) may be relatively high in both human and rodent fetuses, as discussed below.

PHS, formerly known as prostaglandin synthetase, is an enzyme system involved in the bioactivation of many drugs, primarily to reactive **free radical** intermediates. The fetus has significant activity of this enzyme system, and the hydroperoxidase component of PHS may oxidize some drugs to a teratogenic reactive intermediate, as postulated for a number of proteratogens, including benzo[a]pyrene, thalidomide, phenytoin, and related anticonvulsant drugs (Fig 70-9). Drug radicals may react directly with fetal tissues or may react with oxygen to produce toxic reactive oxygen species (ROS), such as superoxide anion radicals, hydrogen peroxide, and hydroxyl radicals. In a process known as **oxidative stress,**

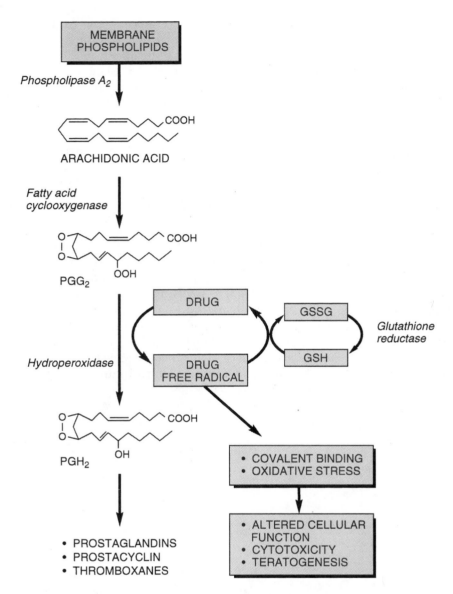

Figure 70-9. Postulated role of prostaglandin H synthase in the bioactivation of drugs to a teratogenic free radical intermediate. Fatty acid cyclooxygenase and hydroperoxidase are catalytic components of prostaglandin H synthase. Free radical intermediates may covalently bind to, and/or initiate the oxidation of, embryonic DNA, protein, and lipid. A similar bioactivation may be catalyzed by lipoxygenases, which also employ arachidonic acid as a substrate in the synthesis of leukotrienes and related hormones. (PGG_2 = prostaglandin G_2; PGH_2 = prostaglandin H_2; GSH = glutathione; GSSG = oxidized glutathione.)

these ROS can oxidize fetal molecular targets such as DNA, protein, and lipid. These oxidative lesions are thought to play a role in teratological initiation.

A similar bioactivation of proteratogens to a teratogenic, free radical intermediate may be catalyzed by lipoxygenases, which are involved in the synthesis of leukotrienes and related hormones. In addition, by acting as the cofactor for reduction of prostaglandin G_2 (PGG_2) to PGH_2, and via a similar role in leukotriene synthesis, drugs may perturb the physiological balance among the fetal synthesis of prostaglandins, prostacyclin, thromboxanes, and leukotrienes, with potential teratological consequences.

The fetus has low concentrations of glutathione and low activities of cytoprotective enzymes such as glutathione reductase, glutathione peroxidase, superoxide dismutase (SOD), catalase, and glucose-6-phosphate dehydrogenase, all of which are critical for cellular protection against free radical damage (Fig. 70-10). Thus, the fetus likely is at increased risk for free-radical-mediated toxicity. In rodent models, inhibition of these cytoprotective enzymes enhances susceptibility to phenytoin teratogenicity, as does the use of a mouse strain with a hereditary deficiency in glucose-6-phosphate dehydrogenase. Conversely, in a rodent embryo culture model, addition of SOD or catalase to the culture medium enhances embryonic antioxidative activity and completely inhibits the embryopathic effects of phenytoin and benzo[*a*]pyrene.

Since many proteratogens are bioactivated to both electrophilic and free radical reactive intermediates, it is difficult to determine their relative teratological contributions, particularly in humans. Interestingly, however, at least for rodents, the ability of SOD and catalase to block the embryopathic effects of phenytoin and benzo[*a*]pyrene suggests an important teratological role for oxidative stress. A secondary principle illustrated by phenytoin is the potential contribution of more than one chemical mechanism to the teratogenicity of drugs—namely, a reversible, receptor-mediated interaction as well as

irreversible interactions of reactive arene oxide and free radical intermediates. Human studies suggest that some particular types of birth defects caused by phenytoin may be due to a reactive intermediate, while others may be due to a receptor-mediated mechanism resulting from excessive maternal plasma concentrations of phenytoin. The relative teratological contributions of these mechanisms may well vary with gestational age, strain, species, and environmental conditions.

Genetic and Environmental Modulation

Modulatory influences, particularly in the case of toxicological mechanisms involving reactive intermediates, generally are complex and poorly understood. In addition to the complicating effects of the maternal and placental systems, modulating factors tend to affect multiple pathways of drug elimination, bioactivation and detoxification, and associated pathways of cytoprotection and molecular repair, with unpredictable teratological consequences.

A number of **genetic determinants** of chemical teratogenesis have been evaluated, primarily on ro-

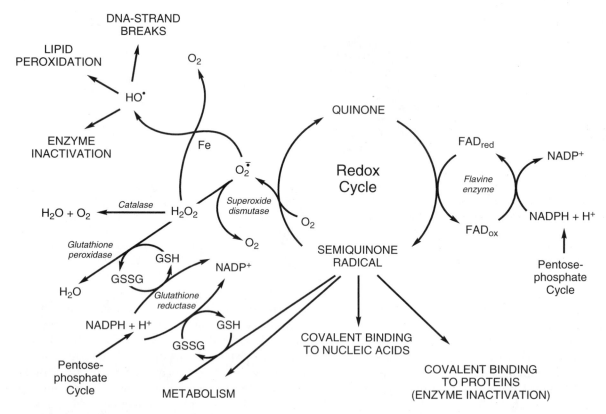

Figure 70-10. The role of cytoprotective pathways in detoxifying reactive oxygen species initiated by xenobiotic free radical intermediates. (GSH = glutathione; GSSG = oxidized glutathione.) (From Kappus 1986.)

dent models, and benzo[*a*]pyrene provides a useful model for discussion. The nonconstitutive P450 CYP1A1, often measured as aryl hydrocarbon hydroxylase (AHH), is controlled genetically by the Ah locus and is involved in the bioactivation of aryl hydrocarbons such as benzo[*a*]pyrene to teratogenic reactive intermediates. Different people, and different strains of mice, genetically are either nonresponsive or responsive to CYP1A1-inducing agents, and only the responsive ones show an increase in CYP1A1. In mouse strains bred to produce both CYP1A1-responsive and -nonresponsive fetuses in the same litter, there is a five- to 15-fold variation in the induction of AHH activity among individual littermates following maternal pretreatment with the CYP1A1 inducer 3-methylcholanthrene. Littermates that are responsive to AHH induction are more susceptible to benzo[*a*]pyrene-initiated malformations, and they have an increased amount of covalent binding of radiolabeled benzo[*a*]pyrene to fetal tissues compared with the AHH-nonresponsive littermates.

In other studies using pregnant inbred B6 mice, which produce only AHH-responsive offspring, benzo[*a*]pyrene causes an incidence of fetal resorptions, stillbirths, and malformations that is fourfold higher than that in inbred AK mice, which produce only AHH-nonresponsive offspring.

In summary, the teratological susceptibility to some chemicals appears to be genetically determined, the determinant can reside within the fetus rather than the mother, and this fetal determinant can be active very early in development. This also might explain why, in humans, it is possible that only one of fraternal (dizygotic) twins may be afflicted with a drug-induced anomaly or how only one of several children from the same mother may demonstrate a teratological response following exposure in utero to a drug that had been taken by the mother in the same doses during all her pregnancies.

The observations above for the Ah locus likely apply to genetic systems that regulate other enzymatic pathways of elimination, bioactivation, detoxification, cytoprotection, and repair. For example, there have been rare cases reported involving patients who are deficient in epoxide hydrolases or enzymes involved in glutathione synthesis and who have experienced life-threatening hepatotoxicity due to their inability to detoxify the reactive intermediates of certain drugs. Such genetically determined deficiencies would be expected to have serious teratological consequences for pregnant women exposed to potential teratogens that are normally detoxified via these pathways. Evidence in humans suggests that a lower activity of fetal epoxide hydrolase may predispose such fetuses to phenytoin teratogenicity. The potential importance of maternal UDP-glucuronosyltransferases in chemical teratogenesis has been demonstrated for benzo[*a*]pyrene, which can be eliminated via glucuronidation prior to its bioactivation to the reactive 7,8-diol-9,10-epoxide intermediate. The embryotoxicity of benzo[*a*]pyrene is significantly increased in Gunn rats, which have a genetic deficiency in UDP-glucuronosyltransferases. With respect to cytoprotection, pregnant mice with hereditary deficiencies in glucose-6-phosphate dehydrogenase are more susceptible to phenytoin teratogenicity. Finally, repair of DNA damage is facilitated by the so-called p53 tumor suppressor gene. Teratogenicity of the DNA-damaging xenobiotics benzo[*a*]pyrene and phenytoin is enhanced in p53-deficient pregnant mice, and p53-deficient fetuses have a higher incidence of in utero death (Fig. 70-11). However, for a few target tissues or other teratogens, a deficiency in p53 in a limited number of cases actually may protect the fetus, although the underlying mechanisms remain to be established.

Relatively little is known about the **environmental determinants** that modulate chemical teratogenicity, particularly with teratogens that are bioactivated to a toxic reactive intermediate. Such determinants could include individual physiological differences, concurrent pathophysiological conditions, and exposure to other drugs or environmental chemicals. For example, in pregnant mice, the teratogenicity of phenytoin and similar drugs is potentiated by pretreatment with the epoxide hydrolase inhibitor trichloropropene oxide, the glutathione depletors diethyl maleate and acetaminophen, the glutathione synthesis inhibitor buthionine sulfoximine, the glutathione reductase inhibitor *bis*-chloroethylnitrosourea (BCNU), and the phospholipase A_2 activator tetradecanoylphorbol acetate. Phenytoin teratogenicity also is enhanced in pregnant mice fed a selenium-deficient diet, which decreases the levels of glutathione peroxidase, a cytoprotective enzyme that detoxifies hydrogen peroxide and lipid hydroperoxidases initiated by free radicals (Fig. 70-10). Conversely, phenytoin teratogenicity in mice is reduced by pretreatment with the prostaglandin cyclooxygenase inhibitor acetylsalicylic acid, the dual cyclooxygenase/lipoxygenase inhibitor eicosatetraynoic acid, the antioxidants caffeic acid and vitamin E, the free radical spin-trapping agent phenylbutylnitrone, and, under some conditions, the glutathione precursor *N*-acetylcysteine.

A variety of physiological and pathological reac-

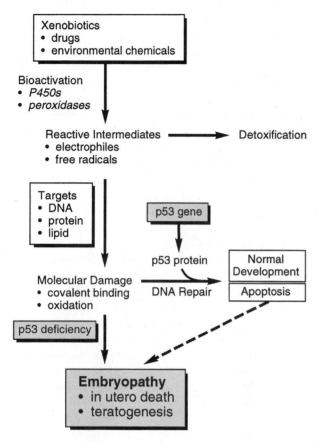

Figure 70-11. Potential embryoprotective role of DNA repair in chemical teratogenesis, exemplified by the p53 tumor suppressor gene. Generally, p53-facilitated DNA repair is embryoprotective for the DNA-damaging teratogens benzo[*a*]pyrene and phenytoin, with teratogenicity increased in p53-deficient dams. However, in some cases, particular fetal anomalies and/or anomalies initiated by different teratogens or mechanisms can be increased in p53-normal dams (dashed arrow), possibly due to the initiation of p53-dependent apoptosis. (From Winn and Wells 1995.)

tions in the body can produce superoxide, which is converted via an iron-catalyzed reaction to highly toxic hydroxyl radicals; hence, iron has been implicated in a number of free-radical-related diseases. In pregnant mice, phenytoin teratogenicity is reduced by pretreatment with the iron chelator deferoxamine. Drug radicals also can react directly or indirectly with oxygen to produce superoxide. As discussed earlier, addition of SOD or catalase, which detoxify superoxide and hydrogen peroxide, to a mouse embryo culture system blocks the embryopathic effects of benzo[*a*]pyrene and phenytoin. Environmental factors with such effects on pathways of xenobiotic elimination, bioactivation, and detoxification, and

associated pathways of cytoprotection and molecular repair, similarly would be expected to modulate the risk of teratogenesis in pregnant women exposed to certain potential teratogens. However, such possibilities have only recently been recognized in animal studies, and there are few data in humans on which to a base any estimate of actual risk. In some cases, knowledge of such modulatory effects ultimately may be employed to therapeutic advantage.

In addition, the complexities of developmental processes and maternal–placental–fetal interdependencies often preclude the straightforward predictions that are possible in other fields of toxicology. For example, in nonpregnant animals, induction of P450s generally will increase, while inhibition will decrease, the toxicity of chemicals that are bioactivated to a reactive intermediate. However, in pregnant mice, the teratogenicity of phenytoin and cyclophosphamide paradoxically is *decreased* by P450 induction and *increased* by inhibition.

Thus it appears that enzyme induction and other environmental perturbations have complex effects in vivo relating both to simultaneous effects on multiple pathways of xenobiotic elimination, bioactivation and detoxification, and to confounding maternal effects. The underlying mechanisms for the most part are not understood, and more studies will be necessary to identify and characterize the environmental determinants of teratogenesis, particularly with regard to human risk.

EXPERIMENTAL TERATOLOGY

The thalidomide tragedy clearly demonstrated the need for improved methods to detect potential chemical teratogens and elucidate their teratological mechanisms. In vivo studies employing more nonrodent animal species are now combined with a battery of in vitro tests. In vivo studies of pregnancy are time-consuming and expensive, however, and are not practical for screening large numbers of drugs and chemicals. Furthermore, the chemical and biological complexities of the maternal–placental–fetal interactions encountered in vivo generally preclude the elucidation of discrete teratological mechanisms. Thus, in vivo studies are most useful for the ultimate teratological testing of chemicals that have been pre-screened in vitro, and for applied aspects of teratological research.

For the above reasons, a large number of in vitro teratological screening methods have been devised, as exemplified in Table 70-3. This discussion will

Table 70-3 In Vitro Tests for Screening Teratogenic Chemicals

Biological Unit	End Points Measured
Virus	Plaque-forming units
Bacteria	Growth rate
Tumor cell	Number attached to surface
Prechondrocytes (chick, rodent)	Colonies formed and staining with Alcian blue
Neural crest cells (chick)	Morphogenesis of cell
Palate mesenchyme (human)	Morphogenesis of cell
Hydra attenuata	Regeneration of adults from tissue fragments
Planaria	Regeneration of organ systems from fragments
Drosophila	Maturation of larvae or colonies formed from disrupted embryo
Xenopus laevis eggs	Malformations in embryos grown from eggs
Fish eggs	Malformations in free-swimming hatchlings
Limb bud	Morphological and biochemical increments
Whole embryo (rodent)	Increase in somites, crown length, protein, DNA, and malformations
Chick embryo	Malformation

Source: Shepard TH et al. In: MacLeod SM, Okey AB, Spielberg SP, eds. *Developmental Pharmacology*. New York: AR Liss, 1983:147.

consider briefly four major categories: cells in culture, embryonic organs in culture, whole embryos in culture, and artificial embryos.

Embryonic **cells** in culture are used to study potential teratogens at various developmental stages, including cellular differentiation, cell–cell interactions, and cellular migration. This method is valuable particularly as a rapid prescreen for chemical teratogenicity and can provide mechanistic information as well.

Numerous types of **organs and tissues** in culture have been used in teratological studies, including palate, limbs, kidneys, sex organs, and skin. This method adds more dimensions to the developmental processes tested in cellular cultures. The explanted organ primordium consists of heterogeneous tissue components that progress through the organogenetic stages, thereby providing a measure of several developmental processes.

Whole embryos from mice or rats can be re-moved from the uterus at various developmental stages and cultured in vitro. This method permits a more comprehensive evaluation of the developmental process than the other in vitro systems. However, substantial facilities are required and the technique is labor-intensive and time-consuming. The embryo culture technique is suited ideally for mechanistic studies of chemical teratogenesis, but is not readily applicable to general teratological screening of large numbers of chemicals.

A number of nonmammalian life forms, such as *Hydra attenuata*, have been developed as **artificial embryos**. The adult *Hydra* are sheared into small pieces of tissue and compressed by centrifugation into an artificial "embryonic pellet." This pellet "embryo" will develop into multiple adults within 1 week, undergoing a remarkable range of complex developmental processes somewhat analogous to mammalian prenatal development. Such model systems are useful in detecting teratogenic potential for large numbers of chemicals in a fairly quick and inexpensive manner.

CLINICAL APPLICATION

There are several textbooks or chapters dealing with the principles and practices relating to clinical pharmacology during pregnancy (e.g., Rubin, 1992) and more particularly to the clinical approach to maternal and fetal toxicology, including teratogenesis (Koren, 1994; Schardein, 1993; Shepard, 1992), some of which are updated regularly. In the clinical setting, often the major dilemma is to determine whether the drug or environmental chemical to which the pregnant woman is or was exposed is potentially teratogenic in humans and, if so, the likelihood of having an abnormal child. Unfortunately, despite the substantial teratological data base for animal models, the human risk is established for only a relatively small number of teratogens which in humans are highly potent and/or cause abnormalities rarely observed in the general population. For less potent human teratogens, which likely includes most xenobiotic exposures, little is known about the human determinants of susceptibility that may render a relatively small number of fetuses highly susceptible.

However, journal reports of individual associations of a xenobiotic with fetal anomalies often are published as case reports or letters to the editor. While useful in identifying important areas requiring more intensive human research, including the use of essential controls, such unsubstantiated reports may be used erroneously as proof of teratogenicity, resulting in unnecessary abortions and lawsuits claiming improper practices of clinicians or the pharmaceutical or chemical industries, and the unwarranted withdrawal of safe drugs from the market.

During a pregnancy, the decision of a family is further complicated by the fact that, even with exposure to a known human teratogen, not all pregnant women will have an abnormal child. Unfortunately, as with weaker teratogens, the determinants of susceptibility in humans are unknown, and hence there are no prenatal tests to guide family decisions. The scientific and practical complexities underlying such decisions, together with a growing public interest in this information, have led to the establishment of several centers around the world composed of multidisciplinary teams of clinicians and biological and social scientists who can provide comprehensive and up-to-date advice to both families and clinicians on the reproductive effects of xenobiotics and physical dangers such as radiation (Koren, 1994).

SUGGESTED READING

Halliwell B, Gutteridge JMC. Free radicals in biology and medicine. 2nd ed. New York: Oxford University Press, 1989.

Juchau MR, ed. The biochemical basis of chemical teratogenesis. New York: Elsevier/North-Holland, 1981.

Juchau MR, Lee QP, Fantel AG. Xenobiotic biotransformation/bioactivation in organogenesis-stage conceptal tissues: implications for embryotoxicity and teratogenesis. Drug Metab Rev 1992; 24:195–238.

Kappus H. Overview of enzyme systems involved in bioreduction of drugs and in redox cycling. Biochem Pharmacol 1986; 35:1–6.

Koren G. Maternal-fetal toxicology: a clinician's guide. 2nd ed. New York: Marcel Dekker, 1994.

Manson JM, Wise LD. Teratogens. In: Amdur MO, Doull J, Klaassen CD, eds. Toxicology: the basic science of poisons. 4th ed. New York: Macmillan, 1991:226–254.

Manson JM, Kang YJ. Test methods for assessing female reproductive and developmental toxicology. In: Hayes AW, ed. Principles and methods of toxicology. 3rd ed. New York: Raven Press, 1994:989–1037.

Marnett LJ. Prostaglandin synthase mediated metabolism of carcinogens and a potential role for peroxyl radicals as reactive intermediates. Environ Health Perspect 1990; 88:5–12.

Neubert D, Barrach HJ, Merker HJ. Drug-induced damage to embryo or fetus. In: Grundmann E, ed. Drug-induced pathology. New York: Springer-Verlag, 1980:242–331.

Rubin PC. Drugs in special patient groups: pregnancy and nursing. In: Melmon KL, Morrelli HF, Hoffman BB, Nierenberg DV, eds. Melmon and Morrelli's clinical pharmacology: basic principles in therapeutics. 3rd ed. New York: McGraw-Hill, 1992: 805–825.

Schardein JL. Chemically induced birth defects. 2nd ed. New York: Marcel Dekker, 1993.

Shepard TH. Catalogue of teratogenic agents. 7th ed. Baltimore: Johns Hopkins University Press, 1992.

Wells PG. Analgesics: direct embryopathic effects, and indirect biochemical effects modulating the teratogenicity of other drugs and chemicals. In: Kacew S, Lock S, eds. Toxicologic and pharmacologic principles in pediatrics. New York: Hemisphere Publishing Corp, 1988:127–166.

Wells PG, Winn LM. Biochemical toxicology of chemical teratogenesis. Crit Rev Biochem Mol Biol 1996; 31:1–40.

Wells PG, Kim PM, Nicol CJ, Parman T, Winn LM. Chapter 17: Reactive intermediates. In: Kavlock RJ, Daston GP, eds. Handbook of experimental pharmacology, vol. 124, part I: Drug toxicity in embryonic development. Heidelberg: Springer-Verlag, 1996:451–516.

Wilson JG. Current status of teratology. In: Wilson JG, Fraser FC, eds. Handbook of teratology, vol. 1. New York: Plenum Press, 1977:47–74.

Winn LM, Wells PG. Free radical-mediated mechanisms of anticonvulsant teratogenicity. Eur J Neurol 1995; 2 (Suppl 4):5–29.

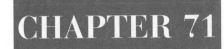

CHAPTER 71

Behavioral Pharmacology

L.A. GRUPP AND H. KALANT

Behavioral pharmacology refers to the study of the changes in behavior produced by a drug and the mechanisms by which the drug produces these changes. Such research draws on the knowledge and techniques of a number of different disciplines including anatomy, biochemistry, pharmacology, physiology, and psychology. Since human behavior differs in important ways from that of laboratory animals, new, behaviorally active drugs must ultimately be tested in humans. However, initial screening is done in various species, including rats, mice, cats, dogs, monkeys, and others. This chapter deals with the procedures used in such animal studies.

The study of drug effects on learned behaviors and on certain instinctive or naturally occurring ones, such as locomotion, food and water intake, aggressive and sexual behavior, requires accurate and reliable methods for quantifying the rates and patterns of these behaviors and sufficient control over the environment to minimize disturbing influences. All these measures are necessary because they provide a stable control or baseline level of performance against which drug effects can be observed and quantified. The following two sections identify some of the behaviors referred to later and describe the techniques used to measure them.

TYPES OF BEHAVIOR STUDIED

Instinctive Behavior

Locomotion

Locomotion refers to simple motor activity that forms part of exploratory behavior or other acts of general movement. It is measured by such means as counting the number of revolutions an animal makes in a running wheel, or the number of sectors traversed during a measured time period in a large open field that has been marked off in a grid pattern.

Sensory function

Since the execution of any behavior requires the use of one or more senses, drugs that affect sensory function can also affect behavior. For example, the sensation of pain has been extensively studied by means of the hot-plate and tail-flick tests. Typically, a rat or mouse is placed with its paws on a metal plate warmed to about 50°C, or the tail is immersed in very warm water, and the latency to retract a paw or the tail, respectively, is measured. The test drug is given, and the procedure is repeated at various times after the dose. The drug effect is measured as the difference in latency between the pre-drug baseline and the post-drug tests.

Food and water intake

Food selection and total amount of food and water consumed, either per day or per meal, are measured. With the aid of computer programs, the pattern of consumption can be analyzed in much finer detail.

Again, the drug effect is measured as the change from pre-drug baseline.

Aggressive behavior

This can be measured by placing two or more animals together in a cage and counting the number of spontaneous attacks or the number of times an animal assumes a dominant or submissive posture. Alternatively, one can induce animals to fight by placing them on an electrified grid. (The electrical current delivered by the grid is irritating, but not damaging.) In this shock-induced aggression model, one can measure posturing and the number of attacks and bites.

Sexual behavior

Receptive females are made available to their male counterparts and the frequency of sexually related behaviors of both the female (the lordosis posture) and the male (mounting, intromission, ejaculation) is measured. Drug-treated animals can be compared with placebo-treated animals with respect to the frequency of these behaviors.

Learned Behavior

Many types of learning tasks have been used to test the effects of drugs. For example, the effect of cannabis has been tested in rats learning to find their way through a series of mazes of increasing complexity to earn a food reward at the exit from each maze. However, two special types of learning that have been very extensively used in drug studies are classical conditioning and operant conditioning.

Classical conditioning

This kind of training or learning procedure is best illustrated by reference to a well-known experiment with dogs by the Russian physiologist I.P. Pavlov. A tuning fork was sounded, followed seconds later by the presentation of some powdered food. Dogs salivate when food is presented to them. Initially the sound did not elicit any salivation; however, after a number of pairings, the sound came to elicit salivation. The dog had learned that the sound predicted the presentation of food and had learned to salivate at the sound in preparation for the food. In the language of learning theory, the sound was the **conditional stimulus**, which initially did not elicit an **unconditional response** (salivation), but which, through repeated association with the food (**unconditional stimulus**), came to elicit the salivation as a **conditional response** in the absence of food. The effect of drugs on the acquisition and maintenance of this conditional response can be studied.

Operant conditioning

This type of learning involves a procedure whereby the probability of occurrence of some particular behavior can be either increased or decreased, depending upon the consequences of the behavior. For example, if a food pellet is presented to a hungry animal every time it presses a lever, it is highly likely that the animal will repeat its lever-pressing behavior and thereby obtain food pellets until its hunger is satisfied. The lever press is termed an **operant response** because the animal operates on its environment to change it in some biologically significant way; the food pellet is termed a **positive reinforcer** because it reinforces or strengthens the behavior that resulted in its presentation (i.e., the lever-press response). The whole process is termed **positive reinforcement.** Similarly, if a lever press *prevents* the presentation of an *unpleasant* stimulus (e.g., an air blast), the lever press is again termed an *operant*; the air blast is termed a **negative reinforcer** because it strengthens the response that prevents the negative or unpleasant event. The whole process is termed **negative reinforcement.** Finally, if the lever press results in the delivery of a painful stimulus (e.g., a foot shock), the animal is reluctant to perform the response again. The process is called **punishment,** and the foot shock is the **punisher.** Note that both positive and negative reinforcement refer to processes that *increase* the probability of the behavior, whereas punishment *decreases* it.

The animal may be required to make the response according to a specific **schedule of reinforcement.** For example, reinforcers can be presented or avoided either after a specified number of lever-press responses (fixed ratio, variable ratio) or after a specified period of time has elapsed (fixed interval, variable interval) since the last presentation of the reinforcer. For example, a fixed-interval 60-second (FI 60s) schedule of food reinforcement indicates that a food pellet will be delivered as a result of the first response that occurs at least 60 seconds following the last food delivery. A fixed-ratio 10 (FR 10) schedule indicates that one food pellet will be delivered for every 10 presses of the response lever. These formulae, which specify the relationship between responding and the delivery of the reinforcer, generate very stable and reliable patterns of responding. Drug effects are easily and effectively measured against such stable control levels of behavior.

The following sections examine (1) the behavioral effects of drugs that alter neurotransmitter function, (2) some of the behavioral factors that determine drug action, (3) the effects of drugs on the processes of learning and memory, (4) the stimulus properties of drugs, (5) behavioral models of mental disorders, and (6) reinforcing properties of drugs.

DRUGS, NEUROTRANSMITTERS, AND BEHAVIOR

When a drug enters the central nervous system, it alters the ongoing activity of the neurotransmitter systems in different ways that produce behavioral effects. The drug action may take various forms, such as a direct effect on ionic permeability; a change in the release, synthesis, or reuptake of a neurotransmitter; or a direct action on receptor sites. Since different neurotransmitter systems coexist in many brain areas, drug-induced changes in the activity of one system may, by shifting the balance of activity, affect behavior as much by altering activity in the other systems as by acting directly on its own target system. Thus, in order to establish a causal relationship between behavior and a particular neurotransmitter system, a number of complementary experimental approaches must be taken.

For example, if a change in behavior follows upon a reduction in the level of a neurotransmitter, then (1) blocking the receptor sites for that transmitter should have a similar effect on behavior and (2) replacing that neurotransmitter should cause behavior to return to normal. The remainder of this section examines the relationships between some neurotransmitter systems and behavior, examines how drugs that modify neurotransmitter function also modify behavior, and examines how similar behaviors can sometimes be related to the activity of a number of different neurotransmitters.

Serotonin (5-HT)

Serotonergic activity is decreased by a number of agents, including synthesis inhibitors (e.g., parachlo-

rophenylalanine, or PCPA), receptor blockers (e.g., methysergide), agents that interfere with storage (e.g., reserpine), and neurotoxins that selectively destroy serotonin-containing cell bodies (e.g., 5,7- or 5,6-dihydroxytryptamine). **When serotonergic activity is decreased,** a number of behavioral changes occur, including the following examples:

1. There is an increase in the sensitivity to a number of different painful stimuli, as shown by a decrease in the threshold stimulus required to make a rat or mouse escape a hot plate or jump in response to an electric shock.

2. The increased sensitivity to painful shock leads to faster acquisition of an avoidance response by animals.

3. Decreasing 5-HT levels by the administration of reserpine or PCPA, or damaging the serotonin-containing cell bodies of the entire brainstem raphe nucleus, leads to a suppression of the electroencephalographic (EEG) signs of both slow-wave and paradoxical sleep, and produces insomnia. This state may last as long as 2 weeks before compensatory mechanisms restore a more balanced sleep function.

4. When two rats are placed on an electrified grid, they tend to approach, attack, and bite each other (shock-induced aggression). When a mouse is introduced into a rat's cage, the rat may suddenly attack the mouse and kill it by breaking the neck (muricide). These are both considered to be experimental models of aggression. Serotonin depletion, produced by PCPA or by raphe lesions, leads to an increase in these aggressive behaviors.

5. In male rats, serotonin depletion leads to an increase in sex-related behaviors such as mutual grooming, scratching, and sniffing of the genitalia. Castrated males will show a temporary increase in sexual behavior after injection of PCPA. After serotonin depletion, males will increase the frequency with which they engage in heterosexual activities if a female rat is present, or mount other males if no female is present.

In general, agents that **increase serotonergic activity** (such as the monoamine oxidase inhibitors or the precursor 5-hydroxytryptophan) antagonize the effects described above.

In addition, **5-HT agonists** have a very marked effect on eating and drinking. They reduce food intake, especially in the form of nonprotein calories, and increase water intake. Serotonin reuptake inhibitors, which increase 5-HT concentration at the receptor, have been used clinically to help obese patients lose weight by inhibiting appetite.

Acetylcholine

Modification of central cholinergic function by agonists (e.g., nicotine, arecoline, carbamylcholine), cholinesterase inhibitors (e.g., physostigmine), and antagonists (e.g., mecamylamine, atropine, scopolamine) (see Chapters 14 and 15) produces a number of characteristic effects on behavior:

1. Both atropine and physostigmine produce a dissociation between behavior and the apparent state of consciousness indicated by the EEG pattern. After atropine, the animal is behaviorally awake but its EEG shows a sleeping pattern. Physostigmine, on the other hand, causes the animal to appear to be sleeping, but its EEG is that of an awake animal.

2. Anticholinergic agents usually increase spontaneous locomotor activity, unless this is already elevated prior to drug administration. In that case, either no change or a decrease in activity results. Conversely, agents such as physostigmine, which increase cholinergic activity by inhibiting cholinesterase, lead to a decrease in general motor activity.

3. Stimulation of cholinergic synapses in the hypothalamus and limbic system has profound effects on feeding and drinking. Direct application of a cholinergic agonist to these areas produces rapid and copious drinking in water-satiated animals and increases drinking by thirsty animals. These effects can be blocked by the administration of atropine.

4. Physostigmine can disrupt the performance of a previously acquired shock avoidance response, and this disruption can be prevented by pretreatment with the receptor blocker atropine.

Catecholamines (Dopamine and Norepinephrine)

Catecholamine levels can be altered by drugs that inhibit synthesis (e.g., α-methyl-p-tyrosine, AMPT) or degradation (e.g., MAO inhibitors) of dopamine (DA) and norepinephrine (NE), block their reuptake (e.g., cocaine), interfere with their storage (e.g., reserpine), or destroy catecholamine-containing cell bodies (e.g., 6-hydroxydopamine, 6-OHDA). Additionally, a large variety of selective DA and NE antagonists (e.g., pimozide and phenoxybenzamine, respectively) and agonists (e.g., apomorphine and clonidine, respectively) are also available (see Chap-

ters 13, 16–18, and 27). The behavioral effects of alteration of catecholamine systems in the brain include the following:

1. Both DA and NE play a role in **locomotor activity**. A decrease in catecholamine levels, as a result of the administration of reserpine or AMPT, leads to a profound decrease in spontaneous locomotor activity, which can be reversed by the administration of their common precursor, L-dopa. L-Dopa given alone produces an increase in locomotor activity. The relative contribution of DA and NE systems to this behavior is the subject of much research.

2. Reduction of catecholamine levels by the administration of 6-OHDA decreases the level of **aggression** in animals tested in the shock-induced fighting paradigm. The increase can be antagonized by the DA agonist apomorphine. The functional relation between catecholamines and 5-HT in the control of aggressive behavior is not yet known.

3. The application of NE directly to certain areas of the hypothalamus elicits **feeding** in a totally satiated animal. Other α-adrenergic agonists also increase feeding, whereas β-adrenergic agonists decrease it, and each effect can be blocked by the corresponding receptor blocker. It is believed that the α system inhibits satiety and thus turns feeding on, while the β system turns feeding off. DA also plays a primary role in feeding: The selective destruction of DA-containing cell bodies in the striatum can result in both **aphagia** and **adipsia,** to the point that the animals must actually be force-fed to insure their survival. The relationship among these two neurotransmitter systems and cholinergic and serotonergic systems in the control of food and water intake is not yet fully understood.

4. A variety of drugs that decrease catecholaminergic activity, including inhibitors of synthesis and those that interfere with storage, attenuate the performance of a previously acquired **shock-avoidance** response. This attenuation can itself be reduced by the administration of the precursor L-dopa.

The foregoing lists of behavioral changes produced by modification of neurotransmitter activity merely scratch the surface. They are intended only to illustrate the wide range of behavioral alterations that have been studied and to indicate the complexity of behavioral interactions among the known neurotransmitter systems.

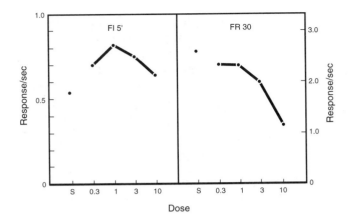

Figure 71-1. Rate of responding on a multiple FI 5-minute, FR 30 schedule of food presentation as a function of four doses of *d*-amphetamine in pigeons. The points at *S* show response rates after a saline injection.

EFFECTS OF DRUGS ON BEHAVIOR CONTROLLED BY SCHEDULES OF REINFORCEMENT

One way to examine the effects of drugs on behavior is to administer a test drug to an animal that is performing a simple, discrete, and easily measurable task and then observe the change in its performance from a pre-drug placebo baseline. The procedures of operant conditioning afford stable behavioral baselines against which drug effects can be meaningfully assessed. Figure 71-1 illustrates this point. Hungry pigeons were trained to peck a key in order to receive brief access to a hopper of grain. The presence of a red light indicated that an FR 30 was in effect, whereas a green light signaled the operation of an FI 5-minute schedule. The appearance of the red and green lights alternated, and the pigeons learned to tailor their response pattern to fit the particular schedule of reinforcement that was signaled by each visual stimulus. They were then tested after an injection of saline and after four different doses of *d*-amphetamine. Under the FI 5-minute schedule all four doses of amphetamine increased the response rate, but under the FR 30 schedule these same doses all reduced responding. Thus, the same dose of *d*-amphetamine produced opposite effects on responding on the two schedules of reinforcement.

The interpretation of such findings depends upon the type of hypothesis from which one starts. The behavioral mechanisms hypothesis states that drugs act on behavior by influencing processes involved in either the learning of a new behavior (such as motivation or memory) or the ability to perform it once it has been learned (e.g., stimulus perception or response output capability). In contrast, the rate-dependency hypothesis states that the *direction* of effect of a drug on the rate of responding (i.e., either increase or decrease) depends on the pre-drug (i.e., saline-tested) rate of occurrence of the behavior and is independent of the mechanism of action of the drug. If the rate of responding is low before drug, a post-drug increase in the rate is likely to ensue at low and intermediate drug doses. If the pre-drug response rate is high, a post-drug decrease in rate will be found even at low and intermediate doses. Rate-dependent effects occur under schedules of both positive and negative reinforcement and have been seen with barbiturates, benzodiazepines, antipsychotics, and stimulants.

Although rate of responding is an important determinant of drug action, it is not the only operative factor and therefore should be considered to *modulate* rather than totally determine the effects of drug action. This is highlighted best by a number of studies on the role of antianxiety agents in punished responding. Specifically, if rate of responding were the sole determinant of the effect of a benzodiazepine such as diazepam, then at equivalent pre-drug response rates this agent should increase responding to the same extent, regardless of whether the responding is being punished or not. However, it reliably increases low rates of punished responding more than equivalently low rates of unpunished responding. Presumably other factors, such as the emotional motivational state of the animal, are operating to produce this result.

DRUG EFFECTS ON LEARNING AND MEMORY

The ability of the brain to modify its output as the result of some previous experience is one of the most important yet least understood of its functions. This process of modification actually involves two separate but related processes: learning and memory. Learning refers to a semipermanent change in behavior as a result of the occurrence of some prior event. Memory refers to the registration of information in some manner that permits its later recall into consciousness. It involves three separate steps: registration of the information in a transitory short-term memory, followed by its consolidation into a more durable long-term trace, and the eventual retrieval from long-term storage when necessary. Some agents that influence the processes of learning and memory are considered briefly below.

Pituitary Peptides

Hypophysectomized animals, which lack ACTH, show deficits in learning a shock-avoidance response and in inhibiting the response once the shock is discontinued (extinction). The administration of ACTH to these animals normalizes both their learning and extinction of the avoidance response. This effect is not necessarily related to the endocrine action of ACTH, since the effect is obtained with fragments of ACTH (α-MSH and β-LPH, see Figs. 23-3 and 51-3) that do not act on the adrenal glands. These peptides are thought to work by modulating neurotransmitter activity in the brain in such a way as to increase arousal and heighten attention to motivationally relevant stimuli.

Vasopressin acts to *delay* extinction of a learned behavior such as a shock-avoidance response. This action can also be dissociated from its pressor and antidiuretic effects (see Chapter 47) and is exerted through specific vasopressin V_1-receptors in the brain.

Drug Effects

Strychnine, which at high doses produces convulsions, acts by blocking postsynaptic inhibition (see Chapter 22), thereby enhancing neuronal transmission. Both pretrial and posttrial injections of low doses of this drug facilitate the acquisition of a visual discrimination task as well as a maze-learning task. Other proconvulsant drugs, such as picrotoxin, bemegride, and pentylenetetrazol, have similar effects.

Amphetamine acts by promoting the release and blocking the reuptake of both DA and NE from nerve endings. Injections of this drug have been reported to improve learning, perhaps through its effects on attentional mechanisms. Yet its ability to reduce fatigue and increase arousal raises the possibility that the improvement is related more to the ability to perform the task than to a real effect on the learning processes.

The turnover of acetylcholine in the rat hippocampus is increased while the animal is learning a new task to obtain a food reward. Conversely, anticholinergic drugs such as atropine and scopolamine impair learning. Drugs that increase cholinergic activity, such as physostigmine, have been reported to facilitate learning. These effects are of central origin, since the quaternary derivatives that do not pass the blood–brain barrier (e.g., atropine methylbromide) are ineffective. As with amphetamine, the facilitation is presumed to be related to improved attention.

Protein Synthesis Inhibitors

Memories appear to be encoded partly by changes in the composition, quantity, or concentration of RNA in nerve cells. In turn, these changes in RNA would direct the synthesis of different amounts or types of protein. The changes in both RNA and protein may be important for memory processes. Indeed, RNA synthesis and metabolism are both increased in trained animals compared to untrained ones. Much evidence suggests that associative learning (Pavlovian conditioning) involves, among other things, increased production of protein kinase C in the cell body and its transport to the specific synapses at which the conditional and unconditional stimuli had coincided. Administration of protein synthesis inhibitors (e.g., puromycin, anisomycin, and cycloheximide) can produce amnesia and impaired retention of a previously learned task. Further research is needed to elaborate fully the role of RNA in memory.

STIMULUS PROPERTIES OF DRUGS

Meaning of "Stimulus Properties"

Discriminative stimuli enable an animal to distinguish between two or more situations in which a particular response will have different outcomes. For example, a rat may be trained in an operant chamber to press one or the other of two levers to obtain a small food pellet as a reward. A signal light can then be added as a discriminative stimulus; e.g., when the light is on, the rat will be rewarded only for pressing on the left-hand lever, while only presses on the right-hand lever will be rewarded when the light is off. The rat soon learns to discriminate correctly according to the presence or absence of the signal light. Responding is then deemed to be under stimulus control. A mundane example in everyday life is the traffic signal: A green light is the discriminative stimulus for removing one's foot from the brake and placing it on the accelerator to proceed through the intersection in relative safety.

Drugs may also be thought of as stimuli that have some properties in common with visual and other sensory stimuli. For example, each acts on specialized stimulus-specific receptors and causes biochemical reactions that initiate or modify a neuroelectrical response in the central nervous system. Both an exteroceptive stimulus such as a light and an interoceptive stimulus such as a drug can act as (1) unconditional stimuli that elicit unconditional reflex responses; (2) conditional stimuli (see section on Classical Conditioning); (3) reinforcing stimuli (see section on Operant Conditioning); or (4) discriminative stimuli that set the occasion for a response. The present section deals with drugs in their role as discriminative stimuli.

Methods of Study

Discriminative stimulus properties of drugs are usually studied by means of the two procedures described below.

State-dependent learning

In this procedure, one group of animals is trained to perform a response in the nondrugged condition, while a second group is trained to make this response while under the influence of a certain drug. Once training is complete, the groups are subdivided. Half of the animals in each group are tested in the drugged condition and the other half in the nondrugged condition. If state-dependent learning has occurred, the animals will perform the task correctly only when tested under the same conditions (either drugged or nondrugged) as were present during training. If the drug simply impaired the animal's ability to perform the response, animals of both groups would do worse when tested under drug than when tested without drug.

In a typical experiment, one group of animals is trained to escape a shock by making a right turn in a T maze while under the influence of pentobarbital, while a second group is trained to turn left when the saline vehicle is given. Upon testing, the first group is observed to make the correct response under pentobarbital but to respond randomly under saline, while the second group responds randomly under pentobarbital and correctly under saline. State-dependent learning has been demonstrated with a wide variety of **drugs,** including ethanol, pentobarbital, scopolamine, morphine, amphetamine, cannabis, and mescaline.

Drug-discrimination procedure

In this procedure animals are trained to make one response after a drug injection and a different response after an injection of either the drug vehicle or a different drug. In effect, the subjective state produced by the effects of the injection gains stimulus control over behavior.

In an experiment typical of this procedure, an animal pressing a lever while under the influence of a given drug obtains food, but if it presses the lever after getting the saline vehicle it receives electric shock. Animals given such differential training eventually learn to press under drug and to withhold pressing under saline. Drug discrimination has been shown with the same drugs as state-dependent learning. The difference between drug-discrimination and state-dependent learning lies in the objectives and the training techniques. In drug-discrimination studies, the purpose is to see whether the subjective effects produced by one drug are similar to, or different from, those produced by another drug. Therefore animals are trained to associate different responses with the different effects of two drugs (or a drug and its vehicle). In state-dependent learning, the purpose is primarily to see how a specific drug interacts with the learning process; therefore the animals are trained under the influence of only one drug and then tested either with the same drug or its vehicle. However, drug-discrimination information can also be obtained by testing with a drug other than that used in training; if it also elicits the same response as the training drug, it must have produced a state similar to that caused by the training drug.

Generalization Gradients

One way to examine the control exerted by drug stimuli is to determine the drug-generalization gradient associated with that drug. Typically a discrimination based on a certain drug and dose is established, and testing is then carried out with a number of different doses of the same drug or with a number of different doses of a different drug. In the former case, the purpose is to find out how strong the drug test stimulus has to be for the animal to react to it in the same way as to the training stimulus. In the latter case, the purpose is to see whether the test drug stimulus is perceived as qualitatively similar to, or different from, the training drug stimulus. The results yield a drug-generalization gradient that indi-

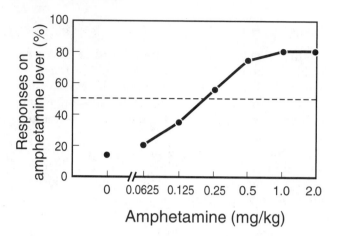

Figure 71-2. Example of drug-generalization gradient obtained in rats for responses on the amphetamine lever as a function of the size of test dose of amphetamine. The animals were trained with a dose of 1.0 mg/kg.

cates the strength of responding to different values of a drug stimulus.

Figure 71-2 illustrates a typical generalization gradient for groups of rats trained to press one lever under the influence of a 1.0-mg/kg dose of *d*-amphetamine and to press a second lever under saline. Typically, drug-generalization gradients show a progressive decrease in responding, the lower the test dose is in relation to the training dose. At test doses higher than the training dose, response gradients do not drop off but tend to plateau. Figure 71-3 gives drug-generalization gradients for animals trained to discriminate alcohol from saline and then tested with alcohol, a barbiturate, and a benzodiazepine. These gradients illustrate that even drugs of different classes can share certain stimulus properties when care is taken to use equivalent doses.

Discriminability

Drug discriminability is defined operationally as those properties of a drug that render it an effective discriminative stimulus. It can be measured in terms of (1) speed of acquisition of discrimination and (2) maximum degree of control of behavior attained by a drug as the dose is increased (i.e., if drug A at any dose does not exert as great a degree of stimulus control as a second drug B after similar training histories, then drug B is a more effective discriminative stimulus). Drugs may differ in their discriminability, just as in other effects, in terms of both potency and efficacy (see Chapter 8).

Mechanisms of Stimulus Control Exerted by Drug Stimuli

A drug must act centrally in order to be readily discriminable. Thus, amphetamine and atropine provide effective discriminative stimuli, but their peripherally acting analogs hydroxyamphetamine and atropine methylbromide do not.

Sensory stimuli may be perceived very differently under the influence of a drug than in its absence, or than under the influence of a different drug. These changes may form the basis of a drug discrimination.

In order to determine the pharmacological systems involved, animals that have been well trained to discriminate a particular agonist may be tested after pretreatment with a general antagonist and with a series of specific antagonists for different receptor subtypes. For example, if morphine has been established as a discriminative stimulus, the performance of the animal can be compared after pretreatment with naloxone and then with specific antagonists of μ-, δ-, and κ-receptor subtypes (see Chapter 23). A difference in the effects of the various antagonists will indicate which receptor subtype is involved in the development of the discrimination. An alternative method is to prevent the acquisition of a drug discrimination by interfering with the presumed neurotransmitter mediating the drug effect. For example, if the acquisition of stimulus control by amphetamine is blocked by pretreatment with the catecholamine-depleting drug α-methyl-*p*-tyrosine (AMPT), this would confirm that the discriminative

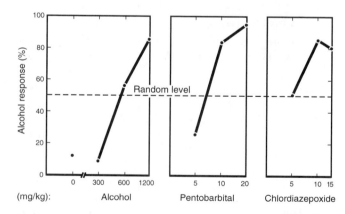

Figure 71-3. Examples of drug- and cross-generalization gradients obtained in rats for responding on the lever appropriate for the alcohol state as a function of various doses of alcohol, pentobarbital, and chlordiazepoxide. The animals were trained with an alcohol dose of 1200 mg/kg.

stimuli produced by amphetamine arise from its action of releasing the catecholamines DA and NE from nerve endings.

BEHAVIORAL MODELS OF MENTAL DISORDERS

In the development of new drugs for treating disorders in humans, it is usually advantageous to have animal models of those disorders. This applies equally to drugs used for treating emotional disorders and psychoses. Examples of the animal models used for screening potential new drugs of these types are described below.

Anxiety

A number of animal models are available that generate anxiety-like behavior and are used to test the anxiolytic properties of drugs.

Elevated plus maze

An elevated plus maze is an apparatus with four long narrow arms in the shape of a plus or cross, mounted on a pedestal about 3–5 feet above the floor. Two of the arms are completely open; the other two have side walls high enough to block the subject's view of the drop to the floor. Rats instinctively explore their environment, but they are normally reticent to "walk the plank" by entering either of the open arms because of the obvious risk of falling. Instead, they prefer to enter the arms that have protective sides. Anxiolytic compounds, such as the **benzodiazepines,** considerably increase the amount of time that animals will spend exploring the open arms; this effect indicates a reduction in fear and appears to be specific, since other types of psychoactive drug do not have this effect.

Conditioned emotional response

Differences in dimensions of the elevated plus maze can produce different results. Therefore, other behavioral models are also used. One of these is the conditioned emotional response or CER. In this model, a hungry animal is placed in a small chamber and trained to press a lever to obtain a food pellet. Once this response is learned and reliably performed, a tone or other sensory stimulus is turned on for a short period (usually 2–5 minutes) at the end of

which one brief foot shock is delivered. Initially, the animal does not associate the stimulus with the imminent foot shock, but after several sessions it shows a consistent pattern of vigorous lever-pressing in the absence of the stimulus and marked reduction of pressing in the presence of the stimulus. The animal has learned to associate the stimulus with the shock, and the resultant "anxiety" deters it from active lever-pressing. In this model, the administration of benzodiazepines (but not other psychoactive agents) results in a reemergence of bar-pressing during the stimulus, which indicates a decrease in the animal's state of anxiety.

A variant of the CER procedure is used to study **conflict.** In this situation, the onset of the stimulus indicates that shocks will be delivered each time a food pellet is obtained. The conflict arises because bar-pressing in the presence of the stimulus brings the inseparable combination of food and foot shock. Under these circumstances the rate of bar-pressing is diminished when the stimulus appears, but anxiolytic agents tend to lessen the conflict and enhance lever-pressing.

Depression

Behavioral despair (Porsolt test)

A rat that is placed in a small glass cylinder partly filled with water will attempt to escape by climbing up the sides but is unsuccessful because the glass is smooth and the top of the cylinder is out of reach. After a period of intense effort, the animal appears to "give up" and curls up and floats on the surface of the water. Antidepressant medications, but not other types of psychoactive drugs, reinstate the escape behavior. This finding led to the use of the test as a screening procedure for new antidepressant medications. The reappearance of the escape behavior following treatment with the antidepressant does not occur immediately but, as in recovery from depression in humans, is seen only after a period of chronic dosing (see Chapter 29).

Olfactory bulbectomy

Bilateral removal of the olfactory bulbs produces a constellation of behavioral, associative, and neurochemical changes that resemble some aspects of human depression (Richardson 1991). Bulbectomized animals are irritable, aggressive, and even hyperactive at times. Their cognitive abilities are impaired, as indicated by difficulty in learning to avoid a foot shock by withholding a response (passive avoidance). These deficits can be significantly attenuated by chronic treatment with antidepressant drugs, but not by other classes of psychoactive drugs. While the olfactory bulbs have obvious important sensory functions, it is thought that their involvement in affective functions is related to their direct synaptic connections with a number of important limbic structures such as the hippocampus, amygdala, and septum (see Chapter 20). These areas are known to modulate the development and expression of emotional behavior. Furthermore, bulbectomy reduces the levels of a number of important neurochemicals in these structures, including dopamine, norepinephrine, serotonin, and acetylcholine. These transmitters are known to be involved in the elaboration of emotional behavior and are important targets for antidepressant medication.

Chronic mild stress

Animals that are continuously exposed to a series of changing and unpredictable low-level stressors develop behavioral deficits that resemble some of the symptoms of endogenous depression. Such stressors include periods of deprivation of food, water, or sleep; cage tilting; introduction of a strange animal; and periods of loud noise or unpredictable mild electric shock. The behavioral deficit is best described as a state of *anhedonia* or flatness of affect, marked by a relative indifference to stimuli that are normally rewarding. For example, rats normally prefer and seek out highly palatable substances such as sucrose or saccharin, or will learn to press a lever to obtain delivery of a low-level electric stimulus to the reward system of the brain (see discussion of reinforcement, below). Animals exposed to chronic mild stress no longer respond as avidly to these stimuli. However, their responses return toward normal during chronic treatment with antidepressant drugs.

Schizophrenia

Of all mental disorders, schizophrenia is undoubtedly the hardest to model in animals, because it is an illness marked by disordered thought, delusions, hallucinations, ambivalence, and incongruous affect. These symptoms appear to be uniquely human and would be very difficult to model in other species. However, the paranoid ideation and hallucinations produced in humans by high doses of amphetamine or cocaine have led to a closer examination of the

effects of high-dose **psychostimulants** in animals. One of the most frequently observed effects is stereotypic behavior, defined as the focused and continuous repetition of apparently purposeless behaviors such as licking, sniffing, gnawing, and repetitive circling activity. These appear to be analogous to certain repetitive behaviors produced by high doses of psychostimulants in humans. In general, antipsychotic drugs that control many of the schizophrenic symptoms in humans also block these stimulant-induced stereotypic behaviors. This finding is the basis for the use of this model to screen potential new antipsychotic drugs.

DRUGS AS REINFORCERS

As seen in the previous sections, psychoactive drugs have stimulus properties of their own, can alter ongoing behavior maintained by positive and negative reinforcement, and can influence basic biological functions such as eating, drinking, sleeping, and learning. However, drugs can also modify behavior by acting as reinforcers or punishers in their own right. If a certain behavior (e.g., pressing a lever) results in the intravenous infusion of a psychoactive drug, the consequences of that drug exposure may reinforce the preceding behavior (i.e., increase the probability that the animal will go back and press the lever again), or may punish it (i.e., decrease the probability of pressing the lever again, or stop it altogether). Psychomotor stimulants (e.g., cocaine, amphetamine), opioids (e.g., heroin, morphine), and some CNS depressants and anxiolytics (e.g., pentobarbital, diazepam) are positive reinforcers and can generate avid self-administration by animals and humans. The reinforcing properties of these drugs are believed to contribute to their risk of generating drug dependence or abuse (see Chapter 72).

In contrast, neuroleptics (e.g., chlorpromazine, haloperidol), tricyclic antidepressants (e.g., amitriptyline), opioid antagonists (e.g., nalorphine) and hallucinogens (e.g., LSD, mescaline, THC) are not self-administered by animals and can act as punishers (i.e., cause avoidance of the behavior that results in self-administration) or negative reinforcers (i.e., strengthen behavior that results in removal of the drug). Caffeine, nicotine, and ethanol under certain circumstances also act as punishers, especially in nonhuman subjects.

These latter examples illustrate an important limitation of the assessment of drug abuse potential in animals: *All drugs that are readily self-administered by animals also show dependence or abuse potential in humans, but not all drugs that generate such problems in humans are readily self-administered by animals.* Ideally, therefore, one would wish to study dependence liability directly in humans, but this is difficult for various reasons, including ethical concerns about administering potentially dangerous or addicting drugs to humans and the presence of confounding variables such as uncontrolled differences in nutritional status, cultural and psychological background, and previous drug experience. For these reasons, studies of drug self-administration in experimental animals are still important in the investigation of abuse or dependence liability of a drug. Various methods have been developed for this purpose.

In the experimental analysis of drug-taking behavior, drug-taking is viewed as an operant response that is reinforced by the effects of the drug. These reinforcing effects may then motivate further drug-taking behavior by themselves, independently of the reasons for the initial drug-taking. However, most drugs also have some unpleasant, punishing (aversive) effects, even in the same range of dosage that produces reinforcement. The strength of reinforcement by a drug in a given individual therefore depends on the balance between reinforcing and punishing effects.

Drugs differ in the strength of their direct positive reinforcing properties. It is much easier for experimental animals to acquire a high level of self-administration of cocaine, amphetamine, or heroin than of alcohol or cannabis, and they are extremely unlikely to acquire such behavior toward LSD or mescaline. Such differences may account for the common but misleading distinction between "hard drugs" and "soft drugs."

Methods of Studying Drug Reinforcement

Oral self-administration can be produced quite simply by putting the drug in the food or the drinking water so that the animal is forced to consume the drug while satisfying its physiological need for food or water. However, such obligatory consumption tells us nothing about the reinforcing properties of the drug and is not relevant to the human situation, in which a choice is almost always available. Therefore the appropriate animal models include a choice between drug solution and water, and consumption is measured in terms of both absolute amount of drug ingested and relative volumes of drug solution and water consumed.

Intravenous self-administration involves the implantation of an indwelling venous catheter, connected via a motor-driven infusion pump to a reservoir of drug solution. When the animal presses a lever that closes the pump circuit, the pump is activated and delivers a preset dose from the reservoir. Automatic programming equipment controls the number and spacing of lever presses required to activate the pump. This setup is illustrated in Figure 71-4. One advantage of the intravenous route is that the taste of the drug, which is often aversive to animals, is no longer a problem. A second advantage is that the drug effect is usually very rapid in onset, so that, if the drug has primary reinforcing properties, they can be demonstrated more easily. A third is that it is not necessary to have a second catheter and pump for water, since the animal can drink water normally.

Both oral and intravenous methods can be used to study the factors that control drug self-administration. Intravenous studies are particularly useful for investigating primary reinforcing properties of drugs, i.e., their ability to generate repeated self-administration without the need for other external inducements. This is often referred to as their "abuse potential." Central stimulants, such as cocaine and amphetamine, are the most potent in this regard. Morphine and heroin are quite effective, but the newer agonist–antagonist opioids (see Chapter 23) are not. Some barbiturates, benzodiazepines, and methaqualone are moderately effective, but alcohol is only weakly and unreliably reinforcing in this type of experiment. Cannabinoids and hallucinogens such as LSD and mescaline are aversive; after experiencing their effects, the animal will not press the lever again.

It is common practice to train the animals to self-administer cocaine and then to substitute a test drug that is under study. If the animal continues to self-administer this drug with a response rate greater than for saline, the drug is considered to be reinforcing. The "relative abuse potential" of different drugs, i.e., their relative strengths of reinforcement, can be assessed by use of the **progressive-ratio method**. After a stable response rate has been established on a fixed-ratio schedule, the ratio is systematically increased in logarithmic steps. This makes the subject work progressively harder for the same amount of drug. The break point, i.e., the ratio value at which drug self-administration ceases or falls below some defined criterion, is a measure of the reinforcing strength of that drug under those particular experimental conditions. The break points for different drugs under the same conditions can then be arranged in order of magnitude to provide a

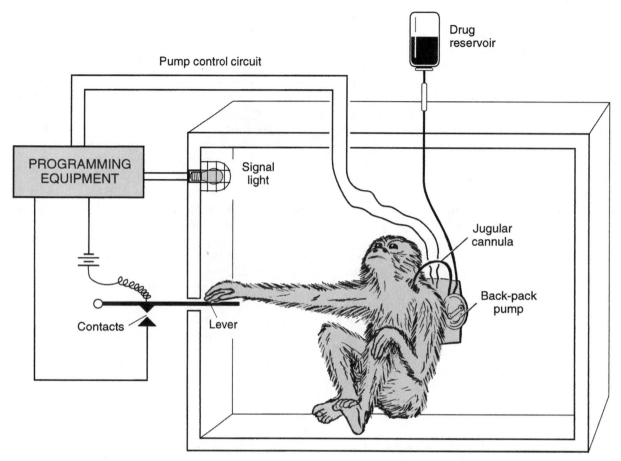

Figure 71-4. Schematic representation of apparatus for investigating reinforcing properties of drugs by the self- administration model in experimental animals (monkeys). Similar setups have been used with rats and other species.

ranking of the relative reinforcing strengths of the drugs.

Neurobiology of Reinforcement

The anatomy of the reinforcement system was first uncovered in 1954 by James Olds and Peter Milner, who were researchers at McGill University in Montreal. They observed that animals would learn to press a lever to self-administer brief trains of low-intensity electric current to the hypothalamic area. At times the rate of lever pressing was so robust that only exhaustion would interrupt further lever pressing. Subsequent research identified the *medial forebrain bundle* (MFB) as the most effective site for this "self-stimulation" and as one of the neural circuits involved in reinforcement.

The MFB is a bundle of axons running from the midbrain to the basal forebrain and connects many limbic, hypothalamic, and midbrain structures with one another. It contains ascending catecholaminergic (i.e., dopamine- and norepinephrine-releasing) and serotonergic neurons. Recently, the midbrain dopaminergic system has been closely linked to the mechanism of reinforcement, particularly the dopaminergic axons in the MFB traveling from the midbrain to the forebrain (Fig. 71-5). These axons arise from cell bodies in the *ventral tegmentum* near the substantia nigra and synapse with cells of the *nucleus accumbens* located just in front of the hypothalamic preoptic area. A variety of studies have shown that reinforcement produced by food, water, drugs of abuse, and even sexual behavior can be modulated by pharmacological manipulation of this tegmental–accumbens dopaminergic circuit.

Such manipulation is possible because the dopaminergic pathway is subject to a wide variety of facilitatory and inhibitory influences exerted by other neurotransmitters that act upon it. Among the most clearly identified are opioid, GABA, and noradrener-

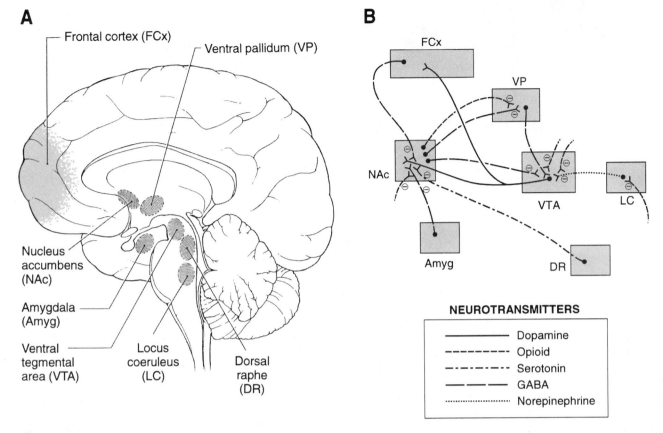

A

— Frontal cortex (FCx)
Ventral pallidum (VP)

Nucleus
accumbens
(NAc)

Amygdala
(Amyg)

Ventral
tegmental
area (VTA)

Locus
coeruleus
(LC)

Dorsal
raphe
(DR)

B

FCx

VP

NAc

VTA

LC

Amyg

DR

NEUROTRANSMITTERS

——————	Dopamine
– – – – – –	Opioid
– · – · – · –	Serotonin
— — — —	GABA
··················	Norepinephrine

Figure 71-5. Schematic representation of the main known elements of the brain "reward system." GABA = aminobutyric acid; ⊖ = inhibitory action; unmarked synapses are excitatory. Adapted from Koob (1992) and McBride et al. (1993).

gic fibers that form synapses at various points in the dopaminergic pathway. Knowledge about this complex interplay of neurotransmitters in the reinforcement process is growing rapidly, and the picture is changing accordingly. A schematic representation of present knowledge is shown in Figure 71-5.

SUGGESTED READING

Grabowski J. Psychopharmacology: basic mechanisms and applied interventions. Washington DC: American Psychological Association, 1993.

Katz RJ. Animal model of depression: pharmacological sensitivity of a hedonic deficit. Pharmacol Biochem Behav 1982; 16:965–968.

Koob GF. Drugs of abuse: anatomy, pharmacology and function of reward pathways. Trends Pharmacol Sci 1992; 13:177–184.

Leonard BE. Fundamentals of psychopharmacology. Chichester: John Wiley, 1993.

McBride WJ, Murphy JM, Gatto GJ, et al. CNS mechanisms of alcohol self-administration. Alcohol Alcohol 1993; Suppl 2:463–467.

Olds J, Milner P. Positive reinforcement produced by electrical stimulation of the septal area and other regions of rat brain. J Comp Physiol Psychol 1954; 47:419–427.

Porsolt RD, Anton G, Blavet N, Jalfre M. Behavioural despair: a new model sensitive to antidepressant treatments. Eur J Pharmacol 1978; 47:379–391.

Richardson JS. The olfactory bulbectomized rat as a model of major depressive disorder. In: Boulton A, Baker G, Martin-Iverson M, eds. Neuromethods, vol 19: Animal models in psychiatry, vol II. Clifton NJ: Humana Press, 1991:61–79.

White NM, Franklin KBJ, eds. The neural basis of reward and reinforcement: a conference in honor of Peter M. Milner. Neurosci Biobehav Rev 1989; 13:59–186.

CHAPTER 72

Drug Abuse and Drug Dependence

H. KALANT AND L.A. GRUPP

Since the beginning of the 20th century the term "addiction" has been applied to certain patterns of heavy use of opioids, alcohol, and other potent CNS drugs. The drugs to which this chapter refers are psychoactive drugs, i.e., those that are used primarily for their effects on consciousness, mood, and perception of the internal and external environments. One rarely, if ever, hears of addiction to digitalis, sulfonamides, or warfarin. No fully satisfactory definition of drug addiction has ever been achieved. An Expert Committee of the World Health Organization made repeated attempts to define it and differentiate it from "habituation" but was unable to produce definitions that were fully consistent with clinical experience.

For various reasons, it became clear that both terms were unsatisfactory, and the WHO committee recommended that they be replaced by the single term drug dependence, which would include all degrees of intensity of desire for the drug, all degrees of damage to both the individual and society, and all degrees of both physical and psychological need to continue using the drug.

In recent years there has been a widespread adoption of the term substance dependence, in which "substance" is really an abbreviation of *psychoactive substance.* The purpose is to avoid the artificial distinction between alcohol and other drugs, since the major features of dependence are found in all types of drug dependence. The fourth edition of the *Diagnostic and Statistical Manual of the American Psychiatric Association (DSM-IV)* defines substance dependence as a maladaptive pattern of substance use, leading to clinically significant impairment or distress, as manifested by three or more of the criteria shown in Table 72-1, occurring at any time in the same 12-month period.

The term *addiction* continues to be widely used, however, both by professionals and by the general public. Because of excessive preoccupation with heroin and other morphine-like drugs, and with the dramatic (but not life-threatening) withdrawal reaction to which they can give rise, there has been a tendency to equate addiction with physical dependence, and even with physical dependence of the opioid type.

In an effort to avoid the confusion caused by these various definitions and concepts, the term hazardous use was introduced. This is an operational term based purely on empirical epidemiological considerations, with no implications regarding dependence. It means use of a drug in such amounts and frequency as to carry a significantly greater risk of physical, mental, or social harm than would be expected in the normal population of the same age, sex, and socioeconomic status. This is a useful term for public-health considerations, but there is still a need for mechanistic terms to describe the processes leading to such levels of consumption.

In contrast to the terms "dependence" and "hazardous use," both of which can be defined operationally, drug abuse is essentially a value judgemental term, with different uses and meanings for different people. Some consider it to be synonymous with nonmedical use, any use of drugs for other than recognized therapeutic purposes being considered abuse. Yet, even though alcohol is rarely employed therapeutically in modern medicine, most use of alcohol is not considered abuse. Others equate the term with heavy or excessive use, but there is no gener-

Table 72-1 DSM-IV Criteria for Diagnosis of Substance Dependence*

1. Tolerance—need for increased amounts of the substance to achieve the desired effect, or markedly decreased effect with the same amount of the substance

2. Withdrawal—occurrence of a withdrawal syndrome characteristic of the substance in question, or use of the same or a closely similar substance to prevent or relieve this syndrome

3. Use of larger amounts, or over longer periods, than intended

4. Persistent desire to cut down or control use, or unsuccessful efforts to do so

5. Spending of a great deal of time getting and using the substance, or recovering from its effects

6. Giving up, or reducing, important social, occupational, or recreational activities because of substance use

7. Continuing use despite knowledge of having persistent or recurrent physical or psychological problems that are likely caused or exacerbated by the substance use

*Specifiers: Indicate whether the dependence is or is not accompanied by physiological dependence (i.e., items 1 or 2 above).

ally accepted definition of "heavy" or "excessive," and in any case it is not clear how these terms differ from "hazardous use." Still others apply the term "drug abuse" to **illicit use,** including *any* use of an illicit drug (such as cannabis or LSD) or **nonapproved use** of a licit but restricted drug (such as amphetamine or cocaine).

In reality, the term *drug abuse means any drug use that the speaker, or society at large, does not approve of.* Because of the subjectivity and vagueness of this concept, many experts in this field believe that the term is useless and should be abandoned. However, like "addiction," "drug abuse" continues to be widely employed even in scientific and clinical publications, and the reader must usually guess what the writer meant by it. Perhaps the best definition (Jaffe, 1985) is:

Drug abuse refers to the use, usually by self-administration, of any drug in a manner that deviates from the approved medical or social patterns within a given culture. The term conveys the notion of social disapproval, and it is not necessarily descriptive of any particular pattern of drug use or its potential adverse consequences.

The term *abuse potential* is used to describe the degree of risk that a drug will be used for nonmedical

purposes. Its operational measurement and significance are described in Chapter 71.

Regardless of whether one talks of addiction or dependence, the essential feature is not tolerance or physical dependence, but compulsive drug-taking, i.e., a behavior rather than a postulated metabolic alteration. This behavior pattern is often referred to as psychological dependence. A somewhat more descriptive term, which will be used in this chapter, is **behavioral dependence** or stimulus-controlled self-administration of drugs, as explained in the section on behavioral dependence. Many people consider this unimportant because one can be "psychologically" dependent on chewing gum, work, television, and so forth. This is totally wrong. It cannot be emphasized enough: *Behavioral dependence is the central problem in drug addiction, while tolerance and physical dependence are secondary features—consequences of the drug-taking.*

If we accept this concept, the terminology becomes a matter of relatively little importance, and classification of drugs as "addictive" or "nonaddictive," or "hard" or "soft," is an oversimplification. It is the interaction among the drug, the user, and the environmental context that determines whether or not dependence arises in a given case. The questions of real concern to the patient and the physician, as well as to society at large, are the following:

1. Why does the user experience a desire or a need to use the drug? In other words, what initiates use, how does dependence arise, and what keeps it going?
2. How intense is the dependence and to what extent does it control the user's lifestyle?
3. What are the consequences of this behavior to the user, to the user's family and immediate associates, and to society at large?

In order to understand abuse and dependence, it is necessary to examine normal or socially accepted patterns of use of psychoactive substances and then see what differentiates these normal patterns from unacceptable or harmful ones.

SOCIALLY APPROVED USE OF PSYCHOACTIVE DRUGS

History of Drug Use

Virtually every society in human history has had at least one psychoactive drug that was used in ways approved by that society and incorporated into its customs and traditions. The type of drug used was originally a matter of chance, depending on what natural products with suitable pharmacological properties were available in the vicinity. The drugs used in preindustrial societies covered the whole spectrum of psychoactive drug categories. A few examples are given in Table 72-2.

With the development of travel and trade between regions and nations, drugs native to one part of the world have become accepted and highly appreciated in other areas. Common examples are coffee, tea, and tobacco. The development of chemistry and industrial technology led to the isolation of pure active ingredients from natural products and the synthesis of highly potent derivatives, analogs, and substitutes. These are generally much less bulky and more stable than the natural products, and their use has spread around the world as a function of travel, commerce, education, communication, and availability of money for nonessentials.

Usually the first members of a society to adopt new drugs from another society are the wealthy and well informed who come into contact with other cultures. Business people, diplomats, performing artists, athletes, and university students on foreign fellowships are frequently involved. If they are prestigious figures in their own societies, their new patterns of drug use tend to be quickly imitated by others.

Social Functions of Psychoactive Drug Use

The universality of drug use and the ease with which one society adopts the drugs of another suggest that drug use must have important social functions. The earliest known role was a **religious** or magical one. The red color of wine has made it a symbolic substitute for blood in the religious sacraments of many societies, both ancient and modern, including our own. The feeling of warmth, due to alcohol-induced vasodilatation, has made it symbolic of the spirit of life itself, as indicated by such names as spirits, eau de vie, akvavit, and even whiskey (from the Gaelic for "water of life"). The hallucinogenic effects of peyote, epena, kaapi, and ololiuqui are used in the religious rites of various South and Central American populations to attain an otherworldly state in which contact with the gods or spirits is sought.

At a later stage, drugs were incorporated into **secular ceremonies,** such as passing around the kava bowl at the start of a Polynesian council meeting, smoking the pipe of peace among North American Indians, passing the "joint" at early marijuana parties before its use became widespread, and drinking toasts with alcohol at weddings or other special events.

Such uses led to drugs being used to induce **conviviality** in social gatherings, to increase pleasure, and to facilitate social interaction. In general, the drugs favored for this type of use have been either stimulants (khat, coffee, coca) or low doses of sedatives that produce disinhibition of behavior and emotional expression (alcohol, cannabis).

With increasing secularization of a society and progressive loosening of social controls over individual behavior, drug use for individual **private pleasure** became steadily more common. The use of wine with meals, smoking a cigarette at coffee break, and drinking caffeine-containing soft drinks as refreshments are among the many examples of such use.

Table 72-2 Examples of Psychoactive Substances with Socially Accepted Uses in Various Parts of the World

Society	Preparation	Pharmacological Agent or Category
Arabia, East Africa	Khat (q̂at)	Cathinone—central stimulant
Bolivian Indians	Coca	Cocaine—central stimulant
North American Indians	Tobacco	Nicotine—ganglionic cholinergic agonist
Indonesia	Betel	Arecoline—like nicotine
Southeast Asia	Opium	Morphine and other opioids
India, North Africa	Cannabis	Tetrahydrocannabinol—sedative
Amazon Indians	Kaapi, epena	Indole derivatives—hallucinogens
Southwest Amerinds	Mescal	Mescaline—hallucinogen
Oceania	Kava	Kavapyrones—sedative, anticonvulsant
Universal	Beer, wine, etc.	Ethanol—sedative

The last stage in the evolution of socially accepted drug use is **utilitarian,** at both individual and corporate levels. Individual utilitarian use is illustrated by the use of alcohol by salesmen who entertain clients during business negotiations, or by tense, nervous, depressed, or angry people who drink to feel better or to be able to release sentiments that they are unable to express when sober. Corporate utilitarian use is illustrated by commercial enterprises that create employment and profits from the manufacture, advertising, and sale of alcohol, tobacco, and other drugs and by the governments that gain large revenues from sale, customs duties, and taxes on these items.

Factors Governing the Extent of Use

The most important factor is the **degree of social acceptance or rejection** of a drug. For example, orthodox Moslems and Mormons do not use alcohol on religious grounds, even though societies around them use large amounts. Moslem society accepted the use of cannabis, whereas European and North American societies still reject it officially, even though large numbers of people use it.

Social upheaval or rapid reorganization may suddenly weaken the conventional attitudes that control alcohol or drug use in stable times. If these substances are readily available, major epidemics of excessive use may occur at such times of crisis and disappear when stability returns. Examples include the "gin epidemic" during the Industrial Revolution in England, the methamphetamine epidemic in Japan after its defeat in 1945, and the heroin epidemic among American troops in Vietnam in the 1960s and 1970s.

Despite common assertions to the contrary, **legal controls** do affect the extent of drug use, but they work best when they are in harmony with the prevailing social values and attitudes. For example, the move to enact Prohibition of alcohol in the United States (by a variety of state and federal measures beginning in 1916, and by Constitutional amendment in 1920) was in keeping with popular sentiment before and during World War I. The female suffrage movement and the temperance movement both saw alcohol-related problems as a major factor working against the well-being of women and children and a threat to young recruits just entering the U.S. armed forces. Therefore Prohibition was at first strongly supported and highly effective in reducing both alcohol consumption and the death rate from alcoholic cirrhosis and other alcohol-related illnesses.

The law also works as an effective deterrent to drug use if it provides severe penalties, is seen to be strictly enforced, and is enforced with a high degree of probability that offenders will be caught and punished. Alcohol rationing was enforced strictly by the German occupation forces in France during World War II, and this brought about a sharp fall in the death rate from cirrhosis, which rose rapidly again after the liberation of Paris in 1944.

In contrast, the law is not an effective deterrent when it is not in keeping with prevailing attitudes or when it is seen to have a low probability of being applied successfully against the majority of offenders. The eventual failure of Prohibition was due largely to public disillusionment with the apparent lack of uniformity, fairness, and effectiveness of enforcement. American and Canadian laws prohibiting the use of cannabis have continued to be supported by the majority of public opinion, and there has been no widespread push for repeal of these laws as there was for repeal of Prohibition.

Another very important factor is **price** in *real* or *constant* units, corrected for inflation and expressed in relation to average income and cost of living. In California, Ontario, Trinidad, and other jurisdictions in which studies have been done, there is almost a mirror-image relationship between the time courses of change in cost of alcohol expressed in these terms and the per capita consumption (Fig. 72-1) as well as the frequency of various alcohol-related problems, such as the cirrhosis death rate or the frequency of alcohol-related driving accidents. The relatively slow increase in alcohol consumption and in cirrhosis death rate in the United States after the repeal of Prohibition in 1933 probably reflects the influence of the severe economic depression at the time.

A closely related factor is **ease of availability.** When liquor stores in Ontario were changed to the self-service type, with all the goods available in open racks rather than held in a stockroom and brought to the counter by the clerk, the volume of sales rose quite substantially.

Occupational factors often relate to ease of access. For example, employees of breweries, distilleries, wineries, and drinking establishments are at higher risk of alcoholism, and physicians, nurses, and pharmacists are at increased risk of dependence on licit opioids, anxiolytics, and other psychoactive drugs.

Travel and mass communication facilitate the spread of drug use by giving large numbers of people the chance to learn about new drug practices. The methamphetamine ("speed") epidemic in Japan was brought to North America by American occupation

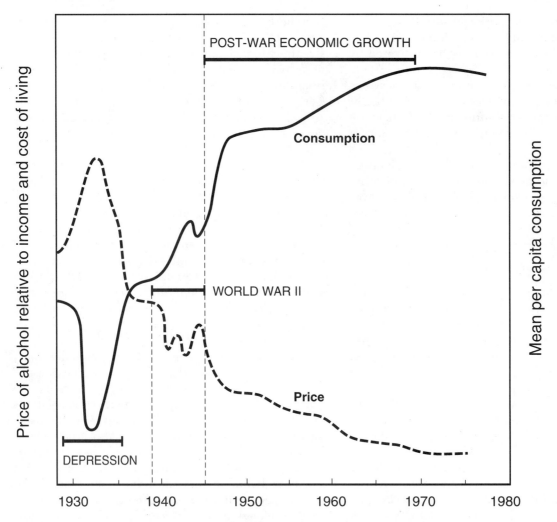

Figure 72-1. Inverse relation between the real price of alcohol and mean per capita consumption in Ontario over a 50-year period. The vertical scales are logarithmic.

(From data provided by R. E. Popham and W. Schmidt, Addiction Research Foundation of Ontario, Canada.)

troops stationed in Japan after 1945. The popularization of cocaine in North America and western Europe in the past three decades has probably been greatly assisted by the enormous publicity and initial glamorization that the drug received in the mass media.

Relation to Individual Use

It is very important to know how the extent of use of a drug by a whole population is related to the level of use by individual members of that population. Theoretically, for example, the average per capita consumption could increase even if the number of heavy users decreased; this would occur if large numbers of former nonusers all began to use small amounts while the smaller numbers of heavy users

all used less. In that case, an increase in per capita consumption might not be a cause for worry. Alternatively, increased per capita consumption might mean that all users, including the heavy users, were consuming more, and this would probably mean a major increase in drug-related problems.

This question is studied by examining the **distribution-of-consumption curve.** If the user population is surveyed and the percentage of users is determined for each interval in a scale of average daily consumption, the results can be plotted in a histogram or on a continuous curve. Conceivably one might find a bimodal curve, with the large majority of moderate users grouped around one mode near the low end of the consumption scale and a small number of heavy users clustered around a second mode near the high end. This would be the case if heavy users were qualitatively different from moderate users and responded to different controlling factors. In reality, however, the distribution-of-consumption curves for different drugs and populations all prove to be unimodal, with a large majority of users in the lower range of the scale and smaller and smaller numbers at progressively higher levels of intake (Fig. 72-2).

Even more important, when there is a change in the mean per capita consumption of the whole population, it comes about through a corresponding displacement of the whole curve. Thus, an increased mean consumption reflects an upward shift of the modal level of use, a decrease in the numbers of users below the mode, and an increase in the numbers above the modal level. This is accompanied by an increased incidence and prevalence of drug-related problems of health, behavior, and economic function. The opposite happens when the mean per capita consumption falls.

This means that heavy users respond in the same direction as light users do to changes in price, legal status, availability, and social attitudes. This has been demonstrated experimentally in a study employing alcoholic and nonalcoholic volunteers. Half of each group were allowed to buy alcoholic drinks at half price during a "happy hour"; the other half were not. The alcoholics drank much more than the nonalcoholics, but within each group the "happy hour" subgroup drank at least twice as much as the regular-price group (Table 72-3).

The conclusion is that *heavy or harmful use of drugs cannot be clearly separated from "normal" drug use.* In other words, the individual and social functions that make psychoactive drug use so universally prevalent carry with them the risk that some individuals or some societies may use too much and encounter the problems resulting from these higher levels of use. Social policy on drugs must take this into account in deciding what level of harm is acceptable in return for what level of social pleasure or functional benefit. At the same time, the goal of research and education is to find ways of reducing the width of the distribution-of-consumption curve so that a given modal value will be accompanied by fewer individuals in the upper part of the consumption range.

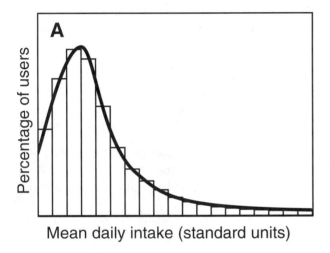

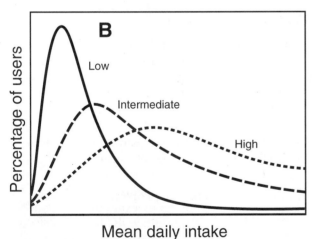

Figure 72-2. Schematic representation of distribution of consumption of alcohol and other psychoactive drugs in a population. A. Distribution shown as a histogram and as a smooth unimodal skewed curve. B. Relation between shape of the curve and mean per capita consumption by three different populations with low, intermediate, and high per capita consumption.

Table 72-3 Effect of Purchase Price on Consumption of Alcohol by Volunteer Subjects in a Long-term "Model Economy" Experiment

Subjects	Mean Number of Drinks Consumed	
	*"Happy Hour" in Effect**	*No "Happy Hour" in Effect*
Moderate drinkers	20.9	10.1
Alcoholics	117.6	49.6

*In the "happy hour" condition, drinks were available at half price for 3 hours each day.
Data from Babor TF et al. (1978).

BEHAVIORAL DEPENDENCE

Although social, legal, economic, and other factors mentioned above appear to have comparable effects on the level of alcohol and other drug use by light users and heavy users, there are nevertheless important quantitative and qualitative differences between dependent and nondependent users. An understanding of these differences is essential for the development of effective means for preventing and treating drug dependence.

Drug-Taking as Reinforced Behavior

People use psychoactive drugs for many different reasons. Some may use alcohol, barbiturates, or opioids for relief of boredom, frustration, tension, anxiety, or pain. Others may use them for a more positive type of pleasure associated with feelings of relaxation, joviality, "euphoria," or even physical visceral sensations that they find intensely gratifying. Still others use amphetamines or other stimulants to achieve feelings of heightened alertness, endurance, and power (also referred to as "euphoria," a rather inadequate word). Others use drugs because their social group does, and there is pressure on them to conform. The only thing common to all these motives is that the use of drugs is somehow **rewarding** to the user, whether by producing pleasure, by relieving displeasure, or by winning approval of the user's peers.

Some of the reward is the result of the pharmacological action of the drugs directly on the "reward system" of the brain, described in Chapter 71. This action is responsible for what is termed direct or primary positive reinforcement of drug-taking behavior. Methods for studying and quantifying this type of reinforcement are also described in Chapter 71. It is important to recognize that reinforcing properties of drugs do not by themselves explain drug dependence. They are an important factor in the acquisition of drug-taking behavior, but the majority of individuals who try psychoactive drugs, and who find the effects pleasing, do not become dependent. Moreover, though the intrinsic reinforcing properties of heroin are much greater than those of alcohol, far more people are dependent on alcohol than on heroin.

In behaviorist terms, drug dependence is the consequence of frequently and strongly reinforced drug-taking behavior, so that this behavior becomes a dominant response that increasingly replaces other possible responses that are less effective in satisfying the individual's drives. It is implicit in this concept that the drug effects must be experienced as a consequence of actively taking the drug. Receiving the drug passively will not give rise to behavioral dependence. Animals or humans can easily be made physically dependent on a drug (e.g., an opioid given by a nurse or physician for relief of severe chronic pain) by being given repeated doses of sufficient size to give rise to withdrawal symptoms when the drug is stopped. Yet, if they have played no role in the drug administration, they will go through the withdrawal reactions without later making any efforts to obtain more drug. For drug-seeking activity to occur, they must experience behavioral conditioning.

In addition to the requirement for self-administration, it is also necessary to examine a number of other internal and external factors that contribute to the differing degrees of risk of dependence in different persons.

Time relations

For the effects of a behavioral response to be reinforcing, those effects must be experienced quite soon after the response is made. Therefore a drug that produces its reinforcing effects rapidly is more likely to give rise to repeated drug-taking than one that has a slow onset of action. Thus, heroin is much more addictive than, for example, methadone (see Chapter 23).

Route of administration

It follows from the preceding point that the route of administration will have an important effect on the speed of reinforcement, and therefore on the probability of producing dependence. For example, heroin is much more likely to produce dependence if taken intravenously than if taken by mouth. The same is true of cannabis or of cocaine when they are smoked, compared to when they are swallowed.

Genetic predisposing or protective factors

In rats and other experimental animals, selective breeding over a number of generations has yielded lines that will voluntarily consume high or low amounts of a drug or that will show high or low sensitivity to some of the drug-induced changes in behavior. Such genetic selection experiments have been carried out repeatedly with alcohol, and there are recent reports of similar genetic selection for high and low intake of opioids. Similarly, in humans, genetic factors may influence the sensitivity of an individual to either the reinforcing or the punishing effects of a drug, or both.

The sons of alcoholic fathers, even when adopted in very early infancy by nonalcoholic families, are three to four times more likely to become alcoholics themselves than the similarly adopted sons of nonalcoholic fathers. What is inherited is almost certainly not a biological *need* for alcohol, but either a greater sensitivity to its reinforcing effects or a greater resistance to its punishing effects, or both. Studies of the nonalcoholic children of alcoholic parents are providing a growing body of evidence that both reinforcing and aversive effects of alcohol are under genetic control and that high-risk and low-risk individuals differ in the intensity of these effects. The evidence for a genetic influence is greater in those alcoholics with early onset, history of juvenile antisocial behavior, rapid progression of the level of alcohol intake, and high frequency of problems associated with intoxication. However, it is important to recognize that *the inheritance of these genetic factors does not inevitably make the person become an alcoholic.* Environmental factors play an essential role; genetic factors affect the degree of susceptibility to them.

Although the evidence is not conclusive, it has been proposed that the dopamine D_2-receptor may be implicated in the genetic vulnerability of this type of alcoholic. The D_2-receptor exists in at least two allelic forms, and the A1 allele is reported to be significantly more common in these patients. However, there is strong evidence that the risk of alcoholism is determined by multiple genes rather than by a single gene. As a result, there are numerous so-called genetic markers (see Chapter 12) of increased risk of alcoholism, such as monoamine oxidase and adenylyl cyclase activities. Some of these are currently being investigated for their possible usefulness in detecting, during childhood, those individuals at greatest risk of becoming dependent on alcohol or other drugs in adult life so that they may be given the benefit of early application of preventive measures. It must be emphasized that genetic factors simply affect the degree of risk; they are not the sole cause of dependence, and the majority of drug-dependent individuals do not have an identifiable genetic predisposition.

Conversely, a high proportion of Oriental people have genetic variants of alcohol dehydrogenase and acetaldehyde dehydrogenase that result in faster oxidation of ethanol to acetaldehyde and slower oxidation of acetaldehyde to acetate (see Chapter 26). Therefore the ingestion of ethanol produces in them a high steady-state level of acetaldehyde that causes very unpleasant effects (flushing, tachycardia, nausea, and dizziness) that greatly decrease the likelihood of further drinking, or at least of heavy drinking. Again, it must be emphasized that these genetic variants *decrease the risk* of alcoholism, but they do not prevent it entirely. If other factors mentioned above are conducive to the development of alcohol dependence, it is possible for people with the atypical form of acetaldehyde dehydrogenase to become dependent in spite of their initially aversive reaction to alcohol.

Motivational factors

In experimental animals, the existence of an aversive motivational state (e.g., fear or approach–avoidance conflict; see Chapter 71) can increase the intake of ethanol and other sedative or anxiolytic drugs (see Chapter 26). Food restriction, leading to chronic weight reduction, can increase the intake of a wide range of drugs of different pharmacological classes, even those that do not provide calories or directly reduce appetite. In humans, periods of heavy drinking or drug use are often triggered by situational changes that produce worry, fear, disappointment, anger, or frustration. Such states presumably increase the negative reinforcing effect of those drugs that are capable of relieving the discomfort.

Numerous studies have shown that situational and personality factors of various kinds are associated with heavy use of psychoactive drugs. Though there is no single pattern of "dependence-prone personality," adolescents with drug problems frequently have histories of parental abuse, long-standing alienation from family and friends, inability to control their impulses, and emotional distress beginning in childhood and preceding the start of drug use. The drugs again appear to act as negative reinforcers by giving temporary relief from the subjective distress caused by these preceding difficulties.

Stimulus control

Environmental stimuli that are regularly associated with the availability and use of a drug can become discriminative stimuli (see Chapter 71), in the presence of which the drug-seeking behavior occurs. The drug-taking is then said to be under stimulus control, rather than being a freely initiated act. Such stimuli, by their repeated association with the reinforcing effects of the drug, can become conditioned reinforcers that produce brief drug-like reinforcing effects. For example, if a light is used regularly to indicate to a rat that it can obtain a drug injection by pressing a lever, the rat will press the lever just to obtain the signal light. Similarly, humans who repeatedly experience the "rush" on self-injecting heroin or amphetamine into a vein often come to feel a brief "rush" on simply inserting a needle into the vein, even if the syringe is empty.

These conditioned responses are eventually extinguished if the conditioned stimuli do not continue to be paired with the drug from time to time. However, as long as they are present they may contribute to the phenomenon of **drug-craving** and the risk of **relapse** into drug use. Addicts who have been in hospital or prison for months or years, without any craving for drugs, can feel a compulsion to take drugs within hours of returning to the environment in which they had regularly taken drugs before.

Intensity and Significance of Behavioral Dependence

Since many different factors, as noted above, can enter into the creation of conditioned drug-taking behavior, and each can vary widely in degree, it is not surprising that the resulting behavioral dependence can also vary greatly in degree from relatively minor to an overwhelming compulsion that dominates all other behavior. It may be directed toward a drug or substance that is intrinsically rather harmless, or to one that is toxic and gives rise to serious physical consequences. The drug selected may be inexpensive and legally available, and so no social harm may result, or it may be expensive or illegal, so simply obtaining the drug may give rise to serious problems. The cost of the drug may deprive the user or the user's family of other necessities, or the user may obtain more money by theft, drug trafficking, or other illegal means and risk arrest and prison. In other words, behavioral dependence is neither harmful nor harmless in itself; the degree of harm depends on what consequences it brings in the individual case.

TOLERANCE AND PHYSICAL DEPENDENCE

Many drugs give rise to the phenomenon of increase in tolerance when they are taken repeatedly or chronically. In other words, it becomes necessary to take progressively larger doses to achieve the same degree of drug effect. This may be illustrated graphically as a shift in the dose–response curve (Fig. 72-3). It may be produced in two quite different ways, referred to as *metabolic* (or *dispositional*, or *pharmacokinetic*) *tolerance* and *functional* (or *target tissue*, or *pharmacodynamic*) *tolerance*.

Metabolic Tolerance

The reactions by which the drug is detoxified, in the liver in most instances, may become more active as a result of enzyme induction (see Chapter 4) following repeated use of the drug. It is then necessary to

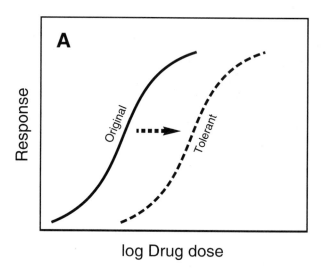

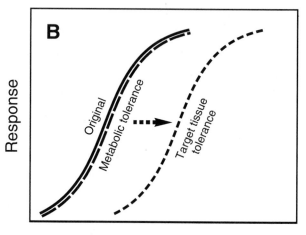

Figure 72-3. A. Shift in *dose*–response curve illustrates tolerance, but gives no indication of the mechanism. B. Metabolic tolerance does not alter the *concentration*–response curve, but target tissue tolerance shows a shift in the concentration–response curve similar to that in the dose–response curve.

take a larger dose in order to maintain effective concentrations of the drug in blood and brain for the same length of time as originally. This form of tolerance is not likely related to physical dependence, because it is really equivalent to taking smaller doses of drug. Common examples include tolerance to numerous barbiturates and, to some extent, alcohol.

Metabolic cross-tolerance is also important for drugs that are biotransformed by hepatic microsomal enzymes. Induction of the cytochrome P450 system by barbiturates, by alcohol, or by phenytoin, for example, can cause increased rates of biotransformation of many other drugs (see Chapters 4 and 26).

Functional Tolerance and Physical Dependence

Tolerance as adaptation

The brain or other tissues on which the drug acts may undergo adaptive changes that tend to offset the effect of the drug. For example, if ethanol, barbiturates, or benzodiazepines cause depression of neuronal excitability, changes in ion fluxes, and impairment of neurotransmission, the adaptation might consist of changes in the cell membrane that facilitate both passive and active ion fluxes and neurotransmitter release and increase the excitability of the neuron. These changes would tend to compensate for the effect of the drug and produce an apparently normal functional state while the drug is present (tolerance).

Such adaptive changes have been found in virtually every type of neuronal function examined, including energy metabolism, spontaneous and evoked electrical activity, neurotransmitter turnover, numbers and affinities of neurotransmitter receptors, intracellular signal transduction systems, and expression of various genes and oncogenes. In most cases, however, it is impossible to know whether the observed changes are necessary for the production of tolerance, or are merely manifestations of tolerance.

Relation to physical dependence

When the drug is withdrawn, the same changes give rise to a "drug-opposite" effect that is recognized as a withdrawal reaction. For example the hyperexcitability that produced tolerance to ethanol, barbiturates, or benzodiazepines now forms the basis of a **withdrawal syndrome**, which may range from sleeplessness, tremor, and irritability to hallucinations and tonic-clonic seizures. The severity depends upon the degree of adaptive change in the nervous system, which in turn depends on the degree and duration of exposure to the drug. Since the withdrawal reaction is abolished by a fresh dose of the drug, it constitutes evidence of **physical dependence** on the drug.

Drug-specific withdrawal patterns

The particular characteristics of the withdrawal syndrome depend on the adaptive changes induced by the drug, which in turn depend on the pharmacological actions of the drug. Thus, morphine suppresses gastrointestinal motility and constricts the pupil; the morphine withdrawal syndrome includes intestinal hypermotility and diarrhea and pupillary dilatation. Cocaine or amphetamine causes hyperactivity and euphoria, and the withdrawal reaction is characterized by profound fatigue and depression. It is a common error to think that a drug does not cause physical dependence if it does not cause a morphine-type withdrawal reaction. This is obviously quite illogical; there is no reason why a central stimulant such as cocaine should produce a withdrawal reaction similar to that of morphine.

Intensity

The intensity of withdrawal reaction is also related to the time-course of action of a drug. For example, a drug that acts for a relatively long time, because of high plasma protein binding and slow biotransformation or excretion, frequently gives rise to less intense withdrawal symptoms than a drug that acts quickly, intensely, and briefly. Presumably the slow elimination of the drug permits some measure of physiological readaptation to occur while the drug concentration is falling. This probably explains the less intense withdrawal reaction after methadone than after heroin or morphine.

Nondrug factors in tolerance

Tolerance is not simply a physiological adaptive response to the physical presence of the drug. Rather, it is a response to the functional disturbance produced by the drug. This depends not only on the kind and amount of drug but on the sensitivity of the individual, on the type and level of the person's ongoing activity at the time the drug is taken, on the environment in which it is taken, and on the user's previous drug history.

Individuals, strains, and species with greater **initial sensitivity** to a drug will experience greater functional disturbance on their first use of the drug than more resistant subjects do, and therefore they will have a greater stimulus to the development of tolerance.

The same dose of a drug produces tolerance more rapidly if the subject is alert and **performing some task** under the influence of the drug than if the drug is taken at rest. This is particularly true if the drug effect causes the **loss of some reinforcer** for which the subject is working.

Tolerance, especially to relatively low doses of a drug, may also be in part a **conditional response.** For example, an animal that receives a dose of morphine every day in the same environment, and has its body temperature taken each time to monitor the hypothermic effect of the drug, shows much greater tolerance in that environment than it does if the drug administration and temperature measurement are then carried out in a different environment. The environmental stimuli become conditional stimuli; they bring on tolerance more rapidly by eliciting a conditional response that is opposite in effect to the action of the drug.

A subject who has a **history of having been tolerant** to a drug previously, and who has then reverted to normal sensitivity after stopping the drug, reacquires tolerance and physical dependence more rapidly on resuming drug use than on the first time around.

These observations show that tolerance is not a simple process, but a complex phenomenon with many components. The same dosage of the same drug can therefore give rise to wide interindividual differences in the degree and rate of development of tolerance and physical dependence, and even within the same individual at different times and with respect to different effects of the drug. Many different biochemical mechanisms have been proposed to explain tolerance; so far, none can account for all the behavioral complexities of the process.

Role of physical dependence in maintaining drug dependence

Physically dependent subjects whose drug use is interrupted for any reason may, on feeling withdrawal symptoms, learn that by taking more drug they obtain rapid relief from these symptoms. This results in a corresponding negative reinforcement of that response that contributes to the strengthening and maintenance of drug-taking and behavioral dependence.

The conditioning of behavior, i.e., learning to take more drug in response to certain stimuli arising during the withdrawal syndrome, may also help to explain the high relapse rate among drug-dependent people. Since these stimuli are not really specific (e.g., intestinal hypermotility, muscle tension, tremor, hyperirritability), they can also be produced by other causes, such as physical illness or emotional disturbance. When they do, even though the person has not been using drugs for some time, these stimuli can evoke the conditioned drug-taking response just as if they were part of a true withdrawal reaction.

CROSS-TOLERANCE AND TRANSFER OF DEPENDENCE

If two drugs cause essentially similar pharmacological effects via essentially the same mechanism, one might anticipate that adaptive changes that arise from the use of one drug will also confer tolerance to the other—i.e., there will be **cross-tolerance.** In fact, it has been noted clinically for many years that alcoholics are unusually resistant to general anesthetics, barbiturates, and other hypnosedatives. In one study, the minimum alveolar concentration of halothane required for anesthesia (see Chapter 24) rose from 0.76% in normal subjects to 1.31% in a group of alcoholics. The same transfer of tolerance is seen from one opioid analgesic to another, and from alcohol and barbiturates to other hypnosedatives and anxiolytics.

Conversely, when one drug in a cross-tolerance group is withdrawn, another in the same group can be used to decrease or abolish the withdrawal symptoms—i.e., there is a **transfer of physical dependence** (i.e., cross-dependence). In fact, new synthetic opioid analgesics are tested for dependence liability by testing their ability to prevent withdrawal symptoms in heroin addicts or in heroin-dependent monkeys. When one treats delirium tremens or other alcohol withdrawal symptoms by giving a benzodiazepine, one is really making therapeutic use of this transfer of dependence. It is still necessary to gradually reduce the dosage of the substitute drug, or nothing will have been accomplished except to replace one drug problem with another.

TREATMENT OF DRUG DEPENDENCE

From the nature of dependence, it is obvious that the goal of treatment is to stop the undesired drug-taking response from continuing to be self-reinforcing. Psychological and social therapy, in the form of counseling and individual and group psychotherapy, are aimed at building up other behavioral responses for problem-solving that are, at the same time, reinforced by social approval and that increase the patient's self-esteem. In other words, long-term treatment of drug dependence requires more than just getting the patient through a withdrawal period with the aid of a tranquilizer—it requires a process of behavioral retraining to enable the patient to make different and more helpful responses to the stimuli that have habitually elicited drug-taking behavior.

Pharmacological agents can help in various ways:

1. *Use of specific blockers to prevent the drug from producing its usual effects, including its reinforcing effect.* The first efforts to do this were directed toward a few drugs for which specific transmitter or receptor mechanisms were known, e.g., naltrexone to block μ-opioid receptors (see Chapter 23), and thus prevent all actions of heroin, including its reinforcing action. Similarly, α-methyl-*p*-tyrosine, an inhibitor of catecholamine synthesis (see Chapter 13), has been used to block the "high" produced by cocaine or amphetamine. There are also blockers of benzodiazepine receptors (e.g., flumazenil; see Chapter 27), but these do not appear to have been used in treating benzodiazepine dependence. In theory, failure of the drug-taking behavior to provide the anticipated reward should lead to **extinction** of this conditioned behavior. In opioid-dependent persons, opioid receptor blockers are not used in this way until withdrawal from the opioid is complete; if used too soon, the blockers will precipitate a severe withdrawal reaction.

2. *Nonspecific blockade of reinforcement.* With increasing recognition of the complexity of the neuronal circuits involved in the reward system (see Chapter 71), which appears to be shared by quite diverse psychoactive substances, it seemed possible that reinforcement by a variety of different drugs might be prevented nonspecifically by the use of agents that interfere with the reinforcement mechanism without being specific antagonists of those drugs.

In view of the important role of dopamine in the reinforcement circuits (see Chapter 71), efforts have been made to block reinforcement by administering dopamine receptor blockers such as butyrophenones and phenothiazines (see Chapter 28). These have been found to decrease alcohol intake but not opioid intake, and the side effects make them unsuitable for treating drug-dependent humans. However, selective dopamine receptor agonists such as bromocriptine and lisuride appear to have some value in reducing alcohol consumption, although the mechanism is not clear.

Serotonin, apparently acting on 5-HT$_2$- and 5-HT$_3$-receptors, is believed to prevent reinforcement by inhibiting the activity of the dopaminergic pathway from the vental tegmental area (VTA) to the nucleus accumbens (see Fig. 71-5). Therefore a number of serotonin reuptake inhibitors (e.g., fluoxetine, citalopram, trazodone) and 5-HT$_{1A}$-receptor agonists (e.g., buspirone) have been tested, in the expectation that they would increase the level of 5-HT inhibitory activity on the VTA dopamine neurons and thus reduce reinforcement by alcohol, nicotine, and other drugs. These agents did produce large and dose-dependent decreases in alcohol intake by rats. Rather surprisingly, however, some *blockers* of 5-HT$_2$-receptors (e.g., ritanserin) and 5-HT$_3$-receptors (e.g., ondansetron) were equally effective in rats, but the effects of all these drugs in humans have been rather modest. It is not yet clear whether they will be more useful when combined with other blockers of reinforcement, or as accessory agents in a program that includes psychosocial and other types of treatment.

Opioid receptors in both the VTA and the nucleus accumbens also play an important role in reinforcement, either by modulating the activity of dopamine neurons or by an independent mechanism (see Chapter 71). Alcohol intake by rats is increased by administration of low doses of opioids, and markedly decreased by opioid receptor blockers such as naloxone and naltrexone. These findings led to clinical studies that have demonstrated a significant beneficial effect of **naltrexone** in reducing the risk of relapse in recovering alcoholics, and in reducing the amount of alcohol consumed if relapse does occur. The use of naltrexone for this purpose has now been approved in the United States and Canada.

3. *Substituting a less reinforcing and legally available drug for a more reinforcing and illicit one,* e.g., **methadone or buprenorphine maintenance** for heroin addicts. Note that *methadone is not a treatment of the dependence.* It simply permits the patient to satisfy the drug need legally, under medical supervision and control. The real treatment component is the social and psychological rehabilitation that should be going on while the patient comes to the clinic regularly to receive the methadone. Since this rehabilitation, when it occurs, usually requires a long time to change the patient's behavior significantly, methadone maintenance treatment is often carried on for periods of many years.

4. *Substituting a less reinforcing drug, in preparation for withdrawal.* The second drug can then be gradually reduced in dosage to avoid a major withdrawal reaction, e.g., methadone withdrawal therapy in heroin dependence, benzodiazepines for withdrawal from alcohol.

5. *Aversive agents* that interact with the drug to produce an unpleasant instead of a rewarding effect, e.g., **disulfiram** or **calcium carbimide** in the treatment of alcoholics (see Chapter 26).

While reinforcement blockers and aversive agents are sound in theory, they have had rather limited success. This is because many patients are unwilling to take them and thus to cut themselves off from the possibility of deriving the desired effects from their drug of dependence. Others may agree to take the blocker or aversive agent but can simply stop taking it if they change their mind. Therefore, the effectiveness of these drugs depends very heavily on the patient's motivation.

Counterconditioning is a behavioral counterpart of this approach, aimed at eliminating stimulus control of drug self-administration. Stimuli that are associated with drug-taking are repeatedly paired with a very aversive stimulus such as electric shock or apomorphine-induced nausea. Unfortunately this technique is also not very successful. It reduces drug self-administration while the aversive conditioning is in progress, but the benefit seldom lasts after the course of conditioning is finished.

6. *Pharmacotherapy of emotional disturbances that may be contributing to the problem drug use,* e.g., lithium or tricyclic antidepressants in many individual cases of alcoholism or barbiturate dependence that may be caused by an underlying depression.

SUGGESTED READING

Babor TF, Mendelson JH, Greenberg I, Kuehnle J. Experimental analysis of the "Happy Hour": effects of purchase price on alcohol consumption. Psychopharmacology 1978; 58:35–41.

Brady JV, Lukas SE, eds. Testing drugs for physical dependence potential and abuse liability. NIDA Research Monograph Series No. 52. Rockville, MD: Nat Inst Drug Abuse, 1984.

Efron DH, Holmstedt B, Kline NS, eds. Ethnopharmacologic search for psychoactive drugs. Washington DC: US Dept HEW, 1967.

Fishman J, ed. The bases of addiction. Berlin-Dahlem Konferenzen: Life Sci Res Rep 8, 1978.

Goldstein A. Addiction—from biology to drug policy. New York: Freeman, 1994.

Jaffe JH. Drug addiction and drug abuse. In: Gilman AG, Goodman LS, Rall TW, Murad F, eds. Goodman and Gilman's the pharmacological basis of therapeutics. 7th ed. New York: Macmillan, 1985:532–581.

Jaffe JH, Naranjo CA, Bremner KE, Kalant H. Pharmacological treatment of dependence on alcohol and other drugs: an overview. In: Approaches to treatment of substance abuse. Geneva: WHO Programme on Substance Abuse, 1993:75–101.

Kalant H, Kalant OJ. Drugs, society and personal choice. Toronto: Addiction Research Foundation, 1971.

Kalant H, LeBlanc AE, Gibbins RJ. Tolerance to, and dependence on, some non-opiate psychotropic drugs. Pharmacol Rev 1971; 23:135–191.

Kissin B, Begleiter H, eds. Social aspects of alcoholism. The biology of alcoholism, vol 4. New York: Plenum Press, 1976. [See especially articles by Schmidt W, deLint J, pp 275–305 and Popham RE, Schmidt W, deLint J, pp 579–625.]

Popham RE, Schmidt W, deLint JE. The prevention of alcoholism; epidemiological study of the effects of government control measures. Br J Addict 1975; 70:125–144.

Tabakoff B, Hoffman P, eds. Biological aspects of alcoholism. Implications for prevention, treatment and policy. Seattle: Hogrefe & Huber, 1995.

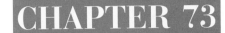

CHAPTER 73

Principles of Toxicology

M.A. McGUIGAN AND P.G. WELLS

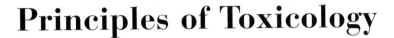

Toxicology is the scientific discipline that is concerned with the adverse effects of chemical agents on biological systems. It is a multidisciplinary field of study that draws from a number of related disciplines, including biology, chemistry, physiology, immunology, pathology, pharmacology, and public health. Because of the vastness of the subject and the specialized approaches to its study, only a general survey of pharmacotoxicological principles can be presented here.

Various classification systems are used to designate specialized areas of interest within the field of toxicology (Table 73-1). One such classification is based on the purpose or application to which the results of the research are to be applied (e.g., forensic toxicology, clinical toxicology). Another classification is on the basis of the organ system primarily affected by the toxic reaction (e.g., cardiovascular, renal, neurotoxicology). A third classification is based on the research methods used to study the toxicity (e.g., biochemical toxicology, behavioral toxicology).

Similarly, the toxic agents themselves are classified in different ways reflecting different special interests. One system classifies agents according to their relative potential for causing poisoning (Table 73-2). Another system, relating specifically to the study of toxic materials of biological origin (toxinology), is based on the source of the toxin (e.g., snake venoms, spider venoms, bee-sting toxins, plant toxins, marine animal toxins). Still other classifications are by chemistry of the toxic agents (e.g., aromatic amines, halogenated hydrocarbons) or by mechanism of toxic action (e.g., sulfhydryl enzyme inhibitors, methemoglobin producers).

Despite these numerous areas of special attention, the objectives are fundamentally the same in all: to understand the mechanisms by which exogenous substances give rise to toxicity in living subjects, to define the quantitative relationships, to identify factors that increase or decrease susceptibility in individuals or populations, and to develop methods for preventing or treating the toxic reactions.

DOSE–RESPONSE RELATIONSHIPS

When investigating the adverse effects of an agent on a biological system, the toxicologist must determine the relationship between the dose and the response. The dose–response concept is defined as a correlative relationship between exposure and effect (see Chapter 8). Three important assumptions are implicit in this definition: (1) the observed response is, in fact, due to the chemical administered; (2) the degree of response is related to the magnitude of the dose; and (3) the response in question is precisely defined and quantifiable.

An important dose–response parameter is the threshold dose, i.e., the lowest dose that evokes a stated all-or-none response. How the response is defined will influence the determination of the threshold dose. For example, for salicylate the threshold dose that causes gastrointestinal bleeding (one to two tablets of ASA [aspirin] in an adult) is different from that which results in tinnitus (20–30 tablets) or that which is associated with systemic acidosis (40–50 tablets).

Responses develop over a period of time, so it is important to establish a fixed observation period. Some toxic effects develop quickly and are reversible

Table 73-1 Classification of Toxicology According to Areas of Application

Field of Toxicology	Area of Application
Environmental	Pollution
	Residues
Economic	Food additives
	Pesticides
Legal	Forensic
	Regulatory
Laboratory	Analytical
Biomedical	Human (clinical)
	Occupational
	Veterinary

$$TI = LD_{50}/ED_{50}$$

The TI provides a rough approximation of the safety of a chemical, bearing in mind both the above limitations and the absence of information on the slopes of the curves for either of the two components of this index. The larger the TI value the safer the drug, with an index of 10 indicating a relatively safe drug. In any event, an acceptable index is relative: In the case of rapidly lethal diseases, such as some cancers and AIDS, for which there is no effective treatment, drugs are tolerated with higher incidences and severities of toxicity than would be acceptable for a drug to treat headaches.

A typical log-dose–response curve is shown in Figure 73-1 and explained in detail in Chapter 8. The dose (e.g., mg/kg) is plotted on a logarithmic

(e.g., inebriation and acidosis due to methanol poisoning), while others develop over several days and are irreversible (e.g., blindness resulting from methanol poisoning).

Another commonly determined dose–response function, which is less susceptible to the above assumptions, is the LD_{50} (the dose causing the death of 50% of the exposed test animals; see Chapter 8). Such parameters should be used with caution for several reasons. First, the LD_{50} often varies substantially depending upon such factors as the species, strain, age, sex, and route of exposure. For example, the LD_{50} for TCDD (dioxin) can vary over 1000-fold between the guinea pig and hamster and does not cause acute lethality in humans, at least at exposure levels encountered to date. Second, some chemicals with relatively negligible acute toxicity, such as the environmental chemical benzo[a]pyrene, nevertheless may initiate other or delayed toxicities, such as cancer or birth defects, and may do so at doses much lower than those necessary to cause lethality or other, less drastic acute toxicities. Finally, the target tissue can vary from strain to strain and species to species, as it does for TCDD, and a particular toxicity such as acute lethality determined in one animal model often is not predictive of the spectrum, let alone the severity, of toxicities expressed in other animal models or humans.

The LD_{50} is sometimes used with the ED_{50}, or effective therapeutic dose for 50% of the population, to calculate the therapeutic index (TI, see Chapter 8):

Table 73-2 Classification of Toxicants According to Poisoning Potential

Toxicity Rating	Example	LD_{50} (mg/kg)*
Slightly toxic (5–15 g/kg)	Ethanol	8000
Moderately toxic (0.5–5 g/kg)	Sodium chloride	4000
	Ferrous sulfate	1500
	Malathion	1300
	Methanol	1000
Very toxic (50–500 mg/kg)	Acetylsalicylic acid	300
	Acetaminophen	300
	Diazinon	200
	Phenobarbital	150
	Imipramine	65
Extremely toxic (5–50 mg/kg)	Theophylline	50
	Diphenhydramine	25
Super toxic (<5 mg/kg)	Potassium cyanide	3
	Methotrexate	3
	Strychnine	2
	Nicotine	1
	Digoxin	0.2
	d-Tubocurarine	0.05
	Tetrodotoxin	0.01
	TCDD (dioxin)	0.001
	Botulinum toxin	0.00001

*LD_{50} is the lethal dose (mg/kg of body weight) for 50% of exposed animals. This list is an approximation, and the relative rank of each chemical may vary substantially depending upon the species tested, as well as other parameters such as strain, age, sex, and route of exposure.

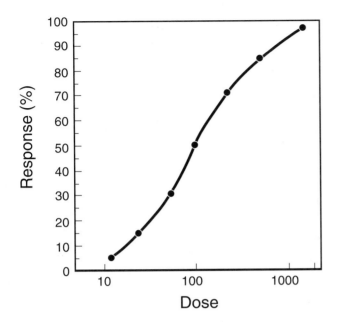

Figure 73-1. Features of the log-dose–response curve (see also Chapter 8).

scale along the horizontal axis, and the response on an arithmetic scale along the vertical axis. The dose–response curves for *effective dose*, *toxic dose*, and *lethal dose* are generally independent of each other. Parallel dose–response curves for two substances indicate that the agents have different LD_{50} values but that this difference is proportional over the whole scale of responses. However, intersecting dose–response curves of two substances may give one substance a lower LD_5 but a higher LD_{50}, analogous to the principle underlying the *certain safety factor* in Chapter 8. The *potency* of a toxin is defined by the position of its dose–response curve along the dose axis. Thus, a substance with an LD_{50} of 8 g/kg is less potent than one with an LD_{50} of 5 g/kg.

MECHANISMS

In general, chemicals initiate adverse effects by one of two mechanisms: (1) the reversible binding of the parent molecule and/or a stable metabolite to a cellular receptor (see Chapter 9) or (2) via bioactivation of a relatively nontoxic chemical to a highly toxic electrophilic or free-radical reactive intermediate that irreversibly (covalently) binds to or oxidizes cellular macromolecules such as DNA, protein, and lipid (see Chapter 70; Fig. 70-7). These two mechanisms differ

in several basic and clinically important ways that are summarized in Table 73-3. Toxicities initiated by reversible, receptor-mediated binding usually are relatively predictable, occurring as a result of drug overdose or exposure to excessive amounts of environmental chemicals, and they can be confirmed by detecting a high plasma or tissue concentration of the chemical. However, toxicities initiated via irreversible macromolecular lesions caused by reactive intermediates may occur at therapeutic plasma drug concentrations or presumably safe exposure levels of environmental chemicals. This toxicological predisposition usually results from individual biochemical imbalances involving one or more of the following: decreased chemical elimination, enhanced chemical bioactivation, decreased detoxification of reactive intermediates, decreased cytoprotective pathways that remove reactive oxygen species, or decreased repair of damaged cellular macromolecules (Chapter 70; Figs. 70-7 to 70-10). In most people, in the absence of excessive exposure levels, bioactivation does not exceed the capacity of the multiple protective pathways, and reactive intermediates are formed and removed with no toxicological consequence.

Most drugs and environmental chemicals can initiate reversible, receptor-mediated toxicities if the exposure level is sufficiently excessive. In the case of drugs, the toxicological sequelae usually will include a predictable exaggeration of the pharmacological effect for which the drug is employed therapeutically; for example, severe hypotension from an overdose of a β-adrenergic-blocking drug given in therapeutic doses to lower blood pressure. Alternatively, bioactivation to a toxic reactive intermediate occurs with a smaller but still substantial number of chemicals, including the analgesic drug acetaminophen, some organophosphate insecticides, and the herbicide paraquat. Many chemicals that cause cancer (carcinogens), birth defects (teratogens), tissue necrosis, neurodegenerative disorders, and immunologically mediated hypersensitivity reactions (allergens or immunogens) are believed to initiate their toxicity at least in part via bioactivation to a reactive intermediate. The target tissue often is determined by the site of bioactivation, because the reactive intermediate is too reactive to travel across membranes to distal tissues without first reacting with more proximal targets. Hence, tissue necrosis caused by higher doses of acetaminophen occurs predominantly in the liver and kidney while that caused by paraquat occurs in the lung.

Table 73-3 Characteristics of Xenobiotic Toxicity Initiated by Reactive Intermediates Compared with Reversible, Receptor-Mediated Interactions

Characteristic	Mechanism of Tissue Interaction	
	Reactive Intermediate	*Receptor-Mediated*
Initiating species	Reactive intermediary metabolite (highly unstable) 　Electrophile 　Free radical Often a minor metabolite amounting only to 1–10% of total xenobiotic/metabolites	Parent compound and/or a stable, major metabolite
Molecular target	Multiple sites within different cellular macromolecules (DNA, protein, lipid, and carbohydrate)	Specific receptor on one type of macromolecule (usually a protein)
Target interaction	Irreversible Covalent binding (arylation/alkylation) Oxidation	Reversible binding (usually)
Duration of target interaction	Cumulative	Transient
Toxic effects*	Unrelated to therapeutic effect†	Generally an extension of the therapeutic effect
Toxic dose/concentration	Toxicity can occur at therapeutic plasma drug concentrations or "safe" concentrations of environmental chemicals	Toxicity occurs when therapeutic or safe plasma concentrations are exceeded
Onset of toxicity	Toxicity occurs well after the time of the peak plasma xenobiotic concentration, and usually after the xenobiotic no longer is detectable in plasma or urine Depending upon both the xenobiotic and the toxicity, this delay can be hours, days, months, or years	Toxicity usually increases with rising plasma xenobiotic concentration, and decreases with or shortly after declining concentrations

*Effect in this case refers to the effect of therapeutic drugs, and is not relevant to environmental chemicals.

†There are some exceptions, such as alkylating anticancer drugs, where drug toxicity does result from the same mechanisms by which tumor cells are killed.

From: Wells PG, Winn LM. *Crit Rev Biochem Mol Biol* 1996; 31:1–40.

MODIFIERS OF TOXICITY

In analogy to the sources of variation in drug response (see Chapter 62), a number of factors can modify the manifestations of toxicity.

These modifiers may alter toxicity via a variety of mechanisms, most often altering chemical biotransformation or disposition. Using toxicological enhancement as an example, likely mechanisms include a reduction in pathways of elimination, allowing the accumulation of excessive concentrations of the chemical, enhanced pathways of bioactivation to a toxic reactive intermediate, or reduced detoxifying or cytoprotective pathways for removing reactive intermediates or reactive oxygen species. For chemicals like aminoglycoside antibiotics that are eliminated by renal excretion without being biotransformed, reduced renal filtration or secretory functions can lead to chemical accumulation and toxicity. For drugs such as the anticoagulant warfarin that have a narrow therapeutic index and are highly bound (over 90%) to plasma carrier proteins such as albumin, exposure to other chemicals or conditions that displace the drug from its carrier protein, or diseases resulting in decreased carrier protein content, will increase the free (active) drug concentration; in the case of warfarin, this leads to internal bleeding. Other potential mechanisms of toxicological enhancement include reduced pathways for repair of cellular macromolecules damaged by reactive intermediates (see Chapter 70). With receptor-mediated effects, toxicity may be altered by the number of receptors and their functional state, particularly in the fetus, neonate, and elderly, and by concomitant exposure to receptor agonists and antagonists, including the unappreciated accumulation of active metabolites that bind to the same receptor as the parent compound.

Age

The age of the subject is an important variable. As shown in Table 73-4 with rats of three distinct age groups, the variability in toxic response to three insecticides may depend on age-related variations in relative organ size, maturation of enzyme systems, and distribution patterns of the toxin. For example, relative toxicity of malathion in different species is inversely related to the rate of biotransformation of malathion by the hepatic cytochrome P450 system (see Chapter 4). Since this system is markedly hypofunctional in the neonatal rat, this may explain the much higher toxicity of malathion in the newborn. However, β-adrenergic receptors are also hypofunctional in the newborn (see Chapter 65). Death by overdose of DDT in the rat is usually attributable to ventricular fibrillation, and immaturity of the catecholaminergic response system may protect the newborn against increase in myocardial irritability by DDT.

This age variability is also present in human responses to poisons. Young children appear to tolerate toxic blood concentrations of acetaminophen, digoxin, and theophylline better than adults do. However, children are more susceptible to severe toxicity from antihistamines, lead, and salicylates than adults are.

Neonates and the elderly have reduced renal function and hence are more susceptible to the accumulation and toxicity of chemicals such as aminoglycoside antibiotics that are predominantly removed via renal elimination.

Route or Site of Administration

The route or site of administration may alter the observed toxicity of a given substance. Routes commonly used for toxicity testing and their influence on the degree of toxicity are shown in Table 73-5. Procaine toxicity depends on the rate and completeness of absorption compared to the rate of hydrolysis by plasma esterases. In most cases, it is probably the variation in bioavailability that accounts for the differences in the LD_{50} found with different routes of administration. Pentobarbital toxicity is related to peak tissue concentrations. Because pentobarbital is primarily absorbed from the intestinal tract rather than from the stomach, absorption is slow and may result in relatively lower tissue levels compared to dosing by the parenteral routes.

Duration or Frequency of Exposure

Another aspect to consider when assessing the toxicity of a substance is the duration and frequency of exposure. In toxicology, acute exposure is defined as exposure lasting less than 24 hours, during which time the substance may have been administered as a single, repeated, or continuous dose. Subacute exposure means exposure for 1 month or less. Subchronic exposure means a duration of 1–3 months, and chronic means more than 3 months. However, these terms are often used loosely; for example, chronic salicylate toxicity is said to develop after use of the drug for more than 2 days.

Different durations of exposure may result in different manifestations of toxicity. For example,

Table 73-4 Effect of Age on Acute Toxicity in Rats*

Age	Malathion	DDT	Dieldrin
Newborn	+ + +	+	+
Preweaning	+ +	+ +	+ + +
Adult	+	+ + +	+ +

*+, + +, + + +: Increasing degrees of toxicity.

Table 73-5 Effect of Route of Administration on LD_{50} in Rats, Relative to Intravenous Injection

Route	Procaine	Isoniazid	Pentobarbital
Intravenous	1.0	1.0	1.0
Intraperitoneal	5.0	0.9	1.6
Intramuscular	14.0	0.9	1.5
Subcutaneous	18.0	1.0	1.6
Oral	11.0	0.9	3.5

acute exposure to benzene results in CNS depression, but chronic exposure may be associated with hematological malignancy.

Nutrition

The role of nutrition in toxicology is complex but must be considered when evaluating the toxicity of a given substance. Variability in nutrition may affect the toxic response through alterations in absorption, distribution, biotransformation, and excretion of drugs and chemicals.

The presence of food in the stomach may enhance the absorption of some drugs (e.g., β-blockers, hydralazine, diazepam, lithium, carbamazepine) but may reduce the absorption of others (e.g., penicillins, isoniazid, rifampin). Malnutrition appears to reduce the absorption of tetracyclines and rifampin.

The biotransformation of drugs and chemicals is affected by nutrition in various ways. Rats that were fasted for 24 hours had a decreased rate of glucuronidation of 7-hydroxycoumarin, which returned to normal after a glucose infusion. Rats fed a diet low in polyunsaturated fats and high in saturated fats had lower than normal activity of cytosolic glutathione transferase. Animals fed a low-fat high-protein diet had lower than normal elimination half-lives for antipyrine and theophylline; this observation suggests that substitution of dietary protein for fat may accelerate some drug transformations. However, children with kwashiorkor (a form of liver damage due to dietary deficiency of certain amino acids) appear to have delayed biotransformation of tetrachloroethylene, which has led to the development of toxicity from this substance when it was used as an antiparasitic agent.

Genetic Variability

A frequent cause of exceptional predisposition to chemical toxicities involves genetic differences in one or more critical biochemical pathways (see Chapters 12 and 70). For receptor-mediated toxicities, this often involves lower levels, or even complete absence, of enzymes or enzymatic activities necessary for drug elimination, such as isoforms or isozymes of the cytochromes P450, UDP-glucuronosyltransferases, and N-acetyltransferases, resulting in the accumulation of a drug and/or its stable metabolite to toxic concentrations. Such deficiencies usually must be great enough to account for a major component of elimination for the xenobiotic, sufficient to substantially decrease clearance and increase plasma and tissue concentrations.

For toxicities produced by reactive intermediates, toxicological predisposition may result from genetically high activity and/or inducibility of bioactivating pathways such as cytochromes P450 (e.g., CYP2D6, CYP1A1), or lower activities of enzymes that detoxify reactive intermediates (e.g., epoxide hydrolases, glutathione S-transferases). Unlike the situation with receptor-mediated toxicity, these pathways often constitute only a minor component of the total elimination of the xenobiotic. However, due to the extraordinary potency of reactive intermediates, pathways that control their formation and detoxification nevertheless have a dramatic effect on toxicological susceptibility, usually without measurably affecting plasma concentrations of the parent compound.

For example, while epoxide hydrolase contributes only about 10% of phenytoin elimination, a genetic deficiency in this enzyme renders such individuals highly susceptible to an otherwise rare but potentially fatal liver necrosis. In another rare case, a genetic deficiency in the enzyme γ-glutamylcysteine synthase results in a marginal ability to synthesize glutathione (GSH), which is essential for the detoxification of both electrophilic and free-radical reactive intermediates, as well as reactive oxygen species. Toxicologically relevant genetic deficiencies in cytoprotective pathways against reactive oxygen species and oxidative stress also have been reported, including GSH peroxidase, GSH reductase, superoxide dismutase, catalase, and glucose-6-phosphate dehydrogenase. Recent evidence suggests that genetic deficiencies in enzymes and other proteins involved directly or indirectly (e.g., DNA damage and the p53 protein) in the repair of cellular macromolecules damaged by reactive intermediates also may enhance toxicological susceptibility.

Genetic susceptibility also can play a further role in immunologically mediated hypersensitivity reactions (see also Chapter 63). For example, everyone taking the antibiotic penicillin has some of this drug covalently bound to their proteins, yet only a relatively small number of these people experience true hypersensitivity reactions. In this case, individual differences in such pathways as antigen recognition and processing, and pathways controlling the immunological cellular response of T and B cells, are the critical determinants of susceptibility.

Environmental Modifiers

All the toxicologically relevant pathways discussed above under Genetic Variability at least theoretically can be either increased or decreased by a multitude of environmental modifiers, including other drugs (both prescription and nonprescription), environmental chemicals (industrial and natural), and microbial agents (e.g., viruses, bacteria). Most of these modifiers alter at least one pathway, and typically more than one. The consequences usually are difficult if not impossible to predict because not all, if any, of the effects of most modifiers are known; toxicity depends upon the net alteration in the balance of several pathways; and the full complement of environmental modifiers to which a patient is exposed usually is not appreciated. Even the relatively circumscribed area of drug interactions often is quite complicated, particularly since the effect of a modifier on a given pathway may be completely opposite in acute compared to chronic exposure. For receptor-mediated and reactive intermediate-mediated toxicities, alterations also can result, respectively, from coexisting agonists/antagonists and macromolecular damage.

Disease

Coexisting diseases often can alter susceptibility to the toxicity of drugs and environmental chemicals. These effects may be readily anticipated, such as in some liver diseases that impair drug metabolism and elimination, and renal diseases that impair the elimination of drugs that are cleared without requiring biotransformation. In either of these cases, the disease would result in excessive drug accumulation. Effects of other diseases may be less apparent. For example, cardiovascular diseases can result in decreased liver blood flow that inhibits the metabolism of so-called high-clearance drugs such as lidocaine and decreased renal blood flow that reduces the elimination of renally cleared drugs. Gastrointestinal diseases also can alter drug metabolism, particularly for chemicals that are extensively metabolized in the intestinal wall during absorption. Via a number of mechanisms, diseases of the kidneys, liver, and gastrointestinal system can alter the amount or binding capacity of carrier proteins in the plasma, thereby altering the free, and potentially toxic, concentration of the chemical. Numerous other effects of these and other diseases in modifying toxicological susceptibility have been reported, and in many cases the underlying mechanisms remain to be fully characterized. An optimal appreciation of even the known possibilities requires an extensive knowledge of the disposition and potential toxicological mechanisms for all drugs and chemicals to which a patient is exposed.

PREDICTIVE TOXICOLOGY

Predictive toxicology assesses the risks (or evaluates the hazards) associated with a situation in which the toxic agent, the subject, and the exposure conditions are defined. The difficulties associated with risk or hazard assessment are compounded by many variables, including the interactions of several agents, the changes in subject population, and differing exposure conditions.

Two concepts are particularly important in predictive toxicology: the "lowest observed effect level" (LOEL) and the "no observed effect level" (NOEL). Increasingly sophisticated analytical techniques have steadily lowered the limits of detection and quantitation for an increasing number of chemicals. Measurable amounts of metals, aflatoxins, dioxins, pesticide residues, and chlorinated hydrocarbons are now found where none were found before, perhaps only because our ability to detect and measure them has improved. Similarly, the degree to which we can detect and observe an effect also depends on the sensitivity of the tests. For example, acceptable levels of lead in the blood of young children have dropped steadily: 40 μ/dL in 1974, 30 μg/dL in 1978, 25 μg/dL in 1985, 15 μg/dL in 1991, and 10 μg/dL in 1993 (respectively, 1.92, 1.44, 1.20, 0.72, 0.48 μmol/L). This reduction in acceptable blood concentrations has occurred as a result of improved ability of complex, sensitive neuropsychological tests to detect subtle defects produced by lower concentrations of lead.

As can be seen in the dose–response curve in Figure 73-1, the curve does not reach either axis. The difficulty at the low ends of the scales lies in extrapolating, for predictive purposes, from high-dose, high-frequency responses to low-dose, low-frequency response. Different approaches in the area of risk assessment are illustrated in Figure 73-2. Once an acceptable risk is defined, the "virtually safe dose" may cover a range of doses depending on the nature of the dose–response curve at the low ends of the scales. Those who believe that very low levels of chemicals in the environment pose significant risks may support the supralinearity concept. Because of the imprecision implicit in measurements at the low end of the scale, arbitrary safety factors may have to be used. For example, when setting a virtually safe dose of a chemical for which good human data and experience of predictive value are available, the NOEL determined in animals may be reduced by a safety factor of 10 for humans; in the absence of human data, however, the NOEL in animals might

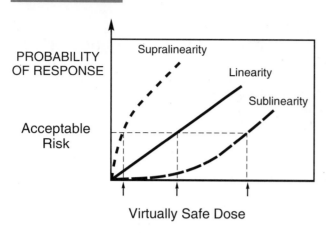

Figure 73-2. Three possible patterns of risk assessment.

have to be reduced by a safety factor of 1000 to be considered virtually safe in humans.

In addition to toxicological data, other factors may need to be considered in establishing acceptable risk levels. A chemical's beneficial effects (in terms of economics, employment, standard of living, quality of life, taxes generated, etc.) must be weighed against its known detrimental effects (e.g., health effects, loss of environmental resources, loss of work, lawsuits). Toxicological risk assessment, therefore, is concerned with promoting the safety of the individual without simultaneously reducing the benefits to contemporary society.

SUGGESTED READING

Ballantyne B, Marrs T, Turner P, eds. General and applied toxicology. New York: Stockton Press, 1993.

Clayson DB, Krewski D, Munro I, eds. Toxicological risk assessment, vols 1 and 2. Boca Raton: CRC Press, 1985.

Klaassen CD, ed. Casarett and Doull's toxicology. The basic science of poisons. 5th ed. New York: McGraw-Hill, 1996.

Lu FC. Basic toxicology. 2nd ed. New York: Hemisphere, 1991.

Marquis J, ed. A guide to general toxicology. 2nd ed. Karger Cont Educ Ser, vol 5. Basel: Karger, 1989.

Timbrell, JA. Principles of biochemical toxicology. 2nd ed. London: Taylor and Francis, 1991.

CHAPTER 74

Poisonings and Antidotal Therapy

M.A. McGUIGAN

CASE HISTORY

A 47-year-old woman weighing about 60 kg was brought to the Emergency Department by ambulance with a verbal history of having ingested about 60 regular-strength acetaminophen tablets (325 mg each) in a suicide attempt approximately 6 hours earlier. The patient was awake and alert on arrival. In the interval, she had vomited twice and was now complaining of nausea. There was no significant past medical history and no medications had recently been used. Her temperature was 37° C, pulse rate 88/min, respirations 20/min, and blood pressure 110/70 mmHg. The rest of the physical examination revealed only mild sweating and slight epigastric distress.

Attempts to empty the stomach (e.g., ipecac-induced vomiting or gastric lavage) were not made because of the significant time delay between acetaminophen ingestion and arrival at the hospital and because the patient had already vomited twice. However, activated charcoal (1 g/kg) was administered through a small-bore nasogastric tube. The activated charcoal was mixed with a sorbitol cathartic. This procedure was tolerated by the patient. Laboratory investigations included determinations of aspartate aminotransferase (AST), alanine aminotransferase (ALT), alkaline phosphatase, bilirubin, and prothrombin time. In addition, blood samples were sent to the laboratory for plasma acetaminophen and salicylate levels.

The results of the laboratory analyses were all within normal ranges. Salicylate was not detected.

However, the acetaminophen level was 1200 μmol/L. When this value was plotted on an acetaminophen nomogram, it fell in the "probable hepatic toxicity" range.

In order to prevent the development of hepatic damage, the patient was started on an intravenous infusion of N-acetylcysteine, which lasted for 21 hours, at which time the hepatic laboratory tests were repeated. The results were normal, and the patient was transferred from the Emergency Department to the Psychiatry service.

Poisonings are a common occurrence. Over the past decade, the number of poisonings reported in Canada and the United States has increased steadily. Nearly 2 million cases of human exposure to poisons were reported in 1993. Approximately 25% of all cases were treated in a health care facility and the mortality rate was 0.07%.

The substances most frequently encountered in poisonings are cleaning substances (10.3%), analgesics (9.6%), cosmetics (8.2%), cough and cold remedies (6%), leaves and other plant materials (5.4%), and bites/envenomations (4.1%). Nondrug substances accounted for 57.6% of all exposures in 1993. Drug categories associated with the largest numbers of fatalities include (in descending order) analgesics, antidepressants, stimulants (including street drugs), hypnotic-sedatives, antipsychotics, cardiovascular drugs, and alcohols.

Poisonings affect people of all ages. In 1993, 56% of cases involved children under 6 years of age; 6% of cases were in children aged 6–12 years; and the teenage and adult groups accounted for 38% of reported cases.

Although most cases of poisoning are classified as inadvertent or accidental, virtually all ingestions by individuals over 10 years of age involve an intentional component.

The specific principles discussed in this chapter will aid in the treatment of a poisoning. In addition, rigorous appropriate supportive care is essential for successful treatment of a poisoned patient.

DEFINITIONS

Poison

A poison may be defined as *any substance which by its chemical action may cause damage to structure or disturbance of function.* Based on this definition, poisons include all types of drugs as well as other synthetic and naturally occurring compounds.

Antidote

An antidote may be defined as *a remedy for counteracting a poison.* Antidotal therapy includes all varieties of therapeutic maneuvers used to prevent, minimize, or reverse the effects of a toxin.

SOURCES OF INFORMATION

It has been recognized that optimal management of a poisoning requires personnel with experience and expertise. This awareness is resulting in the formation, in most countries, of a few large "regional" poison information centers and a decrease in the number of smaller centers. These larger centers are staffed by full-time personnel who are involved with a large number and variety of poisoning cases. Available resources include data bases containing information on product ingredients, medically related toxicological information, and current information on the evaluation and treatment of poisonings. Regional poison information centers are the single best source for accurate up-to-date information on poisonings.

PRINCIPLES OF TREATMENT OF POISONINGS

In order to treat poisonings optimally, the physician must have a clear understanding of some basic prin-

ciples, and therapy should be aimed at a number of specific goals:

- Systemic absorption of the toxin should be minimized.
- The effects of the toxin that has been absorbed should be antagonized.
- Metabolic processes that reduce the overall toxicity should be encouraged, while biotransformation to toxic products should be inhibited.
- Elimination of the toxin from the body should be enhanced.
- Finally, good clinical medical care of the patient must be provided.

Initial treatment should be directed toward decreasing the absorption of a poison. Once the poison is absorbed into the body and distributed to the appropriate sites, termination of its effects usually involves administration of pharmacological agents or biotransformation and excretion from the body. This concept is depicted in Figure 74-1.

MODIFICATION OF ABSORPTION AND DISTRIBUTION

Measures for Decreasing Absorption of Toxins

The most common route by which toxins are absorbed into the body is the gastrointestinal tract (76%), followed in decreasing frequency by the pulmonary system (14%) and the skin (0.7%). Other routes include parenteral (intravenous, intramuscular, subcutaneous), rectal, and vaginal. The route of absorption dictates the initial therapy.

Oral route

Therapeutic interventions affecting absorption of an ingested material include removing the unabsorbed toxins from the stomach and preventing absorption of remaining substances.

Emesis. Induced vomiting has been used to remove most toxins from the stomach, and **ipecac syrup** is the drug of choice. Ipecac is a plant material containing a mixture of alkaloids; cephaeline and emetine are the major ones. It induces emesis through stimulation of the chemoreceptor trigger zone and

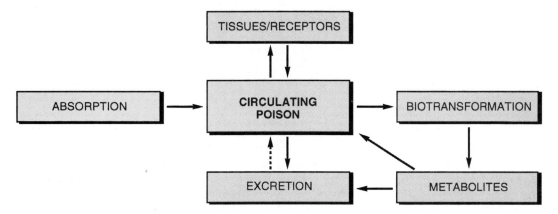

Figure 74-1. Kinetics of poisoning. Note that the various steps are qualitatively identical with those of drug kinetics.

through local irritation of the gastrointestinal tract. The latency period for the induction of emesis by ipecac ranges from 5 to 20 minutes, and a single dose of ipecac produces vomiting in approximately 85% of patients.

Contraindications to the administration of ipecac include the presence of coma or convulsions, and the ingestion of a substance that may result in the rapid onset of coma or convulsions. In addition, ipecac should not be used in patients who have ingested a caustic (corrosive) substance. The use of ipecac syrup is also not routinely recommended in patients who have ingested a petroleum hydrocarbon product (e.g., kerosene), because emesis may lead to a severe aspiration pneumonitis. Other relative contraindications to the use of ipecac include age less than 6 months (no clinical data available), ingestion of a nontoxic quantity of the poison, and prior administration of activated charcoal (which adsorbs the ipecac alkaloids and prevents their pharmacological action).

The ingestion of antiemetic drugs (e.g., phenothiazines) does not affect the efficacy with which ipecac induces vomiting. Passage of the toxin through the pylorus, or systemic absorption of toxin, reduces considerably the value of emesis, so that ipecac is not beneficial if given more than half an hour after ingestion of a liquid or more than 1 hour after ingestion of a solid.

Another pharmacological emetic is **apomorphine.** Subcutaneous administration of apomorphine produces forceful vomiting within 5 minutes, but because it also causes central nervous system and respiratory depression, the clinical usefulness of apomorphine is limited.

Gastric lavage. Lavage is currently the only other acceptable technique used to empty the stomach, but it often is less effective than ipecac-induced emesis in removing solid material. For example, in an animal study, when gastric emptying was carried out 1 hour after the ingestion of a test dose of sodium salicylate tablets, lavage removed an average of 13% while ipecac-induced emesis removed an average of 39% of the ingested salicylate. Lavage may be appropriate when emesis is contraindicated (coma, convulsions), but care must be taken to prevent tracheal aspiration of fluids used in the lavage. The limited clinical efficacy of either ipecac-induced emesis or gastric lavage has led to an increasingly important role of activated charcoal.

Activated charcoal. Activated charcoal is an inert, nonabsorbable, odorless, tasteless, fine black powder that has a high adsorptive capacity. It will bind most toxins within the lumen of the gastrointestinal tract and markedly reduce absorption (Table 74-1). Activated charcoal should be mixed with water (25 g charcoal per 100 mL water) and administered orally or by nasogastric tube. For optimal binding, a charcoal:toxin ratio of 10:1 should be used. When the ingested dose of a toxin is a matter of speculation, the recommended dose of charcoal is 0.5–1 g/kg of body weight. The success with which activated charcoal prevents absorption of a substance depends not only on the substance itself (see Table 74-1) but also on the time between ingestion and administration of charcoal. As an example, the following figures illustrate the progressive decrease in efficacy against ASA (aspirin) with increasing delay in administration of activated charcoal (AC):

Time of AC dosing relative to ASA ingestion	Percent of ASA adsorbed to AC
Simultaneous	59
+ 30 minutes	48
+ 60 minutes	21
+180 minutes	9

When the gastrointestinal absorption of a drug is delayed (e.g., after ingestion of a large quantity or in a sustained-release formulation), the beneficial effects from the use of activated charcoal will be more significant.

Other adsorbents (cholestyramine, etc.) have been evaluated as binding agents, but because they effectively bind only a limited number of toxins, they are not generally useful.

"Local" antidotes. These are compounds that change the ionic form or alter the solubility of the toxin and thus reduce its toxicity. An example is the use of calcium (milk) for fluoride ingestion. The clinical and biochemical efficiency of these techniques remains unproven. Weak acids and alkalis should not be used to neutralize strong alkalis or acids, respectively, because temperatures of up to 100°C may occur during neutralization, which may contribute to tissue damage. (Just flushing with copious amounts of water will dilute and frequently remove acids without causing additional damage.)

Table 74-1 Adsorptive Capacity of Activated Charcoal (AC) in Vitro

Substance	Adsorptive Capacity (g/100 g AC)
Mercuric chloride	180
Imipramine	125
Sulfanilamide	100
Strychnine nitrate	95
Nicotine	70
Barbital	70
Chlorpromazine HCl	36
Phenobarbital	30–35
Malathion (pH 1.0)	31
Aspirin (ASA, pH 1.0)	28
Ferrous sulfate	17
Potassium cyanide	3.5

From Hayden & Comstock 1975.

Pulmonary route

Reduction of absorption of toxic gases is accomplished simply by removing the victim from the site of exposure.

Dermal route

Examples of toxins that are readily absorbed through the unbroken skin are given in Table 74-2.

Minimizing absorption through the skin requires removal of contaminated clothing and gentle washing of the skin with mild soap and cool water. Abrasion of the skin (i.e., removing the keratin barrier) or use of hot water (i.e., increasing local circulation) may enhance absorption of the toxin.

Parenteral route

Application of constricting bands or wraps proximal to the site of injection, combined with restriction of movement of the limb, may retard the systemic distribution of subcutaneously administered toxins. This is applicable primarily to snake bites.

Techniques for Altering Distribution of Toxins

One of the approaches to the therapy of a poisoning involves interruption of gastrointestinal (enterohepatic) recirculation of the substance and limitation of distribution of the toxin within the body.

Limiting recirculation

Some lipid-soluble drugs (e.g., phenobarbital, phencyclidine, tricyclic antidepressants) have long plasma half-lives perhaps in part because they undergo significant recirculation between the gastrointestinal tract and the portal blood. Repeated oral administration of activated charcoal will bind these drugs within

Table 74-2 Toxins Absorbed Through Unbroken Skin

Nerve gas (sarin)
Carbon tetrachloride
Parathion
Phenols
Strychnine
Nicotine
Tetraethyl lead

the gut lumen, cause them to be excreted in the feces, and thus enhance their clearance from the body. For example, administration of repeated oral doses of activated charcoal has reduced the serum half-life of phenobarbital from 110 hours to 45 hours and has shortened the duration of phenobarbital-induced coma.

Some other drugs in which clearance from the body has been affected by repeated oral administration of activated charcoal are carbamazepine, digoxin, methotrexate, salicylates, theophylline, and thyroxine.

Limiting distribution

The distribution of some drugs is partially pH-dependent. Weak acids are less ionized as the pH of the surrounding milieu decreases and will cross membrane barriers more easily. The acidemia (e.g., plasma pH = 7.0) that may occur in a salicylate poisoning affects the salicylate ion in this way, facilitating the entry of salicylate (pK_a = 3.2) into the central nervous system. Normalizing the plasma pH to 7.4 reduces the amount of nonionized salicylate, thus limiting the distribution of this particular toxin into cells.

In the same way, lowering the pH will tend to increase the proportion of the ionized forms of weak bases and thus hinder their diffusion. For example, the nonionized form of morphine can diffuse from the blood into the lumen of the stomach, where gastric acid ionizes it and prevents back-diffusion into the blood (ion trapping). Therefore repeated oral doses of activated charcoal can help to remove morphine even after it has been administered parenterally (see Chapter 2).

PHARMACOLOGICAL MEASURES FOR TERMINATING EFFECTS: ANTIDOTAL THERAPY

The classical antidotes for specific poisons are considered in this section. The antidotes are classified by the mechanism of action.

Competitive Antagonism

Naloxone (Narcan) antagonizes the sedation, respiratory depression, and miosis associated with an overdose of a morphine-like analgesic by reversibly competing with the opioid for μ- and κ-opioid receptors in the brain and spinal cord (see Chapter 23). A critical concentration of naloxone must be achieved and maintained at the receptor site in order for a reversal of narcotic effects to occur and persist.

Naloxone often is administered as an intravenous bolus, and the effects it produces are often of brief duration. This occurs for two reasons: (1) The relatively high central nervous system concentration of naloxone produced by the combination of bolus injection and high blood flow to the brain is rapidly reduced through redistribution of the drug. (2) The half-life of naloxone is short, approximately 30 minutes.

In the clinical setting, the brevity of action of naloxone may be countered by repeated dosing or by continuous infusion of the drug. Alternatively, an analog with longer half-life, such as naltrexone or nalmefene, may be used.

Oxygen may be considered a competitive antagonist to carbon monoxide, and **flumazenil** (a selective $GABA_A$-receptor antagonist) is a competitive antagonist to benzodiazepines.

Noncompetitive Antagonism

Atropine therapy for carbamate or organophosphate insecticide poisoning is an example of noncompetitive antagonism. In other words, the antagonist (atropine) competes with the *effects* of the agonist (insecticide), not against receptor binding of the agonist itself.

Both carbamate and organophosphate insecticides produce clinical effects by inhibiting the enzyme acetylcholinesterase. Because acetylcholine is no longer being degraded, its concentration in nerve synapses increases, producing excessive and persistent stimulation. Clinically, this is a picture of acetylcholine excess, or a "cholinergic syndrome." A sufficiently high concentration of atropine will inhibit the action of acetylcholine on postsynaptic receptors and will reverse the clinical effects (see Chapter 15). Thus, atropine competes with the *effect* of the insecticide but does nothing against the insecticide itself.

Diazepam can be considered a noncompetitive antagonist of strychnine, and **pyrimidine** is a noncompetitive antagonist of isoniazid.

Chemical Neutralization

Cyanide poisoning occurs primarily in the industrial setting, but also in conjunction with therapeutic use of sodium nitroprusside or amygdalin (prussic acid glycoside), which can be hydrolyzed to yield free cyanide. Cyanide combines strongly with ferric iron in various proteins, including cytochrome oxidase, and prevents oxidative metabolism in the mitochondria of all tissues (see Chapter 11):

$$CN^- + \text{cytox-Fe}^{3+} \rightleftharpoons \text{cytox-FeCN}$$

In the treatment of acute cyanide poisoning, the administration of sodium nitrite creates a large circulating pool of ferric iron (methemoglobin), which attracts the cyanide ion away from the cytochrome oxidase, permitting the resumption of oxidative metabolism:

$$NaNO_2 + (O) + HbFe^{2+} \rightarrow HbFe^{3+} + NaNO_3$$
$$HbFe^{3+} + \text{cytox-FeCN} \rightleftharpoons HbFeCN + \text{cytox-Fe}^{3+}$$

The next step in therapy is to supply the mitochondrial enzyme (rhodanese or sulfur transferase), that normally detoxifies cyanide, with its substrate (sodium thiosulfate), so that the enzyme can "neutralize" the cyanide ion by converting it to the nontoxic sodium thiocyanate:

$$HbFeCN + Na_2S_2O_3 \rightleftharpoons HbFe^{3+} + Na_2SO_3 + SCN^-$$

Supplemental oxygen and sodium bicarbonate are also useful in the treatment of cyanide poisoning.

Metabolic Inhibition

Methanol itself is of relatively low toxicity, but when it is metabolized by the enzyme alcohol dehydrogenase to formaldehyde, which is in turn oxidized to formic acid, severe metabolic acidosis (due to the formation of formic, lactic, and α-ketobutyric acids) and blindness (formic acid causes optic nerve demyelination) may result. When ethanol is administered, it competes with methanol for alcohol dehydrogenase, markedly decreasing the rate of oxidation of methanol and the subsequent development of toxicity (see Chapter 26). Another compound that is oxidized by alcohol dehydrogenase, with a resulting increase in toxicity, is **ethylene glycol,** an antifreeze. As with methanol, administration of ethanol prevents the conversion of ethylene glycol to its more toxic metabolites, glycol aldehyde and glycolic acid.

Oxidation-Reduction

Excessive amounts of certain compounds (e.g., benzocaine, nitrites, phenazopyridine) will oxidize hemoglobin (Fe^{2+}) to methemoglobin (Fe^{3+}), resulting in decreased oxygen delivery by the blood.

Administered **methylene blue** (tetramethylthionine) acts as a cofactor to accelerate the conversion of methemoglobin to hemoglobin by methemoglobin reductase. Within 1 hour of administration of methylene blue, most of the methemoglobin will be reduced and tissue oxygenation will be restored.

Chelation

This type of therapy is used to treat metal intoxication. In principle, a chelating agent should be able to bind tightly a specific metal and form a nontoxic chelate that can be excreted from the body. Any chelating agent should be administered as soon as possible following exposure to the toxic metal because the agents are more efficient at preventing enzyme inhibition by the metal than they are at reactivating the enzyme. It is very difficult to evaluate the benefits of therapeutic regimens for metal poisonings. (See also Chapter 46.)

Dimercaprol. Dimercaprol (BAL; British Anti-Lewisite) is used to treat patients with **arsenic poisoning.** It is administered so as to form a chelate with a ratio of two molecules of BAL to one molecule of metal. The 2:1 chelate is more stable and more water-soluble than a 1:1 complex. These chelate complexes are excreted in the urine and bile. BAL increases the urinary excretion of arsenic in the first 24 hours. The magnitude of the increase depends on the "dose" of arsenic and the adequacy of renal function.

Calcium disodium EDTA. Calcium disodium edetate (Versenate), rather than ethylenediaminetetraacetic acid (EDTA) itself, is used as a chelating agent because, although EDTA and Na_2EDTA would chelate many divalent and trivalent metals, they would also chelate calcium. $CaNa_2EDTA$ does not cause hypocalcemia and would chelate metals having a higher affinity for EDTA than calcium does (e.g., lead, zinc). It is now used primarily to treat **lead poisoning.** Following the administration of $CaNa_2EDTA$, lead from soft-tissue depots displaces the calcium ion and forms a stable $PbNa_2EDTA$ complex that is excreted in the urine. Urinary lead levels reach a maximum 6 hours after administration of $CaNa_2EDTA$, and excretion is nearly complete in 18 hours. Lead excretion decreases with subsequent doses. A "rest period" is often recommended between courses of therapy to allow for redistribution of the metal within the body.

Deferoxamine (Desferal). This agent is used to treat

iron poisoning. Following ingestion of excessive amounts of iron, plasma iron concentrations exceed the binding capacity of transferrin, and free (unbound) iron is distributed into cells where it causes disruption of the mitochondria. Deferoxamine not only binds circulating free iron and enhances its elimination in the urine, but it may also remove iron from sites within hepatocytes. Although there are conflicting data on iron excretion, appropriate use of deferoxamine does reduce the mortality rate in acute iron poisoning.

Antigen-Antibody

Serum globulins with specific activity against a given substance have been used in the form of antitoxins (to treat *Clostridium botulinum* poisoning) and antivenins (to treat envenomations from poisonous snakes or spiders). Recently, the development of **antigen binding fragments** (Fab) derived from specific antidigoxin antibodies has improved the treatment of poisoning from the digitalis glycosides. Patients with life-threatening digoxin poisoning who receive intravenous digoxin antibody fragments demonstrate an immediate decrease in free digoxin serum concentrations; favorable changes in cardiac arrhythmias and reduction of hyperkalemia occur within 30 minutes of administration (see Chapter 36).

BIOTRANSFORMATION

Therapeutic interventions in metabolic processes have concentrated on preventing the development or accumulation of toxic metabolites, because there is no safe, effective way to enhance the biotransforma-tion of a toxic substance to nontoxic metabolites rapidly enough to make a clinically important difference in an acute intoxication. The biotransformation of chemicals occurs primarily in the liver, but it also may occur in the kidneys (acetaminophen, carbon tetrachloride), lungs (paraquat), plasma (succinylcholine), or gastrointestinal wall (oral epinephrine). The transformation products are usually intermediates of decreased toxicity and increased excretability (see Chapter 4), but this is not always the case. Many metabolites may be toxicologically active. Examples of compounds that are biotransformed into pharmacologically active or toxic metabolites include imipramine, parathion, methanol, and acetaminophen.

In the case of **acetaminophen** (*N*-acetyl-*p*-aminophenol), small amounts of the drug can be conjugated with glucuronic acid or sulfate; but the major route of biotransformation is oxidation by the hepatic cytochrome P450 system, which forms a reactive metabolite. Normally, this metabolite is "detoxified" through combination with glutathione Figure 74-2. When an overdose of acetaminophen is taken, the reserves of glutathione are depleted, the reactive metabolite accumulates, and hepatocyte damage results (see Chapters 4 and 46). Treatment of acute acetaminophen intoxication currently consists of the administration of *N*-acetylcysteine, which helps to prevent the accumulation of toxic intermediates.

EXCRETION

The liver and the kidneys are the major organs responsible for drug elimination. As noted earlier, elimination of toxins can be accomplished also

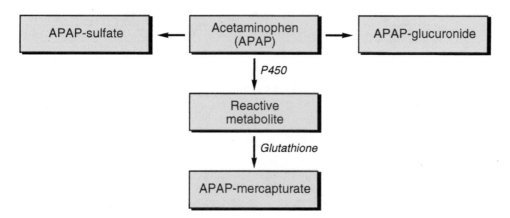

Figure 74-2. Biotransformation of acetaminophen. (APAP = *N*-acetyl-*p*-aminophenol = acetaminophen.)

through the gastrointestinal tract by interrupting gastrointestinal recirculation by the use of repeated doses of activated charcoal. Most techniques used to enhance elimination of toxic substances from the body utilize renal excretion or extracorporeal clearance.

Renal Excretion

Attempts to enhance renal excretion of a toxic substance will be successful only if that substance is excreted to a significant degree in an unchanged or toxic form in the urine, i.e., if a substantial portion of the total body clearance of the substance occurs normally through the kidneys. In order to judge this accurately, it is necessary to know the renal clearance as well as the total body clearance of the substance in the toxic or overdose state. There are relatively few substances encountered in clinical poisonings that have a significant renal excretion following an acute overdose. These compounds are listed in Table 74-3. Although the major part of a dose of amphetamines, phencyclidine, or phenobarbital undergoes biotransformation in the liver, significant portions are excreted through the kidneys. Enhanced renal excretion is accomplished by the systemic administration of drugs that alter the pH of the urine ("ionized diuresis"), i.e., alkalinization of the urine with sodium bicarbonate or acidification of the urine with ammonium chloride, depending on the drug to be eliminated. By the appropriate raising or lowering of the urine pH, the degree of ionization of acidic and basic drugs, respectively, is increased. Because the ionized drug is less able to cross cell membranes and be reabsorbed, it is excreted. Alkalinization of the urine may increase the excretion of salicylates and phenobarbital, whereas excretion of amphetamines and phencyclidine may be increased by acidifying the urine.

Extracorporeal Clearance

Extracorporeal clearance of toxins may take two forms: dialysis or hemoperfusion.

Dialysis (peritoneal dialysis, hemodialysis)

For dialysis to be effective, certain conditions must be met. The dialyzing membrane must be permeable to the toxic molecule, and the toxin should equilibrate rapidly between the circulating plasma and the dialysis fluid. The toxin should be removed in significant quantities compared to the total body burden of toxin or to spontaneous clearance. In addition, ideally, the degree of toxicity from the poison should be a function of its concentration within the body and the length of time that this concentration is maintained. If a toxin produces prompt and irreversible damage, removal of the remaining toxin by dialysis is not likely to be of great therapeutic value. From a clinical perspective, dialysis may be considered in severe intoxications (e.g., deep and prolonged coma), or in the presence of potentially lethal blood concentrations of the toxin. Decreased renal and hepatic clearance and deterioration in the clinical state due to the toxin are also indications for dialysis.

Hemodialysis is usually much more effective than peritoneal dialysis. In practice, the toxins that respond best to hemodialysis are ASA, methanol, and ethylene glycol.

Hemoperfusion

Hemoperfusion consists of passing blood from a blood vessel over a resin or charcoal column and then back into the circulation, leaving the toxin bound to the column. These techniques have essentially the same conditions and criteria for use as dialysis, with the advantage that lipophilic and highly protein-bound drugs are cleared more efficiently.

SUGGESTED READING

Amdur MO, Doull J, Klaassen CD, eds. Casarett and Doull's toxicology. The basic science of poisons. 5th ed. New York: McGraw-Hill, 1995.

American Academy of Pediatrics: Handbook of common poisonings in children. 3rd ed. 1994.

Ellenhorn MF, Barceloux DG. Medical toxicology. Diagnosis and treatment of human poisoning. New York: Elsevier, 1988.

Table 74-3 Renally Excreted Substances

Weak Acids	Ions	Weak Bases	Others
Phenobarbital	Bromide⁻	Phencyclidine	
Salicylates	Iodide⁻	Quinidine	
	Lithium⁺	Amphetamine	Arsenic

Goldfrank LR, Flomenbaum NE, Lewin NA, et al. eds. Toxicologic emergencies. 5th ed. Norwalk, CT: Appleton Lange, 1994.

Hayden JW, Comstock EG. Use of activated charcoal in acute poisoning. [Review] Clin Toxicol 1975; 8:515–533.

Litovitz TL, Felberg L, Soloway RA, et al. 1993 Annual Report of the American Association of Poison Control Centers. Am J Emerg Med 1995; 13(5):551–597.

Olson KR. Poisoning and drug overdose. 2nd ed. Norwalk, CT: Appleton Lange, 1994.

CHAPTER 75

Drug Development and Regulations

C.A. NARANJO AND E. JANECEK

The first documentation of drug use goes back about 4000 years to the Babylonian-Assyrian culture and Egypt. Documents from those times refer to a large number of ingested substances, some pharmacologically active and others inert. The administration of these remedies was often accompanied by incantations, indicating that magic and the supernatural played a major role in the conceptualization and treatment of diseases. The preparation of drugs and the control of their use were usually in the hands of priests who served as exorcists, diviners, and healers. They also functioned as a type of drug regulatory agency.

Medical papers written between 2000 and 1000 B.C. in Egypt contain information on drug formulae and instructions for preparation and use of the remedies. The emphasis on drugs and formulations in these documents suggests that in those times greater attention was paid to the pharmaceutical side of medical care than in Greek times when the emphasis was on the disease process. Hippocrates (fourth century B.C., Greece) changed the concept of disease and stressed simplicity of treatment and freedom from the irrational and supernatural. Galen (second century A.D.) created a system of pathology and therapy that influenced western medicine for 1500 years. Galen classified drugs according to Hippocrates' theory of four humors and described a large number of compounds used at the time.

In ancient Greece and in the Roman empire, the responsibility for the manufacture and use of drugs was still primarily in the hands of physicians, although drug dealers sometimes supplied ready-made medicaments to physicians. The first true pharmacopoeia "Dispensatorium" was published in Germany in 1546. During the 15th, 16th, and 17th centuries many official and unofficial pharmacopoeias were published, most of them for local use only. The first official standard for a whole country was issued in England in 1618. Cellular pathology, medical biology, bacteriology, and experimental pharmacology originated during the 19th century and laid the basis for drug development as we know it today. Now, most new drugs are developed and produced by large international corporations with headquarters primarily in Switzerland, Germany, and the United States. We have no idea how long it took the ancient Egyptians to develop the formulations for their remedies. Now it takes on average about 10 years at a cost of about 150 million dollars, from the time a new drug is synthesized to the time when it can be sold commercially.

This chapter reviews the general concepts regarding drug development, as well as the types of regulation governing it in most countries. Detailed descriptions of the regulations in each country are beyond the scope of the chapter.

METHODS OF DEVELOPING NEW DRUGS

Purification of Drugs from Natural Sources

Natural products were once the only source of drugs. Folk cures often have provided clues to plants with important pharmacological activity. For example, cinchona alkaloids (quinine and quinidine), ephedrine, and *Rauwolfia serpentina* (the active principle of which is the antihypertensive drug reserpine) were all discovered by systematic chemical study of folk remedies. Curare was discovered by similar study of a South American arrowhead poison.

Antibiotics are particularly illustrative of the importance of natural sources. The first step in the identification and development of new antibiotics involved large-scale screening programs in which tens of thousands of samples of soil were assessed systematically for microorganisms with antibacterial or antifungal activity. Cyclosporine, an important immunosuppressant drug, was discovered by a company that required its employees to bring back a sample of soil whenever they traveled to a foreign country. Sometimes the discovery of a drug's activity comes not from a systematic program but from a chance observation, e.g., Fleming's discovery of the antibiotic activity of *Penicillium notatum*. Purification of the culture media and application of modern methods of natural product chemistry are used to isolate, crystallize, and chemically characterize the active ingredients of crude fungal cultures. Antibiotics discovered in this way include streptomycin, chloramphenicol, neomycin, and erythromycin.

The isolation and identification of antileukemic alkaloids in the leaves of the periwinkle plant *(Vinca rosea)* provides another example of the serendipity involved in drug research. Crude preparations of vinca have been used in some parts of the world as antidiabetic agents. Plant extracts were assayed for hypoglycemic activity, but none was found. Some of the experimental animals, however, suffered massive leukopenia, and this effect was used as a bioassay procedure that led to the isolation of an active compound, vinblastine. Routine screening of the crude plant material in an anticancer program revealed activity against experimental leukemia in mice. Using this effect as a bioassay, over 30 different alkaloids were isolated and purified in 3 years. Four, including vinblastine, were found to have antileukemic activity in humans.

Developments in the steroid area are also of interest. Following the discovery in 1949 that cortisone was of value in the treatment of arthritis, intensive industrial competition occurred in the search for an inexpensive way to produce synthetic steroid hormones. After a couple of years of frantic searching, Mexican yams were found to contain a sterol, diosgenin, that could be converted economically to progesterone. The price of progesterone dropped from $80.00 to $1.75 per gram and now is about 15 cents a gram. A *Rhizopus* then was found that could carry out the 11-hydroxylation that was required for production of adrenal cortical hormones from progester-

one, and the road was cleared for low-cost adrenal corticosteroids.

Modification of Chemical Structure

"Molecular manipulation" is widely used to obtain new drugs (see also Chapter 11). Often this is done to produce a patentable product to compete with one already on the market. There may, however, be more important reasons. They include:

1. Modification to improve the desired action. For example, hundreds of modifications of the procaine molecule have been tested as local anesthetics in attempts to produce more stable compounds with longer duration of local anesthesia.

2. Modification to alter absorption, distribution, or elimination. Much effort has been expended in attempts to find drug derivatives that will be absorbed effectively when given orally. Work to develop orally active progestational hormones resulted in the production of oral contraceptives.

3. Modification to improve selectivity of action. For example, conversion of a tertiary nitrogen in atropine to a quaternary nitrogen by adding a methyl group (methatropine) reduces its ability to cross the blood–brain barrier, and thus improves selectivity for peripheral effects.

Drug distribution and hence pharmacological activity may be markedly influenced by molecular modifications. For example, replacement of oxygen in pentobarbital by a sulfur produces thiopental and converts the molecule from a moderately long-lasting anesthetic to an ultra-short-acting one. The reason lies in the extreme lipid solubility of thiopental, which permits it to enter and leave the brain rapidly.

Structural modifications also can influence the length of time a drug is active by altering its biotransformation. Procaine can abolish certain cardiac arrhythmias, but it is an ester and is rapidly hydrolyzed by liver and plasma esterases, limiting its value. Simple substitution of the ester group by an amide group gives rise to procainamide, which has a longer duration of action because of greater resistance to hydrolysis.

Substitution to Reduce Cost

Examples include diethylstilbestrol, an inexpensive nonsteroid substitute for natural estrogens, and methadone, introduced during World War II by the Germans, who needed a cheap replacement for morphine, which was unavailable to them.

De Novo Invention of New Drugs

Although there are exceptions to the rule (e.g., synthesis of H_2-receptor antagonists such as cimetidine), usually new drugs are not produced as a result of highly rational programs based on complete knowledge of structure–activity relationships. Usually, serendipity and chance observations lead to identification of pharmacological activity of a specific molecule. In recent years most pharmaceutical companies have developed systematic programs, using animal models with known predictive value, to screen chemical substances for specific pharmacological activities. For example, several new antidepressants without the anticholinergic side effects of tricyclics (e.g., fluoxetine) have been developed in this fashion. However, recent increases in understanding of the three-dimensional structures of enzymes, receptors and other macromolecules have offered the possibility of designing synthetic molecules that can interact with specific sites in these target molecules. This may become an increasingly important approach to rational drug design in the near future.

Exploitation of Side Effects of Existing Drugs

The most common pattern in the development of new drugs is not de novo invention, but rather the exploitation of side effects of existing drugs. Astute exploitation of the side effects of sulfonamides (see Chapter 11) led to the development of useful drugs that are not antibacterial agents, but rather, diuretics (the carbonic anhydrase inhibitors and thiazides) and antidiabetic agents (the sulfonylureas).

DRUG LEGISLATION AND REGULATIONS

There is wide cross-cultural variation in drug legislation. In general, the requirements for marketing a new drug are more strict in North America (United States, Canada) than in Europe, Asia, Africa, or Latin America. In recent years, however, there has been a trend everywhere to make the requirements for licensing a new drug more stringent. Several factors influence the drug legislation in various countries. In the United States and Canada, major roles are played by multinational drug companies, nonproprietary drug companies, the federal governments, and the public.

An important development has been the action taken by economic blocs, such as the European Community, toward harmonizing their regulatory requirements. However, in the United States, advocacy groups such as the pro-AIDS lobby have forced the Food and Drug Administration (FDA) and legislators to shorten the normal regulatory process and facilitate the early approval of new antiviral medications for the treatment of HIV-positive individuals.

It has been widely claimed that drug legislation impedes the development of new drugs. The "drug lag," the delay in time when a drug becomes available in the United States compared to the United Kingdom, is often cited as an example of how restrictive drug legislation can impede pharmaceutical innovation. In contrast, the less stringent laws in some European countries are cited as encouraging drug investigation and the earlier availability of drugs. However, these arguments are at variance with the experience of developing countries, which, despite minimal or nonexistent legislation, are characterized by limited innovative drug development for lack of adequate resources and of an appropriate academic and/or industrial context. The development of new drugs is a complex matter that depends on a number of factors other than legislation. For example, generic (i.e., nonproprietary) products included in lists such as the Essential Drug List sponsored by the World Health Organization have become dominant in developing countries and more recently have had a major impact on prescribing practices in Health Maintenance Organizations (HMOs). This introduces an important economic factor that a company must take into account in considering the development of a new drug.

PREMARKETING DRUG REGULATIONS

Preclinical Testing of New Drugs

In the United States and Canada, any drug that has not been sold for a sufficient time and in sufficient quantity to establish satisfactorily its safety and effectiveness is defined as a "new drug" by the Regulations of the Food and Drugs Act. This same definition also applies to any new form or use for a drug that is currently on the market. Before a drug can be administered to humans, it must be tested for its pharmacological and toxicological activities in vitro and in animals. Chemical substances must be tested systematically, depending on the type of drug, in biochemical, physiological, behavioral, and pharmacological screening tests designed to identify substances with the desired (expected) activity. If a substance shows such an effect, it is possible to proceed with more detailed studies. However, an enormous amount of research is required to move from initial discovery to finished drug. Chemists may create or isolate up to 5000 different substances in order to come up with one new marketable drug. The active new drug is tested in animals and humans in the sequence shown in Figure 75–1.

Preclinical testing determines the pharmacological actions of the drugs as well as the mechanism of action, the specificity of effect, and the toxicity. Since all drugs have the potential to produce toxic effects, toxicity studies are conducted in animals according to well-defined guidelines. Toxicological tests are used to determine the toxicity of drugs and/or their metabolites in various biological systems in order that predictions may be made regarding the potential risks in humans. Traditionally, toxicity testing has

consisted of acute, subacute, and chronic studies designed to determine the general effects of compounds on animal systems. There is also a requirement to assess the drug effects on reproduction as well as the potential for carcinogenic or genetic damage. The need to conduct *all* the toxicological tests for a new form or for a new use of an existing drug is questionable and is frequently a subject of debate between regulatory agencies and pharmaceutical companies.

Acute toxicity studies are those that involve the administration of a single dose, or a few equally spaced doses, within a 24-hour period. Long-term toxicity studies (subacute and chronic) are those that involve the daily administration of the drug for periods lasting from a few days to several years. In general, it is required that animal tests be carried

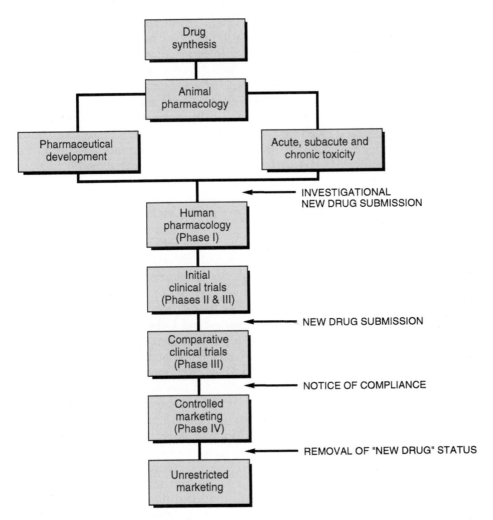

Figure 75-1. New drug development and regulations in most western countries, including the United States and Canada.

out in at least three mammalian species (one of which must be a nonrodent). The acute (single-dose) median lethal dose (LD_{50}) is first determined. Then a series of tests using different dosage routes gives the lethal dose range and the nontoxic range for several species and provides some indication of an approximate dose to use in humans. At the same time the absorption, distribution, metabolism, and elimination of the drug are studied.

The long-term toxicity studies are intended to determine the toxicity (behavioral, physiological, and histopathological effects) when a drug is administered repeatedly and to determine the dose–response relationships of these effects. It is also important to identify clearly the target organ of toxicity, the reversibility, and the factors influencing toxicity (such as sex, age, nutritional status). The first administration of a drug to humans relies heavily on animal data, and it therefore depends on the belief that toxicity or the lack of it, demonstrated in animals, is relevant to humans. However, decisions on specific cases are uncertain. Therefore, it is usual to make conservative decisions, and the appearance of almost any serious toxicity in animals may be considered as sufficient evidence to reject the human administration of a drug. This decision may be faulty, because some toxicity is species-specific, and it is likely that, occasionally, potentially useful new drugs may be unnecessarily rejected. In contrast, animal toxicological tests are usually good predictors of dose-related toxicity in humans, whereas dose-unrelated adverse drug reactions (allergic or genetically determined reactions) are not detected in traditional toxicological tests. Thus, the first administration of a drug to a human still involves some risk, which must be carefully considered.

Evaluation of Clinical Effects (Clinical Trials)

When the new compound passes preclinical screening, clinical investigation can be conducted. The manufacturer must file an **Investigational New Drug Submission** with the respective regulatory agency and request permission to distribute the drug to qualified investigators for clinical testing in order to obtain the necessary evidence concerning the new drug's dosage, efficacy, and safety in humans. The preclinical submission must contain the following information: objectives of proposed clinical testing; name of the drug; chemical structure and source of the new drug; data on its toxicity, pharmacology, and biochemistry (drug metabolism); contraindications and precautions; suggested treatment of overdose;

the methods, equipment, plant, and controls used in the manufacture, processing, and packaging of the new drug; tests for potency, purity, and safety; the names and qualifications of investigators; and the institutions where the studies will be conducted. Once the application is approved, the drug is distributed with a label that states that it is an investigational drug that should be used by qualified investigators only.

Phase I studies

This is the first administration of a drug to humans; it usually follows the completion of pharmacological and toxicological studies in animals. The investigational drug is given to healthy volunteers first in single, increasing doses, and then by multiple administrations to cover the range of therapeutic use. These studies are conducted to obtain data on safety and pharmacokinetics only, since the relevant symptoms on which to test efficacy are rarely present in healthy volunteers. The selection of the initial human dose is difficult. As noted above, animal studies on drug metabolism and toxicity (e.g., LD_{50}) are of limited usefulness for selecting such a dose. A common rule is to begin with one-fifth or one-tenth of the maximum tolerated dose (mg/kg) in the most sensitive animal species, assuming an average human body weight of 70 kg. The drug is then given in some form of increments until the estimated therapeutically effective dose is attained or side effects develop. The protocol usually involves six to nine subjects at each dose level. Placebo and double-blind techniques are used. Multiple-dose tolerance studies are usually conducted in healthy volunteers, but it may be ethically more acceptable, as well as more efficient, to perform them in patients.

Phase I subjects are hospitalized and undergo intensive monitoring, including assessments such as daily physical examinations and determinations of blood pressure, pulse, ECG, EEG, and tests for assessing liver, kidney, and hematological toxicity. A severe adverse event is rare in phase I. For example, in 805 studies, conducted between 1964 and 1976 in 29,000 subjects, only 55 cases of severe, definite, or probable adverse drug reactions occurred.

Phase II studies

This is the first administration of a drug to patients. Elimination of the drug should be assessed, because patients may metabolize it differently than healthy subjects do. These trials are divided into early and late phases. Early phase II trials involve the administration of the drug to patients to observe the potential therapeutic benefits and side effects. An attempt is made to establish a dose range for more definitive therapeutic trials. Late phase II trials are intended to establish the efficacy of the drug in reducing the manifestations of the specific disease and to compare its efficacy and side effects to those of other marketed drugs used for similar purposes.

Phase III studies

These studies include double-blind, randomized, controlled clinical trials on a sufficient number of patients to provide data permitting statistical evaluation of the drug's efficacy and safety. The procedures for assessing clinical toxicity are similar to those used in phase I. However, phase III studies provide better information because of the larger sample size.

If the human studies indicate that the compound may be an efficacious and safe therapeutic agent, the manufacturer can file a **New Drug Submission** (NDS) with the regulatory agency, requesting permission to market the new drug.

The NDS must contain additional information, such as: human data to demonstrate efficacy; recommended use; safety for this use; results of further animal studies; proposed registered name, chemical name, and description; list of all ingredients; product monograph, labels, and package insert; and samples of the finished form of the new drug. An NDS often contains thousands of pages. The data are reviewed by the regulators and outside consultants. NDSs are not always cleared after the first submission of data, and further information or clarifications may be required. If the documentation is acceptable to the regulatory agency, then a **Notice of Compliance** is signed by the regulatory authority. This document indicates that the agency has found the content of the NDS satisfactory and in compliance with regulations. The drug can now enter the market with "new drug" status.

Phase IV studies

These studies occur after the drug has obtained a marketing license. The drug's performance is monitored in the years immediately following marketing, when widespread use may result in the discovery of relatively rare side effects, chronic toxicity developing only after many years of exposure (e.g., cancer), previously unknown drug interactions, or potential new therapeutic use, or the development of more

appropriate dosage recommendations. The drug may remain in new drug status for several years until the regulatory agency is confident that sufficient additional information has accumulated from its general use to justify release from the rigid controls applied to new drugs. While the product still has new drug status, the manufacturer is expected to report any new information concerning safety or efficacy. The regulatory agency reserves the right to suspend the Notice of Compliance for a new drug when it is in the public interest to do so because of such findings as lack of efficacy or serious or frequent toxicity. Thus, the study of the performance of a new drug does not stop with its approval and marketing. Physicians must be constantly and critically assessing the clinical effects of old and new drugs.

POSTMARKETING CONTROLS

In most countries, the availability and use of drugs is controlled by the national governments.

Through legislation and regulations, these governments assume the responsibility for protecting the public against health hazards related to the manufacture and/or sale of drugs, medical devices, cosmetics, and foods. They also control the access of new drugs to the market by requiring that the drugs meet certain standards of efficacy and safety set out in a variety of legislation and regulations covering virtually every aspect of the production, sale, and prescription of drugs. Description of the specific titles and contents of the legislation in each country is beyond the scope of this chapter, but in general the following topics are covered.

Standards of Production, including the purity, efficacy, and safety of the products; these are generally reinforced by the standards set out in the various national or international pharmacopeias.

Packaging, labeling, and advertising of drugs. For example, the proper description of the contents of the package, the nature and prominence of warning labels such as "Keep Out of the Reach of Children," and the veracity of advertising claims about the efficacy, quality, or safety of over-the-counter medications, are all covered by regulations.

Scheduling of drugs, to indicate which ones may be sold over the counter, which are for use only on medical prescription, which are designated as Controlled Drugs, Narcotics, and Restricted Drugs (for investigational use only), and which are prohibited.

The regulations governing the distribution and use of narcotics and controlled drugs are much more stringent than those governing prescription drugs. For example, dealers require a special licence to distribute narcotics and controlled drugs. Pharmacists must keep separate records of purchases and prescriptions filled for these drugs. Both dealers and pharmacists must keep records of inventories and all transactions involving these drugs and make periodic reports to the Bureau of Dangerous Drugs (BDD; in the United States, an agency of the Food and Drug Administration; in Canada, a division of the Health Protection Branch, Department of Health). The records of dealers and pharmacies are also subject to unannounced inspections and audit by the BDD. Unauthorized possession of a narcotic, controlled drug, or restricted drug is a punishable offense. A physician has the onus of proving that any controlled drug or narcotic in his/her possession is for professional use and that the drug was prescribed or administered in accordance with the regulations. The prohibition of unauthorized possession of these drugs applies not only to dealers, pharmacists, and practitioners (physicians, dentists, veterinarians), but also to patients. Patients are required to inform the prescriber if they have received a narcotic from another prescriber. Since this is not a well-known fact (except among the drug-abusing population), it is advisable for the physician prescribing a narcotic to ask whether the patient has been given a prescription for a narcotic in the recent past.

There are also special regulations governing the use and distribution of the narcotic methadone. In many countries, for example, this drug can be prescribed only by a practitioner who is authorized by national health authorities. To receive this authorization, a practitioner is required to provide details of the way methadone will be prescribed in practice or to provide evidence of being associated with an approved drug addiction treatment program. The practitioner or the treatment program must report the use of the drug to the BDD.

SUGGESTED READING

Brown JS, Bienz-Tadmor B, Lasagna L. Availability of anticancer drugs in the United States, Europe, and Japan from 1960 through 1991. Clin Pharmacol Ther 1995; 58:243–256.

Kaitin KI. Pharmaceutical innovation in an era of reform. Am J Ther 1995; 2:730–734.

Kaitin KI, Manocchia M, Seibring M, Lasagna L. The new drug approvals of 1990, 1991, and 1992: trends in drug development. J Clin Pharmacol 1994; 34:120–127.

Orzack LH, Kaitin KI, Lasagna L. Pharmaceutical regulation in the European Community: barriers to a single market integration. J Health Polit Policy Law 1992; 17:847–868.

Sellers EM, Sellers S. Systems for the control of therapeutic drug utilization in Canada. In: Wardell WM, ed. Controlling the use of therapeutic drugs. An international comparison. Washington, DC: American Enterprise Institute, 1978: 71–95.

Shulman SR, Brown JS. The Food and Drug Administration's early access and fast-track approval initiatives: how have they worked? Food Drug Law J 1995; 503–531.

Spilker B, ed. Multinational pharmaceutical companies: Principles and practices. 2nd ed. New York: Raven Press, 1994.

Wardell WM, ed. Controlling the use of therapeutic drugs. An international comparison. Washington, DC: American Enterprise Institute, 1978.

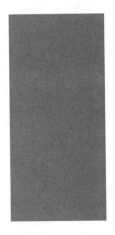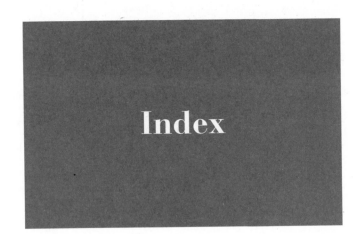

Index

Page numbers in *italics* refer to illustrations, including chemical structures and formulae; page numbers followed by "t" refer to tables; page numbers in **boldface** refer to major discussions and chapter headings.